MAKE THE MOST *of your* PHYSICIAN CODING EXAM Review!

ELSEVIER

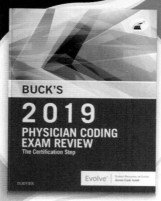

...-Exam

...mpanion
...and
...ed
...ding of
...process.

2. Study!

Use the quizzes in this book to sharpen your skills and build competency.

4. Test! Take the Final Exam

Gauge your readiness for the actual physician coding exam with the Final Exam. Boost your test-taking confidence and ensure certification success.

3. Apply! Take the Post-Exam

After studying, apply your knowledge to the Post-Exam located on the companion Evolve site. When finished, you'll receive scores for both the Pre- and Post-Exams and a breakdown of incorrect answers to help you identify areas where you need more detailed study and review.

ISBN: 978-0-323-58257-5

Perfect *your* **understanding** *and* **prepare for certification**
— START YOUR REVIEW NOW!

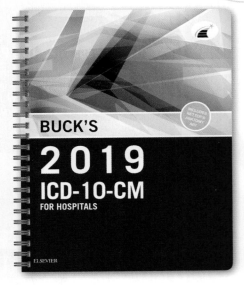
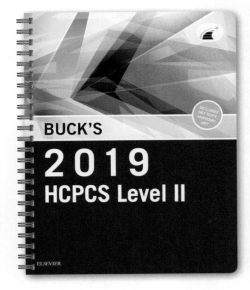
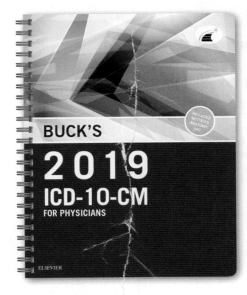

STEP **4:** PROFESSIONAL

"Nothing is particularly hard if you divide it into small jobs."
— HENRY FORD

WE WANT TO APPLAUD YOU FOR TAKING THIS STEP IN YOUR CAREER.
Medical coding is a fine profession that has the ability to intrigue and captivate you for a lifetime. Practice your craft carefully, with due diligence, patience for the process, and always the highest ethical standards.

TRACK YOUR PROGRESS!

See the checklist in the front of this book to learn more about your next step toward coding success!

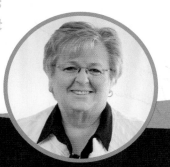

Carol J. Buck, MS, CPC, CCS-P

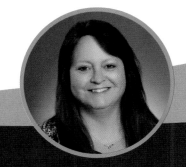

Jackie Grass Koesterman, CPC

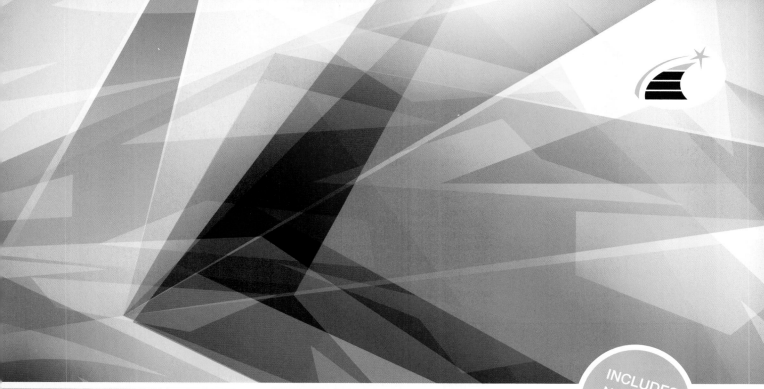

BUCK'S

2019
ICD-10-PCS

INCLUDES NETTER'S ANATOMY ART

ELSEVIER

ELSEVIER

3251 Riverport Lane
St. Louis, Missouri 63043

2019 ICD-10-PCS PROFESSIONAL EDITION

ISBN: 978-0-323-58265-0

Notice

Knowledge and best practice in this field are constantly changing. As new research and experience broaden our understanding, changes in research methods, professional practices, or medical treatment may become necessary.

Practitioners and researchers must always rely on their own experience and knowledge in evaluating and using any information, methods, compounds, or experiments described herein. In using such information or methods they should be mindful of their own safety and the safety of others, including parties for whom they have a professional responsibility.

With respect to any drug or pharmaceutical products identified, readers are advised to check the most current information provided (i) on procedures featured or (ii) by the manufacturer of each product to be administered, to verify the recommended dose or formula, the method and duration of administration, and contraindications. It is the responsibility of practitioners, relying on their own experience and knowledge of their patients, to make diagnoses, to determine dosages and the best treatment for each individual patient, and to take all appropriate safety precautions.

To the fullest extent of the law, neither the Publisher nor the authors, contributors, or editors, assume any liability for any injury and/or damage to persons or property as a matter of products liability, negligence or otherwise, or from any use or operation of any methods, products, instructions, or ideas contained in the material herein.

International Standard Book Number: 978-0-323-58265-0

Content Strategist: Brandi Graham
Content Development Manager: Luke Held
Content Development Specialist: Anna Miller
Publishing Services Manager: Julie Eddy
Project Manager: Abigail Bradberry
Design Manager: Julia Dummitt

Printed in Canada

Last digit is the print number: 9 8 7 6 5 4 3 2 1

Working together
to grow libraries in
developing countries

www.elsevier.com • www.bookaid.org

DEDICATION

To all the brave medical coders who transitioned the nation into a new coding system.
Decades of waiting finally concluded with the implementation of I-10,
and you have been the pioneers leading the way.

With greatest appreciation for your efforts!

Carol J. Buck, MS, CPC, CCS-P

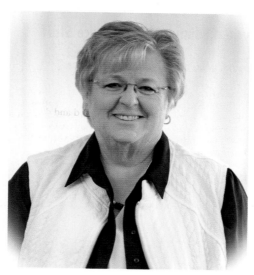

DEVELOPMENT OF THIS EDITION

Lead Technical Collaborator

Jackie Grass Koesterman, CPC
Coding and Reimbursement Specialist
Grand Forks, North Dakota

Query Team

Patricia Cordy Henricksen, MS, CHCA, CPC-I, CPC, CCP-P, ASC-PM
Auditing and Coding Educator
Soterion Medical Services
Lexington, Kentucky

Kathleen Buchda, CPC, CPMA
Revenue Recognition
New Richmond, Wisconsin

Elsevier/MC Strategies Revenue Cycle, Coding and Compliance Staff

"Experts in providing e-learning on revenue cycle, coding and compliance."

Deborah Neville, RHIA, CCS-P
Director

Lynn-Marie D. Wozniak, MS, RHIT
Content Manager

Sandra L. Macica, MS, RHIA, CCS, ROCC
Content Manager

CONTENTS

SYMBOLS AND CONVENTIONS

Annotated

Throughout the manual, revisions, additions, and deleted codes or words are indicated by the following symbols:

New and revised content from the previous edition are indicated by green font.

~~deleted~~ Deletions from the previous edition are struck through.

ICD-10-PCS Table Symbols

Throughout the manual information is indicated by the following symbols:

♀ ♂ **Sex conflict:** *Definitions of Medicare Code Edits* (MCE) detects inconsistencies between a patient's sex and any diagnosis or procedure on the patient's record. For example, a male patient with cervical cancer (diagnosis) or a female patient with a prostatectomy (procedure). In both instances, the indicated diagnosis or the procedure conflicts with the stated sex of the patient. Therefore, either the patient's diagnosis, procedure, or sex is presumed to be incorrect.

Non-covered: There are some procedures for which Medicare does not provide reimbursement. There are also procedures that would normally not be reimbursed by Medicare but due to the presence of certain diagnoses are reimbursed.

Limited Coverage: For certain procedures whose medical complexity and serious nature incur extraordinary associated costs, Medicare limits coverage to a portion of the cost.

DRG Non-OR A **non-operating room procedure that does affect MS-DRG assignment** is indicated by a purple highlight.

Non-OR A **non-operating room procedure that does not affect MS-DRG assignment** is indicated by a yellow highlight.

⊞ **Combination:** Certain combinations of procedures are treated differently than their constituent codes.

Hospital-Acquired Condition: Some procedures are always associated with Hospital Acquired Conditions (HAC) according to the MS-DRG.

Coding Clinic: American Hospital Association's *Coding Clinic®* citations provide reference information to official ICD-10-PCS coding advice.

OGCR The *Official Guidelines for Coding and Reporting* symbol includes the placement of a portion of a guideline as that guideline pertains to the code by which it is located. The complete OGCR are located in the Introduction.

[ ] Brackets below the tables enclose the alphanumeric options for Non-covered, Limited Coverage, DRG Non-OR, Non-OR, and HAC.

Note: The final FY2019 MS-DRG and Medicare Code Edits were unavailable at the time of printing. Proposed new DRG Non-OR procedures were available and have been included below the appropriate tables with "(proposed)" appearing behind the codes. Please check codingupdates.com for final FY2019 MS-DRG and MCE information.

GUIDE TO THE 2019 UPDATES

The ICD-10-PCS codes that have changed are shown in the lists below.
If you would like to see this information in table format, please visit codingupdates.com for a complete listing.

2019 ICD-10-PCS New, Revised, and Deleted Codes.

NEW CODES

001U072	031509T	03724D1	03784D1	041K3JS	041V3JS	05783Z1	057F3Z1	0FD84ZX	0SPD4LZ
001U0J2	03150AT	03724Z1	03784Z1	041L3JQ	041W3JQ	05784D1	057F4D1	0FD88ZX	0SPD4MZ
001U0K2	03150JT	03730D1	03790D1	041L3JS	041W3JS	05784Z1	057F4Z1	0FD93ZX	0SPD4NZ
001U372	03150KT	03730Z1	03790Z1	041M3JQ	05730D1	05790D1	093K7ZZ	0FD94ZX	0SR90EZ
001U3J2	03150ZT	03733D1	03793D1	041M3JS	05730Z1	05790Z1	093K8ZZ	0FD98ZX	0SRB0EZ
001U3K2	031609T	03733Z1	03793Z1	041N3JQ	05733D1	05793D1	0F500ZF	0FDC3ZX	0SRC0EZ
001U472	03160AT	03734D1	03794D1	041N3JS	05733Z1	05793Z1	0F503ZF	0FDC4ZX	0SRC0M9
001U474	03160JT	03734Z1	03794Z1	041P0JQ	05734D1	05794D1	0F504ZF	0FDC8ZX	0SRC0MA
001U476	03160KT	03740D1	037A0D1	041P0JS	05734Z1	05794Z1	0F510ZF	0FDD3ZX	0SRC0MZ
001U477	03160ZT	03740Z1	037A0Z1	041P3JQ	05740D1	057A0D1	0F513ZF	0FDD4ZX	0SRC0N9
001U479	031H09Y	03743D1	037A3D1	041P3JS	05740Z1	057A0Z1	0F514ZF	0FDD8ZX	0SRC0NA
001U4J2	031H0AY	03743Z1	037A3Z1	041P4JQ	05743D1	057A3D1	0F520ZF	0FDF3ZX	0SRC0NZ
001U4J4	031H0JY	03744D1	037A4D1	041P4JS	05743Z1	057A3Z1	0F523ZF	0FDF4ZX	0SRD0EZ
001U4J6	031H0KY	03744Z1	037A4Z1	041Q0JQ	05744D1	057A4D1	0F524ZF	0FDF8ZX	0SRD0M9
001U4J7	031H0ZY	03750D1	037B0D1	041Q0JS	05744Z1	057A4Z1	0F5G0ZF	0FDG3ZX	0SRD0MA
001U4J9	031J09Y	03750Z1	037B0Z1	041Q3JQ	05750D1	057B0D1	0F5G3ZF	0FDG4ZX	0SRD0MZ
001U4K2	031J0AY	03753D1	037B3D1	041Q3JS	05750Z1	057B0Z1	0F5G4ZF	0FDG8ZX	0SRD0N9
001U4K4	031J0JY	03753Z1	037B3Z1	041Q4JQ	05753D1	057B3D1	0FD03ZX	0SP90EZ	0SRD0NA
001U4K6	031J0KY	03754D1	037B4D1	041Q4JS	05753Z1	057B3Z1	0FD04ZX	0SPB0EZ	0SRD0NZ
001U4K7	031J0ZY	03754Z1	037B4Z1	041R0JQ	05754D1	057B4D1	0FD13ZX	0SPC0EZ	0UY90Z0
001U4K9	03700D1	03760D1	037C0D1	041R0JS	05754Z1	057B4Z1	0FD14ZX	0SPC0LZ	0UY90Z1
021W08F	03700Z1	03760Z1	037C0Z1	041R3JQ	05760D1	057C0D1	0FD23ZX	0SPC0MZ	0UY90Z2
021W08G	03703D1	03763D1	037C3D1	041R3JS	05760Z1	057C0Z1	0FD24ZX	0SPC0NZ	0VXT0ZD
021W08H	03703Z1	03763Z1	037C3Z1	041R4JQ	05763D1	057C3D1	0FD43ZX	0SPC3LZ	0VXT0ZS
021W08V	03704D1	03764D1	037C4D1	041R4JS	05763Z1	057C3Z1	0FD44ZX	0SPC3MZ	0VXTXZD
021W09F	03704Z1	03764Z1	037C4Z1	041S0JQ	05764D1	057C4D1	0FD48ZX	0SPC3NZ	0VXTXZS
021W09G	03710D1	03770D1	03CG3Z7	041S0JS	05764Z1	057C4Z1	0FD53ZX	0SPC4LZ	0W190JW
021W09H	03710Z1	03770Z1	03CH3Z7	041S3JQ	05770D1	057D0D1	0FD54ZX	0SPC4MZ	0W193J9
021W09V	03713D1	03773D1	03CJ3Z7	041S3JS	05770Z1	057D0Z1	0FD58ZX	0SPC4NZ	0W193JB
021W0AG	03713Z1	03773Z1	03CK3Z7	041S4JQ	05773D1	057D3D1	0FD63ZX	0SPD0EZ	0W193JG
021W0AH	03714D1	03774D1	03CL3Z7	041S4JS	05773Z1	057D3Z1	0FD64ZX	0SPD0LZ	0W193JJ
021W0AV	03714Z1	03774Z1	03CM3Z7	041T3JQ	05774D1	057D4D1	0FD68ZX	0SPD0MZ	0W193JW
021W0JF	03720D1	03780D1	03CN3Z7	041T3JS	05774Z1	057D4Z1	0FD73ZX	0SPD0NZ	0W193JY
021W0JV	03720Z1	03780Z1	03CP3Z7	041U3JQ	05780D1	057F0D1	0FD74ZX	0SPD3LZ	0W194JW
021W0KF	03723D1	03783D1	03CQ3Z7	041U3JS	05780Z1	057F0Z1	0FD78ZX	0SPD3MZ	0W1B0JW
021W0KV	03723Z1	03783Z1	041K3JQ	041V3JQ	05783D1	057F3D1	0FD83ZX	0SPD3NZ	0W1B3J9

ØW1B3JB	ØW1B3JY	ØW1G3JB	ØW1G3JY	ØW1J3JB	ØW1J3JY	5A1522G	XWØ33H4
ØW1B3JG	ØW1B4JW	ØW1G3JG	ØW1G4JW	ØW1J3JG	ØW1J4JW	5A1522H	XWØ43G4
ØW1B3JJ	ØW1GØJW	ØW1G3JJ	ØW1JØJW	ØW1J3JJ	3EØ234Ø	XV5Ø8A4	XWØ43H4
ØW1B3JW	ØW1G3J9	ØW1G3JW	ØW1J3J9	ØW1J3JW	5A1522F	XWØ33G4	

REVISED CODES

ØSRDØL9	ØSRDØLA	ØSRDØLZ	1ØDØØZØ	1ØDØØZ1	X2A	ØSRCØL9	ØSRCØLA	ØSRCØLZ

DELETED CODES

ØRGØØZØ	ØRG23ZJ	ØRG7ØZØ	ØRGA3Z1	ØRGJØZZ	ØRGR3ZZ	ØSGØØZJ	ØSG34ZØ	ØSGC3ZZ	ØSGL4ZZ
ØRGØØZ1	ØRG24ZØ	ØRG7ØZ1	ØRGA3ZJ	ØRGJ3ZZ	ØRGR4ZZ	ØSGØ3ZØ	ØSG34Z1	ØSGC4ZZ	ØSGMØZZ
ØRGØØZJ	ØRG24Z1	ØRG7ØZJ	ØRGA4ZØ	ØRGJ4ZZ	ØRGSØZZ	ØSGØ3Z1	ØSG34ZJ	ØSGDØZZ	ØSGM3ZZ
ØRGØ3ZØ	ØRG24ZJ	ØRG73ZØ	ØRGA4Z1	ØRGKØZZ	ØRGS3ZZ	ØSGØ3ZJ	ØSG5ØZZ	ØSGD3ZZ	ØSGM4ZZ
ØRGØ3Z1	ØRG4ØZØ	ØRG73Z1	ØRGA4ZJ	ØRGK3ZZ	ØRGS4ZZ	ØSGØ4ZØ	ØSG53ZZ	ØSGD4ZZ	ØSGNØZZ
ØRGØ3ZJ	ØRG4ØZ1	ØRG73ZJ	ØRGCØZZ	ØRGK4ZZ	ØRGTØZZ	ØSGØ4Z1	ØSG54ZZ	ØSGFØZZ	ØSGN3ZZ
ØRGØ4ZØ	ØRG4ØZJ	ØRG74ZØ	ØRGC3ZZ	ØRGLØZZ	ØRGT3ZZ	ØSGØ4ZJ	ØSG6ØZZ	ØSGF3ZZ	ØSGN4ZZ
ØRGØ4Z1	ØRG43ZØ	ØRG74Z1	ØRGC4ZZ	ØRGL3ZZ	ØRGT4ZZ	ØSG1ØZØ	ØSG63ZZ	ØSGF4ZZ	ØSGPØZZ
ØRGØ4ZJ	ØRG43Z1	ØRG74ZJ	ØRGDØZZ	ØRGL4ZZ	ØRGUØZZ	ØSG1ØZ1	ØSG64ZZ	ØSGGØZZ	ØSGP3ZZ
ØRG1ØZØ	ØRG43ZJ	ØRG8ØZØ	ØRGD4ZZ	ØRGMØZZ	ØRGU3ZZ	ØSG1ØZJ	ØSG7ØZZ	ØSGG3ZZ	ØSGP4ZZ
ØRG1ØZ1	ØRG44ZØ	ØRG8ØZ1	ØRGEØZZ	ØRGM3ZZ	ØRGU4ZZ	ØSG13ZØ	ØSG73ZZ	ØSGG4ZZ	ØSGQØZZ
ØRG1ØZJ	ØRG44Z1	ØRG8ØZJ	ØRGE3ZZ	ØRGM4ZZ	ØRGVØZZ	ØSG13Z1	ØSG74ZZ	ØSGHØZZ	ØSGQ3ZZ
ØRG13ZØ	ØRG44ZJ	ØRG83ZØ	ØRGE4ZZ	ØRGNØZZ	ØRGV3ZZ	ØSG13ZJ	ØSG8ØZZ	ØSGH3ZZ	ØSGQ4ZZ
ØRG13Z1	ØRG6ØZØ	ØRG83Z1	ØRGFØZZ	ØRGN3ZZ	ØRGV4ZZ	ØSG14ZØ	ØSG83ZZ	ØSGH4ZZ	ØW4MØZØ
ØRG13ZJ	ØRG6ØZ1	ØRG83ZJ	ØRGF3ZZ	ØRGN4ZZ	ØRGWØZZ	ØSG14Z1	ØSG84ZZ	ØSGJØZZ	ØW4NØZ1
ØRG14ZØ	ØRG6ØZJ	ØRG84ZØ	ØRGF4ZZ	ØRGPØZZ	ØRGW3ZZ	ØSG14ZJ	ØSG9ØZZ	ØSGJ3ZZ	5A15223
ØRG14Z1	ØRG63ZØ	ØRG84Z1	ØRGGØZZ	ØRGP3ZZ	ØRGW4ZZ	ØSG3ØZØ	ØSG93ZZ	ØSGJ4ZZ	
ØRG14ZJ	ØRG63Z1	ØRG84ZJ	ØRGG3ZZ	ØRGP4ZZ	ØRGXØZZ	ØSG3ØZ1	ØSG94ZZ	ØSGKØZZ	
ØRG2ØZ1	ØRG63ZJ	ØRGAØZØ	ØRGG4ZZ	ØRGQØZZ	ØRGX3ZZ	ØSG3ØZJ	ØSGBØZZ	ØSGK3ZZ	
ØRG2ØZJ	ØRG64ZØ	ØRGAØZ1	ØRGHØZZ	ØRGQ3ZZ	ØRGX4ZZ	ØSG33ZØ	ØSGB3ZZ	ØSGK4ZZ	
ØRG23ZØ	ØRG64Z1	ØRGAØZJ	ØRGH3ZZ	ØRGQ4ZZ	ØSGØØZØ	ØSG33Z1	ØSGB4ZZ	ØSGLØZZ	
ØRG23Z1	ØRG64ZJ	ØRGA3ZØ	ØRGH4ZZ	ØRGRØZZ	ØSGØØZ1	ØSG33ZJ	ØSGCØZZ	ØSGL3ZZ	

0HBU022

0UW2422, 0UW7422

041LUXL

0SG10AJ

Introduction

ICD-10-PCS Official Guidelines for Coding and Reporting

2019

The Centers for Medicare and Medicaid Services (CMS) and the National Center for Health Statistics (NCHS), two departments within the U.S. Federal Government's Department of Health and Human Services (DHHS) provide the following guidelines for coding and reporting using the International Classification of Diseases, 10th Revision, Procedure Coding System (ICD-10-PCS). These guidelines should be used as a companion document to the official version of the ICD-10-PCS as published on the CMS website. The ICD-10-PCS is a procedure classification published by the United States for classifying procedures performed in hospital inpatient health care settings.

These guidelines have been approved by the four organizations that make up the Cooperating Parties for the ICD-10-PCS: the American Hospital Association (AHA), the American Health Information Management Association (AHIMA), CMS, and NCHS.

These guidelines are a set of rules that have been developed to accompany and complement the official conventions and instructions provided within the ICD-10-PCS itself. The instructions and conventions of the classification take precedence over guidelines. These guidelines are based on the coding and sequencing instructions in the Tables, Index and Definitions of ICD-10-PCS, but provide additional instruction. Adherence to these guidelines when assigning ICD-10-PCS procedure codes is required under the Health Insurance Portability and Accountability Act (HIPAA). The procedure codes have been adopted under HIPAA for hospital inpatient healthcare settings. A joint effort between the healthcare provider and the coder is essential to achieve complete and accurate documentation, code assignment, and reporting of diagnoses and procedures. These guidelines have been developed to assist both the healthcare provider and the coder in identifying those procedures that are to be reported. The importance of consistent, complete documentation in the medical record cannot be overemphasized. Without such documentation accurate coding cannot be achieved.

Table of Contents

Conventions

A1

ICD-10-PCS codes are composed of seven characters. Each character is an axis of classification that specifies information about the procedure performed. Within a defined code range, a character specifies the same type of information in that axis of classification.

Example: The fifth axis of classification specifies the approach in sections Ø through 4 and 7 through 9 of the system.

A2

One of 34 possible values can be assigned to each axis of classification in the seven-character code: they are the numbers Ø through 9 and the alphabet (except I and O because they are easily confused with the numbers 1 and Ø). The number of unique values used in an axis of classification differs as needed.

Example: Where the fifth axis of classification specifies the approach, seven different approach values are currently used to specify the approach.

A3

The valid values for an axis of classification can be added to as needed.

Example: If a significantly distinct type of device is used in a new procedure, a new device value can be added to the system.

A4

As with words in their context, the meaning of any single value is a combination of its axis of classification and any preceding values on which it may be dependent.

Example: The meaning of a body part value in the Medical and Surgical section is always dependent on the body system value. The body part value Ø in the Central Nervous body system specifies Brain and the body part value Ø in the Peripheral Nervous body system specifies Cervical Plexus.

A5

As the system is expanded to become increasingly detailed, over time more values will depend on preceding values for their meaning.

Example: In the Lower Joints body system, the device value 3 in the root operation Insertion specifies Infusion Device and the device value 3 in the root operation Replacement specifies Ceramic Synthetic Substitute.

A6

The purpose of the alphabetic index is to locate the appropriate table that contains all information necessary to construct a procedure code. The PCS Tables should always be consulted to find the most appropriate valid code.

A7

It is not required to consult the index first before proceeding to the tables to complete the code. A valid code may be chosen directly from the tables.

A8

All seven characters must be specified to be a valid code. If the documentation is incomplete for coding purposes, the physician should be queried for the necessary information.

A9

Within a PCS table, valid codes include all combinations of choices in characters 4 through 7 contained in the same row of the table. In the example below, ØJHT3VZ is a valid code, and ØJHW3VZ is *not* a valid code.

A1Ø

"And," when used in a code description, means "and/or," except when used to describe a combination of multiple body parts for which separate values exist for each body part (e.g., Skin and Subcutaneous Tissue used as a qualifier, where there are separate body part values for "Skin" and "Subcutaneous Tissue").

Example: Lower Arm and Wrist Muscle means lower arm and/or wrist muscle.

A11

Many of the terms used to construct PCS codes are defined within the system. It is the coder's responsibility to determine what the documentation in the medical record equates to in the PCS definitions. The physician is not expected to use the terms used in PCS code descriptions, nor is the coder required to query the physician when the correlation between the documentation and the defined PCS terms is clear.

Example: When the physician documents "partial resection" the coder can independently correlate "partial resection" to the root operation Excision without querying the physician for clarification.

Medical and Surgical Section Guidelines (section Ø)

B2. Body System
General guidelines

B2.1a

The procedure codes in the general anatomical regions body systems can be used when the procedure is performed on an anatomical region rather than a specific body part (e.g., root operations Control and Detachment, Drainage of a body cavity) or on the rare occasion when no information is available to support assignment of a code to a specific body part.

Examples: Control of postoperative hemorrhage is coded to the root operation Control found in the general anatomical regions body systems.

Chest tube drainage of the pleural cavity is coded to the root operation Drainage found in the general anatomical regions body systems. Suture repair of the abdominal wall is coded to the root operation Repair in the general anatomical regions body system.

B2.1b

Where the general body part values "upper" and "lower" are provided as an option in the Upper Arteries, Lower Arteries, Upper Veins, Lower Veins, Muscles and Tendons body systems, "upper" or "lower" specifies body parts located above or below the diaphragm respectively.

Example: Vein body parts above the diaphragm are found in the Upper Veins body system; vein body parts below the diaphragm are found in the Lower Veins body system.

B3. Root Operation
General guidelines

B3.1a

In order to determine the appropriate root operation, the full definition of the root operation as contained in the PCS Tables must be applied.

B3.1b

Components of a procedure specified in the root operation definition and explanation are not coded separately. Procedural steps necessary to reach the operative site and close the operative site, including anastomosis of a tubular body part, are also not coded separately.

Examples: Resection of a joint as part of a joint replacement procedure is included in the root operation definition of Replacement and is not coded separately. Laparotomy performed to reach the site of an open liver biopsy is not coded separately. In a resection of sigmoid colon with anastomosis of descending colon to rectum, the anastomosis is not coded separately.

SECTION: Ø   MEDICAL AND SURGICAL

BODY SYSTEM: J   SUBCUTANEOUS TISSUE AND FASCIA

OPERATION: H   INSERTION: Putting in a nonbiological appliance that monitors, assists, performs, or prevents a physiological function but does not physically take the place of a body part

Body Part	Approach	Device	Qualifier
S Subcutaneous Tissue and Fascia, Head and Neck V Subcutaneous Tissue and Fascia, Upper Extremity W Subcutaneous Tissue and Fascia, Lower Extremity	Ø Open 3 Percutaneous	1 Radioactive Element 3 Infusion Device	Z No Qualifier
T Subcutaneous Tissue and Fascia, Trunk	Ø Open 3 Percutaneous	1 Radioactive Element 3 Infusion Device V Infusion Pump	Z No Qualifier

Multiple procedures
B3.2
During the same operative episode, multiple procedures are coded if:
  a. The same root operation is performed on different body parts as defined by distinct values of the body part character.
    Examples: Diagnostic excision of liver and pancreas are coded separately.
  b. The same root operation is repeated in multiple body parts, and those body parts are separate and distinct body parts classified to a single ICD-10-PCS body part value.
    Examples: Excision of the sartorius muscle and excision of the gracilis muscle are both included in the upper leg muscle body part value, and multiple procedures are coded.
    Extraction of multiple toenails are coded separately.
  c. Multiple root operations with distinct objectives are performed on the same body part.
    Example: Destruction of sigmoid lesion and bypass of sigmoid colon are coded separately.
  d. The intended root operation is attempted using one approach, but is converted to a different approach.
    Example: Laparoscopic cholecystectomy converted to an open cholecystectomy is coded as percutaneous endoscopic Inspection and open Resection.

Discontinued or incomplete procedures
B3.3
If the intended procedure is discontinued or otherwise not completed, code the procedure to the root operation performed. If a procedure is discontinued before any other root operation is performed, code the root operation Inspection of the body part or anatomical region inspected.
Example: A planned aortic valve replacement procedure is discontinued after the initial thoracotomy and before any incision is made in the heart muscle, when the patient becomes hemodynamically unstable. This procedure is coded as an open Inspection of the mediastinum.

Biopsy procedures
B3.4a
Biopsy procedures are coded using the root operations Excision, Extraction, or Drainage and the qualifier Diagnostic.
Examples: Fine needle aspiration biopsy of fluid in the lung is coded to the root operation Drainage with the qualifier Diagnostic. Biopsy of bone marrow is coded to the root operation Extraction with the qualifier Diagnostic. Lymph node sampling for biopsy is coded to the root operation Excision with the qualifier Diagnostic.

Biopsy followed by more definitive treatment
B3.4b
If a diagnostic Excision, Extraction, or Drainage procedure (biopsy) is followed by a more definitive procedure, such as Destruction, Excision or Resection at the same procedure site, both the biopsy and the more definitive treatment are coded.
Example: Biopsy of breast followed by partial mastectomy at the same procedure site, both the biopsy and the partial mastectomy procedure are coded.

Overlapping body layers
B3.5
If the root operations Excision, Repair or Inspection are performed on overlapping layers of the musculoskeletal system, the body part specifying the deepest layer is coded.
Example: Excisional debridement that includes skin and subcutaneous tissue and muscle is coded to the muscle body part.

Bypass procedures
B3.6a
Bypass procedures are coded by identifying the body part bypassed "from" and the body part bypassed "to." The fourth character body part specifies the body part bypassed from, and the qualifier specifies the body part bypassed to.
Example: Bypass from stomach to jejunum, stomach is the body part and jejunum is the qualifier.
B3.6b
Coronary artery bypass procedures are coded differently than other bypass procedures as described in the previous guideline. Rather than identifying the body part bypassed from, the body part identifies the number of coronary arteries bypassed to, and the qualifier specifies the vessel bypassed from.
Example: Aortocoronary artery bypass of the left anterior descending coronary artery and the obtuse marginal coronary artery is classified in the body part axis of classification as two coronary arteries, and the qualifier specifies the aorta as the body part bypassed from.
B3.6c
If multiple coronary arteries are bypassed, a separate procedure is coded for each coronary artery that uses a different device and/or qualifier.
Example: Aortocoronary artery bypass and internal mammary coronary artery bypass are coded separately.

Control vs. more definitive root operations
B3.7
The root operation Control is defined as, "Stopping, or attempting to stop, postprocedural or other acute bleeding." If an attempt to stop postprocedural or other acute bleeding is unsuccessful, and to stop the bleeding requires performing a more definitive root operation, such as Bypass, Detachment, Excision, Extraction, Reposition, Replacement, or Resection, then the more definitive root operation is coded instead of Control.
Example: Resection of spleen to stop bleeding is coded to Resection instead of Control.

Excision vs. Resection
B3.8
PCS contains specific body parts for anatomical subdivisions of a body part, such as lobes of the lungs or liver and regions of the intestine. Resection of the specific body part is coded whenever all of the body part is cut out or off, rather than coding Excision of a less specific body part.
Example: Left upper lung lobectomy is coded to Resection of Upper Lung Lobe, Left rather than Excision of Lung, Left.

Excision for graft
B3.9
If an autograft is obtained from a different procedure site in order to complete the objective of the procedure, a separate procedure is coded.
Example: Coronary bypass with excision of saphenous vein graft, excision of saphenous vein is coded separately.

Fusion procedures of the spine
B3.10a
The body part coded for a spinal vertebral joint(s) rendered immobile by a spinal fusion procedure is classified by the level of the spine (e.g., thoracic). There are distinct body part values for a single vertebral joint and for multiple vertebral joints at each spinal level.
Example: Body part values specify Lumbar Vertebral Joint, Lumbar Vertebral Joints, 2 or More and Lumbosacral Vertebral Joint.

B3.10b

If multiple vertebral joints are fused, a separate procedure is coded for each vertebral joint that uses a different device and/or qualifier.

Example: Fusion of lumbar vertebral joint, posterior approach, anterior column and fusion of lumbar vertebral joint, posterior approach, posterior column are coded separately.

B3.10c

Combinations of devices and materials are often used on a vertebral joint to render the joint immobile. When combinations of devices are used on the same vertebral joint, the device value coded for the procedure is as follows:

- If an interbody fusion device is used to render the joint immobile (alone or containing other material like bone graft), the procedure is coded with the device value Interbody Fusion Device
- If bone graft is the *only* device used to render the joint immobile, the procedure is coded with the device value Nonautologous Tissue Substitute or Autologous Tissue Substitute
- If a mixture of autologous and nonautologous bone graft (with or without biological or synthetic extenders or binders) is used to render the joint immobile, code the procedure with the device value Autologous Tissue Substitute

Examples: Fusion of a vertebral joint using a cage style interbody fusion device containing morsellized bone graft is coded to the device Interbody Fusion Device. Fusion of a vertebral joint using a bone dowel interbody fusion device made of cadaver bone and packed with a mixture of local morsellized bone and demineralized bone matrix is coded to the device Interbody Fusion Device.

Fusion of a vertebral joint using both autologous bone graft and bone bank bone graft is coded to the device Autologous Tissue Substitute.

Inspection procedures

B3.11a

Inspection of a body part(s) performed in order to achieve the objective of a procedure is not coded separately.

Example: Fiberoptic bronchoscopy performed for irrigation of bronchus, only the irrigation procedure is coded.

B3.11b

If multiple tubular body parts are inspected, the most distal body part (the body part furthest from the starting point of the inspection) is coded. If multiple non-tubular body parts in a region are inspected, the body part that specifies the entire area inspected is coded.

Examples: Cystoureteroscopy with inspection of bladder and ureters is coded to the ureter body part value. Exploratory laparotomy with general inspection of abdominal contents is coded to the peritoneal cavity body part value.

B3.11c

When both an Inspection procedure and another procedure are performed on the same body part during the same episode, if the Inspection procedure is performed using a different approach than the other procedure, the Inspection procedure is coded separately.

Example: Endoscopic Inspection of the duodenum is coded separately when open

Excision of the duodenum is performed during the same procedural episode.

Occlusion vs. Restriction for vessel embolization procedures

B3.12

If the objective of an embolization procedure is to completely close a vessel, the root operation Occlusion is coded. If the objective of an embolization procedure is to narrow the lumen of a vessel, the root operation Restriction is coded.

Examples: Tumor embolization is coded to the root operation Occlusion, because the objective of the procedure is to cut off the blood supply to the vessel.

Embolization of a cerebral aneurysm is coded to the root operation Restriction, because the objective of the procedure is not to close off the vessel entirely, but to narrow the lumen of the vessel at the site of the aneurysm where it is abnormally wide.

Release procedures

B3.13

In the root operation Release, the body part value coded is the body part being freed and not the tissue being manipulated or cut to free the body part.

Example: Lysis of intestinal adhesions is coded to the specific intestine body part value.

Release vs. Division

B3.14

If the sole objective of the procedure is freeing a body part without cutting the body part, the root operation is Release. If the sole objective of the procedure is separating or transecting a body part, the root operation is Division.

Examples: Freeing a nerve root from surrounding scar tissue to relieve pain is coded to the root operation Release. Severing a nerve root to relieve pain is coded to the root operation Division.

Reposition for fracture treatment

B3.15

Reduction of a displaced fracture is coded to the root operation Reposition and the application of a cast or splint in conjunction with the Reposition procedure is not coded separately. Treatment of a nondisplaced fracture is coded to the procedure performed.

Examples: Casting of a nondisplaced fracture is coded to the root operation Immobilization in the Placement section. Putting a pin in a nondisplaced fracture is coded to the root operation Insertion.

Transplantation vs. Administration

B3.16

Putting in a mature and functioning living body part taken from another individual or animal is coded to the root operation Transplantation. Putting in autologous or nonautologous cells is coded to the Administration section.

Example: Putting in autologous or nonautologous bone marrow, pancreatic islet cells or stem cells is coded to the Administration section.

Transfer procedures using multiple tissue layers

B3.17

The root operation Transfer contains qualifiers that can be used to specify when a transfer flap is composed of more than one tissue layer, such as a musculocutaneous flap. For procedures involving transfer of multiple tissue layers including skin, subcutaneous tissue, fascia or muscle, the procedure is coded to the body part value that describes the deepest tissue layer in the flap, and the qualifier can be used to describe the other tissue layer(s) in the transfer flap.

Example: A musculocutaneous flap transfer is coded to the appropriate body part value in the body system Muscles, and the qualifier is used to describe the additional tissue layer(s) in the transfer flap.

B4. Body Part

General guidelines

B4.1a

If a procedure is performed on a portion of a body part that does not have a separate body part value, code the body part value corresponding to the whole body part.

Example: A procedure performed on the alveolar process of the mandible is coded to the mandible body part.

4

B4.1b

If the prefix "peri" is combined with a body part to identify the site of the procedure, and the site of the procedure is not further specified, then the procedure is coded to the body part named. This guideline applies only when a more specific body part value is not available.

Examples: A procedure site identified as perirenal is coded to the kidney body part when the site of the procedure is not further specified. A procedure site described in the documentation as peri-urethral, and the documentation also indicates that it is the vulvar tissue and not the urethral tissue that is the site of the procedure, then the procedure is coded to the vulva body part.

B4.1c

If a procedure is performed on a continuous section of a tubular body part, code the body part value corresponding to the furthest anatomical site from the point of entry.

Example: A procedure performed on a continuous section of artery from the femoral artery to the external iliac artery with the point of entry at the femoral artery is coded to the external iliac body part.

Branches of body parts
B4.2

Where a specific branch of a body part does not have its own body part value in PCS, the body part is typically coded to the closest proximal branch that has a specific body part value. In the cardiovascular body systems, if a general body part is available in the correct root operation table, and coding to a proximal branch would require assigning a code in a different body system, the procedure is coded using the general body part value.

Example: A procedure performed on the mandibular branch of the trigeminal nerve is coded to the trigeminal nerve body part value.

Bilateral body part values
B4.3

Bilateral body part values are available for a limited number of body parts. If the identical procedure is performed on contralateral body parts, and a bilateral body part value exists for that body part, a single procedure is coded using the bilateral body part value. If no bilateral body part value exists, each procedure is coded separately using the appropriate body part value.

Examples: The identical procedure performed on both fallopian tubes is coded once using the body part value Fallopian Tube, Bilateral. The identical procedure performed on both knee joints is coded twice using the body part values Knee Joint, Right and Knee Joint, Left.

Coronary arteries
B4.4

The coronary arteries are classified as a single body part that is further specified by number of arteries treated. One procedure code specifying multiple arteries is used when the same procedure is performed, including the same device and qualifier values.

Examples: Angioplasty of two distinct coronary arteries with placement of two stents is coded as Dilation of Coronary Artery, Two Arteries with Two Intraluminal Devices. Angioplasty of two distinct coronary arteries, one with stent placed and one without, is coded separately as Dilation of Coronary Artery, One Artery with Intraluminal Device, and Dilation of Coronary Artery, One Artery with no device.

Tendons, ligaments, bursae and fascia near a joint
B4.5

Procedures performed on tendons, ligaments, bursae and fascia supporting a joint are coded to the body part in the respective body system that is the focus of the procedure. Procedures performed on joint structures themselves are coded to the body part in the joint body systems.

Examples: Repair of the anterior cruciate ligament of the knee is coded to the knee bursae and ligament body part in the bursae and ligaments body system. Knee arthroscopy with shaving of articular cartilage is coded to the knee joint body part in the Lower Joints body system.

Skin, subcutaneous tissue and fascia overlying a joint
B4.6

If a procedure is performed on the skin, subcutaneous tissue or fascia overlying a joint, the procedure is coded to the following body part:

- Shoulder is coded to Upper Arm
- Elbow is coded to Lower Arm
- Wrist is coded to Lower Arm
- Hip is coded to Upper Leg
- Knee is coded to Lower Leg
- Ankle is coded to Foot

Fingers and toes
B4.7

If a body system does not contain a separate body part value for fingers, procedures performed on the fingers are coded to the body part value for the hand. If a body system does not contain a separate body part value for toes, procedures performed on the toes are coded to the body part value for the foot.

Example: Excision of finger muscle is coded to one of the hand muscle body part values in the Muscles body system.

Upper and lower intestinal tract
B4.8

In the Gastrointestinal body system, the general body part values Upper Intestinal Tract and Lower Intestinal Tract are provided as an option for the root operations Change, Inspection, Removal and Revision. Upper Intestinal Tract includes the portion of the gastrointestinal tract from the esophagus down to and including the duodenum, and Lower Intestinal Tract includes the portion of the gastrointestinal tract from the jejunum down to and including the rectum and anus.

Example: In the root operation Change table, change of a device in the jejunum is coded using the body part Lower Intestinal Tract.

B5. Approach

Open approach with percutaneous endoscopic assistance
B5.2

Procedures performed using the open approach with percutaneous endoscopic assistance are coded to the approach Open.

Example: Laparoscopic-assisted sigmoidectomy is coded to the approach Open.

External approach
B5.3a

Procedures performed within an orifice on structures that are visible without the aid of any instrumentation are coded to the approach External.

Example: Resection of tonsils is coded to the approach External.

B5.3b
Procedures performed indirectly by the application of external force through the intervening body layers are coded to the approach External.
Example: Closed reduction of fracture is coded to the approach External.

Percutaneous procedure via device
B5.4
Procedures performed percutaneously via a device placed for the procedure are coded to the approach Percutaneous.
Example: Fragmentation of kidney stone performed via percutaneous nephrostomy is coded to the approach Percutaneous.

B6. Device
General guidelines
B6.1a
A device is coded only if a device remains after the procedure is completed. If no device remains, the device value No Device is coded. In limited root operations, the classification provides the qualifier values Temporary and Intraoperative, for specific procedures involving clinically significant devices, where the purpose of the device is to be utilized for a brief duration during the procedure or current inpatient stay.
If a device that is intended to remain after the procedure is completed requires removal before the end of the operative episode in which it was inserted (for example, the device size is inadequate or a complication occurs), both the insertion and removal of the device should be coded.

B6.1b
Materials such as sutures, ligatures, radiological markers and temporary post-operative wound drains are considered integral to the performance of a procedure and are not coded as devices.
B6.1c
Procedures performed on a device only and not on a body part are specified in the root operations Change, Irrigation, Removal and Revision, and are coded to the procedure performed.
Example: Irrigation of percutaneous nephrostomy tube is coded to the root operation Irrigation of indwelling device in the Administration section.

Drainage device
B6.2
A separate procedure to put in a drainage device is coded to the root operation Drainage with the device value Drainage Device.

Obstetric Section Guidelines (section 1)

C. Obstetrics Section
Products of conception
C1
Procedures performed on the products of conception are coded to the Obstetrics section. Procedures performed on the pregnant female other than the products of conception are coded to the appropriate root operation in the Medical and Surgical section.
Example: Amniocentesis is coded to the products of conception body part in the Obstetrics section. Repair of obstetric urethral laceration is coded to the urethra body part in the Medical and Surgical section.

Procedures following delivery or abortion
C2
Procedures performed following a delivery or abortion for curettage of the endometrium or evacuation of retained products of conception are all coded in the Obstetrics section, to the root operation Extraction and the body part Products of Conception, Retained. Diagnostic or therapeutic dilation and curettage performed during times other than the postpartum or post-abortion period are all coded in the Medical and Surgical section, to the root operation Extraction and the body part Endometrium.

New Technology Section Guidelines (section X)

D. New Technology Section
General guidelines
D1
Section X codes are standalone codes. They are not supplemental codes. Section X codes fully represent the specific procedure described in the code title, and do not require any additional codes from other sections of ICD-10-PCS. When section X contains a code title which describes a specific new technology procedure, only that X code is reported for the procedure. There is no need to report a broader, non-specific code in another section of ICD-10-PCS.
Example: XW04321 Introduction of Ceftazidime-Avibactam Anti-infective into Central Vein, Percutaneous Approach, New Technology Group 1, can be coded to indicate that Ceftazidime-Avibactam Anti-infective was administered via a central vein. A separate code from table 3E0 in the Administration section of ICD-10-PCS is not coded in addition to this code.

Selection of Principal Procedure
The following instructions should be applied in the selection of principal procedure and clarification on the importance of the relation to the principal diagnosis when more than one procedure is performed:
1. Procedure performed for definitive treatment of both principal diagnosis and secondary diagnosis
   a. Sequence procedure performed for definitive treatment most related to principal diagnosis as principal procedure.
2. Procedure performed for definitive treatment and diagnostic procedures performed for both principal diagnosis and secondary diagnosis
   a. Sequence procedure performed for definitive treatment most related to principal diagnosis as principal procedure
3. A diagnostic procedure was performed for the principal diagnosis and a procedure is performed for definitive treatment of a secondary diagnosis.
   a. Sequence diagnostic procedure as principal procedure, since the procedure most related to the principal diagnosis takes precedence.
4. No procedures performed that are related to principal diagnosis; procedures performed for definitive treatment and diagnostic procedures were performed for secondary diagnosis
   a. Sequence procedure performed for definitive treatment of secondary diagnosis as principal procedure, since there are no procedures (definitive or nondefinitive treatment) related to principal diagnosis.

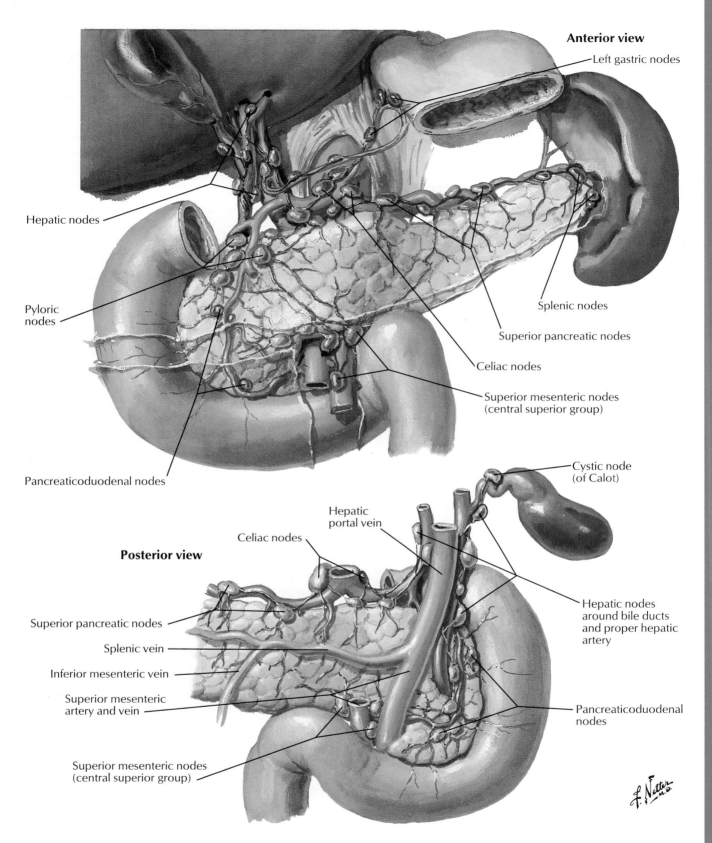

Anterior view

Left gastric nodes

Hepatic nodes

Pyloric nodes

Splenic nodes

Superior pancreatic nodes

Celiac nodes

Superior mesenteric nodes (central superior group)

Pancreaticoduodenal nodes

Cystic node (of Calot)

Hepatic portal vein

Celiac nodes

Posterior view

Hepatic nodes around bile ducts and proper hepatic artery

Superior pancreatic nodes

Splenic vein

Inferior mesenteric vein

Superior mesenteric artery and vein

Pancreaticoduodenal nodes

Superior mesenteric nodes (central superior group)

Plate 315 Lymph Vessels and Nodes of Pancreas. (Netter: Atlas of Human Anatomy, 4 ed, 2006, Saunders.)

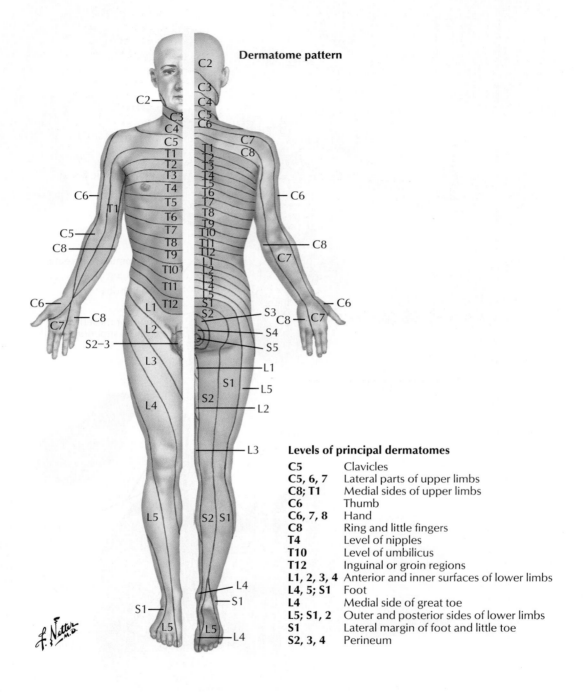

Dermatome pattern

Levels of principal dermatomes

C5	Clavicles
C5, 6, 7	Lateral parts of upper limbs
C8; T1	Medial sides of upper limbs
C6	Thumb
C6, 7, 8	Hand
C8	Ring and little fingers
T4	Level of nipples
T10	Level of umbilicus
T12	Inguinal or groin regions
L1, 2, 3, 4	Anterior and inner surfaces of lower limbs
L4, 5; S1	Foot
L4	Medial side of great toe
L5; S1, 2	Outer and posterior sides of lower limbs
S1	Lateral margin of foot and little toe
S2, 3, 4	Perineum

Plate 164   Dermatomes. (Netter: Atlas of Human Anatomy, 4 ed, 2006, Saunders.)

Female: frontal section

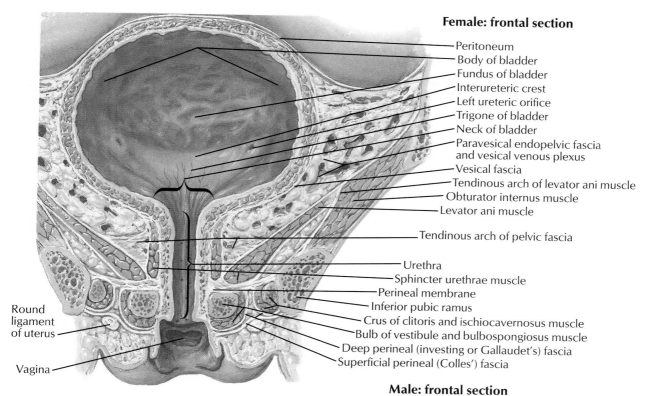

- Peritoneum
- Body of bladder
- Fundus of bladder
- Interureteric crest
- Left ureteric orifice
- Trigone of bladder
- Neck of bladder
- Paravesical endopelvic fascia and vesical venous plexus
- Vesical fascia
- Tendinous arch of levator ani muscle
- Obturator internus muscle
- Levator ani muscle
- Tendinous arch of pelvic fascia
- Urethra
- Sphincter urethrae muscle
- Perineal membrane
- Inferior pubic ramus
- Crus of clitoris and ischiocavernosus muscle
- Bulb of vestibule and bulbospongiosus muscle
- Deep perineal (investing or Gallaudet's) fascia
- Superficial perineal (Colles') fascia

Round ligament of uterus

Vagina

Male: frontal section

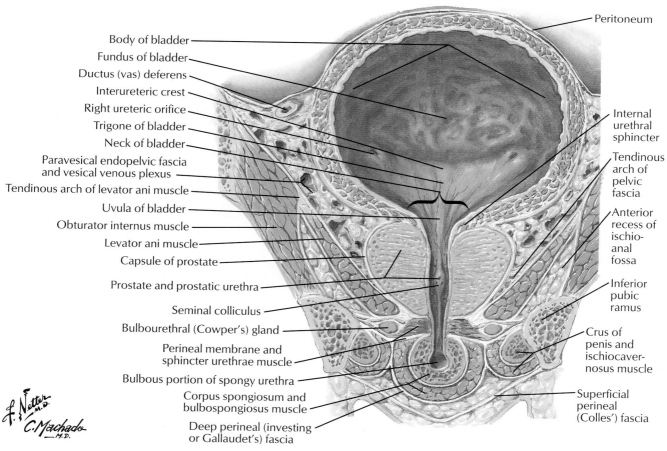

- Body of bladder
- Fundus of bladder
- Ductus (vas) deferens
- Interureteric crest
- Right ureteric orifice
- Trigone of bladder
- Neck of bladder
- Paravesical endopelvic fascia and vesical venous plexus
- Tendinous arch of levator ani muscle
- Uvula of bladder
- Obturator internus muscle
- Levator ani muscle
- Capsule of prostate
- Prostate and prostatic urethra
- Seminal colliculus
- Bulbourethral (Cowper's) gland
- Perineal membrane and sphincter urethrae muscle
- Bulbous portion of spongy urethra
- Corpus spongiosum and bulbospongiosus muscle
- Deep perineal (investing or Gallaudet's) fascia

- Peritoneum
- Internal urethral sphincter
- Tendinous arch of pelvic fascia
- Anterior recess of ischio-anal fossa
- Inferior pubic ramus
- Crus of penis and ischiocavernosus muscle
- Superficial perineal (Colles') fascia

Plate 366 Urinary Bladder: Female and Male. (Netter: Atlas of Human Anatomy, 4 ed, 2006, Saunders.)

NETTER'S ANATOMY ILLUSTRATIONS

9

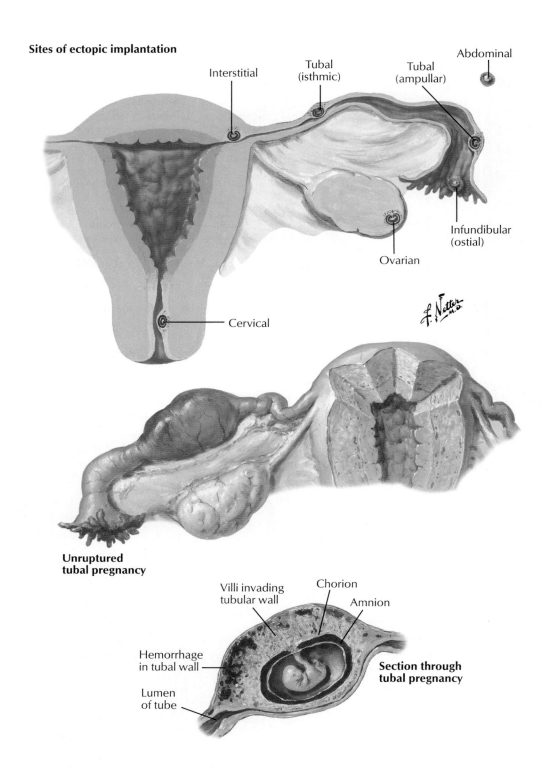

Sites of ectopic implantation

Interstitial

Tubal (isthmic)

Tubal (ampullar)

Abdominal

Infundibular (ostial)

Ovarian

Cervical

Unruptured tubal pregnancy

Villi invading tubular wall

Chorion

Amnion

Hemorrhage in tubal wall

Section through tubal pregnancy

Lumen of tube

Plate 375 Ectopic Pregnancy. (Netter: Atlas of Human Anatomy, 4 ed, 2006, Saunders.)

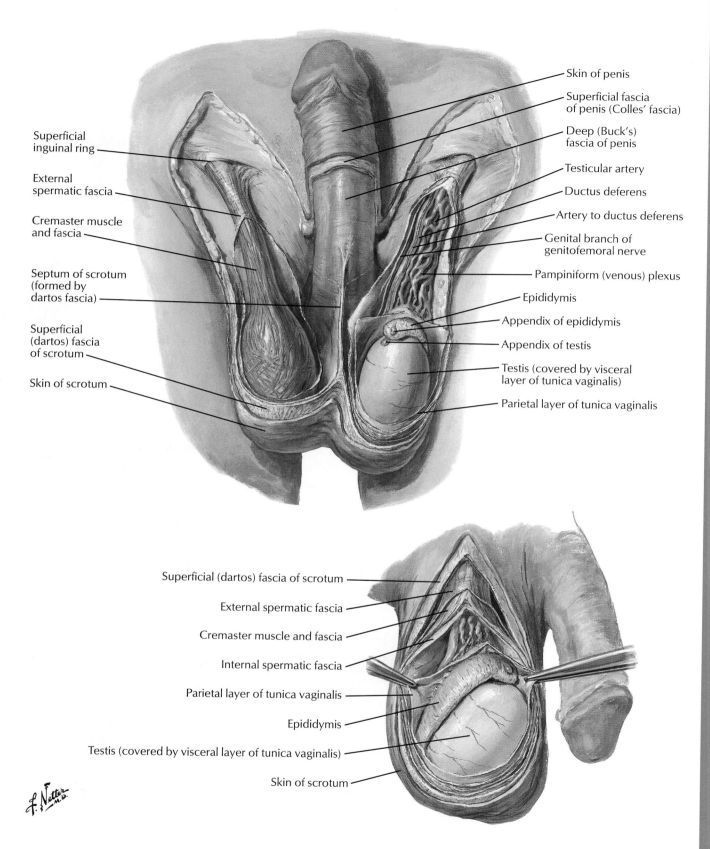

Skin of penis

Superficial fascia
of penis (Colles' fascia)

Deep (Buck's)
fascia of penis

Testicular artery

Ductus deferens

Artery to ductus deferens

Genital branch of
genitofemoral nerve

Pampiniform (venous) plexus

Epididymis

Appendix of epididymis

Appendix of testis

Testis (covered by visceral
layer of tunica vaginalis)

Parietal layer of tunica vaginalis

Superficial
inguinal ring

External
spermatic fascia

Cremaster muscle
and fascia

Septum of scrotum
(formed by
dartos fascia)

Superficial
(dartos) fascia
of scrotum

Skin of scrotum

Superficial (dartos) fascia of scrotum

External spermatic fascia

Cremaster muscle and fascia

Internal spermatic fascia

Parietal layer of tunica vaginalis

Epididymis

Testis (covered by visceral layer of tunica vaginalis)

Skin of scrotum

Plate 387 Scrotum and Contents. (Netter: Atlas of Human Anatomy, 4 ed, 2006, Saunders.)

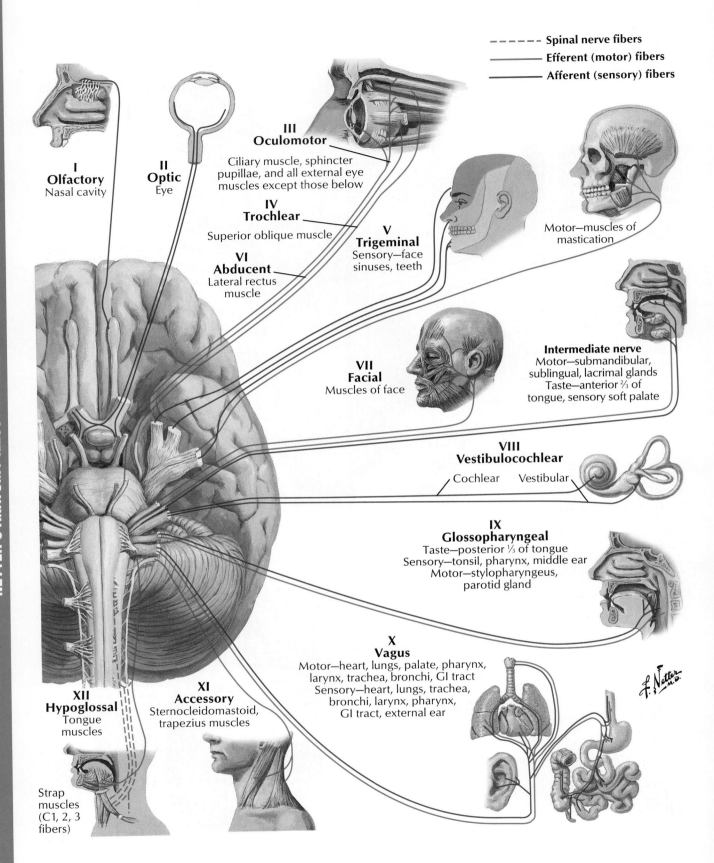

- - - - Spinal nerve fibers
———— Efferent (motor) fibers
———— Afferent (sensory) fibers

**I
Olfactory**
Nasal cavity

**II
Optic**
Eye

**III
Oculomotor**
Ciliary muscle, sphincter pupillae, and all external eye muscles except those below

**IV
Trochlear**
Superior oblique muscle

**V
Trigeminal**
Sensory—face sinuses, teeth

**VI
Abducent**
Lateral rectus muscle

Motor—muscles of mastication

**VII
Facial**
Muscles of face

Intermediate nerve
Motor—submandibular, sublingual, lacrimal glands
Taste—anterior ⅔ of tongue, sensory soft palate

**VIII
Vestibulocochlear**
Cochlear   Vestibular

**IX
Glossopharyngeal**
Taste—posterior ⅓ of tongue
Sensory—tonsil, pharynx, middle ear
Motor—stylopharyngeus, parotid gland

**X
Vagus**
Motor—heart, lungs, palate, pharynx, larynx, trachea, bronchi, GI tract
Sensory—heart, lungs, trachea, bronchi, larynx, pharynx, GI tract, external ear

**XII
Hypoglossal**
Tongue muscles

**XI
Accessory**
Sternocleidomastoid, trapezius muscles

Strap muscles (C1, 2, 3 fibers)

f. Netter m.d.

Plate 118 Cranial Nerves (Motor and Sensory Distribution): Schema. (Netter: Atlas of Human Anatomy, 4 ed, 2006, Saunders.)

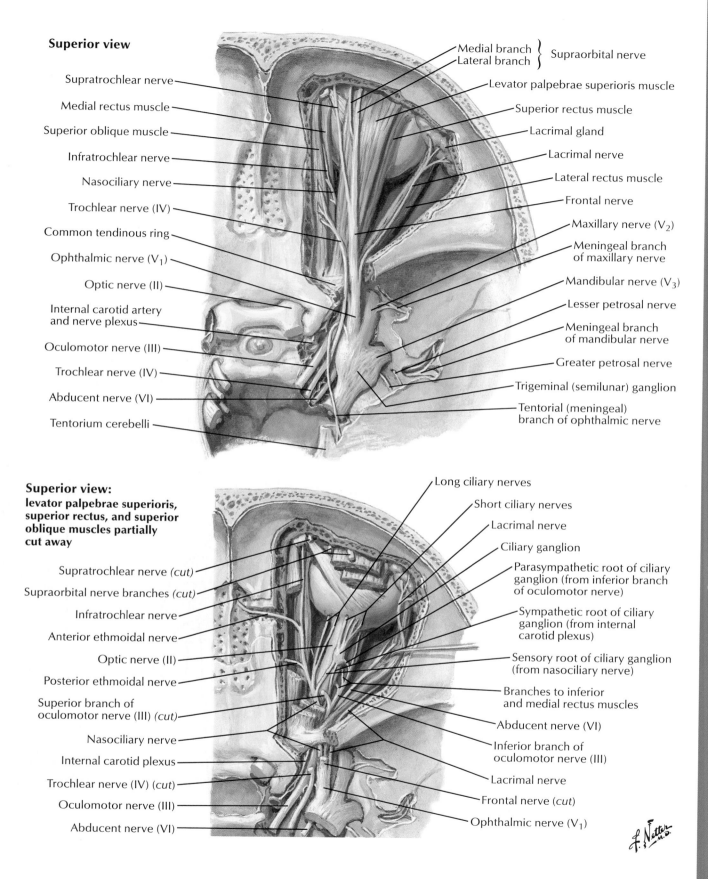

Superior view

Supratrochlear nerve

Medial rectus muscle

Superior oblique muscle

Infratrochlear nerve

Nasociliary nerve

Trochlear nerve (IV)

Common tendinous ring

Ophthalmic nerve (V₁)

Optic nerve (II)

Internal carotid artery and nerve plexus

Oculomotor nerve (III)

Trochlear nerve (IV)

Abducent nerve (VI)

Tentorium cerebelli

Medial branch } Supraorbital nerve
Lateral branch }

Levator palpebrae superioris muscle

Superior rectus muscle

Lacrimal gland

Lacrimal nerve

Lateral rectus muscle

Frontal nerve

Maxillary nerve (V₂)

Meningeal branch of maxillary nerve

Mandibular nerve (V₃)

Lesser petrosal nerve

Meningeal branch of mandibular nerve

Greater petrosal nerve

Trigeminal (semilunar) ganglion

Tentorial (meningeal) branch of ophthalmic nerve

Superior view:
levator palpebrae superioris, superior rectus, and superior oblique muscles partially cut away

Supratrochlear nerve *(cut)*

Supraorbital nerve branches *(cut)*

Infratrochlear nerve

Anterior ethmoidal nerve

Optic nerve (II)

Posterior ethmoidal nerve

Superior branch of oculomotor nerve (III) *(cut)*

Nasociliary nerve

Internal carotid plexus

Trochlear nerve (IV) *(cut)*

Oculomotor nerve (III)

Abducent nerve (VI)

Long ciliary nerves

Short ciliary nerves

Lacrimal nerve

Ciliary ganglion

Parasympathetic root of ciliary ganglion (from inferior branch of oculomotor nerve)

Sympathetic root of ciliary ganglion (from internal carotid plexus)

Sensory root of ciliary ganglion (from nasociliary nerve)

Branches to inferior and medial rectus muscles

Abducent nerve (VI)

Inferior branch of oculomotor nerve (III)

Lacrimal nerve

Frontal nerve *(cut)*

Ophthalmic nerve (V₁)

Plate 86 Nerves of Orbit. (Netter: Atlas of Human Anatomy, 4 ed, 2006, Saunders.)

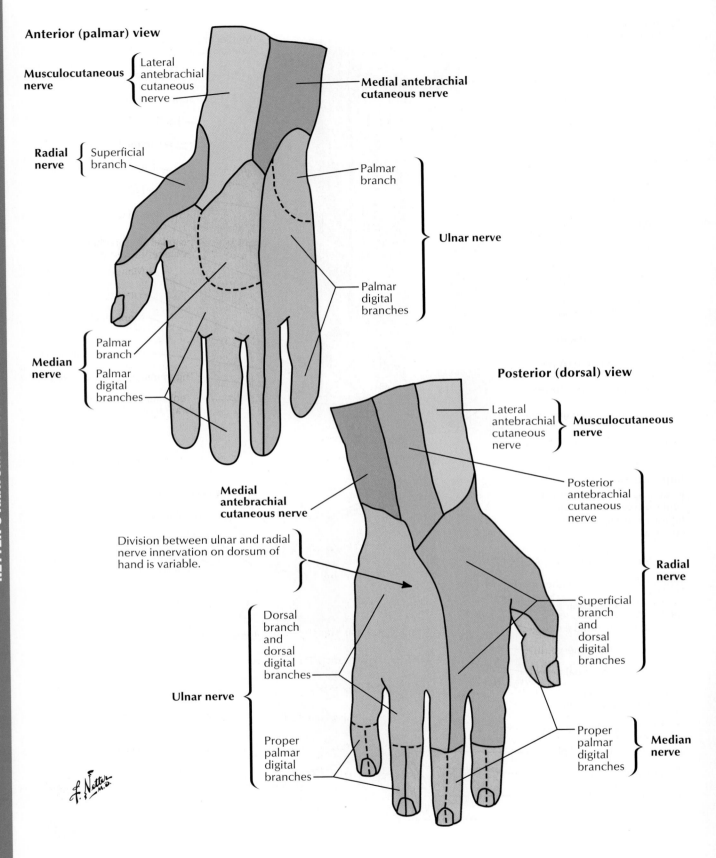

Anterior (palmar) view

Musculocutaneous nerve — Lateral antebrachial cutaneous nerve

Medial antebrachial cutaneous nerve

Radial nerve — Superficial branch

Palmar branch

Ulnar nerve

Palmar digital branches

Median nerve — Palmar branch / Palmar digital branches

Posterior (dorsal) view

Lateral antebrachial cutaneous nerve — Musculocutaneous nerve

Posterior antebrachial cutaneous nerve

Medial antebrachial cutaneous nerve

Division between ulnar and radial nerve innervation on dorsum of hand is variable.

Radial nerve

Superficial branch and dorsal digital branches

Ulnar nerve — Dorsal branch and dorsal digital branches

Proper palmar digital branches

Proper palmar digital branches — Median nerve

Plate 472   Cutaneous Innervation of Wrist and Hand. (Netter: Atlas of Human Anatomy, 4 ed, 2006, Saunders.)

14

NETTER'S ANATOMY ILLUSTRATIONS

Anterior view

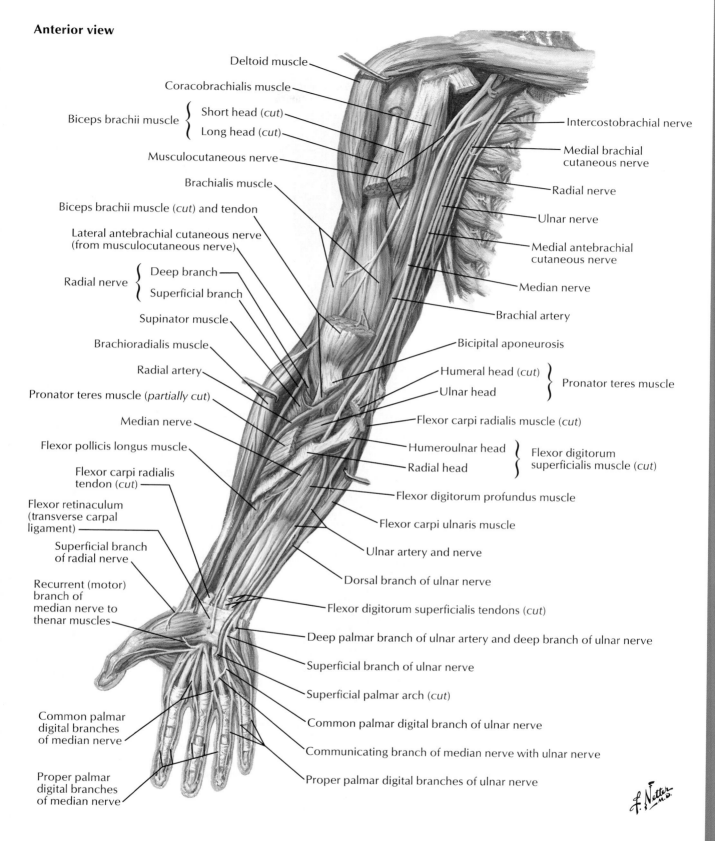

Deltoid muscle

Coracobrachialis muscle

Biceps brachii muscle { Short head (*cut*)
Long head (*cut*)

Musculocutaneous nerve

Brachialis muscle

Biceps brachii muscle (*cut*) and tendon

Lateral antebrachial cutaneous nerve (from musculocutaneous nerve)

Radial nerve { Deep branch
Superficial branch

Supinator muscle

Brachioradialis muscle

Radial artery

Pronator teres muscle (*partially cut*)

Median nerve

Flexor pollicis longus muscle

Flexor carpi radialis tendon (*cut*)

Flexor retinaculum (transverse carpal ligament)

Superficial branch of radial nerve

Recurrent (motor) branch of median nerve to thenar muscles

Common palmar digital branches of median nerve

Proper palmar digital branches of median nerve

Intercostobrachial nerve

Medial brachial cutaneous nerve

Radial nerve

Ulnar nerve

Medial antebrachial cutaneous nerve

Median nerve

Brachial artery

Bicipital aponeurosis

Humeral head (*cut*) }
Ulnar head } Pronator teres muscle

Flexor carpi radialis muscle (*cut*)

Humeroulnar head }
Radial head } Flexor digitorum superficialis muscle (*cut*)

Flexor digitorum profundus muscle

Flexor carpi ulnaris muscle

Ulnar artery and nerve

Dorsal branch of ulnar nerve

Flexor digitorum superficialis tendons (*cut*)

Deep palmar branch of ulnar artery and deep branch of ulnar nerve

Superficial branch of ulnar nerve

Superficial palmar arch (*cut*)

Common palmar digital branch of ulnar nerve

Communicating branch of median nerve with ulnar nerve

Proper palmar digital branches of ulnar nerve

Plate 473 Arteries and Nerves of Upper Limb. (Netter: Atlas of Human Anatomy, 4 ed, 2006, Saunders.)

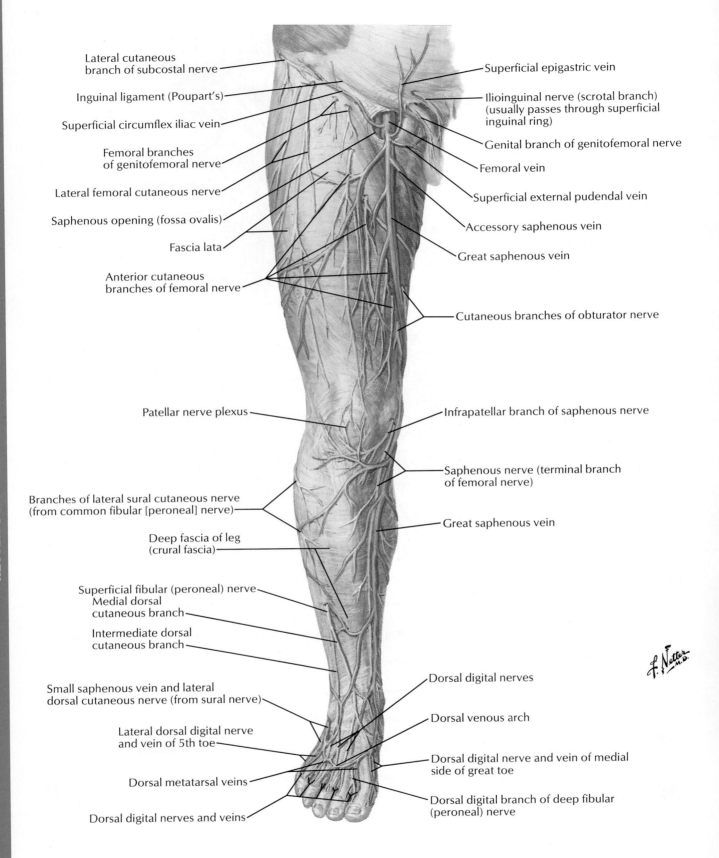

Lateral cutaneous branch of subcostal nerve

Inguinal ligament (Poupart's)

Superficial circumflex iliac vein

Femoral branches of genitofemoral nerve

Lateral femoral cutaneous nerve

Saphenous opening (fossa ovalis)

Fascia lata

Anterior cutaneous branches of femoral nerve

Patellar nerve plexus

Branches of lateral sural cutaneous nerve (from common fibular [peroneal] nerve)

Deep fascia of leg (crural fascia)

Superficial fibular (peroneal) nerve
Medial dorsal cutaneous branch

Intermediate dorsal cutaneous branch

Small saphenous vein and lateral dorsal cutaneous nerve (from sural nerve)

Lateral dorsal digital nerve and vein of 5th toe

Dorsal metatarsal veins

Dorsal digital nerves and veins

Superficial epigastric vein

Ilioinguinal nerve (scrotal branch) (usually passes through superficial inguinal ring)

Genital branch of genitofemoral nerve

Femoral vein

Superficial external pudendal vein

Accessory saphenous vein

Great saphenous vein

Cutaneous branches of obturator nerve

Infrapatellar branch of saphenous nerve

Saphenous nerve (terminal branch of femoral nerve)

Great saphenous vein

Dorsal digital nerves

Dorsal venous arch

Dorsal digital nerve and vein of medial side of great toe

Dorsal digital branch of deep fibular (peroneal) nerve

Plate 544 Superficial Nerves and Veins of Lower Limb: Anterior View. (Netter: Atlas of Human Anatomy, 4 ed, 2006, Saunders.)

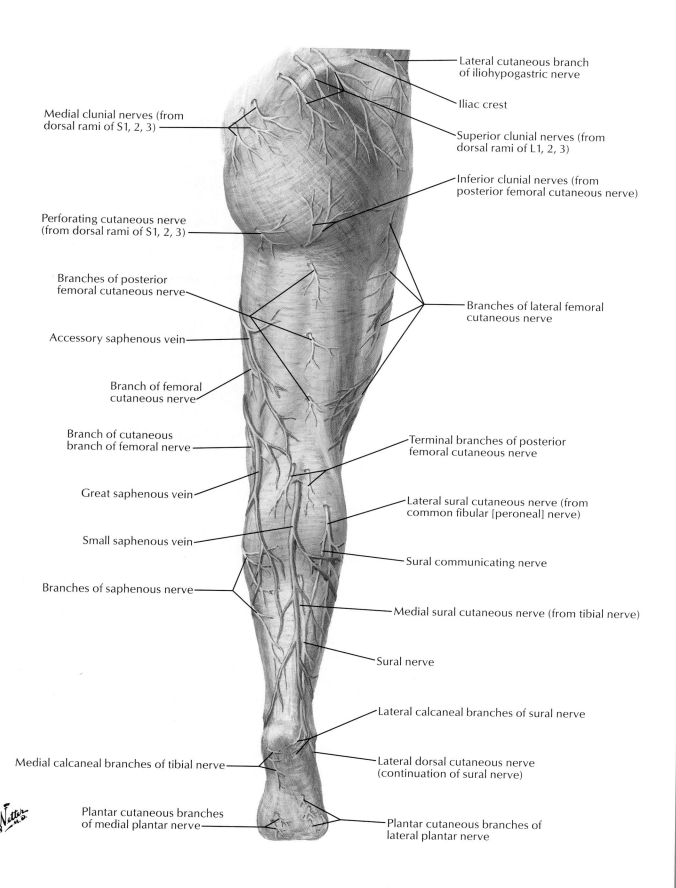

Lateral cutaneous branch of iliohypogastric nerve

Iliac crest

Medial clunial nerves (from dorsal rami of S1, 2, 3)

Superior clunial nerves (from dorsal rami of L1, 2, 3)

Inferior clunial nerves (from posterior femoral cutaneous nerve)

Perforating cutaneous nerve (from dorsal rami of S1, 2, 3)

Branches of posterior femoral cutaneous nerve

Branches of lateral femoral cutaneous nerve

Accessory saphenous vein

Branch of femoral cutaneous nerve

Branch of cutaneous branch of femoral nerve

Terminal branches of posterior femoral cutaneous nerve

Great saphenous vein

Lateral sural cutaneous nerve (from common fibular [peroneal] nerve)

Small saphenous vein

Sural communicating nerve

Branches of saphenous nerve

Medial sural cutaneous nerve (from tibial nerve)

Sural nerve

Lateral calcaneal branches of sural nerve

Medial calcaneal branches of tibial nerve

Lateral dorsal cutaneous nerve (continuation of sural nerve)

Plantar cutaneous branches of medial plantar nerve

Plantar cutaneous branches of lateral plantar nerve

Plate 545 Superficial Nerves and Veins of Lower Limb: Posterior View. (Netter: Atlas of Human Anatomy, 4 ed, 2006, Saunders.)

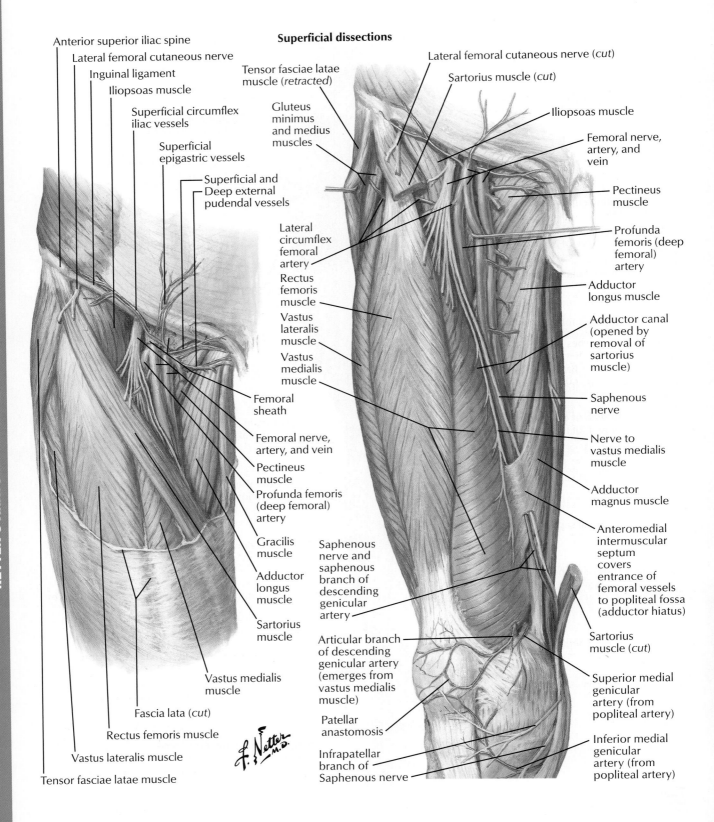

Superficial dissections

Anterior superior iliac spine
Lateral femoral cutaneous nerve
Inguinal ligament
Iliopsoas muscle
Superficial circumflex iliac vessels
Superficial epigastric vessels
Superficial and Deep external pudendal vessels

Tensor fasciae latae muscle (*retracted*)
Gluteus minimus and medius muscles
Lateral circumflex femoral artery
Rectus femoris muscle
Vastus lateralis muscle
Vastus medialis muscle
Femoral sheath
Femoral nerve, artery, and vein
Pectineus muscle
Profunda femoris (deep femoral) artery
Gracilis muscle
Adductor longus muscle
Sartorius muscle

Lateral femoral cutaneous nerve (*cut*)
Sartorius muscle (*cut*)
Iliopsoas muscle
Femoral nerve, artery, and vein
Pectineus muscle
Profunda femoris (deep femoral) artery
Adductor longus muscle
Adductor canal (opened by removal of sartorius muscle)
Saphenous nerve
Nerve to vastus medialis muscle
Adductor magnus muscle
Anteromedial intermuscular septum covers entrance of femoral vessels to popliteal fossa (adductor hiatus)
Sartorius muscle (*cut*)
Superior medial genicular artery (from popliteal artery)
Inferior medial genicular artery (from popliteal artery)

Saphenous nerve and saphenous branch of descending genicular artery
Articular branch of descending genicular artery (emerges from vastus medialis muscle)
Patellar anastomosis
Infrapatellar branch of Saphenous nerve

Vastus medialis muscle
Fascia lata (*cut*)
Rectus femoris muscle
Vastus lateralis muscle
Tensor fasciae latae muscle

F. Netter M.D.

Plate 500   Arteries and Nerves of Thigh: Anterior Views. (Netter: Atlas of Human Anatomy, 4 ed, 2006, Saunders.)

18

NETTER'S ANATOMY ILLUSTRATIONS

Deep dissection

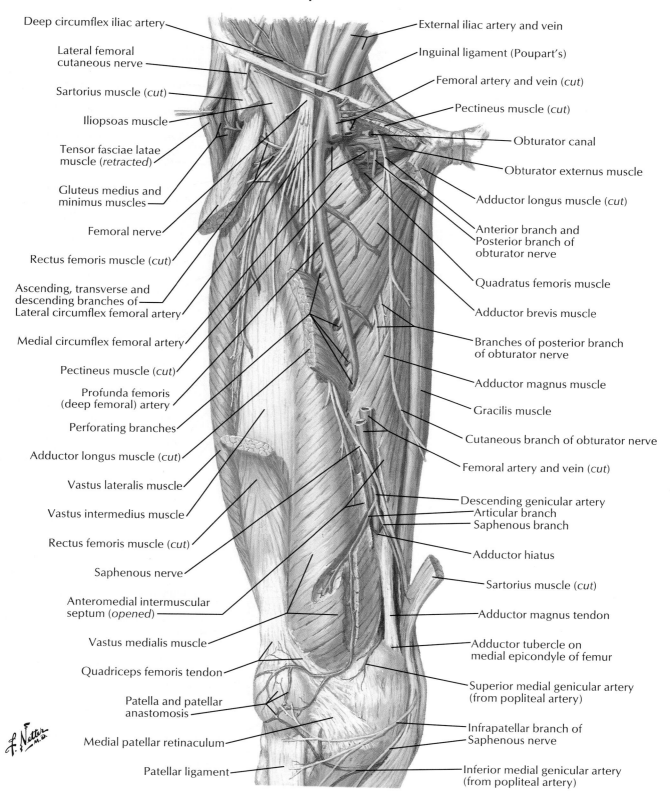

Deep circumflex iliac artery

Lateral femoral cutaneous nerve

Sartorius muscle (cut)

Iliopsoas muscle

Tensor fasciae latae muscle (retracted)

Gluteus medius and minimus muscles

Femoral nerve

Rectus femoris muscle (cut)

Ascending, transverse and descending branches of Lateral circumflex femoral artery

Medial circumflex femoral artery

Pectineus muscle (cut)

Profunda femoris (deep femoral) artery

Perforating branches

Adductor longus muscle (cut)

Vastus lateralis muscle

Vastus intermedius muscle

Rectus femoris muscle (cut)

Saphenous nerve

Anteromedial intermuscular septum (opened)

Vastus medialis muscle

Quadriceps femoris tendon

Patella and patellar anastomosis

Medial patellar retinaculum

Patellar ligament

External iliac artery and vein

Inguinal ligament (Poupart's)

Femoral artery and vein (cut)

Pectineus muscle (cut)

Obturator canal

Obturator externus muscle

Adductor longus muscle (cut)

Anterior branch and Posterior branch of obturator nerve

Quadratus femoris muscle

Adductor brevis muscle

Branches of posterior branch of obturator nerve

Adductor magnus muscle

Gracilis muscle

Cutaneous branch of obturator nerve

Femoral artery and vein (cut)

Descending genicular artery
Articular branch
Saphenous branch

Adductor hiatus

Sartorius muscle (cut)

Adductor magnus tendon

Adductor tubercle on medial epicondyle of femur

Superior medial genicular artery (from popliteal artery)

Infrapatellar branch of Saphenous nerve

Inferior medial genicular artery (from popliteal artery)

Plate 501 Arteries and Nerves of Thigh: Posterior View. (Netter: Atlas of Human Anatomy, 4 ed, 2006, Saunders.)

19

Deep dissection

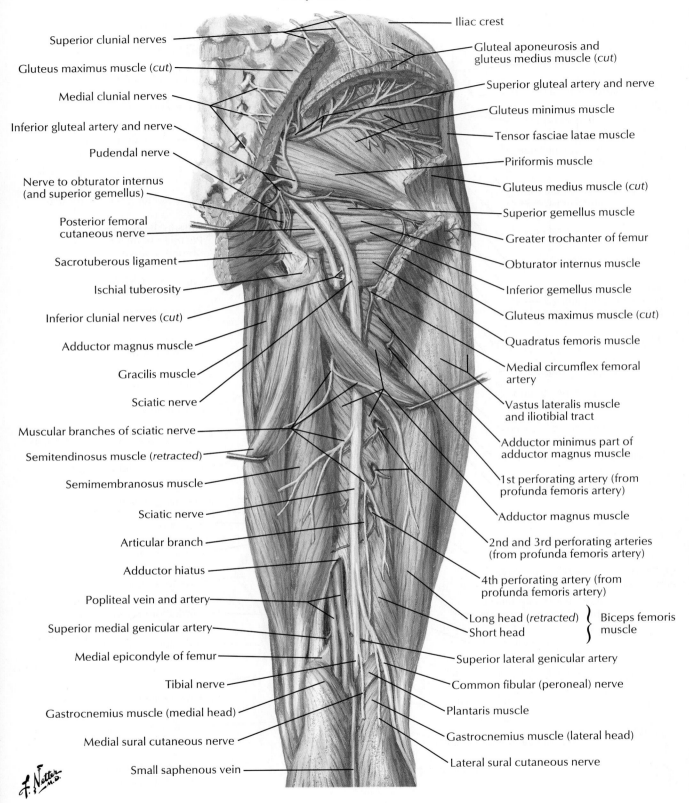

Superior clunial nerves

Gluteus maximus muscle (*cut*)

Medial clunial nerves

Inferior gluteal artery and nerve

Pudendal nerve

Nerve to obturator internus (and superior gemellus)

Posterior femoral cutaneous nerve

Sacrotuberous ligament

Ischial tuberosity

Inferior clunial nerves (*cut*)

Adductor magnus muscle

Gracilis muscle

Sciatic nerve

Muscular branches of sciatic nerve

Semitendinosus muscle (*retracted*)

Semimembranosus muscle

Sciatic nerve

Articular branch

Adductor hiatus

Popliteal vein and artery

Superior medial genicular artery

Medial epicondyle of femur

Tibial nerve

Gastrocnemius muscle (medial head)

Medial sural cutaneous nerve

Small saphenous vein

Iliac crest

Gluteal aponeurosis and gluteus medius muscle (*cut*)

Superior gluteal artery and nerve

Gluteus minimus muscle

Tensor fasciae latae muscle

Piriformis muscle

Gluteus medius muscle (*cut*)

Superior gemellus muscle

Greater trochanter of femur

Obturator internus muscle

Inferior gemellus muscle

Gluteus maximus muscle (*cut*)

Quadratus femoris muscle

Medial circumflex femoral artery

Vastus lateralis muscle and iliotibial tract

Adductor minimus part of adductor magnus muscle

1st perforating artery (from profunda femoris artery)

Adductor magnus muscle

2nd and 3rd perforating arteries (from profunda femoris artery)

4th perforating artery (from profunda femoris artery)

Long head (*retracted*) } Biceps femoris
Short head } muscle

Superior lateral genicular artery

Common fibular (peroneal) nerve

Plantaris muscle

Gastrocnemius muscle (lateral head)

Lateral sural cutaneous nerve

NETTER'S ANATOMY ILLUSTRATIONS

Plate 502 Arteries and Nerves of Thigh: Posterior View. (Netter: Atlas of Human Anatomy, 4 ed, 2006, Saunders.)

20

Horizontal section

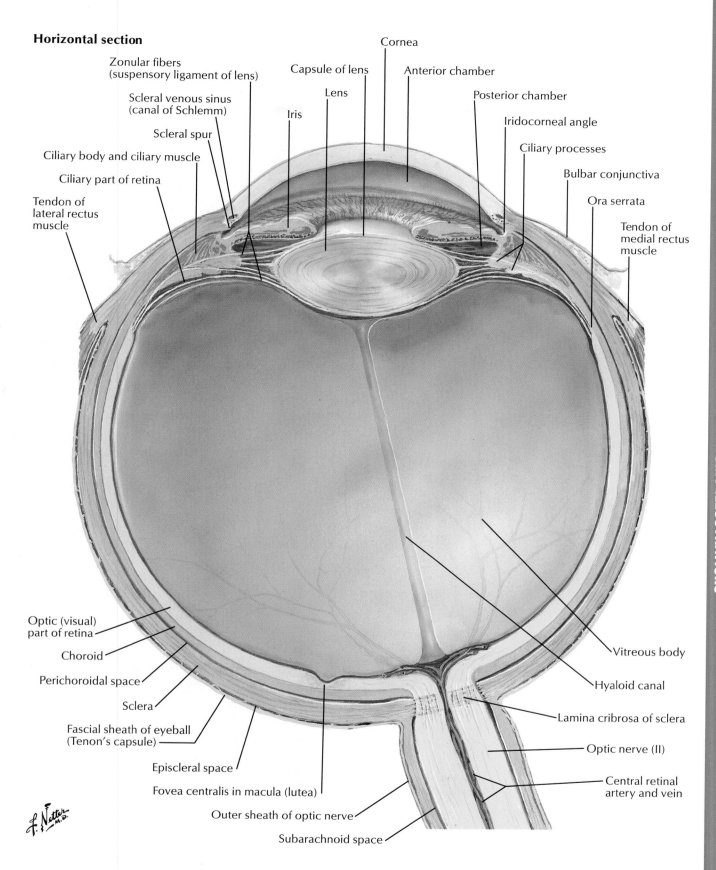

Zonular fibers
(suspensory ligament of lens)

Scleral venous sinus
(canal of Schlemm)

Scleral spur

Ciliary body and ciliary muscle

Ciliary part of retina

Tendon of
lateral rectus
muscle

Iris

Capsule of lens

Lens

Cornea

Anterior chamber

Posterior chamber

Iridocorneal angle

Ciliary processes

Bulbar conjunctiva

Ora serrata

Tendon of
medial rectus
muscle

Optic (visual)
part of retina

Choroid

Perichoroidal space

Sclera

Fascial sheath of eyeball
(Tenon's capsule)

Episcleral space

Fovea centralis in macula (lutea)

Outer sheath of optic nerve

Subarachnoid space

Vitreous body

Hyaloid canal

Lamina cribrosa of sclera

Optic nerve (II)

Central retinal
artery and vein

Plate 87   Eyeball. (Netter: Atlas of Human Anatomy, 4 ed, 2006, Saunders.)

21

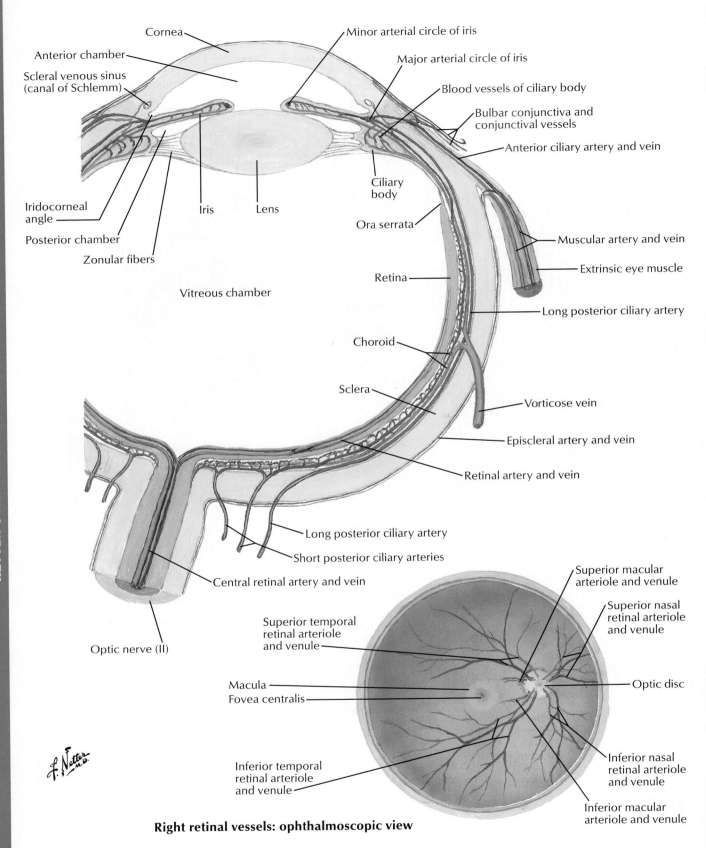

Cornea

Minor arterial circle of iris

Anterior chamber

Major arterial circle of iris

Scleral venous sinus
(canal of Schlemm)

Blood vessels of ciliary body

Bulbar conjunctiva and
conjunctival vessels

Anterior ciliary artery and vein

Ciliary
body

Iridocorneal
angle

Iris

Lens

Ora serrata

Muscular artery and vein

Posterior chamber

Extrinsic eye muscle

Zonular fibers

Retina

Long posterior ciliary artery

Vitreous chamber

Choroid

Sclera

Vorticose vein

Episcleral artery and vein

Retinal artery and vein

Long posterior ciliary artery

Short posterior ciliary arteries

Central retinal artery and vein

Superior macular
arteriole and venule

Superior nasal
retinal arteriole
and venule

Superior temporal
retinal arteriole
and venule

Optic nerve (II)

Macula

Optic disc

Fovea centralis

Inferior nasal
retinal arteriole
and venule

Inferior temporal
retinal arteriole
and venule

Inferior macular
arteriole and venule

Right retinal vessels: ophthalmoscopic view

Plate 90 Intrinsic Arteries and Veins of Eye. (Netter: Atlas of Human Anatomy, 4 ed, 2006, Saunders.)

22

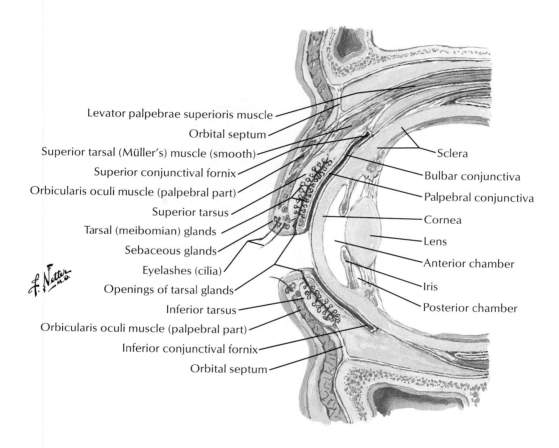

Levator palpebrae superioris muscle

Orbital septum

Superior tarsal (Müller's) muscle (smooth)

Superior conjunctival fornix

Orbicularis oculi muscle (palpebral part)

Superior tarsus

Tarsal (meibomian) glands

Sebaceous glands

Eyelashes (cilia)

Openings of tarsal glands

Inferior tarsus

Orbicularis oculi muscle (palpebral part)

Inferior conjunctival fornix

Orbital septum

Sclera

Bulbar conjunctiva

Palpebral conjunctiva

Cornea

Lens

Anterior chamber

Iris

Posterior chamber

Plate 81, Middle   Eyelids. (Netter: Atlas of Human Anatomy, 4 ed, 2006, Saunders.)

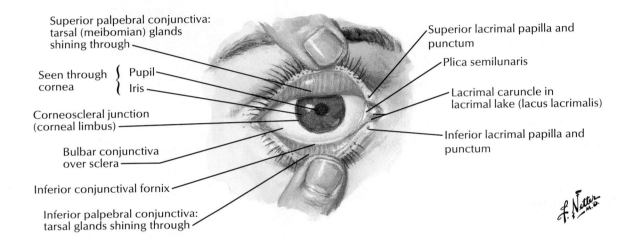

Superior palpebral conjunctiva:
tarsal (meibomian) glands
shining through

Seen through { Pupil
cornea { Iris

Corneoscleral junction
(corneal limbus)

Bulbar conjunctiva
over sclera

Inferior conjunctival fornix

Inferior palpebral conjunctiva:
tarsal glands shining through

Superior lacrimal papilla and
punctum

Plica semilunaris

Lacrimal caruncle in
lacrimal lake (lacus lacrimalis)

Inferior lacrimal papilla and
punctum

Plate 81, Upper   Eyelid. (Netter: Atlas of Human Anatomy, 4 ed, 2006, Saunders.)

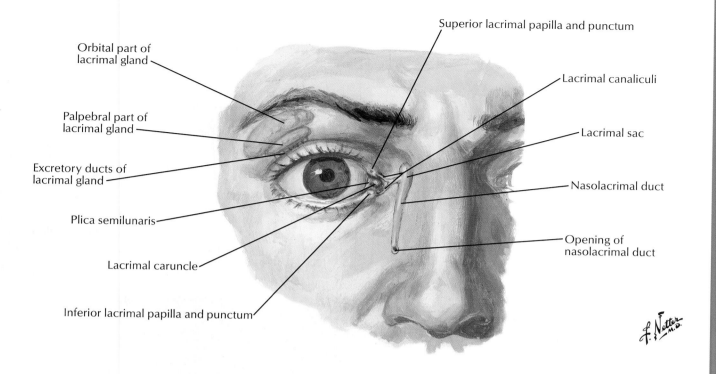

Orbital part of lacrimal gland

Palpebral part of lacrimal gland

Excretory ducts of lacrimal gland

Plica semilunaris

Lacrimal caruncle

Inferior lacrimal papilla and punctum

Superior lacrimal papilla and punctum

Lacrimal canaliculi

Lacrimal sac

Nasolacrimal duct

Opening of nasolacrimal duct

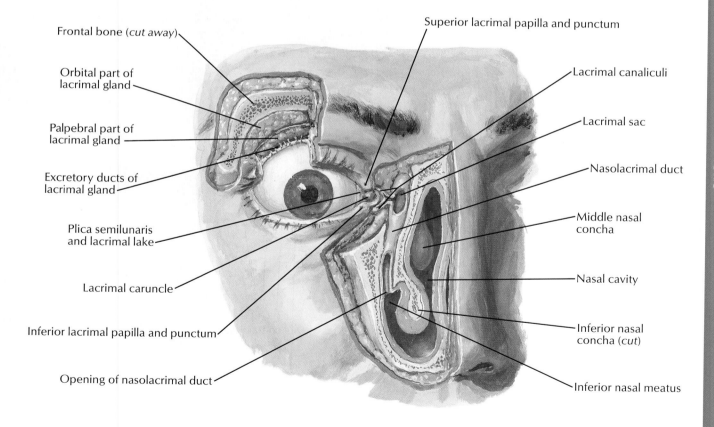

Frontal bone (cut away)

Orbital part of lacrimal gland

Palpebral part of lacrimal gland

Excretory ducts of lacrimal gland

Plica semilunaris and lacrimal lake

Lacrimal caruncle

Inferior lacrimal papilla and punctum

Opening of nasolacrimal duct

Superior lacrimal papilla and punctum

Lacrimal canaliculi

Lacrimal sac

Nasolacrimal duct

Middle nasal concha

Nasal cavity

Inferior nasal concha (cut)

Inferior nasal meatus

Plate 82   Lacrimal Apparatus. (Netter: Atlas of Human Anatomy, 4 ed, 2006, Saunders.)

Frontal section

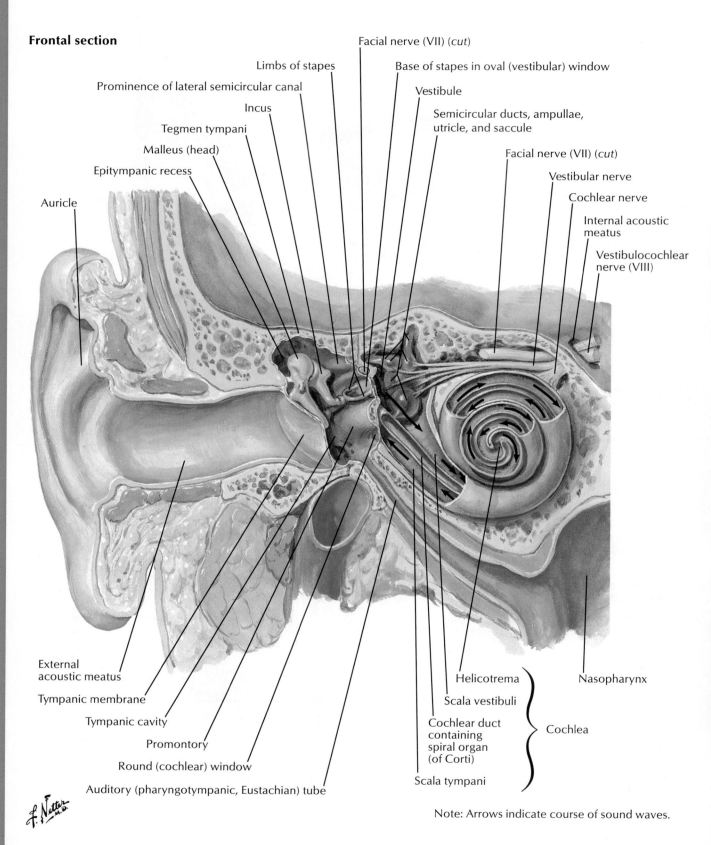

Facial nerve (VII) (*cut*)

Base of stapes in oval (vestibular) window

Limbs of stapes

Vestibule

Prominence of lateral semicircular canal

Semicircular ducts, ampullae, utricle, and saccule

Incus

Tegmen tympani

Facial nerve (VII) (*cut*)

Malleus (head)

Vestibular nerve

Epitympanic recess

Cochlear nerve

Auricle

Internal acoustic meatus

Vestibulocochlear nerve (VIII)

External acoustic meatus

Helicotrema

Nasopharynx

Tympanic membrane

Scala vestibuli

Tympanic cavity

Cochlear duct containing spiral organ (of Corti)

Cochlea

Promontory

Round (cochlear) window

Scala tympani

Auditory (pharyngotympanic, Eustachian) tube

Note: Arrows indicate course of sound waves.

Plate 92   Pathway of Sound Reception. (Netter: Atlas of Human Anatomy, 4 ed, 2006, Saunders.)

Medial wall of tympanic cavity: lateral view

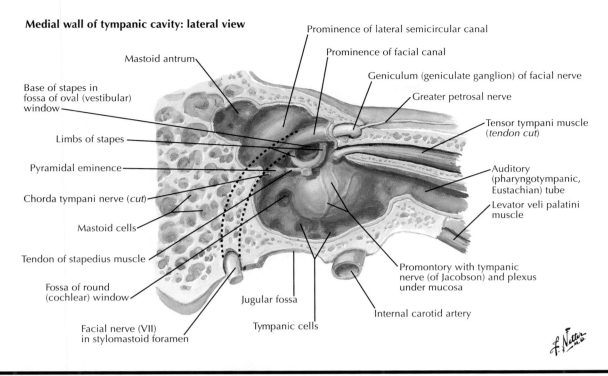

Mastoid antrum

Prominence of lateral semicircular canal

Prominence of facial canal

Geniculum (geniculate ganglion) of facial nerve

Greater petrosal nerve

Base of stapes in fossa of oval (vestibular) window

Tensor tympani muscle (*tendon cut*)

Limbs of stapes

Pyramidal eminence

Auditory (pharyngotympanic, Eustachian) tube

Chorda tympani nerve (*cut*)

Levator veli palatini muscle

Mastoid cells

Tendon of stapedius muscle

Fossa of round (cochlear) window

Promontory with tympanic nerve (of Jacobson) and plexus under mucosa

Jugular fossa

Tympanic cells

Internal carotid artery

Facial nerve (VII) in stylomastoid foramen

Plate 94 Tympanic Cavity. (Netter: Atlas of Human Anatomy, 4 ed, 2006, Saunders.)

Otoscopic view of right tympanic membrane

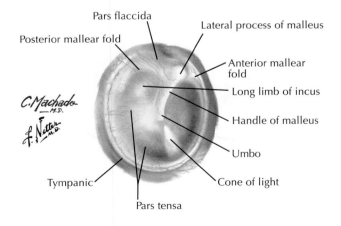

Pars flaccida

Posterior mallear fold

Lateral process of malleus

Anterior mallear fold

Long limb of incus

Handle of malleus

Umbo

Cone of light

Tympanic

Pars tensa

C. Machado M.D.

Plate 93 Tympanic Cavity. (Netter: Atlas of Human Anatomy, 4 ed, 2006, Saunders.)

Dissected right bony labyrinth (otic capsule): membranous labyrinth removed

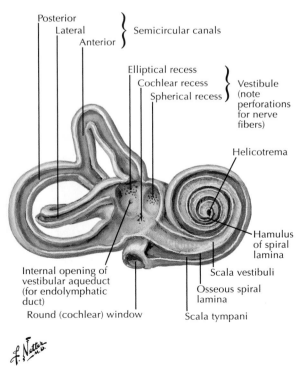

Posterior
Lateral
Anterior } Semicircular canals

Elliptical recess
Cochlear recess
Spherical recess } Vestibule (note perforations for nerve fibers)

Helicotrema

Hamulus of spiral lamina

Scala vestibuli

Osseous spiral lamina

Scala tympani

Internal opening of vestibular aqueduct (for endolymphatic duct)

Round (cochlear) window

Plate 95 Bony Membranous Labyrinth. (Netter: Atlas of Human Anatomy, 4 ed, 2006, Saunders.)

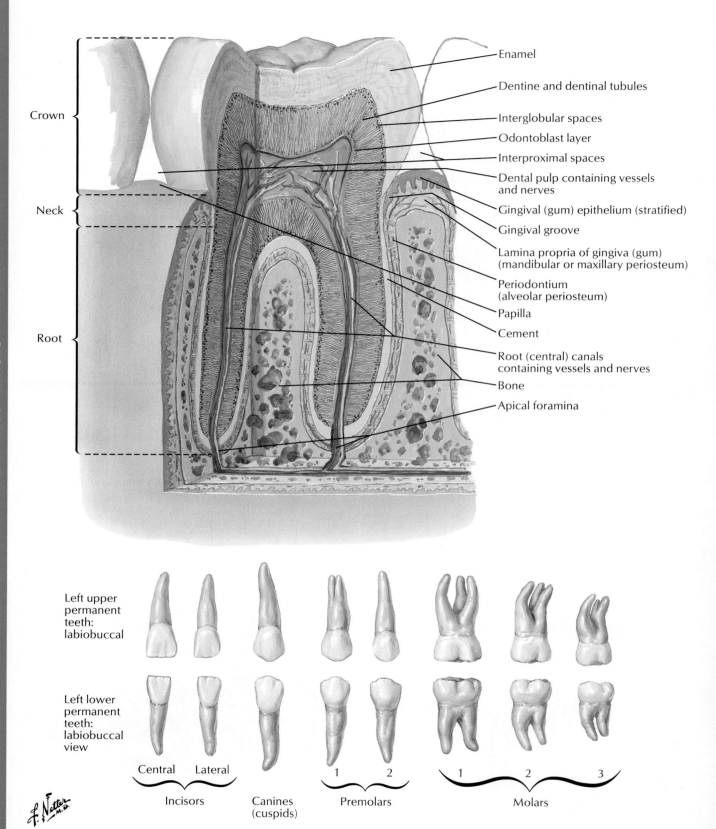

Enamel

Dentine and dentinal tubules

Interglobular spaces

Odontoblast layer

Interproximal spaces

Dental pulp containing vessels and nerves

Gingival (gum) epithelium (stratified)

Gingival groove

Lamina propria of gingiva (gum) (mandibular or maxillary periosteum)

Periodontium (alveolar periosteum)

Papilla

Cement

Root (central) canals containing vessels and nerves

Bone

Apical foramina

Crown

Neck

Root

Left upper permanent teeth: labiobuccal

Left lower permanent teeth: labiobuccal view

Central   Lateral

Incisors

Canines (cuspids)

1   2

Premolars

1   2   3

Molars

Plate 57   Teeth. (Netter: Atlas of Human Anatomy, 4 ed, 2006, Saunders.)

Tongue

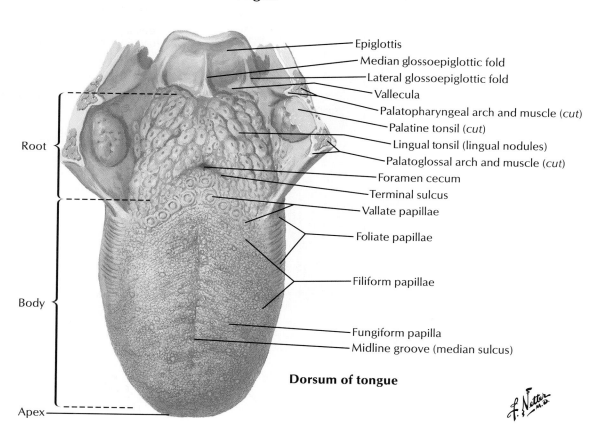

Epiglottis
Median glossoepiglottic fold
Lateral glossoepiglottic fold
Vallecula
Palatopharyngeal arch and muscle (*cut*)
Palatine tonsil (*cut*)
Lingual tonsil (lingual nodules)
Palatoglossal arch and muscle (*cut*)
Foramen cecum
Terminal sulcus
Vallate papillae
Foliate papillae
Filiform papillae
Fungiform papilla
Midline groove (median sulcus)

Root
Body
Apex

Dorsum of tongue

Plate 58   Tongue. (Netter: Atlas of Human Anatomy, 4 ed, 2006, Saunders.)

29

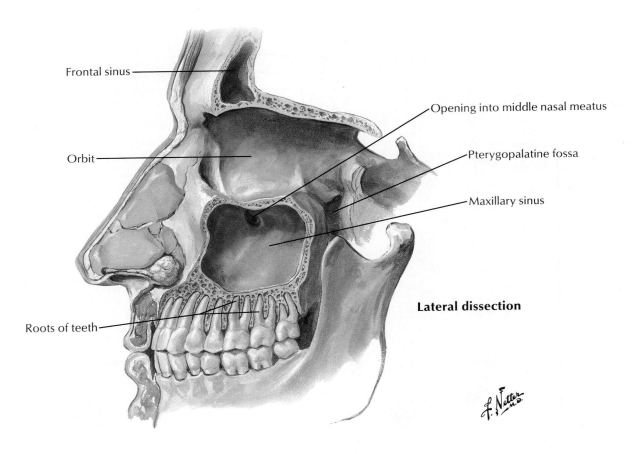

Frontal sinus

Opening into middle nasal meatus

Orbit

Pterygopalatine fossa

Maxillary sinus

Roots of teeth

Lateral dissection

Plate 49   Paranasal Sinuses. (Netter: Atlas of Human Anatomy, 4 ed, 2006, Saunders.)

30

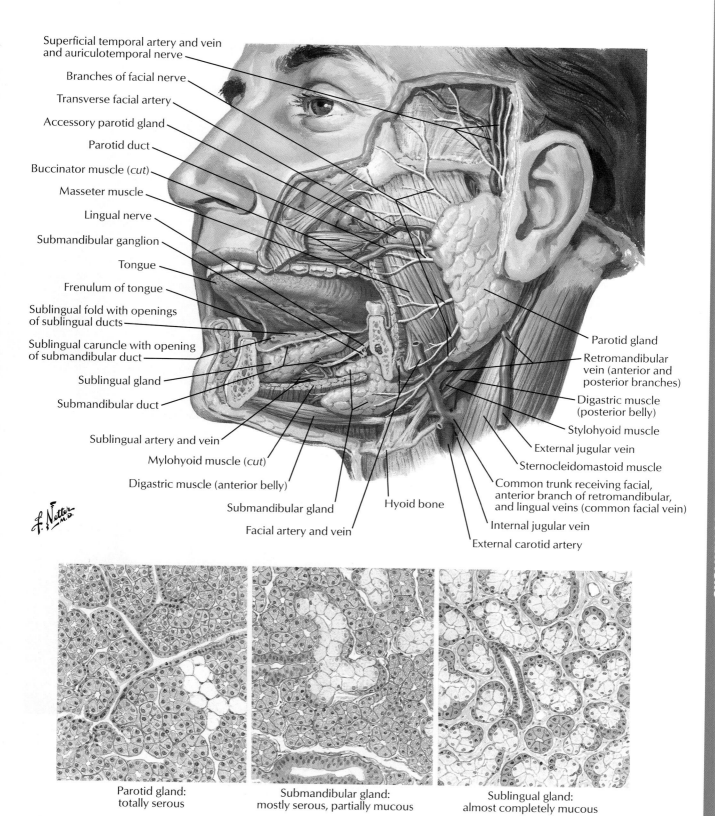

Superficial temporal artery and vein and auriculotemporal nerve

Branches of facial nerve

Transverse facial artery

Accessory parotid gland

Parotid duct

Buccinator muscle (*cut*)

Masseter muscle

Lingual nerve

Submandibular ganglion

Tongue

Frenulum of tongue

Sublingual fold with openings of sublingual ducts

Sublingual caruncle with opening of submandibular duct

Sublingual gland

Submandibular duct

Sublingual artery and vein

Mylohyoid muscle (*cut*)

Digastric muscle (anterior belly)

Submandibular gland

Facial artery and vein

Hyoid bone

Parotid gland

Retromandibular vein (anterior and posterior branches)

Digastric muscle (posterior belly)

Stylohyoid muscle

External jugular vein

Sternocleidomastoid muscle

Common trunk receiving facial, anterior branch of retromandibular, and lingual veins (common facial vein)

Internal jugular vein

External carotid artery

Parotid gland: totally serous

Submandibular gland: mostly serous, partially mucous

Sublingual gland: almost completely mucous

Plate 61 Salivary Glands. (Netter: Atlas of Human Anatomy, 4 ed, 2006, Saunders.)

Coronary Arteries: Arteriographic Views

Right coronary artery: left anterior oblique view

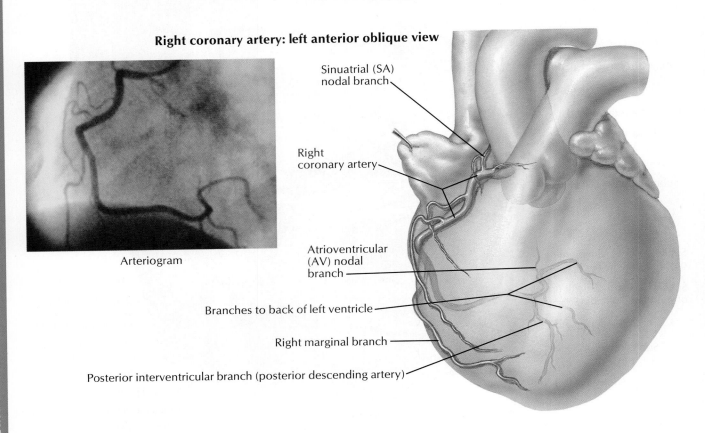

Sinuatrial (SA) nodal branch

Right coronary artery

Atrioventricular (AV) nodal branch

Branches to back of left ventricle

Right marginal branch

Posterior interventricular branch (posterior descending artery)

Arteriogram

Right coronary artery: right anterior oblique view

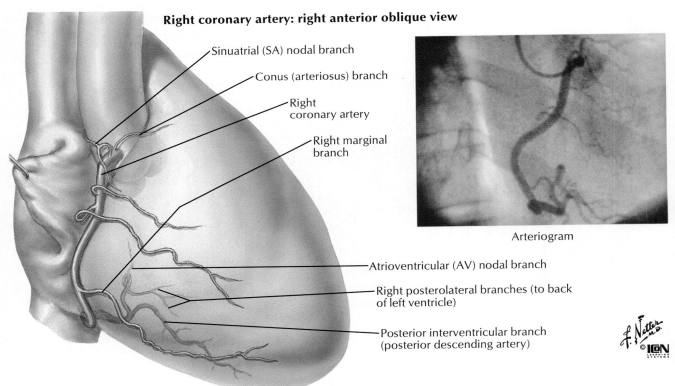

Sinuatrial (SA) nodal branch

Conus (arteriosus) branch

Right coronary artery

Right marginal branch

Atrioventricular (AV) nodal branch

Right posterolateral branches (to back of left ventricle)

Posterior interventricular branch (posterior descending artery)

Arteriogram

Plate 218   Coronary Arteries: Arteriographic Views. (Netter: Atlas of Human Anatomy, 4 ed, 2006, Saunders.)

Left coronary artery: left anterior oblique view

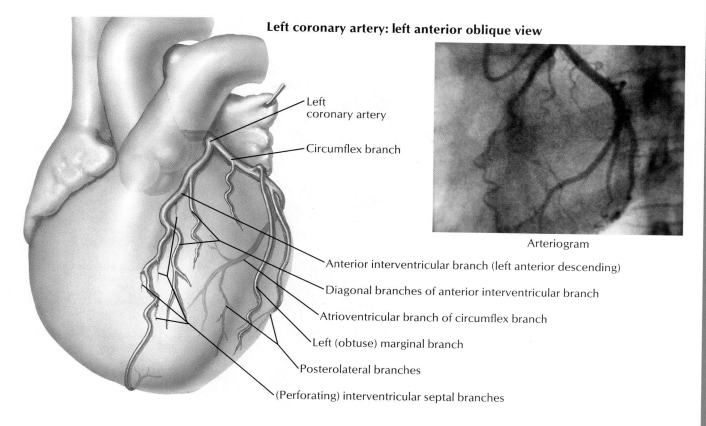

Left coronary artery

Circumflex branch

Arteriogram

Anterior interventricular branch (left anterior descending)

Diagonal branches of anterior interventricular branch

Atrioventricular branch of circumflex branch

Left (obtuse) marginal branch

Posterolateral branches

(Perforating) interventricular septal branches

Left coronary artery: right anterior oblique view

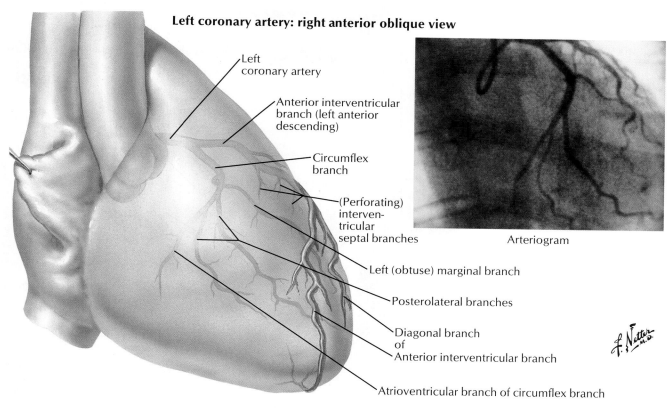

Left coronary artery

Anterior interventricular branch (left anterior descending)

Circumflex branch

(Perforating) interventricular septal branches

Arteriogram

Left (obtuse) marginal branch

Posterolateral branches

Diagonal branch of Anterior interventricular branch

Atrioventricular branch of circumflex branch

Plate 219   Coronary Arteries: Arteriographic Views. (Netter: Atlas of Human Anatomy, 4 ed, 2006, Saunders.)

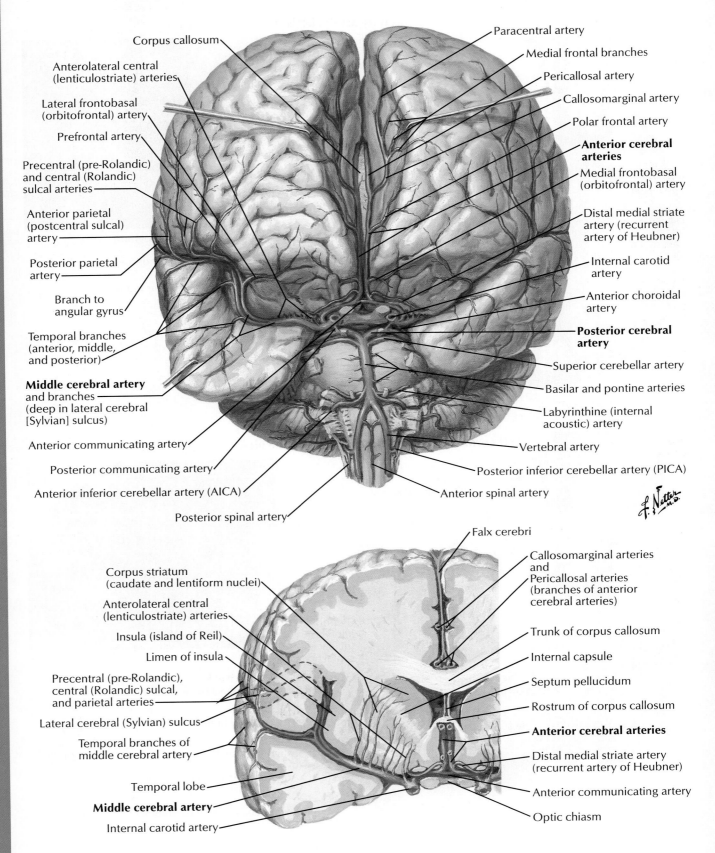

Corpus callosum

Anterolateral central (lenticulostriate) arteries

Lateral frontobasal (orbitofrontal) artery

Prefrontal artery

Precentral (pre-Rolandic) and central (Rolandic) sulcal arteries

Anterior parietal (postcentral sulcal) artery

Posterior parietal artery

Branch to angular gyrus

Temporal branches (anterior, middle, and posterior)

Middle cerebral artery and branches (deep in lateral cerebral [Sylvian] sulcus)

Anterior communicating artery

Posterior communicating artery

Anterior inferior cerebellar artery (AICA)

Posterior spinal artery

Paracentral artery

Medial frontal branches

Pericallosal artery

Callosomarginal artery

Polar frontal artery

Anterior cerebral arteries

Medial frontobasal (orbitofrontal) artery

Distal medial striate artery (recurrent artery of Heubner)

Internal carotid artery

Anterior choroidal artery

Posterior cerebral artery

Superior cerebellar artery

Basilar and pontine arteries

Labyrinthine (internal acoustic) artery

Vertebral artery

Posterior inferior cerebellar artery (PICA)

Anterior spinal artery

Corpus striatum (caudate and lentiform nuclei)

Anterolateral central (lenticulostriate) arteries

Insula (island of Reil)

Limen of insula

Precentral (pre-Rolandic), central (Rolandic) sulcal, and parietal arteries

Lateral cerebral (Sylvian) sulcus

Temporal branches of middle cerebral artery

Temporal lobe

Middle cerebral artery

Internal carotid artery

Falx cerebri

Callosomarginal arteries and Pericallosal arteries (branches of anterior cerebral arteries)

Trunk of corpus callosum

Internal capsule

Septum pellucidum

Rostrum of corpus callosum

Anterior cerebral arteries

Distal medial striate artery (recurrent artery of Heubner)

Anterior communicating artery

Optic chiasm

Plate 141 Arteries of Brain: Frontal View and Section. (Netter: Atlas of Human Anatomy, 4 ed, 2006, Saunders.)

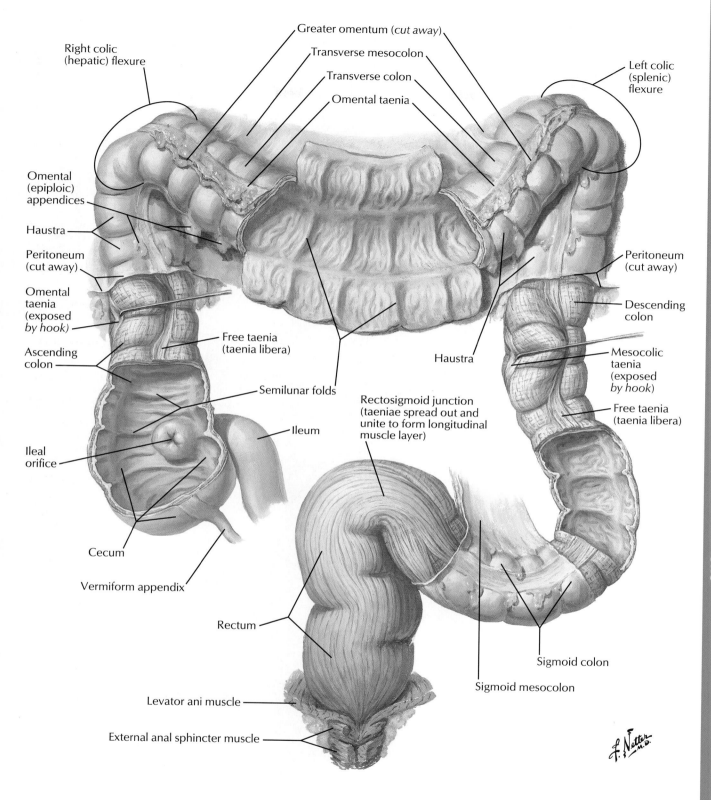

Right colic
(hepatic) flexure

Greater omentum (*cut away*)

Transverse mesocolon

Transverse colon

Omental taenia

Left colic
(splenic)
flexure

Omental
(epiploic)
appendices

Haustra

Peritoneum
(cut away)

Omental
taenia
(exposed
by hook)

Ascending
colon

Ileal
orifice

Cecum

Vermiform appendix

Free taenia
(taenia libera)

Semilunar folds

Ileum

Rectosigmoid junction
(taeniae spread out and
unite to form longitudinal
muscle layer)

Haustra

Peritoneum
(cut away)

Descending
colon

Mesocolic
taenia
(exposed
by hook)

Free taenia
(taenia libera)

Rectum

Levator ani muscle

External anal sphincter muscle

Sigmoid colon

Sigmoid mesocolon

Plate 284 Mucosa and Musculature of Large Intestine. (Netter: Atlas of Human Anatomy, 4 ed, 2006, Saunders.)

Transverse Section: T3–4 Intervertebral Disc, Manubrium

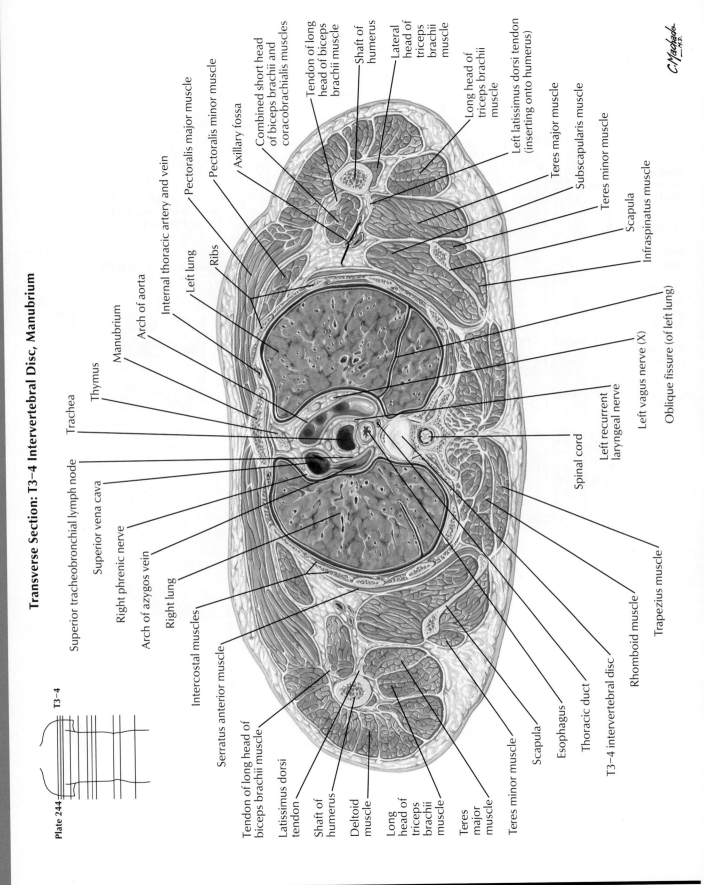

Plate 244

Superior tracheobronchial lymph node

Trachea

Thymus

Manubrium

Arch of aorta

Internal thoracic artery and vein

Left lung

Ribs

Axillary fossa

Pectoralis minor muscle

Pectoralis major muscle

Combined short head of biceps brachii and coracobrachialis muscles

Tendon of long head of biceps brachii muscle

Shaft of humerus

Lateral head of triceps brachii muscle

Long head of triceps brachii muscle

Left latissimus dorsi tendon (inserting onto humerus)

Teres major muscle

Subscapularis muscle

Teres minor muscle

Scapula

Infraspinatus muscle

Oblique fissure (of left lung)

Left vagus nerve (X)

Left recurrent laryngeal nerve

Spinal cord

Trapezius muscle

Rhomboid muscle

T3–4 intervertebral disc

Thoracic duct

Esophagus

Scapula

Teres minor muscle

Teres major muscle

Long head of triceps brachii muscle

Deltoid muscle

Shaft of humerus

Latissimus dorsi tendon

Tendon of long head of biceps brachii muscle

Serratus anterior muscle

Intercostal muscles

Right lung

Arch of azygos vein

Right phrenic nerve

Superior vena cava

Plate 244   Cross Section of Thorax at T3-4 Disc Level. (Netter: Atlas of Human Anatomy, 4 ed, 2006, Saunders.)

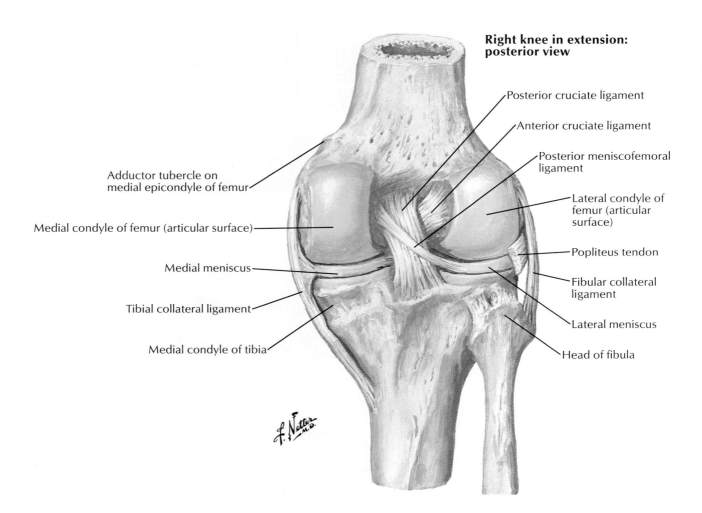

Right knee in extension: posterior view

Posterior cruciate ligament

Anterior cruciate ligament

Posterior meniscofemoral ligament

Lateral condyle of femur (articular surface)

Popliteus tendon

Fibular collateral ligament

Lateral meniscus

Head of fibula

Adductor tubercle on medial epicondyle of femur

Medial condyle of femur (articular surface)

Medial meniscus

Tibial collateral ligament

Medial condyle of tibia

Plate 509   Knee: Cruciate and Collateral Ligaments. (Netter: Atlas of Human Anatomy, 4 ed, 2006, Saunders.)

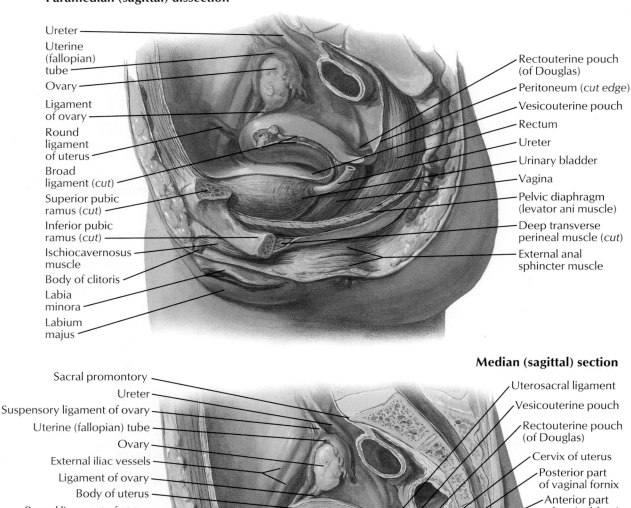

Paramedian (sagittal) dissection

Ureter

Uterine (fallopian) tube

Ovary

Ligament of ovary

Round ligament of uterus

Broad ligament (*cut*)

Superior pubic ramus (*cut*)

Inferior pubic ramus (*cut*)

Ischiocavernosus muscle

Body of clitoris

Labia minora

Labium majus

Rectouterine pouch (of Douglas)

Peritoneum (*cut edge*)

Vesicouterine pouch

Rectum

Ureter

Urinary bladder

Vagina

Pelvic diaphragm (levator ani muscle)

Deep transverse perineal muscle (*cut*)

External anal sphincter muscle

Median (sagittal) section

Sacral promontory

Ureter

Suspensory ligament of ovary

Uterine (fallopian) tube

Ovary

External iliac vessels

Ligament of ovary

Body of uterus

Round ligament of uterus (ligamentum teres)

Fundus of uterus

Urinary bladder

Pubic symphysis

Urethra

Sphincter urethrae

Deep transverse perineal muscle

Deep dorsal vein of clitoris

Crus of clitoris

External urethral orifice

Superficial transverse perineal muscle

Labium minus

Labium majus

Uterosacral ligament

Vesicouterine pouch

Rectouterine pouch (of Douglas)

Cervix of uterus

Posterior part of vaginal fornix

Anterior part of vaginal fornix

Rectum

Vagina

Perineal membrane

Levator ani muscle

Anal canal

External anal sphincter muscle

Anus

Vaginal orifice

Plate 36Ø Pelvic Viscera and Perineum: Female. (Netter: Atlas of Human Anatomy, 4 ed, 2006, Saunders.)

Medical and Surgical

SECTION: Ø MEDICAL AND SURGICAL
BODY SYSTEM: Ø CENTRAL NERVOUS SYSTEM AND CRANIAL NERVES
OPERATION: 1 BYPASS: Altering the route of passage of the contents of a tubular body part

Body Part	Approach	Device	Qualifier
6 Cerebral Ventricle	Ø Open 3 Percutaneous 4 Percutaneous Endoscopic	7 Autologous Tissue Substitute J Synthetic Substitute K Nonautologous Tissue Substitute	Ø Nasopharynx 1 Mastoid Sinus 2 Atrium 3 Blood Vessel 4 Pleural Cavity 5 Intestine 6 Peritoneal Cavity 7 Urinary Tract 8 Bone Marrow B Cerebral Cisterns
6 Cerebral Ventricle	Ø Open 3 Percutaneous 4 Percutaneous Endoscopic	Z No Device	B Cerebral Cisterns
U Spinal Canal	Ø Open 3 Percutaneous 4 Percutaneous Endoscopic	7 Autologous Tissue Substitute J Synthetic Substitute K Nonautologous Tissue Substitute	2 Atrium 4 Pleural Cavity 6 Peritoneal Cavity 7 Urinary Tract 9 Fallopian Tube

Coding Clinic: 2013, Q2, P37 – 00163J6

SECTION: Ø MEDICAL AND SURGICAL
BODY SYSTEM: Ø CENTRAL NERVOUS SYSTEM AND CRANIAL NERVES
OPERATION: 2 CHANGE: Taking out or off a device from a body part and putting back an identical or similar device in or on the same body part without cutting or puncturing the skin or a mucous membrane

Body Part	Approach	Device	Qualifier
Ø Brain E Cranial Nerve U Spinal Canal	X External	Ø Drainage Device Y Other Device	Z No Qualifier

Non-OR All Values

SECTION: 0 MEDICAL AND SURGICAL
BODY SYSTEM: 0 CENTRAL NERVOUS SYSTEM AND CRANIAL NERVES
OPERATION: 5 DESTRUCTION: Physical eradication of all or a portion of a body part by the direct use of energy, force, or a destructive agent

Body Part	Approach	Device	Qualifier
0 Brain 1 Cerebral Meninges 2 Dura Mater 6 Cerebral Ventricle 7 Cerebral Hemisphere 8 Basal Ganglia 9 Thalamus A Hypothalamus B Pons C Cerebellum D Medulla Oblongata F Olfactory Nerve G Optic Nerve H Oculomotor Nerve J Trochlear Nerve K Trigeminal Nerve L Abducens Nerve M Facial Nerve N Acoustic Nerve P Glossopharyngeal Nerve Q Vagus Nerve R Accessory Nerve S Hypoglossal Nerve T Spinal Meninges W Cervical Spinal Cord X Thoracic Spinal Cord Y Lumbar Spinal Cord	0 Open 3 Percutaneous 4 Percutaneous Endoscopic	Z No Device	Z No Qualifier

Non-OR 005[FGHJKLMNPQRS][034]ZZ

SECTION: 0 MEDICAL AND SURGICAL
BODY SYSTEM: 0 CENTRAL NERVOUS SYSTEM AND CRANIAL NERVES
OPERATION: 7 DILATION: Expanding an orifice or the lumen of a tubular body part

Body Part	Approach	Device	Qualifier
6 Cerebral Ventricle	0 Open 3 Percutaneous 4 Percutaneous Endoscopic	Z No Device	Z No Qualifier

Coding Clinic: 2017, Q4, P40 – 00764ZZ

SECTION: Ø MEDICAL AND SURGICAL
BODY SYSTEM: Ø CENTRAL NERVOUS SYSTEM AND CRANIAL NERVES
OPERATION: 8 DIVISION: Cutting into a body part, without draining fluids and/or gases from the body part, in order to separate or transect a body part

Body Part	Approach	Device	Qualifier
Ø Brain 7 Cerebral Hemisphere 8 Basal Ganglia F Olfactory Nerve G Optic Nerve H Oculomotor Nerve J Trochlear Nerve K Trigeminal Nerve L Abducens Nerve M Facial Nerve N Acoustic Nerve P Glossopharyngeal Nerve Q Vagus Nerve R Accessory Nerve S Hypoglossal Nerve W Cervical Spinal Cord X Thoracic Spinal Cord Y Lumbar Spinal Cord	Ø Open 3 Percutaneous 4 Percutaneous Endoscopic	Z No Device	Z No Qualifier

SECTION: Ø MEDICAL AND SURGICAL

BODY SYSTEM: Ø CENTRAL NERVOUS SYSTEM AND CRANIAL NERVES
OPERATION: 9 DRAINAGE: *(on multiple pages)*
Taking or letting out fluids and/or gases from a body part

Body Part	Approach	Device	Qualifier
Ø Brain	Ø Open	Ø Drainage Device	Z No Qualifier
1 Cerebral Meninges	3 Percutaneous		
2 Dura Mater	4 Percutaneous Endoscopic		
3 Epidural Space, Intracranial			
4 Subdural Space, Intracranial			
5 Subarachnoid Space, Intracranial			
6 Cerebral Ventricle			
7 Cerebral Hemisphere			
8 Basal Ganglia			
9 Thalamus			
A Hypothalamus			
B Pons			
C Cerebellum			
D Medulla Oblongata			
F Olfactory Nerve			
G Optic Nerve			
H Oculomotor Nerve			
J Trochlear Nerve			
K Trigeminal Nerve			
L Abducens Nerve			
M Facial Nerve			
N Acoustic Nerve			
P Glossopharyngeal Nerve			
Q Vagus Nerve			
R Accessory Nerve			
S Hypoglossal Nerve			
T Spinal Meninges			
U Spinal Canal			
W Cervical Spinal Cord			
X Thoracic Spinal Cord			
Y Lumbar Spinal Cord			

DRG Non-OR 009[3TWXY]30Z
Non-OR 009U[34]0Z

Coding Clinic: 2015, Q2, P30 – 009W00Z

New/Revised Text in Green deleted Deleted ♀ Females Only ♂ Males Only Coding Clinic
Non-covered Limited Coverage ⊞ Combination (See Appendix E) DRG Non-OR Non-OR Hospital-Acquired Condition

SECTION: Ø MEDICAL AND SURGICAL
BODY SYSTEM: Ø CENTRAL NERVOUS SYSTEM AND CRANIAL NERVES
OPERATION: 9 DRAINAGE: *(continued)*
Taking or letting out fluids and/or gases from a body part

Body Part	Approach	Device	Qualifier
Ø Brain 1 Cerebral Meninges 2 Dura Mater 3 Epidural Space, Intracranial 4 Subdural Space, Intracranial 5 Subarachnoid Space, Intracranial 6 Cerebral Ventricle 7 Cerebral Hemisphere 8 Basal Ganglia 9 Thalamus A Hypothalamus B Pons C Cerebellum D Medulla Oblongata F Olfactory Nerve G Optic Nerve H Oculomotor Nerve J Trochlear Nerve K Trigeminal Nerve L Abducens Nerve M Facial Nerve N Acoustic Nerve P Glossopharyngeal Nerve Q Vagus Nerve R Accessory Nerve S Hypoglossal Nerve T Spinal Meninges U Spinal Canal W Cervical Spinal Cord X Thoracic Spinal Cord Y Lumbar Spinal Cord	Ø Open 3 Percutaneous 4 Percutaneous Endoscopic	Z No Device	X Diagnostic Z No Qualifier

DRG Non-OR 00933ZZ
Non-OR 009[0123456789ABCDFGHJKLMNPQRSU][34]ZX
Non-OR 009U[34]ZZ
Non-OR 009[TWXY]3[XZ]

Coding Clinic: 2015, Q3, P12-13 – 009[46]30Z

SECTION: 0 MEDICAL AND SURGICAL

BODY SYSTEM: 0 CENTRAL NERVOUS SYSTEM AND CRANIAL NERVES

OPERATION: B **EXCISION:** Cutting out or off, without replacement, a portion of a body part

Body Part	Approach	Device	Qualifier
0 Brain	0 Open	Z No Device	X Diagnostic
1 Cerebral Meninges	3 Percutaneous		Z No Qualifier
2 Dura Mater	4 Percutaneous Endoscopic		
6 Cerebral Ventricle			
7 Cerebral Hemisphere			
8 Basal Ganglia			
9 Thalamus			
A Hypothalamus			
B Pons			
C Cerebellum			
D Medulla Oblongata			
F Olfactory Nerve			
G Optic Nerve			
H Oculomotor Nerve			
J Trochlear Nerve			
K Trigeminal Nerve			
L Abducens Nerve			
M Facial Nerve			
N Acoustic Nerve			
P Glossopharyngeal Nerve			
Q Vagus Nerve			
R Accessory Nerve			
S Hypoglossal Nerve			
T Spinal Meninges			
W Cervical Spinal Cord			
X Thoracic Spinal Cord			
Y Lumbar Spinal Cord			

Non-OR 00B[0126789ABCDFGHJKLMNPQRS][34]ZX

Coding Clinic: 2015, Q1, P13 – 00B00ZZ
Coding Clinic: 2016, Q2, P13 – 00B[MRS]0ZZ
Coding Clinic: 2016, Q2, P18 – 00B70ZZ

New/Revised Text in Green   ~~deleted~~ Deleted   ♀ Females Only   ♂ Males Only   **Coding Clinic**

Non-covered   Limited Coverage   ⊞ Combination (See Appendix E)   DRG Non-OR   Non-OR   Hospital-Acquired Condition

SECTION: Ø MEDICAL AND SURGICAL

BODY SYSTEM: Ø CENTRAL NERVOUS SYSTEM AND CRANIAL NERVES

OPERATION: C EXTIRPATION: Taking or cutting out solid matter from a body part

Body Part	Approach	Device	Qualifier
Ø Brain 1 Cerebral Meninges 2 Dura Mater 3 Epidural Space, Intracranial 4 Subdural Space, Intracranial 5 Subarachnoid Space, Intracranial 6 Cerebral Ventricle 7 Cerebral Hemisphere 8 Basal Ganglia 9 Thalamus A Hypothalamus B Pons C Cerebellum D Medulla Oblongata F Olfactory Nerve G Optic Nerve H Oculomotor Nerve J Trochlear Nerve K Trigeminal Nerve L Abducens Nerve M Facial Nerve N Acoustic Nerve P Glossopharyngeal Nerve Q Vagus Nerve R Accessory Nerve S Hypoglossal Nerve T Spinal Meninges U Spinal Canal W Cervical Spinal Cord X Thoracic Spinal Cord Y Lumbar Spinal Cord	Ø Open 3 Percutaneous 4 Percutaneous Endoscopic	Z No Device	Z No Qualifier

Coding Clinic: 2015, Q1, P12 – 00C00ZZ
Coding Clinic: 2016, Q2, P29; 2015, Q3, P11 – 00C40ZZ
Coding Clinic: 2015, Q3, P13 – 00C74ZZ
Coding Clinic: 2016, Q4, P28 – 00C00ZZ
Coding Clinic: 2017, Q4, P48 – 00CU0ZZ

SECTION: Ø MEDICAL AND SURGICAL

BODY SYSTEM: Ø CENTRAL NERVOUS SYSTEM AND CRANIAL NERVES

OPERATION: D **EXTRACTION:** Pulling or stripping out or off all or a portion of a body part by the use of force

Body Part	Approach	Device	Qualifier
1 Cerebral Meninges 2 Dura Mater F Olfactory Nerve G Optic Nerve H Oculomotor Nerve J Trochlear Nerve K Trigeminal Nerve L Abducens Nerve M Facial Nerve N Acoustic Nerve P Glossopharyngeal Nerve Q Vagus Nerve R Accessory Nerve S Hypoglossal Nerve T Spinal Meninges	Ø Open 3 Percutaneous 4 Percutaneous Endoscopic	Z No Device	Z No Qualifier

Coding Clinic: 2015, Q3, P14 – 00D20ZZ

SECTION: Ø MEDICAL AND SURGICAL

BODY SYSTEM: Ø CENTRAL NERVOUS SYSTEM AND CRANIAL NERVES

OPERATION: F **FRAGMENTATION:** Breaking solid matter in a body part into pieces

Body Part	Approach	Device	Qualifier
3 Epidural Space, Intracranial 4 Subdural Space, Intracranial 5 Subarachnoid Space, Intracranial 6 Cerebral Ventricle U Spinal Canal	Ø Open 3 Percutaneous 4 Percutaneous Endoscopic X External	Z No Device	Z No Qualifier

00F[3456]XZZ
Non-OR 00F[3456]XZZ

SECTION: Ø MEDICAL AND SURGICAL

BODY SYSTEM: Ø CENTRAL NERVOUS SYSTEM AND CRANIAL NERVES

OPERATION: H INSERTION: Putting in a nonbiological appliance that monitors, assists, performs, or prevents a physiological function but does not physically take the place of a body part

Body Part	Approach	Device	Qualifier
Ø Brain ⊞	Ø Open	2 Monitoring Device 3 Infusion Device 4 Radioactive Element, Cesium-131 Collagen Implant M Neurostimulator Lead Y Other Device	Z No Qualifier
Ø Brain ⊞	3 Percutaneous 4 Percutaneous Endoscopic	2 Monitoring Device 3 Infusion Device M Neurostimulator Lead Y Other Device	Z No Qualifier
6 Cerebral Ventricle ⊞ E Cranial Nerve ⊞ U Spinal Canal ⊞ V Spinal Cord ⊞	Ø Open 3 Percutaneous 4 Percutaneous Endoscopic	2 Monitoring Device 3 Infusion Device M Neurostimulator Lead Y Other Device	Z No Qualifier

⊞ 00HØ[034]MZ
⊞ 00H[6EUV][034]MZ
DRG Non-OR 00H[O3]3[24]Z
DRG Non-OR 00H[6UV]32Z
Non-OR 00H[UV][034]3Z

SECTION: Ø MEDICAL AND SURGICAL

BODY SYSTEM: Ø CENTRAL NERVOUS SYSTEM AND CRANIAL NERVES

OPERATION: J INSPECTION: Visually and/or manually exploring a body part

Body Part	Approach	Device	Qualifier
Ø Brain E Cranial Nerve U Spinal Canal V Spinal Cord	Ø Open 3 Percutaneous 4 Percutaneous Endoscopic	Z No Device	Z No Qualifier

Non-OR 00JE3ZZ
Non-OR 00J[EUV][03][2Y]Z

Coding Clinic: 2017, Q1, P50 – 00JU3ZZ

SECTION: 0 MEDICAL AND SURGICAL

BODY SYSTEM: 0 CENTRAL NERVOUS SYSTEM AND CRANIAL NERVES

OPERATION: K **MAP:** Locating the route of passage of electrical impulses and/or locating functional areas in a body part

Body Part	Approach	Device	Qualifier
0 Brain	0 Open	Z No Device	Z No Qualifier
7 Cerebral Hemisphere	3 Percutaneous		
8 Basal Ganglia	4 Percutaneous Endoscopic		
9 Thalamus			
A Hypothalamus			
B Pons			
C Cerebellum			
D Medulla Oblongata			

SECTION: 0 MEDICAL AND SURGICAL

BODY SYSTEM: 0 CENTRAL NERVOUS SYSTEM AND CRANIAL NERVES

OPERATION: N **RELEASE:** Freeing a body part from an abnormal physical constraint by cutting or by the use of force

Body Part	Approach	Device	Qualifier
0 Brain	0 Open	Z No Device	Z No Qualifier
1 Cerebral Meninges	3 Percutaneous		
2 Dura Mater	4 Percutaneous Endoscopic		
6 Cerebral Ventricle			
7 Cerebral Hemisphere			
8 Basal Ganglia			
9 Thalamus			
A Hypothalamus			
B Pons			
C Cerebellum			
D Medulla Oblongata			
F Olfactory Nerve			
G Optic Nerve			
H Oculomotor Nerve			
J Trochlear Nerve			
K Trigeminal Nerve			
L Abducens Nerve			
M Facial Nerve			
N Acoustic Nerve			
P Glossopharyngeal Nerve			
Q Vagus Nerve			
R Accessory Nerve			
S Hypoglossal Nerve			
T Spinal Meninges			
W Cervical Spinal Cord			
X Thoracic Spinal Cord			
Y Lumbar Spinal Cord			

Coding Clinic: 2017, Q2, P24; 2015, Q2, P22 – 00NW0ZZ
Coding Clinic: 2016, Q2, P29 – 00N00ZZ
Coding Clinic: 2017, Q3, P10 – 00NC0ZZ

SECTION: Ø MEDICAL AND SURGICAL

BODY SYSTEM: Ø CENTRAL NERVOUS SYSTEM AND CRANIAL NERVES
OPERATION: P REMOVAL: Taking out or off a device from a body part

Body Part	Approach	Device	Qualifier
Ø Brain V Spinal Cord	Ø Open 3 Percutaneous 4 Percutaneous Endoscopic	Ø Drainage Device 2 Monitoring Device 3 Infusion Device 7 Autologous Tissue Substitute J Synthetic Substitute K Nonautologous Tissue Substitute M Neurostimulator Lead Y Other Device	Z No Qualifier
Ø Brain V Spinal Cord	X External	Ø Drainage Device 2 Monitoring Device 3 Infusion Device M Neurostimulator Lead	Z No Qualifier
6 Cerebral Ventricle U Spinal Canal	Ø Open 3 Percutaneous 4 Percutaneous Endoscopic	Ø Drainage Device 2 Monitoring Device 3 Infusion Device J Synthetic Substitute M Neurostimulator Lead Y Other Device	Z No Qualifier
6 Cerebral Ventricle U Spinal Canal	X External	Ø Drainage Device 2 Monitoring Device 3 Infusion Device M Neurostimulator Lead	Z No Qualifier
E Cranial Nerve	Ø Open 3 Percutaneous 4 Percutaneous Endoscopic	Ø Drainage Device 2 Monitoring Device 3 Infusion Device 7 Autologous Tissue Substitute M Neurostimulator Lead Y Other Device	Z No Qualifier
E Cranial Nerve	X External	Ø Drainage Device 2 Monitoring Device 3 Infusion Device M Neurostimulator Lead	Z No Qualifier

Non-OR ØØP[ØV]X[Ø23M]Z
Non-OR ØØP6X[Ø3]Z
Non-OR ØØPEX[Ø23]Z
Non-OR ØØPUX[Ø23M]Z
Non-OR ØØP[Ø6EUV][3X][Ø23M]Z

Ø: M/S

Ø: CENTRAL NERVOUS SYSTEM AND CRANIAL NERVES

P: REMOVAL

SECTION: 0 MEDICAL AND SURGICAL

BODY SYSTEM: 0 CENTRAL NERVOUS SYSTEM AND CRANIAL NERVES

OPERATION: Q REPAIR: Restoring, to the extent possible, a body part to its normal anatomic structure and function

Body Part	Approach	Device	Qualifier
0 Brain	0 Open	Z No Device	Z No Qualifier
1 Cerebral Meninges	3 Percutaneous		
2 Dura Mater	4 Percutaneous Endoscopic		
6 Cerebral Ventricle			
7 Cerebral Hemisphere			
8 Basal Ganglia			
9 Thalamus			
A Hypothalamus			
B Pons			
C Cerebellum			
D Medulla Oblongata			
F Olfactory Nerve			
G Optic Nerve			
H Oculomotor Nerve			
J Trochlear Nerve			
K Trigeminal Nerve			
L Abducens Nerve			
M Facial Nerve			
N Acoustic Nerve			
P Glossopharyngeal Nerve			
Q Vagus Nerve			
R Accessory Nerve			
S Hypoglossal Nerve			
T Spinal Meninges			
W Cervical Spinal Cord			
X Thoracic Spinal Cord			
Y Lumbar Spinal Cord			

Coding Clinic: 2013, Q3, P25 – 00Q20ZZ

New/Revised Text in Green ~~deleted~~ Deleted ♀ Females Only ♂ Males Only **Coding Clinic**

Non-covered Limited Coverage ⊞ Combination (See Appendix E) DRG Non-OR Non-OR Hospital-Acquired Condition

SECTION: Ø MEDICAL AND SURGICAL

BODY SYSTEM: Ø CENTRAL NERVOUS SYSTEM AND CRANIAL NERVES

OPERATION: R REPLACEMENT: Putting in or on biological or synthetic material that physically takes the place and/or function of all or a portion of a body part

Body Part	Approach	Device	Qualifier
1 Cerebral Meninges 2 Dura Mater 6 Cerebral Ventricle F Olfactory Nerve G Optic Nerve H Oculomotor Nerve J Trochlear Nerve K Trigeminal Nerve L Abducens Nerve M Facial Nerve N Acoustic Nerve P Glossopharyngeal Nerve Q Vagus Nerve R Accessory Nerve S Hypoglossal Nerve T Spinal Meninges	Ø Open 4 Percutaneous Endoscopic	7 Autologous Tissue Substitute J Synthetic Substitute K Nonautologous Tissue Substitute	Z No Qualifier

SECTION: Ø MEDICAL AND SURGICAL

BODY SYSTEM: Ø CENTRAL NERVOUS SYSTEM AND CRANIAL NERVES

OPERATION: S REPOSITION: Moving to its normal location, or other suitable location, all or a portion of a body part

Body Part	Approach	Device	Qualifier
F Olfactory Nerve G Optic Nerve H Oculomotor Nerve J Trochlear Nerve K Trigeminal Nerve L Abducens Nerve M Facial Nerve N Acoustic Nerve P Glossopharyngeal Nerve Q Vagus Nerve R Accessory Nerve S Hypoglossal Nerve W Cervical Spinal Cord X Thoracic Spinal Cord Y Lumbar Spinal Cord	Ø Open 3 Percutaneous 4 Percutaneous Endoscopic	Z No Device	Z No Qualifier

SECTION: Ø MEDICAL AND SURGICAL
BODY SYSTEM: Ø CENTRAL NERVOUS SYSTEM AND CRANIAL NERVES
OPERATION: T RESECTION: Cutting out or off, without replacement, all of a body part

Body Part	Approach	Device	Qualifier
7 Cerebral Hemisphere	Ø Open 3 Percutaneous 4 Percutaneous Endoscopic	Z No Device	Z No Qualifier

SECTION: Ø MEDICAL AND SURGICAL
BODY SYSTEM: Ø CENTRAL NERVOUS SYSTEM AND CRANIAL NERVES
OPERATION: U SUPPLEMENT: Putting in or on biological or synthetic material that physically reinforces and/or augments the function of a portion of a body part

Body Part	Approach	Device	Qualifier
1 Cerebral Meninges 2 Dura Mater 6 Cerebral Ventricle F Olfactory Nerve G Optic Nerve H Oculomotor Nerve J Trochlear Nerve K Trigeminal Nerve L Abducens Nerve M Facial Nerve N Acoustic Nerve P Glossopharyngeal Nerve Q Vagus Nerve R Accessory Nerve S Hypoglossal Nerve T Spinal Meninges	Ø Open 3 Percutaneous 4 Percutaneous Endoscopic	7 Autologous Tissue Substitute J Synthetic Substitute K Nonautologous Tissue Substitute	Z No Qualifier

Coding Clinic: 2018, Q1, P9; 2017, Q3, P11 – 00U20KZ

New/Revised Text in Green   ~~deleted~~ Deleted   ♀ Females Only   ♂ Males Only   **Coding Clinic**

Non-covered   Limited Coverage   ⊞ Combination (See Appendix E)   DRG Non-OR   Non-OR   Hospital-Acquired Condition

SECTION: Ø MEDICAL AND SURGICAL

BODY SYSTEM: Ø CENTRAL NERVOUS SYSTEM AND CRANIAL NERVES
OPERATION: W REVISION: Correcting, to the extent possible, a portion of a malfunctioning device or the position of a displaced device

Body Part	Approach	Device	Qualifier
Ø Brain V Spinal Cord	Ø Open 3 Percutaneous 4 Percutaneous Endoscopic	Ø Drainage Device 2 Monitoring Device 3 Infusion Device 7 Autologous Tissue Substitute J Synthetic Substitute K Nonautologous Tissue Substitute M Neurostimulator Lead Y Other Device	Z No Qualifier
Ø Brain V Spinal Cord	X External	Ø Drainage Device 2 Monitoring Device 3 Infusion Device 7 Autologous Tissue Substitute J Synthetic Substitute K Nonautologous Tissue Substitute M Neurostimulator Lead	Z No Qualifier
6 Cerebral Ventricle U Spinal Canal	Ø Open 3 Percutaneous 4 Percutaneous Endoscopic	Ø Drainage Device 2 Monitoring Device 3 Infusion Device J Synthetic Substitute M Neurostimulator Lead Y Other Device	Z No Qualifier
6 Cerebral Ventricle U Spinal Canal	X External	Ø Drainage Device 2 Monitoring Device 3 Infusion Device J Synthetic Substitute M Neurostimulator Lead	Z No Qualifier
E Cranial Nerve	Ø Open 3 Percutaneous 4 Percutaneous Endoscopic	Ø Drainage Device 2 Monitoring Device 3 Infusion Device 7 Autologous Tissue Substitute M Neurostimulator Lead Y Other Device	Z No Qualifier
E Cranial Nerve	X External	Ø Drainage Device 2 Monitoring Device 3 Infusion Device 7 Autologous Tissue Substitute M Neurostimulator Lead	Z No Qualifier

Non-OR ØØW[ØV]X[Ø237JKM]Z
Non-OR ØØW[6U]X[Ø23JM]Z
Non-OR ØØWEX[Ø237M]Z

New/Revised Text in Green ~~deleted~~ Deleted ♀ Females Only ♂ Males Only **Coding Clinic**
Non-covered Limited Coverage Combination (See Appendix E) DRG Non-OR Non-OR Hospital-Acquired Condition

SECTION: Ø MEDICAL AND SURGICAL
BODY SYSTEM: Ø **CENTRAL NERVOUS SYSTEM AND CRANIAL NERVES**
OPERATION: **X TRANSFER:** Moving, without taking out, all or a portion of a body part to another location to take over the function of all or a portion of a body part

Body Part	Approach	Device	Qualifier
F Olfactory Nerve G Optic Nerve H Oculomotor Nerve J Trochlear Nerve K Trigeminal Nerve L Abducens Nerve M Facial Nerve N Acoustic Nerve P Glossopharyngeal Nerve Q Vagus Nerve R Accessory Nerve S Hypoglossal Nerve	Ø Open 4 Percutaneous Endoscopic	Z No Device	F Olfactory Nerve G Optic Nerve H Oculomotor Nerve J Trochlear Nerve K Trigeminal Nerve L Abducens Nerve M Facial Nerve N Acoustic Nerve P Glossopharyngeal Nerve Q Vagus Nerve R Accessory Nerve S Hypoglossal Nerve

New/Revised Text in Green ~~deleted~~ Deleted ♀ Females Only ♂ Males Only **Coding Clinic**
⬥ Non-covered ⬥ Limited Coverage ⊞ Combination (See Appendix E) DRG Non-OR Non-OR ⬥ Hospital-Acquired Condition

Ø1. Peripheral Nervous System

SECTION: Ø MEDICAL AND SURGICAL
BODY SYSTEM: 1 PERIPHERAL NERVOUS SYSTEM
OPERATION: 2 CHANGE: Taking out or off a device from a body part and putting back an identical or similar device in or on the same body part without cutting or puncturing the skin or a mucous membrane

Body Part	Approach	Device	Qualifier
Y Peripheral Nerve	X External	Ø Drainage Device Y Other Device	Z No Qualifier

Non-OR Ø12YX[ØY]Z

SECTION: Ø MEDICAL AND SURGICAL
BODY SYSTEM: 1 PERIPHERAL NERVOUS SYSTEM
OPERATION: 5 DESTRUCTION: Physical eradication of all or a portion of a body part by the direct use of energy, force, or a destructive agent

Body Part	Approach	Device	Qualifier
Ø Cervical Plexus 1 Cervical Nerve 2 Phrenic Nerve 3 Brachial Plexus 4 Ulnar Nerve 5 Median Nerve 6 Radial Nerve 8 Thoracic Nerve 9 Lumbar Plexus A Lumbosacral Plexus B Lumbar Nerve C Pudendal Nerve D Femoral Nerve F Sciatic Nerve G Tibial Nerve H Peroneal Nerve K Head and Neck Sympathetic Nerve L Thoracic Sympathetic Nerve M Abdominal Sympathetic Nerve N Lumbar Sympathetic Nerve P Sacral Sympathetic Nerve Q Sacral Plexus R Sacral Nerve	Ø Open 3 Percutaneous 4 Percutaneous Endoscopic	Z No Device	Z No Qualifier

Non-OR Ø15[Ø234569ACDFGHQ][Ø34]ZZ
Non-OR Ø15[18BR]3ZZ

SECTION: Ø **MEDICAL AND SURGICAL**

BODY SYSTEM: 1 **PERIPHERAL NERVOUS SYSTEM**

OPERATION: 8 **DIVISION:** Cutting into a body part, without draining fluids and/or gases from the body part, in order to separate or transect a body part

Body Part	Approach	Device	Qualifier
Ø Cervical Plexus	Ø Open	Z No Device	Z No Qualifier
1 Cervical Nerve	3 Percutaneous		
2 Phrenic Nerve	4 Percutaneous Endoscopic		
3 Brachial Plexus			
4 Ulnar Nerve			
5 Median Nerve			
6 Radial Nerve			
8 Thoracic Nerve			
9 Lumbar Plexus			
A Lumbosacral Plexus			
B Lumbar Nerve			
C Pudendal Nerve			
D Femoral Nerve			
F Sciatic Nerve			
G Tibial Nerve			
H Peroneal Nerve			
K Head and Neck Sympathetic Nerve			
L Thoracic Sympathetic Nerve			
M Abdominal Sympathetic Nerve			
N Lumbar Sympathetic Nerve			
P Sacral Sympathetic Nerve			
Q Sacral Plexus			
R Sacral Nerve			

Ø: M/S

1: PERIPHERAL NERVOUS SYSTEM

8: DIVISION

SECTION: Ø MEDICAL AND SURGICAL
BODY SYSTEM: 1 PERIPHERAL NERVOUS SYSTEM
OPERATION: 9 DRAINAGE: Taking or letting out fluids and/or gases from a body part

Body Part	Approach	Device	Qualifier
Ø Cervical Plexus 1 Cervical Nerve 2 Phrenic Nerve 3 Brachial Plexus 4 Ulnar Nerve 5 Median Nerve 6 Radial Nerve 8 Thoracic Nerve 9 Lumbar Plexus A Lumbosacral Plexus B Lumbar Nerve C Pudendal Nerve D Femoral Nerve F Sciatic Nerve G Tibial Nerve H Peroneal Nerve K Head and Neck Sympathetic Nerve L Thoracic Sympathetic Nerve M Abdominal Sympathetic Nerve N Lumbar Sympathetic Nerve P Sacral Sympathetic Nerve Q Sacral Plexus R Sacral Nerve	Ø Open 3 Percutaneous 4 Percutaneous Endoscopic	Ø Drainage Device	Z No Qualifier
Ø Cervical Plexus 1 Cervical Nerve 2 Phrenic Nerve 3 Brachial Plexus 4 Ulnar Nerve 5 Median Nerve 6 Radial Nerve 8 Thoracic Nerve 9 Lumbar Plexus A Lumbosacral Plexus B Lumbar Nerve C Pudendal Nerve D Femoral Nerve F Sciatic Nerve G Tibial Nerve H Peroneal Nerve K Head and Neck Sympathetic Nerve L Thoracic Sympathetic Nerve M Abdominal Sympathetic Nerve N Lumbar Sympathetic Nerve P Sacral Sympathetic Nerve Q Sacral Plexus R Sacral Nerve	Ø Open 3 Percutaneous 4 Percutaneous Endoscopic	Z No Device	X Diagnostic Z No Qualifier

Non-OR Ø19[Ø12345689ABCDFGHKLMNPQR]3ØZ
Non-OR Ø19[Ø12345689ABCDFGHKLMNPQR]3ZZ
Non-OR Ø19[Ø12345689ABCDFGHQR][34]ZX

New/Revised Text in Green   deleted Deleted   ♀ Females Only   ♂ Males Only   **Coding Clinic**
Non-covered   Limited Coverage   ⊞ Combination (See Appendix E)   DRG Non-OR   Non-OR   Hospital-Acquired Condition

Left margin: 9: DRAINAGE   1: PERIPHERAL NERVOUS SYSTEM   Ø: M/S

SECTION: Ø MEDICAL AND SURGICAL
BODY SYSTEM: 1 PERIPHERAL NERVOUS SYSTEM
OPERATION: B EXCISION: Cutting out or off, without replacement, a portion of a body part

Body Part	Approach	Device	Qualifier
Ø Cervical Plexus 1 Cervical Nerve 2 Phrenic Nerve 3 Brachial Plexus ⊕ 4 Ulnar Nerve 5 Median Nerve 6 Radial Nerve 8 Thoracic Nerve 9 Lumbar Plexus A Lumbosacral Plexus B Lumbar Nerve C Pudendal Nerve D Femoral Nerve F Sciatic Nerve G Tibial Nerve H Peroneal Nerve K Head and Neck Sympathetic Nerve L Thoracic Sympathetic Nerve ⊕ M Abdominal Sympathetic Nerve N Lumbar Sympathetic Nerve P Sacral Sympathetic Nerve Q Sacral Plexus R Sacral Nerve	Ø Open 3 Percutaneous 4 Percutaneous Endoscopic	Z No Device	X Diagnostic Z No Qualifier

⊕ Ø1B[3L]ØZZ

Non-OR Ø1B[Ø12345689ABCDFGHQR][34]ZX

Coding Clinic: 2017, Q2, P19 – Ø1BLØZZ

New/Revised Text in Green   deleted Deleted   ♀ Females Only   ♂ Males Only   **Coding Clinic**
Non-covered   Limited Coverage   ⊕ Combination (See Appendix E)   DRG Non-OR   Non-OR   Hospital-Acquired Condition

SECTION: 0 MEDICAL AND SURGICAL
BODY SYSTEM: 1 PERIPHERAL NERVOUS SYSTEM
OPERATION: C EXTIRPATION: Taking or cutting out solid matter from a body part

Body Part	Approach	Device	Qualifier
0 Cervical Plexus 1 Cervical Nerve 2 Phrenic Nerve 3 Brachial Plexus 4 Ulnar Nerve 5 Median Nerve 6 Radial Nerve 8 Thoracic Nerve 9 Lumbar Plexus A Lumbosacral Plexus B Lumbar Nerve C Pudendal Nerve D Femoral Nerve F Sciatic Nerve G Tibial Nerve H Peroneal Nerve K Head and Neck Sympathetic Nerve L Thoracic Sympathetic Nerve M Abdominal Sympathetic Nerve N Lumbar Sympathetic Nerve P Sacral Sympathetic Nerve Q Sacral Plexus R Sacral Nerve	0 Open 3 Percutaneous 4 Percutaneous Endoscopic	Z No Device	Z No Qualifier

C: EXTIRPATION — 1: PERIPHERAL NERVOUS SYSTEM — 0: M/S

SECTION: Ø MEDICAL AND SURGICAL
BODY SYSTEM: 1 PERIPHERAL NERVOUS SYSTEM
OPERATION: D **EXTRACTION:** Pulling or stripping out or off all or a portion of a body part by the use of force

Body Part	Approach	Device	Qualifier
Ø Cervical Plexus 1 Cervical Nerve 2 Phrenic Nerve 3 Brachial Plexus 4 Ulnar Nerve 5 Median Nerve 6 Radial Nerve 8 Thoracic Nerve 9 Lumbar Plexus A Lumbosacral Plexus B Lumbar Nerve C Pudendal Nerve D Femoral Nerve F Sciatic Nerve G Tibial Nerve H Peroneal Nerve K Head and Neck Sympathetic Nerve L Thoracic Sympathetic Nerve M Abdominal Sympathetic Nerve N Lumbar Sympathetic Nerve P Sacral Sympathetic Nerve Q Sacral Plexus R Sacral Nerve	Ø Open 3 Percutaneous 4 Percutaneous Endoscopic	Z No Device	Z No Qualifier

SECTION: Ø MEDICAL AND SURGICAL
BODY SYSTEM: 1 PERIPHERAL NERVOUS SYSTEM
OPERATION: H **INSERTION:** Putting in a nonbiological appliance that monitors, assists, performs, or prevents a physiological function but does not physically take the place of a body part

Body Part	Approach	Device	Qualifier
Y Peripheral Nerve ⊞	Ø Open 3 Percutaneous 4 Percutaneous Endoscopic	2 Monitoring Device M Neurostimulator Lead Y Other Device	Z No Qualifier

⊞ Ø1HY[Ø34]MZ

SECTION: Ø MEDICAL AND SURGICAL
BODY SYSTEM: 1 PERIPHERAL NERVOUS SYSTEM
OPERATION: J **INSPECTION:** Visually and/or manually exploring a body part

Body Part	Approach	Device	Qualifier
Y Peripheral Nerve	Ø Open 3 Percutaneous 4 Percutaneous Endoscopic	Z No Device	Z No Qualifier

Non-OR   Ø1JY3ZZ

New/Revised Text in Green   ~~deleted~~ Deleted   ♀ Females Only   ♂ Males Only   **Coding Clinic**
🔖 Non-covered   🔖 Limited Coverage   ⊞ Combination (See Appendix E)   DRG Non-OR   Non-OR   🔖 Hospital-Acquired Condition

SECTION: Ø MEDICAL AND SURGICAL
BODY SYSTEM: 1 PERIPHERAL NERVOUS SYSTEM
OPERATION: N RELEASE: Freeing a body part from an abnormal physical constraint by cutting or by the use of force

Body Part	Approach	Device	Qualifier
Ø Cervical Plexus 1 Cervical Nerve 2 Phrenic Nerve 3 Brachial Plexus 4 Ulnar Nerve 5 Median Nerve 6 Radial Nerve 8 Thoracic Nerve 9 Lumbar Plexus A Lumbosacral Plexus B Lumbar Nerve C Pudendal Nerve D Femoral Nerve F Sciatic Nerve G Tibial Nerve H Peroneal Nerve K Head and Neck Sympathetic Nerve L Thoracic Sympathetic Nerve M Abdominal Sympathetic Nerve N Lumbar Sympathetic Nerve P Sacral Sympathetic Nerve Q Sacral Plexus R Sacral Nerve	Ø Open 3 Percutaneous 4 Percutaneous Endoscopic	Z No Device	Z No Qualifier

Coding Clinic: 2016, Q2, P16; 2015, Q2, P34 – 01NBØZZ
Coding Clinic: 2016, Q2, P17 – 01N10ZZ
Coding Clinic: 2016, Q2, P23 – 01N30ZZ
Coding Clinic: 2018, Q2, P23 – 01NBØZZ

SECTION: Ø MEDICAL AND SURGICAL
BODY SYSTEM: 1 PERIPHERAL NERVOUS SYSTEM
OPERATION: P REMOVAL: Taking out or off a device from a body part

Body Part	Approach	Device	Qualifier
Y Peripheral Nerve	Ø Open 3 Percutaneous 4 Percutaneous Endoscopic	Ø Drainage Device 2 Monitoring Device 7 Autologous Tissue Substitute M Neurostimulator Lead Y Other Device	Z No Qualifier
Y Peripheral Nerve	X External	Ø Drainage Device 2 Monitoring Device M Neurostimulator Lead	Z No Qualifier

Non-OR 01PY[3X][02M]Z

Left margin: N: RELEASE   P: REMOVAL
Left margin: 1: PERIPHERAL NERVOUS SYSTEM
Left margin: Ø: M/S

New/Revised Text in Green   ~~deleted~~ Deleted   ♀ Females Only   ♂ Males Only   **Coding Clinic**
Non-covered   Limited Coverage   ⊞ Combination (See Appendix E)   DRG Non-OR   Non-OR   Hospital-Acquired Condition

SECTION: Ø MEDICAL AND SURGICAL

BODY SYSTEM: 1 PERIPHERAL NERVOUS SYSTEM

OPERATION: Q REPAIR: Restoring, to the extent possible, a body part to its normal anatomic structure and function

Body Part	Approach	Device	Qualifier
Ø Cervical Plexus 1 Cervical Nerve 2 Phrenic Nerve 3 Brachial Plexus 4 Ulnar Nerve 5 Median Nerve 6 Radial Nerve 8 Thoracic Nerve 9 Lumbar Plexus A Lumbosacral Plexus B Lumbar Nerve C Pudendal Nerve D Femoral Nerve F Sciatic Nerve G Tibial Nerve H Peroneal Nerve K Head and Neck Sympathetic Nerve L Thoracic Sympathetic Nerve M Abdominal Sympathetic Nerve N Lumbar Sympathetic Nerve P Sacral Sympathetic Nerve Q Sacral Plexus R Sacral Nerve	Ø Open 3 Percutaneous 4 Percutaneous Endoscopic	Z No Device	Z No Qualifier

SECTION: Ø MEDICAL AND SURGICAL

BODY SYSTEM: 1 PERIPHERAL NERVOUS SYSTEM

OPERATION: R REPLACEMENT: Putting in or on biological or synthetic material that physically takes the place and/or function of all or a portion of a body part

Body Part	Approach	Device	Qualifier
1 Cervical Nerve 2 Phrenic Nerve 4 Ulnar Nerve 5 Median Nerve 6 Radial Nerve 8 Thoracic Nerve B Lumbar Nerve C Pudendal Nerve D Femoral Nerve F Sciatic Nerve G Tibial Nerve H Peroneal Nerve R Sacral Nerve	Ø Open 4 Percutaneous Endoscopic	7 Autologous Tissue Substitute J Synthetic Substitute K Nonautologous Tissue Substitute	Z No Qualifier

Ø: M/S 1: PERIPHERAL NERVOUS SYSTEM Q: REPAIR R: REPLACEMENT

SECTION: 0 MEDICAL AND SURGICAL

BODY SYSTEM: 1 PERIPHERAL NERVOUS SYSTEM

OPERATION: S REPOSITION: Moving to its normal location, or other suitable location, all or a portion of a body part

Body Part	Approach	Device	Qualifier
0 Cervical Plexus 1 Cervical Nerve 2 Phrenic Nerve 3 Brachial Plexus 4 Ulnar Nerve 5 Median Nerve 6 Radial Nerve 8 Thoracic Nerve 9 Lumbar Plexus A Lumbosacral Plexus B Lumbar Nerve C Pudendal Nerve D Femoral Nerve F Sciatic Nerve G Tibial Nerve H Peroneal Nerve Q Sacral Plexus R Sacral Nerve	0 Open 3 Percutaneous 4 Percutaneous Endoscopic	Z No Device	Z No Qualifier

SECTION: 0 MEDICAL AND SURGICAL

BODY SYSTEM: 1 PERIPHERAL NERVOUS SYSTEM

OPERATION: U SUPPLEMENT: Putting in or on biological or synthetic material that physically reinforces and/or augments the function of a portion of a body part

Body Part	Approach	Device	Qualifier
1 Cervical Nerve 2 Phrenic Nerve 4 Ulnar Nerve 5 Median Nerve 6 Radial Nerve 8 Thoracic Nerve B Lumbar Nerve C Pudendal Nerve D Femoral Nerve F Sciatic Nerve G Tibial Nerve H Peroneal Nerve R Sacral Nerve	0 Open 3 Percutaneous 4 Percutaneous Endoscopic	7 Autologous Tissue Substitute J Synthetic Substitute K Nonautologous Tissue Substitute	Z No Qualifier

Coding Clinic: 2017, Q4, P62 – 01U50KZ

SECTION: Ø MEDICAL AND SURGICAL

BODY SYSTEM: 1 PERIPHERAL NERVOUS SYSTEM

OPERATION: W REVISION: Correcting, to the extent possible, a portion of a malfunctioning device or the position of a displaced device

Body Part	Approach	Device	Qualifier
Y Peripheral Nerve	Ø Open 3 Percutaneous 4 Percutaneous Endoscopic	Ø Drainage Device 2 Monitoring Device 7 Autologous Tissue Substitute M Neurostimulator Lead Y Other Device	Z No Qualifier
Y Peripheral Nerve	X External	Ø Drainage Device 2 Monitoring Device 7 Autologous Tissue Substitute M Neurostimulator Lead	Z No Qualifier

Non-OR   Ø1WY[ØX][Ø27M]Z

SECTION: Ø MEDICAL AND SURGICAL

BODY SYSTEM: 1 PERIPHERAL NERVOUS SYSTEM

OPERATION: X TRANSFER: Moving, without taking out, all or a portion of a body part to another location to take over the function of all or a portion of a body part

Body Part	Approach	Device	Qualifier
1 Cervical Nerve 2 Phrenic Nerve	Ø Open 4 Percutaneous Endoscopic	Z No Device	1 Cervical Nerve 2 Phrenic Nerve
4 Ulnar Nerve 5 Median Nerve 6 Radial Nerve	Ø Open 4 Percutaneous Endoscopic	Z No Device	4 Ulnar Nerve 5 Median Nerve 6 Radial Nerve
8 Thoracic Nerve	Ø Open 4 Percutaneous Endoscopic	Z No Device	8 Thoracic Nerve
B Lumbar Nerve C Pudendal Nerve	Ø Open 4 Percutaneous Endoscopic	Z No Device	B Lumbar Nerve C Pudendal Nerve
D Femoral Nerve F Sciatic Nerve G Tibial Nerve H Peroneal Nerve	Ø Open 4 Percutaneous Endoscopic	Z No Device	D Femoral Nerve F Sciatic Nerve G Tibial Nerve H Peroneal Nerve

SECTION: 0 MEDICAL AND SURGICAL

BODY SYSTEM: 2 HEART AND GREAT VESSELS

OPERATION: 1 BYPASS: *(on multiple pages)*
Altering the route of passage of the contents of a tubular body part

Body Part	Approach	Device	Qualifier
0 Coronary Artery, One Artery 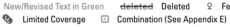Ⓠ 1 Coronary Artery, Two Arteries Ⓠ 2 Coronary Artery, Three Arteries Ⓠ 3 Coronary Artery, Four or More Arteries Ⓠ	0 Open	8 Zooplastic Tissue 9 Autologous Venous Tissue A Autologous Arterial Tissue J Synthetic Substitute K Nonautologous Tissue Substitute	3 Coronary Artery 8 Internal Mammary, Right 9 Internal Mammary, Left C Thoracic Artery F Abdominal Artery W Aorta
0 Coronary Artery, One Artery Ⓠ 1 Coronary Artery, Two Arteries Ⓠ 2 Coronary Artery, Three Arteries Ⓠ 3 Coronary Artery, Four or More Arteries Ⓠ	0 Open	Z No Device	3 Coronary Artery 8 Internal Mammary, Right 9 Internal Mammary, Left C Thoracic Artery F Abdominal Artery
0 Coronary Artery, One Artery 1 Coronary Artery, Two Arteries 2 Coronary Artery, Three Arteries 3 Coronary Artery, Four or More Arteries	3 Percutaneous	4 Drug-eluting Intraluminal Device D Intraluminal Device	4 Coronary Vein
0 Coronary Artery, One Artery 1 Coronary Artery, Two Arteries 2 Coronary Artery, Three Arteries 3 Coronary Artery, Four or More Arteries	4 Percutaneous Endoscopic	4 Drug-eluting Intraluminal Device D Intraluminal Device	4 Coronary Vein
0 Coronary Artery, One Artery Ⓠ 1 Coronary Artery, Two Arteries Ⓠ 2 Coronary Artery, Three Arteries Ⓠ 3 Coronary Artery, Four or More Arteries Ⓠ	4 Percutaneous Endoscopic	8 Zooplastic Tissue 9 Autologous Venous Tissue A Autologous Arterial Tissue J Synthetic Substitute K Nonautologous Tissue Substitute	3 Coronary Artery 8 Internal Mammary, Right 9 Internal Mammary, Left C Thoracic Artery F Abdominal Artery W Aorta
0 Coronary Artery, One Artery Ⓠ 1 Coronary Artery, Two Arteries Ⓠ 2 Coronary Artery, Three Arteries Ⓠ 3 Coronary Artery, Four or More Arteries Ⓠ	4 Percutaneous Endoscopic	Z No Device	3 Coronary Artery 8 Internal Mammary, Right 9 Internal Mammary, Left C Thoracic Artery F Abdominal Artery
6 Atrium, Right	0 Open 4 Percutaneous Endoscopic	8 Zooplastic Tissue 9 Autologous Venous Tissue A Autologous Arterial Tissue J Synthetic Substitute K Nonautologous Tissue Substitute	P Pulmonary Trunk Q Pulmonary Artery, Right R Pulmonary Artery, Left
6 Atrium, Right	0 Open 4 Percutaneous Endoscopic	Z No Device	7 Atrium, Left P Pulmonary Trunk Q Pulmonary Artery, Right R Pulmonary Artery, Left
6 Atrium, Right	3 Percutaneous	Z No Device	7 Atrium, Left

Ⓠ 02170Z[PQR]
Non-OR 021[0123]4[4D]4
Non-OR 021[0123]3[4D]4
Ⓠ 021[0123]0[89AJK][389CFW] when reported with Secondary Diagnosis J98.5
Ⓠ 021[0123]0Z[389CF] when reported with Secondary Diagnosis J98.5
Ⓠ 021[0123]4[89AJK][389CFW] when reported with Secondary Diagnosis J98.5

Ⓠ 021[0123]4Z[389CF] when reported with Secondary Diagnosis J98.5

Coding Clinic: 2015, Q4, P23 P25, Q3, P17 – 021K0KP
Coding Clinic: 2016, Q1, P28 – 02100Z9, 021209W
Coding Clinic: 2016, Q4, P81-82, 102, 108-109 – 021
Coding Clinic: 2016, Q4, P83 – 02100AW, 021109W

Coding Clinic: 2016, Q4, P84 – 02100Z9
Coding Clinic: 2016, Q4, P108 – 02170ZU
Coding Clinic: 2016, Q4, P102 – 021W0JQ
Coding Clinic: 2016, Q4, P103 – 021Q0JA
Coding Clinic: 2016, Q4, P107 – 021K0KP
Coding Clinic: 2016, Q4, P144 – 021V09S
Coding Clinic: 2016, Q4, P145 – 021V08S
Coding Clinic: 2017, Q1, P19 – 021K0JP
Coding Clinic: 2017, Q4, P56 – 02163Z7

New/Revised Text in Green   ~~deleted~~ Deleted   ♀ Females Only   ♂ Males Only   **Coding Clinic**

Ⓠ Non-covered   Ⓠ Limited Coverage   ⊡ Combination (See Appendix E)   DRG Non-OR   Non-OR   Ⓠ Hospital-Acquired Condition

0: M/S   2: HEART AND GREAT VESSELS   1: BYPASS

SECTION: 0 MEDICAL AND SURGICAL
BODY SYSTEM: 2 HEART AND GREAT VESSELS
OPERATION: 1 BYPASS: (continued)
Altering the route of passage of the contents of a tubular body part

1: BYPASS

2: HEART AND GREAT VESSELS

0: M/S

Body Part	Approach	Device	Qualifier
7 Atrium, Left ⊞ V Superior Vena Cava	0 Open 4 Percutaneous Endoscopic	8 Zooplastic Tissue 9 Autologous Venous Tissue A Autologous Arterial Tissue J Synthetic Substitute K Nonautologous Tissue Substitute Z No Device	P Pulmonary Trunk Q Pulmonary Artery, Right R Pulmonary Artery, Left S Pulmonary Vein, Right T Pulmonary Vein, Left U Pulmonary Vein, Confluence
K Ventricle, Right L Ventricle, Left	0 Open 4 Percutaneous Endoscopic	8 Zooplastic Tissue 9 Autologous Venous Tissue A Autologous Arterial Tissue J Synthetic Substitute K Nonautologous Tissue Substitute	P Pulmonary Trunk Q Pulmonary Artery, Right R Pulmonary Artery, Left
K Ventricle, Right L Ventricle, Left	0 Open 4 Percutaneous Endoscopic	Z No Device	5 Coronary Circulation 8 Internal Mammary, Right 9 Internal Mammary, Left C Thoracic Artery F Abdominal Artery P Pulmonary Trunk Q Pulmonary Artery, Right R Pulmonary Artery, Left W Aorta
P Pulmonary Trunk Q Pulmonary Artery, Right R Pulmonary Artery, Left	0 Open 4 Percutaneous Endoscopic	8 Zooplastic Tissue 9 Autologous Venous Tissue A Autologous Arterial Tissue J Synthetic Substitute K Nonautologous Tissue Substitute Z No Device	A Innominate Artery B Subclavian D Carotid
W Thoracic Aorta, Descending	0 Open	8 Zooplastic Tissue 9 Autologous Venous Tissue A Autologous Arterial Tissue J Synthetic Substitute K Nonautologous Tissue Substitute Z No Device	B Subclavian D Carotid F Abdominal Artery G Axillary Artery H Brachial Artery P Pulmonary Trunk Q Pulmonary Artery, Right R Pulmonary Artery, Left V Lower Extremity Artery
W Thoracic Aorta, Descending	0 Open	J Synthetic Substitute K Nonautologous Tissue Substitute Z No Device	B Subclavian D Carotid G Axillary Artery H Brachial Artery P Pulmonary Trunk Q Pulmonary Artery, Right R Pulmonary Artery, Left
W Thoracic Aorta, Descending	4 Percutaneous Endoscopic	8 Zooplastic Tissue 9 Autologous Venous Tissue A Autologous Arterial Tissue J Synthetic Substitute K Nonautologous Tissue Substitute Z No Device	B Subclavian D Carotid P Pulmonary Trunk Q Pulmonary Artery, Right R Pulmonary Artery, Left
X Thoracic Aorta, Ascending/Arch	0 Open 4 Percutaneous Endoscopic	8 Zooplastic Tissue 9 Autologous Venous Tissue A Autologous Arterial Tissue J Synthetic Substitute K Nonautologous Tissue Substitute Z No Device	B Subclavian D Carotid P Pulmonary Trunk Q Pulmonary Artery, Right R Pulmonary Artery, Left

New/Revised Text in Green ~~deleted~~ Deleted ♀ Females Only ♂ Males Only **Coding Clinic**

🚫 Non-covered 🚫 Limited Coverage ⊞ Combination (See Appendix E) DRG Non-OR Non-OR 🚫 Hospital-Acquired Condition

SECTION: Ø MEDICAL AND SURGICAL
BODY SYSTEM: 2 HEART AND GREAT VESSELS
OPERATION: 4 **CREATION:** Putting in or on biological or synthetic material to form a new body part that to the extent possible replicates the anatomic structure or function of an absent body part

Body Part	Approach	Device	Qualifier
F Aortic Valve	Ø Open	7 Autologous Tissue Substitute 8 Zooplastic Tissue J Synthetic Substitute K Nonautologous Tissue Substitute	J Truncal Valve
G Mitral Valve J Tricuspid Valve	Ø Open	7 Autologous Tissue Substitute 8 Zooplastic Tissue J Synthetic Substitute K Nonautologous Tissue Substitute	2 Common Atrioventricular Valve

Coding Clinic: 2Ø16, Q4, P1Ø1-1Ø2, 1Ø6 – Ø24
Coding Clinic: 2Ø16, Q4, P1Ø5 – ØØ2[GJ]Ø[JK]2
Coding Clinic: 2Ø16, Q4, P1Ø7 – Ø24FØ[8J]J

SECTION: Ø MEDICAL AND SURGICAL
BODY SYSTEM: 2 HEART AND GREAT VESSELS
OPERATION: 5 **DESTRUCTION:** Physical eradication of all or a portion of a body part by the direct use of energy, force, or a destructive agent

Body Part	Approach	Device	Qualifier
4 Coronary Vein 5 Atrial Septum 6 Atrium, Right 7 Atrium, Left 8 Conduction Mechanism 9 Chordae Tendineae D Papillary Muscle F Aortic Valve G Mitral Valve H Pulmonary Valve J Tricuspid Valve K Ventricle, Right L Ventricle, Left M Ventricular Septum N Pericardium P Pulmonary Trunk Q Pulmonary Artery, Right R Pulmonary Artery, Left S Pulmonary Vein, Right T Pulmonary Vein, Left V Superior Vena Cava W Thoracic Aorta, Descending X Thoracic Aorta, Ascending/Arch	Ø Open 3 Percutaneous 4 Percutaneous Endoscopic	Z No Device	Z No Qualifier
7 Atrium, Left	Ø Open 3 Percutaneous 4 Percutaneous Endoscopic	Z No Device	K Left Atrial Appendage Z No Qualifier

DRG Non-OR   Ø257[Ø34]ZK

Coding Clinic: 2Ø13, Q2, P39 – Ø25S3ZZ, Ø25T3ZZ   Coding Clinic: 2Ø16, Q3, P44 – Ø258ØZZ
Coding Clinic: 2Ø16, Q2, P18 – Ø25NØZZ   Coding Clinic: 2Ø16, Q3, P44 – Ø257ØZK
Coding Clinic: 2Ø16, Q3, P43 – Ø2583ZZ   Coding Clinic: 2Ø16, Q4, P81 – Ø25

New/Revised Text in Green   ~~deleted~~ Deleted   ♀ Females Only   ♂ Males Only   **Coding Clinic**
 Non-covered   Limited Coverage   ⊞ Combination (See Appendix E)   DRG Non-OR   Non-OR   Hospital-Acquired Condition

SECTION: 0 MEDICAL AND SURGICAL
BODY SYSTEM: 2 HEART AND GREAT VESSELS
OPERATION: 7 DILATION: Expanding an orifice or the lumen of a tubular body part

Body Part	Approach	Device	Qualifier
0 Coronary Artery, One Artery 1 Coronary Artery, Two Arteries 2 Coronary Artery, Three Arteries 3 Coronary Artery, Four or More Arteries	0 Open 3 Percutaneous 4 Percutaneous Endoscopic	4 Drug-eluting Intraluminal Device 5 Intraluminal Device, Drug-eluting, Two 6 Intraluminal Device, Drug-eluting, Three 7 Intraluminal Device, Drug-eluting, Four or More D Intraluminal Device E Intraluminal Device, Two F Intraluminal Device, Three G Intraluminal Device, Four or More T Radioactive Intraluminal Device Z No Device	6 Bifurcation Z No Qualifier
F Aortic Valve G Mitral Valve H Pulmonary Valve J Tricuspid Valve K Ventricle, Right L Ventricle, Left P Pulmonary Trunk Q Pulmonary Artery, Right S Pulmonary Vein, Right T Pulmonary Vein, Left V Superior Vena Cava W Thoracic Aorta, Descending X Thoracic Aorta, Ascending/Arch	0 Open 3 Percutaneous 4 Percutaneous Endoscopic	4 Drug-eluting Intraluminal Device D Intraluminal Device Z No Device	Z No Qualifier
R Pulmonary Artery, Left	0 Open 3 Percutaneous 4 Percutaneous Endoscopic	4 Drug-eluting Intraluminal Device D Intraluminal Device Z No Device	T Ductus Arteriosus Z No Qualifier

Coding Clinic: 2015, Q2, P3-5 – 027234Z, 02703[4D]Z, 0270346, 027134Z
Coding Clinic: 2015, Q3, P10, P17 – 02703ZZ, 027Q0DZ
Coding Clinic: 2015, Q4, P14 – 027034Z
Coding Clinic: 2016, Q1, P17 – 027H0ZZ
Coding Clinic: 2016, Q4, P81-82 – 027
Coding Clinic: 2016, Q4, P85 – 02703EZ, 027136Z
Coding Clinic: 2016, Q4, P86 – 027037Z
Coding Clinic: 2016, Q4, P87 – 0271356
Coding Clinic: 2016, Q4, P88 – 0270346, 02703ZZ
Coding Clinic: 2017, Q4, P33 – 027L0ZZ

SECTION: Ø **MEDICAL AND SURGICAL**

BODY SYSTEM: 2 HEART AND GREAT VESSELS

OPERATION: 8 **DIVISION:** Cutting into a body part, without draining fluids and/or gases from the body part, in order to separate or transect a body part

Body Part	Approach	Device	Qualifier
8 Conduction Mechanism 9 Chordae Tendineae D Papillary Muscle	Ø Open 3 Percutaneous 4 Percutaneous Endoscopic	Z No Device	Z No Qualifier

SECTION: Ø **MEDICAL AND SURGICAL**

BODY SYSTEM: 2 HEART AND GREAT VESSELS

OPERATION: B **EXCISION:** Cutting out or off, without replacement, a portion of a body part

Body Part	Approach	Device	Qualifier
4 Coronary Vein 5 Atrial Septum 6 Atrium, Right 8 Conduction Mechanism 9 Chordae Tendineae D Papillary Muscle F Aortic Valve G Mitral Valve H Pulmonary Valve J Tricuspid Valve K Ventricle, Right 🦠 ⊞ L Ventricle, Left 🦠 M Ventricular Septum N Pericardium P Pulmonary Trunk Q Pulmonary Artery, Right R Pulmonary Artery, Left S Pulmonary Vein, Right T Pulmonary Vein, Left V Superior Vena Cava W Thoracic Aorta, Descending X Thoracic Aorta, Ascending/Arch	Ø Open 3 Percutaneous 4 Percutaneous Endoscopic	Z No Device	X Diagnostic Z No Qualifier
7 Atrium, Left	Ø Open 3 Percutaneous 4 Percutaneous Endoscopic	Z No Device	K Left Atrial Appendage X Diagnostic Z No Qualifier

🦠 Ø2B[KL][Ø34]ZZ
⊞ Ø2BKØZZ
DRG Non-OR Ø2B7[Ø34]ZK
Non-OR Ø2B[45689DFGHJKLM][Ø34]ZX
Non-OR Ø2B7[Ø34]ZX

Coding Clinic: 2Ø15, Q2, P24 – Ø2BGØZZ
Coding Clinic: 2Ø16, Q4, P81 – Ø2B

SECTION: Ø MEDICAL AND SURGICAL
BODY SYSTEM: 2   HEART AND GREAT VESSELS
OPERATION: C EXTIRPATION: Taking or cutting out solid matter from a body part

Body Part	Approach	Device	Qualifier
Ø Coronary Artery, One Artery 1 Coronary Artery, Two Arteries 2 Coronary Artery, Three Arteries 3 Coronary Artery, Four or More Arteries	Ø Open 3 Percutaneous 4 Percutaneous Endoscopic	Z No Device	6 Bifurcation Z No Qualifier
4 Coronary Vein 5 Atrial Septum 6 Atrium, Right 7 Atrium, Left 8 Conduction Mechanism 9 Chordae Tendineae D Papillary Muscle F Aortic Valve G Mitral Valve H Pulmonary Valve J Tricuspid Valve K Ventricle, Right L Ventricle, Left M Ventricular Septum N Pericardium P Pulmonary Trunk Q Pulmonary Artery, Right R Pulmonary Artery, Left S Pulmonary Vein, Right T Pulmonary Vein, Left V Superior Vena Cava W Thoracic Aorta, Descending X Thoracic Aorta, Ascending/Arch	Ø Open 3 Percutaneous 4 Percutaneous Endoscopic	Z No Device	Z No Qualifier

Coding Clinic: 2Ø16, Q2, P25 – Ø2CGØZZ
Coding Clinic: 2Ø16, Q4, P81-82, 87 – Ø2C

SECTION: Ø MEDICAL AND SURGICAL
BODY SYSTEM: 2   HEART AND GREAT VESSELS
OPERATION: F FRAGMENTATION: Breaking solid matter in a body part into pieces

Body Part	Approach	Device	Qualifier
N Pericardium 🔖	Ø Open 3 Percutaneous 4 Percutaneous Endoscopic X External	Z No Device	Z No Qualifier

🔖 Ø2FNXZZ
Non-OR Ø2FNXZZ

New/Revised Text in Green   ~~deleted~~ Deleted   ♀ Females Only   ♂ Males Only   **Coding Clinic**
🔖 Non-covered   🔖 Limited Coverage   ⊟ Combination (See Appendix E)   DRG Non-OR   Non-OR   🔖 Hospital-Acquired Condition

SECTION: 0 MEDICAL AND SURGICAL

BODY SYSTEM: 2 HEART AND GREAT VESSELS

OPERATION: H INSERTION: *(on multiple pages)*
Putting in a nonbiological appliance that monitors, assists, performs, or prevents a physiological function but does not physically take the place of a body part

Body Part	Approach	Device	Qualifier
4 Coronary Vein ⊞ ◔ 6 Atrium, Right ⊞ ◔ 7 Atrium, Left ⊞ ◔ K Ventricle, Right ⊞ ◔ L Ventricle, Left ⊞ ◔	0 Open 3 Percutaneous 4 Percutaneous Endoscopic	0 Monitoring Device, Pressure Sensor 2 Monitoring Device 3 Infusion Device D Intraluminal Device J Cardiac Lead, Pacemaker K Cardiac Lead, Defibrillator M Cardiac Lead N Intracardiac Pacemaker Y Other Device	Z No Qualifier
A Heart ◔ ◔	0 Open 3 Percutaneous 4 Percutaneous Endoscopic	Q Implantable Heart Assist System Y Other Device	Z No Qualifier
A Heart ⊞	0 Open 3 Percutaneous 4 Percutaneous Endoscopic	R Short-term External Heart Assist System	J Intraoperative S Biventricular Z No Qualifier
N Pericardium ⊞ ◔	0 Open 3 Percutaneous 4 Percutaneous Endoscopic	0 Monitoring Device, Pressure Sensor 2 Monitoring Device J Cardiac Lead, Pacemaker K Cardiac Lead, Defibrillator M Cardiac Lead Y Other Device	Z No Qualifier

◔ 02HA[34]QZ
◔ 02HA0QZ
⊞ 02H4[04]KZ
⊞ 02H43[JKM]Z
⊞ 02H[67][034]KZ
⊞ 02HK[034][02K]Z
⊞ 02HL[034][KM]Z
⊞ 02HA[04]R[SZ]
⊞ 02HA3RS
⊞ 02HN[034][JKM]Z
DRG Non-OR 02H[467][04][JM]Z
DRG Non-OR 02H[67]3JZ
DRG Non-OR 02H[KL][034][JM]Z
DRG Non-OR 02HK3[2JM]Z
DRG Non-OR 02H[467KL]3DZ
DRG Non-OR 02H[PQRSTVW]3DZ
Non-OR 02H[467KL]3[23M]Z
Non-OR 02HK33Z

◔ 02H43[JKM]Z when reported with Secondary Diagnosis K68.11, T81.4XXA, T82.6XXA, or T82.7XXA
◔ 02H[6K]33Z when reported with Secondary Diagnosis J95.811
◔ 02H[67]3[JM]Z when reported with Secondary Diagnosis K68.11, T81.4XXA, T82.6XXA, or T82.7XXA
◔ 02H[KL]3JZ when reported with Secondary Diagnosis K68.11, T81.4XXA, T82.6XXA, or T82.7XXA
◔ 02HN[034][JM]Z when reported with Secondary Diagnosis K68.11, T81.4XXA, T82.6XXA, or T82.7XXA

Coding Clinic: 2013, Q3, P18 – 02HV33Z
Coding Clinic: 2015, Q2, P32-33 – 02HK3DZ, 02HV33Z
Coding Clinic: 2015, Q3, P35 – 02HP32Z
Coding Clinic: 2017, Q4, P63; 2015, Q4, P14, P28-32 – 02HV33Z
Coding Clinic: 2016, Q2, P15 – 02H633Z
Coding Clinic: 2017, Q1, P10; 2016, Q4, P81, 95, 137 – 02H
Coding Clinic: 2017, Q1, P11-12; 2016, Q4, P139 – 02HA3RS
Coding Clinic: 2017, Q2, P25 – 02H633Z
Coding Clinic: 2017, Q4, P44-45 – 02HA3E[JZ]
Coding Clinic: 2017, Q4, P105 – 02H73DZ
Coding Clinic: 2018, Q2, P19 – 02H63KZ

New/Revised Text in Green   ~~deleted~~ Deleted   ♀ Females Only   ♂ Males Only   **Coding Clinic**
◔ Non-covered   ◔ Limited Coverage   ⊞ Combination (See Appendix E)   DRG Non-OR   Non-OR   ◔ Hospital-Acquired Condition

75

SECTION: Ø MEDICAL AND SURGICAL

BODY SYSTEM: 2 HEART AND GREAT VESSELS

OPERATION: H INSERTION: *(continued)*

Putting in a nonbiological appliance that monitors, assists, performs, or prevents a physiological function but does not physically take the place of a body part

Body Part	Approach	Device	Qualifier
P Pulmonary Trunk Q Pulmonary Artery, Right R Pulmonary Artery, Left S Pulmonary Vein, Right 🕭 T Pulmonary Vein, Left 🕭 V Superior Vena Cava 🕭 W Thoracic Aorta, Descending	Ø Open 3 Percutaneous 4 Percutaneous Endoscopic	Ø Monitoring Device, Pressure Sensor 2 Monitoring Device 3 Infusion Device D Intraluminal Device Y Other Device	Z No Qualifier
X Thoracic Aorta, Ascending/Arch	Ø Open 3 Percutaneous 4 Percutaneous Endoscopic	Ø Monitoring Device, Pressure Sensor 2 Monitoring Device 3 Infusion Device D Intraluminal Device	Z No Qualifier

Non-OR   02HP[034][023]Z
Non-OR   02H[QR][034][23]Z
Non-OR   02H[STV][034]3Z
Non-OR   02H[STVW]32Z
Non-OR   02HW[034][03]Z
🕭 02H[STV][34]3Z when reported with Secondary Diagnosis J95.811

SECTION: Ø MEDICAL AND SURGICAL

BODY SYSTEM: 2 HEART AND GREAT VESSELS

OPERATION: J INSPECTION: Visually and/or manually exploring a body part

Body Part	Approach	Device	Qualifier
A Heart Y Great Vessel	Ø Open 3 Percutaneous 4 Percutaneous Endoscopic	Z No Device	Z No Qualifier

Non-OR   02J[AY]3ZZ

Coding Clinic: 2Ø15, Q3, P9 – Ø2JA3ZZ

SECTION: Ø **MEDICAL AND SURGICAL**

BODY SYSTEM: 2 HEART AND GREAT VESSELS

OPERATION: **K MAP:** Locating the route of passage of electrical impulses and/or locating functional areas in a body part

Body Part	Approach	Device	Qualifier
8 Conduction Mechanism	Ø Open 3 Percutaneous 4 Percutaneous Endoscopic	Z No Device	Z No Qualifier

DRG Non-OR 02K8[034]ZZ

SECTION: Ø **MEDICAL AND SURGICAL**

BODY SYSTEM: 2 HEART AND GREAT VESSELS

OPERATION: **L OCCLUSION:** Completely closing an orifice or the lumen of a tubular body part

Body Part	Approach	Device	Qualifier
7 Atrium, Left	Ø Open 3 Percutaneous 4 Percutaneous Endoscopic	C Extraluminal Device D Intraluminal Device Z No Device	K Left Atrial Appendage
H Pulmonary Valve P Pulmonary Trunk Q Pulmonary Artery, Right S Pulmonary Vein, Right T Pulmonary Vein, Left V Superior Vena Cava	Ø Open 3 Percutaneous 4 Percutaneous Endoscopic	C Extraluminal Device D Intraluminal Device Z No Device	Z No Qualifier
R Pulmonary Artery, Left	Ø Open 3 Percutaneous 4 Percutaneous Endoscopic	C Extraluminal Device D Intraluminal Device Z No Device	T Ductus Arteriosus Z No Qualifier
W Thoracic Aorta, Descending	3 Percutaneous	D Intraluminal Device	J Temporary

DRG Non-OR 02L7[034][CDZ]K

Coding Clinic: 2015, Q4, P24 – 02LRØZT
Coding Clinic: 2016, Q2, P26 – 02LS3DZ
Coding Clinic: 2016, Q4, P102, 104 – 02L
Coding Clinic: 2017, Q4, P34 – 02L[QS]3DZ

0: M/S 2: HEART AND GREAT VESSELS K: MAP L: OCCLUSION

New/Revised Text in Green   deleted Deleted   ♀ Females Only   ♂ Males Only   **Coding Clinic**
Non-covered   Limited Coverage   Combination (See Appendix E)   DRG Non-OR   Non-OR   Hospital-Acquired Condition

77

SECTION: 0 MEDICAL AND SURGICAL

BODY SYSTEM: 2 HEART AND GREAT VESSELS

OPERATION: N RELEASE: Freeing a body part from an abnormal physical constraint by cutting or by the use of force

Body Part	Approach	Device	Qualifier
0 Coronary Artery, One Artery	0 Open	Z No Device	Z No Qualifier
1 Coronary Artery, Two Arteries	3 Percutaneous		
2 Coronary Artery, Three Arteries	4 Percutaneous Endoscopic		
3 Coronary Artery, Four or More Arteries			
4 Coronary Vein			
5 Atrial Septum			
6 Atrium, Right			
7 Atrium, Left			
8 Conduction Mechanism			
9 Chordae Tendineae			
D Papillary Muscle			
F Aortic Valve			
G Mitral Valve			
H Pulmonary Valve			
J Tricuspid Valve			
K Ventricle, Right			
L Ventricle, Left			
M Ventricular Septum			
N Pericardium			
P Pulmonary Trunk			
Q Pulmonary Artery, Right			
R Pulmonary Artery, Left			
S Pulmonary Vein, Right			
T Pulmonary Vein, Left			
V Superior Vena Cava			
W Thoracic Aorta, Descending			
X Thoracic Aorta, Ascending/Arch			

Coding Clinic: 2016, Q4, P81 – 02N

SECTION: Ø MEDICAL AND SURGICAL
BODY SYSTEM: 2 HEART AND GREAT VESSELS
OPERATION: P REMOVAL: Taking out or off a device from a body part

Body Part	Approach	Device	Qualifier
A Heart 🔖	Ø Open 3 Percutaneous 4 Percutaneous Endoscopic	2 Monitoring Device 3 Infusion Device 7 Autologous Tissue Substitute 8 Zooplastic Tissue C Extraluminal Device D Intraluminal Device J Synthetic Substitute K Nonautologous Tissue Substitute M Cardiac Lead N Intracardiac Pacemaker Q Implantable Heart Assist System Y Other Device	Z No Qualifier
A Heart ⊞	Ø Open 3 Percutaneous 4 Percutaneous Endoscopic	R Short-term External Heart Assist System	S Biventricular Z No Qualifier
A Heart ⊞ 🔖	X External	2 Monitoring Device 3 Infusion Device D Intraluminal Device M Cardiac Lead	Z No Qualifier
Y Great Vessel	Ø Open 3 Percutaneous 4 Percutaneous Endoscopic	2 Monitoring Device 3 Infusion Device 7 Autologous Tissue Substitute 8 Zooplastic Tissue C Extraluminal Device D Intraluminal Device J Synthetic Substitute K Nonautologous Tissue Substitute Y Other Device	Z No Qualifier
Y Great Vessel	X External	2 Monitoring Device 3 Infusion Device D Intraluminal Device	Z No Qualifier

⊞ 02PA[034]RZ
⊞ 02PAXMZ
Non-OR 02PAX[23DM]Z
Non-OR 02PA3[23D]Z
Non-OR 02PY3[23D]Z
Non-OR 02PYX[23D]Z
🔖 02PA[034]MZ when reported with Secondary Diagnosis K68.11, T81.4XXA, T82.6XXA, or T82.7XXA
🔖 02PAXMZ when reported with Secondary Diagnosis K68.11, T81.4XXA, T82.6XXA, or T82.7XXA

Coding Clinic: 2015, Q3, P33 – 02PA3MZ
Coding Clinic: 2016, Q2, P15; 2015, Q4, P32 – 02PY33Z
Coding Clinic: 2016, Q3, P19 – 02PYX3Z
Coding Clinic: 2016, Q4, P95 – 02P
Coding Clinic: 2016, Q4, P97 – 02PA3NZ
Coding Clinic: 2017, Q1, P11-21; 2016, Q4, P139 – 02PA3RZ
Coding Clinic: 2017, Q1, P14 – 02PA0RZ
Coding Clinic: 2017, Q2, P25 – 02PY33Z
Coding Clinic: 2017, Q4, P45, 105 – 02PA[DQ]Z

New/Revised Text in Green   ~~deleted~~ Deleted   ♀ Females Only   ♂ Males Only   **Coding Clinic**
🔖 Non-covered   🔖 Limited Coverage   ⊞ Combination (See Appendix E)   DRG Non-OR   Non-OR   🔖 Hospital-Acquired Condition

SECTION: Ø MEDICAL AND SURGICAL

BODY SYSTEM: 2 HEART AND GREAT VESSELS

OPERATION: **Q REPAIR:** Restoring, to the extent possible, a body part to its normal anatomic structure and function

Body Part	Approach	Device	Qualifier
Ø Coronary Artery, One Artery 1 Coronary Artery, Two Arteries 2 Coronary Artery, Three Arteries 3 Coronary Artery, Four or More Arteries 4 Coronary Vein 5 Atrial Septum 6 Atrium, Right 7 Atrium, Left 8 Conduction Mechanism 9 Chordae Tendineae A Heart B Heart, Right C Heart, Left D Papillary Muscle H Pulmonary Valve K Ventricle, Right L Ventricle, Left M Ventricular Septum N Pericardium P Pulmonary Trunk Q Pulmonary Artery, Right R Pulmonary Artery, Left S Pulmonary Vein, Right T Pulmonary Vein, Left V Superior Vena Cava W Thoracic Aorta, Descending X Thoracic Aorta, Ascending/Arch	Ø Open 3 Percutaneous 4 Percutaneous Endoscopic	Z No Device	Z No Qualifier
F Aortic Valve	Ø Open 3 Percutaneous 4 Percutaneous Endoscopic	Z No Device	J Truncal Valve Z No Qualifier
G Mitral Valve	Ø Open 3 Percutaneous 4 Percutaneous Endoscopic	Z No Device	E Atrioventricular Valve, Left Z No Qualifier
J Tricuspid Valve	Ø Open 3 Percutaneous 4 Percutaneous Endoscopic	Z No Device	G Atrioventricular Valve, Right Z No Qualifier

Non-OR 02Q[WX][034]ZZ

Coding Clinic: 2015, Q3, P16 – 02QWØZZ
Coding Clinic: 2015, Q4, P24 – 02Q5ØZZ
Coding Clinic: 2016, Q4, P81, 83, 102 – 02Q
Coding Clinic: 2016, Q4, P106 – 02QGØZE, 02QJØZG
Coding Clinic: 2016, Q4, P107 – 02QFØZJ
Coding Clinic: 2017, Q18, P10 – 02Q[ST]ØZZ

Left margin: Q: REPAIR   2: HEART AND GREAT VESSELS   Ø: M/S

New/Revised Text in Green   deleted Deleted   ♀ Females Only   ♂ Males Only   **Coding Clinic**
Non-covered   Limited Coverage   ⊞ Combination (See Appendix E)   DRG Non-OR   Non-OR   Hospital-Acquired Condition

SECTION: 0 MEDICAL AND SURGICAL
BODY SYSTEM: 2 HEART AND GREAT VESSELS
OPERATION: R REPLACEMENT: Putting in or on biological or synthetic material that physically takes the place and/or function of all or a portion of a body part

Body Part	Approach	Device	Qualifier
5 Atrial Septum 6 Atrium, Right 7 Atrium, Left 9 Chordae Tendineae D Papillary Muscle K Ventricle, Right 🔖 🔖 ⊞ L Ventricle, Left 🔖 🔖 ⊞ M Ventricular Septum N Pericardium P Pulmonary Trunk Q Pulmonary Artery, Right R Pulmonary Artery, Left S Pulmonary Vein, Right T Pulmonary Vein, Left V Superior Vena Cava W Thoracic Aorta, Descending X Thoracic Aorta, Ascending/Arch	0 Open 4 Percutaneous Endoscopic	7 Autologous Tissue Substitute 8 Zooplastic Tissue J Synthetic Substitute K Nonautologous Tissue Substitute	Z No Qualifier
F Aortic Valve G Mitral Valve H Pulmonary Valve J Tricuspid Valve	0 Open 4 Percutaneous Endoscopic	7 Autologous Tissue Substitute 8 Zooplastic Tissue J Synthetic Substitute K Nonautologous Tissue Substitute	Z No Qualifier
F Aortic Valve G Mitral Valve H Pulmonary Valve J Tricuspid Valve	3 Percutaneous	7 Autologous Tissue Substitute 8 Zooplastic Tissue J Synthetic Substitute K Nonautologous Tissue Substitute	H Transapical Z No Qualifier

🔖 02R[KL]0JZ except when combined with diagnosis code Z00.6
🔖 02R[KL]0JZ when combined with Z00.6
⊞ 02R[KL]0JZ

Coding Clinic: 2016, Q3, P32 – 02RJ48Z
Coding Clinic: 2016, Q4, P81 – 02R
Coding Clinic: 2017, Q1, P13 – 02R[KL]0JZ
Coding Clinic: 2017, Q4, P56 – 02RJ3JZ

SECTION: Ø MEDICAL AND SURGICAL

BODY SYSTEM: 2 HEART AND GREAT VESSELS

OPERATION: S REPOSITION: Moving to its normal location, or other suitable location, all or a portion of a body part

Body Part	Approach	Device	Qualifier
Ø Coronary Artery, One Artery	Ø Open	Z No Device	Z No Qualifier
1 Coronary Artery, Two Arteries			
P Pulmonary Trunk			
Q Pulmonary Artery, Right			
R Pulmonary Artery, Left			
S Pulmonary Vein, Right			
T Pulmonary Vein, Left			
V Superior Vena Cava			
W Thoracic Aorta, Descending			
X Thoracic Aorta, Ascending/Arch			

Coding Clinic: 2015, Q4, P24 – 02S[PW]ØZZ
Coding Clinic: 2016, Q4, P81, 83, 102 – 02S
Coding Clinic: 2016, Q4, P103-104 – 02S[1PX]ØZZ

SECTION: Ø MEDICAL AND SURGICAL

BODY SYSTEM: 2 HEART AND GREAT VESSELS

OPERATION: T RESECTION: Cutting out or off, without replacement, all of a body part

Body Part	Approach	Device	Qualifier
5 Atrial Septum	Ø Open	Z No Device	Z No Qualifier
8 Conduction Mechanism	3 Percutaneous		
9 Chordae Tendineae	4 Percutaneous Endoscopic		
D Papillary Muscle			
H Pulmonary Valve			
M Ventricular Septum			
N Pericardium			

New/Revised Text in Green   ~~deleted~~ Deleted   ♀ Females Only   ♂ Males Only   **Coding Clinic**
Non-covered   Limited Coverage   Combination (See Appendix E)   DRG Non-OR   Non-OR   Hospital-Acquired Condition

SECTION: Ø MEDICAL AND SURGICAL
BODY SYSTEM: 2 HEART AND GREAT VESSELS
OPERATION: U SUPPLEMENT: Putting in or on biological or synthetic material that physically reinforces and/or augments the function of a portion of a body part

Body Part	Approach	Device	Qualifier
5 Atrial Septum 6 Atrium, Right 7 Atrium, Left 9 Chordae Tendineae A Heart D Papillary Muscle H Pulmonary Valve K Ventricle, Right L Ventricle, Left M Ventricular Septum N Pericardium P Pulmonary Trunk Q Pulmonary Artery, Right R Pulmonary Artery, Left S Pulmonary Vein, Right T Pulmonary Vein, Left V Superior Vena Cava W Thoracic Aorta, Descending X Thoracic Aorta, Ascending/Arch	Ø Open 3 Percutaneous 4 Percutaneous Endoscopic	7 Autologous Tissue Substitute 8 Zooplastic Tissue J Synthetic Substitute K Nonautologous Tissue Substitute	Z No Qualifier
F Aortic Valve	Ø Open 3 Percutaneous 4 Percutaneous Endoscopic	7 Autologous Tissue Substitute 8 Zooplastic Tissue J Synthetic Substitute K Nonautologous Tissue Substitute	J Truncal Valve Z No Qualifier
G Mitral Valve	Ø Open 3 Percutaneous 4 Percutaneous Endoscopic	7 Autologous Tissue Substitute 8 Zooplastic Tissue J Synthetic Substitute K Nonautologous Tissue Substitute	E Atrioventricular Valve, Left Z No Qualifier
J Tricuspid Valve	Ø Open 3 Percutaneous 4 Percutaneous Endoscopic	7 Autologous Tissue Substitute 8 Zooplastic Tissue J Synthetic Substitute K Nonautologous Tissue Substitute	G Atrioventricular Valve, Right Z No Qualifier

DRG Non-OR Ø2U7[34]JZ

Coding Clinic: 2015, Q2, P24 – Ø2UGØJZ
Coding Clinic: 2015, Q3, P17 – Ø2U[QR]ØKZ
Coding Clinic: 2015, Q4, P23-25 – Ø2UFØ8Z, Ø2UMØJZ, Ø2UMØ8Z, Ø2UWØ7Z
Coding Clinic: 2016, Q2, P24 – Ø2U[PR]Ø7Z
Coding Clinic: 2016, Q2, P27 – Ø2UWØJZ
Coding Clinic: 2016, Q4, P81, 102 – Ø2U
Coding Clinic: 2016, Q4, P1Ø6 – Ø2UGØJE, Ø2UJØKG
Coding Clinic: 2016, Q4, P1Ø7 – Ø2UMØ8Z, Ø2UFØKJ
Coding Clinic: 2017, Q1, P2Ø – Ø2UXØKZ
Coding Clinic: 2017, Q3, P7 - Ø2U[67]Ø7Z
Coding Clinic: 2017, Q4, P36 - Ø2UGØ8Z

SECTION: Ø MEDICAL AND SURGICAL
BODY SYSTEM: 2 HEART AND GREAT VESSELS
OPERATION: V RESTRICTION: Partially closing an orifice or the lumen of a tubular body part

Body Part	Approach	Device	Qualifier
A Heart	Ø Open 3 Percutaneous 4 Percutaneous Endoscopic	C Extraluminal Device Z No Device	Z No Qualifier
G Mitral Valve	Ø Open 3 Percutaneous 4 Percutaneous Endoscopic	Z No Device	Z No Qualifier
P Pulmonary Trunk Q Pulmonary Artery, Right S Pulmonary Vein, Right T Pulmonary Vein, Left V Superior Vena Cava	Ø Open 3 Percutaneous 4 Percutaneous Endoscopic	C Extraluminal Device D Intraluminal Device Z No Device	Z No Qualifier
R Pulmonary Artery, Left	Ø Open 3 Percutaneous 4 Percutaneous Endoscopic	C Extraluminal Device D Intraluminal Device Z No Device	T Ductus Arteriosus Z No Qualifier
W Thoracic Aorta, Descending X Thoracic Aorta, Ascending/Arch	Ø Open 3 Percutaneous 4 Percutaneous Endoscopic	C Extraluminal Device D Intraluminal Device E Intraluminal Device, Branched or Fenestrated, One or Two Arteries F Intraluminal Device, Branched or Fenestrated, Three or More Arteries Z No Device	Z No Qualifier

Coding Clinic: 2016, Q4, P81, 89 – 02V
Coding Clinic: 2016, Q4, P93 – 02VW3DZ
Coding Clinic: 2017, Q4, P36 – 02VG0ZZ

V: RESTRICTION

2: HEART AND GREAT VESSELS

Ø: M/S

New/Revised Text in Green   ~~deleted~~ Deleted   ♀ Females Only   ♂ Males Only   **Coding Clinic**

Non-covered   Limited Coverage   Combination (See Appendix E)   DRG Non-OR   Non-OR   Hospital-Acquired Condition

SECTION: Ø MEDICAL AND SURGICAL

BODY SYSTEM: 2 HEART AND GREAT VESSELS

OPERATION: W REVISION: *(on multiple pages)*

Correcting, to the extent possible, a portion of a malfunctioning device or the position of a displaced device

Body Part	Approach	Device	Qualifier
5 Atrial Septum M Ventricular Septum	Ø Open 4 Percutaneous Endoscopic	J Synthetic Substitute	Z No Qualifier
A Heart 🦠 🦠 ⊡ 🦠	Ø Open 3 Percutaneous 4 Percutaneous Endoscopic	2 Monitoring Device 3 Infusion Device 7 Autologous Tissue Substitute 8 Zooplastic Tissue C Extraluminal Device D Intraluminal Device J Synthetic Substitute K Nonautologous Tissue Substitute M Cardiac Lead N Intracardiac Pacemaker Q Implantable Heart Assist System Y Other Device	Z No Qualifier
A Heart	Ø Open 3 Percutaneous 4 Percutaneous Endoscopic	R Short-term External Heart Assist System	S Biventricular Z No Qualifier
A Heart	X External	2 Monitoring Device 3 Infusion Device 7 Autologous Tissue Substitute 8 Zooplastic Tissue C Extraluminal Device D Intraluminal Device J Synthetic Substitute K Nonautologous Tissue Substitute M Cardiac Lead N Intracardiac Pacemaker Q Implantable Heart Assist System	Z No Qualifier
A Heart	X External	R Short-term External Heart Assist System	S Biventricular Z No Qualifier
F Aortic Valve G Mitral Valve H Pulmonary Valve J Tricuspid Valve	Ø Open 3 Percutaneous 4 Percutaneous Endoscopic	7 Autologous Tissue Substitute 8 Zooplastic Tissue J Synthetic Substitute K Nonautologous Tissue Substitute	Z No Qualifier

🦠 02WA[34]QZ
🦠 02WA0[JQ]Z
⊡ 02WA[034][QR]Z
Non-OR 02WAX[2378CDJKMQ]Z
Non-OR 02WAXRZ
Non-OR 02WA3[23D]Z

🦠 02WA[034]MZ when reported with Secondary Diagnosis K68.11, T81.4XXA, T82.6XXA, or T82.7XXA

Coding Clinic: 2015, Q3, P32 – 02WA3MZ
Coding Clinic: 2016, Q4, P95 – 02W
Coding Clinic: 2016, Q4, P96 – 02WA3NZ
Coding Clinic: 2018, Q1, P17 – 02WAXRZ

New/Revised Text in Green   deleted Deleted   ♀ Females Only   ♂ Males Only   **Coding Clinic**
🦠 Non-covered   🦠 Limited Coverage   ⊡ Combination (See Appendix E)   DRG Non-OR   Non-OR   🦠 Hospital-Acquired Condition

SECTION: 0 MEDICAL AND SURGICAL

BODY SYSTEM: 2 HEART AND GREAT VESSELS

OPERATION: W REVISION: *(continued)*

Correcting, to the extent possible, a portion of a malfunctioning device or the position of a displaced device

Body Part	Approach	Device	Qualifier
Y Great Vessel	0 Open 3 Percutaneous 4 Percutaneous Endoscopic	2 Monitoring Device 3 Infusion Device 7 Autologous Tissue Substitute 8 Zooplastic Tissue C Extraluminal Device D Intraluminal Device J Synthetic Substitute K Nonautologous Tissue Substitute Y Other Device	Z No Qualifier
Y Great Vessel	X External	2 Monitoring Device 3 Infusion Device 7 Autologous Tissue Substitute 8 Zooplastic Tissue C Extraluminal Device D Intraluminal Device J Synthetic Substitute K Nonautologous Tissue Substitute	Z No Qualifier

Non-OR   02WY[3X][2378CDJK]Z

SECTION: 0 MEDICAL AND SURGICAL

BODY SYSTEM: 2 HEART AND GREAT VESSELS

OPERATION: Y TRANSPLANTATION: Putting in or on all or a portion of a living body part taken from another individual or animal to physically take the place and/or function of all or a portion of a similar body part

Body Part	Approach	Device	Qualifier
A Heart 🗞	0 Open	Z No Device	0 Allogeneic 1 Syngeneic 2 Zooplastic

🗞 02YA0Z[012]

Coding Clinic: 2013, Q3, P19 – 02YA0Z0

SECTION: Ø MEDICAL AND SURGICAL
BODY SYSTEM: 3 **UPPER ARTERIES**
OPERATION: 1 **BYPASS:** *(on multiple pages)*
Altering the route of passage of the contents of a tubular body part

1: BYPASS

3: UPPER ARTERIES

Ø: M/S

Body Part	Approach	Device	Qualifier
2 Innominate Artery	Ø Open	9 Autologous Venous Tissue A Autologous Arterial Tissue J Synthetic Substitute K Nonautologous Tissue Substitute Z No Device	Ø Upper Arm Artery, Right 1 Upper Arm Artery, Left 2 Upper Arm Artery, Bilateral 3 Lower Arm Artery, Right 4 Lower Arm Artery, Left 5 Lower Arm Artery, Bilateral 6 Upper Leg Artery, Right 7 Upper Leg Artery, Left 8 Upper Leg Artery, Bilateral 9 Lower Leg Artery, Right B Lower Leg Artery, Left C Lower Leg Artery, Bilateral D Upper Arm Vein F Lower Arm Vein J Extracranial Artery, Right K Extracranial Artery, Left
3 Subclavian Artery, Right 4 Subclavian Artery, Left	Ø Open	9 Autologous Venous Tissue A Autologous Arterial Tissue J Synthetic Substitute K Nonautologous Tissue Substitute Z No Device	Ø Upper Arm Artery, Right 1 Upper Arm Artery, Left 2 Upper Arm Artery, Bilateral 3 Lower Arm Artery, Right 4 Lower Arm Artery, Left 5 Lower Arm Artery, Bilateral 6 Upper Leg Artery, Right 7 Upper Leg Artery, Left 8 Upper Leg Artery, Bilateral 9 Lower Leg Artery, Right B Lower Leg Artery, Left C Lower Leg Artery, Bilateral D Upper Arm Vein F Lower Arm Vein J Extracranial Artery, Right K Extracranial Artery, Left M Pulmonary Artery, Right N Pulmonary Artery, Left
5 Axillary Artery, Right 6 Axillary Artery, Left	Ø Open	9 Autologous Venous Tissue A Autologous Arterial Tissue J Synthetic Substitute K Nonautologous Tissue Substitute Z No Device	Ø Upper Arm Artery, Right 1 Upper Arm Artery, Left 2 Upper Arm Artery, Bilateral 3 Lower Arm Artery, Right 4 Lower Arm Artery, Left 5 Lower Arm Artery, Bilateral 6 Upper Leg Artery, Right 7 Upper Leg Artery, Left 8 Upper Leg Artery, Bilateral 9 Lower Leg Artery, Right B Lower Leg Artery, Left C Lower Leg Artery, Bilateral D Upper Arm Vein F Lower Arm Vein J Extracranial Artery, Right K Extracranial Artery, Left T Abdominal Artery V Superior Vena Cava

Coding Clinic: 2Ø16, Q3, P38 – Ø318ØJD

New/Revised Text in Green   ~~deleted~~ Deleted   ♀ Females Only   ♂ Males Only   **Coding Clinic**

⊘ Non-covered   ⊘ Limited Coverage   ⊞ Combination (See Appendix E)   DRG Non-OR   Non-OR   ⊘ Hospital-Acquired Condition

SECTION: Ø MEDICAL AND SURGICAL

BODY SYSTEM: 3 UPPER ARTERIES
OPERATION: 1 BYPASS: *(continued)*
Altering the route of passage of the contents of a tubular body part

Body Part	Approach	Device	Qualifier
7 Brachial Artery, Right	Ø Open	9 Autologous Venous Tissue A Autologous Arterial Tissue J Synthetic Substitute K Nonautologous Tissue Substitute Z No Device	Ø Upper Arm Artery, Right 3 Lower Arm Artery, Right D Upper Arm Vein F Lower Arm Vein V Superior Vena Cava
8 Brachial Artery, Left	Ø Open	9 Autologous Venous Tissue A Autologous Arterial Tissue J Synthetic Substitute K Nonautologous Tissue Substitute Z No Device	1 Upper Arm Artery, Left 4 Lower Arm Artery, Left D Upper Arm Vein F Lower Arm Vein V Superior Vena Cava
9 Ulnar Artery, Right B Radial Artery, Right	Ø Open	9 Autologous Venous Tissue A Autologous Arterial Tissue J Synthetic Substitute K Nonautologous Tissue Substitute Z No Device	3 Lower Arm Artery, Right F Lower Arm Vein
A Ulnar Artery, Left C Radial Artery, Left	Ø Open	9 Autologous Venous Tissue A Autologous Arterial Tissue J Synthetic Substitute K Nonautologous Tissue Substitute Z No Device	4 Lower Arm Artery, Left F Lower Arm Vein
G Intracranial Artery S Temporal Artery, Right T Temporal Artery, Left	Ø Open	9 Autologous Venous Tissue A Autologous Arterial Tissue J Synthetic Substitute K Nonautologous Tissue Substitute Z No Device	G Intracranial Artery
H Common Carotid Artery, Right J Common Carotid Artery, Left	Ø Open	9 Autologous Venous Tissue A Autologous Arterial Tissue J Synthetic Substitute K Nonautologous Tissue Substitute Z No Device	G Intracranial Artery J Extracranial Artery, Right K Extracranial Artery, Left Y Upper Artery
K Internal Carotid Artery, Right L Internal Carotid Artery, Left M External Carotid Artery, Right N External Carotid Artery, Left	Ø Open	9 Autologous Venous Tissue A Autologous Arterial Tissue J Synthetic Substitute K Nonautologous Tissue Substitute Z No Device	J Extracranial Artery, Right K Extracranial Artery, Left

Non-OR Ø31[789ABCGHJ]Ø[9AJKZ][Ø134DFGJK]

Coding Clinic: 2Ø13, Q1, P228 – Ø31CØZF
Coding Clinic: 2Ø17, Q2, P22 – Ø31JØZK
Coding Clinic: 2Ø17, Q4, P65 – Ø31JØJJ

Ø: M/S

3: UPPER ARTERIES

1: BYPASS

SECTION: Ø MEDICAL AND SURGICAL
BODY SYSTEM: 3 UPPER ARTERIES
OPERATION: 5 DESTRUCTION: Physical eradication of all or a portion of a body part by the direct use of energy, force, or a destructive agent

Body Part	Approach	Device	Qualifier
Ø Internal Mammary Artery, Right	Ø Open	Z No Device	Z No Qualifier
1 Internal Mammary Artery, Left	3 Percutaneous		
2 Innominate Artery	4 Percutaneous Endoscopic		
3 Subclavian Artery, Right			
4 Subclavian Artery, Left			
5 Axillary Artery, Right			
6 Axillary Artery, Left			
7 Brachial Artery, Right			
8 Brachial Artery, Left			
9 Ulnar Artery, Right			
A Ulnar Artery, Left			
B Radial Artery, Right			
C Radial Artery, Left			
D Hand Artery, Right			
F Hand Artery, Left			
G Intracranial Artery			
H Common Carotid Artery, Right			
J Common Carotid Artery, Left			
K Internal Carotid Artery, Right			
L Internal Carotid Artery, Left			
M External Carotid Artery, Right			
N External Carotid Artery, Left			
P Vertebral Artery, Right			
Q Vertebral Artery, Left			
R Face Artery			
S Temporal Artery, Right			
T Temporal Artery, Left			
U Thyroid Artery, Right			
V Thyroid Artery, Left			
Y Upper Artery			

New/Revised Text in Green deleted Deleted ♀ Females Only ♂ Males Only **Coding Clinic**
Non-covered Limited Coverage ⊞ Combination (See Appendix E) DRG Non-OR Non-OR Hospital-Acquired Condition

SECTION: Ø MEDICAL AND SURGICAL
BODY SYSTEM: 3 UPPER ARTERIES
OPERATION: 7 DILATION: Expanding an orifice or the lumen of a tubular body part

Body Part	Approach	Device	Qualifier
Ø Internal Mammary Artery, Right 1 Internal Mammary Artery, Left 2 Innominate Artery 3 Subclavian Artery, Right 4 Subclavian Artery, Left 5 Axillary Artery, Right 6 Axillary Artery, Left 7 Brachial Artery, Right 8 Brachial Artery, Left 9 Ulnar Artery, Right A Ulnar Artery, Left B Radial Artery, Right C Radial Artery, Left	Ø Open 3 Percutaneous 4 Percutaneous Endoscopic	4 Intraluminal Device, Drug-eluting 5 Intraluminal Device, Drug-eluting, Two 6 Intraluminal Device, Drug-eluting, Three 7 Intraluminal Device, Drug-eluting, Four or More E Intraluminal Device, Two F Intraluminal Device, Three G Intraluminal Device, Four or More	6 Bifurcation Z No Qualifier
Ø Internal Mammary Artery, Right 1 Internal Mammary Artery, Left 2 Innominate Artery 3 Subclavian Artery, Right 4 Subclavian Artery, Left 5 Axillary Artery, Right 6 Axillary Artery, Left 7 Brachial Artery, Right 8 Brachial Artery, Left 9 Ulnar Artery, Right A Ulnar Artery, Left B Radial Artery, Right C Radial Artery, Left	Ø Open 3 Percutaneous 4 Percutaneous Endoscopic	D Intraluminal Device Z No Device	1 Drug-Coated Balloon 6 Bifurcation Z No Qualifier
D Hand Artery, Right F Hand Artery, Left G Intracranial Artery 🐾 H Common Carotid Artery, Right J Common Carotid Artery, Left K Internal Carotid Artery, Right L Internal Carotid Artery, Left M External Carotid Artery, Right N External Carotid Artery, Left P Vertebral Artery, Right Q Vertebral Artery, Left R Face Artery S Temporal Artery, Right T Temporal Artery, Left U Thyroid Artery, Right V Thyroid Artery, Left Y Upper Artery	Ø Open 3 Percutaneous 4 Percutaneous Endoscopic	4 Intraluminal Device, Drug-eluting 5 Intraluminal Device, Drug-eluting, Two 6 Intraluminal Device, Drug-eluting, Three 7 Intraluminal Device, Drug-eluting, Four or More D Intraluminal Device E Intraluminal Device, Two F Intraluminal Device, Three G Intraluminal Device, Four or More Z No Device	6 Bifurcation Z No Qualifier

🐾 Ø37G[34]Z[6Z]

Coding Clinic: 2Ø16, Q4, P87 – Ø37

SECTION: Ø MEDICAL AND SURGICAL

BODY SYSTEM: 3 UPPER ARTERIES

OPERATION: 9 DRAINAGE: *(on multiple pages)*
Taking or letting out fluids and/or gases from a body part

Body Part	Approach	Device	Qualifier
Ø Internal Mammary Artery, Right	Ø Open	Ø Drainage Device	Z No Qualifier
1 Internal Mammary Artery, Left	3 Percutaneous		
2 Innominate Artery	4 Percutaneous Endoscopic		
3 Subclavian Artery, Right			
4 Subclavian Artery, Left			
5 Axillary Artery, Right			
6 Axillary Artery, Left			
7 Brachial Artery, Right			
8 Brachial Artery, Left			
9 Ulnar Artery, Right			
A Ulnar Artery, Left			
B Radial Artery, Right			
C Radial Artery, Left			
D Hand Artery, Right			
F Hand Artery, Left			
G Intracranial Artery			
H Common Carotid Artery, Right			
J Common Carotid Artery, Left			
K Internal Carotid Artery, Right			
L Internal Carotid Artery, Left			
M External Carotid Artery, Right			
N External Carotid Artery, Left			
P Vertebral Artery, Right			
Q Vertebral Artery, Left			
R Face Artery			
S Temporal Artery, Right			
T Temporal Artery, Left			
U Thyroid Artery, Right			
V Thyroid Artery, Left			
Y Upper Artery			

Non-OR   Ø39[Ø123456789ABCDFGHJKLMNPQRSTUVY][Ø34]ØZ

Left sidebar: 9: DRAINAGE   3: UPPER ARTERIES   Ø: M/S

SECTION: Ø MEDICAL AND SURGICAL
BODY SYSTEM: 3 UPPER ARTERIES
OPERATION: 9 DRAINAGE: *(continued)*

Taking or letting out fluids and/or gases from a body part

Body Part	Approach	Device	Qualifier
Ø Internal Mammary Artery, Right	Ø Open	Z No Device	X Diagnostic
1 Internal Mammary Artery, Left	3 Percutaneous		Z No Qualifier
2 Innominate Artery	4 Percutaneous Endoscopic		
3 Subclavian Artery, Right			
4 Subclavian Artery, Left			
5 Axillary Artery, Right			
6 Axillary Artery, Left			
7 Brachial Artery, Right			
8 Brachial Artery, Left			
9 Ulnar Artery, Right			
A Ulnar Artery, Left			
B Radial Artery, Right			
C Radial Artery, Left			
D Hand Artery, Right			
F Hand Artery, Left			
G Intracranial Artery			
H Common Carotid Artery, Right			
J Common Carotid Artery, Left			
K Internal Carotid Artery, Right			
L Internal Carotid Artery, Left			
M External Carotid Artery, Right			
N External Carotid Artery, Left			
P Vertebral Artery, Right			
Q Vertebral Artery, Left			
R Face Artery			
S Temporal Artery, Right			
T Temporal Artery, Left			
U Thyroid Artery, Right			
V Thyroid Artery, Left			
Y Upper Artery			

Non-OR Ø39[Ø123456789ABCDFGHJKLMNPQRSTUVY][Ø34]Z[3XZ]

SECTION: Ø MEDICAL AND SURGICAL
BODY SYSTEM: 3 UPPER ARTERIES
OPERATION: B EXCISION: Cutting out or off, without replacement, a portion of a body part

Body Part	Approach	Device	Qualifier
Ø Internal Mammary Artery, Right 1 Internal Mammary Artery, Left 2 Innominate Artery 3 Subclavian Artery, Right 4 Subclavian Artery, Left 5 Axillary Artery, Right 6 Axillary Artery, Left 7 Brachial Artery, Right 8 Brachial Artery, Left 9 Ulnar Artery, Right A Ulnar Artery, Left B Radial Artery, Right C Radial Artery, Left D Hand Artery, Right F Hand Artery, Left G Intracranial Artery H Common Carotid Artery, Right J Common Carotid Artery, Left K Internal Carotid Artery, Right L Internal Carotid Artery, Left M External Carotid Artery, Right N External Carotid Artery, Left P Vertebral Artery, Right Q Vertebral Artery, Left R Face Artery S Temporal Artery, Right T Temporal Artery, Left U Thyroid Artery, Right V Thyroid Artery, Left Y Upper Artery	Ø Open 3 Percutaneous 4 Percutaneous Endoscopic	Z No Device	X Diagnostic Z No Qualifier

Coding Clinic: 2016, Q2, P13 – Ø3BNØZZ

B: EXCISION 3: UPPER ARTERIES Ø: M/S

New/Revised Text in Green deleted Deleted ♀ Females Only ♂ Males Only Coding Clinic Non-covered Limited Coverage Combination (See Appendix E) DRG Non-OR Non-OR Hospital-Acquired Condition

SECTION: 0 MEDICAL AND SURGICAL
BODY SYSTEM: 3 UPPER ARTERIES
OPERATION: C EXTIRPATION: Taking or cutting out solid matter from a body part

Body Part	Approach	Device	Qualifier
0 Internal Mammary Artery, Right 1 Internal Mammary Artery, Left 2 Innominate Artery 3 Subclavian Artery, Right 4 Subclavian Artery, Left 5 Axillary Artery, Right 6 Axillary Artery, Left 7 Brachial Artery, Right 8 Brachial Artery, Left 9 Ulnar Artery, Right A Ulnar Artery, Left B Radial Artery, Right C Radial Artery, Left D Hand Artery, Right F Hand Artery, Left R Face Artery S Temporal Artery, Right T Temporal Artery, Left U Thyroid Artery, Right V Thyroid Artery, Left Y Upper Artery	0 Open 3 Percutaneous 4 Percutaneous Endoscopic	Z No Device	6 Bifurcation Z No Qualifier
G Intracranial Artery H Common Carotid Artery, Right J Common Carotid Artery, Left K Internal Carotid Artery, Right L Internal Carotid Artery, Left M External Carotid Artery, Right N External Carotid Artery, Left P Vertebral Artery, Right Q Vertebral Artery, Left	0 Open 4 Percutaneous Endoscopic	Z No Device	6 Bifurcation Z No Qualifier
G Intracranial Artery H Common Carotid Artery, Right J Common Carotid Artery, Left K Internal Carotid Artery, Right L Internal Carotid Artery, Left M External Carotid Artery, Right N External Carotid Artery, Left P Vertebral Artery, Right Q Vertebral Artery, Left	3 Percutaneous	Z No Device	6 Bifurcation 7 Stent Retriever Z No Qualifier

Coding Clinic: 2016, Q2, P12 – 03CK0ZZ
Coding Clinic: 2016, Q4, P87 – 03C
Coding Clinic: 2017, Q4, P65 – 03CN0ZZ

SECTION: Ø MEDICAL AND SURGICAL

BODY SYSTEM: 3 UPPER ARTERIES

OPERATION: **H INSERTION:** Putting in a nonbiological appliance that monitors, assists, performs, or prevents a physiological function but does not physically take the place of a body part

Body Part	Approach	Device	Qualifier
Ø Internal Mammary Artery, Right 1 Internal Mammary Artery, Left 2 Innominate Artery 3 Subclavian Artery, Right 4 Subclavian Artery, Left 5 Axillary Artery, Right 6 Axillary Artery, Left 7 Brachial Artery, Right 8 Brachial Artery, Left 9 Ulnar Artery, Right A Ulnar Artery, Left B Radial Artery, Right C Radial Artery, Left D Hand Artery, Right F Hand Artery, Left G Intracranial Artery H Common Carotid Artery, Right J Common Carotid Artery, Left M External Carotid Artery, Right N External Carotid Artery, Left P Vertebral Artery, Right Q Vertebral Artery, Left R Face Artery S Temporal Artery, Right T Temporal Artery, Left U Thyroid Artery, Right V Thyroid Artery, Left	Ø Open 3 Percutaneous 4 Percutaneous Endoscopic	3 Infusion Device D Intraluminal Device	Z No Qualifier
K Internal Carotid Artery, Right L Internal Carotid Artery, Left	Ø Open 3 Percutaneous 4 Percutaneous Endoscopic	3 Infusion Device D Intraluminal Device M Stimulator Lead	Z No Qualifier
Y Upper Artery	Ø Open 3 Percutaneous 4 Percutaneous Endoscopic	2 Monitoring Device 3 Infusion Device D Intraluminal Device Y Other Device	Z No Qualifier

Non-OR   Ø3H[Ø123456789ABCDFGHJMNPQRSTUV][Ø34]3Z
Non-OR   Ø3H[KL][Ø34]3Z
Non-OR   Ø3HY[Ø34]3Z
Non-OR   Ø3HY32Z

Coding Clinic: 2Ø16, Q2, P32 – Ø3HY32Z

Sidebar: H: INSERTION   3: UPPER ARTERIES   Ø: M/S

SECTION: 0   MEDICAL AND SURGICAL

BODY SYSTEM: 3   UPPER ARTERIES
OPERATION: J   INSPECTION: Visually and/or manually exploring a body part

Body Part	Approach	Device	Qualifier
Y Upper Artery	0 Open 3 Percutaneous 4 Percutaneous Endoscopic X External	Z No Device	Z No Qualifier

Non-OR   03JY[34X]ZZ

Coding Clinic: 2015, Q1, P29 – 03JY0ZZ

SECTION: 0   MEDICAL AND SURGICAL

BODY SYSTEM: 3   UPPER ARTERIES
OPERATION: L   OCCLUSION: Completely closing an orifice or the lumen of a tubular body part

Body Part	Approach	Device	Qualifier
0 Internal Mammary Artery, Right 1 Internal Mammary Artery, Left 2 Innominate Artery 3 Subclavian Artery, Right 4 Subclavian Artery, Left 5 Axillary Artery, Right 6 Axillary Artery, Left 7 Brachial Artery, Right 8 Brachial Artery, Left 9 Ulnar Artery, Right A Ulnar Artery, Left B Radial Artery, Right C Radial Artery, Left D Hand Artery, Right F Hand Artery, Left R Face Artery S Temporal Artery, Right T Temporal Artery, Left U Thyroid Artery, Right V Thyroid Artery, Left Y Upper Artery	0 Open 3 Percutaneous 4 Percutaneous Endoscopic	C Extraluminal Device D Intraluminal Device Z No Device	Z No Qualifier
G Intracranial Artery H Common Carotid Artery, Right J Common Carotid Artery, Left K Internal Carotid Artery, Right L Internal Carotid Artery, Left M External Carotid Artery, Right N External Carotid Artery, Left P Vertebral Artery, Right Q Vertebral Artery, Left	0 Open 3 Percutaneous 4 Percutaneous Endoscopic	B Intraluminal Device, Bioactive C Extraluminal Device D Intraluminal Device Z No Device	Z No Qualifier

Coding Clinic: 2016, Q2, P30 – 03LG0CZ

SECTION: Ø MEDICAL AND SURGICAL
BODY SYSTEM: 3 UPPER ARTERIES

OPERATION: **N RELEASE:** Freeing a body part from an abnormal physical constraint by cutting or by the use of force

Body Part	Approach	Device	Qualifier
Ø Internal Mammary Artery, Right 1 Internal Mammary Artery, Left 2 Innominate Artery 3 Subclavian Artery, Right 4 Subclavian Artery, Left 5 Axillary Artery, Right 6 Axillary Artery, Left 7 Brachial Artery, Right 8 Brachial Artery, Left 9 Ulnar Artery, Right A Ulnar Artery, Left B Radial Artery, Right C Radial Artery, Left D Hand Artery, Right F Hand Artery, Left G Intracranial Artery H Common Carotid Artery, Right J Common Carotid Artery, Left K Internal Carotid Artery, Right L Internal Carotid Artery, Left M External Carotid Artery, Right N External Carotid Artery, Left P Vertebral Artery, Right Q Vertebral Artery, Left R Face Artery S Temporal Artery, Right T Temporal Artery, Left U Thyroid Artery, Right V Thyroid Artery, Left Y Upper Artery	Ø Open 3 Percutaneous 4 Percutaneous Endoscopic	Z No Device	Z No Qualifier

SECTION: Ø MEDICAL AND SURGICAL

BODY SYSTEM: 3 UPPER ARTERIES
OPERATION: P REMOVAL: Taking out or off a device from a body part

Body Part	Approach	Device	Qualifier
Y Upper Artery	Ø Open 3 Percutaneous 4 Percutaneous Endoscopic	Ø Drainage Device 2 Monitoring Device 3 Infusion Device 7 Autologous Tissue Substitute C Extraluminal Device D Intraluminal Device J Synthetic Substitute K Nonautologous Tissue Substitute M Stimulator Lead Y Other Device	Z No Qualifier
Y Upper Artery	X External	Ø Drainage Device 2 Monitoring Device 3 Infusion Device D Intraluminal Device M Stimulator Lead	Z No Qualifier

Non-OR Ø3PY3[Ø23D]Z
Non-OR Ø3PYX[Ø23DM]Z

SECTION: Ø MEDICAL AND SURGICAL
BODY SYSTEM: 3 UPPER ARTERIES
OPERATION: Q REPAIR: Restoring, to the extent possible, a body part to its normal anatomic structure and function

Body Part	Approach	Device	Qualifier
Ø Internal Mammary Artery, Right	Ø Open	Z No Device	Z No Qualifier
1 Internal Mammary Artery, Left	3 Percutaneous		
2 Innominate Artery	4 Percutaneous Endoscopic		
3 Subclavian Artery, Right			
4 Subclavian Artery, Left			
5 Axillary Artery, Right			
6 Axillary Artery, Left			
7 Brachial Artery, Right			
8 Brachial Artery, Left			
9 Ulnar Artery, Right			
A Ulnar Artery, Left			
B Radial Artery, Right			
C Radial Artery, Left			
D Hand Artery, Right			
F Hand Artery, Left			
G Intracranial Artery			
H Common Carotid Artery, Right			
J Common Carotid Artery, Left			
K Internal Carotid Artery, Right			
L Internal Carotid Artery, Left			
M External Carotid Artery, Right			
N External Carotid Artery, Left			
P Vertebral Artery, Right			
Q Vertebral Artery, Left			
R Face Artery			
S Temporal Artery, Right			
T Temporal Artery, Left			
U Thyroid Artery, Right			
V Thyroid Artery, Left			
Y Upper Artery			

Coding Clinic: 2Ø17, Q1, P32 – Ø3QHØZZ

New/Revised Text in Green   ~~deleted~~ Deleted   ♀ Females Only   ♂ Males Only   **Coding Clinic**
🏷 Non-covered   🏷 Limited Coverage   ⊡ Combination (See Appendix E)   DRG Non-OR   Non-OR   🏷 Hospital-Acquired Condition

SECTION: Ø MEDICAL AND SURGICAL
BODY SYSTEM: 3 UPPER ARTERIES
OPERATION: R REPLACEMENT: Putting in or on biological or synthetic material that physically takes the place and/or function of all or a portion of a body part

Body Part	Approach	Device	Qualifier
Ø Internal Mammary Artery, Right 1 Internal Mammary Artery, Left 2 Innominate Artery 3 Subclavian Artery, Right 4 Subclavian Artery, Left 5 Axillary Artery, Right 6 Axillary Artery, Left 7 Brachial Artery, Right 8 Brachial Artery, Left 9 Ulnar Artery, Right A Ulnar Artery, Left B Radial Artery, Right C Radial Artery, Left D Hand Artery, Right F Hand Artery, Left G Intracranial Artery H Common Carotid Artery, Right J Common Carotid Artery, Left K Internal Carotid Artery, Right L Internal Carotid Artery, Left M External Carotid Artery, Right N External Carotid Artery, Left P Vertebral Artery, Right Q Vertebral Artery, Left R Face Artery S Temporal Artery, Right T Temporal Artery, Left U Thyroid Artery, Right V Thyroid Artery, Left Y Upper Artery	Ø Open 4 Percutaneous Endoscopic	7 Autologous Tissue Substitute J Synthetic Substitute K Nonautologous Tissue Substitute	Z No Qualifier

SECTION: Ø MEDICAL AND SURGICAL
BODY SYSTEM: 3 UPPER ARTERIES
OPERATION: S REPOSITION: Moving to its normal location, or other suitable location, all or a portion of a body part

Body Part	Approach	Device	Qualifier
Ø Internal Mammary Artery, Right 1 Internal Mammary Artery, Left 2 Innominate Artery 3 Subclavian Artery, Right 4 Subclavian Artery, Left 5 Axillary Artery, Right 6 Axillary Artery, Left 7 Brachial Artery, Right 8 Brachial Artery, Left 9 Ulnar Artery, Right A Ulnar Artery, Left B Radial Artery, Right C Radial Artery, Left D Hand Artery, Right F Hand Artery, Left G Intracranial Artery H Common Carotid Artery, Right J Common Carotid Artery, Left K Internal Carotid Artery, Right L Internal Carotid Artery, Left M External Carotid Artery, Right N External Carotid Artery, Left P Vertebral Artery, Right Q Vertebral Artery, Left R Face Artery S Temporal Artery, Right T Temporal Artery, Left U Thyroid Artery, Right V Thyroid Artery, Left Y Upper Artery	Ø Open 3 Percutaneous 4 Percutaneous Endoscopic	Z No Device	Z No Qualifier

Coding Clinic: 2015, Q3, P28 – 03SS0ZZ

New/Revised Text in Green   ~~deleted~~ Deleted   ♀ Females Only   ♂ Males Only   **Coding Clinic**
Non-covered   Limited Coverage   Combination (See Appendix E)   DRG Non-OR   Non-OR   Hospital-Acquired Condition

S: REPOSITION   3: UPPER ARTERIES   Ø: M/S

SECTION: Ø MEDICAL AND SURGICAL
BODY SYSTEM: 3 UPPER ARTERIES
OPERATION: **U SUPPLEMENT:** Putting in or on biological or synthetic material that physically reinforces and/or augments the function of a portion of a body part

Body Part	Approach	Device	Qualifier
Ø Internal Mammary Artery, Right	Ø Open	7 Autologous Tissue Substitute	Z No Qualifier
1 Internal Mammary Artery, Left	3 Percutaneous	J Synthetic Substitute	
2 Innominate Artery	4 Percutaneous Endoscopic	K Nonautologous Tissue Substitute	
3 Subclavian Artery, Right			
4 Subclavian Artery, Left			
5 Axillary Artery, Right			
6 Axillary Artery, Left			
7 Brachial Artery, Right			
8 Brachial Artery, Left			
9 Ulnar Artery, Right			
A Ulnar Artery, Left			
B Radial Artery, Right			
C Radial Artery, Left			
D Hand Artery, Right			
F Hand Artery, Left			
G Intracranial Artery			
H Common Carotid Artery, Right			
J Common Carotid Artery, Left			
K Internal Carotid Artery, Right			
L Internal Carotid Artery, Left			
M External Carotid Artery, Right			
N External Carotid Artery, Left			
P Vertebral Artery, Right			
Q Vertebral Artery, Left			
R Face Artery			
S Temporal Artery, Right			
T Temporal Artery, Left			
U Thyroid Artery, Right			
V Thyroid Artery, Left			
Y Upper Artery			

Coding Clinic: 2Ø16, Q2, P12 – Ø3UKØJZ

New/Revised Text in Green   ~~deleted~~ Deleted   ♀ Females Only   ♂ Males Only   **Coding Clinic**

Non-covered   Limited Coverage   Combination (See Appendix E)   DRG Non-OR   Non-OR   Hospital-Acquired Condition

SECTION: Ø MEDICAL AND SURGICAL

BODY SYSTEM: 3 UPPER ARTERIES

OPERATION: V RESTRICTION: Partially closing an orifice or the lumen of a tubular body part

V: RESTRICTION

3: UPPER ARTERIES

Ø: M/S

Body Part	Approach	Device	Qualifier
Ø Internal Mammary Artery, Right 1 Internal Mammary Artery, Left 2 Innominate Artery 3 Subclavian Artery, Right 4 Subclavian Artery, Left 5 Axillary Artery, Right 6 Axillary Artery, Left 7 Brachial Artery, Right 8 Brachial Artery, Left 9 Ulnar Artery, Right A Ulnar Artery, Left B Radial Artery, Right C Radial Artery, Left D Hand Artery, Right F Hand Artery, Left R Face Artery S Temporal Artery, Right T Temporal Artery, Left U Thyroid Artery, Right V Thyroid Artery, Left Y Upper Artery	Ø Open 3 Percutaneous 4 Percutaneous Endoscopic	C Extraluminal Device D Intraluminal Device Z No Device	Z No Qualifier
G Intracranial Artery H Common Carotid Artery, Right J Common Carotid Artery, Left K Internal Carotid Artery, Right L Internal Carotid Artery, Left M External Carotid Artery, Right N External Carotid Artery, Left P Vertebral Artery, Right Q Vertebral Artery, Left	Ø Open 3 Percutaneous 4 Percutaneous Endoscopic	B Intraluminal Device, Bioactive C Extraluminal Device D Intraluminal Device Z No Device	Z No Qualifier

Coding Clinic: 2016, Q1, P20 – 03VG3DZ
Coding Clinic: 2016, Q4, P26 – 03VM3DZ

SECTION: Ø MEDICAL AND SURGICAL
BODY SYSTEM: 3 UPPER ARTERIES
OPERATION: W **REVISION:** Correcting, to the extent possible, a portion of a malfunctioning device or the position of a displaced device

Body Part	Approach	Device	Qualifier
Y Upper Artery	Ø Open 3 Percutaneous 4 Percutaneous Endoscopic	Ø Drainage Device 2 Monitoring Device 3 Infusion Device 7 Autologous Tissue Substitute C Extraluminal Device D Intraluminal Device J Synthetic Substitute K Nonautologous Tissue Substitute M Stimulator Lead Y Other Device	Z No Qualifier
Y Upper Artery	X External	Ø Drainage Device 2 Monitoring Device 3 Infusion Device 7 Autologous Tissue Substitute C Extraluminal Device D Intraluminal Device J Synthetic Substitute K Nonautologous Tissue Substitute M Stimulator Lead	Z No Qualifier

Non-OR   Ø3WY3[Ø23D]Z
Non-OR   Ø3WYX[Ø237CDJKM]Z

Coding Clinic: 2Ø15, Q1, P33 – ØØWY3DZ
Coding Clinic: 2Ø16, Q3, P4Ø – Ø3WYØJZ

New/Revised Text in Green   ~~deleted~~ Deleted   ♀ Females Only   ♂ Males Only   **Coding Clinic**
🚫 Non-covered   🚫 Limited Coverage   ⊞ Combination (See Appendix E)   DRG Non-OR   Non-OR   🚫 Hospital-Acquired Condition

Ø: M/S   3: UPPER ARTERIES   W: REVISION

1Ø5

SECTION: 0 MEDICAL AND SURGICAL
BODY SYSTEM: 4 LOWER ARTERIES
OPERATION: 1 BYPASS: *(on multiple pages)*
Altering the route of passage of the contents of a tubular body part

Body Part	Approach	Device	Qualifier
0 Abdominal Aorta C Common Iliac Artery, Right D Common Iliac Artery, Left	0 Open 4 Percutaneous Endoscopic	9 Autologous Venous Tissue A Autologous Arterial Tissue J Synthetic Substitute K Nonautologous Tissue Substitute Z No Device	0 Abdominal Aorta 1 Celiac Artery 2 Mesenteric Artery 3 Renal Artery, Right 4 Renal Artery, Left 5 Renal Artery, Bilateral 6 Common Iliac Artery, Right 7 Common Iliac Artery, Left 8 Common Iliac Arteries, Bilateral 9 Internal Iliac Artery, Right B Internal Iliac Artery, Left C Internal Iliac Arteries, Bilateral D External Iliac Artery, Right F External Iliac Artery, Left G External Iliac Arteries, Bilateral H Femoral Artery, Right J Femoral Artery, Left K Femoral Arteries, Bilateral Q Lower Extremity Artery R Lower Artery
3 Hepatic Artery 4 Splenic Artery	0 Open 4 Percutaneous Endoscopic	9 Autologous Venous Tissue A Autologous Arterial Tissue J Synthetic Substitute K Nonautologous Tissue Substitute Z No Device	3 Renal Artery, Right 4 Renal Artery, Left 5 Renal Artery, Bilateral
E Internal Iliac Artery, Right F Internal Iliac Artery, Left H External Iliac Artery, Right J External Iliac Artery, Left	0 Open 4 Percutaneous Endoscopic	9 Autologous Venous Tissue A Autologous Arterial Tissue J Synthetic Substitute K Nonautologous Tissue Substitute Z No Device	9 Internal Iliac Artery, Right B Internal Iliac Artery, Left C Internal Iliac Arteries, Bilateral D External Iliac Artery, Right F External Iliac Artery, Left G External Iliac Arteries, Bilateral H Femoral Artery, Right J Femoral Artery, Left K Femoral Arteries, Bilateral P Foot Artery Q Lower Extremity Artery
K Femoral Artery, Right L Femoral Artery, Left	0 Open 4 Percutaneous Endoscopic	9 Autologous Venous Tissue A Autologous Arterial Tissue J Synthetic Substitute K Nonautologous Tissue Substitute Z No Device	H Femoral Artery, Right J Femoral Artery, Left K Femoral Arteries, Bilateral L Popliteal Artery M Peroneal Artery N Posterior Tibial Artery P Foot Artery Q Lower Extremity Artery S Lower Extremity Vein
K Femoral Artery, Right L Femoral Artery, Left	3 Percutaneous	J Synthetic Substitute	Q Lower Extremity Artery S Lower Extremity Vein
M Popliteal Artery, Right N Popliteal Artery, Left	0 Open 4 Percutaneous Endoscopic	9 Autologous Venous Tissue A Autologous Arterial Tissue J Synthetic Substitute K Nonautologous Tissue Substitute Z No Device	L Popliteal Artery M Peroneal Artery P Foot Artery Q Lower Extremity Artery S Lower Extremity Vein

Coding Clinic: 2015, Q3, P28 – 04100Z3, 04140Z4
Coding Clinic: 2016, Q2, P19 – 041K0JN
Coding Clinic: 2017, Q3, P6 – 041K09N, 041K0JN

Coding Clinic: 2017, Q3, P16 – 041C0J[25]
Coding Clinic: 2017, Q4, P47 – 041[34]0Z[34]

0: M/S

4: LOWER ARTERIES

1: BYPASS

New/Revised Text in Green   ~~deleted~~ Deleted   ♀ Females Only   ♂ Males Only   **Coding Clinic**
🔖 Non-covered   🔖 Limited Coverage   ⊞ Combination (See Appendix E)   DRG Non-OR   Non-OR   🔖 Hospital-Acquired Condition

107

SECTION: Ø MEDICAL AND SURGICAL
BODY SYSTEM: 4 LOWER ARTERIES
OPERATION: 1 BYPASS: *(continued)*
Altering the route of passage of the contents of a tubular body part

Body Part	Approach	Device	Qualifier
M Popliteal Artery, Right N Popliteal Artery, Left	3 Percutaneous	J Synthetic Substitute	Q Lower Extremity Artery S Lower Extremity Vein
P Anterior Tibial Artery, Right Q Anterior Tibial Artery, Left R Posterior Tibial Artery, Right S Posterior Tibial Artery, Left	Ø Open 3 Percutaneous 4 Percutaneous Endoscopic	J Synthetic Substitute	Q Lower Extremity Artery S Lower Extremity Vein
T Peroneal Artery, Right U Peroneal Artery, Left V Foot Artery, Right W Foot Artery, Left	Ø Open 4 Percutaneous Endoscopic	9 Autologous Venous Tissue A Autologous Arterial Tissue J Synthetic Substitute K Nonautologous Tissue Substitute Z No Device	P Foot Artery Q Lower Extremity Artery S Lower Extremity Vein
T Peroneal Artery, Right U Peroneal Artery, Left V Foot Artery, Right W Foot Artery, Left	3 Percutaneous	J Synthetic Substitute	Q Lower Extremity Artery S Lower Extremity Vein

Coding Clinic: 2Ø17, Q1, P33 – Ø41MØ9P

SECTION: Ø MEDICAL AND SURGICAL
BODY SYSTEM: 4 LOWER ARTERIES
OPERATION: 5 DESTRUCTION: Physical eradication of all or a portion of a body part by the direct use of energy, force, or a destructive agent

Body Part	Approach	Device	Qualifier
Ø Abdominal Aorta 1 Celiac Artery 2 Gastric Artery 3 Hepatic Artery 4 Splenic Artery 5 Superior Mesenteric Artery 6 Colic Artery, Right 7 Colic Artery, Left 8 Colic Artery, Middle 9 Renal Artery, Right A Renal Artery, Left B Inferior Mesenteric Artery C Common Iliac Artery, Right D Common Iliac Artery, Left E Internal Iliac Artery, Right F Internal Iliac Artery, Left H External Iliac Artery, Right J External Iliac Artery, Left K Femoral Artery, Right L Femoral Artery, Left M Popliteal Artery, Right N Popliteal Artery, Left P Anterior Tibial Artery, Right Q Anterior Tibial Artery, Left R Posterior Tibial Artery, Right S Posterior Tibial Artery, Left T Peroneal Artery, Right U Peroneal Artery, Left V Foot Artery, Right W Foot Artery, Left Y Lower Artery	Ø Open 3 Percutaneous 4 Percutaneous Endoscopic	Z No Device	Z No Qualifier

1: BYPASS   5: DESTRUCTION

4: LOWER ARTERIES   Ø: M/S

SECTION: Ø MEDICAL AND SURGICAL
BODY SYSTEM: 4 LOWER ARTERIES
OPERATION: 7 **DILATION:** *(on multiple pages)*
Expanding an orifice or the lumen of a tubular body part

Body Part	Approach	Device	Qualifier
Ø Abdominal Aorta	Ø Open	4 Intraluminal Device, Drug-eluting	1 Drug-Coated Balloon
1 Celiac Artery	3 Percutaneous		6 Bifurcation
2 Gastric Artery	4 Percutaneous Endoscopic	D Intraluminal Device	Z No Qualifier
3 Hepatic Artery		Z No Device	
4 Splenic Artery			
5 Superior Mesenteric Artery			
6 Colic Artery, Right			
7 Colic Artery, Left			
8 Colic Artery, Middle			
9 Renal Artery, Right			
A Renal Artery, Left			
B Inferior Mesenteric Artery			
C Common Iliac Artery, Right			
D Common Iliac Artery, Left			
E Internal Iliac Artery, Right			
F Internal Iliac Artery, Left			
H External Iliac Artery, Right			
J External Iliac Artery, Left			
K Femoral Carotid Artery, Right			
L Femoral Carotid Artery, Left			
M Popliteal Carotid Artery, Right			
N Popliteal Carotid Artery, Left			
P Anterior Tibial Artery, Right			
Q Anterior Tibial Artery, Left			
R Posterior Tibial Artery, Right			
S Posterior Tibial Artery, Left			
T Peroneal Artery, Right			
U Peroneal Artery, Left			
V Foot Artery, Right			
W Foot Artery, Left			
Y Lower Artery			

Non-OR   Ø47[59A]4DZ

Coding Clinic: 2015, Q4, P7 – Ø47K3D1
Coding Clinic: 2015, Q4, P15 – Ø47K3D1, Ø47L3Z1
Coding Clinic: 2016, Q3, P39 – Ø47C3DZ
Coding Clinic: 2016, Q4, P87 – Ø47
Coding Clinic: 2016, Q4, P89 – Ø47K3Z6

SECTION: Ø MEDICAL AND SURGICAL
BODY SYSTEM: 4 LOWER ARTERIES
OPERATION: 7 DILATION: *(continued)*
Expanding an orifice or the lumen of a tubular body part

Body Part	Approach	Device	Qualifier
Ø Abdominal Aorta 1 Celiac Artery 2 Gastric Artery 3 Hepatic Artery 4 Splenic Artery 5 Superior Mesenteric Artery 6 Colic Artery, Right 7 Colic Artery, Left 8 Colic Artery, Middle 9 Renal Artery, Right A Renal Artery, Left B Inferior Mesenteric Artery C Common Iliac Artery, Right D Common Iliac Artery, Left E Internal Iliac Artery, Right F Internal Iliac Artery, Left H External Iliac Artery, Right J External Iliac Artery, Left K Femoral Carotid Artery, Right L Femoral Carotid Artery, Left M Popliteal Carotid Artery, Right N Popliteal Carotid Artery, Left P Anterior Tibial Artery, Right Q Anterior Tibial Artery, Left R Posterior Tibial Artery, Right S Posterior Tibial Artery, Left T Peroneal Artery, Right U Peroneal Artery, Left V Foot Artery, Right W Foot Artery, Left Y Lower Artery	Ø Open 3 Percutaneous 4 Percutaneous Endoscopic	5 Intraluminal Device, Drug-eluting, Two 6 Intraluminal Device, Drug-eluting, Three 7 Intraluminal Device, Drug-eluting, Four or More E Intraluminal Device, Two F Intraluminal Device, Three G Intraluminal Device, Four or More	6 Bifurcation Z No Qualifier

7: DILATION

4: LOWER ARTERIES

Ø: M/S

SECTION: Ø MEDICAL AND SURGICAL
BODY SYSTEM: 4 LOWER ARTERIES
OPERATION: 9 DRAINAGE: *(on multiple pages)*

Taking or letting out fluids and/or gases from a body part

Body Part	Approach	Device	Qualifier
Ø Abdominal Aorta	Ø Open	Ø Drainage Device	Z No Qualifier
1 Celiac Artery	3 Percutaneous		
2 Gastric Artery	4 Percutaneous Endoscopic		
3 Hepatic Artery			
4 Splenic Artery			
5 Superior Mesenteric Artery			
6 Colic Artery, Right			
7 Colic Artery, Left			
8 Colic Artery, Middle			
9 Renal Artery, Right			
A Renal Artery, Left			
B Inferior Mesenteric Artery			
C Common Iliac Artery, Right			
D Common Iliac Artery, Left			
E Internal Iliac Artery, Right			
F Internal Iliac Artery, Left			
H External Iliac Artery, Right			
J External Iliac Artery, Left			
K Femoral Artery, Right			
L Femoral Artery, Left			
M Popliteal Artery, Right			
N Popliteal Artery, Left			
P Anterior Tibial Artery, Right			
Q Anterior Tibial Artery, Left			
R Posterior Tibial Artery, Right			
S Posterior Tibial Artery, Left			
T Peroneal Artery, Right			
U Peroneal Artery, Left			
V Foot Artery, Right			
W Foot Artery, Left			
Y Lower Artery			

Non-OR   Ø49[Ø123456789ABCDEFHJKLMNPQRSTUVWY][Ø34]ØZ

SECTION: Ø MEDICAL AND SURGICAL
BODY SYSTEM: 4 LOWER ARTERIES
OPERATION: 9 DRAINAGE: *(continued)*

Taking or letting out fluids and/or gases from a body part

Body Part	Approach	Device	Qualifier
Ø Abdominal Aorta	Ø Open	Z No Device	X Diagnostic
1 Celiac Artery	3 Percutaneous		Z No Qualifier
2 Gastric Artery	4 Percutaneous Endoscopic		
3 Hepatic Artery			
4 Splenic Artery			
5 Superior Mesenteric Artery			
6 Colic Artery, Right			
7 Colic Artery, Left			
8 Colic Artery, Middle			
9 Renal Artery, Right			
A Renal Artery, Left			
B Inferior Mesenteric Artery			
C Common Iliac Artery, Right			
D Common Iliac Artery, Left			
E Internal Iliac Artery, Right			
F Internal Iliac Artery, Left			
H External Iliac Artery, Right			
J External Iliac Artery, Left			
K Femoral Artery, Right			
L Femoral Artery, Left			
M Popliteal Artery, Right			
N Popliteal Artery, Left			
P Anterior Tibial Artery, Right			
Q Anterior Tibial Artery, Left			
R Posterior Tibial Artery, Right			
S Posterior Tibial Artery, Left			
T Peroneal Artery, Right			
U Peroneal Artery, Left			
V Foot Artery, Right			
W Foot Artery, Left			
Y Lower Artery			

Non-OR   Ø49[Ø123456789ABCDEFHJKLMNPQRSTUVWY][Ø34]Z[XZ]

9: DRAINAGE

4: LOWER ARTERIES

Ø: M/S

New/Revised Text in Green   ~~deleted~~ Deleted   ♀ Females Only   ♂ Males Only   **Coding Clinic**

Non-covered   Limited Coverage   ⊞ Combination (See Appendix E)   DRG Non-OR   Non-OR   Hospital-Acquired Condition

SECTION: Ø MEDICAL AND SURGICAL

BODY SYSTEM: 4 LOWER ARTERIES

OPERATION: B EXCISION: Cutting out or off, without replacement, a portion of a body part

Body Part	Approach	Device	Qualifier
Ø Abdominal Aorta	Ø Open	Z No Device	X Diagnostic
1 Celiac Artery	3 Percutaneous		Z No Qualifier
2 Gastric Artery	4 Percutaneous Endoscopic		
3 Hepatic Artery			
4 Splenic Artery			
5 Superior Mesenteric Artery			
6 Colic Artery, Right			
7 Colic Artery, Left			
8 Colic Artery, Middle			
9 Renal Artery, Right			
A Renal Artery, Left			
B Inferior Mesenteric Artery			
C Common Iliac Artery, Right			
D Common Iliac Artery, Left			
E Internal Iliac Artery, Right			
F Internal Iliac Artery, Left			
H External Iliac Artery, Right			
J External Iliac Artery, Left			
K Femoral Artery, Right			
L Femoral Artery, Left			
M Popliteal Artery, Right			
N Popliteal Artery, Left			
P Anterior Tibial Artery, Right			
Q Anterior Tibial Artery, Left			
R Posterior Tibial Artery, Right			
S Posterior Tibial Artery, Left			
T Peroneal Artery, Right			
U Peroneal Artery, Left			
V Foot Artery, Right			
W Foot Artery, Left			
Y Lower Artery			

SECTION: Ø MEDICAL AND SURGICAL
BODY SYSTEM: 4 LOWER ARTERIES
OPERATION: C EXTIRPATION: Taking or cutting out solid matter from a body part

Body Part	Approach	Device	Qualifier
Ø Abdominal Aorta	Ø Open	Z No Device	6 Bifurcation
1 Celiac Artery	3 Percutaneous		Z No Qualifier
2 Gastric Artery	4 Percutaneous Endoscopic		
3 Hepatic Artery			
4 Splenic Artery			
5 Superior Mesenteric Artery			
6 Colic Artery, Right			
7 Colic Artery, Left			
8 Colic Artery, Middle			
9 Renal Artery, Right			
A Renal Artery, Left			
B Inferior Mesenteric Artery			
C Common Iliac Artery, Right			
D Common Iliac Artery, Left			
E Internal Iliac Artery, Right			
F Internal Iliac Artery, Left			
H External Iliac Artery, Right			
J External Iliac Artery, Left			
K Femoral Artery, Right			
L Femoral Artery, Left			
M Popliteal Artery, Right			
N Popliteal Artery, Left			
P Anterior Tibial Artery, Right			
Q Anterior Tibial Artery, Left			
R Posterior Tibial Artery, Right			
S Posterior Tibial Artery, Left			
T Peroneal Artery, Right			
U Peroneal Artery, Left			
V Foot Artery, Right			
W Foot Artery, Left			
Y Lower Artery			

Coding Clinic: 2015, Q1, P36 – 04CL3ZZ
Coding Clinic: 2016, Q1, P31 – 04CJ0ZZ
Coding Clinic: 2016, Q4, P89 – 04CK3Z6

C: EXTIRPATION

4: LOWER ARTERIES

Ø: M/S

SECTION: Ø MEDICAL AND SURGICAL

BODY SYSTEM: 4 LOWER ARTERIES

OPERATION: H INSERTION: Putting in a nonbiological appliance that monitors, assists, performs, or prevents a physiological function but does not physically take the place of a body part

Body Part	Approach	Device	Qualifier
Ø Abdominal Aorta	Ø Open 3 Percutaneous 4 Percutaneous Endoscopic	2 Monitoring Device 3 Infusion Device D Intraluminal Device	Z No Qualifier
1 Celiac Artery 2 Gastric Artery 3 Hepatic Artery 4 Splenic Artery 5 Superior Mesenteric Artery 6 Colic Artery, Right 7 Colic Artery, Left 8 Colic Artery, Middle 9 Renal Artery, Right A Renal Artery, Left B Inferior Mesenteric Artery C Common Iliac Artery, Right D Common Iliac Artery, Left E Internal Iliac Artery, Right F Internal Iliac Artery, Left H External Iliac Artery, Right J External Iliac Artery, Left K Femoral Artery, Right L Femoral Artery, Left M Popliteal Artery, Right N Popliteal Artery, Left P Anterior Tibial Artery, Right Q Anterior Tibial Artery, Left R Posterior Tibial Artery, Right S Posterior Tibial Artery, Left T Peroneal Artery, Right U Peroneal Artery, Left V Foot Artery, Right W Foot Artery, Left	Ø Open 3 Percutaneous 4 Percutaneous Endoscopic	3 Infusion Device D Intraluminal Device	Z No Qualifier
Y Lower Artery	Ø Open 3 Percutaneous 4 Percutaneous Endoscopic	2 Monitoring Device 3 Infusion Device D Intraluminal Device Y Other Device	Z No Qualifier

DRG Non-OR   Ø4HY32Z
Non-OR   Ø4HØ[Ø34][23]Z
Non-OR   Ø4H[123456789ABCDEFHJKLMNPQRSTUVW][Ø34]3Z
Non-OR   Ø4HY[Ø34]3Z

Coding Clinic: 2017, Q1, P21 – Ø4HY32Z

Ø: M/S   4: LOWER ARTERIES   H: INSERTION

SECTION: Ø MEDICAL AND SURGICAL
BODY SYSTEM: 4 LOWER ARTERIES
OPERATION: J INSPECTION: Visually and/or manually exploring a body part

Body Part	Approach	Device	Qualifier
Y Lower Artery	Ø Open 3 Percutaneous 4 Percutaneous Endoscopic X External	Z No Device	Z No Qualifier

Non-OR   04JY[34X]ZZ

SECTION: Ø MEDICAL AND SURGICAL

BODY SYSTEM: 4 LOWER ARTERIES

OPERATION: L OCCLUSION: Completely closing an orifice or the lumen of a tubular body part

Body Part	Approach	Device	Qualifier
Ø Abdominal Aorta	Ø Open 4 Percutaneous Endoscopic	C Extraluminal Device D Intraluminal Device Z No Device	Z No Qualifier
Ø Abdominal Aorta	3 Percutaneous	C Extraluminal Device Z No Device	Z No Qualifier
Ø Abdominal Aorta	3 Percutaneous	D Intraluminal Device	J Temporary Z No Qualifier
1 Celiac Artery 2 Gastric Artery 3 Hepatic Artery 4 Splenic Artery 5 Superior Mesenteric Artery 6 Colic Artery, Right 7 Colic Artery, Left 8 Colic Artery, Middle 9 Renal Artery, Right A Renal Artery, Left B Inferior Mesenteric Artery C Common Iliac Artery, Right D Common Iliac Artery, Left H External Iliac Artery, Right J External Iliac Artery, Left K Femoral Artery, Right L Femoral Artery, Left M Popliteal Artery, Right N Popliteal Artery, Left P Anterior Tibial Artery, Right Q Anterior Tibial Artery, Left R Posterior Tibial Artery, Right S Posterior Tibial Artery, Left T Peroneal Artery, Right U Peroneal Artery, Left V Foot Artery, Right W Foot Artery, Left Y Lower Artery	Ø Open 3 Percutaneous 4 Percutaneous Endoscopic	C Extraluminal Device D Intraluminal Device Z No Device	Z No Qualifier
E Internal Iliac Artery, Right	Ø Open 3 Percutaneous 4 Percutaneous Endoscopic	C Extraluminal Device D Intraluminal Device Z No Device	T Uterine Artery, Right ♀ Z No Qualifier
F Internal Iliac Artery, Left	Ø Open 3 Percutaneous 4 Percutaneous Endoscopic	C Extraluminal Device D Intraluminal Device Z No Device	U Uterine Artery, Left ♀ Z No Qualifier

Non-OR 04L23DZ

Coding Clinic: 2015, Q2, P27 – 04LE3DT
Coding Clinic: 2018, Q2, P18 – 04L[HJ]ØCZ

New/Revised Text in Green ~~deleted~~ Deleted ♀ Females Only ♂ Males Only **Coding Clinic**
🐾 Non-covered 🐾 Limited Coverage ⊡ Combination (See Appendix E) DRG Non-OR Non-OR 🐾 Hospital-Acquired Condition

SECTION: 0 MEDICAL AND SURGICAL
BODY SYSTEM: 4 LOWER ARTERIES

OPERATION: N RELEASE: Freeing a body part from an abnormal physical constraint by cutting or by the use of force

Body Part	Approach	Device	Qualifier
0 Abdominal Aorta 1 Celiac Artery 2 Gastric Artery 3 Hepatic Artery 4 Splenic Artery 5 Superior Mesenteric Artery 6 Colic Artery, Right 7 Colic Artery, Left 8 Colic Artery, Middle 9 Renal Artery, Right A Renal Artery, Left B Inferior Mesenteric Artery C Common Iliac Artery, Right D Common Iliac Artery, Left E Internal Iliac Artery, Right F Internal Iliac Artery, Left H External Iliac Artery, Right J External Iliac Artery, Left K Femoral Artery, Right L Femoral Artery, Left M Popliteal Artery, Right N Popliteal Artery, Left P Anterior Tibial Artery, Right Q Anterior Tibial Artery, Left R Posterior Tibial Artery, Right S Posterior Tibial Artery, Left T Peroneal Artery, Right U Peroneal Artery, Left V Foot Artery, Right W Foot Artery, Left Y Lower Artery	0 Open 3 Percutaneous 4 Percutaneous Endoscopic	Z No Device	Z No Qualifier

Coding Clinic: 2015, Q2, P28 – 04N10ZZ

N: RELEASE

4: LOWER ARTERIES

0: M/S

New/Revised Text in Green   ~~deleted~~ Deleted   ♀ Females Only   ♂ Males Only   **Coding Clinic**
Non-covered   Limited Coverage   ⊞ Combination (See Appendix E)   DRG Non-OR   Non-OR   Hospital-Acquired Condition

SECTION: Ø MEDICAL AND SURGICAL
BODY SYSTEM: 4 LOWER ARTERIES
OPERATION: P REMOVAL: Taking out or off a device from a body part

Body Part	Approach	Device	Qualifier
Y Lower Artery	Ø Open 3 Percutaneous 4 Percutaneous Endoscopic	Ø Drainage Device 2 Monitoring Device 3 Infusion Device 7 Autologous Tissue Substitute C Extraluminal Device D Intraluminal Device J Synthetic Substitute K Nonautologous Tissue Substitute Y Other Device	Z No Qualifier
Y Lower Artery	X External	Ø Drainage Device 1 Radioactive Element 2 Monitoring Device 3 Infusion Device D Intraluminal Device	Z No Qualifier

Non-OR   04PYX[0123D]Z

SECTION: 0 MEDICAL AND SURGICAL

BODY SYSTEM: 4 LOWER ARTERIES

OPERATION: Q REPAIR: Restoring, to the extent possible, a body part to its normal anatomic structure and function

Body Part	Approach	Device	Qualifier
0 Abdominal Aorta	0 Open	Z No Device	Z No Qualifier
1 Celiac Artery	3 Percutaneous		
2 Gastric Artery	4 Percutaneous Endoscopic		
3 Hepatic Artery			
4 Splenic Artery			
5 Superior Mesenteric Artery			
6 Colic Artery, Right			
7 Colic Artery, Left			
8 Colic Artery, Middle			
9 Renal Artery, Right			
A Renal Artery, Left			
B Inferior Mesenteric Artery			
C Common Iliac Artery, Right			
D Common Iliac Artery, Left			
E Internal Iliac Artery, Right			
F Internal Iliac Artery, Left			
H External Iliac Artery, Right			
J External Iliac Artery, Left			
K Femoral Artery, Right			
L Femoral Artery, Left			
M Popliteal Artery, Right			
N Popliteal Artery, Left			
P Anterior Tibial Artery, Right			
Q Anterior Tibial Artery, Left			
R Posterior Tibial Artery, Right			
S Posterior Tibial Artery, Left			
T Peroneal Artery, Right			
U Peroneal Artery, Left			
V Foot Artery, Right			
W Foot Artery, Left			
Y Lower Artery			

Q: REPAIR

4: LOWER ARTERIES

0: M/S

New/Revised Text in Green   deleted Deleted   ♀ Females Only   ♂ Males Only   **Coding Clinic**

Non-covered   Limited Coverage   ⊕ Combination (See Appendix E)   DRG Non-OR   Non-OR   Hospital-Acquired Condition

SECTION: Ø MEDICAL AND SURGICAL

BODY SYSTEM: 4 LOWER ARTERIES

OPERATION: R **REPLACEMENT:** Putting in or on biological or synthetic material that physically takes the place and/or function of all or a portion of a body part

Body Part	Approach	Device	Qualifier
Ø Abdominal Aorta 1 Celiac Artery 2 Gastric Artery 3 Hepatic Artery 4 Splenic Artery 5 Superior Mesenteric Artery 6 Colic Artery, Right 7 Colic Artery, Left 8 Colic Artery, Middle 9 Renal Artery, Right A Renal Artery, Left B Inferior Mesenteric Artery C Common Iliac Artery, Right D Common Iliac Artery, Left E Internal Iliac Artery, Right F Internal Iliac Artery, Left H External Iliac Artery, Right J External Iliac Artery, Left K Femoral Artery, Right L Femoral Artery, Left M Popliteal Artery, Right N Popliteal Artery, Left P Anterior Tibial Artery, Right Q Anterior Tibial Artery, Left R Posterior Tibial Artery, Right S Posterior Tibial Artery, Left T Peroneal Artery, Right U Peroneal Artery, Left V Foot Artery, Right W Foot Artery, Left Y Lower Artery	Ø Open 4 Percutaneous Endoscopic	7 Autologous Tissue Substitute J Synthetic Substitute K Nonautologous Tissue Substitute	Z No Qualifier

Coding Clinic: 2015, Q2, P28 – 04R10JZ

SECTION: 0 MEDICAL AND SURGICAL
BODY SYSTEM: 4 LOWER ARTERIES
OPERATION: S REPOSITION: Moving to its normal location, or other suitable location, all or a portion of a body part

Body Part	Approach	Device	Qualifier
0 Abdominal Aorta	0 Open	Z No Device	Z No Qualifier
1 Celiac Artery	3 Percutaneous		
2 Gastric Artery	4 Percutaneous Endoscopic		
3 Hepatic Artery			
4 Splenic Artery			
5 Superior Mesenteric Artery			
6 Colic Artery, Right			
7 Colic Artery, Left			
8 Colic Artery, Middle			
9 Renal Artery, Right			
A Renal Artery, Left			
B Inferior Mesenteric Artery			
C Common Iliac Artery, Right			
D Common Iliac Artery, Left			
E Internal Iliac Artery, Right			
F Internal Iliac Artery, Left			
H External Iliac Artery, Right			
J External Iliac Artery, Left			
K Femoral Artery, Right			
L Femoral Artery, Left			
M Popliteal Artery, Right			
N Popliteal Artery, Left			
P Anterior Tibial Artery, Right			
Q Anterior Tibial Artery, Left			
R Posterior Tibial Artery, Right			
S Posterior Tibial Artery, Left			
T Peroneal Artery, Right			
U Peroneal Artery, Left			
V Foot Artery, Right			
W Foot Artery, Left			
Y Lower Artery			

S: REPOSITION

4: LOWER ARTERIES

0: M/S

New/Revised Text in Green   deleted Deleted   ♀ Females Only   ♂ Males Only   **Coding Clinic**
Non-covered   Limited Coverage   ⊞ Combination (See Appendix E)   DRG Non-OR   Non-OR   Hospital-Acquired Condition

SECTION: 0 MEDICAL AND SURGICAL

BODY SYSTEM: 4 LOWER ARTERIES

OPERATION: U SUPPLEMENT: Putting in or on biological or synthetic material that physically reinforces and/or augments the function of a portion of a body part

Body Part	Approach	Device	Qualifier
0 Abdominal Aorta	0 Open	7 Autologous Tissue Substitute	Z No Qualifier
1 Celiac Artery	3 Percutaneous	J Synthetic Substitute	
2 Gastric Artery	4 Percutaneous Endoscopic	K Nonautologous Tissue	
3 Hepatic Artery		Substitute	
4 Splenic Artery			
5 Superior Mesenteric Artery			
6 Colic Artery, Right			
7 Colic Artery, Left			
8 Colic Artery, Middle			
9 Renal Artery, Right			
A Renal Artery, Left			
B Inferior Mesenteric Artery			
C Common Iliac Artery, Right			
D Common Iliac Artery, Left			
E Internal Iliac Artery, Right			
F Internal Iliac Artery, Left			
H External Iliac Artery, Right			
J External Iliac Artery, Left			
K Femoral Artery, Right			
L Femoral Artery, Left			
M Popliteal Artery, Right			
N Popliteal Artery, Left			
P Anterior Tibial Artery, Right			
Q Anterior Tibial Artery, Left			
R Posterior Tibial Artery, Right			
S Posterior Tibial Artery, Left			
T Peroneal Artery, Right			
U Peroneal Artery, Left			
V Foot Artery, Right			
W Foot Artery, Left			
Y Lower Artery			

Coding Clinic: 2016, Q1, P31 – 04UJ0KZ
Coding Clinic: 2016, Q2, P19 – 04UR07Z

New/Revised Text in Green   ~~deleted~~ Deleted   ♀ Females Only   ♂ Males Only   **Coding Clinic**
Non-covered   Limited Coverage   ⊞ Combination (See Appendix E)   DRG Non-OR   Non-OR   Hospital-Acquired Condition

SECTION: Ø MEDICAL AND SURGICAL
BODY SYSTEM: 4 LOWER ARTERIES
OPERATION: V RESTRICTION: Partially closing an orifice or the lumen of a tubular body part

Body Part	Approach	Device	Qualifier
Ø Abdominal Aorta	Ø Open 3 Percutaneous 4 Percutaneous Endoscopic	C Extraluminal Device E Intraluminal Device, Branched or Fenestrated, One or Two Arteries F Intraluminal Device, Branched or Fenestrated, Three or More Arteries Z No Device	6 Bifurcation Z No Qualifier
Ø Abdominal Aorta	Ø Open 3 Percutaneous 4 Percutaneous Endoscopic	D Intraluminal Device	6 Bifurcation J Temporary Z No Qualifier
1 Celiac Artery 2 Gastric Artery 3 Hepatic Artery 4 Splenic Artery 5 Superior Mesenteric Artery 6 Colic Artery, Right 7 Colic Artery, Left 8 Colic Artery, Middle 9 Renal Artery, Right A Renal Artery, Left B Inferior Mesenteric Artery E Internal Iliac Artery, Right F Internal Iliac Artery, Left H External Iliac Artery, Right J External Iliac Artery, Left K Femoral Artery, Right L Femoral Artery, Left M Popliteal Artery, Right N Popliteal Artery, Left P Anterior Tibial Artery, Right Q Anterior Tibial Artery, Left R Posterior Tibial Artery, Right S Posterior Tibial Artery, Left T Peroneal Artery, Right U Peroneal Artery, Left V Foot Artery, Right W Foot Artery, Left Y Lower Artery	Ø Open 3 Percutaneous 4 Percutaneous Endoscopic	C Extraluminal Device D Intraluminal Device Z No Device	Z No Qualifier
C Common Iliac Artery, Right D Common Iliac Artery, Left	Ø Open 3 Percutaneous 4 Percutaneous Endoscopic	C Extraluminal Device D Intraluminal Device E Intraluminal Device, Branched or Fenestrated, One or Two Arteries F Intraluminal Device, Branched or Fenestrated, Three or More Arteries Z No Device	Z No Qualifier

Non-OR   04V[CDY][034][023F]Z

Coding Clinic: 2016, Q3, P39 – 04V03DZ
Coding Clinic: 2016, Q4, P87, 89-90 – 04V
Coding Clinic: 2016, Q4, P91 – 04V03E6
Coding Clinic: 2016, Q4, P93-94 – 04V03F6
Coding Clinic: 2016, Q4, P94 – 04V[CD]3EZ

New/Revised Text in Green   deleted Deleted   ♀ Females Only   ♂ Males Only   **Coding Clinic**
🝆 Non-covered   🝆 Limited Coverage   ⊞ Combination (See Appendix E)   DRG Non-OR   Non-OR   🝆 Hospital-Acquired Condition

SECTION: Ø MEDICAL AND SURGICAL
BODY SYSTEM: 4 LOWER ARTERIES
OPERATION: W REVISION: Correcting, to the extent possible, a portion of a malfunctioning device or the position of a displaced device

Body Part	Approach	Device	Qualifier
Y Lower Artery	Ø Open 3 Percutaneous 4 Percutaneous Endoscopic	Ø Drainage Device 2 Monitoring Device 3 Infusion Device 7 Autologous Tissue Substitute C Extraluminal Device D Intraluminal Device J Synthetic Substitute K Nonautologous Tissue Substitute Y Other Device	Z No Qualifier
Y Lower Artery	X External	Ø Drainage Device 2 Monitoring Device 3 Infusion Device 7 Autologous Tissue Substitute C Extraluminal Device D Intraluminal Device J Synthetic Substitute K Nonautologous Tissue Substitute	Z No Qualifier

DRG Non-OR Ø4WY3[Ø23D]Z (proposed)
Non-OR Ø4WYX[Ø237CDJK]Z

Coding Clinic: 2015, Q1, P37 – Ø4WYØ7Z

SECTION: Ø MEDICAL AND SURGICAL

BODY SYSTEM: 5 UPPER VEINS

OPERATION: 1 **BYPASS:** Altering the route of passage of the contents of a tubular body part

Body Part	Approach	Device	Qualifier
Ø Azygos Vein	Ø Open	7 Autologous Tissue Substitute	Y Upper Vein
1 Hemiazygos Vein	4 Percutaneous Endoscopic	9 Autologous Venous Tissue	
3 Innominate Vein, Right		A Autologous Arterial Tissue	
4 Innominate Vein, Left		J Synthetic Substitute	
5 Subclavian Vein, Right		K Nonautologous Tissue Substitute	
6 Subclavian Vein, Left		Z No Device	
7 Axillary Vein, Right			
8 Axillary Vein, Left			
9 Brachial Vein, Right			
A Brachial Vein, Left			
B Basilic Vein, Right			
C Basilic Vein, Left			
D Cephalic Vein, Right			
F Cephalic Vein, Left			
G Hand Vein, Right			
H Hand Vein, Left			
L Intracranial Vein			
M Internal Jugular Vein, Right			
N Internal Jugular Vein, Left			
P External Jugular Vein, Right			
Q External Jugular Vein, Left			
R Vertebral Vein, Right			
S Vertebral Vein, Left			
T Face Vein, Right			
V Face Vein, Left			

Ø: M/S

5: UPPER VEINS

1: BYPASS

SECTION: Ø MEDICAL AND SURGICAL

BODY SYSTEM: 5 UPPER VEINS

OPERATION: 5 DESTRUCTION: Physical eradication of all or a portion of a body part by the direct use of energy, force, or a destructive agent

Body Part	Approach	Device	Qualifier
Ø Azygos Vein 1 Hemiazygos Vein 3 Innominate Vein, Right 4 Innominate Vein, Left 5 Subclavian Vein, Right 6 Subclavian Vein, Left 7 Axillary Vein, Right 8 Axillary Vein, Left 9 Brachial Vein, Right A Brachial Vein, Left B Basilic Vein, Right C Basilic Vein, Left D Cephalic Vein, Right F Cephalic Vein, Left G Hand Vein, Right H Hand Vein, Left L Intracranial Vein M Internal Jugular Vein, Right N Internal Jugular Vein, Left P External Jugular Vein, Right Q External Jugular Vein, Left R Vertebral Vein, Right S Vertebral Vein, Left T Face Vein, Right V Face Vein, Left Y Upper Vein	Ø Open 3 Percutaneous 4 Percutaneous Endoscopic	Z No Device	Z No Qualifier

New/Revised Text in Green   ~~deleted~~ Deleted   ♀ Females Only   ♂ Males Only   **Coding Clinic**

⚕ Non-covered   ⚕ Limited Coverage   ⊞ Combination (See Appendix E)   DRG Non-OR   Non-OR   ⚕ Hospital-Acquired Condition

SECTION: Ø MEDICAL AND SURGICAL

BODY SYSTEM: 5 UPPER VEINS

OPERATION: 7 DILATION: Expanding an orifice or the lumen of a tubular body part

Body Part	Approach	Device	Qualifier
Ø Azygos Vein 1 Hemiazygos Vein G Hand Vein, Right H Hand Vein, Left L Intracranial Vein 🔖 M Internal Jugular Vein, Right N Internal Jugular Vein, Left P External Jugular Vein, Right Q External Jugular Vein, Left R Vertebral Vein, Right S Vertebral Vein, Left T Face Vein, Right V Face Vein, Left Y Upper Vein	Ø Open 3 Percutaneous 4 Percutaneous Endoscopic	D Intraluminal Device Z No Device	Z No Qualifier
3 Innominate Vein, Right 4 Innominate Vein, Left 5 Subclavian Vein, Right 6 Subclavian Vein, Left 7 Axillary Vein, Right 8 Axillary Vein, Left 9 Brachial Vein, Right A Brachial Vein, Left B Basilic Vein, Right C Basilic Vein, Left D Cephalic Vein, Right F Cephalic Vein, Left	Ø Open 3 Percutaneous 4 Percutaneous Endoscopic	D Intraluminal Device Z No Device	1 Drug-Coated Balloon Z No Qualifier

🔖 Ø57L[34]ZZ

SECTION: Ø MEDICAL AND SURGICAL
BODY SYSTEM: 5 UPPER VEINS
OPERATION: 9 DRAINAGE: Taking or letting out fluids and/or gases from a body part

Body Part	Approach	Device	Qualifier
Ø Azygos Vein 1 Hemiazygos Vein 3 Innominate Vein, Right 4 Innominate Vein, Left 5 Subclavian Vein, Right 6 Subclavian Vein, Left 7 Axillary Vein, Right 8 Axillary Vein, Left 9 Brachial Vein, Right A Brachial Vein, Left B Basilic Vein, Right C Basilic Vein, Left D Cephalic Vein, Right F Cephalic Vein, Left G Hand Vein, Right H Hand Vein, Left L Intracranial Vein M Internal Jugular Vein, Right N Internal Jugular Vein, Left P External Jugular Vein, Right Q External Jugular Vein, Left R Vertebral Vein, Right S Vertebral Vein, Left T Face Vein, Right V Face Vein, Left Y Upper Vein	Ø Open 3 Percutaneous 4 Percutaneous Endoscopic	Ø Drainage Device	Z No Qualifier
Ø Azygos Vein 1 Hemiazygos Vein 3 Innominate Vein, Right 4 Innominate Vein, Left 5 Subclavian Vein, Right 6 Subclavian Vein, Left 7 Axillary Vein, Right 8 Axillary Vein, Left 9 Brachial Vein, Right A Brachial Vein, Left B Basilic Vein, Right C Basilic Vein, Left D Cephalic Vein, Right F Cephalic Vein, Left G Hand Vein, Right H Hand Vein, Left L Intracranial Vein M Internal Jugular Vein, Right N Internal Jugular Vein, Left P External Jugular Vein, Right Q External Jugular Vein, Left R Vertebral Vein, Right S Vertebral Vein, Left T Face Vein, Right V Face Vein, Left Y Upper Vein	Ø Open 3 Percutaneous 4 Percutaneous Endoscopic	Z No Device	X Diagnostic Z No Qualifier

Non-OR Ø59[Ø13456789ABCDFGHLMNPQRSTVY][Ø34]ØZ
Non-OR Ø59[Ø13456789ABCDFGHLMNPQRSTVY][Ø34]Z[XZ]

New/Revised Text in Green   deleted Deleted   ♀ Females Only   ♂ Males Only   **Coding Clinic**
Non-covered   Limited Coverage   ⊞ Combination (See Appendix E)   DRG Non-OR   Non-OR   Hospital-Acquired Condition

SECTION: Ø MEDICAL AND SURGICAL
BODY SYSTEM: 5 UPPER VEINS
OPERATION: B EXCISION: Cutting out or off, without replacement, a portion of a body part

Body Part	Approach	Device	Qualifier
Ø Azygos Vein 1 Hemiazygos Vein 3 Innominate Vein, Right 4 Innominate Vein, Left 5 Subclavian Vein, Right 6 Subclavian Vein, Left 7 Axillary Vein, Right 8 Axillary Vein, Left 9 Brachial Vein, Right A Brachial Vein, Left B Basilic Vein, Right C Basilic Vein, Left D Cephalic Vein, Right F Cephalic Vein, Left G Hand Vein, Right H Hand Vein, Left L Intracranial Vein M Internal Jugular Vein, Right N Internal Jugular Vein, Left P External Jugular Vein, Right Q External Jugular Vein, Left R Vertebral Vein, Right S Vertebral Vein, Left T Face Vein, Right V Face Vein, Left Y Upper Vein	Ø Open 3 Percutaneous 4 Percutaneous Endoscopic	Z No Device	X Diagnostic Z No Qualifier

Coding Clinic: 2Ø16, Q2, P13-14 — Ø5B[NQ]ØZZ

SECTION: Ø MEDICAL AND SURGICAL

BODY SYSTEM: 5 UPPER VEINS

OPERATION: C EXTIRPATION: Taking or cutting out solid matter from a body part

Body Part	Approach	Device	Qualifier
Ø Azygos Vein 1 Hemiazygos Vein 3 Innominate Vein, Right 4 Innominate Vein, Left 5 Subclavian Vein, Right 6 Subclavian Vein, Left 7 Axillary Vein, Right 8 Axillary Vein, Left 9 Brachial Vein, Right A Brachial Vein, Left B Basilic Vein, Right C Basilic Vein, Left D Cephalic Vein, Right F Cephalic Vein, Left G Hand Vein, Right H Hand Vein, Left L Intracranial Vein M Internal Jugular Vein, Right N Internal Jugular Vein, Left P External Jugular Vein, Right Q External Jugular Vein, Left R Vertebral Vein, Right S Vertebral Vein, Left T Face Vein, Right V Face Vein, Left Y Upper Vein	Ø Open 3 Percutaneous 4 Percutaneous Endoscopic	Z No Device	Z No Qualifier

SECTION: Ø MEDICAL AND SURGICAL

BODY SYSTEM: 5 UPPER VEINS

OPERATION: D EXTRACTION: Pulling or stripping out or off all or a portion of a body part by the use of force

Body Part	Approach	Device	Qualifier
9 Brachial Vein, Right A Brachial Vein, Left B Basilic Vein, Right C Basilic Vein, Left D Cephalic Vein, Right F Cephalic Vein, Left G Hand Vein, Right H Hand Vein, Left Y Upper Vein	Ø Open 3 Percutaneous	Z No Device	Z No Qualifier

C: EXTIRPATION   D: EXTRACTION

5: UPPER VEINS

Ø: M/S

New/Revised Text in Green   deleted Deleted   ♀ Females Only   ♂ Males Only   **Coding Clinic**

Non-covered   Limited Coverage   Combination (See Appendix E)   DRG Non-OR   Non-OR   Hospital-Acquired Condition

SECTION: Ø MEDICAL AND SURGICAL

BODY SYSTEM: 5 UPPER VEINS

OPERATION: **H INSERTION:** Putting in a nonbiological appliance that monitors, assists, performs, or prevents a physiological function but does not physically take the place of a body part

Body Part	Approach	Device	Qualifier
Ø Azygos Vein ⊞ 🐾	Ø Open 3 Percutaneous 4 Percutaneous Endoscopic	2 Monitoring Device 3 Infusion Device D Intraluminal Device M Neurostimulator Lead	Z No Qualifier
1 Hemiazygos Vein 🐾 5 Subclavian Vein, Right 🐾 6 Subclavian Vein, Left 🐾 7 Axillary Vein, Right 8 Axillary Vein, Left 9 Brachial Vein, Right A Brachial Vein, Left B Basilic Vein, Right C Basilic Vein, Left D Cephalic Vein, Right F Cephalic Vein, Left G Hand Vein, Right H Hand Vein, Left L Intracranial Vein M Internal Jugular Vein, Right 🐾 N Internal Jugular Vein, Left 🐾 P External Jugular Vein, Right 🐾 Q External Jugular Vein, Left 🐾 R Vertebral Vein, Right S Vertebral Vein, Left T Face Vein, Right V Face Vein, Left	Ø Open 3 Percutaneous 4 Percutaneous Endoscopic	3 Infusion Device D Intraluminal Device	Z No Qualifier
3 Innominate Vein, Right ⊞ 🐾 4 Innominate Vein, Left ⊞ 🐾	Ø Open 3 Percutaneous 4 Percutaneous Endoscopic	3 Infusion Device D Intraluminal Device M Neurostimulator Lead	Z No Qualifier
Y Upper Vein	Ø Open 3 Percutaneous 4 Percutaneous Endoscopic	2 Monitoring Device 3 Infusion Device D Intraluminal Device Y Other Device	Z No Qualifier

⊞ Ø5HØ[Ø34]MZ
⊞ Ø5H[34][Ø34]MZ
Non-OR Ø5HØ[Ø34]3Z
Non-OR Ø5H[13789ABCDFGHLRSTV][Ø34]3Z
Non-OR Ø5H[56MNPQ][Ø34]3Z
Non-OR Ø5H[34][Ø34]3Z
Non-OR Ø5HY[Ø34]3Z
Non-OR Ø5HY32Z
🐾 Ø5HØ[34]3Z when reported with Secondary Diagnosis J95.811
🐾 Ø5H[156][34]3Z when reported with Secondary Diagnosis J95.811
🐾 Ø5H[34][34]3Z when reported with Secondary Diagnosis J95.811
🐾 Ø5H[MNPQ]33Z when reported with Secondary Diagnosis J95.811

Coding Clinic: 2Ø16, Q4, P98 – Ø5H, Ø5HØ32Z
Coding Clinic: 2Ø16, Q4, P99 – Ø5H43MZ

New/Revised Text in Green   deleted Deleted   ♀ Females Only   ♂ Males Only   **Coding Clinic**
🐾 Non-covered   🐾 Limited Coverage   ⊞ Combination (See Appendix E)   DRG Non-OR   Non-OR   🐾 Hospital-Acquired Condition

133

SECTION: Ø MEDICAL AND SURGICAL
BODY SYSTEM: 5 UPPER VEINS
OPERATION: **J** INSPECTION: Visually and/or manually exploring a body part

Body Part	Approach	Device	Qualifier
Y Upper Vein	Ø Open 3 Percutaneous 4 Percutaneous Endoscopic X External	Z No Device	Z No Qualifier

Non-OR Ø5JY[3X]ZZ

SECTION: Ø MEDICAL AND SURGICAL
BODY SYSTEM: 5 UPPER VEINS
OPERATION: **L** OCCLUSION: Completely closing an orifice or the lumen of a tubular body part

Body Part	Approach	Device	Qualifier
Ø Azygos Vein 1 Hemiazygos Vein 3 Innominate Vein, Right 4 Innominate Vein, Left 5 Subclavian Vein, Right 6 Subclavian Vein, Left 7 Axillary Vein, Right 8 Axillary Vein, Left 9 Brachial Vein, Right A Brachial Vein, Left B Basilic Vein, Right C Basilic Vein, Left D Cephalic Vein, Right F Cephalic Vein, Left G Hand Vein, Right H Hand Vein, Left L Intracranial Vein M Internal Jugular Vein, Right N Internal Jugular Vein, Left P External Jugular Vein, Right Q External Jugular Vein, Left R Vertebral Vein, Right S Vertebral Vein, Left T Face Vein, Right V Face Vein, Left Y Upper Vein	Ø Open 3 Percutaneous 4 Percutaneous Endoscopic	C Extraluminal Device D Intraluminal Device Z No Device	Z No Qualifier

SECTION: Ø MEDICAL AND SURGICAL

BODY SYSTEM: 5 UPPER VEINS

OPERATION: N RELEASE: Freeing a body part from an abnormal physical constraint

Body Part	Approach	Device	Qualifier
Ø Azygos Vein 1 Hemiazygos Vein 3 Innominate Vein, Right 4 Innominate Vein, Left 5 Subclavian Vein, Right 6 Subclavian Vein, Left 7 Axillary Vein, Right 8 Axillary Vein, Left 9 Brachial Vein, Right A Brachial Vein, Left B Basilic Vein, Right C Basilic Vein, Left D Cephalic Vein, Right F Cephalic Vein, Left G Hand Vein, Right H Hand Vein, Left L Intracranial Vein M Internal Jugular Vein, Right N Internal Jugular Vein, Left P External Jugular Vein, Right Q External Jugular Vein, Left R Vertebral Vein, Right S Vertebral Vein, Left T Face Vein, Right V Face Vein, Left Y Upper Vein	Ø Open 3 Percutaneous 4 Percutaneous Endoscopic	Z No Device	Z No Qualifier

SECTION: Ø MEDICAL AND SURGICAL

BODY SYSTEM: 5 UPPER VEINS

OPERATION: P REMOVAL: Taking out or off a device from a body part

Body Part	Approach	Device	Qualifier
Ø Azygos Vein	Ø Open 3 Percutaneous 4 Percutaneous Endoscopic X External	2 Monitoring Device M Neurostimulator Lead	Z No Qualifier
3 Innominate Vein, Right 4 Innominate Vein, Left	Ø Open 3 Percutaneous 4 Percutaneous Endoscopic X External	M Neurostimulator Lead	Z No Qualifier
Y Upper Vein	Ø Open 3 Percutaneous 4 Percutaneous Endoscopic	Ø Drainage Device 2 Monitoring Device 3 Infusion Device 7 Autologous Tissue Substitute C Extraluminal Device D Intraluminal Device J Synthetic Substitute K Nonautologous Tissue Substitute Y Other Device	Z No Qualifier
Y Upper Vein	X External	Ø Drainage Device 2 Monitoring Device 3 Infusion Device D Intraluminal Device	Z No Qualifier

Non-OR Ø5PØ[Ø3X]2Z
Non-OR Ø5PY3[Ø23D]Z
Non-OR Ø5PYX[Ø23D]Z

Coding Clinic: 2Ø16, Q4, P98 – Ø5P

SECTION: Ø MEDICAL AND SURGICAL

BODY SYSTEM: 5 UPPER VEINS

OPERATION: Q REPAIR: Restoring, to the extent possible, a body part to its normal anatomic structure and function

Body Part	Approach	Device	Qualifier
Ø Azygos Vein	Ø Open	Z No Device	Z No Qualifier
1 Hemiazygos Vein	3 Percutaneous		
3 Innominate Vein, Right	4 Percutaneous Endoscopic		
4 Innominate Vein, Left			
5 Subclavian Vein, Right			
6 Subclavian Vein, Left			
7 Axillary Vein, Right			
8 Axillary Vein, Left			
9 Brachial Vein, Right			
A Brachial Vein, Left			
B Basilic Vein, Right			
C Basilic Vein, Left			
D Cephalic Vein, Right			
F Cephalic Vein, Left			
G Hand Vein, Right			
H Hand Vein, Left			
L Intracranial Vein			
M Internal Jugular Vein, Right			
N Internal Jugular Vein, Left			
P External Jugular Vein, Right			
Q External Jugular Vein, Left			
R Vertebral Vein, Right			
S Vertebral Vein, Left			
T Face Vein, Right			
V Face Vein, Left			
Y Upper Vein			

Coding Clinic: 2017, Q3, P16 – 05Q40ZZ

SECTION: Ø MEDICAL AND SURGICAL
BODY SYSTEM: 5 UPPER VEINS

OPERATION: **R REPLACEMENT:** Putting in or on biological or synthetic material that physically takes the place and/or function of all or a portion of a body part

Body Part	Approach	Device	Qualifier
Ø Azygos Vein 1 Hemiazygos Vein 3 Innominate Vein, Right 4 Innominate Vein, Left 5 Subclavian Vein, Right 6 Subclavian Vein, Left 7 Axillary Vein, Right 8 Axillary Vein, Left 9 Brachial Vein, Right A Brachial Vein, Left B Basilic Vein, Right C Basilic Vein, Left D Cephalic Vein, Right F Cephalic Vein, Left G Hand Vein, Right H Hand Vein, Left L Intracranial Vein M Internal Jugular Vein, Right N Internal Jugular Vein, Left P External Jugular Vein, Right Q External Jugular Vein, Left R Vertebral Vein, Right S Vertebral Vein, Left T Face Vein, Right V Face Vein, Left Y Upper Vein	Ø Open 4 Percutaneous Endoscopic	7 Autologous Tissue Substitute J Synthetic Substitute K Nonautologous Tissue Substitute	Z No Qualifier

Sidebar: R: REPLACEMENT   5: UPPER VEINS   Ø: M/S

SECTION: Ø MEDICAL AND SURGICAL

BODY SYSTEM: 5 UPPER VEINS

OPERATION: S **REPOSITION:** Moving to its normal location, or other suitable location, all or a portion of a body part

Body Part	Approach	Device	Qualifier
Ø Azygos Vein	Ø Open	Z No Device	Z No Qualifier
1 Hemiazygos Vein	3 Percutaneous		
3 Innominate Vein, Right	4 Percutaneous Endoscopic		
4 Innominate Vein, Left			
5 Subclavian Vein, Right			
6 Subclavian Vein, Left			
7 Axillary Vein, Right			
8 Axillary Vein, Left			
9 Brachial Vein, Right			
A Brachial Vein, Left			
B Basilic Vein, Right			
C Basilic Vein, Left			
D Cephalic Vein, Right			
F Cephalic Vein, Left			
G Hand Vein, Right			
H Hand Vein, Left			
L Intracranial Vein			
M Internal Jugular Vein, Right			
N Internal Jugular Vein, Left			
P External Jugular Vein, Right			
Q External Jugular Vein, Left			
R Vertebral Vein, Right			
S Vertebral Vein, Left			
T Face Vein, Right			
V Face Vein, Left			
Y Upper Vein			

Ø: M/S

5: UPPER VEINS

S: REPOSITION

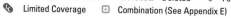

SECTION: Ø MEDICAL AND SURGICAL

BODY SYSTEM: 5 UPPER VEINS

OPERATION: U SUPPLEMENT: Putting in or on biological or synthetic material that physically reinforces and/or augments the function of a portion of a body part

Body Part	Approach	Device	Qualifier
Ø Azygos Vein	Ø Open	7 Autologous Tissue Substitute	Z No Qualifier
1 Hemiazygos Vein	3 Percutaneous	J Synthetic Substitute	
3 Innominate Vein, Right	4 Percutaneous Endoscopic	K Nonautologous Tissue Substitute	
4 Innominate Vein, Left			
5 Subclavian Vein, Right			
6 Subclavian Vein, Left			
7 Axillary Vein, Right			
8 Axillary Vein, Left			
9 Brachial Vein, Right			
A Brachial Vein, Left			
B Basilic Vein, Right			
C Basilic Vein, Left			
D Cephalic Vein, Right			
F Cephalic Vein, Left			
G Hand Vein, Right			
H Hand Vein, Left			
L Intracranial Vein			
M Internal Jugular Vein, Right			
N Internal Jugular Vein, Left			
P External Jugular Vein, Right			
Q External Jugular Vein, Left			
R Vertebral Vein, Right			
S Vertebral Vein, Left			
T Face Vein, Right			
V Face Vein, Left			
Y Upper Vein			

U: SUPPLEMENT

5: UPPER VEINS

Ø: M/S

New/Revised Text in Green   deleted Deleted   ♀ Females Only   ♂ Males Only   **Coding Clinic**

Non-covered   Limited Coverage   Combination (See Appendix E)   DRG Non-OR   Non-OR   Hospital-Acquired Condition

SECTION: Ø MEDICAL AND SURGICAL
BODY SYSTEM: 5 UPPER VEINS
OPERATION: **V RESTRICTION:** Partially closing an orifice or the lumen of a tubular body part

Body Part	Approach	Device	Qualifier
Ø Azygos Vein	Ø Open	C Extraluminal Device	Z No Qualifier
1 Hemiazygos Vein	3 Percutaneous	D Intraluminal Device	
3 Innominate Vein, Right	4 Percutaneous Endoscopic	Z No Device	
4 Innominate Vein, Left			
5 Subclavian Vein, Right			
6 Subclavian Vein, Left			
7 Axillary Vein, Right			
8 Axillary Vein, Left			
9 Brachial Vein, Right			
A Brachial Vein, Left			
B Basilic Vein, Right			
C Basilic Vein, Left			
D Cephalic Vein, Right			
F Cephalic Vein, Left			
G Hand Vein, Right			
H Hand Vein, Left			
L Intracranial Vein			
M Internal Jugular Vein, Right			
N Internal Jugular Vein, Left			
P External Jugular Vein, Right			
Q External Jugular Vein, Left			
R Vertebral Vein, Right			
S Vertebral Vein, Left			
T Face Vein, Right			
V Face Vein, Left			
Y Upper Vein			

Ø: M/S

5: UPPER VEINS

V: RESTRICTION

SECTION: Ø MEDICAL AND SURGICAL
BODY SYSTEM: 5 UPPER VEINS
OPERATION: **W REVISION:** Correcting, to the extent possible, a portion of a malfunctioning device or the position of a displaced device

Body Part	Approach	Device	Qualifier
Ø Azygos Vein	Ø Open 3 Percutaneous 4 Percutaneous Endoscopic X External	2 Monitoring Device M Neurostimulator Lead	Z No Qualifier
3 Innominate Vein, Right 4 Innominate Vein, Left	Ø Open 3 Percutaneous 4 Percutaneous Endoscopic X External	M Neurostimulator Lead	Z No Qualifier
Y Upper Vein	Ø Open 3 Percutaneous 4 Percutaneous Endoscopic	Ø Drainage Device 2 Monitoring Device 3 Infusion Device 7 Autologous Tissue Substitute C Extraluminal Device D Intraluminal Device J Synthetic Substitute K Nonautologous Tissue Substitute Y Other Device	Z No Qualifier
Y Upper Vein	X External	Ø Drainage Device 2 Monitoring Device 3 Infusion Device 7 Autologous Tissue Substitute C Extraluminal Device D Intraluminal Device J Synthetic Substitute K Nonautologous Tissue Substitute	Z No Qualifier

Non-OR Ø5WY3[Ø23D]Z
Non-OR Ø5WØXMZ
Non-OR Ø5W[34]XMZ
Non-OR Ø5WYX[Ø237CDJK]Z

Coding Clinic: 2Ø16, Q4, P98 – Ø5W

SECTION: Ø MEDICAL AND SURGICAL

BODY SYSTEM: 6 LOWER VEINS

OPERATION: 1 BYPASS: Altering the route of passage of the contents of a tubular body part

Body Part	Approach	Device	Qualifier
Ø Inferior Vena Cava	Ø Open 4 Percutaneous Endoscopic	7 Autologous Tissue Substitute 9 Autologous Venous Tissue A Autologous Arterial Tissue J Synthetic Substitute K Nonautologous Tissue Substitute Z No Device	5 Superior Mesenteric Vein 6 Inferior Mesenteric Vein P Pulmonary Trunk Q Pulmonary Artery, Right R Pulmonary Artery, Left Y Lower Vein
1 Splenic Vein	Ø Open 4 Percutaneous Endoscopic	7 Autologous Tissue Substitute 9 Autologous Venous Tissue A Autologous Arterial Tissue J Synthetic Substitute K Nonautologous Tissue Substitute Z No Device	9 Renal Vein, Right B Renal Vein, Left Y Lower Vein
2 Gastric Vein 3 Esophageal Vein 4 Hepatic Vein 5 Superior Mesenteric Vein 6 Inferior Mesenteric Vein 7 Colic Vein 9 Renal Vein, Right B Renal Vein, Left C Common Iliac Vein, Right D Common Iliac Vein, Left F External Iliac Vein, Right G External Iliac Vein, Left H Hypogastric Vein, Right J Hypogastric Vein, Left M Femoral Vein, Right N Femoral Vein, Left P Saphenous Vein, Right Q Saphenous Vein, Left T Foot Vein, Right V Foot Vein, Left	Ø Open 4 Percutaneous Endoscopic	7 Autologous Tissue Substitute 9 Autologous Venous Tissue A Autologous Arterial Tissue J Synthetic Substitute K Nonautologous Tissue Substitute Z No Device	Y Lower Vein
8 Portal Vein	Ø Open	7 Autologous Tissue Substitute 9 Autologous Venous Tissue A Autologous Arterial Tissue J Synthetic Substitute K Nonautologous Tissue Substitute Z No Device	9 Renal Vein, Right B Renal Vein, Left Y Lower Vein
8 Portal Vein	3 Percutaneous	J Synthetic Substitute	4 Hepatic Vein Y Lower Vein
8 Portal Vein	4 Percutaneous Endoscopic	7 Autologous Tissue Substitute 9 Autologous Venous Tissue A Autologous Arterial Tissue K Nonautologous Tissue Substitute Z No Device	9 Renal Vein, Right B Renal Vein, Left Y Lower Vein
8 Portal Vein	4 Percutaneous Endoscopic	J Synthetic Substitute	4 Hepatic Vein 9 Renal Vein, Right B Renal Vein, Left Y Lower Vein

Coding Clinic: 2017, Q4, P38 – 06100JP

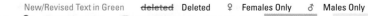
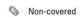

New/Revised Text in Green ~~deleted~~ Deleted ♀ Females Only ♂ Males Only **Coding Clinic**

🅠 Non-covered 🅠 Limited Coverage ⊕ Combination (See Appendix E) DRG Non-OR Non-OR 🅠 Hospital-Acquired Condition

SECTION: Ø MEDICAL AND SURGICAL

BODY SYSTEM: 6 LOWER VEINS

OPERATION: 5 DESTRUCTION: Physical eradication of all or a portion of a body part by the direct use of energy, force, or a destructive agent

Body Part	Approach	Device	Qualifier
Ø Inferior Vena Cava 1 Splenic Vein 2 Gastric Vein 3 Esophageal Vein 4 Hepatic Vein 5 Superior Mesenteric Vein 6 Inferior Mesenteric Vein 7 Colic Vein 8 Portal Vein 9 Renal Vein, Right B Renal Vein, Left C Common Iliac Vein, Right D Common Iliac Vein, Left F External Iliac Vein, Right G External Iliac Vein, Left H Hypogastric Vein, Right J Hypogastric Vein, Left M Femoral Vein, Right N Femoral Vein, Left P Saphenous Vein, Right Q Saphenous Vein, Left T Foot Vein, Right V Foot Vein, Left	Ø Open 3 Percutaneous 4 Percutaneous Endoscopic	Z No Device	Z No Qualifier
Y Lower Vein	Ø Open 3 Percutaneous 4 Percutaneous Endoscopic	Z No Device	C Hemorrhoidal Plexus Z No Qualifier

Ø: M/S

6: LOWER VEINS

5: DESTRUCTION

SECTION: Ø MEDICAL AND SURGICAL

BODY SYSTEM: 6 LOWER VEINS

OPERATION: 7 **DILATION:** Expanding an orifice or the lumen of a tubular body part

Body Part	Approach	Device	Qualifier
Ø Inferior Vena Cava	Ø Open	D Intraluminal Device	Z No Qualifier
1 Splenic Vein	3 Percutaneous	Z No Device	
2 Gastric Vein	4 Percutaneous Endoscopic		
3 Esophageal Vein			
4 Hepatic Vein			
5 Superior Mesenteric Vein			
6 Inferior Mesenteric Vein			
7 Colic Vein			
8 Portal Vein			
9 Renal Vein, Right			
B Renal Vein, Left			
C Common Iliac Vein, Right			
D Common Iliac Vein, Left			
F External Iliac Vein, Right			
G External Iliac Vein, Left			
H Hypogastric Vein, Right			
J Hypogastric Vein, Left			
M Femoral Vein, Right			
N Femoral Vein, Left			
P Saphenous Vein, Right			
Q Saphenous Vein, Left			
T Foot Vein, Right			
V Foot Vein, Left			
Y Lower Vein			

7: DILATION

6: LOWER VEINS

Ø: M/S

New/Revised Text in Green   ~~deleted~~ Deleted   ♀ Females Only   ♂ Males Only   **Coding Clinic**
🝠 Non-covered   🝠 Limited Coverage   ⊕ Combination (See Appendix E)   DRG Non-OR   Non-OR   🝠 Hospital-Acquired Condition

SECTION: Ø MEDICAL AND SURGICAL
BODY SYSTEM: 6 LOWER VEINS
OPERATION: 9 **DRAINAGE:** *(on multiple pages)*
Taking or letting out fluids and/or gases from a body part

Body Part	Approach	Device	Qualifier
Ø Inferior Vena Cava 1 Splenic Vein 2 Gastric Vein 3 Esophageal Vein 4 Hepatic Vein 5 Superior Mesenteric Vein 6 Inferior Mesenteric Vein 7 Colic Vein 8 Portal Vein 9 Renal Vein, Right B Renal Vein, Left C Common Iliac Vein, Right D Common Iliac Vein, Left F External Iliac Vein, Right G External Iliac Vein, Left H Hypogastric Vein, Right J Hypogastric Vein, Left M Femoral Vein, Right N Femoral Vein, Left P Saphenous Vein, Right Q Saphenous Vein, Left T Foot Vein, Right V Foot Vein, Left Y Lower Vein	Ø Open 3 Percutaneous 4 Percutaneous Endoscopic	Ø Drainage Device	Z No Qualifier

Non-OR Ø69330Z
Non-OR Ø69[Ø12456789BCDFGHJMNPQTVY][Ø34]ØZ

SECTION: Ø MEDICAL AND SURGICAL

BODY SYSTEM: 6 LOWER VEINS
OPERATION: 9 DRAINAGE: *(continued)*
Taking or letting out fluids and/or gases from a body part

Body Part	Approach	Device	Qualifier
Ø Inferior Vena Cava	Ø Open	Z No Device	X Diagnostic
1 Splenic Vein	3 Percutaneous		Z No Qualifier
2 Gastric Vein	4 Percutaneous Endoscopic		
3 Esophageal Vein			
4 Hepatic Vein			
5 Superior Mesenteric Vein			
6 Inferior Mesenteric Vein			
7 Colic Vein			
8 Portal Vein			
9 Renal Vein, Right			
B Renal Vein, Left			
C Common Iliac Vein, Right			
D Common Iliac Vein, Left			
F External Iliac Vein, Right			
G External Iliac Vein, Left			
H Hypogastric Vein, Right			
J Hypogastric Vein, Left			
M Femoral Vein, Right			
N Femoral Vein, Left			
P Saphenous Vein, Right			
Q Saphenous Vein, Left			
T Foot Vein, Right			
V Foot Vein, Left			
Y Lower Vein			

Non-OR   Ø6933ZZ
Non-OR   Ø69[Ø123456789BCDFGHJMNPQRSTVY][Ø34]Z[XZ]

New/Revised Text in Green   ~~deleted~~ Deleted   ♀ Females Only   ♂ Males Only   **Coding Clinic**
Non-covered   Limited Coverage   ⊞ Combination (See Appendix E)   DRG Non-OR   Non-OR   Hospital-Acquired Condition

(side tab) 9: DRAINAGE   6: LOWER VEINS   Ø: M/S

SECTION: Ø MEDICAL AND SURGICAL
BODY SYSTEM: 6 LOWER VEINS
OPERATION: B EXCISION: Cutting out or off, without replacement, a portion of a body part

Body Part	Approach	Device	Qualifier
Ø Inferior Vena Cava 1 Splenic Vein 2 Gastric Vein 3 Esophageal Vein 4 Hepatic Vein 5 Superior Mesenteric Vein 6 Inferior Mesenteric Vein 7 Colic Vein 8 Portal Vein 9 Renal Vein, Right B Renal Vein, Left C Common Iliac Vein, Right D Common Iliac Vein, Left F External Iliac Vein, Right G External Iliac Vein, Left H Hypogastric Vein, Right J Hypogastric Vein, Left M Femoral Vein, Right N Femoral Vein, Left P Saphenous Vein, Right Q Saphenous Vein, Left T Foot Vein, Right V Foot Vein, Left	Ø Open 3 Percutaneous 4 Percutaneous Endoscopic	Z No Device	X Diagnostic Z No Qualifier
Y Lower Vein	Ø Open 3 Percutaneous 4 Percutaneous Endoscopic	Z No Device	C Hemorrhoidal Plexus X Diagnostic Z No Qualifier

Coding Clinic: 2016, Q1, P28 – 06BQ4ZZ
Coding Clinic: 2016, Q2, P19 – 06B90ZZ
Coding Clinic: 2017, Q1, P32 – 06BP0ZZ
Coding Clinic: 2017, Q1, P33 – 06BQ0ZZ
Coding Clinic: 2017, Q3, P6 – 06BP0ZZ

Ø: M/S

6: LOWER VEINS

B: EXCISION

SECTION: 0 MEDICAL AND SURGICAL
BODY SYSTEM: 6 LOWER VEINS
OPERATION: C EXTIRPATION: Taking or cutting out solid matter from a body part

Body Part	Approach	Device	Qualifier
0 Inferior Vena Cava 1 Splenic Vein 2 Gastric Vein 3 Esophageal Vein 4 Hepatic Vein 5 Superior Mesenteric Vein 6 Inferior Mesenteric Vein 7 Colic Vein 8 Portal Vein 9 Renal Vein, Right B Renal Vein, Left C Common Iliac Vein, Right D Common Iliac Vein, Left F External Iliac Vein, Right G External Iliac Vein, Left H Hypogastric Vein, Right J Hypogastric Vein, Left M Femoral Vein, Right N Femoral Vein, Left P Saphenous Vein, Right Q Saphenous Vein, Left T Foot Vein, Right V Foot Vein, Left Y Lower Vein	0 Open 3 Percutaneous 4 Percutaneous Endoscopic	Z No Device	Z No Qualifier

SECTION: 0 MEDICAL AND SURGICAL
BODY SYSTEM: 6 LOWER VEINS
OPERATION: D EXTRACTION: Pulling or stripping out or off all or a portion of a body part by the use of force

Body Part	Approach	Device	Qualifier
M Femoral Vein, Right N Femoral Vein, Left P Saphenous Vein, Right Q Saphenous Vein, Left T Foot Vein, Right V Foot Vein, Left Y Lower Vein	0 Open 3 Percutaneous 4 Percutaneous Endoscopic	Z No Device	Z No Qualifier

SECTION: Ø MEDICAL AND SURGICAL
BODY SYSTEM: 6 LOWER VEINS
OPERATION: H **INSERTION:** Putting in a nonbiological appliance that monitors, assists, performs, or prevents a physiological function but does not physically take the place of a body part

Body Part	Approach	Device	Qualifier
Ø Inferior Vena Cava	Ø Open 3 Percutaneous	3 Infusion Device	T Via Unbilical Vein Z No Qualifier
Ø Inferior Vena Cava	Ø Open 3 Percutaneous	D Intraluminal Device	Z No Qualifier
Ø Inferior Vena Cava	4 Percutaneous Endoscopic	3 Infusion Device D Intraluminal Device	Z No Qualifier
1 Splenic Vein 2 Gastric Vein 3 Esophageal Vein 4 Hepatic Vein 5 Superior Mesenteric Vein 6 Inferior Mesenteric Vein 7 Colic Vein 8 Portal Vein 9 Renal Vein, Right B Renal Vein, Left C Common Iliac Vein, Right D Common Iliac Vein, Left F External Iliac Vein, Right G External Iliac Vein, Left H Hypogastric Vein, Right J Hypogastric Vein, Left M Femoral Vein, Right N Femoral Vein, Left P Saphenous Vein, Right Q Saphenous Vein, Left T Foot Vein, Right V Foot Vein, Left	Ø Open 3 Percutaneous 4 Percutaneous Endoscopic	3 Infusion Device D Intraluminal Device	Z No Qualifier
Y Lower Vein	Ø Open 3 Percutaneous 4 Percutaneous Endoscopic	2 Monitoring Device 3 Infusion Device D Intraluminal Device Y Other Device	Z No Qualifier

Non-OR 06HØ[Ø3]3[DTZ]
Non-OR 06HØ43Z
Non-OR 06H[123456789BCDFGHJPQTV][Ø34]3Z
Non-OR 06H[MN][Ø34]3Z
Non-OR 06HY32Z
Non-OR 06HY[Ø34]3Z

Coding Clinic: 2013, Q3, P19 – 06HØ33Z
Coding Clinic: 2017, Q1, P31 – 06HØ33T, 06HY33Z

Ø: M/S

6: LOWER VEINS

H: INSERTION

SECTION: Ø MEDICAL AND SURGICAL
BODY SYSTEM: 6 LOWER VEINS
OPERATION: J INSPECTION: Visually and/or manually exploring a body part

Body Part	Approach	Device	Qualifier
Y Lower Vein	Ø Open 3 Percutaneous 4 Percutaneous Endoscopic X External	Z No Device	Z No Qualifier

Non-OR Ø6JY[3X]ZZ

SECTION: Ø MEDICAL AND SURGICAL
BODY SYSTEM: 6 LOWER VEINS
OPERATION: L OCCLUSION: Completely closing an orifice or the lumen of a tubular body part

Body Part	Approach	Device	Qualifier
Ø Inferior Vena Cava 1 Splenic Vein 2 Gastric Vein 4 Hepatic Vein 5 Superior Mesenteric Vein 6 Inferior Mesenteric Vein 7 Colic Vein 8 Portal Vein 9 Renal Vein, Right B Renal Vein, Left C Common Iliac Vein, Right D Common Iliac Vein, Left F External Iliac Vein, Right G External Iliac Vein, Left H Hypogastric Vein, Right J Hypogastric Vein, Left M Femoral Vein, Right N Femoral Vein, Left P Saphenous Vein, Right Q Saphenous Vein, Left T Foot Vein, Right V Foot Vein, Left	Ø Open 3 Percutaneous 4 Percutaneous Endoscopic	C Extraluminal Device D Intraluminal Device Z No Device	Z No Qualifier
3 Esophageal Vein	Ø Open 3 Percutaneous 4 Percutaneous Endoscopic 7 Via Natural or Artificial Opening 8 Via Natural or Artificial Opening Endoscopic	C Extraluminal Device D Intraluminal Device Z No Device	Z No Qualifier
Y Lower Vein	Ø Open 3 Percutaneous 4 Percutaneous Endoscopic	C Extraluminal Device D Intraluminal Device Z No Device	C Hemorrhoidal Plexus Z No Qualifier

Non-OR Ø6L3[34][CDZ]Z

Coding Clinic: 2017, Q4, P57 – ØØ6L38CZ
Coding Clinic: 2018, Q2, P19 – Ø6LFØCZ

SECTION: Ø MEDICAL AND SURGICAL

BODY SYSTEM: 6 LOWER VEINS

OPERATION: N RELEASE: Freeing a body part from an abnormal physical constraint by cutting or by the use of force

Body Part	Approach	Device	Qualifier
Ø Inferior Vena Cava 1 Splenic Vein 2 Gastric Vein 3 Esophageal Vein 4 Hepatic Vein 5 Superior Mesenteric Vein 6 Inferior Mesenteric Vein 7 Colic Vein 8 Portal Vein 9 Renal Vein, Right B Renal Vein, Left C Common Iliac Vein, Right D Common Iliac Vein, Left F External Iliac Vein, Right G External Iliac Vein, Left H Hypogastric Vein, Right J Hypogastric Vein, Left M Femoral Vein, Right N Femoral Vein, Left P Saphenous Vein, Right Q Saphenous Vein, Left T Foot Vein, Right V Foot Vein, Left Y Lower Vein	Ø Open 3 Percutaneous 4 Percutaneous Endoscopic	Z No Device	Z No Qualifier

SECTION: Ø MEDICAL AND SURGICAL

BODY SYSTEM: 6 LOWER VEINS

OPERATION: P REMOVAL: Taking out or off a device from a body part

Body Part	Approach	Device	Qualifier
Y Lower Vein	Ø Open 3 Percutaneous 4 Percutaneous Endoscopic	Ø Drainage Device 2 Monitoring Device 3 Infusion Device 7 Autologous Tissue Substitute C Extraluminal Device D Intraluminal Device J Synthetic Substitute K Nonautologous Tissue Substitute Y Other Device	Z No Qualifier
Y Lower Vein	X External	Ø Drainage Device 2 Monitoring Device 3 Infusion Device D Intraluminal Device	Z No Qualifier

Non-OR 06PY3[023D]Z
Non-OR 06PYX[023D]Z

SECTION: 0 MEDICAL AND SURGICAL
BODY SYSTEM: 6 LOWER VEINS

OPERATION: Q **REPAIR:** Restoring, to the extent possible, a body part to its normal anatomic structure and function

Body Part	Approach	Device	Qualifier
0 Inferior Vena Cava 1 Splenic Vein 2 Gastric Vein 3 Esophageal Vein 4 Hepatic Vein 5 Superior Mesenteric Vein 6 Inferior Mesenteric Vein 7 Colic Vein 8 Portal Vein 9 Renal Vein, Right B Renal Vein, Left C Common Iliac Vein, Right D Common Iliac Vein, Left F External Iliac Vein, Right G External Iliac Vein, Left H Hypogastric Vein, Right J Hypogastric Vein, Left M Femoral Vein, Right N Femoral Vein, Left P Saphenous Vein, Right Q Saphenous Vein, Left T Foot Vein, Right V Foot Vein, Left Y Lower Vein	0 Open 3 Percutaneous 4 Percutaneous Endoscopic	Z No Device	Z No Qualifier

Q: REPAIR   6: LOWER VEINS   0: M/S

SECTION: Ø MEDICAL AND SURGICAL
BODY SYSTEM: 6 LOWER VEINS
OPERATION: R **REPLACEMENT:** Putting in or on biological or synthetic material that physically takes the place and/or function of all or a portion of a body part

Body Part	Approach	Device	Qualifier
Ø Inferior Vena Cava 1 Splenic Vein 2 Gastric Vein 3 Esophageal Vein 4 Hepatic Vein 5 Superior Mesenteric Vein 6 Inferior Mesenteric Vein 7 Colic Vein 8 Portal Vein 9 Renal Vein, Right B Renal Vein, Left C Common Iliac Vein, Right D Common Iliac Vein, Left F External Iliac Vein, Right G External Iliac Vein, Left H Hypogastric Vein, Right J Hypogastric Vein, Left M Femoral Vein, Right N Femoral Vein, Left P Saphenous Vein, Right Q Saphenous Vein, Left T Foot Vein, Right V Foot Vein, Left Y Lower Vein	Ø Open 4 Percutaneous Endoscopic	7 Autologous Tissue Substitute J Synthetic Substitute K Nonautologous Tissue Substitute	Z No Qualifier

Ø: M/S

6: LOWER VEINS

R: REPLACEMENT

SECTION: 0 MEDICAL AND SURGICAL

BODY SYSTEM: 6 LOWER VEINS

OPERATION: S REPOSITION: Moving to its normal location, or other suitable location, all or a portion of a body part

Body Part	Approach	Device	Qualifier
0 Inferior Vena Cava 1 Splenic Vein 2 Gastric Vein 3 Esophageal Vein 4 Hepatic Vein 5 Superior Mesenteric Vein 6 Inferior Mesenteric Vein 7 Colic Vein 8 Portal Vein 9 Renal Vein, Right B Renal Vein, Left C Common Iliac Vein, Right D Common Iliac Vein, Left F External Iliac Vein, Right G External Iliac Vein, Left H Hypogastric Vein, Right J Hypogastric Vein, Left M Femoral Vein, Right N Femoral Vein, Left P Saphenous Vein, Right Q Saphenous Vein, Left T Foot Vein, Right V Foot Vein, Left Y Lower Vein	0 Open 3 Percutaneous 4 Percutaneous Endoscopic	Z No Device	Z No Qualifier

S: REPOSITION

6: LOWER VEINS

0: M/S

New/Revised Text in Green ~~deleted~~ Deleted ♀ Females Only ♂ Males Only **Coding Clinic**
🚫 Non-covered 🚫 Limited Coverage ⊞ Combination (See Appendix E) DRG Non-OR Non-OR 🚫 Hospital-Acquired Condition

SECTION: Ø MEDICAL AND SURGICAL
BODY SYSTEM: 6 LOWER VEINS
OPERATION: U SUPPLEMENT: Putting in or on biological or synthetic material that physically reinforces and/or augments the function of a portion of a body part

Body Part	Approach	Device	Qualifier
Ø Inferior Vena Cava	Ø Open	7 Autologous Tissue Substitute	Z No Qualifier
1 Splenic Vein	3 Percutaneous	J Synthetic Substitute	
2 Gastric Vein	4 Percutaneous Endoscopic	K Nonautologous Tissue Substitute	
3 Esophageal Vein			
4 Hepatic Vein			
5 Superior Mesenteric Vein			
6 Inferior Mesenteric Vein			
7 Colic Vein			
8 Portal Vein			
9 Renal Vein, Right			
B Renal Vein, Left			
C Common Iliac Vein, Right			
D Common Iliac Vein, Left			
F External Iliac Vein, Right			
G External Iliac Vein, Left			
H Hypogastric Vein, Right			
J Hypogastric Vein, Left			
M Femoral Vein, Right			
N Femoral Vein, Left			
P Saphenous Vein, Right			
Q Saphenous Vein, Left			
T Foot Vein, Right			
V Foot Vein, Left			
Y Lower Vein			

SECTION: 0 MEDICAL AND SURGICAL
BODY SYSTEM: 6 LOWER VEINS
OPERATION: V RESTRICTION: Partially closing an orifice or the lumen of a tubular body part

Body Part	Approach	Device	Qualifier
0 Inferior Vena Cava	0 Open	C Extraluminal Device	Z No Qualifier
1 Splenic Vein	3 Percutaneous	D Intraluminal Device	
2 Gastric Vein	4 Percutaneous Endoscopic	Z No Device	
3 Esophageal Vein			
4 Hepatic Vein			
5 Superior Mesenteric Vein			
6 Inferior Mesenteric Vein			
7 Colic Vein			
8 Portal Vein			
9 Renal Vein, Right			
B Renal Vein, Left			
C Common Iliac Vein, Right			
D Common Iliac Vein, Left			
F External Iliac Vein, Right			
G External Iliac Vein, Left			
H Hypogastric Vein, Right			
J Hypogastric Vein, Left			
M Femoral Vein, Right			
N Femoral Vein, Left			
P Saphenous Vein, Right			
Q Saphenous Vein, Left			
T Foot Vein, Right			
V Foot Vein, Left			
Y Lower Vein			

New/Revised Text in Green   ~~deleted~~ Deleted   ♀ Females Only   ♂ Males Only   **Coding Clinic**

Non-covered   Limited Coverage   ⊕ Combination (See Appendix E)   DRG Non-OR   Non-OR   Hospital-Acquired Condition

SECTION: Ø MEDICAL AND SURGICAL
BODY SYSTEM: 6 LOWER VEINS
OPERATION: W REVISION: Correcting, to the extent possible, a portion of a malfunctioning device or the position of a displaced device

Body Part	Approach	Device	Qualifier
Y Lower Vein	Ø Open 3 Percutaneous 4 Percutaneous Endoscopic	Ø Drainage Device 2 Monitoring Device 3 Infusion Device 7 Autologous Tissue Substitute C Extraluminal Device D Intraluminal Device J Synthetic Substitute K Nonautologous Tissue Substitute Y Other Device	Z No Qualifier
Y Lower Vein	X External	Ø Drainage Device 2 Monitoring Device 3 Infusion Device 7 Autologous Tissue Substitute C Extraluminal Device D Intraluminal Device J Synthetic Substitute K Nonautologous Tissue Substitute	Z No Qualifier

Non-OR Ø6WY[3X][Ø237CDJK]Z

Coding Clinic: 2Ø18, Q1, P11 – Ø6WY3DZ

New/Revised Text in Green   deleted Deleted   ♀ Females Only   ♂ Males Only   **Coding Clinic**
Non-covered   Limited Coverage   Combination (See Appendix E)   DRG Non-OR   Non-OR   Hospital-Acquired Condition

159

New/Revised Text in Green   ~~deleted~~ Deleted   ♀ Females Only   ♂ Males Only   **Coding Clinic**

Non-covered   Limited Coverage   ⊞ Combination (See Appendix E)   DRG Non-OR   Non-OR   Hospital-Acquired Condition

SECTION: Ø MEDICAL AND SURGICAL
BODY SYSTEM: 7 LYMPHATIC AND HEMIC SYSTEMS
OPERATION: 2 CHANGE: Taking out or off a device from a body part and putting back an identical or similar device in or on the same body part without cutting or puncturing the skin or a mucous membrane

Body Part	Approach	Device	Qualifier
K Thoracic Duct L Cisterna Chyli M Thymus N Lymphatic P Spleen T Bone Marrow	X External	Ø Drainage Device Y Other Device	Z No Qualifier

Non-OR All Values

Coding Clinic: 2016, Q1, P30 – 07T50ZZ

SECTION: Ø MEDICAL AND SURGICAL
BODY SYSTEM: 7 LYMPHATIC AND HEMIC SYSTEMS
OPERATION: 5 DESTRUCTION: Physical eradication of all or a portion of a body part by the direct use of energy, force, or a destructive agent

Body Part	Approach	Device	Qualifier
Ø Lymphatic, Head 1 Lymphatic, Right Neck 2 Lymphatic, Left Neck 3 Lymphatic, Right Upper Extremity 4 Lymphatic, Left Upper Extremity 5 Lymphatic, Right Axillary 6 Lymphatic, Left Axillary 7 Lymphatic, Thorax 8 Lymphatic, Internal Mammary, Right 9 Lymphatic, Internal Mammary, Left B Lymphatic, Mesenteric C Lymphatic, Pelvis D Lymphatic, Aortic F Lymphatic, Right Lower Extremity G Lymphatic, Left Lower Extremity H Lymphatic, Right Inguinal J Lymphatic, Left Inguinal K Thoracic Duct L Cisterna Chyli M Thymus P Spleen	Ø Open 3 Percutaneous 4 Percutaneous Endoscopic	Z No Device	Z No Qualifier

SECTION: Ø MEDICAL AND SURGICAL

BODY SYSTEM: 7 LYMPHATIC AND HEMIC SYSTEMS

OPERATION: 9 DRAINAGE: Taking or letting out fluids and/or gases from a body part

Body Part	Approach	Device	Qualifier
Ø Lymphatic, Head 1 Lymphatic, Right Neck 2 Lymphatic, Left Neck 3 Lymphatic, Right Upper Extremity 4 Lymphatic, Left Upper Extremity 5 Lymphatic, Right Axillary 6 Lymphatic, Left Axillary 7 Lymphatic, Thorax 8 Lymphatic, Internal Mammary, Right 9 Lymphatic, Internal Mammary, Left B Lymphatic, Mesenteric C Lymphatic, Pelvis D Lymphatic, Aortic F Lymphatic, Right Lower Extremity G Lymphatic, Left Lower Extremity H Lymphatic, Right Inguinal J Lymphatic, Left Inguinal K Thoracic Duct L Cisterna Chyli	Ø Open 3 Percutaneous 4 Percutaneous Endoscopic 8 Via Natural or Artificial Opening Endoscopic	Ø Drainage Device	Z No Qualifier
Ø Lymphatic, Head 1 Lymphatic, Right Neck 2 Lymphatic, Left Neck 3 Lymphatic, Right Upper Extremity 4 Lymphatic, Left Upper Extremity 5 Lymphatic, Right Axillary 6 Lymphatic, Left Axillary 7 Lymphatic, Thorax 8 Lymphatic, Internal Mammary, Right 9 Lymphatic, Internal Mammary, Left B Lymphatic, Mesenteric C Lymphatic, Pelvis D Lymphatic, Aortic F Lymphatic, Right Lower Extremity G Lymphatic, Left Lower Extremity H Lymphatic, Right Inguinal J Lymphatic, Left Inguinal K Thoracic Duct L Cisterna Chyli	Ø Open 3 Percutaneous 4 Percutaneous Endoscopic 8 Via Natural or Artificial Opening Endoscopic	Z No Device	X Diagnostic Z No Qualifier
M Thymus P Spleen T Bone Marrow	Ø Open 3 Percutaneous 4 Percutaneous Endoscopic	Ø Drainage Device	Z No Qualifier
M Thymus P Spleen T Bone Marrow	Ø Open 3 Percutaneous 4 Percutaneous Endoscopic	Z No Device	X Diagnostic Z No Qualifier

Non-OR Ø79[123456789BCDEFGHJKL]3ØZ
Non-OR Ø79P[34]ØZ
Non-OR Ø79T[Ø34]ØZ

Non-OR Ø79[123456789BCDEFGHJKL]3ZZ
Non-OR Ø79P[34]Z[XZ]
Non-OR Ø79T[Ø34]Z[XZ]

9: DRAINAGE

7: LYMPHATIC AND HEMIC SYSTEMS

Ø: M/S

New/Revised Text in Green ~~deleted~~ Deleted ♀ Females Only ♂ Males Only **Coding Clinic**
Non-covered Limited Coverage ⊞ Combination (See Appendix E) DRG Non-OR Non-OR   Hospital-Acquired Condition

SECTION: Ø MEDICAL AND SURGICAL

BODY SYSTEM: 7 LYMPHATIC AND HEMIC SYSTEMS
OPERATION: B EXCISION: Cutting out or off, without replacement, a portion of a body part

Body Part	Approach	Device	Qualifier
Ø Lymphatic, Head	Ø Open	Z No Device	X Diagnostic
1 Lymphatic, Right Neck	3 Percutaneous		Z No Qualifier
2 Lymphatic, Left Neck	4 Percutaneous Endoscopic		
3 Lymphatic, Right Upper Extremity			
4 Lymphatic, Left Upper Extremity			
5 Lymphatic, Right Axillary			
6 Lymphatic, Left Axillary			
7 Lymphatic, Thorax			
8 Lymphatic, Internal Mammary, Right			
9 Lymphatic, Internal Mammary, Left			
B Lymphatic, Mesenteric			
C Lymphatic, Pelvis			
D Lymphatic, Aortic			
F Lymphatic, Right Lower Extremity			
G Lymphatic, Left Lower Extremity			
H Lymphatic, Right Inguinal ⊞			
J Lymphatic, Left Inguinal ⊞			
K Thoracic Duct			
L Cisterna Chyli			
M Thymus			
P Spleen			

⊞ Ø7B[HJ][Ø4]ZZ
Non-OR Ø7BP[34]ZX

SECTION: Ø MEDICAL AND SURGICAL

BODY SYSTEM: 7 LYMPHATIC AND HEMIC SYSTEMS
OPERATION: C EXTIRPATION: Taking or cutting out solid matter from a body part

Body Part	Approach	Device	Qualifier
Ø Lymphatic, Head	Ø Open	Z No Device	Z No Qualifier
1 Lymphatic, Right Neck	3 Percutaneous		
2 Lymphatic, Left Neck	4 Percutaneous Endoscopic		
3 Lymphatic, Right Upper Extremity			
4 Lymphatic, Left Upper Extremity			
5 Lymphatic, Right Axillary			
6 Lymphatic, Left Axillary			
7 Lymphatic, Thorax			
8 Lymphatic, Internal Mammary, Right			
9 Lymphatic, Internal Mammary, Left			
B Lymphatic, Mesenteric			
C Lymphatic, Pelvis			
D Lymphatic, Aortic			
F Lymphatic, Right Lower Extremity			
G Lymphatic, Left Lower Extremity			
H Lymphatic, Right Inguinal			
J Lymphatic, Left Inguinal			
K Thoracic Duct			
L Cisterna Chyli			
M Thymus			
P Spleen			

Non-OR Ø7CP[34]ZZ

SECTION: Ø MEDICAL AND SURGICAL
BODY SYSTEM: 7 LYMPHATIC AND HEMIC SYSTEMS
OPERATION: D EXTRACTION: Pulling or stripping out or off all or a portion of a body part by the use of force

Body Part	Approach	Device	Qualifier
Ø Lymphatic, Head 1 Lymphatic, Right Neck 2 Lymphatic, Left Neck 3 Lymphatic, Right Upper Extremity 4 Lymphatic, Left Upper Extremity 5 Lymphatic, Right Axillary 6 Lymphatic, Left Axillary 7 Lymphatic, Thorax 8 Lymphatic, Internal Mammary, Right 9 Lymphatic, Internal Mammary, Left B Lymphatic, Mesenteric C Lymphatic, Pelvis D Lymphatic, Aortic F Lymphatic, Right Lower Extremity G Lymphatic, Left Lower Extremity H Lymphatic, Right Inguinal J Lymphatic, Left Inguinal K Thoracic Duct L Cisterna Chyli	3 Percutaneous 4 Percutaneous Endoscopic 8 Via Natural or Artificial Opening Endoscopic	Z No Device	X Diagnostic
M Thymus P Spleen	3 Percutaneous 4 Percutaneous Endoscopic	Z No Device	X Diagnostic
Q Bone Marrow, Sternum R Bone Marrow, Iliac S Bone Marrow, Vertebral	Ø Open 3 Percutaneous	Z No Device	X Diagnostic Z No Qualifier

Non-OR Ø7D[QRS][Ø3]Z[XZ]

SECTION: Ø MEDICAL AND SURGICAL
BODY SYSTEM: 7 LYMPHATIC AND HEMIC SYSTEMS
OPERATION: H INSERTION: Putting in a nonbiological appliance that monitors, assists, performs, or prevents a physiological function but does not physically take the place of a body part

Body Part	Approach	Device	Qualifier
K Thoracic Duct L Cisterna Chyli M Thymus N Lymphatic P Spleen	Ø Open 3 Percutaneous 4 Percutaneous Endoscopic	3 Infusion Device Y Other Device	Z No Qualifier

DRG Non-OR Ø7H[KLMNP][Ø34]3Z

SECTION: Ø MEDICAL AND SURGICAL
BODY SYSTEM: 7 LYMPHATIC AND HEMIC SYSTEMS
OPERATION: J INSPECTION: Visually and/or manually exploring a body part

Body Part	Approach	Device	Qualifier
K Thoracic Duct L Cisterna Chyli M Thymus T Bone Marrow	Ø Open 3 Percutaneous 4 Percutaneous Endoscopic	Z No Device	Z No Qualifier
N Lymphatic	Ø Open 3 Percutaneous 4 Percutaneous Endoscopic 8 Via Natural or Artificial Opening Endoscopic X External	Z No Device	Z No Qualifier
P Spleen	Ø Open 3 Percutaneous 4 Percutaneous Endoscopic X External	Z No Device	Z No Qualifier

Non-OR 07J[KLM]3ZZ
Non-OR 07JN[3X]ZZ
Non-OR 07JP[34X]ZZ
Non-OR 07JT[Ø34]ZZ

SECTION: Ø MEDICAL AND SURGICAL
BODY SYSTEM: 7 LYMPHATIC AND HEMIC SYSTEMS
OPERATION: L OCCLUSION: Completely closing an orifice or the lumen of a tubular body part

Body Part	Approach	Device	Qualifier
Ø Lymphatic, Head 1 Lymphatic, Right Neck 2 Lymphatic, Left Neck 3 Lymphatic, Right Upper Extremity 4 Lymphatic, Left Upper Extremity 5 Lymphatic, Right Axillary 6 Lymphatic, Left Axillary 7 Lymphatic, Thorax 8 Lymphatic, Internal Mammary, Right 9 Lymphatic, Internal Mammary, Left B Lymphatic, Mesenteric C Lymphatic, Pelvis D Lymphatic, Aortic F Lymphatic, Right Lower Extremity G Lymphatic, Left Lower Extremity H Lymphatic, Right Inguinal J Lymphatic, Left Inguinal K Thoracic Duct L Cisterna Chyli	Ø Open 3 Percutaneous 4 Percutaneous Endoscopic	C Extraluminal Device D Intraluminal Device Z No Device	Z No Qualifier

SECTION: Ø MEDICAL AND SURGICAL
BODY SYSTEM: 7 LYMPHATIC AND HEMIC SYSTEMS
OPERATION: N RELEASE: Freeing a body part from an abnormal physical constraint by cutting or by the use of force

Body Part	Approach	Device	Qualifier
Ø Lymphatic, Head 1 Lymphatic, Right Neck 2 Lymphatic, Left Neck 3 Lymphatic, Right Upper Extremity 4 Lymphatic, Left Upper Extremity 5 Lymphatic, Right Axillary 6 Lymphatic, Left Axillary 7 Lymphatic, Thorax 8 Lymphatic, Internal Mammary, Right 9 Lymphatic, Internal Mammary, Left B Lymphatic, Mesenteric C Lymphatic, Pelvis D Lymphatic, Aortic F Lymphatic, Right Lower Extremity G Lymphatic, Left Lower Extremity H Lymphatic, Right Inguinal J Lymphatic, Left Inguinal K Thoracic Duct L Cisterna Chyli M Thymus P Spleen	Ø Open 3 Percutaneous 4 Percutaneous Endoscopic	Z No Device	Z No Qualifier

SECTION: Ø MEDICAL AND SURGICAL
BODY SYSTEM: 7 LYMPHATIC AND HEMIC SYSTEMS
OPERATION: P REMOVAL: Taking out or off a device from a body part

Body Part	Approach	Device	Qualifier
K Thoracic Duct L Cisterna Chyli N Lymphatic	Ø Open 3 Percutaneous 4 Percutaneous Endoscopic	Ø Drainage Device 3 Infusion Device 7 Autologous Tissue Substitute C Extraluminal Device D Intraluminal Device J Synthetic Substitute K Nonautologous Tissue Substitute Y Other Device	Z No Qualifier
K Thoracic Duct L Cisterna Chyli N Lymphatic	X External	Ø Drainage Device 3 Infusion Device D Intraluminal Device	Z No Qualifier
M Thymus P Spleen	Ø Open 3 Percutaneous 4 Percutaneous Endoscopic	Ø Drainage Device 3 Infusion Device Y Other Device	Z No Qualifier
M Thymus P Spleen	X External	Ø Drainage Device 3 Infusion Device	Z No Qualifier
T Bone Marrow	Ø Open 3 Percutaneous 4 Percutaneous Endoscopic X External	Ø Drainage Device	Z No Qualifier

Non-OR 07P[KLN]X[03D]Z   Non-OR 07P[MP]X[03]Z   Non-OR 07PT[034X]0Z

N: RELEASE   P: REMOVAL
7: LYMPHATIC AND HEMIC SYSTEMS
Ø: M/S

New/Revised Text in Green   deleted Deleted   ♀ Females Only   ♂ Males Only   Coding Clinic
Non-covered   Limited Coverage   Combination (See Appendix E)   DRG Non-OR   Non-OR   Hospital-Acquired Condition

SECTION: Ø MEDICAL AND SURGICAL
BODY SYSTEM: 7 LYMPHATIC AND HEMIC SYSTEMS
OPERATION: Q REPAIR: Restoring, to the extent possible, a body part to its normal anatomic structure and function

Body Part	Approach	Device	Qualifier
Ø Lymphatic, Head 1 Lymphatic, Right Neck 2 Lymphatic, Left Neck 3 Lymphatic, Right Upper Extremity 4 Lymphatic, Left Upper Extremity 5 Lymphatic, Right Axillary 6 Lymphatic, Left Axillary 7 Lymphatic, Thorax 8 Lymphatic, Internal Mammary, Right 9 Lymphatic, Internal Mammary, Left B Lymphatic, Mesenteric C Lymphatic, Pelvis D Lymphatic, Aortic F Lymphatic, Right Lower Extremity G Lymphatic, Left Lower Extremity H Lymphatic, Right Inguinal J Lymphatic, Left Inguinal K Thoracic Duct L Cisterna Chyli	Ø Open 3 Percutaneous 4 Percutaneous Endoscopic 8 Via Natural or Artificial Opening Endoscopic	Z No Device	Z No Qualifier
M Thymus P Spleen	Ø Open 3 Percutaneous 4 Percutaneous Endoscopic	Z No Device	Z No Qualifier

Coding Clinic: 2017, Q1, P34 – 07Q60ZZ

SECTION: Ø MEDICAL AND SURGICAL
BODY SYSTEM: 7 LYMPHATIC AND HEMIC SYSTEMS
OPERATION: S REPOSITION: Moving to its normal location, or other suitable location, all or a portion of a body part

Body Part	Approach	Device	Qualifier
M Thymus P Spleen	Ø Open	Z No Device	Z No Qualifier

SECTION: Ø MEDICAL AND SURGICAL
BODY SYSTEM: 7 LYMPHATIC AND HEMIC SYSTEMS
OPERATION: **T RESECTION:** Cutting out or off, without replacement, all of a body part

Body Part	Approach	Device	Qualifier
Ø Lymphatic, Head	Ø Open	Z No Device	Z No Qualifier
1 Lymphatic, Right Neck	4 Percutaneous Endoscopic		
2 Lymphatic, Left Neck			
3 Lymphatic, Right Upper Extremity			
4 Lymphatic, Left Upper Extremity			
5 Lymphatic, Right Axillary ⊞			
6 Lymphatic, Left Axillary ⊞			
7 Lymphatic, Thorax ⊞			
8 Lymphatic, Internal Mammary, Right ⊞			
9 Lymphatic, Internal Mammary, Left ⊞			
B Lymphatic, Mesenteric			
C Lymphatic, Pelvis			
D Lymphatic, Aortic			
F Lymphatic, Right Lower Extremity			
G Lymphatic, Left Lower Extremity			
H Lymphatic, Right Inguinal			
J Lymphatic, Left Inguinal			
K Thoracic Duct			
L Cisterna Chyli			
M Thymus			
P Spleen			

⊞ Ø7T[56789]ØZZ

Coding Clinic: 2Ø15, Q4, P13 – Ø7TPØZZ
Coding Clinic: 2Ø16, Q2, P13 – Ø7T2ØZZ

New/Revised Text in Green   ~~deleted~~ Deleted   ♀ Females Only   ♂ Males Only   **Coding Clinic**
🚫 Non-covered   🚫 Limited Coverage   ⊞ Combination (See Appendix E)   DRG Non-OR   Non-OR   🚫 Hospital-Acquired Condition

T: RESECTION
7: LYMPHATIC AND HEMIC SYSTEMS
Ø: M/S

SECTION: Ø MEDICAL AND SURGICAL

BODY SYSTEM: 7 LYMPHATIC AND HEMIC SYSTEMS

OPERATION: U SUPPLEMENT: Putting in or on biological or synthetic material that physically reinforces and/or augments the function of a portion of a body part

Body Part	Approach	Device	Qualifier
Ø Lymphatic, Head 1 Lymphatic, Right Neck 2 Lymphatic, Left Neck 3 Lymphatic, Right Upper Extremity 4 Lymphatic, Left Upper Extremity 5 Lymphatic, Right Axillary 6 Lymphatic, Left Axillary 7 Lymphatic, Thorax 8 Lymphatic, Internal Mammary, Right 9 Lymphatic, Internal Mammary, Left B Lymphatic, Mesenteric C Lymphatic, Pelvis D Lymphatic, Aortic F Lymphatic, Right Lower Extremity G Lymphatic, Left Lower Extremity H Lymphatic, Right Inguinal J Lymphatic, Left Inguinal K Thoracic Duct L Cisterna Chyli	Ø Open 4 Percutaneous Endoscopic	7 Autologous Tissue Substitute J Synthetic Substitute K Nonautologous Tissue Substitute	Z No Qualifier

SECTION: Ø MEDICAL AND SURGICAL

BODY SYSTEM: 7 LYMPHATIC AND HEMIC SYSTEMS

OPERATION: V RESTRICTION: Partially closing an orifice or the lumen of a tubular body part

Body Part	Approach	Device	Qualifier
Ø Lymphatic, Head 1 Lymphatic, Right Neck 2 Lymphatic, Left Neck 3 Lymphatic, Right Upper Extremity 4 Lymphatic, Left Upper Extremity 5 Lymphatic, Right Axillary 6 Lymphatic, Left Axillary 7 Lymphatic, Thorax 8 Lymphatic, Internal Mammary, Right 9 Lymphatic, Internal Mammary, Left B Lymphatic, Mesenteric C Lymphatic, Pelvis D Lymphatic, Aortic F Lymphatic, Right Lower Extremity G Lymphatic, Left Lower Extremity H Lymphatic, Right Inguinal J Lymphatic, Left Inguinal K Thoracic Duct L Cisterna Chyli	Ø Open 3 Percutaneous 4 Percutaneous Endoscopic	C Extraluminal Device D Intraluminal Device Z No Device	Z No Qualifier

SECTION: Ø MEDICAL AND SURGICAL

BODY SYSTEM: 7 LYMPHATIC AND HEMIC SYSTEMS

OPERATION: W REVISION: Correcting, to the extent possible, a portion of a malfunctioning device or the position of a displaced device

Body Part	Approach	Device	Qualifier
K Thoracic Duct L Cisterna Chyli N Lymphatic	Ø Open 3 Percutaneous 4 Percutaneous Endoscopic	Ø Drainage Device 3 Infusion Device 7 Autologous Tissue Substitute C Extraluminal Device D Intraluminal Device J Synthetic Substitute K Nonautologous Tissue Substitute Y Other Device	Z No Qualifier
K Thoracic Duct L Cisterna Chyli N Lymphatic	X External	Ø Drainage Device 3 Infusion Device 7 Autologous Tissue Substitute C Extraluminal Device D Intraluminal Device J Synthetic Substitute K Nonautologous Tissue Substitute	Z No Qualifier
M Thymus P Spleen	Ø Open 3 Percutaneous 4 Percutaneous Endoscopic	Ø Drainage Device 3 Infusion Device Y Other Device	Z No Qualifier
M Thymus P Spleen	X External	Ø Drainage Device 3 Infusion Device	Z No Qualifier
T Bone Marrow	Ø Open 3 Percutaneous 4 Percutaneous Endoscopic X External	Ø Drainage Device	Z No Qualifier

Non-OR Ø7W[KLN]X[Ø37CDJK]Z
Non-OR Ø7W[MP]X[Ø3]Z
Non-OR Ø7WT[Ø34X]ØZ

SECTION: Ø MEDICAL AND SURGICAL

BODY SYSTEM: 7 LYMPHATIC AND HEMIC SYSTEMS

OPERATION: Y TRANSPLANTATION: Putting in or on all or a portion of a living body part taken from another individual or animal to physically take the place and/or function of all or a portion of a similar body part

Body Part	Approach	Device	Qualifier
M Thymus P Spleen	Ø Open	Z No Device	Ø Allogeneic 1 Syngeneic 2 Zooplastic

New/Revised Text in Green ~~deleted~~ Deleted ♀ Females Only ♂ Males Only **Coding Clinic**
Non-covered Limited Coverage Combination (See Appendix E) DRG Non-OR Non-OR Hospital-Acquired Condition

SECTION: Ø MEDICAL AND SURGICAL

BODY SYSTEM: 8 EYE

OPERATION: Ø **ALTERATION:** Modifying the anatomic structure of a body part without affecting the function of the body part

Body Part	Approach	Device	Qualifier
N Upper Eyelid, Right P Upper Eyelid, Left Q Lower Eyelid, Right R Lower Eyelid, Left	Ø Open 3 Percutaneous X External	7 Autologous Tissue Substitute J Synthetic Substitute K Nonautologous Tissue Substitute Z No Device	Z No Qualifier

Non-OR   All Values

SECTION: Ø MEDICAL AND SURGICAL

BODY SYSTEM: 8 EYE

OPERATION: 1 **BYPASS:** Altering the route of passage of the contents of a tubular body part

Body Part	Approach	Device	Qualifier
2 Anterior Chamber, Right 3 Anterior Chamber, Left	3 Percutaneous	J Synthetic Substitute K Nonautologous Tissue Substitute Z No Device	4 Sclera
X Lacrimal Duct, Right Y Lacrimal Duct, Left	Ø Open 3 Percutaneous	J Synthetic Substitute K Nonautologous Tissue Substitute Z No Device	3 Nasal Cavity

SECTION: Ø MEDICAL AND SURGICAL

BODY SYSTEM: 8 EYE

OPERATION: 2 **CHANGE:** Taking out or off a device from a body part and putting back an identical or similar device in or on the same body part without cutting or puncturing the skin or a mucous membrane

Body Part	Approach	Device	Qualifier
Ø Eye, Right 1 Eye, Left	X External	Ø Drainage Device Y Other Device	Z No Qualifier

Non-OR   All Values

Side tab: 2: CHANGE   1: BYPASS   Ø: ALTERATION   8: EYE   Ø: M/S

SECTION: Ø MEDICAL AND SURGICAL

BODY SYSTEM: 8 EYE

OPERATION: 5 DESTRUCTION: Physical eradication of all or a portion of a body part by the direct use of energy, force, or a destructive agent

Body Part	Approach	Device	Qualifier
Ø Eye, Right 1 Eye, Left 6 Sclera, Right 7 Sclera, Left 8 Cornea, Right 9 Cornea, Left S Conjunctiva, Right T Conjunctiva, Left	X External	Z No Device	Z No Qualifier
2 Anterior Chamber, Right 3 Anterior Chamber, Left 4 Vitreous, Right 5 Vitreous, Left C Iris, Right D Iris, Left E Retina, Right F Retina, Left G Retinal Vessel, Right H Retinal Vessel, Left J Lens, Right K Lens, Left	3 Percutaneous	Z No Device	Z No Qualifier
A Choroid, Right B Choroid, Left L Extraocular Muscle, Right M Extraocular Muscle, Left V Lacrimal Gland, Right W Lacrimal Gland, Left	Ø Open 3 Percutaneous	Z No Device	Z No Qualifier
N Upper Eyelid, Right P Upper Eyelid, Left Q Lower Eyelid, Right R Lower Eyelid, Left	Ø Open 3 Percutaneous X External	Z No Device	Z No Qualifier
X Lacrimal Duct, Right Y Lacrimal Duct, Left	Ø Open 3 Percutaneous 7 Via Natural or Artificial Opening 8 Via Natural or Artificial Opening Endoscopic	Z No Device	Z No Qualifier

SECTION: Ø MEDICAL AND SURGICAL

BODY SYSTEM: 8 EYE

OPERATION: 7 DILATION: Expanding an orifice or the lumen of a tubular body part

Body Part	Approach	Device	Qualifier
X Lacrimal Duct, Right Y Lacrimal Duct, Left	Ø Open 3 Percutaneous 7 Via Natural or Artificial Opening 8 Via Natural or Artificial Opening Endoscopic	D Intraluminal Device Z No Device	Z No Qualifier

Ø: M/S   8: EYE   5: DESTRUCTION   7: DILATION

SECTION: Ø MEDICAL AND SURGICAL
BODY SYSTEM: 8 EYE
OPERATION: 9 DRAINAGE: *(on multiple pages)*
Taking or letting out fluids and/or gases from a body part

9: DRAINAGE

8: EYE

Ø: M/S

Body Part	Approach	Device	Qualifier
Ø Eye, Right 1 Eye, Left 6 Sclera, Right 7 Sclera, Left 8 Cornea, Right 9 Cornea, Left S Conjunctiva, Right T Conjunctiva, Left	X External	Ø Drainage Device	Z No Qualifier
Ø Eye, Right 1 Eye, Left 6 Sclera, Right 7 Sclera, Left 8 Cornea, Right 9 Cornea, Left S Conjunctiva, Right T Conjunctiva, Left	X External	Z No Device	X Diagnostic Z No Qualifier
2 Anterior Chamber, Right 3 Anterior Chamber, Left 4 Vitreous, Right 5 Vitreous, Left C Iris, Right D Iris, Left E Retina, Right F Retina, Left G Retinal Vessel, Right H Retinal Vessel, Left J Lens, Right K Lens, Left	3 Percutaneous	Ø Drainage Device	Z No Qualifier
2 Anterior Chamber, Right 3 Anterior Chamber, Left 4 Vitreous, Right 5 Vitreous, Left C Iris, Right D Iris, Left E Retina, Right F Retina, Left G Retinal Vessel, Right H Retinal Vessel, Left J Lens, Right K Lens, Left	3 Percutaneous	Z No Device	X Diagnostic Z No Qualifier
A Choroid, Right B Choroid, Left L Extraocular Muscle, Right M Extraocular Muscle, Left V Lacrimal Gland, Right W Lacrimal Gland, Left	Ø Open 3 Percutaneous	Ø Drainage Device	Z No Qualifier

DRG Non-OR Ø89[Ø16789ST]XZ[XZ] *(proposed)*

Coding Clinic: 2016, Q2, P21 – Ø8923ZZ

SECTION: Ø MEDICAL AND SURGICAL
BODY SYSTEM: 8 EYE
OPERATION: 9 DRAINAGE: *(continued)*
Taking or letting out fluids and/or gases from a body part

Body Part	Approach	Device	Qualifier
A Choroid, Right B Choroid, Left L Extraocular Muscle, Right M Extraocular Muscle, Left V Lacrimal Gland, Right W Lacrimal Gland, Left	Ø Open 3 Percutaneous	Z No Device	X Diagnostic Z No Qualifier
N Upper Eyelid, Right P Upper Eyelid, Left Q Lower Eyelid, Right R Lower Eyelid, Left	Ø Open 3 Percutaneous X External	Ø Drainage Device	Z No Qualifier
N Upper Eyelid, Right P Upper Eyelid, Left Q Lower Eyelid, Right R Lower Eyelid, Left	Ø Open 3 Percutaneous X External	Z No Device	X Diagnostic Z No Qualifier
X Lacrimal Duct, Right Y Lacrimal Duct, Left	Ø Open 3 Percutaneous 7 Via Natural or Artificial Opening 8 Via Natural or Artificial Opening Endoscopic	Ø Drainage Device	Z No Qualifier
X Lacrimal Duct, Right Y Lacrimal Duct, Left	Ø Open 3 Percutaneous 7 Via Natural or Artificial Opening 8 Via Natural or Artificial Opening Endoscopic	Z No Device	X Diagnostic Z No Qualifier

DRG Non-OR   Ø89[NPQR]XZX *(proposed)*
Non-OR   Ø89[NPQR][Ø3X]ØZ
Non-OR   Ø89[NPQR][Ø3X]ZZ

New/Revised Text in Green   ~~deleted~~ Deleted   ♀ Females Only   ♂ Males Only   **Coding Clinic**
Non-covered   Limited Coverage   Combination (See Appendix E)   DRG Non-OR   Non-OR   Hospital-Acquired Condition

175

SECTION: Ø MEDICAL AND SURGICAL
BODY SYSTEM: 8 EYE
OPERATION: B **EXCISION:** Cutting out or off, without replacement, a portion of a body part

Body Part	Approach	Device	Qualifier
Ø Eye, Right 1 Eye, Left N Upper Eyelid, Right P Upper Eyelid, Left Q Lower Eyelid, Right R Lower Eyelid, Left	Ø Open 3 Percutaneous X External	Z No Device	X Diagnostic Z No Qualifier
4 Vitreous, Right 5 Vitreous, Left C Iris, Right D Iris, Left E Retina, Right F Retina, Left J Lens, Right K Lens, Left	3 Percutaneous	Z No Device	X Diagnostic Z No Qualifier
6 Sclera, Right 7 Sclera, Left 8 Cornea, Right 9 Cornea, Left S Conjunctiva, Right T Conjunctiva, Left	X External	Z No Device	X Diagnostic Z No Qualifier
A Choroid, Right B Choroid, Left L Extraocular Muscle, Right M Extraocular Muscle, Left V Lacrimal Gland, Right W Lacrimal Gland, Left	Ø Open 3 Percutaneous	Z No Device	X Diagnostic Z No Qualifier
X Lacrimal Duct, Right Y Lacrimal Duct, Left	Ø Open 3 Percutaneous 7 Via Natural or Artificial Opening 8 Via Natural or Artificial Opening Endoscopic	Z No Device	X Diagnostic Z No Qualifier

SECTION: 0 MEDICAL AND SURGICAL

BODY SYSTEM: 8 EYE

OPERATION: C EXTIRPATION: Taking or cutting out solid matter from a body part

Body Part	Approach	Device	Qualifier
0 Eye, Right 1 Eye, Left 6 Sclera, Right 7 Sclera, Left 8 Cornea, Right 9 Cornea, Left S Conjunctiva, Right T Conjunctiva, Left	X External	Z No Device	Z No Qualifier
2 Anterior Chamber, Right 3 Anterior Chamber, Left 4 Vitreous, Right 5 Vitreous, Left C Iris, Right D Iris, Left E Retina, Right F Retina, Left G Retinal Vessel, Right H Retinal Vessel, Left J Lens, Right K Lens, Left	3 Percutaneous X External	Z No Device	Z No Qualifier
A Choroid, Right B Choroid, Left L Extraocular Muscle, Right M Extraocular Muscle, Left N Upper Eyelid, Right P Upper Eyelid, Left Q Lower Eyelid, Right R Lower Eyelid, Left V Lacrimal Gland, Right W Lacrimal Gland, Left	0 Open 3 Percutaneous X External	Z No Device	Z No Qualifier
X Lacrimal Duct, Right Y Lacrimal Duct, Left	0 Open 3 Percutaneous 7 Via Natural or Artificial Opening 8 Via Natural or Artificial Opening Endoscopic	Z No Device	Z No Qualifier

Non-OR 08C[23]XZZ
Non-OR 08C[67]XZZ
Non-OR 08C[NPQR][03X]ZZ

SECTION: 0 MEDICAL AND SURGICAL

BODY SYSTEM: 8 EYE

OPERATION: D EXTRACTION: Pulling or stripping out or off all or a portion of a body part by the use of force

Body Part	Approach	Device	Qualifier
8 Cornea, Right 9 Cornea, Left	X External	Z No Device	X Diagnostic Z No Qualifier
J Lens, Right K Lens, Left	3 Percutaneous	Z No Device	Z No Qualifier

SECTION: Ø MEDICAL AND SURGICAL
BODY SYSTEM: 8 EYE

OPERATION: F FRAGMENTATION: Breaking solid matter in a body part into pieces

Body Part	Approach	Device	Qualifier
4 Vitreous, Right 🔖 5 Vitreous, Left 🔖	3 Percutaneous X External	Z No Device	Z No Qualifier

🔖 Ø8F[45]XZZ
Non-OR Ø8F[45]XZZ

SECTION: Ø MEDICAL AND SURGICAL
BODY SYSTEM: 8 EYE

OPERATION: H INSERTION: Putting in a nonbiological appliance that monitors, assists, performs, or prevents a physiological function but does not physically take the place of a body part

Body Part	Approach	Device	Qualifier
Ø Eye, Right 1 Eye, Left	Ø Open	5 Epiretinal Visual Prosthesis Y Other Device	Z No Qualifier
Ø Eye, Right 1 Eye, Left	3 Percutaneous	1 Radioactive Element 3 Infusion Device Y Other Device	Z No Qualifier
Ø Eye, Right 1 Eye, Left	7 Via Natural or Artificial Opening 8 Via Natural or Artificial Opening Endoscopic	Y Other Device	Z No Qualifier
Ø Eye, Right 1 Eye, Left	X External	1 Radioactive Element 3 Infusion Device	Z No Qualifier

SECTION: Ø MEDICAL AND SURGICAL
BODY SYSTEM: 8 EYE

OPERATION: J INSPECTION: Visually and/or manually exploring a body part

Body Part	Approach	Device	Qualifier
Ø Eye, Right 1 Eye, Left J Lens, Right K Lens, Left	X External	Z No Device	Z No Qualifier
L Extraocular Muscle, Right M Extraocular Muscle, Left	Ø Open X External	Z No Device	Z No Qualifier

Non-OR Ø8J[Ø1JK]XZZ
Non-OR Ø8J[LM]XZZ

Coding Clinic: 2Ø15, Q1, P36 – Ø8JØXZZ

New/Revised Text in Green   ~~deleted~~ Deleted   ♀ Females Only   ♂ Males Only   **Coding Clinic**
🔖 Non-covered   🔖 Limited Coverage   ⊡ Combination (See Appendix E)   DRG Non-OR   Non-OR   🔖 Hospital-Acquired Condition

SECTION: Ø MEDICAL AND SURGICAL

BODY SYSTEM: 8 EYE

OPERATION: L OCCLUSION: Completely closing an orifice or the lumen of a tubular body part

Body Part	Approach	Device	Qualifier
X Lacrimal Duct, Right Y Lacrimal Duct, Left	Ø Open 3 Percutaneous	C Extraluminal Device D Intraluminal Device Z No Device	Z No Qualifier
X Lacrimal Duct, Right Y Lacrimal Duct, Left	7 Via Natural or Artificial Opening 8 Via Natural or Artificial Opening Endoscopic	D Intraluminal Device Z No Device	Z No Qualifier

SECTION: Ø MEDICAL AND SURGICAL

BODY SYSTEM: 8 EYE

OPERATION: M REATTACHMENT: Putting back in or on all or a portion of a separated body part to its normal location or other suitable location

Body Part	Approach	Device	Qualifier
N Upper Eyelid, Right P Upper Eyelid, Left Q Lower Eyelid, Right R Lower Eyelid, Left	X External	Z No Device	Z No Qualifier

SECTION: 0 MEDICAL AND SURGICAL
BODY SYSTEM: 8 EYE
OPERATION: N RELEASE: Freeing a body part from an abnormal physical constraint by cutting or by the use of force

Body Part	Approach	Device	Qualifier
0 Eye, Right 1 Eye, Left 6 Sclera, Right 7 Sclera, Left 8 Cornea, Right 9 Cornea, Left S Conjunctiva, Right T Conjunctiva, Left	X External	Z No Device	Z No Qualifier
2 Anterior Chamber, Right 3 Anterior Chamber, Left 4 Vitreous, Right 5 Vitreous, Left C Iris, Right D Iris, Left E Retina, Right F Retina, Left G Retinal Vessel, Right H Retinal Vessel, Left J Lens, Right K Lens, Left	3 Percutaneous	Z No Device	Z No Qualifier
A Choroid, Right B Choroid, Left L Extraocular Muscle, Right M Extraocular Muscle, Left V Lacrimal Gland, Right W Lacrimal Gland, Left	0 Open 3 Percutaneous	Z No Device	Z No Qualifier
N Upper Eyelid, Right P Upper Eyelid, Left Q Lower Eyelid, Right R Lower Eyelid, Left	0 Open 3 Percutaneous X External	Z No Device	Z No Qualifier
X Lacrimal Duct, Right Y Lacrimal Duct, Left	0 Open 3 Percutaneous 7 Via Natural or Artificial Opening 8 Via Natural or Artificial Opening Endoscopic	Z No Device	Z No Qualifier

Coding Clinic: 2015, Q2, P25 – 08NC3ZZ

N: RELEASE   8: EYE   0: M/S

SECTION: Ø MEDICAL AND SURGICAL

BODY SYSTEM: 8 EYE

OPERATION: P REMOVAL: Taking out or off a device from a body part

Body Part	Approach	Device	Qualifier
Ø Eye, Right 1 Eye, Left	Ø Open 3 Percutaneous 7 Via Natural or Artificial Opening 8 Via Natural or Artificial Opening Endoscopic	Ø Drainage Device 1 Radioactive Element 3 Infusion Device 7 Autologous Tissue Substitute C Extraluminal Device D Intraluminal Device J Synthetic Substitute K Nonautologous Tissue Substitute Y Other Device	Z No Qualifier
Ø Eye, Right 1 Eye, Left	X External	Ø Drainage Device 1 Radioactive Element 3 Infusion Device 7 Autologous Tissue Substitute C Extraluminal Device D Intraluminal Device J Synthetic Substitute K Nonautologous Tissue Substitute	Z No Qualifier
J Lens, Right K Lens, Left	3 Percutaneous	J Synthetic Substitute Y Other Device	Z No Qualifier
L Extraocular Muscle, Right M Extraocular Muscle, Left	Ø Open 3 Percutaneous	Ø Drainage Device 7 Autologous Tissue Substitute J Synthetic Substitute K Nonautologous Tissue Substitute Y Other Device	Z No Qualifier

Non-OR 08P[Ø1][78][Ø3D]Z

Non-OR 08PØX[Ø3CD]Z

Non-OR 08P1X[Ø13CD]Z

SECTION: Ø MEDICAL AND SURGICAL
BODY SYSTEM: 8 EYE

OPERATION: Q REPAIR: Restoring, to the extent possible, a body part to its normal anatomic structure and function

Body Part	Approach	Device	Qualifier
Ø Eye, Right 1 Eye, Left 6 Sclera, Right 7 Sclera, Left 8 Cornea, Right 🜊 9 Cornea, Left 🜊 S Conjunctiva, Right T Conjunctiva, Left	X External	Z No Device	Z No Qualifier
2 Anterior Chamber, Right 3 Anterior Chamber, Left 4 Vitreous, Right 5 Vitreous, Left C Iris, Right D Iris, Left E Retina, Right F Retina, Left G Retinal Vessel, Right H Retinal Vessel, Left J Lens, Right K Lens, Left	3 Percutaneous	Z No Device	Z No Qualifier
A Choroid, Right B Choroid, Left L Extraocular Muscle, Right M Extraocular Muscle, Left V Lacrimal Gland, Right W Lacrimal Gland, Left	Ø Open 3 Percutaneous	Z No Device	Z No Qualifier
N Upper Eyelid, Right P Upper Eyelid, Left Q Lower Eyelid, Right R Lower Eyelid, Left	Ø Open 3 Percutaneous X External	Z No Device	Z No Qualifier
X Lacrimal Duct, Right Y Lacrimal Duct, Left	Ø Open 3 Percutaneous 7 Via Natural or Artificial Opening 8 Via Natural or Artificial Opening Endoscopic	Z No Device	Z No Qualifier

🜊 Ø8Q[89]XZZ

Non-OR Ø8Q[NPQR][Ø3X]ZZ

Q: REPAIR 8: EYE Ø: M/S

SECTION: 0 MEDICAL AND SURGICAL

BODY SYSTEM: 8 EYE

OPERATION: R REPLACEMENT: Putting in or on biological or synthetic material that physically takes the place and/or function of all or a portion of a body part

Body Part	Approach	Device	Qualifier
0 Eye, Right 1 Eye, Left A Choroid, Right B Choroid, Left	0 Open 3 Percutaneous	7 Autologous Tissue Substitute J Synthetic Substitute K Nonautologous Tissue Substitute	Z No Qualifier
4 Vitreous, Right 5 Vitreous, Left C Iris, Right D Iris, Left G Retinal Vessel, Right H Retinal Vessel, Left	3 Percutaneous	7 Autologous Tissue Substitute J Synthetic Substitute K Nonautologous Tissue Substitute	Z No Qualifier
6 Sclera, Right 7 Sclera, Left S Conjunctiva, Right T Conjunctiva, Left	X External	7 Autologous Tissue Substitute J Synthetic Substitute K Nonautologous Tissue Substitute	Z No Qualifier
8 Cornea, Right 9 Cornea, Left	3 Percutaneous X External	7 Autologous Tissue Substitute J Synthetic Substitute K Nonautologous Tissue Substitute	Z No Qualifier
J Lens, Right K Lens, Left	3 Percutaneous	0 Synthetic Substitute, Intraocular Telescope 7 Autologous Tissue Substitute J Synthetic Substitute K Nonautologous Tissue Substitute	Z No Qualifier
N Upper Eyelid, Right P Upper Eyelid, Left Q Lower Eyelid, Right R Lower Eyelid, Left	0 Open 3 Percutaneous X External	7 Autologous Tissue Substitute J Synthetic Substitute K Nonautologous Tissue Substitute	Z No Qualifier
X Lacrimal Duct, Right Y Lacrimal Duct, Left	0 Open 3 Percutaneous 7 Via Natural or Artificial Opening 8 Via Natural or Artificial Opening Endoscopic	7 Autologous Tissue Substitute J Synthetic Substitute K Nonautologous Tissue Substitute	Z No Qualifier

Coding Clinic: 2015, Q2, P25-26 – 08R8XKZ

New/Revised Text in Green · ~~deleted~~ Deleted · ♀ Females Only · ♂ Males Only · **Coding Clinic**

🚫 Non-covered · 🚫 Limited Coverage · ⊕ Combination (See Appendix E) · DRG Non-OR · Non-OR · 🚫 Hospital-Acquired Condition

183

0: M/S 8: EYE R: REPLACEMENT

SECTION: Ø MEDICAL AND SURGICAL

BODY SYSTEM: 8 EYE

OPERATION: S **REPOSITION:** Moving to its normal location, or other suitable location, all or a portion of a body part

Body Part	Approach	Device	Qualifier
C Iris, Right D Iris, Left G Retinal Vessel, Right H Retinal Vessel, Left J Lens, Right K Lens, Left	3 Percutaneous	Z No Device	Z No Qualifier
L Extraocular Muscle, Right M Extraocular Muscle, Left V Lacrimal Gland, Right W Lacrimal Gland, Left	Ø Open 3 Percutaneous	Z No Device	Z No Qualifier
N Upper Eyelid, Right P Upper Eyelid, Left Q Lower Eyelid, Right R Lower Eyelid, Left	Ø Open 3 Percutaneous X External	Z No Device	Z No Qualifier
X Lacrimal Duct, Right Y Lacrimal Duct, Left	Ø Open 3 Percutaneous 7 Via Natural or Artificial Opening 8 Via Natural or Artificial Opening Endoscopic	Z No Device	Z No Qualifier

S: REPOSITION

8: EYE

Ø: M/S

SECTION: Ø MEDICAL AND SURGICAL
BODY SYSTEM: 8 EYE
OPERATION: T RESECTION: Cutting out or off, without replacement, all of a body part

Body Part	Approach	Device	Qualifier
Ø Eye, Right 1 Eye, Left 8 Cornea, Right 9 Cornea, Left	X External	Z No Device	Z No Qualifier
4 Vitreous, Right 5 Vitreous, Left C Iris, Right D Iris, Left J Lens, Right K Lens, Left	3 Percutaneous	Z No Device	Z No Qualifier
L Extraocular Muscle, Right M Extraocular Muscle, Left V Lacrimal Gland, Right W Lacrimal Gland, Left	Ø Open 3 Percutaneous	Z No Device	Z No Qualifier
N Upper Eyelid, Right P Upper Eyelid, Left Q Lower Eyelid, Right R Lower Eyelid, Left	Ø Open X External	Z No Device	Z No Qualifier
X Lacrimal Duct, Right Y Lacrimal Duct, Left	Ø Open 3 Percutaneous 7 Via Natural or Artificial Opening 8 Via Natural or Artificial Opening Endoscopic	Z No Device	Z No Qualifier

Coding Clinic: 2Ø15, Q2, P13 – Ø8T1XZZ, Ø8T[MR]ØZZ

SECTION: Ø MEDICAL AND SURGICAL
BODY SYSTEM: 8 EYE
OPERATION: U SUPPLEMENT: Putting in or on biological or synthetic material that physically reinforces and/or augments the function of a portion of a body part

Body Part	Approach	Device	Qualifier
Ø Eye, Right 1 Eye, Left C Iris, Right D Iris, Left E Retina, Right F Retina, Left G Retinal Vessel, Right H Retinal Vessel, Left L Extraocular Muscle, Right M Extraocular Muscle, Left	Ø Open 3 Percutaneous	7 Autologous Tissue Substitute J Synthetic Substitute K Nonautologous Tissue Substitute	Z No Qualifier
8 Cornea, Right 🐾 9 Cornea, Left 🐾 N Upper Eyelid, Right P Upper Eyelid, Left Q Lower Eyelid, Right R Lower Eyelid, Left	Ø Open 3 Percutaneous X External	7 Autologous Tissue Substitute J Synthetic Substitute K Nonautologous Tissue Substitute	Z No Qualifier
X Lacrimal Duct, Right Y Lacrimal Duct, Left	Ø Open 3 Percutaneous 7 Via Natural or Artificial Opening 8 Via Natural or Artificial Opening Endoscopic	7 Autologous Tissue Substitute J Synthetic Substitute K Nonautologous Tissue Substitute	Z No Qualifier

🐾 Ø8U[89][Ø3X]KZ

SECTION: Ø MEDICAL AND SURGICAL
BODY SYSTEM: 8 EYE
OPERATION: V RESTRICTION: Partially closing an orifice or the lumen of a tubular body part

Body Part	Approach	Device	Qualifier
X Lacrimal Duct, Right Y Lacrimal Duct, Left	Ø Open 3 Percutaneous	C Extraluminal Device D Intraluminal Device Z No Device	Z No Qualifier
X Lacrimal Duct, Right Y Lacrimal Duct, Left	7 Via Natural or Artificial Opening 8 Via Natural or Artificial Opening Endoscopic	D Intraluminal Device Z No Device	Z No Qualifier

Left margin: U: SUPPLEMENT　V: RESTRICTION　　8: EYE　　Ø: M/S

SECTION: Ø MEDICAL AND SURGICAL

BODY SYSTEM: 8 EYE

OPERATION: W REVISION: Correcting, to the extent possible, a portion of a malfunctioning device or the positon of a displaced device

Body Part	Approach	Device	Qualifier
Ø Eye, Right 1 Eye, Left	Ø Open 3 Percutaneous 7 Via Natural or Artificial Opening 8 Via Natural or Artificial Opening Endoscopic	Ø Drainage Device 3 Infusion Device 7 Autologous Tissue Substitute C Extraluminal Device D Intraluminal Device J Synthetic Substitute K Nonautologous Tissue Substitute Y Other Device	Z No Qualifier
Ø Eye, Right 1 Eye, Left	X External	Ø Drainage Device 3 Infusion Device 7 Autologous Tissue Substitute C Extraluminal Device D Intraluminal Device J Synthetic Substitute K Nonautologous Tissue Substitute	Z No Qualifier
J Lens, Right K Lens, Left	3 Percutaneous	J Synthetic Substitute Y Other Device	Z No Qualifier
J Lens, Right K Lens, Left	X External	J Synthetic Substitute	Z No Qualifier
L Extraocular Muscle, Right M Extraocular Muscle, Left	Ø Open 3 Percutaneous	Ø Drainage Device 7 Autologous Tissue Substitute J Synthetic Substitute K Nonautologous Tissue Substitute Y Other Device	Z No Qualifier

Non-OR Ø8W[Ø1]X[Ø37CDJK]Z

Non-OR Ø8W[JK]XJZ

SECTION: Ø MEDICAL AND SURGICAL

BODY SYSTEM: 8 EYE

OPERATION: X TRANSFER: Moving, without taking out, all or a portion of a body part to another location to take over the function of all or a portion of a body part

Body Part	Approach	Device	Qualifier
L Extraocular Muscle, Right M Extraocular Muscle, Left	Ø Open 3 Percutaneous	Z No Device	Z No Qualifier

SECTION: Ø MEDICAL AND SURGICAL
BODY SYSTEM: 9 EAR, NOSE, SINUS
OPERATION: Ø ALTERATION: Modifying the anatomic structure of a body part without affecting the function of the body part

Body Part	Approach	Device	Qualifier
Ø External Ear, Right 1 External Ear, Left 2 External Ear, Bilateral K Nasal Mucosa and Soft Tissue	Ø Open 3 Percutaneous 4 Percutaneous Endoscopic X External	7 Autologous Tissue Substitute J Synthetic Substitute K Nonautologous Tissue Substitute Z No Device	Z No Qualifier

SECTION: Ø MEDICAL AND SURGICAL
BODY SYSTEM: 9 EAR, NOSE, SINUS
OPERATION: 1 BYPASS: Altering the route of passage of the contents of a tubular body part

Body Part	Approach	Device	Qualifier
D Inner Ear, Right E Inner Ear, Left	Ø Open	7 Autologous Tissue Substitute J Synthetic Substitute K Nonautologous Tissue Substitute Z No Device	Ø Endolymphatic

SECTION: Ø MEDICAL AND SURGICAL
BODY SYSTEM: 9 EAR, NOSE, SINUS
OPERATION: 2 CHANGE: Taking out or off a device from a body part and putting back an identical or similar device in or on the same body part without cutting or puncturing the skin or a mucous membrane

Body Part	Approach	Device	Qualifier
H Ear, Right J Ear, Left K Nasal Mucosa and Soft Tissue Y Sinus	X External	Ø Drainage Device Y Other Device	Z No Qualifier

Non-OR All Values

SECTION: Ø MEDICAL AND SURGICAL
BODY SYSTEM: 9 EAR, NOSE, SINUS
OPERATION: 3 CONTROL: Stopping, or attempting to stop, postprocedural or other acute bleeding

Body Part	Approach	Device	Qualifier
K Nasal Mucosa and Soft Tissue	7 Via Natural or Artificial Opening 8 Via Natural or Artificial Opening Endoscopic	Z No Device	Z No Qualifier

SECTION: Ø MEDICAL AND SURGICAL
BODY SYSTEM: 9 EAR, NOSE, SINUS
OPERATION: 5 DESTRUCTION: Physical eradication of all or a portion of a body part by the direct use of energy, force, or a destructive agent

Body Part	Approach	Device	Qualifier
Ø External Ear, Right 1 External Ear, Left	Ø Open 3 Percutaneous 4 Percutaneous Endoscopic X External	Z No Device	Z No Qualifier
3 External Auditory Canal, Right 4 External Auditory Canal, Left	Ø Open 3 Percutaneous 4 Percutaneous Endoscopic 7 Via Natural or Artificial Opening 8 Via Natural or Artificial Opening Endoscopic X External	Z No Device	Z No Qualifier
5 Middle Ear, Right 6 Middle Ear, Left 9 Auditory Ossicle, Right A Auditory Ossicle, Left D Inner Ear, Right E Inner Ear, Left	Ø Open 8 Via Natural or Artificial Opening Endoscopic	Z No Device	Z No Qualifier
7 Tympanic Membrane, Right 8 Tympanic Membrane, Left F Eustachian Tube, Right G Eustachian Tube, Left L Nasal Turbinate N Nasopharynx	Ø Open 3 Percutaneous 4 Percutaneous Endoscopic 7 Via Natural or Artificial Opening 8 Via Natural or Artificial Opening Endoscopic	Z No Device	Z No Qualifier
B Mastoid Sinus, Right C Mastoid Sinus, Left M Nasal Septum P Accessory Sinus Q Maxillary Sinus, Right R Maxillary Sinus, Left S Frontal Sinus, Right T Frontal Sinus, Left U Ethmoid Sinus, Right V Ethmoid Sinus, Left W Sphenoid Sinus, Right X Sphenoid Sinus, Left	Ø Open 3 Percutaneous 4 Percutaneous Endoscopic 8 Via Natural or Artificial Opening Endoscopic	Z No Device	Z No Qualifier
K Nasal Mucosa and Soft Tissue	Ø Open 3 Percutaneous 4 Percutaneous Endoscopic 8 Via Natural or Artificial Opening Endoscopic X External	Z No Device	Z No Qualifier

Non-OR Ø95[Ø1][Ø34X]ZZ
Non-OR Ø95[34][Ø3478X]ZZ
Non-OR Ø95[FG][Ø3478]ZZ
Non-OR Ø95M[Ø34]ZZ
Non-OR Ø95K[Ø34X]ZZ

5: DESTRUCTION

9: EAR, NOSE, SINUS

Ø: M/S

SECTION: Ø MEDICAL AND SURGICAL
BODY SYSTEM: 9 EAR, NOSE, SINUS
OPERATION: 7 DILATION: Expanding an orifice or the lumen of a tubular body part

Body Part	Approach	Device	Qualifier
F Eustachian Tube, Right G Eustachian Tube, Left	Ø Open 7 Via Natural or Artificial Opening 8 Via Natural or Artificial Opening Endoscopic	D Intraluminal Device Z No Device	Z No Qualifier
F Eustachian Tube, Right G Eustachian Tube, Left	3 Percutaneous 4 Percutaneous Endoscopic	Z No Device	Z No Qualifier

Non-OR All Values

SECTION: Ø MEDICAL AND SURGICAL
BODY SYSTEM: 9 EAR, NOSE, SINUS
OPERATION: 8 DIVISION: Cutting into a body part, without draining fluids and/or gases from the body part, in order to separate or transect a body part

Body Part	Approach	Device	Qualifier
L Nasal Turbinate	Ø Open 3 Percutaneous 4 Percutaneous Endoscopic 7 Via Natural or Artificial Opening 8 Via Natural or Artificial Opening Endoscopic	Z No Device	Z No Qualifier

Ø: M/S   9: EAR, NOSE, SINUS   7: DILATION   8: DIVISION

SECTION: Ø MEDICAL AND SURGICAL
BODY SYSTEM: 9 EAR, NOSE, SINUS
OPERATION: 9 DRAINAGE: *(on multiple pages)*
　　　　　　　Taking or letting out fluids and/or gases from a body part

Body Part	Approach	Device	Qualifier
Ø External Ear, Right 1 External Ear, Left	Ø Open 3 Percutaneous 4 Percutaneous Endoscopic X External	Ø Drainage Device	Z No Qualifier
Ø External Ear, Right 1 External Ear, Left	Ø Open 3 Percutaneous 4 Percutaneous Endoscopic X External	Z No Device	X Diagnostic Z No Qualifier
3 External Auditory Canal, Right 4 External Auditory Canal, Left K Nasal Mucosa and Soft Tissue	Ø Open 3 Percutaneous 4 Percutaneous Endoscopic 7 Via Natural or Artificial Opening 8 Via Natural or Artificial Opening Endoscopic X External	Ø Drainage Device	Z No Qualifier
3 External Auditory Canal, Right 4 External Auditory Canal, Left K Nasal Mucosa and Soft Tissue	Ø Open 3 Percutaneous 4 Percutaneous Endoscopic 7 Via Natural or Artificial Opening 8 Via Natural or Artificial Opening Endoscopic X External	Z No Device	X Diagnostic Z No Qualifier
5 Middle Ear, Right 6 Middle Ear, Left 9 Auditory Ossicle, Right A Auditory Ossicle, Left D Inner Ear, Right E Inner Ear, Left	Ø Open 7 Via Natural or Artificial Opening 8 Via Natural or Artificial Opening Endoscopic	Ø Drainage Device	Z No Qualifier
5 Middle Ear, Right 6 Middle Ear, Left 9 Auditory Ossicle, Right A Auditory Ossicle, Left D Inner Ear, Right E Inner Ear, Left	Ø Open 7 Via Natural or Artificial Opening 8 Via Natural or Artificial Opening Endoscopic	Z No Device	X Diagnostic Z No Qualifier

Non-OR　Ø99[Ø1][Ø34X]ØZ
Non-OR　Ø99[Ø1][Ø34X]Z[XZ]
Non-OR　Ø99[34][Ø3478X]ØZ
Non-OR　Ø99K[Ø34X]ØZ
Non-OR　Ø99[34][Ø3478X]Z[XZ]
Non-OR　Ø99K[Ø34X]Z[XZ]
Non-OR　Ø99[56]ØZZ

Side margin: 9: DRAINAGE　　9: EAR, NOSE, SINUS　　Ø: M/S

New/Revised Text in Green　~~deleted~~ Deleted　♀ Females Only　♂ Males Only　**Coding Clinic**
🔖 Non-covered　🔖 Limited Coverage　⊟ Combination (See Appendix E)　DRG Non-OR　Non-OR　🔖 Hospital-Acquired Condition

SECTION: Ø MEDICAL AND SURGICAL
BODY SYSTEM: 9 EAR, NOSE, SINUS
OPERATION: 9 DRAINAGE: *(continued)*
Taking or letting out fluids and/or gases from a body part

Body Part	Approach	Device	Qualifier
7 Tympanic Membrane, Right 8 Tympanic Membrane, Left B Mastoid Sinus, Right C Mastoid Sinus, Left F Eustachian Tube, Right G Eustachian Tube, Left L Nasal Turbinate M Nasal Septum N Nasopharynx P Accessory Sinus Q Maxillary Sinus, Right R Maxillary Sinus, Left S Frontal Sinus, Right T Frontal Sinus, Left U Ethmoid Sinus, Right V Ethmoid Sinus, Left W Sphenoid Sinus, Right X Sphenoid Sinus, Left	Ø Open 3 Percutaneous 4 Percutaneous Endoscopic 7 Via Natural or Artificial Opening 8 Via Natural or Artificial Opening Endoscopic	Ø Drainage Device	Z No Qualifier
7 Tympanic Membrane, Right 8 Tympanic Membrane, Left B Mastoid Sinus, Right C Mastoid Sinus, Left F Eustachian Tube, Right G Eustachian Tube, Left L Nasal Turbinate M Nasal Septum N Nasopharynx P Accessory Sinus Q Maxillary Sinus, Right R Maxillary Sinus, Left S Frontal Sinus, Right T Frontal Sinus, Left U Ethmoid Sinus, Right V Ethmoid Sinus, Left W Sphenoid Sinus, Right X Sphenoid Sinus, Left	Ø Open 3 Percutaneous 4 Percutaneous Endoscopic 7 Via Natural or Artificial Opening 8 Via Natural or Artificial Opening Endoscopic	Z No Device	X Diagnostic Z No Qualifier

Non-OR Ø99[FGL][Ø3478]ØZ
Non-OR Ø99N3ØZ
Non-OR Ø99[78FG][Ø3478]ZZ
Non-OR Ø99L[Ø3478]Z[XZ]
Non-OR Ø99N[Ø3478]ZX
Non-OR Ø99N3ZZ

Non-OR Ø99[BC]3ØZ
Non-OR Ø99M[Ø34]ØZ
Non-OR Ø99[PQRSTUVWX][34]ØZ
Non-OR Ø99[BC]3ZZ
Non-OR Ø99M[Ø34]Z[XZ]
Non-OR Ø99[PQRSTUVWX][34]Z[XZ]

New/Revised Text in Green ~~deleted~~ Deleted ♀ Females Only ♂ Males Only **Coding Clinic**
Non-covered Limited Coverage ⊞ Combination (See Appendix E) DRG Non-OR Non-OR Hospital-Acquired Condition

B: EXCISION

9: EAR, NOSE, SINUS

0: M/S

SECTION: Ø MEDICAL AND SURGICAL
BODY SYSTEM: 9 EAR, NOSE, SINUS
OPERATION: B EXCISION: Cutting out or off, without replacement, a portion of a body part

Body Part	Approach	Device	Qualifier
Ø External Ear, Right 1 External Ear, Left	Ø Open 3 Percutaneous 4 Percutaneous Endoscopic X External	Z No Device	X Diagnostic Z No Qualifier

3 External Auditory Canal, Right
4 External Auditory Canal, Left
	Ø Open
	3 Percutaneous
	4 Percutaneous Endoscopic
	7 Via Natural or Artificial
	   Opening
	8 Via Natural or Artificial
	   Opening Endoscopic
	X External
		Z No Device	X Diagnostic
			Z No Qualifier

5 Middle Ear, Right 6 Middle Ear, Left 9 Auditory Ossicle, Right A Auditory Ossicle, Left D Inner Ear, Right E Inner Ear, Left	Ø Open 8 Via Natural or Artificial Opening Endoscopic	Z No Device	X Diagnostic Z No Qualifier

7 Tympanic Membrane, Right
8 Tympanic Membrane, Left
F Eustachian Tube, Right
G Eustachian Tube, Left
L Nasal Turbinate
N Nasopharynx
	Ø Open
	3 Percutaneous
	4 Percutaneous Endoscopic
	7 Via Natural or Artificial
	   Opening
	8 Via Natural or Artificial
	   Opening Endoscopic
		Z No Device	X Diagnostic
			Z No Qualifier

B Mastoid Sinus, Right C Mastoid Sinus, Left M Nasal Septum P Accessory Sinus Q Maxillary Sinus, Right R Maxillary Sinus, Left S Frontal Sinus, Right T Frontal Sinus, Left U Ethmoid Sinus, Right V Ethmoid Sinus, Left W Sphenoid Sinus, Right X Sphenoid Sinus, Left	Ø Open 3 Percutaneous 4 Percutaneous Endoscopic 8 Via Natural or Artificial Opening Endoscopic	Z No Device	X Diagnostic Z No Qualifier
K Nasal Mucosa and Soft Tissue	Ø Open 3 Percutaneous 4 Percutaneous Endoscopic 8 Via Natural or Artificial Opening Endoscopic X External	Z No Device	X Diagnostic Z No Qualifier

Non-OR   09B[Ø1][Ø34X]Z[XZ]
Non-OR   09B[34][Ø3478X]Z[XZ]
Non-OR   09B[FG][Ø3478]Z[XZ]
Non-OR   09B[LN][Ø3478]ZX
Non-OR   09BM[Ø34]ZX
Non-OR   09B[PQRSTUVWX][34]ZX
Non-OR   09BK[Ø34X]Z[XZ]

New/Revised Text in Green   ~~deleted~~ Deleted   ♀ Females Only   ♂ Males Only   **Coding Clinic**
   Non-covered   Limited Coverage   ⊡ Combination (See Appendix E)   DRG Non-OR   Non-OR   Hospital-Acquired Condition

SECTION: 0 MEDICAL AND SURGICAL
BODY SYSTEM: 9 EAR, NOSE, SINUS
OPERATION: C EXTIRPATION: Taking or cutting out solid matter from a body part

Body Part	Approach	Device	Qualifier
0 External Ear, Right 1 External Ear, Left	0 Open 3 Percutaneous 4 Percutaneous Endoscopic X External	Z No Device	Z No Qualifier
3 External Auditory Canal, Right 4 External Auditory Canal, Left	0 Open 3 Percutaneous 4 Percutaneous Endoscopic 7 Via Natural or Artificial Opening 8 Via Natural or Artificial Opening Endoscopic X External	Z No Device	Z No Qualifier
5 Middle Ear, Right 6 Middle Ear, Left 9 Auditory Ossicle, Right A Auditory Ossicle, Left D Inner Ear, Right E Inner Ear, Left	0 Open 8 Via Natural or Artificial Opening Endoscopic	Z No Device	Z No Qualifier
7 Tympanic Membrane, Right 8 Tympanic Membrane, Left F Eustachian Tube, Right G Eustachian Tube, Left L Nasal Turbinate N Nasopharynx	0 Open 3 Percutaneous 4 Percutaneous Endoscopic 7 Via Natural or Artificial Opening 8 Via Natural or Artificial Opening Endoscopic	Z No Device	Z No Qualifier
B Mastoid Sinus, Right C Mastoid Sinus, Left M Nasal Septum P Accessory Sinus Q Maxillary Sinus, Right R Maxillary Sinus, Left S Frontal Sinus, Right T Frontal Sinus, Left U Ethmoid Sinus, Right V Ethmoid Sinus, Left W Sphenoid Sinus, Right X Sphenoid Sinus, Left	0 Open 3 Percutaneous 4 Percutaneous Endoscopic 8 Via Natural or Artificial Opening Endoscopic	Z No Device	Z No Qualifier
K Nasal Mucosa and Soft Tissue	0 Open 3 Percutaneous 4 Percutaneous Endoscopic 8 Via Natural or Artificial Opening Endoscopic X External	Z No Device	Z No Qualifier

Non-OR 09C[01][034X]ZZ
Non-OR 09C[34][03478X]ZZ
Non-OR 09C[78FGL][03478]ZZ
Non-OR 09CM[034]ZZ
Non-OR 09BK[034X]ZZ

SECTION: Ø MEDICAL AND SURGICAL
BODY SYSTEM: 9 EAR, NOSE, SINUS
OPERATION: D EXTRACTION: Pulling or stripping out or off all or a portion of a body part by the use of force

Body Part	Approach	Device	Qualifier
7 Tympanic Membrane, Right 8 Tympanic Membrane, Left L Nasal Turbinate	Ø Open 3 Percutaneous 4 Percutaneous Endoscopic 7 Via Natural or Artificial Opening 8 Via Natural or Artificial Opening Endoscopic	Z No Device	Z No Qualifier
9 Auditory Ossicle, Right A Auditory Ossicle, Left	Ø Open	Z No Device	Z No Qualifier
B Mastoid Sinus, Right C Mastoid Sinus, Left M Nasal Septum P Accessory Sinus Q Maxillary Sinus, Right R Maxillary Sinus, Left S Frontal Sinus, Right T Frontal Sinus, Left U Ethmoid Sinus, Right V Ethmoid Sinus, Left W Sphenoid Sinus, Right X Sphenoid Sinus, Left	Ø Open 3 Percutaneous 4 Percutaneous Endoscopic	Z No Device	Z No Qualifier

SECTION: Ø MEDICAL AND SURGICAL
BODY SYSTEM: 9 EAR, NOSE, SINUS
OPERATION: H INSERTION: Putting in a nonbiological appliance that monitors, assists, performs, or prevents a physiological function but does not physically take the place of a body part

Body Part	Approach	Device	Qualifier
D Inner Ear, Right E Inner Ear, Left	Ø Open 3 Percutaneous 4 Percutaneous Endoscopic	4 Hearing Device, Bone Conduction 5 Hearing Device, Single Channel Cochlear Prosthesis 6 Hearing Device, Multiple Channel Cochlear Prosthesis S Hearing Device	Z No Qualifier
H Ear, Right J Ear, Left K Nasal Mucosa and Soft Tissue Y Sinus	Ø Open 3 Percutaneous 4 Percutaneous Endoscopic 7 Via Natural or Artificial Opening 8 Via Natural or Artificial Opening Endoscopic	Y Other Device	Z No Qualifier
N Nasopharynx	7 Via Natural or Artificial Opening 8 Via Natural or Artificial Opening Endoscopic	B Intraluminal Device, Airway	Z No Qualifier

Non-OR Ø9HN[78]BZ

Side tab: **D: EXTRACTION   H: INSERTION**
Side tab: **9: EAR, NOSE, SINUS   Ø: M/S**

SECTION: Ø MEDICAL AND SURGICAL
BODY SYSTEM: 9 EAR, NOSE, SINUS
OPERATION: J INSPECTION: Visually and/or manually exploring a body part

Body Part	Approach	Device	Qualifier
7 Tympanic Membrane, Right 8 Tympanic Membrane, Left H Ear, Right J Ear, Left	Ø Open 3 Percutaneous 4 Percutaneous Endoscopic 7 Via Natural or Artificial Opening 8 Via Natural or Artificial Opening Endoscopic X External	Z No Device	Z No Qualifier
D Inner Ear, Right E Inner Ear, Left K Nasal Mucosa and Soft Tissue Y Sinus	Ø Open 3 Percutaneous 4 Percutaneous Endoscopic 8 Via Natural or Artificial Opening Endoscopic X External	Z No Device	Z No Qualifier

Non-OR Ø9J[78][378X]ZZ
Non-OR Ø9J[HJ][Ø3478X]ZZ
Non-OR Ø9J[DE][3X]ZZ
Non-OR Ø9J[KY][Ø34X]ZZ

SECTION: Ø MEDICAL AND SURGICAL
BODY SYSTEM: 9 EAR, NOSE, SINUS
OPERATION: M REATTACHMENT: Putting back in or on all or a portion of a separated body part to its normal location or other suitable location

Body Part	Approach	Device	Qualifier
Ø External Ear, Right 1 External Ear, Left K Nasal Mucosa and Soft Tissue	X External	Z No Device	Z No Qualifier

New/Revised Text in Green ~~deleted~~ Deleted ♀ Females Only ♂ Males Only **Coding Clinic**

Non-covered Limited Coverage Combination (See Appendix E) DRG Non-OR Non-OR Hospital-Acquired Condition

SECTION: Ø MEDICAL AND SURGICAL

BODY SYSTEM: 9 EAR, NOSE, SINUS

OPERATION: N RELEASE: Freeing a body part from an abnormal physical constraint

Body Part	Approach	Device	Qualifier
Ø External Ear, Right 1 External Ear, Left	Ø Open 3 Percutaneous 4 Percutaneous Endoscopic X External	Z No Device	Z No Qualifier
3 External Auditory Canal, Right 4 External Auditory Canal, Left	Ø Open 3 Percutaneous 4 Percutaneous Endoscopic 7 Via Natural or Artificial Opening 8 Via Natural or Artificial Opening Endoscopic X External	Z No Device	Z No Qualifier
5 Middle Ear, Right 6 Middle Ear, Left 9 Auditory Ossicle, Right A Auditory Ossicle, Left D Inner Ear, Right E Inner Ear, Left	Ø Open 8 Via Natural or Artificial Opening Endoscopic	Z No Device	Z No Qualifier
7 Tympanic Membrane, Right 8 Tympanic Membrane, Left F Eustachian Tube, Right G Eustachian Tube, Left L Nasal Turbinate N Nasopharynx	Ø Open 3 Percutaneous 4 Percutaneous Endoscopic 7 Via Natural or Artificial Opening 8 Via Natural or Artificial Opening Endoscopic	Z No Device	Z No Qualifier
B Mastoid Sinus, Right C Mastoid Sinus, Left M Nasal Septum P Accessory Sinus Q Maxillary Sinus, Right R Maxillary Sinus, Left S Frontal Sinus, Right T Frontal Sinus, Left U Ethmoid Sinus, Right V Ethmoid Sinus, Left W Sphenoid Sinus, Right X Sphenoid Sinus, Left	Ø Open 3 Percutaneous 4 Percutaneous Endoscopic 8 Via Natural or Artificial Opening Endoscopic	Z No Device	Z No Qualifier
K Nasal Mucosa and Soft Tissue	Ø Open 3 Percutaneous 4 Percutaneous Endoscopic 8 Via Natural or Artificial Opening Endoscopic X External	Z No Device	Z No Qualifier

Non-OR 09N[FGL][03478]ZZ
Non-OR 09NM[034]ZZ
Non-OR 09NK[034X]ZZ

SECTION: Ø MEDICAL AND SURGICAL
BODY SYSTEM: 9 EAR, NOSE, SINUS
OPERATION: P REMOVAL: Taking out or off a device from a body part

Body Part	Approach	Device	Qualifier
7 Tympanic Membrane, Right 8 Tympanic Membrane, Left	Ø Open 7 Via Natural or Artificial Opening 8 Via Natural or Artificial Opening Endoscopic X External	Ø Drainage Device	Z No Qualifier
D Inner Ear, Right E Inner Ear, Left	Ø Open 7 Via Natural or Artificial Opening 8 Via Natural or Artificial Opening Endoscopic	S Hearing Device	Z No Qualifier
H Ear, Right J Ear, Left K Nasal Mucosa and Soft Tissue	Ø Open 3 Percutaneous 4 Percutaneous Endoscopic 7 Via Natural or Artificial Opening 8 Via Natural or Artificial Opening Endoscopic	Ø Drainage Device 7 Autologous Tissue Substitute D Intraluminal Device J Synthetic Substitute K Nonautologous Tissue Substitute Y Other Device	Z No Qualifier
H Ear, Right J Ear, Left K Nasal Mucosa and Soft Tissue	X External	Ø Drainage Device 7 Autologous Tissue Substitute D Intraluminal Device J Synthetic Substitute K Nonautologous Tissue Substitute	Z No Qualifier
Y Sinus	Ø Open 3 Percutaneous 4 Percutaneous Endoscopic	Ø Drainage Device Y Other Device	Z No Qualifier
Y Sinus	7 Via Natural or Artificial Opening 8 Via Natural or Artificial Opening Endoscopic	Y Other Device	Z No Qualifier
Y Sinus	X External	Ø Drainage Device	Z No Qualifier

Non-OR Ø9P[78][Ø78X]ØZ
Non-OR Ø9P[HJ][34][ØJK]Z
Non-OR Ø9P[HJ][78][ØD]Z
Non-OR Ø9P[HJ]X[Ø7DJK]Z
Non-OR Ø9PK[Ø3478][Ø7DJK]Z
Non-OR Ø9PYXØZ
Non-OR Ø9PKX[Ø7DJK]Z

SECTION: Ø MEDICAL AND SURGICAL

BODY SYSTEM: 9 EAR, NOSE, SINUS
OPERATION: Q REPAIR: Restoring, to the extent possible, a body part to its normal anatomic structure and function

Body Part	Approach	Device	Qualifier
Ø External Ear, Right 1 External Ear, Left 2 External Ear, Bilateral	Ø Open 3 Percutaneous 4 Percutaneous Endoscopic X External	Z No Device	Z No Qualifier
3 External Auditory Canal, Right 4 External Auditory Canal, Left F Eustachian Tube, Right G Eustachian Tube, Left	Ø Open 3 Percutaneous 4 Percutaneous Endoscopic 7 Via Natural or Artificial Opening 8 Via Natural or Artificial Opening Endoscopic X External	Z No Device	Z No Qualifier
5 Middle Ear, Right 6 Middle Ear, Left 9 Auditory Ossicle, Right A Auditory Ossicle, Left D Inner Ear, Right E Inner Ear, Left	Ø Open 8 Via Natural or Artificial Opening Endoscopic	Z No Device	Z No Qualifier
7 Tympanic Membrane, Right 8 Tympanic Membrane, Left L Nasal Turbinate N Nasopharynx	Ø Open 3 Percutaneous 4 Percutaneous Endoscopic 7 Via Natural or Artificial Opening 8 Via Natural or Artificial Opening Endoscopic	Z No Device	Z No Qualifier
B Mastoid Sinus, Right C Mastoid Sinus, Left M Nasal Septum P Accessory Sinus Q Maxillary Sinus, Right R Maxillary Sinus, Left S Frontal Sinus, Right T Frontal Sinus, Left U Ethmoid Sinus, Right V Ethmoid Sinus, Left W Sphenoid Sinus, Right X Sphenoid Sinus, Left	Ø Open 3 Percutaneous 4 Percutaneous Endoscopic 8 Via Natural or Artificial Opening Endoscopic	Z No Device	Z No Qualifier
K Nasal Mucosa and Soft Tissue	Ø Open 3 Percutaneous 4 Percutaneous Endoscopic 8 Via Natural or Artificial Opening Endoscopic X External	Z No Device	Z No Qualifier

Non-OR 09Q[Ø12]XZZ
Non-OR 09Q[34]XZZ
Non-OR 09Q[FG][Ø3478X]ZZ

Q: REPAIR   **9: EAR, NOSE, SINUS**   **Ø: M/S**

New/Revised Text in Green   deleted Deleted   ♀ Females Only   ♂ Males Only   **Coding Clinic**
Non-covered   Limited Coverage   ⊕ Combination (See Appendix E)   DRG Non-OR   Non-OR   Hospital-Acquired Condition

SECTION: Ø MEDICAL AND SURGICAL
BODY SYSTEM: 9 EAR, NOSE, SINUS
OPERATION: R REPLACEMENT: Putting in or on biological or synthetic material that physically takes the place and/or function of all or a portion of a body part

Body Part	Approach	Device	Qualifier
Ø External Ear, Right 1 External Ear, Left 2 External Ear, Bilateral K Nasal Mucosa and Soft Tissue	Ø Open X External	7 Autologous Tissue Substitute J Synthetic Substitute K Nonautologous Tissue Substitute	Z No Qualifier
5 Middle Ear, Right 6 Middle Ear, Left 9 Auditory Ossicle, Right A Auditory Ossicle, Left D Inner Ear, Right E Inner Ear, Left	Ø Open	7 Autologous Tissue Substitute J Synthetic Substitute K Nonautologous Tissue Substitute	Z No Qualifier
7 Tympanic Membrane, Right 8 Tympanic Membrane, Left N Nasopharynx	Ø Open 7 Via Natural or Artificial Opening 8 Via Natural or Artificial Opening Endoscopic	7 Autologous Tissue Substitute J Synthetic Substitute K Nonautologous Tissue Substitute	Z No Qualifier
L Nasal Turbinate	Ø Open 3 Percutaneous 4 Percutaneous Endoscopic 7 Via Natural or Artificial Opening 8 Via Natural or Artificial Opening Endoscopic	7 Autologous Tissue Substitute J Synthetic Substitute K Nonautologous Tissue Substitute	Z No Qualifier
M Nasal Septum	Ø Open 3 Percutaneous 4 Percutaneous Endoscopic	7 Autologous Tissue Substitute J Synthetic Substitute K Nonautologous Tissue Substitute	Z No Qualifier

SECTION: Ø MEDICAL AND SURGICAL
BODY SYSTEM: 9 EAR, NOSE, SINUS
OPERATION: S REPOSITION: Moving to its normal location, or other suitable location, all or a portion of a body part

Body Part	Approach	Device	Qualifier
Ø External Ear, Right 1 External Ear, Left 2 External Ear, Bilateral K Nasal Mucosa and Soft Tissue	Ø Open 4 Percutaneous Endoscopic X External	Z No Device	Z No Qualifier
7 Tympanic Membrane, Right 8 Tympanic Membrane, Left F Eustachian Tube, Right G Eustachian Tube, Left L Nasal Turbinate	Ø Open 4 Percutaneous Endoscopic 7 Via Natural or Artificial Opening 8 Via Natural or Artificial Opening Endoscopic	Z No Device	Z No Qualifier
9 Auditory Ossicle, Right A Auditory Ossicle, Left M Nasal Septum	Ø Open 4 Percutaneous Endoscopic	Z No Device	Z No Qualifier

Non-OR   Ø9S[FG][Ø478]ZZ

S: REPOSITION

9: EAR, NOSE, SINUS

Ø: M/S

SECTION: Ø MEDICAL AND SURGICAL
BODY SYSTEM: 9 EAR, NOSE, SINUS
OPERATION: T RESECTION: Cutting out or off, without replacement, all of a body part

Body Part	Approach	Device	Qualifier
Ø External Ear, Right 1 External Ear, Left	Ø Open 4 Percutaneous Endoscopic X External	Z No Device	Z No Qualifier
5 Middle Ear, Right 6 Middle Ear, Left 9 Auditory Ossicle, Right A Auditory Ossicle, Left D Inner Ear, Right E Inner Ear, Left	Ø Open 8 Via Natural or Artificial Opening Endoscopic	Z No Device	Z No Qualifier
7 Tympanic Membrane, Right 8 Tympanic Membrane, Left F Eustachian Tube, Right G Eustachian Tube, Left L Nasal Turbinate N Nasopharynx	Ø Open 4 Percutaneous Endoscopic 7 Via Natural or Artificial Opening 8 Via Natural or Artificial Opening Endoscopic	Z No Device	Z No Qualifier
B Mastoid Sinus, Right C Mastoid Sinus, Left M Nasal Septum P Accessory Sinus Q Maxillary Sinus, Right R Maxillary Sinus, Left S Frontal Sinus, Right T Frontal Sinus, Left U Ethmoid Sinus, Right V Ethmoid Sinus, Left W Sphenoid Sinus, Right X Sphenoid Sinus, Left	Ø Open 4 Percutaneous Endoscopic 8 Via Natural or Artificial Opening Endoscopic	Z No Device	Z No Qualifier
K Nasal Mucosa and Soft Tissue	Ø Open 4 Percutaneous Endoscopic 8 Via Natural or Artificial Opening Endoscopic X External	Z No Device	Z No Qualifier

Non-OR 09T[FG][0478]ZZ

New/Revised Text in Green   ~~deleted~~ Deleted   ♀ Females Only   ♂ Males Only   **Coding Clinic**
Non-covered   Limited Coverage   Combination (See Appendix E)   DRG Non-OR   Non-OR   Hospital-Acquired Condition

SECTION: Ø MEDICAL AND SURGICAL

BODY SYSTEM: 9 EAR, NOSE, SINUS

OPERATION: U SUPPLEMENT: Putting in or on biological or synthetic material that physically reinforces and/or augments the function of a portion of a body part

U: SUPPLEMENT

9: EAR, NOSE, SINUS

Ø: M/S

Body Part	Approach	Device	Qualifier
Ø External Ear, Right 1 External Ear, Left 2 External Ear, Bilateral	Ø Open X External	7 Autologous Tissue Substitute J Synthetic Substitute K Nonautologous Tissue Substitute	Z No Qualifier
5 Middle Ear, Right 6 Middle Ear, Left 9 Auditory Ossicle, Right A Auditory Ossicle, Left D Inner Ear, Right E Inner Ear, Left	Ø Open 8 Via Natural or Artificial Opening Endoscopic	7 Autologous Tissue Substitute J Synthetic Substitute K Nonautologous Tissue Substitute	Z No Qualifier
7 Tympanic Membrane, Right 8 Tympanic Membrane, Left N Nasopharynx	Ø Open 7 Via Natural or Artificial Opening 8 Via Natural or Artificial Opening Endoscopic	7 Autologous Tissue Substitute J Synthetic Substitute K Nonautologous Tissue Substitute	Z No Qualifier
K Nasal Mucosa and Soft Tissue	Ø Open 8 Via Natural or Artificial Opening Endoscopic X External	7 Autologous Tissue Substitute J Synthetic Substitute K Nonautologous Tissue Substitute	Z No Qualifier
L Nasal Turbinate	Ø Open 3 Percutaneous 4 Percutaneous Endoscopic 7 Via Natural or Artificial Opening 8 Via Natural or Artificial Opening Endoscopic	7 Autologous Tissue Substitute J Synthetic Substitute K Nonautologous Tissue Substitute	Z No Qualifier
M Nasal Septum	Ø Open 3 Percutaneous 4 Percutaneous Endoscopic 8 Via Natural or Artificial Opening Endoscopic	7 Autologous Tissue Substitute J Synthetic Substitute K Nonautologous Tissue Substitute	Z No Qualifier

SECTION: Ø MEDICAL AND SURGICAL
BODY SYSTEM: 9 EAR, NOSE, SINUS
OPERATION: W REVISION: Correcting, to the extent possible, a portion of a malfunctioning device or the position of a displaced device

Body Part	Approach	Device	Qualifier
7 Tympanic Membrane, Right 8 Tympanic Membrane, Left 9 Auditory Ossicle, Right A Auditory Ossicle, Left	Ø Open 7 Via Natural or Artificial Opening 8 Via Natural or Artificial Opening Endoscopic	7 Autologous Tissue Substitute J Synthetic Substitute K Nonautologous Tissue Substitute	Z No Qualifier
D Inner Ear, Right E Inner Ear, Left	Ø Open 7 Via Natural or Artificial Opening 8 Via Natural or Artificial Opening Endoscopic	S Hearing Device	Z No Qualifier
H Ear, Right J Ear, Left K Nasal Mucosa and Soft Tissue	Ø Open 3 Percutaneous 4 Percutaneous Endoscopic 7 Via Natural or Artificial Opening 8 Via Natural or Artificial Opening Endoscopic	Ø Drainage Device 7 Autologous Tissue Substitute D Intraluminal Device J Synthetic Substitute K Nonautologous Tissue Substitute Y Other Device	Z No Qualifier
H Ear, Right J Ear, Left K Nasal Mucosa and Soft Tissue	X External	Ø Drainage Device 7 Autologous Tissue Substitute D Intraluminal Device J Synthetic Substitute K Nonautologous Tissue Substitute	Z No Qualifier
Y Sinus	Ø Open 3 Percutaneous 4 Percutaneous Endoscopic	Ø Drainage Device Y Other Device	Z No Qualifier
Y Sinus	7 Via Natural or Artificial Opening 8 Via Natural or Artificial Opening Endoscopic	Y Other Device	Z No Qualifier
Y Sinus	X External	Ø Drainage Device	Z No Qualifier

Non-OR 09W[HJ][34][JK]Z
Non-OR 09W[HJ][78]DZ
Non-OR 09W[HJ]X[Ø7DJK]Z
Non-OR 09WK[Ø3478][Ø7DJK]Z
Non-OR 09WYXØZ
Non-OR 09QKX[Ø7DJK]Z

SECTION: Ø MEDICAL AND SURGICAL

BODY SYSTEM: B RESPIRATORY SYSTEM

OPERATION: 1 BYPASS: Altering the route of passage of the contents of a tubular body part

Body Part	Approach	Device	Qualifier
1 Trachea	Ø Open	D Intraluminal Device	6 Esophagus
1 Trachea	Ø Open	F Tracheostomy Device Z No Device	4 Cutaneous
1 Trachea	3 Percutaneous 4 Percutaneous Endoscopic	F Tracheostomy Device Z No Device	4 Cutaneous

DRG Non-OR ØB113[FZ]4
Non-OR ØB110D6

SECTION: Ø MEDICAL AND SURGICAL

BODY SYSTEM: B RESPIRATORY SYSTEM

OPERATION: 2 CHANGE: Taking out or off a device from a body part and putting back an identical or similar device in or on the same body part without cutting or puncturing the skin or a mucous membrane

Body Part	Approach	Device	Qualifier
Ø Tracheobronchial Tree K Lung, Right L Lung, Left Q Pleura T Diaphragm	X External	Ø Drainage Device Y Other Device	Z No Qualifier
1 Trachea	X External	Ø Drainage Device E Intraluminal Device, Endotracheal Airway F Tracheostomy Device Y Other Device	Z No Qualifier

Non-OR All Values

New/Revised Text in Green   ~~deleted~~ Deleted   ♀ Females Only   ♂ Males Only   **Coding Clinic**

Non-covered   Limited Coverage   ⊡ Combination (See Appendix E)   DRG Non-OR   Non-OR   Hospital-Acquired Condition

SECTION: Ø MEDICAL AND SURGICAL
BODY SYSTEM: B RESPIRATORY SYSTEM
OPERATION: 5 **DESTRUCTION:** Physical eradication of all or a portion of a body part by the direct use of energy, force, or a destructive agent

Body Part	Approach	Device	Qualifier
1 Trachea 2 Carina 3 Main Bronchus, Right 4 Upper Lobe Bronchus, Right 5 Middle Lobe Bronchus, Right 6 Lower Lobe Bronchus, Right 7 Main Bronchus, Left 8 Upper Lobe Bronchus, Left 9 Lingula Bronchus B Lower Lobe Bronchus, Left C Upper Lung Lobe, Right D Middle Lung Lobe, Right F Lower Lung Lobe, Right G Upper Lung Lobe, Left H Lung Lingula J Lower Lung Lobe, Left K Lung, Right L Lung, Left M Lungs, Bilateral	Ø Open 3 Percutaneous 4 Percutaneous Endoscopic 7 Via Natural or Artificial Opening 8 Via Natural or Artificial Opening Endoscopic	Z No Device	Z No Qualifier
N Pleura, Right P Pleura, Left T Diaphragm	Ø Open 3 Percutaneous 4 Percutaneous Endoscopic	Z No Device	Z No Qualifier

Non-OR   ØB5[3456789B]4ZZ
Non-OR   ØB5[CDFGHJKLM]8ZZ

Coding Clinic: 2016, Q2, P18 – ØB5[PS]ØZZ

SECTION: Ø MEDICAL AND SURGICAL
BODY SYSTEM: B RESPIRATORY SYSTEM
OPERATION: 7 **DILATION:** Expanding an orifice or the lumen of a tubular body part

Body Part	Approach	Device	Qualifier
1 Trachea 2 Carina 3 Main Bronchus, Right 4 Upper Lobe Bronchus, Right 5 Middle Lobe Bronchus, Right 6 Lower Lobe Bronchus, Right 7 Main Bronchus, Left 8 Upper Lobe Bronchus, Left 9 Lingula Bronchus B Lower Lobe Bronchus, Left	Ø Open 3 Percutaneous 4 Percutaneous Endoscopic 7 Via Natural or Artificial Opening 8 Via Natural or Artificial Opening Endoscopic	D Intraluminal Device Z No Device	Z No Qualifier

Non-OR   ØB5[3456789B][03478][DZ]Z

SECTION: Ø MEDICAL AND SURGICAL
BODY SYSTEM: B RESPIRATORY SYSTEM
OPERATION: 9 DRAINAGE: *(on multiple pages)*
Taking or letting out fluids and/or gases from a body part

Body Part	Approach	Device	Qualifier
1 Trachea 2 Carina 3 Main Bronchus, Right 4 Upper Lobe Bronchus, Right 5 Middle Lobe Bronchus, Right 6 Lower Lobe Bronchus, Right 7 Main Bronchus, Left 8 Upper Lobe Bronchus, Left 9 Lingula Bronchus B Lower Lobe Bronchus, Left C Upper Lung Lobe, Right D Middle Lung Lobe, Right F Lower Lung Lobe, Right G Upper Lung Lobe, Left H Lung Lingula J Lower Lung Lobe, Left K Lung, Right L Lung, Left M Lungs, Bilateral	Ø Open 3 Percutaneous 4 Percutaneous Endoscopic 7 Via Natural or Artificial Opening 8 Via Natural or Artificial Opening Endoscopic	Ø Drainage Device	Z No Qualifier
1 Trachea 2 Carina 3 Main Bronchus, Right 4 Upper Lobe Bronchus, Right 5 Middle Lobe Bronchus, Right 6 Lower Lobe Bronchus, Right 7 Main Bronchus, Left 8 Upper Lobe Bronchus, Left 9 Lingula Bronchus B Lower Lobe Bronchus, Left C Upper Lung Lobe, Right D Middle Lung Lobe, Right F Lower Lung Lobe, Right G Upper Lung Lobe, Left H Lung Lingula J Lower Lung Lobe, Left K Lung, Right L Lung, Left M Lungs, Bilateral	Ø Open 3 Percutaneous 4 Percutaneous Endoscopic 7 Via Natural or Artificial Opening 8 Via Natural or Artificial Opening Endoscopic	Z No Device	X Diagnostic Z No Qualifier
N Pleura, Right P Pleura, Left	Ø Open 3 Percutaneous 4 Percutaneous Endoscopic 8 Via Natural or Artificial Opening Endoscopic	Ø Drainage Device	Z No Qualifier

DRG Non-OR ØB9[123456789B][78]ØZ *(proposed)*
DRG Non-OR ØB9[123456789B][78]ZZ *(proposed)*
Non-OR ØB9[123456789B][3478]ZX
Non-OR ØB9[CDFGHJKLM][347]ZX
Non-OR ØB9[NP][Ø3]ØZ

Coding Clinic: 2016, Q1, P26 – ØB948ZX, ØB9B8ZX
Coding Clinic: 2016, Q1, P27 – ØB988ZX
Coding Clinic: 2017, Q1, P51 – ØB9[BJ]8ZX
Coding Clinic: 2017, Q3, P15 – ØB9M8ZZ

New/Revised Text in Green   deleted Deleted   ♀ Females Only   ♂ Males Only   **Coding Clinic**
Non-covered   Limited Coverage   ⊞ Combination (See Appendix E)   DRG Non-OR   Non-OR   Hospital-Acquired Condition

SECTION: Ø MEDICAL AND SURGICAL

BODY SYSTEM: B RESPIRATORY SYSTEM

OPERATION: 9 DRAINAGE: *(continued)*
Taking or letting out fluids and/or gases from a body part

Body Part	Approach	Device	Qualifier
N Pleura, Right P Pleura, Left	Ø Open 3 Percutaneous 4 Percutaneous Endoscopic 8 Via Natural or Artificial Opening Endoscopic	Z No Device	X Diagnostic Z No Qualifier
T Diaphragm	Ø Open 3 Percutaneous 4 Percutaneous Endoscopic	Ø Drainage	Z No Qualifier
T Diaphragm	Ø Open 3 Percutaneous 4 Percutaneous Endoscopic	Z No Device	X Diagnostic Z No Qualifier

Non-OR　ØB9[NP][Ø3]Z[XZ]　　　Non-OR　ØB9[NP]4ZX　　　Non-OR　ØB9T3ZZ

SECTION: Ø MEDICAL AND SURGICAL

BODY SYSTEM: B RESPIRATORY SYSTEM

OPERATION: B EXCISION: Cutting out or off, without replacement, a portion of a body part

Body Part	Approach	Device	Qualifier
1 Trachea 2 Carina 3 Main Bronchus, Right 4 Upper Lobe Bronchus, Right 5 Middle Lobe Bronchus, Right 6 Lower Lobe Bronchus, Right 7 Main Bronchus, Left 8 Upper Lobe Bronchus, Left 9 Lingula Bronchus B Lower Lobe Bronchus, Left C Upper Lung Lobe, Right D Middle Lung Lobe, Right F Lower Lung Lobe, Right G Upper Lung Lobe, Left H Lung Lingula J Lower Lung Lobe, Left K Lung, Right L Lung, Left M Lungs, Bilateral	Ø Open 3 Percutaneous 4 Percutaneous Endoscopic 7 Via Natural or Artificial Opening 8 Via Natural or Artificial Opening Endoscopic	Z No Device	X Diagnostic Z No Qualifier
N Pleura, Right P Pleura, Left	Ø Open 3 Percutaneous 4 Percutaneous Endoscopic 8 Via Natural or Artificial Opening Endoscopic	Z No Device	X Diagnostic Z No Qualifier
T Diaphragm	Ø Open 3 Percutaneous 4 Percutaneous Endoscopic	Z No Device	X Diagnostic Z No Qualifier

Non-OR　ØBB[123456789B][3478]ZX
Non-OR　ØBB[3456789BM][48]ZZ
Non-OR　ØBB[CDFGHJKLM]3ZX

Non-OR　ØBB[CDFGHJKL]8ZZ
Non-OR　ØBB[NP][Ø3]ZX

Coding Clinic: 2015, Q1, P16 – ØBB1ØZZ
Coding Clinic: 2016, Q1, P26 – ØBB48ZX, ØBBC8ZX
Coding Clinic: 2016, Q1, P27 – ØBB88ZX

New/Revised Text in Green　　deleted Deleted　　♀ Females Only　　♂ Males Only　　**Coding Clinic**
🗐 Non-covered　　🗐 Limited Coverage　　⊞ Combination (See Appendix E)　　DRG Non-OR　　Non-OR　　🗐 Hospital-Acquired Condition

Left margin (rotated): 9: DRAINAGE　B: EXCISION　B: RESPIRATORY SYSTEM　Ø: M/S

SECTION: Ø MEDICAL AND SURGICAL

BODY SYSTEM: B RESPIRATORY SYSTEM

OPERATION: C **EXTIRPATION:** Taking or cutting out solid matter from a body part

Body Part	Approach	Device	Qualifier
1 Trachea 2 Carina 3 Main Bronchus, Right 4 Upper Lobe Bronchus, Right 5 Middle Lobe Bronchus, Right 6 Lower Lobe Bronchus, Right 7 Main Bronchus, Left 8 Upper Lobe Bronchus, Left 9 Lingula Bronchus B Lower Lobe Bronchus, Left C Upper Lung Lobe, Right D Middle Lung Lobe, Right F Lower Lung Lobe, Right G Upper Lung Lobe, Left H Lung Lingula J Lower Lung Lobe, Left K Lung, Right L Lung, Left M Lungs, Bilateral	Ø Open 3 Percutaneous 4 Percutaneous Endoscopic 7 Via Natural or Artificial Opening 8 Via Natural or Artificial Opening Endoscopic	Z No Device	Z No Qualifier
N Pleura, Right P Pleura, Left T Diaphragm	Ø Open 3 Percutaneous 4 Percutaneous Endoscopic	Z No Device	Z No Qualifier

Non-OR ØBC[123456789B][78]ZZ
Non-OR ØBC[NP][Ø34]ZZ

Coding Clinic: 2Ø17, Q3, P15 – ØBC58ZZ

SECTION: Ø MEDICAL AND SURGICAL

BODY SYSTEM: B RESPIRATORY SYSTEM

OPERATION: D **EXTRACTION:** Pulling or stripping out or off all or a portion of a body part by the use of force

Body Part	Approach	Device	Qualifier
1 Trachea 2 Carina 3 Main Bronchus, Right 4 Upper Lobe Bronchus, Right 5 Middle Lobe Bronchus, Right 6 Lower Lobe Bronchus, Right 7 Main Bronchus, Left 8 Upper Lobe Bronchus, Left 9 Lingula Bronchus B Lower Lobe Bronchus, Left C Upper Lung Lobe, Right D Middle Lung Lobe, Right F Lower Lung Lobe, Right G Upper Lung Lobe, Left H Lung Lingula J Lower Lung Lobe, Left K Lung, Right L Lung, Left M Lungs, Bilateral	4 Percutaneous Endoscopic 8 Via Natural or Artificial Opening Endoscopic	Z No Device	X Diagnostic
N Pleura, Right P Pleura, Left	Ø Open 3 Percutaneous 4 Percutaneous Endoscopic	Z No Device	X Diagnostic Z No Qualifier

SECTION: Ø MEDICAL AND SURGICAL

BODY SYSTEM: B RESPIRATORY SYSTEM

OPERATION: F FRAGMENTATION: Breaking solid matter in a body part into pieces

Body Part	Approach	Device	Qualifier
1 Trachea 🐾 2 Carina 🐾 3 Main Bronchus, Right 🐾 4 Upper Lobe Bronchus, Right 🐾 5 Middle Lobe Bronchus, Right 🐾 6 Lower Lobe Bronchus, Right 🐾 7 Main Bronchus, Left 🐾 8 Upper Lobe Bronchus, Left 🐾 9 Lingula Bronchus 🐾 B Lower Lobe Bronchus, Left 🐾	Ø Open 3 Percutaneous 4 Percutaneous Endoscopic 7 Via Natural or Artificial Opening 8 Via Natural or Artificial Opening Endoscopic X External	Z No Device	Z No Qualifier

🐾 ØBF[123456789B]XZZ

Non-OR ØBF[123456789B]XZZ

SECTION: Ø MEDICAL AND SURGICAL

BODY SYSTEM: B RESPIRATORY SYSTEM

OPERATION: H INSERTION: *(on multiple pages)*
Putting in a nonbiological appliance that monitors, assists, performs, or prevents a physiological function but does not physically take the place of a body part

Body Part	Approach	Device	Qualifier
Ø Tracheobronchial Tree	Ø Open 3 Percutaneous 4 Percutaneous Endoscopic 7 Via Natural or Artificial Opening 8 Via Natural or Artificial Opening Endoscopic	1 Radioactive Element 2 Monitoring Device 3 Infusion Device D Intraluminal Device Y Other Device	Z No Qualifier
1 Trachea	Ø Open	2 Monitoring Device D Intraluminal Device Y Other Device	Z No Qualifier
1 Trachea	3 Percutaneous	D Intraluminal Device E Intraluminal Device, Endotracheal Airway Y Other Device	Z No Qualifier
1 Trachea	4 Percutaneous Endoscopic	D Intraluminal Device Y Other Device	Z No Qualifier

Non-OR ØBHØ[78][23D]Z

Non-OR ØBH13EZ

New/Revised Text in Green   ~~deleted~~ Deleted   ♀ Females Only   ♂ Males Only   **Coding Clinic**

🐾 Non-covered   🐾 Limited Coverage   ⊞ Combination (See Appendix E)   DRG Non-OR   Non-OR   🐾 Hospital-Acquired Condition

SECTION: Ø MEDICAL AND SURGICAL

BODY SYSTEM: B RESPIRATORY SYSTEM
OPERATION: H INSERTION: *(continued)*

Putting in a nonbiological appliance that monitors, assists, performs, or prevents a physiological function but does not physically take the place of a body part

Body Part	Approach	Device	Qualifier
1 Trachea	7 Via Natural or Artificial Opening 8 Via Natural or Artificial Opening Endoscopic	2 Monitoring Device D Intraluminal Device E Intraluminal Device, Endotracheal Airway Y Other Device	Z No Qualifier
3 Main Bronchus, Right 4 Upper Lobe Bronchus, Right 5 Middle Lobe Bronchus, Right 6 Lower Lobe Bronchus, Right 7 Main Bronchus, Left 8 Upper Lobe Bronchus, Left 9 Lingula Bronchus B Lower Lobe Bronchus, Left	Ø Open 3 Percutaneous 4 Percutaneous Endoscopic 7 Via Natural or Artificial Opening 8 Via Natural or Artificial Opening Endoscopic	G Endobronchial Device, Endobronchial Valve	Z No Qualifier
K Lung, Right L Lung, Left	Ø Open 3 Percutaneous 4 Percutaneous Endoscopic 7 Via Natural or Artificial Opening 8 Via Natural or Artificial Opening Endoscopic	1 Radioactive Element 2 Monitoring Device 3 Infusion Device Y Other Device	Z No Qualifier
Q Pleura	Ø Open 3 Percutaneous 4 Percutaneous Endoscopic 7 Via Natural or Artificial Opening 8 Via Natural or Artificial Opening Endoscopic	Y Other Device	Z No Qualifier
T Diaphragm	Ø Open 3 Percutaneous 4 Percutaneous Endoscopic	2 Monitoring Device M Diaphragmatic Pacemaker Lead Y Other Device	Z No Qualifier
T Diaphragm	7 Via Natural or Artificial Opening 8 Via Natural or Artificial Opening Endoscopic	Y Other Device	Z No Qualifier

Non-OR ØBH1[78]2Z
Non-OR ØBH1[78]EZ
Non-OR ØBH[3456789B]8GZ
Non-OR ØBH[KL][78][23]Z

New/Revised Text in Green ~~deleted~~ Deleted ♀ Females Only ♂ Males Only **Coding Clinic**
Non-covered Limited Coverage ⊞ Combination (See Appendix E) DRG Non-OR Non-OR Hospital-Acquired Condition

213

Ø: M/S

B: RESPIRATORY SYSTEM

H: INSERTION

SECTION: Ø MEDICAL AND SURGICAL
BODY SYSTEM: B RESPIRATORY SYSTEM
OPERATION: J INSPECTION: Visually and/or manually exploring a body part

Body Part	Approach	Device	Qualifier
Ø Tracheobronchial Tree 1 Trachea K Lung, Right L Lung, Left Q Pleura T Diaphragm	Ø Open 3 Percutaneous 4 Percutaneous Endoscopic 7 Via Natural or Artificial Opening 8 Via Natural or Artificial Opening Endoscopic X External	Z No Device	Z No Qualifier

Non-OR ØBJ[ØKL][378X]ZZ
Non-OR ØBJ1[3478X]ZZ
Non-OR ØBJ[QT][378X]ZZ

Coding Clinic: 2Ø15, Q2, P31 – ØBJQ4ZZ

SECTION: Ø MEDICAL AND SURGICAL
BODY SYSTEM: B RESPIRATORY SYSTEM
OPERATION: L OCCLUSION: Completely closing an orifice or the lumen of a tubular body part

Body Part	Approach	Device	Qualifier
1 Trachea 2 Carina 3 Main Bronchus, Right 4 Upper Lobe Bronchus, Right 5 Middle Lobe Bronchus, Right 6 Lower Lobe Bronchus, Right 7 Main Bronchus, Left 8 Upper Lobe Bronchus, Left 9 Lingula Bronchus B Lower Lobe Bronchus, Left	Ø Open 3 Percutaneous 4 Percutaneous Endoscopic	C Extraluminal Device D Intraluminal Device Z No Device	Z No Qualifier
1 Trachea 2 Carina 3 Main Bronchus, Right 4 Upper Lobe Bronchus, Right 5 Middle Lobe Bronchus, Right 6 Lower Lobe Bronchus, Right 7 Main Bronchus, Left 8 Upper Lobe Bronchus, Left 9 Lingula Bronchus B Lower Lobe Bronchus, Left	7 Via Natural or Artificial Opening 8 Via Natural or Artificial Opening Endoscopic	D Intraluminal Device Z No Device	Z No Qualifier

Side tab: J: INSPECTION   L: OCCLUSION   B: RESPIRATORY SYSTEM   Ø: M/S

SECTION: Ø MEDICAL AND SURGICAL

BODY SYSTEM: B RESPIRATORY SYSTEM

OPERATION: M REATTACHMENT: Putting back in or on all or a portion of a separated body part to its normal location or other suitable location

Body Part	Approach	Device	Qualifier
1 Trachea	Ø Open	Z No Device	Z No Qualifier
2 Carina			
3 Main Bronchus, Right			
4 Upper Lobe Bronchus, Right			
5 Middle Lobe Bronchus, Right			
6 Lower Lobe Bronchus, Right			
7 Main Bronchus, Left			
8 Upper Lobe Bronchus, Left			
9 Lingula Bronchus			
B Lower Lobe Bronchus, Left			
C Upper Lung Lobe, Right			
D Middle Lung Lobe, Right			
F Lower Lung Lobe, Right			
G Upper Lung Lobe, Left			
H Lung Lingula			
J Lower Lung Lobe, Left			
K Lung, Right			
L Lung, Left			
T Diaphragm			

SECTION: Ø MEDICAL AND SURGICAL

BODY SYSTEM: B RESPIRATORY SYSTEM

OPERATION: N RELEASE: Freeing a body part from an abnormal physical constraint by cutting or by the use of force

Body Part	Approach	Device	Qualifier
1 Trachea	Ø Open	Z No Device	Z No Qualifier
2 Carina	3 Percutaneous		
3 Main Bronchus, Right	4 Percutaneous Endoscopic		
4 Upper Lobe Bronchus, Right	7 Via Natural or Artificial Opening		
5 Middle Lobe Bronchus, Right	8 Via Natural or Artificial Opening Endoscopic		
6 Lower Lobe Bronchus, Right			
7 Main Bronchus, Left			
8 Upper Lobe Bronchus, Left			
9 Lingula Bronchus			
B Lower Lobe Bronchus, Left			
C Upper Lung Lobe, Right			
D Middle Lung Lobe, Right			
F Lower Lung Lobe, Right			
G Upper Lung Lobe, Left			
H Lung Lingula			
J Lower Lung Lobe, Left			
K Lung, Right			
L Lung, Left			
M Lungs, Bilateral			
N Pleura, Right	Ø Open	Z No Device	Z No Qualifier
P Pleura, Left	3 Percutaneous		
T Diaphragm	4 Percutaneous Endoscopic		

Coding Clinic: 2015, Q3, P15 – ØBN1ØZZ

New/Revised Text in Green   ~~deleted~~ Deleted   ♀ Females Only   ♂ Males Only   **Coding Clinic**
 Non-covered   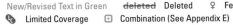 Limited Coverage   ⊡ Combination (See Appendix E)   DRG Non-OR   Non-OR   Hospital-Acquired Condition

215

SECTION: Ø MEDICAL AND SURGICAL
BODY SYSTEM: B RESPIRATORY SYSTEM
OPERATION: P REMOVAL: *(on multiple pages)*
Taking out or off a device from a body part

Body Part	Approach	Device	Qualifier
Ø Tracheobronchial Tree	Ø Open 3 Percutaneous 4 Percutaneous Endoscopic 7 Via Natural or Artificial Opening 8 Via Natural or Artificial Opening Endoscopic	Ø Drainage Device 1 Radioactive Element 2 Monitoring Device 3 Infusion Device 7 Autologous Tissue Substitute C Extraluminal Device D Intraluminal Device J Synthetic Substitute K Nonautologous Tissue Substitute Y Other Device	Z No Qualifier
Ø Tracheobronchial Tree	X External	Ø Drainage Device 1 Radioactive Element 2 Monitoring Device 3 Infusion Device D Intraluminal Device	Z No Qualifier
1 Trachea	Ø Open 3 Percutaneous 4 Percutaneous Endoscopic 7 Via Natural or Artificial Opening 8 Via Natural or Artificial Opening Endoscopic	Ø Drainage Device 2 Monitoring Device 7 Autologous Tissue Substitute C Extraluminal Device D Intraluminal Device F Tracheostomy Device J Synthetic Substitute K Nonautologous Tissue Substitute	Z No Qualifier
1 Trachea	X External	Ø Drainage Device 2 Monitoring Device D Intraluminal Device F Tracheostomy Device	Z No Qualifier
K Lung, Right L Lung, Left	Ø Open 3 Percutaneous 4 Percutaneous Endoscopic 7 Via Natural or Artificial Opening 8 Via Natural or Artificial Opening Endoscopic	Ø Drainage Device 1 Radioactive Element 2 Monitoring Device 3 Infusion Device Y Other Device	Z No Qualifier

Non-OR   ØBPØ[78][Ø23D]Z
Non-OR   ØBPØX[Ø123D]Z
Non-OR   ØBP1[Ø34]FZ
Non-OR   ØBP1[78][Ø2DF]Z
Non-OR   ØBP1X[Ø2DF]Z
Non-OR   ØBP[KL][78][Ø23]Z
Non-OR   ØBP[KL]X[Ø123]Z

P: REMOVAL

B: RESPIRATORY SYSTEM

Ø: M/S

SECTION: Ø MEDICAL AND SURGICAL
BODY SYSTEM: B RESPIRATORY SYSTEM
OPERATION: P REMOVAL: *(continued)*
Taking out or off a device from a body part

Body Part	Approach	Device	Qualifier
K Lung, Right L Lung, Left	X External	Ø Drainage Device 1 Radioactive Element 2 Monitoring Device 3 Infusion Device	Z No Qualifier
Q Pleura	Ø Open 3 Percutaneous 4 Percutaneous Endoscopic 7 Via Natural or Artificial Opening 8 Via Natural or Artificial Opening Endoscopic	Ø Drainage Device 1 Radioactive Element 2 Monitoring Device Y Other Device	Z No Qualifier
Q Pleura	X External	Ø Drainage Device 1 Radioactive Element 2 Monitoring Device	Z No Qualifier
T Diaphragm	Ø Open 3 Percutaneous 4 Percutaneous Endoscopic 7 Via Natural or Artificial Opening 8 Via Natural or Artificial Opening Endoscopic	Ø Drainage Device 2 Monitoring Device 7 Autologous Tissue Substitute J Synthetic Substitute K Nonautologous Tissue Substitute M Diaphragmatic Pacemaker Lead Y Other Device	Z No Qualifier
T Diaphragm	X External	Ø Drainage Device 2 Monitoring Device M Diaphragmatic Pacemaker Lead	Z No Qualifier

Non-OR ØBPQ[Ø3478X][Ø12]Z
Non-OR ØBPQX[Ø12]Z
Non-OR ØBPT[78][Ø2]Z
Non-OR ØBPTX[Ø2M]Z

Ø: M/S

B: RESPIRATORY SYSTEM

P: REMOVAL

SECTION: Ø MEDICAL AND SURGICAL

BODY SYSTEM: B RESPIRATORY SYSTEM

OPERATION: Q **REPAIR:** Restoring, to the extent possible, a body part to its normal anatomic structure and function

Body Part	Approach	Device	Qualifier
1 Trachea 2 Carina 3 Main Bronchus, Right 4 Upper Lobe Bronchus, Right 5 Middle Lobe Bronchus, Right 6 Lower Lobe Bronchus, Right 7 Main Bronchus, Left 8 Upper Lobe Bronchus, Left 9 Lingula Bronchus B Lower Lobe Bronchus, Left C Upper Lung Lobe, Right D Middle Lung Lobe, Right F Lower Lung Lobe, Right G Upper Lung Lobe, Left H Lung Lingula J Lower Lung Lobe, Left K Lung, Right L Lung, Left M Lungs, Bilateral	Ø Open 3 Percutaneous 4 Percutaneous Endoscopic 7 Via Natural or Artificial Opening 8 Via Natural or Artificial Opening Endoscopic	Z No Device	Z No Qualifier
N Pleura, Right P Pleura, Left T Diaphragm	Ø Open 3 Percutaneous 4 Percutaneous Endoscopic	Z No Device	Z No Qualifier

Coding Clinic: 2016, Q2, P23 – ØBQ[RS]ØZZ

SECTION: Ø MEDICAL AND SURGICAL

BODY SYSTEM: B RESPIRATORY SYSTEM

OPERATION: R **REPLACEMENT:** Putting in or on biological or synthetic material that physically takes the place and/or function of all or a portion of a body part

Body Part	Approach	Device	Qualifier
1 Trachea 2 Carina 3 Main Bronchus, Right 4 Upper Lobe Bronchus, Right 5 Middle Lobe Bronchus, Right 6 Lower Lobe Bronchus, Right 7 Main Bronchus, Left 8 Upper Lobe Bronchus, Left 9 Lingula Bronchus B Lower Lobe Bronchus, Left T Diaphragm	Ø Open 4 Percutaneous Endoscopic	7 Autologous Tissue Substitute J Synthetic Substitute K Nonautologous Tissue Substitute	Z No Qualifier

New/Revised Text in Green   ~~deleted~~ Deleted   ♀ Females Only   ♂ Males Only   **Coding Clinic**

Non-covered   Limited Coverage   ⊞ Combination (See Appendix E)   DRG Non-OR   Non-OR   Hospital-Acquired Condition

Q: REPAIR   R: REPLACEMENT

B: RESPIRATORY SYSTEM

Ø: M/S

SECTION: Ø MEDICAL AND SURGICAL

BODY SYSTEM: B RESPIRATORY SYSTEM

OPERATION: S REPOSITION: Moving to its normal location, or other suitable location, all or a portion of a body part

Body Part	Approach	Device	Qualifier
1 Trachea	Ø Open	Z No Device	Z No Qualifier
2 Carina			
3 Main Bronchus, Right			
4 Upper Lobe Bronchus, Right			
5 Middle Lobe Bronchus, Right			
6 Lower Lobe Bronchus, Right			
7 Main Bronchus, Left			
8 Upper Lobe Bronchus, Left			
9 Lingula Bronchus			
B Lower Lobe Bronchus, Left			
C Upper Lung Lobe, Right			
D Middle Lung Lobe, Right			
F Lower Lung Lobe, Right			
G Upper Lung Lobe, Left			
H Lung Lingula			
J Lower Lung Lobe, Left			
K Lung, Right			
L Lung, Left			
T Diaphragm			

SECTION: Ø MEDICAL AND SURGICAL

BODY SYSTEM: B RESPIRATORY SYSTEM

OPERATION: T RESECTION: Cutting out or off, without replacement, all of a body part

Body Part	Approach	Device	Qualifier
1 Trachea	Ø Open	Z No Device	Z No Qualifier
2 Carina	4 Percutaneous Endoscopic		
3 Main Bronchus, Right			
4 Upper Lobe Bronchus, Right			
5 Middle Lobe Bronchus, Right			
6 Lower Lobe Bronchus, Right			
7 Main Bronchus, Left			
8 Upper Lobe Bronchus, Left			
9 Lingula Bronchus			
B Lower Lobe Bronchus, Left			
C Upper Lung Lobe, Right			
D Middle Lung Lobe, Right			
F Lower Lung Lobe, Right			
G Upper Lung Lobe, Left			
H Lung Lingula			
J Lower Lung Lobe, Left			
K Lung, Right			
L Lung, Left			
M Lungs, Bilateral			
T Diaphragm			

SECTION: Ø MEDICAL AND SURGICAL

BODY SYSTEM: B RESPIRATORY SYSTEM

OPERATION: U SUPPLEMENT: Putting in or on biological or synthetic material that physically reinforces and/or augments the function of a portion of a body part

Body Part	Approach	Device	Qualifier
1 Trachea 2 Carina 3 Main Bronchus, Right 4 Upper Lobe Bronchus, Right 5 Middle Lobe Bronchus, Right 6 Lower Lobe Bronchus, Right 7 Main Bronchus, Left 8 Upper Lobe Bronchus, Left 9 Lingula Bronchus B Lower Lobe Bronchus, Left	Ø Open 4 Percutaneous Endoscopic 8 Via Natural or Artificial Opening Endoscopic	7 Autologous Tissue Substitute J Synthetic Substitute K Nonautologous Tissue Substitute	Z No Qualifier
T Diaphragm	Ø Open 4 Percutaneous Endoscopic	7 Autologous Tissue Substitute J Synthetic Substitute K Nonautologous Tissue Substitute	Z No Qualifier

Coding Clinic: 2015, Q1, P28 – ØBU3Ø7Z

SECTION: Ø MEDICAL AND SURGICAL

BODY SYSTEM: B RESPIRATORY SYSTEM

OPERATION: V RESTRICTION: Partially closing an orifice or the lumen of a tubular body part

Body Part	Approach	Device	Qualifier
1 Trachea 2 Carina 3 Main Bronchus, Right 4 Upper Lobe Bronchus, Right 5 Middle Lobe Bronchus, Right 6 Lower Lobe Bronchus, Right 7 Main Bronchus, Left 8 Upper Lobe Bronchus, Left 9 Lingula Bronchus B Lower Lobe Bronchus, Left	Ø Open 3 Percutaneous 4 Percutaneous Endoscopic	C Extraluminal Device D Intraluminal Device Z No Device	Z No Qualifier
1 Trachea 2 Carina 3 Main Bronchus, Right 4 Upper Lobe Bronchus, Right 5 Middle Lobe Bronchus, Right 6 Lower Lobe Bronchus, Right 7 Main Bronchus, Left 8 Upper Lobe Bronchus, Left 9 Lingula Bronchus B Lower Lobe Bronchus, Left	7 Via Natural or Artificial Opening 8 Via Natural or Artificial Opening Endoscopic	D Intraluminal Device Z No Device	Z No Qualifier

SECTION: Ø MEDICAL AND SURGICAL
BODY SYSTEM: B RESPIRATORY SYSTEM
OPERATION: W REVISION: *(on multiple pages)*
Correcting, to the extent possible, a portion of a malfunctioning device or the position of a displaced device

Body Part	Approach	Device	Qualifier
Ø Tracheobronchial Tree	Ø Open 3 Percutaneous 4 Percutaneous Endoscopic 7 Via Natural or Artificial Opening 8 Via Natural or Artificial Opening Endoscopic	Ø Drainage Device 2 Monitoring Device 3 Infusion Device 7 Autologous Tissue Substitute C Extraluminal Device D Intraluminal Device J Synthetic Substitute K Nonautologous Tissue Substitute Y Other Device	Z No Qualifier
Ø Tracheobronchial Tree	X External	Ø Drainage Device 2 Monitoring Device 3 Infusion Device 7 Autologous Tissue Substitute C Extraluminal Device D Intraluminal Device J Synthetic Substitute K Nonautologous Tissue Substitute	Z No Qualifier
1 Trachea	Ø Open 3 Percutaneous 4 Percutaneous Endoscopic 7 Via Natural or Artificial Opening 8 Via Natural or Artificial Opening Endoscopic X External	Ø Drainage Device 2 Monitoring Device 7 Autologous Tissue Substitute C Extraluminal Device D Intraluminal Device F Tracheostomy Device J Synthetic Substitute K Nonautologous Tissue Substitute	Z No Qualifier
K Lung, Right L Lung, Left	Ø Open 3 Percutaneous 4 Percutaneous Endoscopic 7 Via Natural or Artificial Opening 8 Via Natural or Artificial Opening Endoscopic	Ø Drainage Device 2 Monitoring Device 3 Infusion Device Y Other Device	Z No Qualifier
K Lung, Right L Lung, Left	X External	Ø Drainage Device 2 Monitoring Device 3 Infusion Device	Z No Qualifier
Q Pleura	Ø Open 3 Percutaneous 4 Percutaneous Endoscopic 7 Via Natural or Artificial Opening 8 Via Natural or Artificial Opening Endoscopic	Ø Drainage Device 2 Monitoring Device Y Other Device	Z No Qualifier
Q Pleura	X External	Ø Drainage Device 2 Monitoring Device	Z No Qualifier

DRG Non-OR ØBWØ[78][23D]Z *(proposed)*
DRG Non-OR ØBWK[78][Ø23D]Z *(proposed)*
DRG Non-OR ØBWL[78][Ø23]Z *(proposed)*

Non-OR ØBWØX[Ø237CDJK]Z
Non-OR ØBW1X[Ø27CDFJK]Z
Non-OR ØBW[KL]X[Ø23]Z
Non-OR ØBWQ[Ø3478][Ø2]Z

New/Revised Text in Green   ~~deleted~~ Deleted   ♀ Females Only   ♂ Males Only   **Coding Clinic**
🚫 Non-covered   🚫 Limited Coverage   ⊞ Combination (See Appendix E)   DRG Non-OR   Non-OR   🚫 Hospital-Acquired Condition

SECTION: Ø MEDICAL AND SURGICAL
BODY SYSTEM: B RESPIRATORY SYSTEM
OPERATION: W REVISION: *(continued)*
Correcting, to the extent possible, a portion of a malfunctioning device or the position of a displaced device

Body Part	Approach	Device	Qualifier
T Diaphragm	Ø Open 3 Percutaneous 4 Percutaneous Endoscopic 7 Via Natural or Artificial Opening 8 Via Natural or Artificial Opening Endoscopic	Ø Drainage Device 2 Monitoring Device 7 Autologous Tissue Substitute J Synthetic Substitute K Nonautologous Tissue Substitute M Diaphragmatic Pacemaker Lead Y Other Device	Z No Qualifier
T Diaphragm	X External	Ø Drainage Device 2 Monitoring Device 7 Autologous Tissue Substitute J Synthetic Substitute K Nonautologous Tissue Substitute M Diaphragmatic Pacemaker Lead	Z No Qualifier

Non-OR   ØBWQX[Ø2]Z
Non-OR   ØBWTX[Ø27JKM]Z

SECTION: Ø MEDICAL AND SURGICAL
BODY SYSTEM: B RESPIRATORY SYSTEM
OPERATION: Y TRANSPLANTATION: Putting in or on all or a portion of a living body part taken from another individual or animal to physically take the place and/or function of all or a portion of a similar body part

Body Part	Approach	Device	Qualifier
C Upper Lung Lobe, Right ◐ D Middle Lung Lobe, Right ◐ F Lower Lung Lobe, Right ◐ G Upper Lung Lobe, Left ◐ H Lung Lingula ◐ J Lower Lung Lobe, Left ◐ K Lung, Right ◐ L Lung, Left ◐ M Lungs, Bilateral ◐	Ø Open	Z No Device	Ø Allogeneic 1 Syngeneic 2 Zooplastic

◐ All Values

W: REVISION   Y: TRANSPLANTATION
B: RESPIRATORY SYSTEM
Ø: M/S

SECTION: 0 MEDICAL AND SURGICAL
BODY SYSTEM: C MOUTH AND THROAT
OPERATION: 0 **ALTERATION:** Modifying the anatomic structure of a body part without affecting the function of the body part

Body Part	Approach	Device	Qualifier
0 Upper Lip 1 Lower Lip	X External	7 Autologous Tissue Substitute J Synthetic Substitute K Nonautologous Tissue Substitute Z No Device	Z No Qualifier

SECTION: 0 MEDICAL AND SURGICAL
BODY SYSTEM: C MOUTH AND THROAT
OPERATION: 2 **CHANGE:** Taking out or off a device from a body part and putting back an identical or similar device in or on the same body part without cutting or puncturing the skin or a mucous membrane

Body Part	Approach	Device	Qualifier
A Salivary Gland S Larynx Y Mouth and Throat	X External	0 Drainage Device Y Other Device	Z No Qualifier

Non-OR All Values

SECTION: 0 MEDICAL AND SURGICAL
BODY SYSTEM: C MOUTH AND THROAT
OPERATION: 5 **DESTRUCTION:** *(on multiple pages)*
Physical eradication of all or a portion of a body part by the use of direct energy, force, or a destructive agent

Body Part	Approach	Device	Qualifier
0 Upper Lip 1 Lower Lip 2 Hard Palate 3 Soft Palate 4 Buccal Mucosa 5 Upper Gingiva 6 Lower Gingiva 7 Tongue N Uvula P Tonsils Q Adenoids	0 Open 3 Percutaneous X External	Z No Device	Z No Qualifier

Non-OR 0C5[56][03X]ZZ

Side tab: 0: ALTERATION 2: CHANGE 5: DESTRUCTION

Side tab: C: MOUTH AND THROAT 0: M/S

New/Revised Text in Green   ~~deleted~~ Deleted   ♀ Females Only   ♂ Males Only   **Coding Clinic**
Non-covered   Limited Coverage   Combination (See Appendix E)   DRG Non-OR   Non-OR   Hospital-Acquired Condition

SECTION: Ø MEDICAL AND SURGICAL

BODY SYSTEM: C MOUTH AND THROAT
OPERATION: 5 DESTRUCTION: *(continued)*
Physical eradication of all or a portion of a body part by the use of direct energy, force, or a destructive agent

Body Part	Approach	Device	Qualifier
8 Parotid Gland, Right 9 Parotid Gland, Left B Parotid Duct, Right C Parotid Duct, Left D Sublingual Gland, Right F Sublingual Gland, Left G Submaxillary Gland, Right H Submaxillary Gland, Left J Minor Salivary Gland	Ø Open 3 Percutaneous	Z No Device	Z No Qualifier
M Pharynx R Epiglottis S Larynx T Vocal Cord, Right V Vocal Cord, Left	Ø Open 3 Percutaneous 4 Percutaneous Endoscopic 7 Via Natural or Artificial Opening 8 Via Natural or Artificial Opening Endoscopic	Z No Device	Z No Qualifier
W Upper Tooth X Lower Tooth	Ø Open X External	Z No Device	Ø Single 1 Multiple 2 All

Non-OR   ØC5[WX][ØX]Z[Ø12]

SECTION: Ø MEDICAL AND SURGICAL

BODY SYSTEM: C MOUTH AND THROAT
OPERATION: 7 DILATION: Expanding an orifice or the lumen of a tubular body part

Body Part	Approach	Device	Qualifier
B Parotid Duct, Right C Parotid Duct, Left	Ø Open 3 Percutaneous 7 Via Natural or Artificial Opening	D Intraluminal Device Z No Device	Z No Qualifier
M Pharynx	7 Via Natural or Artificial Opening 8 Via Natural or Artificial Opening Endoscopic	D Intraluminal Device Z No Device	Z No Qualifier
S Larynx	Ø Open 3 Percutaneous 4 Percutaneous Endoscopic 7 Via Natural or Artificial Opening 8 Via Natural or Artificial Opening Endoscopic	D Intraluminal Device Z No Device	Z No Qualifier

Non-OR   ØC7[BC][Ø37][DZ]Z
Non-OR   ØC7M[78][DZ]Z

New/Revised Text in Green   ~~deleted~~ Deleted   ♀ Females Only   ♂ Males Only   **Coding Clinic**
🚫 Non-covered   🚫 Limited Coverage   ⊡ Combination (See Appendix E)   DRG Non-OR   Non-OR   🚫 Hospital-Acquired Condition

225

SECTION: Ø MEDICAL AND SURGICAL
BODY SYSTEM: C MOUTH AND THROAT
OPERATION: 9 DRAINAGE: *(on multiple pages)*
Taking or letting out fluids and/or gases from a body part

Body Part	Approach	Device	Qualifier
Ø Upper Lip 1 Lower Lip 2 Hard Palate 3 Soft Palate 4 Buccal Mucosa 5 Upper Gingiva 6 Lower Gingiva 7 Tongue N Uvula P Tonsils Q Adenoids	Ø Open 3 Percutaneous X External	Ø Drainage Device	Z No Qualifier
Ø Upper Lip 1 Lower Lip 2 Hard Palate 3 Soft Palate 4 Buccal Mucosa 5 Upper Gingiva 6 Lower Gingiva 7 Tongue N Uvula P Tonsils Q Adenoids	Ø Open 3 Percutaneous X External	Z No Device	X Diagnostic Z No Qualifier
8 Parotid Gland, Right 9 Parotid Gland, Left B Parotid Duct, Right C Parotid Duct, Left D Sublingual Gland, Right F Sublingual Gland, Left G Submaxillary Gland, Right H Submaxillary Gland, Left J Minor Salivary Gland	Ø Open 3 Percutaneous	Ø Drainage Device	Z No Qualifier
8 Parotid Gland, Right 9 Parotid Gland, Left B Parotid Duct, Right C Parotid Duct, Left D Sublingual Gland, Right F Sublingual Gland, Left G Submaxillary Gland, Right H Submaxillary Gland, Left J Minor Salivary Gland	Ø Open 3 Percutaneous	Z No Device	X Diagnostic Z No Qualifier
M Pharynx R Epiglottis S Larynx T Vocal Cord, Right V Vocal Cord, Left	Ø Open 3 Percutaneous 4 Percutaneous Endoscopic 7 Via Natural or Artificial Opening 8 Via Natural or Artificial Opening Endoscopic	Ø Drainage Device	Z No Qualifier

Non-OR　0C9[012347NPQ]30Z
Non-OR　0C9[012347NPQ]3ZZ
Non-OR　0C9[56][03X]0Z
Non-OR　0C9[01456][03X]ZX
Non-OR　0C9[56][03X]ZZ

Non-OR　0C97[3X]ZX
Non-OR　0C9[89BCDFGHJ][03]0Z
Non-OR　0C9[89BCDFGHJ]3ZX
Non-OR　0C9[89BCDFGHJ][03]ZZ
Non-OR　0C9[MRSTV]30Z

SECTION: 0 MEDICAL AND SURGICAL
BODY SYSTEM: C MOUTH AND THROAT
OPERATION: 9 DRAINAGE: *(continued)*

Taking or letting out fluids and/or gases from a body part

Body Part	Approach	Device	Qualifier
M Pharynx R Epiglottis S Larynx T Vocal Cord, Right V Vocal Cord, Left	0 Open 3 Percutaneous 4 Percutaneous Endoscopic 7 Via Natural or Artificial Opening 8 Via Natural or Artificial Opening Endoscopic	Z No Device	X Diagnostic Z No Qualifier
W Upper Tooth X Lower Tooth	0 Open X External	0 Drainage Device Z No Device	0 Single 1 Multiple 2 All

Non-OR 0C9[MRSTV]3ZZ
Non-OR 0C9M[03478]ZX

Non-OR 0C9[RSTV][3478]ZX
Non-OR 0C9[WX][0X][0Z][012]

SECTION: 0 MEDICAL AND SURGICAL
BODY SYSTEM: C MOUTH AND THROAT
OPERATION: B EXCISION: Cutting out or off, without replacement, a portion of a body part

Body Part	Approach	Device	Qualifier
0 Upper Lip 1 Lower Lip 2 Hard Palate 3 Soft Palate 4 Buccal Mucosa 5 Upper Gingiva 6 Lower Gingiva 7 Tongue N Uvula P Tonsils Q Adenoids	0 Open 3 Percutaneous X External	Z No Device	X Diagnostic Z No Qualifier
8 Parotid Gland, Right 9 Parotid Gland, Left B Parotid Duct, Right C Parotid Duct, Left D Sublingual Gland, Right F Sublingual Gland, Left G Submaxillary Gland, Right H Submaxillary Gland, Left J Minor Salivary Gland	0 Open 3 Percutaneous	Z No Device	X Diagnostic Z No Qualifier
M Pharynx R Epiglottis S Larynx T Vocal Cord, Right V Vocal Cord, Left	0 Open 3 Percutaneous 4 Percutaneous Endoscopic 7 Via Natural or Artificial Opening 8 Via Natural or Artificial Opening Endoscopic	Z No Device	X Diagnostic Z No Qualifier
W Upper Tooth X Lower Tooth	0 Open X External	Z No Device	0 Single 1 Multiple 2 All

Non-OR 0CB[01456][03X]ZX
Non-OR 0CB[56][03X]ZZ
Non-OR 0CB7[3X]ZX
Non-OR 0CB[89BCDFGHJ]3ZX
Non-OR 0CBM[03478]ZX

Non-OR 0CB[RSTV][3478]ZX
Non-OR 0CB[WX][0X]Z[012]

Coding Clinic: 2016, Q2, P20 – 0CBM8ZX
Coding Clinic: 2016, Q3, P28 – 0CBM8ZZ

New/Revised Text in Green   ~~deleted~~ Deleted   ♀ Females Only   ♂ Males Only   **Coding Clinic**
🏷 Non-covered   🏷 Limited Coverage   ⊞ Combination (See Appendix E)   `DRG Non-OR`   Non-OR   🏷 Hospital-Acquired Condition

SECTION: 0 MEDICAL AND SURGICAL
BODY SYSTEM: C MOUTH AND THROAT
OPERATION: C EXTIRPATION: Taking or cutting out solid matter from a body part

Body Part	Approach	Device	Qualifier
0 Upper Lip 1 Lower Lip 2 Hard Palate 3 Soft Palate 4 Buccal Mucosa 5 Upper Gingiva 6 Lower Gingiva 7 Tongue N Uvula P Tonsils Q Adenoids	0 Open 3 Percutaneous X External	Z No Device	Z No Qualifier
8 Parotid Gland, Right 9 Parotid Gland, Left B Parotid Duct, Right C Parotid Duct, Left D Sublingual Gland, Right F Sublingual Gland, Left G Submaxillary Gland, Right H Submaxillary Gland, Left J Minor Salivary Gland	0 Open 3 Percutaneous	Z No Device	Z No Qualifier
M Pharynx R Epiglottis S Larynx T Vocal Cord, Right V Vocal Cord, Left	0 Open 3 Percutaneous 4 Percutaneous Endoscopic 7 Via Natural or Artificial Opening 8 Via Natural or Artificial Opening Endoscopic	Z No Device	Z No Qualifier
W Upper Tooth X Lower Tooth	0 Open X External	Z No Device	0 Single 1 Multiple 2 All

Non-OR   0CC[012347NPQ]XZZ
Non-OR   0CC[56][03X]ZZ
Non-OR   0CC[89BCDFGHJ][03]ZZ

Non-OR   0CC[MS][78]ZZ
Non-OR   0CC[WX][0X]Z[012]

Coding Clinic: 2016, Q2, P20 – 0CCH3ZZ

SECTION: 0 MEDICAL AND SURGICAL
BODY SYSTEM: C MOUTH AND THROAT
OPERATION: D EXTRACTION: Pulling or stripping out or off all or a portion of a body part by the use of force

Body Part	Approach	Device	Qualifier
T Vocal Cord, Right V Vocal Cord, Left	0 Open 3 Percutaneous 4 Percutaneous Endoscopic 7 Via Natural or Artificial Opening 8 Via Natural or Artificial Opening Endoscopic	Z No Device	Z No Qualifier
W Upper Tooth X Lower Tooth	X External	Z No Device	0 Single 1 Multiple 2 All

Non-OR   0CD[WX]XZ[012]

New/Revised Text in Green   ~~deleted~~ Deleted   ♀ Females Only   ♂ Males Only   **Coding Clinic**
Non-covered   Limited Coverage   ⊞ Combination (See Appendix E)   DRG Non-OR   Non-OR   Hospital-Acquired Condition

(side tab) D: EXTRACTION   C: EXTIRPATION   C: MOUTH AND THROAT   0: M/S

SECTION: 0 MEDICAL AND SURGICAL

BODY SYSTEM: C MOUTH AND THROAT
OPERATION: F FRAGMENTATION: Breaking solid matter in a body part into pieces

Body Part	Approach	Device	Qualifier
B Parotid Duct, Right 🖉 C Parotid Duct, Left 🖉	0 Open 3 Percutaneous 7 Via Natural or Artificial Opening X External	Z No Device	Z No Qualifier

🖉 0CF[BC]XZZ   Non-OR   All Values

SECTION: 0 MEDICAL AND SURGICAL

BODY SYSTEM: C MOUTH AND THROAT
OPERATION: H INSERTION: Putting in a nonbiological appliance that monitors, assists, performs, or prevents a physiological function but does not physically take the place of a body part

Body Part	Approach	Device	Qualifier
7 Tongue	0 Open 3 Percutaneous X External	1 Radioactive Element	Z No Qualifier
A Salivary Gland S Larynx	0 Open 3 Percutaneous 7 Via Natural or Artificial Opening 8 Via Natural or Artificial Opening Endoscopic	Y Other Device	Z No Qualifier
Y Mouth and Throat	0 Open 3 Percutaneous	Y Other Device	Z No Qualifier
Y Mouth and Throat	7 Via Natural or Artificial Opening 8 Via Natural or Artificial Opening Endoscopic	B Intraluminal Device, Airway Y Other Device	Z No Qualifier

Non-OR   0CHY[78]BZ

SECTION: 0 MEDICAL AND SURGICAL

BODY SYSTEM: C MOUTH AND THROAT
OPERATION: J INSPECTION: Visually and/or manually exploring a body part

Body Part	Approach	Device	Qualifier
A Salivary Gland	0 Open 3 Percutaneous X External	Z No Device	Z No Qualifier
S Larynx Y Mouth and Throat	0 Open 3 Percutaneous 4 Percutaneous Endoscopic 7 Via Natural or Artificial Opening 8 Via Natural or Artificial Opening Endoscopic X External	Z No Device	Z No Qualifier

Non-OR   All Values

0: M/S   C: MOUTH AND THROAT   F: FRAGMENTATION   H: INSERTION   J: INSPECTION

SECTION: Ø MEDICAL AND SURGICAL
BODY SYSTEM: C MOUTH AND THROAT
OPERATION: L OCCLUSION: Completely closing an orifice or the lumen of a tubular body part

Body Part	Approach	Device	Qualifier
B Parotid Duct, Right C Parotid Duct, Left	Ø Open 3 Percutaneous 4 Percutaneous Endoscopic	C Extraluminal Device D Intraluminal Device Z No Device	Z No Qualifier
B Parotid Duct, Right C Parotid Duct, Left	7 Via Natural or Artificial Opening 8 Via Natural or Artificial Opening Endoscopic	D Intraluminal Device Z No Device	Z No Qualifier

SECTION: Ø MEDICAL AND SURGICAL
BODY SYSTEM: C MOUTH AND THROAT
OPERATION: M REATTACHMENT: Putting back in or on all or a portion of a separated body part to its normal location or other suitable location

Body Part	Approach	Device	Qualifier
Ø Upper Lip 1 Lower Lip 3 Soft Palate 7 Tongue N Uvula	Ø Open	Z No Device	Z No Qualifier
W Upper Tooth X Lower Tooth	Ø Open X External	Z No Device	Ø Single 1 Multiple 2 All

Non-OR   ØCM[WX][ØX]Z[Ø12]

SECTION: Ø MEDICAL AND SURGICAL

BODY SYSTEM: C MOUTH AND THROAT

OPERATION: N RELEASE: Freeing a body part from an abnormal physical constraint by cutting or by the use of force

Body Part	Approach	Device	Qualifier
Ø Upper Lip 1 Lower Lip 2 Hard Palate 3 Soft Palate 4 Buccal Mucosa 5 Upper Gingiva 6 Lower Gingiva 7 Tongue N Uvula P Tonsils Q Adenoids	Ø Open 3 Percutaneous X External	Z No Device	Z No Qualifier
8 Parotid Gland, Right 9 Parotid Gland, Left B Parotid Duct, Right C Parotid Duct, Left D Sublingual Gland, Right F Sublingual Gland, Left G Submaxillary Gland, Right H Submaxillary Gland, Left J Minor Salivary Gland	Ø Open 3 Percutaneous	Z No Device	Z No Qualifier
M Pharynx R Epiglottis S Larynx T Vocal Cord, Right V Vocal Cord, Left	Ø Open 3 Percutaneous 4 Percutaneous Endoscopic 7 Via Natural or Artificial Opening 8 Via Natural or Artificial Opening Endoscopic	Z No Device	Z No Qualifier
W Upper Tooth X Lower Tooth	Ø Open X External	Z No Device	Ø Single 1 Multiple 2 All

Non-OR ØCN[Ø1567][Ø3X]ZZ
Non-OR ØCN[WX][ØX]Z[Ø12]

SECTION: 0 MEDICAL AND SURGICAL

BODY SYSTEM: C MOUTH AND THROAT

OPERATION: P REMOVAL: Taking out or off a device from a body part

Body Part	Approach	Device	Qualifier
A Salivary Gland	0 Open 3 Percutaneous	0 Drainage Device C Extraluminal Device Y Other Device	Z No Qualifier
A Salivary Gland	7 Via Natural or Artificial Opening 8 Via Natural or Artificial Opening Endoscopic	Y Other Device	Z No Qualifier
S Larynx	0 Open 3 Percutaneous 7 Via Natural or Artificial Opening 8 Via Natural or Artificial Opening Endoscopic	0 Drainage Device 7 Autologous Tissue Substitute D Intraluminal Device J Synthetic Substitute K Nonautologous Tissue Substitute Y Other Device	Z No Qualifier
S Larynx	X External	0 Drainage Device 7 Autologous Tissue Substitute D Intraluminal Device J Synthetic Substitute K Nonautologous Tissue Substitute	Z No Qualifier
Y Mouth and Throat	0 Open 3 Percutaneous 7 Via Natural or Artificial Opening 8 Via Natural or Artificial Opening Endoscopic	0 Drainage Device 1 Radioactive Element 7 Autologous Tissue Substitute D Intraluminal Device J Synthetic Substitute K Nonautologous Tissue Substitute Y Other Device	Z No Qualifier
Y Mouth and Throat	X External	0 Drainage Device 1 Radioactive Element 7 Autologous Tissue Substitute D Intraluminal Device J Synthetic Substitute K Nonautologous Tissue Substitute	Z No Qualifier

Non-OR 0CPA[03][0C]Z
Non-OR 0CPS[78][0D]Z
Non-OR 0CPSX[07DJK]Z
Non-OR 0CPY[78][0D]Z
Non-OR 0CPYX[017DJK]Z

New/Revised Text in Green   ~~deleted~~ Deleted   ♀ Females Only   ♂ Males Only   **Coding Clinic**
Non-covered   Limited Coverage   ⊡ Combination (See Appendix E)   DRG Non-OR   Non-OR   Hospital-Acquired Condition

SECTION: Ø MEDICAL AND SURGICAL

BODY SYSTEM: C MOUTH AND THROAT

OPERATION: **Q REPAIR:** Restoring, to the extent possible, a body part to its normal anatomic structure and function

Body Part	Approach	Device	Qualifier
Ø Upper Lip 1 Lower Lip 2 Hard Palate 3 Soft Palate 4 Buccal Mucosa 5 Upper Gingiva 6 Lower Gingiva 7 Tongue N Uvula P Tonsils Q Adenoids	Ø Open 3 Percutaneous X External	Z No Device	Z No Qualifier
8 Parotid Gland, Right 9 Parotid Gland, Left B Parotid Duct, Right C Parotid Duct, Left D Sublingual Gland, Right F Sublingual Gland, Left G Submaxillary Gland, Right H Submaxillary Gland, Left J Minor Salivary Gland	Ø Open 3 Percutaneous	Z No Device	Z No Qualifier
M Pharynx R Epiglottis S Larynx T Vocal Cord, Right V Vocal Cord, Left	Ø Open 3 Percutaneous 4 Percutaneous Endoscopic 7 Via Natural or Artificial Opening 8 Via Natural or Artificial Opening Endoscopic	Z No Device	Z No Qualifier
W Upper Tooth X Lower Tooth	Ø Open X External	Z No Device	Ø Single 1 Multiple 2 All

Non-OR   ØCQ[Ø1]XZZ
Non-OR   ØCQ[56][Ø3X]ZZ
Non-OR   ØCQ[WX][ØX]Z[Ø12]

Coding Clinic: 2017, Q1, P21 – ØCQ5ØZZ

SECTION: 0 MEDICAL AND SURGICAL
BODY SYSTEM: C MOUTH AND THROAT
OPERATION: R REPLACEMENT: Putting in or on biological or synthetic material that physically takes the place and/or function of all or a portion of a body part

Body Part	Approach	Device	Qualifier
0 Upper Lip 1 Lower Lip 2 Hard Palate 3 Soft Palate 4 Buccal Mucosa 5 Upper Gingiva 6 Lower Gingiva 7 Tongue N Uvula	0 Open 3 Percutaneous X External	7 Autologous Tissue Substitute J Synthetic Substitute K Nonautologous Tissue Substitute	Z No Qualifier
B Parotid Duct, Right C Parotid Duct, Left	0 Open 3 Percutaneous	7 Autologous Tissue Substitute J Synthetic Substitute K Nonautologous Tissue Substitute	Z No Qualifier
M Pharynx R Epiglottis S Larynx T Vocal Cord, Right V Vocal Cord, Left	0 Open 7 Via Natural or Artificial Opening 8 Via Natural or Artificial Opening Endoscopic	7 Autologous Tissue Substitute J Synthetic Substitute K Nonautologous Tissue Substitute	Z No Qualifier
W Upper Tooth X Lower Tooth	0 Open X External	7 Autologous Tissue Substitute J Synthetic Substitute K Nonautologous Tissue Substitute	0 Single 1 Multiple 2 All

Non-OR   0CR[WX][0X][7JK][012]

SECTION: 0 MEDICAL AND SURGICAL
BODY SYSTEM: C MOUTH AND THROAT
OPERATION: S REPOSITION: Moving to its normal location, or other suitable location, all or a portion of a body part

Body Part	Approach	Device	Qualifier
0 Upper Lip 1 Lower Lip 2 Hard Palate 3 Soft Palate 7 Tongue N Uvula	0 Open X External	Z No Device	Z No Qualifier
B Parotid Duct, Right C Parotid Duct, Left	0 Open 3 Percutaneous	Z No Device	Z No Qualifier
R Epiglottis T Vocal Cord, Right V Vocal Cord, Left	0 Open 7 Via Natural or Artificial Opening 8 Via Natural or Artificial Opening Endoscopic	Z No Device	Z No Qualifier
W Upper Tooth X Lower Tooth	0 Open X External	5 External Fixation Device Z No Device	0 Single 1 Multiple 2 All

Non-OR   0CS[WX][0X][5Z][012]

Coding Clinic: 2016, Q3, P29 – 0CSR8ZZ

SECTION: Ø MEDICAL AND SURGICAL

BODY SYSTEM: C MOUTH AND THROAT

OPERATION: T RESECTION: Cutting out or off, without replacement, all of a body part

Body Part	Approach	Device	Qualifier
Ø Upper Lip 1 Lower Lip 2 Hard Palate 3 Soft Palate 7 Tongue N Uvula P Tonsils Q Adenoids	Ø Open X External	Z No Device	Z No Qualifier
8 Parotid Gland, Right 9 Parotid Gland, Left B Parotid Duct, Right C Parotid Duct, Left D Sublingual Gland, Right F Sublingual Gland, Left G Submaxillary Gland, Right H Submaxillary Gland, Left J Minor Salivary Gland	Ø Open	Z No Device	Z No Qualifier
M Pharynx R Epiglottis S Larynx T Vocal Cord, Right V Vocal Cord, Left	Ø Open 4 Percutaneous Endoscopic 7 Via Natural or Artificial Opening 8 Via Natural or Artificial Opening Endoscopic	Z No Device	Z No Qualifier
W Upper Tooth X Lower Tooth	Ø Open	Z No Device	Ø Single 1 Multiple 2 All

Non-OR ØCT[WX]ØZ[Ø12]

Coding Clinic: 2Ø16, Q2, P13 – ØCT9ØZZ

SECTION: Ø MEDICAL AND SURGICAL

BODY SYSTEM: C MOUTH AND THROAT

OPERATION: U SUPPLEMENT: Putting in or on biological or synthetic material that physically reinforces and/or augments the function of a portion of a body part

Body Part	Approach	Device	Qualifier
Ø Upper Lip 1 Lower Lip 2 Hard Palate 3 Soft Palate 4 Buccal Mucosa 5 Upper Gingiva 6 Lower Gingiva 7 Tongue N Uvula	Ø Open 3 Percutaneous X External	7 Autologous Tissue Substitute J Synthetic Substitute K Nonautologous Tissue Substitute	Z No Qualifier
M Pharynx R Epiglottis S Larynx T Vocal Cord, Right V Vocal Cord, Left	Ø Open 7 Via Natural or Artificial Opening 8 Via Natural or Artificial Opening Endoscopic	7 Autologous Tissue Substitute J Synthetic Substitute K Nonautologous Tissue Substitute	Z No Qualifier

Non-OR ØCU2[Ø3]JZ

New/Revised Text in Green ~~deleted~~ Deleted ♀ Females Only ♂ Males Only **Coding Clinic**

🔖 Non-covered 🔖 Limited Coverage ⊞ Combination (See Appendix E) DRG Non-OR Non-OR 🔖 Hospital-Acquired Condition

SECTION: 0 MEDICAL AND SURGICAL
BODY SYSTEM: C MOUTH AND THROAT
OPERATION: V RESTRICTION: Partially closing an orifice or the lumen of a tubular body part

Body Part	Approach	Device	Qualifier
B Parotid Duct, Right C Parotid Duct, Left	0 Open 3 Percutaneous	C Extraluminal Device D Intraluminal Device Z No Device	Z No Qualifier
B Parotid Duct, Right C Parotid Duct, Left	7 Via Natural or Artificial Opening 8 Via Natural or Artificial Opening Endoscopic	D Intraluminal Device Z No Device	Z No Qualifier

SECTION: 0 MEDICAL AND SURGICAL
BODY SYSTEM: C MOUTH AND THROAT
OPERATION: W REVISION: (on multiple pages)
Correcting, to the extent possible, a portion of a malfunctioning device or the position of a displaced device

Body Part	Approach	Device	Qualifier
A Salivary Gland	0 Open 3 Percutaneous	0 Drainage Device C Extraluminal Device Y Other Device	Z No Qualifier
A Salivary Gland	7 Via Natural or Artificial Opening 8 Via Natural or Artificial Opening Endoscopic	Y Other Device	Z No Qualifier
A Salivary Gland	X External	0 Drainage Device C Extraluminal Device	Z No Qualifier
S Larynx	0 Open 3 Percutaneous 7 Via Natural or Artificial Opening 8 Via Natural or Artificial Opening Endoscopic	0 Drainage Device 7 Autologous Tissue Substitute D Intraluminal Device J Synthetic Substitute K Nonautologous Tissue Substitute Y Other Device	Z No Qualifier
S Larynx	X External	0 Drainage Device 7 Autologous Tissue Substitute D Intraluminal Device J Synthetic Substitute K Nonautologous Tissue Substitute	Z No Qualifier

Non-OR 0CWA[03X][0C]Z
Non-OR 0CWSX[07DHJ]Z

New/Revised Text in Green ~~deleted~~ Deleted ♀ Females Only ♂ Males Only **Coding Clinic**
Non-covered Limited Coverage ⊡ Combination (See Appendix E) DRG Non-OR Non-OR Hospital-Acquired Condition

SECTION: Ø MEDICAL AND SURGICAL

BODY SYSTEM: C MOUTH AND THROAT

OPERATION: W REVISION: *(continued)*
Correcting, to the extent possible, a portion of a malfunctioning device or the position of a displaced device

Body Part	Approach	Device	Qualifier
Y Mouth and Throat	Ø Open 3 Percutaneous 7 Via Natural or Artificial Opening 8 Via Natural or Artificial Opening Endoscopic	Ø Drainage Device 1 Radioactive Element 7 Autologous Tissue Substitute D Intraluminal Device J Synthetic Substitute K Nonautologous Tissue Substitute Y Other Device	Z No Qualifier
Y Mouth and Throat	X External	Ø Drainage Device 1 Radioactive Element 7 Autologous Tissue Substitute D Intraluminal Device J Synthetic Substitute K Nonautologous Tissue Substitute	Z No Qualifier

Non-OR ØCWYØ7Z
Non-OR ØCWYX[Ø17DJK]Z

SECTION: Ø MEDICAL AND SURGICAL

BODY SYSTEM: C MOUTH AND THROAT

OPERATION: X TRANSFER: Moving, without taking out, all or a portion of a body part to another location to take over the function of all or a portion of a body part

Body Part	Approach	Device	Qualifier
Ø Upper Lip 1 Lower Lip 3 Soft Palate 4 Buccal Mucosa 5 Upper Gingiva 6 Lower Gingiva 7 Tongue	Ø Open X External	Z No Device	Z No Qualifier

SECTION: Ø MEDICAL AND SURGICAL
BODY SYSTEM: D GASTROINTESTINAL SYSTEM
OPERATION: 1 BYPASS: *(on multiple pages)*
Altering the route of passage of the contents of a tubular body part

Body Part	Approach	Device	Qualifier
1 Esophagus, Upper 2 Esophagus, Middle 3 Esophagus, Lower 5 Esophagus	Ø Open 4 Percutaneous Endoscopic 8 Via Natural or Artificial Opening Endoscopic	7 Autologous Tissue Substitute J Synthetic Substitute K Nonautologous Tissue Substitute Z No Device	4 Cutaneous 6 Stomach 9 Duodenum A Jejunum B Ileum
1 Esophagus, Upper 2 Esophagus, Middle 3 Esophagus, Lower 5 Esophagus	3 Percutaneous	J Synthetic Substitute	4 Cutaneous
6 Stomach 🗞 9 Duodenum	Ø Open 4 Percutaneous Endoscopic 8 Via Natural or Artificial Opening Endoscopic	7 Autologous Tissue Substitute J Synthetic Substitute K Nonautologous Tissue Substitute Z No Device	4 Cutaneous 9 Duodenum A Jejunum B Ileum L Transverse Colon
6 Stomach 9 Duodenum	3 Percutaneous	J Synthetic Substitute	4 Cutaneous
A Jejunum	Ø Open 4 Percutaneous Endoscopic 8 Via Natural or Artificial Opening Endoscopic	7 Autologous Tissue Substitute J Synthetic Substitute K Nonautologous Tissue Substitute Z No Device	4 Cutaneous A Jejunum B Ileum H Cecum K Ascending Colon L Transverse Colon M Descending Colon N Sigmoid Colon P Rectum Q Anus
A Jejunum	3 Percutaneous	J Synthetic Substitute	4 Cutaneous
B Ileum	Ø Open 4 Percutaneous Endoscopic 8 Via Natural or Artificial Opening Endoscopic	7 Autologous Tissue Substitute J Synthetic Substitute K Nonautologous Tissue Substitute Z No Device	4 Cutaneous B Ileum H Cecum K Ascending Colon L Transverse Colon M Descending Colon N Sigmoid Colon P Rectum Q Anus
B Ileum	3 Percutaneous	J Synthetic Substitute	4 Cutaneous
H Cecum	Ø Open 4 Percutaneous Endoscopic 8 Via Natural or Artificial Opening Endoscopic	7 Autologous Tissue Substitute J Synthetic Substitute K Nonautologous Tissue Substitute Z No Device	4 Cutaneous H Cecum K Ascending Colon L Transverse Colon M Descending Colon N Sigmoid Colon P Rectum
H Cecum	3 Percutaneous	J Synthetic Substitute	4 Cutaneous

Non-OR ØD16[Ø48][7JKZ]4
Non-OR ØD163J4

🗞 ØD16[Ø48][7JKZ][9ABL] when reported with Principal Diagnosis E66.Ø1 and Secondary Diagnosis K68.11, K95.Ø1, K95.81, or T81.4XXA

Coding Clinic: 2Ø16, Q2, P31 – ØD194ZB
Coding Clinic: 2Ø17, Q2, P18 – ØD16ØZA

New/Revised Text in Green   ~~deleted~~ Deleted   ♀ Females Only   ♂ Males Only   **Coding Clinic**

🗞 Non-covered   Limited Coverage   ⊞ Combination (See Appendix E)   DRG Non-OR   Non-OR   🗞 Hospital-Acquired Condition

SECTION: Ø MEDICAL AND SURGICAL

BODY SYSTEM: D GASTROINTESTINAL SYSTEM

OPERATION: 1 **BYPASS:** *(continued)*
Altering the route of passage of the contents of a tubular body part

Body Part	Approach	Device	Qualifier
K Ascending Colon	Ø Open 4 Percutaneous Endoscopic 8 Via Natural or Artificial Opening Endoscopic	7 Autologous Tissue Substitute J Synthetic Substitute K Nonautologous Tissue Substitute Z No Device	4 Cutaneous K Ascending Colon L Transverse Colon M Descending Colon N Sigmoid Colon P Rectum
K Ascending Colon	3 Percutaneous	J Synthetic Substitute	4 Cutaneous
L Transverse Colon	Ø Open 4 Percutaneous Endoscopic 8 Via Natural or Artificial Opening Endoscopic	7 Autologous Tissue Substitute J Synthetic Substitute K Nonautologous Tissue Substitute Z No Device	4 Cutaneous L Transverse Colon M Descending Colon N Sigmoid Colon P Rectum
L Transverse Colon	3 Percutaneous	J Synthetic Substitute	4 Cutaneous
M Descending Colon	Ø Open 4 Percutaneous Endoscopic 8 Via Natural or Artificial Opening Endoscopic	7 Autologous Tissue Substitute J Synthetic Substitute K Nonautologous Tissue Substitute Z No Device	4 Cutaneous M Descending Colon N Sigmoid Colon P Rectum
M Descending Colon	3 Percutaneous	J Synthetic Substitute	4 Cutaneous
N Sigmoid Colon	Ø Open 4 Percutaneous Endoscopic 8 Via Natural or Artificial Opening Endoscopic	7 Autologous Tissue Substitute J Synthetic Substitute K Nonautologous Tissue Substitute Z No Device	4 Cutaneous N Sigmoid Colon P Rectum
N Sigmoid Colon	3 Percutaneous	J Synthetic Substitute	4 Cutaneous

SECTION: Ø MEDICAL AND SURGICAL

BODY SYSTEM: D GASTROINTESTINAL SYSTEM

OPERATION: 2 **CHANGE:** Taking out or off a device from a body part and putting back an identical or similar device in or on the same body part without cutting or puncturing the skin or a mucous membrane

Body Part	Approach	Device	Qualifier
Ø Upper Intestinal Tract D Lower Intestinal Tract	X External	Ø Drainage Device U Feeding Device Y Other Device	Z No Qualifier
U Omentum V Mesentery W Peritoneum	X External	Ø Drainage Device Y Other Device	Z No Qualifier

Non-OR   All Values

New/Revised Text in Green   ~~deleted~~ Deleted   ♀ Females Only   ♂ Males Only   **Coding Clinic**

🏷 Non-covered   🏷 Limited Coverage   ⊟ Combination (See Appendix E)   DRG Non-OR   Non-OR   🏷 Hospital-Acquired Condition

SECTION: Ø MEDICAL AND SURGICAL
BODY SYSTEM: D GASTROINTESTINAL SYSTEM
OPERATION: 5 DESTRUCTION: Physical eradication of all or a portion of a body part by the direct use of energy, force, or a destructive agent

Body Part	Approach	Device	Qualifier
1 Esophagus, Upper 2 Esophagus, Middle 3 Esophagus, Lower 4 Esophagogastric Junction 5 Esophagus 6 Stomach 7 Stomach, Pylorus 8 Small Intestine 9 Duodenum A Jejunum B Ileum C Ileocecal Valve E Large Intestine F Large Intestine, Right G Large Intestine, Left H Cecum J Appendix K Ascending Colon L Transverse Colon M Descending Colon N Sigmoid Colon P Rectum	Ø Open 3 Percutaneous 4 Percutaneous Endoscopic 7 Via Natural or Artificial Opening 8 Via Natural or Artificial Opening Endoscopic	Z No Device	Z No Qualifier
Q Anus	Ø Open 3 Percutaneous 4 Percutaneous Endoscopic 7 Via Natural or Artificial Opening 8 Via Natural or Artificial Opening Endoscopic X External	Z No Device	Z No Qualifier
R Anal Sphincter U Omentum V Mesentery W Peritoneum	Ø Open 3 Percutaneous 4 Percutaneous Endoscopic	Z No Device	Z No Qualifier

Non-OR ØD5[12345679EFGHKLMN][48]ZZ
Non-OR ØD5P[Ø3478]ZZ
Non-OR ØD5Q[48]ZZ
Non-OR ØD5R4ZZ

Coding Clinic: 2017, Q1, P35 – ØD5WØZZ

SECTION: 0 MEDICAL AND SURGICAL

BODY SYSTEM: D GASTROINTESTINAL SYSTEM
OPERATION: 7 DILATION: Expanding an orifice or the lumen of a tubular body part

Body Part	Approach	Device	Qualifier
1 Esophagus, Upper 2 Esophagus, Middle 3 Esophagus, Lower 4 Esophagogastric Junction 5 Esophagus 6 Stomach 7 Stomach, Pylorus 8 Small Intestine 9 Duodenum A Jejunum B Ileum C Ileocecal Valve E Large Intestine F Large Intestine, Right G Large Intestine, Left H Cecum K Ascending Colon L Transverse Colon M Descending Colon N Sigmoid Colon P Rectum Q Anus	0 Open 3 Percutaneous 4 Percutaneous Endoscopic 7 Via Natural or Artificial Opening 8 Via Natural or Artificial Opening Endoscopic	D Intraluminal Device Z No Device	Z No Qualifier

Non-OR	0D7[12345689ABCEFGHKLMNPQ][78][DZ]Z
Non-OR	0D77[478]DZ
Non-OR	0D778ZZ
Non-OR	0D7[89ABCEFGHKLMN][034]DZ

SECTION: 0 MEDICAL AND SURGICAL

BODY SYSTEM: D GASTROINTESTINAL SYSTEM
OPERATION: 8 DIVISION: Cutting into a body part, without draining fluids and/or gases from the body part, in order to separate or transect a body part

Body Part	Approach	Device	Qualifier
4 Esophagogastric Junction 7 Stomach, Pylorus	0 Open 3 Percutaneous 4 Percutaneous Endoscopic 7 Via Natural or Artificial Opening 8 Via Natural or Artificial Opening Endoscopic	Z No Device	Z No Qualifier
R Anal Sphincter	0 Open 3 Percutaneous	Z No Device	Z No Qualifier

Coding Clinic: 2017, Q3, P23-24 – 0D8[47]4ZZ

New/Revised Text in Green   deleted Deleted   ♀ Females Only   ♂ Males Only   Coding Clinic
Non-covered   Limited Coverage   Combination (See Appendix E)   DRG Non-OR   Non-OR   Hospital-Acquired Condition

SECTION: Ø MEDICAL AND SURGICAL

BODY SYSTEM: D GASTROINTESTINAL SYSTEM

OPERATION: 9 DRAINAGE: *(on multiple pages)*
Taking or letting out fluids and/or gases from a body part

Body Part	Approach	Device	Qualifier
1 Esophagus, Upper 2 Esophagus, Middle 3 Esophagus, Lower 4 Esophagogastric Junction 5 Esophagus 6 Stomach 7 Stomach, Pylorus 8 Small Intestine 9 Duodenum A Jejunum B Ileum C Ileocecal Valve E Large Intestine F Large Intestine, Right G Large Intestine, Left H Cecum J Appendix K Ascending Colon L Transverse Colon M Descending Colon N Sigmoid Colon P Rectum	Ø Open 3 Percutaneous 4 Percutaneous Endoscopic 7 Via Natural or Artificial Opening 8 Via Natural or Artificial Opening Endoscopic	Ø Drainage Device	Z No Qualifier
1 Esophagus, Upper 2 Esophagus, Middle 3 Esophagus, Lower 4 Esophagogastric Junction 5 Esophagus 6 Stomach 7 Stomach, Pylorus 8 Small Intestine 9 Duodenum A Jejunum B Ileum C Ileocecal Valve E Large Intestine F Large Intestine, Right G Large Intestine, Left H Cecum J Appendix K Ascending Colon L Transverse Colon M Descending Colon N Sigmoid Colon P Rectum	Ø Open 3 Percutaneous 4 Percutaneous Endoscopic 7 Via Natural or Artificial Opening 8 Via Natural or Artificial Opening Endoscopic	Z No Device	X Diagnostic Z No Qualifier

DRG Non-OR ØD9[8ABC]3ØZ
DRG Non-OR ØD9[ABC]3ZZ
Non-OR ØD9[12345679EFGHJKLMNP]3ØZ
Non-OR ØD9[6789ABEFGHKLMNP][78]ØZ
Non-OR ØD9[123456789ABCEFGHKLMNP][3478]ZX
Non-OR ØD9[12345679EFGHJKLMNP]3ZZ

Coding Clinic: 2015, Q2, P29 – ØD967ØZ

SECTION: Ø MEDICAL AND SURGICAL
BODY SYSTEM: D GASTROINTESTINAL SYSTEM
OPERATION: 9 DRAINAGE: *(continued)*
Taking or letting out fluids and/or gases from a body part

Body Part	Approach	Device	Qualifier
Q Anus	Ø Open 3 Percutaneous 4 Percutaneous Endoscopic 7 Via Natural or Artificial Opening 8 Via Natural or Artificial Opening Endoscopic X External	Ø Drainage Device	Z No Qualifier
Q Anus	Ø Open 3 Percutaneous 4 Percutaneous Endoscopic 7 Via Natural or Artificial Opening 8 Via Natural or Artificial Opening Endoscopic X External	Z No Device	X Diagnostic Z No Qualifier
R Anal Sphincter U Omentum V Mesentery W Peritoneum	Ø Open 3 Percutaneous 4 Percutaneous Endoscopic	Ø Drainage Device	Z No Qualifier
R Anal Sphincter U Omentum V Mesentery W Peritoneum	Ø Open 3 Percutaneous 4 Percutaneous Endoscopic	Z No Device	X Diagnostic Z No Qualifier

DRG Non-OR   ØD9[UVW]3ZX *(proposed)*
Non-OR   ØD9Q3ØZ
Non-OR   ØD9Q[Ø3478X]ZX
Non-OR   ØD9Q3ZZ
Non-OR   ØD9R3ØZ
Non-OR   ØD9R3ZZ
Non-OR   ØD9[UVW][34]ØZ
Non-OR   ØD9R[Ø34]ZX
Non-OR   ØD9[UVW][34]ZZ

New/Revised Text in Green   ~~deleted~~ Deleted   ♀ Females Only   ♂ Males Only   **Coding Clinic**
Non-covered   Limited Coverage   ⊞ Combination (See Appendix E)   DRG Non-OR   Non-OR   Hospital-Acquired Condition

SECTION: Ø MEDICAL AND SURGICAL
BODY SYSTEM: D GASTROINTESTINAL SYSTEM
OPERATION: B EXCISION: *(on multiple pages)*
Cutting out or off, without replacement, a portion of a body part

Body Part	Approach	Device	Qualifier
1 Esophagus, Upper 2 Esophagus, Middle 3 Esophagus, Lower 4 Esophagogastric Junction 5 Esophagus 7 Stomach, Pylorus 8 Small Intestine 9 Duodenum A Jejunum B Ileum C Ileocecal Valve E Large Intestine F Large Intestine, Right H Cecum J Appendix K Ascending Colon P Rectum	Ø Open 3 Percutaneous 4 Percutaneous Endoscopic 7 Via Natural or Artificial Opening 8 Via Natural or Artificial Opening Endoscopic	Z No Device	X Diagnostic Z No Qualifier
6 Stomach	Ø Open 3 Percutaneous 4 Percutaneous Endoscopic 7 Via Natural or Artificial Opening 8 Via Natural or Artificial Opening Endoscopic	Z No Device	3 Vertical X Diagnostic Z No Qualifier
G Large Intestine, Left L Transverse Colon M Descending Colon N Sigmoid Colon	Ø Open 3 Percutaneous 4 Percutaneous Endoscopic 7 Via Natural or Artificial Opening 8 Via Natural or Artificial Opening Endoscopic	Z No Device	X Diagnostic Z No Qualifier

Non-OR ØDB[12345789ABCEFHKP][3478]ZX
Non-OR ØDB[123579][48]ZZ
Non-OR ØDB[4EFHKP]8ZZ
Non-OR ØDB6[3478]ZX
Non-OR ØDB6[48]ZZ
Non-OR ØDB[GLMN][3478]ZX
Non-OR ØDB[GLMN]8ZZ

Coding Clinic: 2016, Q1, P22 – ØDBP7ZZ
Coding Clinic: 2016, Q1, P24 – ØDB28ZX
Coding Clinic: 2016, Q2, P31 – ØDB64Z3
Coding Clinic: 2016, Q3, P5-7 – ØDBBØZZ
Coding Clinic: 2017, Q1, P16 – ØDBK8ZZ
Coding Clinic: 2017, Q2, P17 – ØDB6ØZZ

New/Revised Text in Green ~~deleted~~ Deleted ♀ Females Only ♂ Males Only **Coding Clinic**
🔲 Non-covered 🔲 Limited Coverage ⊞ Combination (See Appendix E) DRG Non-OR Non-OR 🔲 Hospital-Acquired Condition

B: EXCISION

D: GASTROINTESTINAL SYSTEM

Ø: M/S

SECTION: Ø MEDICAL AND SURGICAL

BODY SYSTEM: D GASTROINTESTINAL SYSTEM

OPERATION: B EXCISION: *(continued)* Cutting out or off, without replacement, a portion of a body part

Body Part	Approach	Device	Qualifier
G Large Intestine, Left L Transverse Colon M Descending Colon N Sigmoid Colon	F Via Natural or Artificial Opening With Percutaneous Endoscopic Assistance	Z No Device	Z No Qualifier
Q Anus	Ø Open 3 Percutaneous 4 Percutaneous Endoscopic 7 Via Natural or Artificial Opening 8 Via Natural or Artificial Opening Endoscopic X External	Z No Device	X Diagnostic Z No Qualifier
R Anal Sphincter U Omentum V Mesentery W Peritoneum	Ø Open 3 Percutaneous 4 Percutaneous Endoscopic	Z No Device	X Diagnostic Z No Qualifier

Non-OR ØDBQ[03478X]ZX
Non-OR ØDBR[034]ZX
Non-OR ØDB[UVW][34]ZX

New/Revised Text in Green ~~deleted~~ Deleted ♀ Females Only ♂ Males Only **Coding Clinic**
Non-covered Limited Coverage ⊞ Combination (See Appendix E) DRG Non-OR Non-OR Hospital-Acquired Condition

SECTION: Ø MEDICAL AND SURGICAL
BODY SYSTEM: D GASTROINTESTINAL SYSTEM
OPERATION: C **EXTIRPATION:** Taking or cutting out solid matter from a body part

Body Part	Approach	Device	Qualifier
1 Esophagus, Upper 2 Esophagus, Middle 3 Esophagus, Lower 4 Esophagogastric Junction 5 Esophagus 6 Stomach 7 Stomach, Pylorus 8 Small Intestine 9 Duodenum A Jejunum B Ileum C Ileocecal Valve E Large Intestine F Large Intestine, Right G Large Intestine, Left H Cecum J Appendix K Ascending Colon L Transverse Colon M Descending Colon N Sigmoid Colon P Rectum	Ø Open 3 Percutaneous 4 Percutaneous Endoscopic 7 Via Natural or Artificial Opening 8 Via Natural or Artificial Opening Endoscopic	Z No Device	Z No Qualifier
Q Anus	Ø Open 3 Percutaneous 4 Percutaneous Endoscopic 7 Via Natural or Artificial Opening 8 Via Natural or Artificial Opening Endoscopic X External	Z No Device	Z No Qualifier
R Anal Sphincter U Omentum V Mesentery W Peritoneum	Ø Open 3 Percutaneous 4 Percutaneous Endoscopic	Z No Device	Z No Qualifier

Non-OR ØDC[123456789ABCEFGHKLMNP][78]ZZ
Non-OR ØDCQ[78X]ZZ

SECTION: Ø MEDICAL AND SURGICAL

BODY SYSTEM: D GASTROINTESTINAL SYSTEM

OPERATION: D EXTRACTION: Pulling or stripping out or off all or a portion of a body part by the use of force

Body Part	Approach	Device	Qualifier
1 Esophagus, Upper 2 Esophagus, Middle 3 Esophagus, Lower 4 Esophagogastric Junction 5 Esophagus 6 Stomach 7 Stomach, Pylorus 8 Small Intestine 9 Duodenum A Jejunum B Ileum C Ileocecal Valve E Large Intestine F Large Intestine, Right G Large Intestine, Left H Cecum J Appendix K Ascending Colon L Transverse Colon M Descending Colon N Sigmoid Colon P Rectum	3 Percutaneous 4 Percutaneous Endoscopic 8 Via Natural or Artificial Opening Endoscopic	Z No Device	X Diagnostic
Q Anus	3 Percutaneous 4 Percutaneous Endoscopic 8 Via Natural or Artificial Opening Endoscopic X External	Z No Device	X Diagnostic

Coding Clinic: 2017, Q4, P42 – ØDD68ZX

SECTION: Ø MEDICAL AND SURGICAL

BODY SYSTEM: D GASTROINTESTINAL SYSTEM

OPERATION: F FRAGMENTATION: Breaking solid matter in a body part into pieces

Body Part	Approach	Device	Qualifier

5 Esophagus 🜲
6 Stomach 🜲
8 Small Intestine 🜲
9 Duodenum 🜲
A Jejunum 🜲
B Ileum 🜲
E Large Intestine 🜲
F Large Intestine, Right 🜲
G Large Intestine, Left 🜲
H Cecum 🜲
J Appendix 🜲
K Ascending Colon 🜲
L Transverse Colon 🜲
M Descending Colon 🜲
N Sigmoid Colon 🜲
P Rectum 🜲
Q Anus 🜲
	0 Open
	3 Percutaneous
	4 Percutaneous Endoscopic
	7 Via Natural or Artificial
	  Opening
	8 Via Natural or Artificial
	  Opening Endoscopic
	X External
		Z No Device	Z No Qualifier

🜲 ØDF[5689ABEFGHJKLMNPQ]XZZ   Non-OR ØDF[5689ABEFGHJKLMNPQ]XZZ

New/Revised Text in Green   ~~deleted~~ Deleted   ♀ Females Only   ♂ Males Only   **Coding Clinic**

🜲 Non-covered   🜲 Limited Coverage   ⊞ Combination (See Appendix E)   DRG Non-OR   Non-OR   🜲 Hospital-Acquired Condition

SECTION: Ø MEDICAL AND SURGICAL

BODY SYSTEM: D GASTROINTESTINAL SYSTEM
OPERATION: H INSERTION: *(on multiple pages)*
Putting in a nonbiological appliance that monitors, assists, performs, or prevents a physiological function but does not physically take the place of a body part

Body Part	Approach	Device	Qualifier
Ø Upper Intestinal Tract D Lower Intestinal Tract	Ø Open 3 Percutaneous 4 Percutaneous Endoscopic 7 Via Natural or Artificial Opening 8 Via Natural or Artificial Opening Endoscopic	Y Other Device	Z No Qualifier
5 Esophagus	Ø Open 3 Percutaneous 4 Percutaneous Endoscopic	1 Radioactive Element 2 Monitoring Device 3 Infusion Device D Intraluminal Device U Feeding Device Y Other Device	Z No Qualifier
5 Esophagus	7 Via Natural or Artificial Opening 8 Via Natural or Artificial Opening Endoscopic	1 Radioactive Element 2 Monitoring Device 3 Infusion Device B Airway D Intraluminal Device U Feeding Device Y Other Device	Z No Qualifier
6 Stomach ⊞	Ø Open 3 Percutaneous 4 Percutaneous Endoscopic	2 Monitoring Device 3 Infusion Device D Intraluminal Device M Stimulator Lead U Feeding Device Y Other Device	Z No Qualifier
6 Stomach	7 Via Natural or Artificial Opening 8 Via Natural or Artificial Opening Endoscopic	2 Monitoring Device 3 Infusion Device D Intraluminal Device U Feeding Device Y Other Device	Z No Qualifier
8 Small Intestine 9 Duodenum A Jejunum B Ileum	Ø Open 3 Percutaneous 4 Percutaneous Endoscopic 7 Via Natural or Artificial Opening 8 Via Natural or Artificial Opening Endoscopic	2 Monitoring Device 3 Infusion Device D Intraluminal Device U Feeding Device	Z No Qualifier
E Large Intestine	Ø Open 3 Percutaneous 4 Percutaneous Endoscopic 7 Via Natural or Artificial Opening 8 Via Natural or Artificial Opening Endoscopic	D Intraluminal Device	Z No Qualifier

⊞ ØDH6[Ø34]MZ
Non-OR ØDH5[Ø34][DU]Z
Non-OR ØDH5[78][23BDU]Z
Non-OR ØDH6[34]UZ
Non-OR ØDH6[78][23U]Z

Non-OR ØDH[89AB][Ø3478][DU]Z
Non-OR ØDH[89AB][78][23]Z
Non-OR ØDHE[Ø3478]DZ
Non-OR ØDHP[Ø3478]DZ

Coding Clinic: 2Ø16, Q26, P5 – ØDH67UZ

New/Revised Text in Green ~~deleted~~ Deleted ♀ Females Only ♂ Males Only **Coding Clinic**
🞲 Non-covered 🞲 Limited Coverage ⊞ Combination (See Appendix E) DRG Non-OR Non-OR 🞲 Hospital-Acquired Condition

SECTION: Ø MEDICAL AND SURGICAL

BODY SYSTEM: D GASTROINTESTINAL SYSTEM

OPERATION: H INSERTION: *(continued)*
Putting in a nonbiological appliance that monitors, assists, performs, or prevents a physiological function but does not physically take the place of a body part

Body Part	Approach	Device	Qualifier
P Rectum	Ø Open 3 Percutaneous 4 Percutaneous Endoscopic 7 Via Natural or Artificial Opening 8 Via Natural or Artificial Opening Endoscopic	1 Radioactive Element D Intraluminal Device	Z No Qualifier
Q Anus	Ø Open 3 Percutaneous 4 Percutaneous Endoscopic	D Intraluminal Device L Artificial Sphincter	Z No Qualifier
Q Anus	7 Via Natural or Artificial Opening 8 Via Natural or Artificial Opening Endoscopic	D Intraluminal Device	Z No Qualifier
R Anal Sphincter	Ø Open 3 Percutaneous 4 Percutaneous Endoscopic	M Stimulator Lead	Z No Qualifier

SECTION: Ø MEDICAL AND SURGICAL

BODY SYSTEM: D GASTROINTESTINAL SYSTEM

OPERATION: J INSPECTION: Visually and/or manually exploring a body part

Body Part	Approach	Device	Qualifier
Ø Upper Intestinal Tract 6 Stomach D Lower Intestinal Tract	Ø Open 3 Percutaneous 4 Percutaneous Endoscopic 7 Via Natural or Artificial Opening 8 Via Natural or Artificial Opening Endoscopic X External	Z No Device	Z No Qualifier
U Omentum V Mesentery W Peritoneum	Ø Open 3 Percutaneous 4 Percutaneous Endoscopic X External	Z No Device	Z No Qualifier

DRG Non-OR ØDJ[UVW]3ZZ
Non-OR ØDJ[Ø6D][378X]ZZ
Non-OR ØDJ[UVW]XZZ

Coding Clinic: 2015, Q3, P25 – ØDJØ8ZZ
Coding Clinic: 2016, Q2, P21 – ØDJØ7ZZ
Coding Clinic: 2017, Q2, P15 – ØDJD8ZZ

SECTION: Ø MEDICAL AND SURGICAL
BODY SYSTEM: D GASTROINTESTINAL SYSTEM
OPERATION: L OCCLUSION: Completely closing an orifice or the lumen of a tubular body part

Body Part	Approach	Device	Qualifier
1 Esophagus, Upper 2 Esophagus, Middle 3 Esophagus, Lower 4 Esophagogastric Junction 5 Esophagus 6 Stomach 7 Stomach, Pylorus 8 Small Intestine 9 Duodenum A Jejunum B Ileum C Ileocecal Valve E Large Intestine F Large Intestine, Right G Large Intestine, Left H Cecum K Ascending Colon L Transverse Colon M Descending Colon N Sigmoid Colon P Rectum	Ø Open 3 Percutaneous 4 Percutaneous Endoscopic	C Extraluminal Device D Intraluminal Device Z No Device	Z No Qualifier
1 Esophagus, Upper 2 Esophagus, Middle 3 Esophagus, Lower 4 Esophagogastric Junction 5 Esophagus 6 Stomach 7 Stomach, Pylorus 8 Small Intestine 9 Duodenum A Jejunum B Ileum C Ileocecal Valve E Large Intestine F Large Intestine, Right G Large Intestine, Left H Cecum K Ascending Colon L Transverse Colon M Descending Colon N Sigmoid Colon P Rectum	7 Via Natural or Artificial Opening 8 Via Natural or Artificial Opening Endoscopic	D Intraluminal Device Z No Device	Z No Qualifier
Q Anus	Ø Open 3 Percutaneous 4 Percutaneous Endoscopic X External	C Extraluminal Device D Intraluminal Device Z No Device	Z No Qualifier
Q Anus	7 Via Natural or Artificial Opening 8 Via Natural or Artificial Opening Endoscopic	D Intraluminal Device Z No Device	Z No Qualifier

Non-OR ØDL[12345][Ø34][CDZ]Z
Non-OR ØDL[12345][78][DZ]Z

Ø: M/S

D: GASTROINTESTINAL SYSTEM

L: OCCLUSION

New/Revised Text in Green ~~deleted~~ Deleted ♀ Females Only ♂ Males Only **Coding Clinic**
Non-covered Limited Coverage ⊞ Combination (See Appendix E) DRG Non-OR Non-OR Hospital-Acquired Condition

SECTION: Ø MEDICAL AND SURGICAL
BODY SYSTEM: D GASTROINTESTINAL SYSTEM
OPERATION: M REATTACHMENT: Putting back in or on all or a portion of a separated body part to its normal location or other suitable location

Body Part	Approach	Device	Qualifier
5 Esophagus 6 Stomach 8 Small Intestine 9 Duodenum A Jejunum B Ileum E Large Intestine F Large Intestine, Right G Large Intestine, Left H Cecum K Ascending Colon L Transverse Colon M Descending Colon N Sigmoid Colon P Rectum	Ø Open 4 Percutaneous Endoscopic	Z No Device	Z No Qualifier

SECTION: Ø MEDICAL AND SURGICAL

BODY SYSTEM: D GASTROINTESTINAL SYSTEM

OPERATION: N RELEASE: Freeing a body part from an abnormal physical constraint by cutting or by the use of force

Body Part	Approach	Device	Qualifier

1 Esophagus, Upper
2 Esophagus, Middle
3 Esophagus, Lower
4 Esophagogastric Junction
5 Esophagus
6 Stomach
7 Stomach, Pylorus
8 Small Intestine
9 Duodenum
A Jejunum
B Ileum
C Ileocecal Valve
E Large Intestine
F Large Intestine, Right
G Large Intestine, Left
H Cecum
J Appendix
K Ascending Colon
L Transverse Colon
M Descending Colon
N Sigmoid Colon
P Rectum
	Ø Open
	3 Percutaneous
	4 Percutaneous Endoscopic
	7 Via Natural or Artificial
	   Opening
	8 Via Natural or Artificial
	   Opening Endoscopic
		Z No Device	Z No Qualifier

Q Anus	Ø Open
	3 Percutaneous
	4 Percutaneous Endoscopic
	7 Via Natural or Artificial
	   Opening
	8 Via Natural or Artificial
	   Opening Endoscopic
	X External
		Z No Device	Z No Qualifier

R Anal Sphincter U Omentum V Mesentery W Peritoneum	Ø Open 3 Percutaneous 4 Percutaneous Endoscopic	Z No Device	Z No Qualifier

Non-OR ØDN[89ABEFGHKLMN][78]ZZ

Coding Clinic: 2015, Q3, P15-16 – ØDN5ØZZ
Coding Clinic: 2017, Q1, P35 – ØDNWØZZ
Coding Clinic: 2017, Q4, P5Ø – ØDN8ØZZ

SECTION: Ø MEDICAL AND SURGICAL
BODY SYSTEM: D GASTROINTESTINAL SYSTEM
OPERATION: P REMOVAL: *(on multiple pages)*
Taking out or off a device from a body part

P: REMOVAL

D: GASTROINTESTINAL SYSTEM

Ø: M/S

Body Part	Approach	Device	Qualifier
Ø Upper Intestinal Tract D Lower Intestinal Tract	Ø Open 3 Percutaneous 4 Percutaneous Endoscopic 7 Via Natural or Artificial Opening 8 Via Natural or Artificial Opening Endoscopic	Ø Drainage Device 2 Monitoring Device 3 Infusion Device 7 Autologous Tissue Substitute C Extraluminal Device D Intraluminal Device J Synthetic Substitute K Nonautologous Tissue Substitute U Feeding Device Y Other Device	Z No Qualifier
Ø Upper Intestinal Tract D Lower Intestinal Tract	X External	Ø Drainage Device 2 Monitoring Device 3 Infusion Device D Intraluminal Device U Feeding Device	Z No Qualifier
5 Esophagus	Ø Open 3 Percutaneous 4 Percutaneous Endoscopic	1 Radioactive Element 2 Monitoring Device 3 Infusion Device U Feeding Device Y Other Device	Z No Qualifier
5 Esophagus	7 Via Natural or Artificial Opening 8 Via Natural or Artificial Opening Endoscopic	1 Radioactive Element D Intraluminal Device Y Other Device	Z No Qualifier
5 Esophagus	X External	1 Radioactive Element 2 Monitoring Device 3 Infusion Device D Intraluminal Device U Feeding Device	Z No Qualifier
6 Stomach	Ø Open 3 Percutaneous 4 Percutaneous Endoscopic	Ø Drainage Device 2 Monitoring Device 3 Infusion Device 7 Autologous Tissue Substitute C Extraluminal Device D Intraluminal Device J Synthetic Substitute K Nonautologous Tissue Substitute M Stimulator Lead U Feeding Device Y Other Device	Z No Qualifier

Non-OR ØDP[ØD][78][Ø23D]Z
Non-OR ØDP[ØD]X[Ø23DU]Z
Non-OR ØDP5[78][1D]Z
Non-OR ØDP5X[123DU]Z

New/Revised Text in Green ~~deleted~~ Deleted ♀ Females Only ♂ Males Only **Coding Clinic**
Non-covered Limited Coverage ⊕ Combination (See Appendix E) DRG Non-OR Non-OR Hospital-Acquired Condition

SECTION: Ø MEDICAL AND SURGICAL
BODY SYSTEM: D GASTROINTESTINAL SYSTEM
OPERATION: P REMOVAL: *(continued)*
Taking out or off a device from a body part

Body Part	Approach	Device	Qualifier
6 Stomach	7 Via Natural or Artificial Opening 8 Via Natural or Artificial Opening Endoscopic	Ø Drainage Device 2 Monitoring Device 3 Infusion Device 7 Autologous Tissue Substitute C Extraluminal Device D Intraluminal Device J Synthetic Substitute K Nonautologous Tissue Substitute U Feeding Device Y Other Device	Z No Qualifier
6 Stomach	X External	Ø Drainage Device 2 Monitoring Device 3 Infusion Device D Intraluminal Device U Feeding Device	Z No Qualifier
P Rectum	Ø Open 3 Percutaneous 4 Percutaneous Endoscopic 7 Via Natural or Artificial Opening 8 Via Natural or Artificial Opening Endoscopic X External	1 Radioactive Element	Z No Qualifier
Q Anus	Ø Open 3 Percutaneous 4 Percutaneous Endoscopic 7 Via Natural or Artificial Opening 8 Via Natural or Artificial Opening Endoscopic	L Artificial Sphincter	Z No Qualifier
R Anal Sphincter	Ø Open 3 Percutaneous 4 Percutaneous Endoscopic	M Stimulator Lead	Z No Qualifier
U Omentum V Mesentery W Peritoneum	Ø Open 3 Percutaneous 4 Percutaneous Endoscopic	Ø Drainage Device 1 Radioactive Element 7 Autologous Tissue Substitute J Synthetic Substitute K Nonautologous Tissue Substitute	Z No Qualifier

Non-OR ØDP6[78][Ø23D]Z
Non-OR ØDP6X[Ø23DU]Z
Non-OR ØDPP[78X]1Z

New/Revised Text in Green   ~~deleted~~ Deleted   ♀ Females Only   ♂ Males Only   **Coding Clinic**

Non-covered   Limited Coverage   ⊕ Combination (See Appendix E)   DRG Non-OR   Non-OR   Hospital-Acquired Condition

SECTION: Ø MEDICAL AND SURGICAL
BODY SYSTEM: D GASTROINTESTINAL SYSTEM
OPERATION: Q REPAIR: Restoring, to the extent possible, a body part to its normal anatomic structure and function

Body Part	Approach	Device	Qualifier
1 Esophagus, Upper 2 Esophagus, Middle 3 Esophagus, Lower 4 Esophagogastric Junction 5 Esophagus 6 Stomach 7 Stomach, Pylorus 8 Small Intestine ⊞ 9 Duodenum ⊞ A Jejunum ⊞ B Ileum ⊞ C Ileocecal Valve E Large Intestine ⊞ F Large Intestine, Right ⊞ G Large Intestine, Left ⊞ H Cecum ⊞ J Appendix K Ascending Colon ⊞ L Transverse Colon ⊞ M Descending Colon ⊞ N Sigmoid Colon ⊞ P Rectum	Ø Open 3 Percutaneous 4 Percutaneous Endoscopic 7 Via Natural or Artificial Opening 8 Via Natural or Artificial Opening Endoscopic	Z No Device	Z No Qualifier
Q Anus	Ø Open 3 Percutaneous 4 Percutaneous Endoscopic 7 Via Natural or Artificial Opening 8 Via Natural or Artificial Opening Endoscopic X External	Z No Device	Z No Qualifier
R Anal Sphincter U Omentum V Mesentery W Peritoneum	Ø Open 3 Percutaneous 4 Percutaneous Endoscopic	Z No Device	Z No Qualifier

⊞ ØDQ[89ABEFGHKLMN]ØZZ
⊞ ØDQW[Ø34]ZZ

Coding Clinic: 2016, Q1, P7-8 – ØDQRØZZ, ØDQPØZZ
Coding Clinic: 2018, Q1, P11 – ØDQV4ZZ

SECTION: Ø MEDICAL AND SURGICAL

BODY SYSTEM: D GASTROINTESTINAL SYSTEM

OPERATION: R REPLACEMENT: Putting in or on biological or synthetic material that physically takes the place and/or function of all or a portion of a body part

Body Part	Approach	Device	Qualifier
5 Esophagus	Ø Open 4 Percutaneous Endoscopic 7 Via Natural or Artificial Opening 8 Via Natural or Artificial Opening Endoscopic	7 Autologous Tissue Substitute J Synthetic Substitute K Nonautologous Tissue Substitute	Z No Qualifier
R Anal Sphincter U Omentum V Mesentery W Peritoneum	Ø Open 4 Percutaneous Endoscopic	7 Autologous Tissue Substitute J Synthetic Substitute K Nonautologous Tissue Substitute	Z No Qualifier

SECTION: Ø MEDICAL AND SURGICAL

BODY SYSTEM: D GASTROINTESTINAL SYSTEM

OPERATION: S REPOSITION: Moving to its normal location, or other suitable location, all or a portion of a body part

Body Part	Approach	Device	Qualifier
5 Esophagus 6 Stomach 9 Duodenum A Jejunum B Ileum H Cecum K Ascending Colon L Transverse Colon M Descending Colon N Sigmoid Colon P Rectum Q Anus	Ø Open 4 Percutaneous Endoscopic 7 Via Natural or Artificial Opening 8 Via Natural or Artificial Opening Endoscopic X External	Z No Device	Z No Qualifier
8 Small Intestine E Large Intestine	Ø Open 4 Percutaneous Endoscopic 7 Via Natural or Artificial Opening 8 Via Natural or Artificial Opening Endoscopic	Z No Device	Z No Qualifier

Non-OR ØDS[69ABHKLMNP]XZZ

Coding Clinic: 2016, Q3, P5 – ØDSM4ZZ
Coding Clinic: 2017, Q3, P10 – ØDS[BK]7ZZ
Coding Clinic: 2017, Q3, P18 – ØDSPØZZ
Coding Clinic: 2017, Q4, P50 – ØDS[8E]ØZZ

SECTION: Ø MEDICAL AND SURGICAL
BODY SYSTEM: D GASTROINTESTINAL SYSTEM
OPERATION: T RESECTION: Cutting out or off, without replacement, all of a body part

Body Part	Approach	Device	Qualifier
1 Esophagus, Upper 2 Esophagus, Middle 3 Esophagus, Lower 4 Esophagogastric Junction 5 Esophagus 6 Stomach 7 Stomach, Pylorus 8 Small Intestine 9 Duodenum ⊞ A Jejunum B Ileum C Ileocecal Valve E Large Intestine F Large Intestine, Right H Cecum J Appendix K Ascending Colon P Rectum Q Anus	Ø Open 4 Percutaneous Endoscopic 7 Via Natural or Artificial Opening 8 Via Natural or Artificial Opening Endoscopic	Z No Device	Z No Qualifier
G Large Intestine, Left L Transverse Colon M Descending Colon N Sigmoid Colon	Ø Open 4 Percutaneous Endoscopic 7 Via Natural or Artificial Opening 8 Via Natural or Artificial Opening Endoscopic F Via Natural or Artificial Opening With Percutaneous Endoscopic Assistance	Z No Device	Z No Qualifier
R Anal Sphincter U Omentum	Ø Open 4 Percutaneous Endoscopic	Z No Device	Z No Qualifier

⊞ ØDT9ØZZ

Coding Clinic: 2017, Q4, P5Ø – ØDTJØZZ

SECTION: Ø MEDICAL AND SURGICAL
BODY SYSTEM: D GASTROINTESTINAL SYSTEM
OPERATION: U SUPPLEMENT: Putting in or on biological or synthetic material that physically reinforces and/or augments the function of a portion of a body part

Body Part	Approach	Device	Qualifier
1 Esophagus, Upper 2 Esophagus, Middle 3 Esophagus, Lower 4 Esophagogastric Junction 5 Esophagus 6 Stomach 7 Stomach, Pylorus 8 Small Intestine 9 Duodenum A Jejunum B Ileum C Ileocecal Valve E Large Intestine F Large Intestine, Right G Large Intestine, Left H Cecum K Ascending Colon L Transverse Colon M Descending Colon N Sigmoid Colon P Rectum	Ø Open 4 Percutaneous Endoscopic 7 Via Natural or Artificial Opening 8 Via Natural or Artificial Opening Endoscopic	7 Autologous Tissue Substitute J Synthetic Substitute K Nonautologous Tissue Substitute	Z No Qualifier
Q Anus	Ø Open 4 Percutaneous Endoscopic 7 Via Natural or Artificial Opening 8 Via Natural or Artificial Opening Endoscopic X External	7 Autologous Tissue Substitute J Synthetic Substitute K Nonautologous Tissue Substitute	Z No Qualifier
R Anal Sphincter U Omentum V Mesentery W Peritoneum	Ø Open 4 Percutaneous Endoscopic	7 Autologous Tissue Substitute J Synthetic Substitute K Nonautologous Tissue Substitute	Z No Qualifier

Ø: M/S

D: GASTROINTESTINAL SYSTEM

U: SUPPLEMENT

SECTION: Ø MEDICAL AND SURGICAL
BODY SYSTEM: D GASTROINTESTINAL SYSTEM
OPERATION: V RESTRICTION: Partially closing an orifice or the lumen of a tubular body part

Body Part	Approach	Device	Qualifier
1 Esophagus, Upper 2 Esophagus, Middle 3 Esophagus, Lower 4 Esophagogastric Junction 5 Esophagus 6 Stomach 7 Stomach, Pylorus 8 Small Intestine 9 Duodenum A Jejunum B Ileum C Ileocecal Valve E Large Intestine F Large Intestine, Right G Large Intestine, Left H Cecum K Ascending Colon L Transverse Colon M Descending Colon N Sigmoid Colon P Rectum	Ø Open 3 Percutaneous 4 Percutaneous Endoscopic	C Extraluminal Device D Intraluminal Device Z No Device	Z No Qualifier
1 Esophagus, Upper 2 Esophagus, Middle 3 Esophagus, Lower 4 Esophagogastric Junction 5 Esophagus 6 Stomach 7 Stomach, Pylorus 8 Small Intestine 9 Duodenum A Jejunum B Ileum C Ileocecal Valve E Large Intestine F Large Intestine, Right G Large Intestine, Left H Cecum K Ascending Colon L Colon M Descending Colon N Sigmoid Colon P Rectum	7 Via Natural or Artificial Opening 8 Via Natural or Artificial Opening Endoscopic	D Intraluminal Device Z No Device	Z No Qualifier
Q Anus	Ø Open 3 Percutaneous 4 Percutaneous Endoscopic X External	C Extraluminal Device D Intraluminal Device Z No Device	Z No Qualifier
Q Anus	7 Via Natural or Artificial Opening 8 Via Natural or Artificial Opening Endoscopic	D Intraluminal Device Z No Device	Z No Qualifier

ØDV6[78]DZ
Non-OR ØDV6[78]DZ
ØDV64CZ when reported with Principal Diagnosis E66.01 and Secondary Diagnosis K68.11, K95.01, K95.81, or T81.4XXA

Coding Clinic: 2016, Q2, P23 – ØDV4ØZZ   Coding Clinic: 2017, Q3, P23 – ØDV44ZZ

New/Revised Text in Green   deleted Deleted   ♀ Females Only   ♂ Males Only   **Coding Clinic**
Non-covered   Limited Coverage   ⊞ Combination (See Appendix E)   DRG Non-OR   Non-OR   Hospital-Acquired Condition

SECTION: Ø MEDICAL AND SURGICAL
BODY SYSTEM: D GASTROINTESTINAL SYSTEM
OPERATION: W REVISION: *(on multiple pages)*
Correcting, to the extent possible, a portion of a malfunctioning device or the position of a displaced device

Body Part	Approach	Device	Qualifier
Ø Upper Intestinal Tract D Lower Intestinal Tract	Ø Open 3 Percutaneous 4 Percutaneous Endoscopic 7 Via Natural or Artificial Opening 8 Via Natural or Artificial Opening Endoscopic	Ø Drainage Device 2 Monitoring Device 3 Infusion Device 7 Autologous Tissue Substitute C Extraluminal Device D Intraluminal Device J Synthetic Substitute K Nonautologous Tissue Substitute U Feeding Device Y Other Device	Z No Qualifier
Ø Upper Intestinal Tract D Lower Intestinal Tract	X External	Ø Drainage Device 2 Monitoring Device 3 Infusion Device 7 Autologous Tissue Substitute C Extraluminal Device D Intraluminal Device J Synthetic Substitute K Nonautologous Tissue Substitute U Feeding Device	Z No Qualifier
5 Esophagus	Ø Open 3 Percutaneous 4 Percutaneous Endoscopic	Y Other Device	Z No Qualifier
5 Esophagus	7 Via Natural or Artificial Opening 8 Via Natural or Artificial Opening Endoscopic	D Intraluminal Device Y Other Device	Z No Qualifier
5 Esophagus	X External	D Intraluminal Device	Z No Qualifier
6 Stomach	Ø Open 3 Percutaneous 4 Percutaneous Endoscopic	Ø Drainage Device 2 Monitoring Device 3 Infusion Device 7 Autologous Tissue Substitute C Extraluminal Device D Intraluminal Device J Synthetic Substitute K Nonautologous Tissue Substitute M Stimulator Lead U Feeding Device Y Other Device	Z No Qualifier
6 Stomach	7 Via Natural or Artificial Opening 8 Via Natural or Artificial Opening Endoscopic	Ø Drainage Device 2 Monitoring Device 3 Infusion Device 7 Autologous Tissue Substitute C Extraluminal Device D Intraluminal Device J Synthetic Substitute K Nonautologous Tissue Substitute U Feeding Device Y Other Device	Z No Qualifier

Non-OR ØDW[ØD]X[Ø237CDJKU]Z
Non-OR ØDW5XDZ
Non-OR ØDW6X[Ø237CDJKU]Z
Non-OR ØDW[UVW][Ø34]ØZ

Coding Clinic: 2Ø18, Q1, P2Ø – ØDW63CZ

New/Revised Text in Green   ~~deleted~~ Deleted   ♀ Females Only   ♂ Males Only   **Coding Clinic**
🔷 Non-covered   🔷 Limited Coverage   ⊞ Combination (See Appendix E)   DRG Non-OR   Non-OR   🔷 Hospital-Acquired Condition

261

SECTION: Ø MEDICAL AND SURGICAL
BODY SYSTEM: D GASTROINTESTINAL SYSTEM
OPERATION: W REVISION: *(continued)*
Correcting, to the extent possible, a portion of a malfunctioning device or the position of a displaced device

Body Part	Approach	Device	Qualifier
6 Stomach	X External	Ø Drainage Device 2 Monitoring Device 3 Infusion Device 7 Autologous Tissue Substitute C Extraluminal Device D Intraluminal Device J Synthetic Substitute K Nonautologous Tissue Substitute U Feeding Device	Z No Qualifier
8 Small Intestine E Large Intestine	Ø Open 4 Percutaneous Endoscopic 7 Via Natural or Artificial Opening 8 Via Natural or Artificial Opening Endoscopic	7 Autologous Tissue Substitute J Synthetic Substitute K Nonautologous Tissue Substitute	Z No Qualifier
Q Anus	Ø Open 3 Percutaneous 4 Percutaneous Endoscopic 7 Via Natural or Artificial Opening 8 Via Natural or Artificial Opening Endoscopic	L Artificial Sphincter	Z No Qualifier
R Anal Sphincter	Ø Open 3 Percutaneous 4 Percutaneous Endoscopic	M Stimulator Lead	Z No Qualifier
U Omentum V Mesentery W Peritoneum	Ø Open 3 Percutaneous 4 Percutaneous Endoscopic	Ø Drainage Device 7 Autologous Tissue Substitute J Synthetic Substitute K Nonautologous Tissue Substitute	Z No Qualifier

W: REVISION

D: GASTROINTESTINAL SYSTEM

Ø: M/S

New/Revised Text in Green   deleted Deleted   ♀ Females Only   ♂ Males Only   **Coding Clinic**
🖢 Non-covered   🖢 Limited Coverage   ⊞ Combination (See Appendix E)   DRG Non-OR   Non-OR   🖢 Hospital-Acquired Condition

SECTION: Ø MEDICAL AND SURGICAL

BODY SYSTEM: D GASTROINTESTINAL SYSTEM

OPERATION: X TRANSFER: Moving, without taking out, all or a portion of a body part to another location to take over the function of all or a portion of a body part

Body Part	Approach	Device	Qualifier
6 Stomach 8 Small Intestine E Large Intestine	Ø Open 4 Percutaneous Endoscopic	Z No Device	5 Esophagus

Coding Clinic: 2017, Q2, P18; 2016, Q2, P24 – ØDX60Z5

SECTION: Ø MEDICAL AND SURGICAL

BODY SYSTEM: D GASTROINTESTINAL SYSTEM

OPERATION: Y TRANSPLANTATION: Putting in or on all or a portion of a living body part taken from another individual or animal to physically take the place and/or function of all or a portion of a similar body part

Body Part	Approach	Device	Qualifier
5 Esophagus 6 Stomach 8 Small Intestine 🐾 E Large Intestine 🐾	Ø Open	Z No Device	0 Allogeneic 1 Syngeneic 2 Zooplastic

🐾 ØDY[8E]ØZ[012]
Non-OR ØDY5ØZ[012]

New/Revised Text in Green   ~~deleted~~ Deleted   ♀ Females Only   ♂ Males Only   **Coding Clinic**

Non-covered   Limited Coverage   Combination (See Appendix E)   DRG Non-OR   Non-OR   Hospital-Acquired Condition

SECTION: Ø MEDICAL AND SURGICAL

BODY SYSTEM: F HEPATOBILIARY SYSTEM AND PANCREAS

OPERATION: 1 **BYPASS:** Altering the route of passage of the contents of a tubular body part

Body Part	Approach	Device	Qualifier
4 Gallbladder 5 Hepatic Duct, Right 6 Hepatic Duct, Left 7 Hepatic Duct, Common 8 Cystic Duct 9 Common Bile Duct	Ø Open 4 Percutaneous Endoscopic	D Intraluminal Device Z No Device	3 Duodenum 4 Stomach 5 Hepatic Duct, Right 6 Hepatic Duct, Left 7 Hepatic Duct, Caudate 8 Cystic Duct 9 Common Bile Duct B Small Intestine
D Pancreatic Duct F Pancreatic Duct, Accessory G Pancreas	Ø Open 4 Percutaneous Endoscopic	D Intraluminal Device Z No Device	3 Duodenum B Small Intestine C Large Intestine

SECTION: Ø MEDICAL AND SURGICAL

BODY SYSTEM: F HEPATOBILIARY SYSTEM AND PANCREAS

OPERATION: 2 **CHANGE:** Taking out or off a device from a body part and putting back an identical or similar device in or on the same body part without cutting or puncturing the skin or a mucous membrane

Body Part	Approach	Device	Qualifier
Ø Liver 4 Gallbladder B Hepatobiliary Duct D Pancreatic Duct G Pancreas	X External	Ø Drainage Device Y Other Device	Z No Qualifier

Non-OR All Values

SECTION: Ø MEDICAL AND SURGICAL
BODY SYSTEM: F HEPATOBILIARY SYSTEM AND PANCREAS
OPERATION: 5 **DESTRUCTION:** Physical eradication of all or a portion of a body part by the direct use of energy, force, or a destructive agent

Body Part	Approach	Device	Qualifier
Ø Liver 1 Liver, Right Lobe 2 Liver, Left Lobe	Ø Open 3 Percutaneous 4 Percutaneous Endoscopic	Z No Device	F Irreversible Electroporation Z No Qualifier
4 Gallbladder G Pancreas	Ø Open 3 Percutaneous 4 Percutaneous Endoscopic 8 Via Natural or Artificial Opening Endoscopic	Z No Device	Z No Qualifier
5 Hepatic Duct, Right 6 Hepatic Duct, Left 7 Hepatic Duct, Common 8 Cystic Duct 9 Common Bile Duct C Ampulla of Vater D Pancreatic Duct F Pancreatic Duct, Accessory	Ø Open 3 Percutaneous 4 Percutaneous Endoscopic 7 Via Natural or Artificial Opening 8 Via Natural or Artificial Opening Endoscopic	Z No Device	Z No Qualifier
G Pancreas	Ø Open 3 Percutaneous 4 Percutaneous Endoscopic	Z No Device	F Irreversible Electroporation Z No Qualifier
G Pancreas	8 Via Natural or Artificial Opening Endoscopic	Z No Device	Z No Qualifier

Non-OR ØF5G4ZZ
Non-OR ØF5[5689CDF][48]ZZ

New/Revised Text in Green   ~~deleted~~ Deleted   ♀ Females Only   ♂ Males Only   **Coding Clinic**
🞕 Non-covered   🞕 Limited Coverage   ⊕ Combination (See Appendix E)   DRG Non-OR   Non-OR   🞕 Hospital-Acquired Condition

SECTION:　Ø　MEDICAL AND SURGICAL

BODY SYSTEM: F　HEPATOBILIARY SYSTEM AND PANCREAS

OPERATION:　7　**DILATION:** Expanding an orifice or the lumen of a tubular body part

Body Part	Approach	Device	Qualifier
5 Hepatic Duct, Right 6 Hepatic Duct, Left 7 Hepatic Duct, Common 8 Cystic Duct 9 Common Bile Duct C Ampulla of Vater D Pancreatic Duct F Pancreatic Duct, Accessory	Ø Open 3 Percutaneous 4 Percutaneous Endoscopic 7 Via Natural or Artificial Opening 8 Via Natural or Artificial Opening 　 Endoscopic	D Intraluminal Device Z No Device	Z No Qualifier

Non-OR　ØF7[5689][34][DZ]Z
Non-OR　ØF7[5689D][78]DZ
Non-OR　ØF7[CF]8DZ
Non-OR　ØF7[DF]4[DZ]Z
Non-OR　ØF7[5689CDF]8ZZ

Coding Clinic: 2016, Q1, P25 – ØF798DZ, ØF7D8DZ
Coding Clinic: 2016, Q3, P28 – ØF7D8DZ

SECTION:　Ø　MEDICAL AND SURGICAL

BODY SYSTEM: F　HEPATOBILIARY SYSTEM AND PANCREAS

OPERATION:　8　**DIVISION:** Cutting into a body part, without draining fluids and/or gases from the body part, in order to separate or transect a body part

Body Part	Approach	Device	Qualifier
G Pancreas	Ø Open 3 Percutaneous 4 Percutaneous Endoscopic	Z No Device	Z No Qualifier

SECTION: Ø MEDICAL AND SURGICAL
BODY SYSTEM: F HEPATOBILIARY SYSTEM AND PANCREAS
OPERATION: 9 DRAINAGE: Taking or letting out fluids and/or gases from a body part

Body Part	Approach	Device	Qualifier
Ø Liver 1 Liver, Right Lobe 2 Liver, Left Lobe	Ø Open 3 Percutaneous 4 Percutaneous Endoscopic	Ø Drainage Device	Z No Qualifier
Ø Liver 1 Liver, Right Lobe 2 Liver, Left Lobe	Ø Open 3 Percutaneous 4 Percutaneous Endoscopic	Z No Device	X Diagnostic Z No Qualifier
4 Gallbladder G Pancreas	Ø Open 3 Percutaneous 4 Percutaneous Endoscopic 8 Via Natural or Artificial Opening Endoscopic	Ø Drainage Device	Z No Qualifier
4 Gallbladder G Pancreas	Ø Open 3 Percutaneous 4 Percutaneous Endoscopic 8 Via Natural or Artificial Opening Endoscopic	Z No Device	X Diagnostic Z No Qualifier
5 Hepatic Duct, Right 6 Hepatic Duct, Left 7 Hepatic Duct, Common 8 Cystic Duct 9 Common Bile Duct C Ampulla of Vater D Pancreatic Duct F Pancreatic Duct, Accessory	Ø Open 3 Percutaneous 4 Percutaneous Endoscopic 7 Via Natural or Artificial Opening 8 Via Natural or Artificial Opening Endoscopic	Ø Drainage Device	Z No Qualifier
5 Hepatic Duct, Right 6 Hepatic Duct, Left 7 Hepatic Duct, Common 8 Cystic Duct 9 Common Bile Duct C Ampulla of Vater D Pancreatic Duct F Pancreatic Duct, Accessory	Ø Open 3 Percutaneous 4 Percutaneous Endoscopic 7 Via Natural or Artificial Opening 8 Via Natural or Artificial Opening Endoscopic	Z No Device	X Diagnostic Z No Qualifier

Non-OR ØF9[Ø12][34]ØZ
Non-OR ØF9[4G]3ØZ
Non-OR ØF944ØZ
Non-OR ØF9G3ZZ
Non-OR ØF9[Ø124][34]Z[XZ]
Non-OR ØF9G[34]ZX
Non-OR ØF9[5689CDF]3ØZ
Non-OR ØF9[9DF]8ØZ
Non-OR ØF9C[48]ØZ

Non-OR ØF9[568][3478]ZX
Non-OR ØF99[3478]Z[XZ]
Non-OR ØF9[CDF][347]ZX
Non-OR ØF9[568CDF]3ZZ
Non-OR ØF994ZZ
Non-OR ØF9C8Z[XZ]
Non-OR ØF9[DF]8ZX

Coding Clinic: 2Ø15, Q1, P32 – ØF963ØZ

New/Revised Text in Green deleted Deleted ♀ Females Only ♂ Males Only **Coding Clinic**
Non-covered Limited Coverage Combination (See Appendix E) DRG Non-OR Non-OR Hospital-Acquired Condition

9: DRAINAGE
F: HEPATOBILIARY SYSTEM AND PANCREAS
Ø: M/S

SECTION: Ø MEDICAL AND SURGICAL
BODY SYSTEM: F HEPATOBILIARY SYSTEM AND PANCREAS
OPERATION: B EXCISION: Cutting out or off, without replacement, a portion of a body part

Body Part	Approach	Device	Qualifier
Ø Liver 1 Liver, Right Lobe 2 Liver, Left Lobe	Ø Open 3 Percutaneous 4 Percutaneous Endoscopic	Z No Device	X Diagnostic Z No Qualifier
4 Gallbladder G Pancreas	Ø Open 3 Percutaneous 4 Percutaneous Endoscopic 8 Via Natural or Artificial Opening Endoscopic	Z No Device	X Diagnostic Z No Qualifier
5 Hepatic Duct, Right 6 Hepatic Duct, Left 7 Hepatic Duct, Common 8 Cystic Duct 9 Common Bile Duct C Ampulla of Vater D Pancreatic Duct F Pancreatic Duct, Accessory	Ø Open 3 Percutaneous 4 Percutaneous Endoscopic 7 Via Natural or Artificial Opening 8 Via Natural or Artificial Opening Endoscopic	Z No Device	X Diagnostic Z No Qualifier

Non-OR ØFB[Ø12]3ZX
Non-OR ØFB[4G][34]ZX
Non-OR ØFB[5689CDF][3478]ZX
Non-OR ØFB[5689CDF][48]ZZ

Coding Clinic: 2016, Q1, P23, P25 – ØFB98ZX
Coding Clinic: 2016, Q1, P25 – ØFBD8ZX
Coding Clinic: 2016, Q3, P41 – ØFBØØZX

SECTION: Ø MEDICAL AND SURGICAL
BODY SYSTEM: F HEPATOBILIARY SYSTEM AND PANCREAS
OPERATION: C EXTIRPATION: Taking or cutting out solid matter from a body part

Body Part	Approach	Device	Qualifier
Ø Liver 1 Liver, Right Lobe 2 Liver, Left Lobe	Ø Open 3 Percutaneous 4 Percutaneous Endoscopic	Z No Device	Z No Qualifier
4 Gallbladder G Pancreas	Ø Open 3 Percutaneous 4 Percutaneous Endoscopic 8 Via Natural or Artificial Opening Endoscopic	Z No Device	Z No Qualifier
5 Hepatic Duct, Right 6 Hepatic Duct, Left 7 Hepatic Duct, Common 8 Cystic Duct 9 Common Bile Duct C Ampulla of Vater D Pancreatic Duct F Pancreatic Duct, Accessory	Ø Open 3 Percutaneous 4 Percutaneous Endoscopic 7 Via Natural or Artificial Opening 8 Via Natural or Artificial Opening Endoscopic	Z No Device	Z No Qualifier

Non-OR ØFC[5689][3478]ZZ
Non-OR ØFCC[48]ZZ
Non-OR ØFC[DF][348]ZZ

Ø: M/S

F: HEPATOBILIARY SYSTEM AND PANCREAS

B: EXCISION   C: EXTIRPATION

New/Revised Text in Green   ~~deleted~~ Deleted   ♀ Females Only   ♂ Males Only   **Coding Clinic**
🚫 Non-covered   🚫 Limited Coverage   ⊞ Combination (See Appendix E)   DRG Non-OR   Non-OR   🚫 Hospital-Acquired Condition

269

SECTION: Ø MEDICAL AND SURGICAL
BODY SYSTEM: F HEPATOBILIARY SYSTEM AND PANCREAS
OPERATION: D EXTRACTION: Pulling or stripping out or off all or a portion of a body part by the use of force

Body Part	Approach	Device	Qualifier
Ø Liver 1 Liver, Right Lobe 2 Liver, Left Lobe	3 Percutaneous 4 Percutaneous Endoscopic	Z No Device	X Diagnostic
4 Gallbladder 5 Hepatic Duct, Right 6 Hepatic Duct, Left 7 Hepatic Duct, Common 8 Cystic Duct 9 Common Bile Duct C Ampulla of Vater D Pancreatic Duct F Pancreatic Duct, Accessory G Pancreas	3 Percutaneous 4 Percutaneous Endoscopic 8 Via Natural or Artificial Opening Endoscopic	Z No Device	X Diagnostic

SECTION: Ø MEDICAL AND SURGICAL
BODY SYSTEM: F HEPATOBILIARY SYSTEM AND PANCREAS
OPERATION: F FRAGMENTATION: Breaking solid matter in a body part into pieces

Body Part	Approach	Device	Qualifier
4 Gallbladder ☜ 5 Hepatic Duct, Right ☜ 6 Hepatic Duct, Left ☜ 7 Hepatic Duct, Common 8 Cystic Duct ☜ 9 Common Bile Duct ☜ C Ampulla of Vater ☜ D Pancreatic Duct ☜ F Pancreatic Duct, Acessory ☜	Ø Open 3 Percutaneous 4 Percutaneous Endoscopic 7 Via Natural or Artificial Opening 8 Via Natural or Artificial Opening Endoscopic X External	Z No Device	Z No Qualifier

☜ ØFF[45689CDF]XZZ   Non-OR ØFF[45689C][8X]ZZ   Non-OR ØFF[DF]XZZ

SECTION: Ø MEDICAL AND SURGICAL
BODY SYSTEM: F HEPATOBILIARY SYSTEM AND PANCREAS
OPERATION: H INSERTION: Putting in a nonbiological appliance that monitors, assists, performs, or prevents a physiological function but does not physically take the place of a body part

Body Part	Approach	Device	Qualifier
Ø Liver 4 Gallbladder G Pancreas	Ø Open 3 Percutaneous 4 Percutaneous Endoscopic	2 Monitoring Device 3 Infusion Device Y Other Device	Z No Qualifier
1 Liver, Right Lobe 2 Liver, Left Lobe	Ø Open 3 Percutaneous 4 Percutaneous Endoscopic	2 Monitoring Device 3 Infusion Device	Z No Qualifier
B Hepatobiliary Duct D Pancreatic Duct	Ø Open 3 Percutaneous 4 Percutaneous Endoscopic 7 Via Natural or Artificial Opening 8 Via Natural or Artificial Opening Endoscopic	1 Radioactive Element 2 Monitoring Device 3 Infusion Device D Intraluminal Device Y Other Device	Z No Qualifier

Non-OR ØFH[04G][034]3Z   Non-OR ØFH[BD][78][23]Z   Non-OR ØFH[BD]4DZ
Non-OR ØFH[12][034]3Z   Non-OR ØFH[BD][03478]3Z   Non-OR ØFH[BD]8DZ

New/Revised Text in Green   ~~deleted~~ Deleted   ♀ Females Only   ♂ Males Only   **Coding Clinic**
☜ Non-covered   ☜ Limited Coverage   ⊡ Combination (See Appendix E)   DRG Non-OR   Non-OR   ☜ Hospital-Acquired Condition

SECTION: Ø MEDICAL AND SURGICAL
BODY SYSTEM: F HEPATOBILIARY SYSTEM AND PANCREAS
OPERATION: J INSPECTION: Visually and/or manually exploring a body part

Body Part	Approach	Device	Qualifier
Ø Liver	Ø Open 3 Percutaneous 4 Percutaneous Endoscopic X External	Z No Device	Z No Qualifier
4 Gallbladder G Pancreas	Ø Open 3 Percutaneous 4 Percutaneous Endoscopic 8 Via Natural or Artificial Opening Endoscopic X External	Z No Device	Z No Qualifier

B Hepatobiliary Duct
D Pancreatic Duct
	Ø Open
	3 Percutaneous
	4 Percutaneous Endoscopic
	7 Via Natural or Artificial
	   Opening
	8 Via Natural or Artificial
	   Opening Endoscopic
		Z No Device	Z No Qualifier

DRG Non-OR	ØFJØ3ZZ
DRG Non-OR	ØFJG3ZZ
DRG Non-OR	ØFJD[378]ZZ
Non-OR	ØFJØXZZ
Non-OR	ØFJ[4G]XZZ
Non-OR	ØFJ43ZZ
Non-OR	ØFJB[378]ZZ

SECTION: Ø MEDICAL AND SURGICAL
BODY SYSTEM: F HEPATOBILIARY SYSTEM AND PANCREAS
OPERATION: L OCCLUSION: Completely closing an orifice or the lumen of a tubular body part

Body Part	Approach	Device	Qualifier
5 Hepatic Duct, Right 6 Hepatic Duct, Left 7 Hepatic Duct, Common 8 Cystic Duct 9 Common Bile Duct C Ampulla of Vater D Pancreatic Duct F Pancreatic Duct, Accessory	Ø Open 3 Percutaneous 4 Percutaneous Endoscopic	C Extraluminal Device D Intraluminal Device Z No Device	Z No Qualifier

5 Hepatic Duct, Right
6 Hepatic Duct, Left
7 Hepatic Duct, Common
8 Cystic Duct
9 Common Bile Duct
C Ampulla of Vater
D Pancreatic Duct
F Pancreatic Duct, Accessory
	7 Via Natural or Artificial
	   Opening
	8 Via Natural or Artificial
	   Opening Endoscopic
		D Intraluminal Device
		Z No Device
			Z No Qualifier

Non-OR	ØFL[5689][34][CDZ]Z
Non-OR	ØFL[5689][78][DZ]Z

Ø: M/S   F: HEPATOBILIARY SYSTEM AND PANCREAS   J: INSPECTION   L: OCCLUSION

SECTION: **Ø MEDICAL AND SURGICAL**

BODY SYSTEM: F HEPATOBILIARY SYSTEM AND PANCREAS

OPERATION: **M REATTACHMENT:** Putting back in or on all or a portion of a separated body part to its normal location or other suitable location

Body Part	Approach	Device	Qualifier
Ø Liver 1 Liver, Right Lobe 2 Liver, Left Lobe 4 Gallbladder 5 Hepatic Duct, Right 6 Hepatic Duct, Left 7 Hepatic Duct, Common 8 Cystic Duct 9 Common Bile Duct C Ampulla of Vater D Pancreatic Duct F Pancreatic Duct, Accessory G Pancreas	Ø Open 4 Percutaneous Endoscopic	Z No Device	Z No Qualifier

Non-OR ØFM[45689]4ZZ

SECTION: **Ø MEDICAL AND SURGICAL**

BODY SYSTEM: F HEPATOBILIARY SYSTEM AND PANCREAS

OPERATION: **N RELEASE:** Freeing a body part from an abnormal physical constraint by cutting or by the use of force

Body Part	Approach	Device	Qualifier
Ø Liver 1 Liver, Right Lobe 2 Liver, Left Lobe	Ø Open 3 Percutaneous 4 Percutaneous Endoscopic	Z No Device	Z No Qualifier
4 Gallbladder G Pancreas	Ø Open 3 Percutaneous 4 Percutaneous Endoscopic 8 Via Natural or Artificial Opening Endoscopic	Z No Device	Z No Qualifier
5 Hepatic Duct, Right 6 Hepatic Duct, Left 7 Hepatic Duct, Common 8 Cystic Duct 9 Common Bile Duct C Ampulla of Vater D Pancreatic Duct F Pancreatic Duct, Accessory	Ø Open 3 Percutaneous 4 Percutaneous Endoscopic 7 Via Natural or Artificial Opening 8 Via Natural or Artificial Opening Endoscopic	Z No Device	Z No Qualifier

New/Revised Text in Green   ~~deleted~~ Deleted   ♀ Females Only   ♂ Males Only   **Coding Clinic**

🇶 Non-covered   🇶 Limited Coverage   ⊕ Combination (See Appendix E)   DRG Non-OR   Non-OR   🇶 Hospital-Acquired Condition

SECTION: Ø MEDICAL AND SURGICAL
BODY SYSTEM: F HEPATOBILIARY SYSTEM AND PANCREAS
OPERATION: P REMOVAL: Taking out or off a device from a body part

Body Part	Approach	Device	Qualifier
Ø Liver	Ø Open 3 Percutaneous 4 Percutaneous Endoscopic	Ø Drainage Device 2 Monitoring Device 3 Infusion Device Y Other Device	Z No Qualifier
Ø Liver	X External	Ø Drainage Device 2 Monitoring Device 3 Infusion Device	Z No Qualifier
4 Gallbladder G Pancreas	Ø Open 3 Percutaneous 4 Percutaneous Endoscopic	Ø Drainage Device 2 Monitoring Device 3 Infusion Device D Intraluminal Device Y Other Device	Z No Qualifier
4 Gallbladder G Pancreas	X External	Ø Drainage Device 2 Monitoring Device 3 Infusion Device D Intraluminal Device	Z No Qualifier
B Hepatobiliary Duct D Pancreatic Duct	Ø Open 3 Percutaneous 4 Percutaneous Endoscopic 7 Via Natural or Artificial Opening 8 Via Natural or Artificial Opening Endoscopic	Ø Drainage Device 1 Radioactive Element 2 Monitoring Device 3 Infusion Device 7 Autologous Tissue Substitute C Extraluminal Device D Intraluminal Device J Synthetic Substitute K Nonautologous Tissue Substitute Y Other Device	Z No Qualifier
B Hepatobiliary Duct D Pancreatic Duct	X External	Ø Drainage Device 1 Radioactive Element 2 Monitoring Device 3 Infusion Device D Intraluminal Device	Z No Qualifier

Non-OR ØFPØX[Ø23]Z
Non-OR ØFP4X[Ø23D]Z
Non-OR ØFPGX[Ø23]Z
Non-OR ØFP[BD][78][Ø23D]Z
Non-OR ØFP[BD]X[Ø123D]Z

Ø: M/S

F: HEPATOBILIARY SYSTEM AND PANCREAS

P: REMOVAL

SECTION: Ø MEDICAL AND SURGICAL

BODY SYSTEM: F HEPATOBILIARY SYSTEM AND PANCREAS

OPERATION: Q REPAIR: Restoring, to the extent possible, a body part to its normal anatomic structure and function

Body Part	Approach	Device	Qualifier
Ø Liver 1 Liver, Right Lobe 2 Liver, Left Lobe	Ø Open 3 Percutaneous 4 Percutaneous Endoscopic	Z No Device	Z No Qualifier
4 Gallbladder G Pancreas	Ø Open 3 Percutaneous 4 Percutaneous Endoscopic 8 Via Natural or Artificial Opening Endoscopic	Z No Device	Z No Qualifier
5 Hepatic Duct, Right 6 Hepatic Duct, Left 7 Hepatic Duct, Common 8 Cystic Duct 9 Common Bile Duct C Ampulla of Vater D Pancreatic Duct F Pancreatic Duct, Accessory	Ø Open 3 Percutaneous 4 Percutaneous Endoscopic 7 Via Natural or Artificial Opening 8 Via Natural or Artificial Opening Endoscopic	Z No Device	Z No Qualifier

Coding Clinic: 2016, Q3, P27 – ØFQ9ØZZ

SECTION: Ø MEDICAL AND SURGICAL

BODY SYSTEM: F HEPATOBILIARY SYSTEM AND PANCREAS

OPERATION: R REPLACEMENT: Putting in or on biological or synthetic material that physically takes the place and/or function of all or a portion of a body part

Body Part	Approach	Device	Qualifier
5 Hepatic Duct, Right 6 Hepatic Duct, Left 7 Hepatic Duct, Common 8 Cystic Duct 9 Common Bile Duct C Ampulla of Vater D Pancreatic Duct F Pancreatic Duct, Accessory	Ø Open 4 Percutaneous Endoscopic 8 Via Natural or Artificial Opening Endoscopic	7 Autologous Tissue Substitute J Synthetic Substitute K Nonautologous Tissue Substitute	Z No Qualifier

Q: REPAIR   R: REPLACEMENT

F: HEPATOBILIARY SYSTEM AND PANCREAS

Ø: M/S

New/Revised Text in Green   ~~deleted~~ Deleted   ♀ Females Only   ♂ Males Only   **Coding Clinic**

Non-covered   Limited Coverage   ⊟ Combination (See Appendix E)   DRG Non-OR   Non-OR   Hospital-Acquired Condition

SECTION: Ø MEDICAL AND SURGICAL

BODY SYSTEM: F HEPATOBILIARY SYSTEM AND PANCREAS

OPERATION: S REPOSITION: Moving to its normal location, or other suitable location, all or a portion of a body part

Body Part	Approach	Device	Qualifier
Ø Liver 4 Gallbladder 5 Hepatic Duct, Right 6 Hepatic Duct, Left 7 Hepatic Duct, Common 8 Cystic Duct 9 Common Bile Duct C Ampulla of Vater D Pancreatic Duct F Pancreatic Duct, Accessory G Pancreas	Ø Open 4 Percutaneous Endoscopic	Z No Device	Z No Qualifier

SECTION: Ø MEDICAL AND SURGICAL

BODY SYSTEM: F HEPATOBILIARY SYSTEM AND PANCREAS

OPERATION: T RESECTION: Cutting out or off, without replacement, all of a body part

Body Part	Approach	Device	Qualifier
Ø Liver 1 Liver, Right Lobe 2 Liver, Left Lobe 4 Gallbladder G Pancreas ⊞	Ø Open 4 Percutaneous Endoscopic	Z No Device	Z No Qualifier
5 Hepatic Duct, Right 6 Hepatic Duct, Left 7 Hepatic Duct, Common 8 Cystic Duct 9 Common Bile Duct C Ampulla of Vater D Pancreatic Duct F Pancreatic Duct, Accessory	Ø Open 4 Percutaneous Endoscopic 7 Via Natural or Artificial Opening 8 Via Natural or Artificial Opening Endoscopic	Z No Device	Z No Qualifier

⊞ ØFTGØZZ

Non-OR ØFT[DF][48]ZZ

Coding Clinic: 2012, Q4, P100 – ØFT00ZZ

SECTION: Ø MEDICAL AND SURGICAL

BODY SYSTEM: F HEPATOBILIARY SYSTEM AND PANCREAS

OPERATION: U SUPPLEMENT: Putting in or on biological or synthetic material that physically reinforces and/or augments the function of a portion of a body part

Body Part	Approach	Device	Qualifier
5 Hepatic Duct, Right 6 Hepatic Duct, Left 7 Hepatic Duct, Common 8 Cystic Duct 9 Common Bile Duct C Ampulla of Vater D Pancreatic Duct F Pancreatic Duct, Accessory	Ø Open 3 Percutaneous 4 Percutaneous Endoscopic 8 Via Natural or Artificial Opening Endoscopic	7 Autologous Tissue Substitute J Synthetic Substitute K Nonautologous Tissue Substitute	Z No Qualifier

SECTION: Ø MEDICAL AND SURGICAL

BODY SYSTEM: F HEPATOBILIARY SYSTEM AND PANCREAS

OPERATION: V RESTRICTION: Partially closing an orifice or the lumen of a tubular body part

Body Part	Approach	Device	Qualifier
5 Hepatic Duct, Right 6 Hepatic Duct, Left 7 Hepatic Duct, Common 8 Cystic Duct 9 Common Bile Duct C Ampulla of Vater D Pancreatic Duct F Pancreatic Duct, Accessory	Ø Open 3 Percutaneous 4 Percutaneous Endoscopic	C Extraluminal Device D Intraluminal Device Z No Device	Z No Qualifier
5 Hepatic Duct, Right 6 Hepatic Duct, Left 7 Hepatic Duct, Common 8 Cystic Duct 9 Common Bile Duct C Ampulla of Vater D Pancreatic Duct F Pancreatic Duct, Accessory	7 Via Natural or Artificial Opening 8 Via Natural or Artificial Opening Endoscopic	D Intraluminal Device Z No Device	Z No Qualifier

Non-OR   ØFV[5689][34][CDZ]Z
Non-OR   ØFV[5689][78][DZ]Z

SECTION: Ø MEDICAL AND SURGICAL
BODY SYSTEM: F HEPATOBILIARY SYSTEM AND PANCREAS
OPERATION: W REVISION: Correcting, to the extent possible, a portion of a malfunctioning device or the position of a displaced device

Body Part	Approach	Device	Qualifier
Ø Liver	Ø Open 3 Percutaneous 4 Percutaneous Endoscopic	Ø Drainage Device 2 Monitoring Device 3 Infusion Device Y Other Device	Z No Qualifier
Ø Liver	X External	Ø Drainage Device 2 Monitoring Device 3 Infusion Device	Z No Qualifier
4 Gallbladder G Pancreas	Ø Open 3 Percutaneous 4 Percutaneous Endoscopic	Ø Drainage Device 2 Monitoring Device 3 Infusion Device D Intraluminal Device Y Other Device	Z No Qualifier
4 Gallbladder G Pancreas	X External	Ø Drainage Device 2 Monitoring Device 3 Infusion Device D Intraluminal Device	Z No Qualifier
B Hepatobiliary Duct D Pancreatic Duct	Ø Open 3 Percutaneous 4 Percutaneous Endoscopic 7 Via Natural or Artificial Opening 8 Via Natural or Artificial Opening Endoscopic	Ø Drainage Device 2 Monitoring Device 3 Infusion Device 7 Autologous Tissue Substitute C Extraluminal Device D Intraluminal Device J Synthetic Substitute K Nonautologous Tissue Substitute Y Other Device	Z No Qualifier
B Hepatobiliary Duct D Pancreatic Duct	X External	Ø Drainage Device 2 Monitoring Device 3 Infusion Device 7 Autologous Tissue Substitute C Extraluminal Device D Intraluminal Device J Synthetic Substitute K Nonautologous Tissue Substitute	Z No Qualifier

Non-OR   ØFWØX[Ø23]Z
Non-OR   ØFW[4G]X[Ø23D]Z
Non-OR   ØFW[BD]X[Ø237CDJK]Z

Ø: M/S

F: HEPATOBILIARY SYSTEM AND PANCREAS

W: REVISION

SECTION: Ø MEDICAL AND SURGICAL

BODY SYSTEM: F HEPATOBILIARY SYSTEM AND PANCREAS

OPERATION: Y TRANSPLANTATION: Putting in or on all or a portion of a living body part taken from another individual or animal to physically take the place and/or function of all or a portion of a similar body part

Body Part	Approach	Device	Qualifier
Ø Liver 🦠 G Pancreas 🦠 🦠 ⊞	Ø Open	Z No Device	Ø Allogeneic 1 Syngeneic 2 Zooplastic

🦠 ØFYGØZ2

🦠 ØFYGØZØ, ØFYGØZ1 alone [without kidney transplant codes (ØTYØØZ[Ø1], ØTY1ØZ[Ø12])], except when ØFYGØZØ or ØFYGØZ1 is combined with at least one principal or secondary diagnosis code from the following list:

E10.10	E10.321	E10.359	E10.44	E10.620	E10.649
E10.11	E10.329	E10.36	E10.49	E10.621	E10.65
E10.21	E10.331	E10.39	E10.51	E10.622	E10.69
E10.22	E10.339	E10.40	E10.52	E10.628	E10.8
E10.29	E10.341	E10.41	E10.59	E10.630	E10.9
E10.311	E10.349	E10.42	E10.610	E10.638	E89.1
E10.319	E10.351	E10.43	E10.618	E10.641	

🦠 ØFYØØZ[Ø12]

🦠 ØFYGØZ[Ø1]

⊞ ØFYGØZ[Ø12]

Coding Clinic: 2012, Q4, P100 – ØFYØØZØ

New/Revised Text in Green   ~~deleted~~ Deleted   ♀ Females Only   ♂ Males Only   **Coding Clinic**
🦠 Non-covered   🦠 Limited Coverage   ⊞ Combination (See Appendix E)   DRG Non-OR   Non-OR   🦠 Hospital-Acquired Condition

SECTION: Ø MEDICAL AND SURGICAL

BODY SYSTEM: G ENDOCRINE SYSTEM

OPERATION: 2 CHANGE: Taking out or off a device from a body part and putting back an identical or similar device in or on the same body part without cutting or puncturing the skin or a mucous membrane

Body Part	Approach	Device	Qualifier
Ø Pituitary Gland 1 Pineal Body 5 Adrenal Gland K Thyroid Gland R Parathyroid Gland S Endocrine Gland	X External	Ø Drainage Device Y Other Device	Z No Qualifier

Non-OR All Values

SECTION: Ø MEDICAL AND SURGICAL

BODY SYSTEM: G ENDOCRINE SYSTEM

OPERATION: 5 DESTRUCTION: Physical eradication of all or a portion of a body part by the direct use of energy, force, or a destructive agent

Body Part	Approach	Device	Qualifier
Ø Pituitary Gland 1 Pineal Body 2 Adrenal Gland, Left 3 Adrenal Gland, Right 4 Adrenal Glands, Bilateral 6 Carotid Body, Left 7 Carotid Body, Right 8 Carotid Bodies, Bilateral 9 Para-aortic Body B Coccygeal Glomus C Glomus Jugulare D Aortic Body F Paraganglion Extremity G Thyroid Gland Lobe, Left H Thyroid Gland Lobe, Right K Thyroid Gland L Superior Parathyroid Gland, Right M Superior Parathyroid Gland, Left N Inferior Parathyroid Gland, Right P Inferior Parathyroid Gland, Left Q Parathyroid Glands, Multiple R Parathyroid Gland	Ø Open 3 Percutaneous 4 Percutaneous Endoscopic	Z No Device	Z No Qualifier

SECTION: Ø MEDICAL AND SURGICAL

BODY SYSTEM: G ENDOCRINE SYSTEM

OPERATION: 8 DIVISION: Cutting into a body part, without draining fluids and/or gases from the body part, in order to separate or transect a body part

Body Part	Approach	Device	Qualifier
Ø Pituitary Gland J Thyroid Gland Isthmus	Ø Open 3 Percutaneous 4 Percutaneous Endoscopic	Z No Device	Z No Qualifier

New/Revised Text in Green   deleted Deleted   ♀ Females Only   ♂ Males Only   **Coding Clinic**

🚫 Non-covered   🚫 Limited Coverage   ⊡ Combination (See Appendix E)   DRG Non-OR   Non-OR   🚫 Hospital-Acquired Condition

Sidebar: 2: CHANGE 5: DESTRUCTION 8: DIVISION G: ENDOCRINE SYSTEM Ø: M/S

SECTION: 0 MEDICAL AND SURGICAL

BODY SYSTEM: G ENDOCRINE SYSTEM

OPERATION: 9 DRAINAGE: Taking or letting out fluids and/or gases from a body part

Body Part	Approach	Device	Qualifier
0 Pituitary Gland 1 Pineal Body 2 Adrenal Gland, Left 3 Adrenal Gland, Right 4 Adrenal Glands, Bilateral 6 Carotid Body, Left 7 Carotid Body, Right 8 Carotid Bodies, Bilateral 9 Para-aortic Body B Coccygeal Glomus C Glomus Jugulare D Aortic Body F Paraganglion Extremity G Thyroid Gland Lobe, Left H Thyroid Gland Lobe, Right K Thyroid Gland L Superior Parathyroid Gland, Right M Superior Parathyroid Gland, Left N Inferior Parathyroid Gland, Right P Inferior Parathyroid Gland, Left Q Parathyroid Glands, Multiple R Parathyroid Gland	0 Open 3 Percutaneous 4 Percutaneous Endoscopic	0 Drainage Device	Z No Qualifier
0 Pituitary Gland 1 Pineal Body 2 Adrenal Gland, Left 3 Adrenal Gland, Right 4 Adrenal Glands, Bilateral 6 Carotid Body, Left 7 Carotid Body, Right 8 Carotid Bodies, Bilateral 9 Para-aortic Body B Coccygeal Glomus C Glomus Jugulare D Aortic Body F Paraganglion Extremity G Thyroid Gland Lobe, Left H Thyroid Gland Lobe, Right K Thyroid Gland L Superior Parathyroid Gland, Right M Superior Parathyroid Gland, Left N Inferior Parathyroid Gland, Right P Inferior Parathyroid Gland, Left Q Parathyroid Glands, Multiple R Parathyroid Gland	0 Open 3 Percutaneous 4 Percutaneous Endoscopic	Z No Device	X Diagnostic Z No Qualifier

Non-OR 0G9[012346789BCDF]30Z
Non-OR 0G9[GHKLMNPQR][34]0Z
Non-OR 0G9[234GHK][34]ZX
Non-OR 0G9[012346789BCDF]3ZZ
Non-OR 0G9[GHKLMNPQR][34]ZZ

SECTION: 0 MEDICAL AND SURGICAL
BODY SYSTEM: G ENDOCRINE SYSTEM
OPERATION: B EXCISION: Cutting out or off, without replacement, a portion of a body part

Body Part	Approach	Device	Qualifier
0 Pituitary Gland 1 Pineal Body 2 Adrenal Gland, Left 3 Adrenal Gland, Right 4 Adrenal Glands, Bilateral 6 Carotid Body, Left 7 Carotid Body, Right 8 Carotid Bodies, Bilateral 9 Para-aortic Body B Coccygeal Glomus C Glomus Jugulare D Aortic Body F Paraganglion Extremity G Thyroid Gland Lobe, Left H Thyroid Gland Lobe, Right J Thyroid Gland Isthmus L Superior Parathyroid Gland, Right M Superior Parathyroid Gland, Left N Inferior Parathyroid Gland, Right P Inferior Parathyroid Gland, Left Q Parathyroid Glands, Multiple R Parathyroid Gland	0 Open 3 Percutaneous 4 Percutaneous Endoscopic	Z No Device	X Diagnostic Z No Qualifier

Non-OR 0GB[234GH][34]ZX

Coding Clinic: 2017, Q2, P20 – 0GB[GH]0ZZ

SECTION: 0 MEDICAL AND SURGICAL
BODY SYSTEM: G ENDOCRINE SYSTEM
OPERATION: C EXTIRPATION: Taking or cutting out solid matter from a body part

Body Part	Approach	Device	Qualifier
0 Pituitary Gland 1 Pineal Body 2 Adrenal Gland, Left 3 Adrenal Gland, Right 4 Adrenal Glands, Bilateral 6 Carotid Body, Left 7 Carotid Body, Right 8 Carotid Bodies, Bilateral 9 Para-aortic Body B Coccygeal Glomus C Glomus Jugulare D Aortic Body F Paraganglion Extremity G Thyroid Gland Lobe, Left H Thyroid Gland Lobe, Right K Thyroid Gland L Superior Parathyroid Gland, Right M Superior Parathyroid Gland, Left N Inferior Parathyroid Gland, Right P Inferior Parathyroid Gland, Left Q Parathyroid Glands, Multiple R Parathyroid Gland	0 Open 3 Percutaneous 4 Percutaneous Endoscopic	Z No Device	Z No Qualifier

Non-covered   New/Revised Text in Green   deleted Deleted   ♀ Females Only   ♂ Males Only   **Coding Clinic**
Limited Coverage   ⊕ Combination (See Appendix E)   DRG Non-OR   Non-OR   Hospital-Acquired Condition

Side tab (left margin): B: EXCISION   C: EXTIRPATION   G: ENDOCRINE SYSTEM   0: M/S

SECTION: Ø MEDICAL AND SURGICAL

BODY SYSTEM: G ENDOCRINE SYSTEM

OPERATION: H INSERTION: Putting in a nonbiological appliance that monitors, assists, performs, or prevents a physiological function but does not physically take the place of a body part

Body Part	Approach	Device	Qualifier
S Endocrine Gland	Ø Open 3 Percutaneous 4 Percutaneous Endoscopic	2 Monitoring Device 3 Infusion Device Y Other Device	Z No Qualifier

SECTION: Ø MEDICAL AND SURGICAL

BODY SYSTEM: G ENDOCRINE SYSTEM

OPERATION: J INSPECTION: Visually and/or manually exploring a body part

Body Part	Approach	Device	Qualifier
Ø Pituitary Gland 1 Pineal Body 5 Adrenal Gland K Thyroid Gland R Parathyroid Gland S Endocrine Gland	Ø Open 3 Percutaneous 4 Percutaneous Endoscopic	Z No Device	Z No Qualifier

Non-OR ØGJ[Ø15KRS]3ZZ

SECTION: Ø MEDICAL AND SURGICAL

BODY SYSTEM: G ENDOCRINE SYSTEM

OPERATION: M REATTACHMENT: Putting back in or on all or a portion of a separated body part to its normal location or other suitable location

Body Part	Approach	Device	Qualifier
2 Adrenal Gland, Left 3 Adrenal Gland, Right G Thyroid Gland Lobe, Left H Thyroid Gland Lobe, Right L Superior Parathyroid Gland, Right M Superior Parathyroid Gland, Left N Inferior Parathyroid Gland, Right P Inferior Parathyroid Gland, Left Q Parathyroid Glands, Multiple R Parathyroid Gland	Ø Open 4 Percutaneous Endoscopic	Z No Device	Z No Qualifier

SECTION: 0 MEDICAL AND SURGICAL

BODY SYSTEM: G ENDOCRINE SYSTEM
OPERATION: N RELEASE: Freeing a body part from an abnormal physical constraint by cutting or by the use of force

Body Part	Approach	Device	Qualifier
0 Pituitary Gland 1 Pineal Body 2 Adrenal Gland, Left 3 Adrenal Gland, Right 4 Adrenal Glands, Bilateral 6 Carotid Body, Left 7 Carotid Body, Right 8 Carotid Bodies, Bilateral 9 Para-aortic Body B Coccygeal Glomus C Glomus Jugulare D Aortic Body F Paraganglion Extremity G Thyroid Gland Lobe, Left H Thyroid Gland Lobe, Right K Thyroid Gland L Superior Parathyroid Gland, Right M Superior Parathyroid Gland, Left N Inferior Parathyroid Gland, Right P Inferior Parathyroid Gland, Left Q Parathyroid Glands, Multiple R Parathyroid Gland	0 Open 3 Percutaneous 4 Percutaneous Endoscopic	Z No Device	Z No Qualifier

SECTION: 0 MEDICAL AND SURGICAL

BODY SYSTEM: G ENDOCRINE SYSTEM
OPERATION: P REMOVAL: Taking out or off a device from a body part

Body Part	Approach	Device	Qualifier
0 Pituitary Gland 1 Pineal Body 5 Adrenal Gland K Thyroid Gland R Parathyroid Gland	0 Open 3 Percutaneous 4 Percutaneous Endoscopic X External	0 Drainage Device	Z No Qualifier
S Endocrine Gland	0 Open 3 Percutaneous 4 Percutaneous Endoscopic	0 Drainage Device 2 Monitoring Device 3 Infusion Device Y Other Device	Z No Qualifier
S Endocrine Gland	X External	0 Drainage Device 2 Monitoring Device 3 Infusion Device	Z No Qualifier

Non-OR 0GP[015KR]X0Z
Non-OR 0GPSX[023]Z

New/Revised Text in Green   ~~deleted~~ Deleted   ♀ Females Only   ♂ Males Only   **Coding Clinic**
Non-covered   Limited Coverage   ⊕ Combination (See Appendix E)   DRG Non-OR   Non-OR   Hospital-Acquired Condition

SECTION: 0 MEDICAL AND SURGICAL
BODY SYSTEM: G ENDOCRINE SYSTEM
OPERATION: **Q REPAIR:** Restoring, to the extent possible, a body part to its normal anatomic structure and function

Body Part	Approach	Device	Qualifier
0 Pituitary Gland 1 Pineal Body 2 Adrenal Gland, Left 3 Adrenal Gland, Right 4 Adrenal Glands, Bilateral 6 Carotid Body, Left 7 Carotid Body, Right 8 Carotid Bodies, Bilateral 9 Para-aortic Body B Coccygeal Glomus C Glomus Jugulare D Aortic Body F Paraganglion Extremity G Thyroid Gland Lobe, Left H Thyroid Gland Lobe, Right J Thyroid Gland Isthmus K Thyroid Gland L Superior Parathyroid Gland, Right M Superior Parathyroid Gland, Left N Inferior Parathyroid Gland, Right P Inferior Parathyroid Gland, Left Q Parathyroid Glands, Multiple R Parathyroid Gland	0 Open 3 Percutaneous 4 Percutaneous Endoscopic	Z No Device	Z No Qualifier

SECTION: 0 MEDICAL AND SURGICAL
BODY SYSTEM: G ENDOCRINE SYSTEM
OPERATION: **S REPOSITION:** Moving to its normal location, or other suitable location, all or a portion of a body part

Body Part	Approach	Device	Qualifier
2 Adrenal Gland, Left 3 Adrenal Gland, Right G Thyroid Gland Lobe, Left H Thyroid Gland Lobe, Right L Superior Parathyroid Gland, Right M Superior Parathyroid Gland, Left N Inferior Parathyroid Gland, Right P Inferior Parathyroid Gland, Left Q Parathyroid Glands, Multiple R Parathyroid Gland	0 Open 4 Percutaneous Endoscopic	Z No Device	Z No Qualifier

SECTION: Ø MEDICAL AND SURGICAL

BODY SYSTEM: G ENDOCRINE SYSTEM

OPERATION: T RESECTION: Cutting out or off, without replacement, all of a body part

Body Part	Approach	Device	Qualifier
Ø Pituitary Gland 1 Pineal Body 2 Adrenal Gland, Left 3 Adrenal Gland, Right 4 Adrenal Glands, Bilateral 6 Carotid Body, Left 7 Carotid Body, Right 8 Carotid Bodies, Bilateral 9 Para-aortic Body B Coccygeal Glomus C Glomus Jugulare D Aortic Body F Paraganglion Extremity G Thyroid Gland Lobe, Left H Thyroid Gland Lobe, Right J Thyroid Gland Isthmus K Thyroid Gland L Superior Parathyroid Gland, Right M Superior Parathyroid Gland, Left N Inferior Parathyroid Gland, Right P Inferior Parathyroid Gland, Left Q Parathyroid Glands, Multiple R Parathyroid Gland	Ø Open 4 Percutaneous Endoscopic	Z No Device	Z No Qualifier

SECTION: Ø MEDICAL AND SURGICAL

BODY SYSTEM: G ENDOCRINE SYSTEM

OPERATION: W REVISION: Correcting, to the extent possible, a portion of a malfunctioning device or the position of a displaced device

Body Part	Approach	Device	Qualifier
Ø Pituitary Gland 1 Pineal Body 5 Adrenal Gland K Thyroid Gland R Parathyroid Gland	Ø Open 3 Percutaneous 4 Percutaneous Endoscopic X External	Ø Drainage Device	Z No Qualifier
S Endocrine Gland	Ø Open 3 Percutaneous 4 Percutaneous Endoscopic	Ø Drainage Device 2 Monitoring Device 3 Infusion Device Y Other Device	Z No Qualifier
S Endocrine Gland	X External	Ø Drainage Device 2 Monitoring Device 3 Infusion Device	Z No Qualifier

Non-OR   ØGW[Ø15KR]XØZ
Non-OR   ØGWSX[Ø23]Z

Ø: ALTERATION   2: CHANGE

H: SKIN AND BREAST

Ø: M/S

SECTION: Ø MEDICAL AND SURGICAL
BODY SYSTEM: H SKIN AND BREAST
OPERATION: Ø **ALTERATION:** Modifying the anatomic structure of a body part without affecting the function of the body part

Body Part	Approach	Device	Qualifier
T Breast, Right U Breast, Left V Breast, Bilateral	Ø Open 3 Percutaneous X External	7 Autologous Tissue Substitute J Synthetic Substitute K Nonautologous Tissue Substitute Z No Device	Z No Qualifier

SECTION: Ø MEDICAL AND SURGICAL
BODY SYSTEM: H SKIN AND BREAST
OPERATION: 2 **CHANGE:** Taking out or off a device from a body part and putting back an identical or similar device in or on the same body part without cutting or puncturing the skin or a mucous membrane

Body Part	Approach	Device	Qualifier
P Skin T Breast, Right U Breast, Left	X External	Ø Drainage Device Y Other Device	Z No Qualifier

Non-OR **All Values**

SECTION: Ø MEDICAL AND SURGICAL
BODY SYSTEM: H SKIN AND BREAST
OPERATION: 5 **DESTRUCTION:** Physical eradication of all or a portion of a body part by the direct use of energy, force, or a destructive agent

Body Part	Approach	Device	Qualifier
Ø Skin, Scalp 1 Skin, Face 2 Skin, Right Ear 3 Skin, Left Ear 4 Skin, Neck 5 Skin, Chest 6 Skin, Back 7 Skin, Abdomen 8 Skin, Buttock 9 Skin, Perineum A Skin, Inguinal B Skin, Right Upper Arm C Skin, Left Upper Arm D Skin, Right Lower Arm E Skin, Left Lower Arm F Skin, Right Hand G Skin, Left Hand H Skin, Right Upper Leg J Skin, Left Upper Leg K Skin, Right Lower Leg L Skin, Left Lower Leg M Skin, Right Foot N Skin, Left Foot	X External	Z No Device	D Multiple Z No Qualifier
Q Finger Nail R Toe Nail	X External	Z No Device	Z No Qualifier
T Breast, Right U Breast, Left V Breast, Bilateral W Nipple, Right X Nipple, Left	Ø Open 3 Percutaneous 7 Via Natural or Artificial Opening 8 Via Natural or Artificial Opening Endoscopic X External	Z No Device	Z No Qualifier

DRG Non-OR ØH5[Ø1456789ABCDEFGHJKLMN]XZ[DZ]
DRG Non-OR ØH5[QR]XZZ
Non-OR ØH5[23]XZ[DZ]

SECTION: Ø MEDICAL AND SURGICAL
BODY SYSTEM: H SKIN AND BREAST
OPERATION: 8 DIVISION: Cutting into a body part, without draining fluids and/or gases from the body part, in order to separate or transect a body part

Body Part	Approach	Device	Qualifier
Ø Skin, Scalp	X External	Z No Device	Z No Qualifier
1 Skin, Face			
2 Skin, Right Ear			
3 Skin, Left Ear			
4 Skin, Neck			
5 Skin, Chest			
6 Skin, Back			
7 Skin, Abdomen			
8 Skin, Buttock			
9 Skin, Perineum			
A Skin, Inguinal			
B Skin, Right Upper Arm			
C Skin, Left Upper Arm			
D Skin, Right Lower Arm			
E Skin, Left Lower Arm			
F Skin, Right Hand			
G Skin, Left Hand			
H Skin, Right Upper Leg			
J Skin, Left Upper Leg			
K Skin, Right Lower Leg			
L Skin, Left Lower Leg			
M Skin, Right Foot			
N Skin, Left Foot			

DRG Non-OR   ØH8[01456789ABCDEFGHJKLMN]XZZ
Non-OR   ØH8[23]XZZ

8: DIVISION

H: SKIN AND BREAST

Ø: M/S

New/Revised Text in Green   deleted Deleted   ♀ Females Only   ♂ Males Only   **Coding Clinic**
Non-covered   Limited Coverage   ⊕ Combination (See Appendix E)   DRG Non-OR   Non-OR   Hospital-Acquired Condition

SECTION: Ø MEDICAL AND SURGICAL

BODY SYSTEM: H SKIN AND BREAST

OPERATION: 9 DRAINAGE: *(on multiple pages)*

Taking or letting out fluids and/or gases from a body part

Body Part	Approach	Device	Qualifier
Ø Skin, Scalp	X External	Ø Drainage Device	Z No Qualifier
1 Skin, Face			
2 Skin, Right Ear			
3 Skin, Left Ear			
4 Skin, Neck			
5 Skin, Chest			
6 Skin, Back			
7 Skin, Abdomen			
8 Skin, Buttock			
9 Skin, Perineum			
A Skin, Inguinal			
B Skin, Right Upper Arm			
C Skin, Left Upper Arm			
D Skin, Right Lower Arm			
E Skin, Left Lower Arm			
F Skin, Right Hand			
G Skin, Left Hand			
H Skin, Right Upper Leg			
J Skin, Left Upper Leg			
K Skin, Right Lower Leg			
L Skin, Left Lower Leg			
M Skin, Right Foot			
N Skin, Left Foot			
Q Finger Nail			
R Toe Nail			
Ø Skin, Scalp	X External	Z No Device	X Diagnostic
1 Skin, Face			Z No Qualifier
2 Skin, Right Ear			
3 Skin, Left Ear			
4 Skin, Neck			
5 Skin, Chest			
6 Skin, Back			
7 Skin, Abdomen			
8 Skin, Buttock			
9 Skin, Perineum			
A Skin, Inguinal			
B Skin, Right Upper Arm			
C Skin, Left Upper Arm			
D Skin, Right Lower Arm			
E Skin, Left Lower Arm			
F Skin, Right Hand			
G Skin, Left Hand			
H Skin, Right Upper Leg			
J Skin, Left Upper Leg			
K Skin, Right Lower Leg			
L Skin, Left Lower Leg			
M Skin, Right Foot			
N Skin, Left Foot			
Q Finger Nail			
R Toe Nail			

Non-OR ØH9[Ø12345678ABCDEFGHJKLMNQR]XØZ
Non-OR ØH9[Ø123456789ABCDEFGHJKLMNQR]XZX
Non-OR ØH9[Ø12345678ABCDEFGHJKLMNQR]XZZ

Ø: M/S

H: SKIN AND BREAST

9: DRAINAGE

New/Revised Text in Green ~~deleted~~ Deleted ♀ Females Only ♂ Males Only **Coding Clinic**

Non-covered Limited Coverage ⊞ Combination (See Appendix E) DRG Non-OR Non-OR Hospital-Acquired Condition

9: DRAINAGE   B: EXCISION

H: SKIN AND BREAST

Ø: M/S

SECTION: Ø MEDICAL AND SURGICAL

BODY SYSTEM: H SKIN AND BREAST

OPERATION: 9 DRAINAGE: *(continued)*
Taking or letting out fluids and/or gases from a body part

Body Part	Approach	Device	Qualifier
T Breast, Right U Breast, Left V Breast, Bilateral W Nipple, Right X Nipple, Left	Ø Open 3 Percutaneous 7 Via Natural or Artificial Opening 8 Via Natural or Artificial Opening Endoscopic X External	Ø Drainage Device	Z No Qualifier
T Breast, Right U Breast, Left V Breast, Bilateral W Nipple, Right X Nipple, Left	Ø Open 3 Percutaneous 7 Via Natural or Artificial Opening 8 Via Natural or Artificial Opening Endoscopic X External	Z No Device	X Diagnostic Z No Qualifier

Non-OR   ØH9[TUVWX][Ø378X]ØZ
Non-OR   ØH9[TUVWX][378X]ZX
Non-OR   ØH9[TUVWX][Ø378X]ZZ

SECTION: Ø MEDICAL AND SURGICAL

BODY SYSTEM: H SKIN AND BREAST

OPERATION: B EXCISION: *(on multiple pages)*
Cutting out or off, without replacement, a portion of a body part

Body Part	Approach	Device	Qualifier
Ø Skin, Scalp 1 Skin, Face 2 Skin, Right Ear 3 Skin, Left Ear 4 Skin, Neck 5 Skin, Chest 6 Skin, Back 7 Skin, Abdomen 8 Skin, Buttock 9 Skin, Perineum A Skin, Inguinal B Skin, Right Upper Arm C Skin, Left Upper Arm D Skin, Right Lower Arm E Skin, Left Lower Arm F Skin, Right Hand G Skin, Left Hand H Skin, Right Upper Leg J Skin, Left Upper Leg K Skin, Right Lower Leg L Skin, Left Lower Leg M Skin, Right Foot N Skin, Left Foot Q Finger Nail R Toe Nail	X External	Z No Device	X Diagnostic Z No Qualifier

DRG Non-OR   ØHB9XZZ
DRG Non-OR   ØHB[Ø145678ABCDEFGHJKLMN]XZZ
Non-OR   ØHB[Ø12456789ABCDEFGHJKLMNQR]XZX

Non-OR   ØHB[23QR]XZZ

Coding Clinic: 2Ø16, Q3, P29 – ØHBJXZZ

New/Revised Text in Green   ~~deleted~~ Deleted   ♀ Females Only   ♂ Males Only   **Coding Clinic**
Non-covered   Limited Coverage   Combination (See Appendix E)   DRG Non-OR   Non-OR   Hospital-Acquired Condition

SECTION: Ø MEDICAL AND SURGICAL
BODY SYSTEM: H SKIN AND BREAST
OPERATION: B EXCISION: *(continued)*

Cutting out or off, without replacement, a portion of a body part

Body Part	Approach	Device	Qualifier
T Breast, Right U Breast, Left V Breast, Bilateral W Nipple, Right X Nipple, Left Y Supernumerary Breast	Ø Open 3 Percutaneous 7 Via Natural or Artificial Opening 8 Via Natural or Artificial Opening Endoscopic X External	Z No Device	X Diagnostic Z No Qualifier

Non-OR ØHB[TUVWXY][378X]ZX

Coding Clinic: 2015, Q3, P3 – ØHB8XZZ
Coding Clinic: 2018, Q1, P15 – ØHBTØZZ

SECTION: Ø MEDICAL AND SURGICAL
BODY SYSTEM: H SKIN AND BREAST
OPERATION: C EXTIRPATION: Taking or cutting out solid matter from a body part

Body Part	Approach	Device	Qualifier
Ø Skin, Scalp 1 Skin, Face 2 Skin, Right Ear 3 Skin, Left Ear 4 Skin, Neck 5 Skin, Chest 6 Skin, Back 7 Skin, Abdomen 8 Skin, Buttock 9 Skin, Perineum A Skin, Inguinal B Skin, Right Upper Arm C Skin, Left Upper Arm D Skin, Right Lower Arm E Skin, Left Lower Arm F Skin, Right Hand G Skin, Left Hand H Skin, Right Upper Leg J Skin, Left Upper Leg K Skin, Right Lower Leg L Skin, Left Lower Leg M Skin, Right Foot N Skin, Left Foot Q Finger Nail R Toe Nail	X External	Z No Device	Z No Qualifier
T Breast, Right U Breast, Left V Breast, Bilateral W Nipple, Right X Nipple, Left	Ø Open 3 Percutaneous 7 Via Natural or Artificial Opening 8 Via Natural or Artificial Opening Endoscopic X External	Z No Device	Z No Qualifier

Non-OR All Values

Ø: M/S   H: SKIN AND BREAST   B: EXCISION   C: EXTIRPATION

SECTION: Ø MEDICAL AND SURGICAL
BODY SYSTEM: H SKIN AND BREAST
OPERATION: D EXTRACTION: Pulling or stripping out or off all or a portion of a body part by the use of force

Body Part	Approach	Device	Qualifier
Ø Skin, Scalp	X External	Z No Device	Z No Qualifier
1 Skin, Face			
2 Skin, Right Ear			
3 Skin, Left Ear			
4 Skin, Neck			
5 Skin, Chest			
6 Skin, Back			
7 Skin, Abdomen			
8 Skin, Buttock			
9 Skin, Perineum			
A Skin, Inguinal			
B Skin, Right Upper Arm			
C Skin, Left Upper Arm			
D Skin, Right Lower Arm			
E Skin, Left Lower Arm			
F Skin, Right Hand			
G Skin, Left Hand			
H Skin, Right Upper Leg			
J Skin, Left Upper Leg			
K Skin, Right Lower Leg			
L Skin, Left Lower Leg			
M Skin, Right Foot			
N Skin, Left Foot			
Q Finger Nail			
R Toe Nail			
S Hair			

Non-OR   All Values

Coding Clinic: 2015, Q3, P5-6 – ØHD[6H]XZZ

New/Revised Text in Green   ~~deleted~~ Deleted   ♀ Females Only   ♂ Males Only   **Coding Clinic**
⬡ Non-covered   ⬡ Limited Coverage   ⊞ Combination (See Appendix E)   DRG Non-OR   Non-OR   ⬡ Hospital-Acquired Condition

SECTION: Ø MEDICAL AND SURGICAL
BODY SYSTEM: H SKIN AND BREAST
OPERATION: H **INSERTION:** Putting in a nonbiological appliance that monitors, assists, performs, or prevents a physiological function but does not physically take the place of a body part

Body Part	Approach	Device	Qualifier
P Skin	X External	Y Other Device	Z No Qualifier
T Breast, Right U Breast, Left	Ø Open 3 Percutaneous 7 Via Natural or Artificial Opening 8 Via Natural or Artificial Opening Endoscopic	1 Radioactive Element N Tissue Expander Y Other Device	Z No Qualifier
T Breast, Right U Breast, Left	X External	1 Radioactive Element	Z No Qualifier
V Breast, Bilateral W Nipple, Right X Nipple, Left	Ø Open 3 Percutaneous 7 Via Natural or Artificial Opening 8 Via Natural or Artificial Opening Endoscopic	1 Radioactive Element N Tissue Expander	Z No Qualifier
V Breast, Bilateral W Nipple, Right X Nipple, Left	X External	1 Radioactive Element	Z No Qualifier

Coding Clinic: 2017, Q4, P67 – ØHHTØNZ

SECTION: Ø MEDICAL AND SURGICAL
BODY SYSTEM: H SKIN AND BREAST
OPERATION: J **INSPECTION:** Visually and/or manually exploring a body part

Body Part	Approach	Device	Qualifier
P Skin Q Finger Nail R Toe Nail	X External	Z No Device	Z No Qualifier
T Breast, Right U Breast, Left	Ø Open 3 Percutaneous 7 Via Natural or Artificial Opening 8 Via Natural or Artificial Opening Endoscopic X External	Z No Device	Z No Qualifier

Non-OR All Values

SECTION: Ø MEDICAL AND SURGICAL
BODY SYSTEM: H SKIN AND BREAST
OPERATION: M REATTACHMENT: Putting back in or on all or a portion of a separated body part to its normal location or other suitable location

Body Part	Approach	Device	Qualifier
Ø Skin, Scalp	X External	Z No Device	Z No Qualifier
1 Skin, Face			
2 Skin, Right Ear			
3 Skin, Left Ear			
4 Skin, Neck			
5 Skin, Chest			
6 Skin, Back			
7 Skin, Abdomen			
8 Skin, Buttock			
9 Skin, Perineum			
A Skin, Inguinal			
B Skin, Right Upper Arm			
C Skin, Left Upper Arm			
D Skin, Right Lower Arm			
E Skin, Left Lower Arm			
F Skin, Right Hand			
G Skin, Left Hand			
H Skin, Right Upper Leg			
J Skin, Left Upper Leg			
K Skin, Right Lower Leg			
L Skin, Left Lower Leg			
M Skin, Right Foot			
N Skin, Left Foot			
T Breast, Right			
U Breast, Left			
V Breast, Bilateral			
W Nipple, Right			
X Nipple, Left			

Non-OR ØHMØXZZ

M: REATTACHMENT

H: SKIN AND BREAST

Ø: M/S

New/Revised Text in Green   ~~deleted~~ Deleted   ♀ Females Only   ♂ Males Only   **Coding Clinic**
Non-covered   Limited Coverage   ⊞ Combination (See Appendix E)   DRG Non-OR   Non-OR   Hospital-Acquired Condition

SECTION: Ø MEDICAL AND SURGICAL
BODY SYSTEM: H SKIN AND BREAST
OPERATION: N RELEASE: Freeing a body part from an abnormal physical constraint by cutting or by the use of force

Body Part	Approach	Device	Qualifier
Ø Skin, Scalp 1 Skin, Face 2 Skin, Right Ear 3 Skin, Left Ear 4 Skin, Neck 5 Skin, Chest 6 Skin, Back 7 Skin, Abdomen 8 Skin, Buttock 9 Skin, Perineum A Skin, Inguinal B Skin, Right Upper Arm C Skin, Left Upper Arm D Skin, Right Lower Arm E Skin, Left Lower Arm F Skin, Right Hand G Skin, Left Hand H Skin, Right Upper Leg J Skin, Left Upper Leg K Skin, Right Lower Leg L Skin, Left Lower Leg M Skin, Right Foot N Skin, Left Foot Q Finger Nail R Toe Nail	X External	Z No Device	Z No Qualifier
T Breast, Right U Breast, Left V Breast, Bilateral W Nipple, Right X Nipple, Left	Ø Open 3 Percutaneous 7 Via Natural or Artificial Opening 8 Via Natural or Artificial Opening Endoscopic X External	Z No Device	Z No Qualifier

SECTION: Ø MEDICAL AND SURGICAL
BODY SYSTEM: H SKIN AND BREAST

OPERATION: P REMOVAL: Taking out or off a device from a body part

Body Part	Approach	Device	Qualifier
P Skin	X External	Ø Drainage Device 7 Autologous Tissue Substitute J Synthetic Substitute K Nonautologous Tissue Substitute Y Other Device	Z No Qualifier
Q Finger Nail R Toe Nail	X External	Ø Drainage Device 7 Autologous Tissue Substitute J Synthetic Substitute K Nonautologous Tissue Substitute	Z No Qualifier
S Hair	X External	7 Autologous Tissue Substitute J Synthetic Substitute K Nonautologous Tissue Substitute	Z No Qualifier
T Breast, Right U Breast, Left	Ø Open 3 Percutaneous 7 Via Natural or Artificial Opening 8 Via Natural or Artificial Opening Endoscopic	Ø Drainage Device 1 Radioactive Element 7 Autologous Tissue Substitute J Synthetic Substitute K Nonautologous Tissue Substitute N Tissue Expander Y Other Device	Z No Qualifier
T Breast, Right U Breast, Left	X External	Ø Drainage Device 1 Radioactive Element 7 Autologous Tissue Substitute J Synthetic Substitute K Nonautologous Tissue Substitute	Z No Qualifier

Non-OR ØPHPX[Ø7JK]Z
Non-OR ØHP[QR]X[Ø7JK]Z
Non-OR ØHPSX[7JK]Z
Non-OR ØHP[TU][Ø3][Ø17K]Z
Non-OR ØHP[TU][78][Ø17JKN]Z
Non-OR ØHP[TU]X[Ø17JK]Z

Coding Clinic: 2016, Q2, P27 – ØHP[TU]Ø7Z

New/Revised Text in Green   deleted Deleted   ♀ Females Only   ♂ Males Only   **Coding Clinic**
Non-covered   Limited Coverage   Combination (See Appendix E)   DRG Non-OR   Non-OR   Hospital-Acquired Condition

P: REMOVAL   H: SKIN AND BREAST   Ø: M/S

SECTION: Ø MEDICAL AND SURGICAL

BODY SYSTEM: H SKIN AND BREAST

OPERATION: **Q REPAIR:** Restoring, to the extent possible, a body part to its normal anatomic structure and function

Body Part	Approach	Device	Qualifier
Ø Skin, Scalp 1 Skin, Face 2 Skin, Right Ear 3 Skin, Left Ear 4 Skin, Neck 5 Skin, Chest 6 Skin, Back 7 Skin, Abdomen 8 Skin, Buttock 9 Skin, Perineum A Skin, Inguinal B Skin, Right Upper Arm C Skin, Left Upper Arm D Skin, Right Lower Arm E Skin, Left Lower Arm F Skin, Right Hand G Skin, Left Hand H Skin, Right Upper Leg J Skin, Left Upper Leg K Skin, Right Lower Leg L Skin, Left Lower Leg M Skin, Right Foot N Skin, Left Foot Q Finger Nail R Toe Nail	X External	Z No Device	Z No Qualifier
T Breast, Right U Breast, Left V Breast, Bilateral W Nipple, Right X Nipple, Left Y Supernumerary Breast	Ø Open 3 Percutaneous 7 Via Natural or Artificial Opening 8 Via Natural or Artificial Opening Endoscopic X External	Z No Device	Z No Qualifier

DRG Non-OR ØHQ9XZZ
Non-OR ØHQ[Ø12345678ABCDEFGHJKLMN]XZZ
Non-OR ØHQ[TUVY]XZZ

Coding Clinic: 2016, Q1, P7 – ØHQ9XZZ

SECTION: Ø MEDICAL AND SURGICAL
BODY SYSTEM: H SKIN AND BREAST
OPERATION: R REPLACEMENT: *(on multiple pages)*
Putting in or on biological or synthetic material that physically takes the place and/or function of all or a portion of a body part

Body Part	Approach	Device	Qualifier
Ø Skin, Scalp 1 Skin, Face 2 Skin, Right Ear 3 Skin, Left Ear 4 Skin, Neck 5 Skin, Chest 6 Skin, Back 7 Skin, Abdomen 8 Skin, Buttock 9 Skin, Perineum A Skin, Inguinal B Skin, Right Upper Arm C Skin, Left Upper Arm D Skin, Right Lower Arm E Skin, Left Lower Arm F Skin, Right Hand G Skin, Left Hand H Skin, Right Upper Leg J Skin, Left Upper Leg K Skin, Right Lower Leg L Skin, Left Lower Leg M Skin, Right Foot N Skin, Left Foot	X External	7 Autologous Tissue Substitute K Nonautologous Tissue Substitute	3 Full Thickness 4 Partial Thickness
Ø Skin, Scalp 1 Skin, Face 2 Skin, Right Ear 3 Skin, Left Ear 4 Skin, Neck 5 Skin, Chest 6 Skin, Back 7 Skin, Abdomen 8 Skin, Buttock 9 Skin, Perineum A Skin, Inguinal B Skin, Right Upper Arm C Skin, Left Upper Arm D Skin, Right Lower Arm E Skin, Left Lower Arm F Skin, Right Hand G Skin, Left Hand H Skin, Right Upper Leg J Skin, Left Upper Leg K Skin, Right Lower Leg L Skin, Left Lower Leg M Skin, Right Foot N Skin, Left Foot	X External	J Synthetic Substitute	3 Full Thickness 4 Partial Thickness Z No Qualifier
Q Finger Nail R Toe Nail S Hair	X External	7 Autologous Tissue Substitute J Synthetic Substitute K Nonautologous Tissue Substitute	Z No Qualifier

Non-OR ØHRSX7Z

Coding Clinic: 2Ø17, Q1, P36 – ØHRMXK3

New/Revised Text in Green ~~deleted~~ Deleted ♀ Females Only ♂ Males Only **Coding Clinic**
🦋 Non-covered 🦋 Limited Coverage ⊞ Combination (See Appendix E) DRG Non-OR Non-OR 🦋 Hospital-Acquired Condition

(side margin) R: REPLACEMENT H: SKIN AND BREAST Ø: M/S

SECTION: Ø MEDICAL AND SURGICAL

BODY SYSTEM: H **SKIN AND BREAST**

OPERATION: R **REPLACEMENT:** *(continued)*
Putting in or on biological or synthetic material that physically takes the place and/or function of all or a portion of a body part

Body Part	Approach	Device	Qualifier
T Breast, Right U Breast, Left V Breast, Bilateral	Ø Open	7 Autologous Tissue Substitute	5 Latissimus Dorsi Myocutaneous Flap 6 Transverse Rectus Abdominis Myocutaneous Flap 7 Deep Inferior Epigastric Artery Perforator Flap 8 Superficial Inferior Epigastric Artery Flap 9 Gluteal Artery Perforator Flap Z No Qualifier
T Breast, Right U Breast, Left V Breast, Bilateral	Ø Open	J Synthetic Substitute K Nonautologous Tissue Substitute	Z No Qualifier
T Breast, Right ⊞ U Breast, Left ⊞ V Breast, Bilateral ⊞	3 Percutaneous X External	7 Autologous Tissue Substitute J Synthetic Substitute K Nonautologous Tissue Substitute	Z No Qualifier
W Nipple, Right X Nipple, Left	Ø Open 3 Percutaneous X External	7 Autologous Tissue Substitute J Synthetic Substitute K Nonautologous Tissue Substitute	Z No Qualifier

⊞ ØHR[TUV]37Z

SECTION: Ø MEDICAL AND SURGICAL

BODY SYSTEM: H **SKIN AND BREAST**

OPERATION: S **REPOSITION:** Moving to its normal location, or other suitable location, all or a portion of a body part

Body Part	Approach	Device	Qualifier
S Hair W Nipple, Right X Nipple, Left	X External	Z No Device	Z No Qualifier
T Breast, Right U Breast, Left V Breast, Bilateral	Ø Open	Z No Device	Z No Qualifier

Non-OR ØHSSXZZ

SECTION: Ø MEDICAL AND SURGICAL

BODY SYSTEM: H SKIN AND BREAST

OPERATION: T RESECTION: Cutting out or off, without replacement, all of a body part

Body Part	Approach	Device	Qualifier
Q Finger Nail R Toe Nail W Nipple, Right X Nipple, Left	X External	Z No Device	Z No Qualifier
T Breast, Right ⊞ U Breast, Left ⊞ V Breast, Bilateral ⊞ Y Supernumerary Breast	Ø Open	Z No Device	Z No Qualifier

⊞ ØHT[TUV]ØZZ

Non-OR ØHT[QR]XZZ

SECTION: Ø MEDICAL AND SURGICAL

BODY SYSTEM: H SKIN AND BREAST

OPERATION: U SUPPLEMENT: Putting in or on biological or synthetic material that physically reinforces and/or augments the function of a portion of a body part

Body Part	Approach	Device	Qualifier
T Breast, Right U Breast, Left V Breast, Bilateral W Nipple, Right X Nipple, Left	Ø Open 3 Percutaneous 7 Via Natural of Artificial Opening 8 Via Natural or Artificial Opening Endoscopic X External	7 Autologous Tissue Substitute J Synthetic Substitute K Nonautologous Tissue Substitute	Z No Qualifier

New/Revised Text in Green ~~deleted~~ Deleted ♀ Females Only ♂ Males Only **Coding Clinic**

Non-covered Limited Coverage ⊞ Combination (See Appendix E) DRG Non-OR Non-OR Hospital-Acquired Condition

T: RESECTION U: SUPPLEMENT

H: SKIN AND BREAST

Ø: M/S

SECTION: Ø MEDICAL AND SURGICAL
BODY SYSTEM: H SKIN AND BREAST
OPERATION: W REVISION: Correcting, to the extent possible, a portion of a malfunctioning device or the position of a displaced device

Body Part	Approach	Device	Qualifier
P Skin	X External	Ø Drainage Device 7 Autologous Tissue Substitute J Synthetic Substitute K Nonautologous Tissue Substitute Y Other Device	Z No Qualifier
Q Finger Nail R Toe Nail	X External	Ø Drainage Device 7 Autologous Tissue Substitute J Synthetic Substitute K Nonautologous Tissue Substitute	Z No Qualifier
S Hair	X External	7 Autologous Tissue Substitute J Synthetic Substitute K Nonautologous Tissue Substitute	Z No Qualifier
T Breast, Right U Breast, Left	Ø Open 3 Percutaneous 7 Via Natural or Artificial Opening 8 Via Natural or Artificial Opening Endoscopic	Ø Drainage Device 7 Autologous Tissue Substitute J Synthetic Substitute K Nonautologous Tissue Substitute N Tissue Expander Y Other Device	Z No Qualifier
T Breast, Right U Breast, Left	X External	Ø Drainage Device 7 Autologous Tissue Substitute J Synthetic Substitute K Nonautologous Tissue Substitute	Z No Qualifier

Non-OR ØHWPX[Ø7JK]Z
Non-OR ØHW[QR]X[Ø7JK]Z
Non-OR ØHWSX[7JK]Z
Non-OR ØHW[TU][Ø3][Ø7KN]Z
Non-OR ØHW[TU][78][Ø7JKN]Z
Non-OR ØHW[TU]X[Ø7JK]Z

New/Revised Text in Green ~~deleted~~ Deleted ♀ Females Only ♂ Males Only **Coding Clinic**
Non-covered Limited Coverage ⊡ Combination (See Appendix E) DRG Non-OR Non-OR Hospital-Acquired Condition

SECTION: Ø MEDICAL AND SURGICAL
BODY SYSTEM: H SKIN AND BREAST
OPERATION: X TRANSFER: Moving, without taking out, all or a portion of a body part to another location to take over the function of all or a portion of a body part

Body Part	Approach	Device	Qualifier
Ø Skin, Scalp	X External	Z No Device	Z No Qualifier
1 Skin, Face			
2 Skin, Right Ear			
3 Skin, Left Ear			
4 Skin, Neck			
5 Skin, Chest			
6 Skin, Back			
7 Skin, Abdomen			
8 Skin, Buttock			
9 Skin, Perineum			
A Skin, Inguinal			
B Skin, Right Upper Arm			
C Skin, Left Upper Arm			
D Skin, Right Lower Arm			
E Skin, Left Lower Arm			
F Skin, Right Hand			
G Skin, Left Hand			
H Skin, Right Upper Leg			
J Skin, Left Upper Leg			
K Skin, Right Lower Leg			
L Skin, Left Lower Leg			
M Skin, Right Foot			
N Skin, Left Foot			

X: TRANSFER

H: SKIN AND BREAST

Ø: M/S

	New/Revised Text in Green	~~deleted~~ Deleted	♀ Females Only	♂ Males Only	**Coding Clinic**	
🔖 Non-covered	🔖 Limited Coverage	⊞ Combination (See Appendix E)	DRG Non-OR	Non-OR	🔖 Hospital-Acquired Condition	

305

SECTION: Ø MEDICAL AND SURGICAL

BODY SYSTEM: J SUBCUTANEOUS TISSUE AND FASCIA
OPERATION: Ø **ALTERATION:** Modifying the anatomic structure of a body part without affecting the function of the body part

Body Part	Approach	Device	Qualifier
1 Subcutaneous Tissue and Fascia, Face 4 Subcutaneous Tissue and Fascia, Right Neck 5 Subcutaneous Tissue and Fascia, Left Neck 6 Subcutaneous Tissue and Fascia, Chest 7 Subcutaneous Tissue and Fascia, Back 8 Subcutaneous Tissue and Fascia, Abdomen 9 Subcutaneous Tissue and Fascia, Buttock D Subcutaneous Tissue and Fascia, Right Upper Arm F Subcutaneous Tissue and Fascia, Left Upper Arm G Subcutaneous Tissue and Fascia, Right Lower Arm H Subcutaneous Tissue and Fascia, Left Lower Arm L Subcutaneous Tissue and Fascia, Right Upper Leg M Subcutaneous Tissue and Fascia, Left Upper Leg N Subcutaneous Tissue and Fascia, Right Lower Leg P Subcutaneous Tissue and Fascia, Left Lower Leg	Ø Open 3 Percutaneous	Z No Device	Z No Qualifier

SECTION: Ø MEDICAL AND SURGICAL

BODY SYSTEM: J SUBCUTANEOUS TISSUE AND FASCIA
OPERATION: 2 **CHANGE:** Taking out or off a device from a body part and putting back an identical or similar device in or on the same body part without cutting or puncturing the skin or a mucous membrane

Body Part	Approach	Device	Qualifier
S Subcutaneous Tissue and Fascia, Head and Neck T Subcutaneous Tissue and Fascia, Trunk V Subcutaneous Tissue and Fascia, Upper Extremity W Subcutaneous Tissue and Fascia, Lower Extremity	X External	Ø Drainage Device Y Other Device	Z No Qualifier

Non-OR   All Values

Coding Clinic: 2017, Q2, P25 – ØJ2TXYZ

SECTION: Ø MEDICAL AND SURGICAL

BODY SYSTEM: J SUBCUTANEOUS TISSUE AND FASCIA

OPERATION: 5 DESTRUCTION: Physical eradication of all or a portion of a body part by the direct use of energy, force, or a destructive agent

Body Part	Approach	Device	Qualifier
Ø Subcutaneous Tissue and Fascia, Scalp 1 Subcutaneous Tissue and Fascia, Face 4 Subcutaneous Tissue and Fascia, Right Neck 5 Subcutaneous Tissue and Fascia, Left Neck 6 Subcutaneous Tissue and Fascia, Chest 7 Subcutaneous Tissue and Fascia, Back 8 Subcutaneous Tissue and Fascia, Abdomen 9 Subcutaneous Tissue and Fascia, Buttock B Subcutaneous Tissue and Fascia, Perineum C Subcutaneous Tissue and Fascia, Pelvic Region D Subcutaneous Tissue and Fascia, Right Upper Arm F Subcutaneous Tissue and Fascia, Left Upper Arm G Subcutaneous Tissue and Fascia, Right Lower Arm H Subcutaneous Tissue and Fascia, Left Lower Arm J Subcutaneous Tissue and Fascia, Right Hand K Subcutaneous Tissue and Fascia, Left Hand L Subcutaneous Tissue and Fascia, Right Upper Leg M Subcutaneous Tissue and Fascia, Left Upper Leg N Subcutaneous Tissue and Fascia, Right Lower Leg P Subcutaneous Tissue and Fascia, Left Lower Leg Q Subcutaneous Tissue and Fascia, Right Foot R Subcutaneous Tissue and Fascia, Left Foot	Ø Open 3 Percutaneous	Z No Device	Z No Qualifier

`DRG Non-OR` All Values

SECTION: Ø MEDICAL AND SURGICAL

BODY SYSTEM: J SUBCUTANEOUS TISSUE AND FASCIA

OPERATION: 8 DIVISION: Cutting into a body part, without draining fluids and/or gases from the body part, in order to separate or transect a body part

Body Part	Approach	Device	Qualifier
Ø Subcutaneous Tissue and Fascia, Scalp 1 Subcutaneous Tissue and Fascia, Face 4 Subcutaneous Tissue and Fascia, Right Neck 5 Subcutaneous Tissue and Fascia, Left Neck 6 Subcutaneous Tissue and Fascia, Chest 7 Subcutaneous Tissue and Fascia, Back 8 Subcutaneous Tissue and Fascia, Abdomen 9 Subcutaneous Tissue and Fascia, Buttock B Subcutaneous Tissue and Fascia, Perineum C Subcutaneous Tissue and Fascia, Pelvic Region D Subcutaneous Tissue and Fascia, Right Upper Arm F Subcutaneous Tissue and Fascia, Left Upper Arm G Subcutaneous Tissue and Fascia, Right Lower Arm H Subcutaneous Tissue and Fascia, Left Lower Arm J Subcutaneous Tissue and Fascia, Right Hand K Subcutaneous Tissue and Fascia, Left Hand L Subcutaneous Tissue and Fascia, Right Upper Leg M Subcutaneous Tissue and Fascia, Left Upper Leg N Subcutaneous Tissue and Fascia, Right Lower Leg P Subcutaneous Tissue and Fascia, Left Lower Leg Q Subcutaneous Tissue and Fascia, Right Foot R Subcutaneous Tissue and Fascia, Left Foot S Subcutaneous Tissue and Fascia, Head and Neck T Subcutaneous Tissue and Fascia, Trunk V Subcutaneous Tissue and Fascia, Upper Extremity W Subcutaneous Tissue and Fascia, Lower Extremity	Ø Open 3 Percutaneous	Z No Device	Z No Qualifier

New/Revised Text in Green ~~deleted~~ Deleted ♀ Females Only ♂ Males Only **Coding Clinic**
Non-covered Limited Coverage ⊞ Combination (See Appendix E) DRG Non-OR Non-OR Hospital-Acquired Condition

SECTION: Ø MEDICAL AND SURGICAL
BODY SYSTEM: J SUBCUTANEOUS TISSUE AND FASCIA
OPERATION: 9 DRAINAGE: *(on multiple pages)*
Taking or letting out fluids and/or gases from a body part

Body Part	Approach	Device	Qualifier
Ø Subcutaneous Tissue and Fascia, Scalp	Ø Open	Ø Drainage Device	Z No Qualifier
1 Subcutaneous Tissue and Fascia, Face	3 Percutaneous		
4 Subcutaneous Tissue and Fascia, Right Neck			
5 Subcutaneous Tissue and Fascia, Left Neck			
6 Subcutaneous Tissue and Fascia, Chest			
7 Subcutaneous Tissue and Fascia, Back			
8 Subcutaneous Tissue and Fascia, Abdomen			
9 Subcutaneous Tissue and Fascia, Buttock			
B Subcutaneous Tissue and Fascia, Perineum			
C Subcutaneous Tissue and Fascia, Pelvic Region			
D Subcutaneous Tissue and Fascia, Right Upper Arm			
F Subcutaneous Tissue and Fascia, Left Upper Arm			
G Subcutaneous Tissue and Fascia, Right Lower Arm			
H Subcutaneous Tissue and Fascia, Left Lower Arm			
J Subcutaneous Tissue and Fascia, Right Hand			
K Subcutaneous Tissue and Fascia, Left Hand			
L Subcutaneous Tissue and Fascia, Right Upper Leg			
M Subcutaneous Tissue and Fascia, Left Upper Leg			
N Subcutaneous Tissue and Fascia, Right Lower Leg			
P Subcutaneous Tissue and Fascia, Left Lower Leg			
Q Subcutaneous Tissue and Fascia, Right Foot			
R Subcutaneous Tissue and Fascia, Left Foot			

DRG Non-OR ØJ9[1]ØØZ
Non-OR ØJ9[1JK]3ØZ
Non-OR ØJ9[0456789BCDFGHJKLMNPQR][Ø3]ØZ

Ø: M/S

J: SUBCUTANEOUS TISSUE AND FASCIA

9: DRAINAGE

New/Revised Text in Green ~~deleted~~ Deleted ♀ Females Only ♂ Males Only **Coding Clinic**
Non-covered Limited Coverage Combination (See Appendix E) DRG Non-OR Non-OR Hospital-Acquired Condition

SECTION: Ø MEDICAL AND SURGICAL

BODY SYSTEM: J SUBCUTANEOUS TISSUE AND FASCIA
OPERATION: 9 DRAINAGE: *(continued)*
Taking or letting out fluids and/or gases from a body part

Body Part	Approach	Device	Qualifier
Ø Subcutaneous Tissue and Fascia, Scalp 1 Subcutaneous Tissue and Fascia, Face 4 Subcutaneous Tissue and Fascia, Right Neck 5 Subcutaneous Tissue and Fascia, Left Neck 6 Subcutaneous Tissue and Fascia, Chest 7 Subcutaneous Tissue and Fascia, Back 8 Subcutaneous Tissue and Fascia, Abdomen 9 Subcutaneous Tissue and Fascia, Buttock B Subcutaneous Tissue and Fascia, Perineum C Subcutaneous Tissue and Fascia, Pelvic Region D Subcutaneous Tissue and Fascia, Right Upper Arm F Subcutaneous Tissue and Fascia, Left Upper Arm G Subcutaneous Tissue and Fascia, Right Lower Arm H Subcutaneous Tissue and Fascia, Left Lower Arm J Subcutaneous Tissue and Fascia, Right Hand K Subcutaneous Tissue and Fascia, Left Hand L Subcutaneous Tissue and Fascia, Right Upper Leg M Subcutaneous Tissue and Fascia, Left Upper Leg N Subcutaneous Tissue and Fascia, Right Lower Leg P Subcutaneous Tissue and Fascia, Left Lower Leg Q Subcutaneous Tissue and Fascia, Right Foot R Subcutaneous Tissue and Fascia, Left Foot	Ø Open 3 Percutaneous	Z No Device	X Diagnostic Z No Qualifier

DRG Non-OR   ØJ9[Ø1456789BCDFGHLMNPQR]ØZZ
Non-OR   ØJ9[Ø1456789BCDFGHJKLMNPQR][Ø3]ZX
Non-OR   ØJ9[Ø1456789BCDFGHJKLMNPQR]3ZZ

Coding Clinic: 2Ø15, Q3, P24 – ØJ9[6CDFLM]ØZZ

New/Revised Text in Green   ~~deleted~~ Deleted   ♀ Females Only   ♂ Males Only   **Coding Clinic**
Non-covered   Limited Coverage   ⊞ Combination (See Appendix E)   DRG Non-OR   Non-OR   Hospital-Acquired Condition

Sidebar: 9: DRAINAGE   J: SUBCUTANEOUS TISSUE AND FASCIA   Ø: M/S

SECTION: Ø MEDICAL AND SURGICAL

BODY SYSTEM: J SUBCUTANEOUS TISSUE AND FASCIA

OPERATION: B EXCISION: Cutting out or off, without replacement, a portion of a body part

Body Part	Approach	Device	Qualifier
Ø Subcutaneous Tissue and Fascia, Scalp 1 Subcutaneous Tissue and Fascia, Face 4 Subcutaneous Tissue and Fascia, Right Neck 5 Subcutaneous Tissue and Fascia, Left Neck 6 Subcutaneous Tissue and Fascia, Chest 7 Subcutaneous Tissue and Fascia, Back 8 Subcutaneous Tissue and Fascia, Abdomen 9 Subcutaneous Tissue and Fascia, Buttock B Subcutaneous Tissue and Fascia, Perineum C Subcutaneous Tissue and Fascia, Pelvic Region D Subcutaneous Tissue and Fascia, Right Upper Arm F Subcutaneous Tissue and Fascia, Left Upper Arm G Subcutaneous Tissue and Fascia, Right Lower Arm H Subcutaneous Tissue and Fascia, Left Lower Arm J Subcutaneous Tissue and Fascia, Right Hand K Subcutaneous Tissue and Fascia, Left Hand L Subcutaneous Tissue and Fascia, Right Upper Leg M Subcutaneous Tissue and Fascia, Left Upper Leg N Subcutaneous Tissue and Fascia, Right Lower Leg P Subcutaneous Tissue and Fascia, Left Lower Leg Q Subcutaneous Tissue and Fascia, Right Foot R Subcutaneous Tissue and Fascia, Left Foot	Ø Open 3 Percutaneous	Z No Device	X Diagnostic Z No Qualifier

DRG Non-OR   ØJB[Ø456789BCDFGHLMNPQR]3ZZ

Non-OR   ØJB[Ø1456789BCDFGHJKLMNPQR][Ø3]ZX

Coding Clinic: 2015, Q1, P3Ø – ØJBBØZZ
Coding Clinic: 2015, Q2, P13 – ØJBHØZZ
Coding Clinic: 2015, Q3, P7 – ØJB9ØZZ
Coding Clinic: 2018, Q1, P7 – ØJB7ØZZ

Ø: M/S

J: SUBCUTANEOUS TISSUE AND FASCIA

B: EXCISION

SECTION: Ø MEDICAL AND SURGICAL

BODY SYSTEM: J SUBCUTANEOUS TISSUE AND FASCIA
OPERATION: C EXTIRPATION: Taking or cutting out solid matter from a body part

Body Part	Approach	Device	Qualifier
Ø Subcutaneous Tissue and Fascia, Scalp 1 Subcutaneous Tissue and Fascia, Face 4 Subcutaneous Tissue and Fascia, Right Neck 5 Subcutaneous Tissue and Fascia, Left Neck 6 Subcutaneous Tissue and Fascia, Chest 7 Subcutaneous Tissue and Fascia, Back 8 Subcutaneous Tissue and Fascia, Abdomen 9 Subcutaneous Tissue and Fascia, Buttock B Subcutaneous Tissue and Fascia, Perineum C Subcutaneous Tissue and Fascia, Pelvic Region D Subcutaneous Tissue and Fascia, Right Upper Arm F Subcutaneous Tissue and Fascia, Left Upper Arm G Subcutaneous Tissue and Fascia, Right Lower Arm H Subcutaneous Tissue and Fascia, Left Lower Arm J Subcutaneous Tissue and Fascia, Right Hand K Subcutaneous Tissue and Fascia, Left Hand L Subcutaneous Tissue and Fascia, Right Upper Leg M Subcutaneous Tissue and Fascia, Left Upper Leg N Subcutaneous Tissue and Fascia, Right Lower Leg P Subcutaneous Tissue and Fascia, Left Lower Leg Q Subcutaneous Tissue and Fascia, Right Foot R Subcutaneous Tissue and Fascia, Left Foot	Ø Open 3 Percutaneous	Z No Device	Z No Qualifier

Non-OR   All Values

Coding Clinic: 2017, Q3, P22 – ØJC8ØZZ

New/Revised Text in Green   ~~deleted~~ Deleted   ♀ Females Only   ♂ Males Only   **Coding Clinic**
🚫 Non-covered   🚫 Limited Coverage   ⊞ Combination (See Appendix E)   DRG Non-OR   Non-OR   🚫 Hospital-Acquired Condition

SECTION: Ø MEDICAL AND SURGICAL

BODY SYSTEM: J SUBCUTANEOUS TISSUE AND FASCIA

OPERATION: D EXTRACTION: Pulling or stripping out or off all or a portion of a body part by the use of force

Body Part	Approach	Device	Qualifier
Ø Subcutaneous Tissue and Fascia, Scalp	Ø Open	Z No Device	Z No Qualifier
1 Subcutaneous Tissue and Fascia, Face	3 Percutaneous		
4 Subcutaneous Tissue and Fascia, Right Neck			
5 Subcutaneous Tissue and Fascia, Left Neck			
6 Subcutaneous Tissue and Fascia, Chest ⊕			
7 Subcutaneous Tissue and Fascia, Back ⊕			
8 Subcutaneous Tissue and Fascia, Abdomen ⊕			
9 Subcutaneous Tissue and Fascia, Buttock ⊕			
B Subcutaneous Tissue and Fascia, Perineum			
C Subcutaneous Tissue and Fascia, Pelvic Region			
D Subcutaneous Tissue and Fascia, Right Upper Arm			
F Subcutaneous Tissue and Fascia, Left Upper Arm			
G Subcutaneous Tissue and Fascia, Right Lower Arm			
H Subcutaneous Tissue and Fascia, Left Lower Arm			
J Subcutaneous Tissue and Fascia, Right Hand			
K Subcutaneous Tissue and Fascia, Left Hand			
L Subcutaneous Tissue and Fascia, Right Upper Leg ⊕			
M Subcutaneous Tissue and Fascia, Left Upper Leg ⊕			
N Subcutaneous Tissue and Fascia, Right Lower Leg			
P Subcutaneous Tissue and Fascia, Left Lower Leg			
Q Subcutaneous Tissue and Fascia, Right Foot			
R Subcutaneous Tissue and Fascia, Left Foot			

⊕ ØJD[6789LM]3ZZ

DRG Non-OR ØJD[01456789BCDFGHJKLMNPQR][03]ZZ

Coding Clinic: 2015, Q1, P23 – ØJDCØZZ
Coding Clinic: 2016, Q1, P40 – ØJDLØZZ
Coding Clinic: 2016, Q3, P21-22 – ØJD[7NR]ØZZ

SECTION: Ø MEDICAL AND SURGICAL
BODY SYSTEM: J SUBCUTANEOUS TISSUE AND FASCIA
OPERATION: H INSERTION: *(on multiple pages)*
Putting in a nonbiological appliance that monitors, assists, performs, or prevents a physiological function but does not physically take the place of a body part

Body Part	Approach	Device	Qualifier
Ø Subcutaneous Tissue and Fascia, Scalp 1 Subcutaneous Tissue and Fascia, Face 4 Subcutaneous Tissue and Fascia, Right Neck 5 Subcutaneous Tissue and Fascia, Left Neck 9 Subcutaneous Tissue and Fascia, Buttock B Subcutaneous Tissue and Fascia, Perineum C Subcutaneous Tissue and Fascia, Pelvic Region J Subcutaneous Tissue and Fascia, Right Hand K Subcutaneous Tissue and Fascia, Left Hand Q Subcutaneous Tissue and Fascia, Right Foot R Subcutaneous Tissue and Fascia, Left Foot	Ø Open 3 Percutaneous	N Tissue Expander	Z No Qualifer
6 Subcutaneous Tissue and Fascia, Chest ⊞ ⍟ 8 Subcutaneous Tissue and Fascia, Abdomen ⍟ ⊞ ⍟	Ø Open 3 Percutaneous	Ø Monitoring Device, Hemodynamic 2 Monitoring Device 4 Pacemaker, Single Chamber 5 Pacemaker, Single Chamber Rate Responsive 6 Pacemaker, Dual Chamber 7 Cardiac Resynchronization Pacemaker Pulse Generator 8 Defibrillator Generator 9 Cardiac Resynchronization Defibrillator Pulse Generator A Contractility Modulation Device B Stimulator Generator, Single Array C Stimulator Generator, Single Array Rechargeable D Stimulator Generator, Multiple Array E Stimulator Generator, Multiple Array Rechargeable H Contraceptive Device M Stimulator Generator N Tissue Expander P Cardiac Rhythm Related Device V Infusion Device, Pump W Vascular Access Device, Totally Implantable X Vascular Access Device, Tunneled	Z No Qualifier

⍟ ØJH8[Ø3]MZ
⊞ ØJH[68][Ø3][Ø89ABCDE]Z
DRG Non-OR ØJH[68][Ø3][456HWX]Z
DRG Non-OR ØJH8[Ø3]2Z
⍟ ØJH[68][Ø3][456789P]Z when reported with Secondary Diagnosis K68.11, T81.4XXA, T82.6XXA, or T82.7XXA, except ØJH63XZ
⍟ ØJH63XZ when reported with Secondary Diagnosis J95.811

Coding Clinic: 2015, Q2, P33 – ØJH6ØXZ
Coding Clinic: 2015, Q4, P15 – ØJH63VZ
Coding Clinic: 2017, Q2, P25; 2016, Q2, P16; 2015, Q4, P31-32 – ØJH63XZ
Coding Clinic: 2016, Q4, P99 – ØJH6ØMZ
Coding Clinic: 2017, Q4, P64 – ØJH6ØWZ

New/Revised Text in Green ~~deleted~~ Deleted ♀ Females Only ♂ Males Only **Coding Clinic**
⍟ Non-covered ⍟ Limited Coverage ⊞ Combination (See Appendix E) **DRG Non-OR** Non-OR ⍟ Hospital-Acquired Condition

SECTION: Ø MEDICAL AND SURGICAL
BODY SYSTEM: J SUBCUTANEOUS TISSUE AND FASCIA
OPERATION: H INSERTION: *(continued)*

Putting in a nonbiological appliance that monitors, assists, performs, or prevents a physiological function but does not physically take the place of a body part

Body Part	Approach	Device	Qualifier
7 Subcutaneous Tissue and Fascia, Back 🔖 ⊞	Ø Open 3 Percutaneous	B Stimulator Generator, Single Array C Stimulator Generator, Single Array Rechargeable D Stimulator Generator, Multiple Array E Stimulator Generator, Multiple Array Rechargeable M Stimulator Generator N Tissue Expander V Infusion Device, Pump	Z No Qualifier
D Subcutaneous Tissue and Fascia, Right Upper Arm F Subcutaneous Tissue and Fascia, Left Upper Arm G Subcutaneous Tissue and Fascia, Right Lower Arm H Subcutaneous Tissue and Fascia, Left Lower Arm L Subcutaneous Tissue and Fascia, Right Upper Leg M Subcutaneous Tissue and Fascia, Left Upper Leg N Subcutaneous Tissue and Fascia, Right Lower Leg P Subcutaneous Tissue and Fascia, Left Lower Leg	Ø Open 3 Percutaneous	H Contraceptive Device N Tissue Expander V Infusion Device, Pump W Vascular Access Device, Totally Implantable X Vascular Access Device, Tunneled	Z No Qualifier
S Subcutaneous Tissue and Fascia, Head and Neck V Subcutaneous Tissue and Fascia, Upper Extremity W Subcutaneous Tissue and Fascia, Lower Extremity	Ø Open 3 Percutaneous	1 Radioactive Element 3 Infusion Device Y Other Device	Z No Qualifier
T Subcutaneous Tissue and Fascia, Trunk	Ø Open 3 Percutaneous	1 Radioactive Element 3 Infusion Device V Infusion Device, Pump Y Other Device	Z No Qualifier

🔖 ØJH7[Ø3]MZ
⊞ ØJH7[Ø3][BCDE]Z
DRG Non-OR ØJH[DFGHLM][Ø3][WX]Z
DRG Non-OR ØJHNØ[WX]Z
DRG Non-OR ØJHN3[HWX]Z
DRG Non-OR ØJHP[Ø3][HWX]Z
DRG Non-OR ØJH[SVW][Ø3]3Z
DRG Non-OR ØJHT[Ø3]3Z
Non-OR ØJH[DFGHLM][Ø3]HZ
Non-OR ØJHNØHZ
Non-OR ØJH[SVW][Ø3]3Z
Non-OR ØJHT[Ø3]3Z

Coding Clinic: 2012, Q4, P105 – ØJH6Ø8Z & ØJH6ØPZ
Coding Clinic: 2016, Q2, P14 – ØJH8ØWZ

New/Revised Text in Green ~~deleted~~ Deleted ♀ Females Only ♂ Males Only **Coding Clinic**
🔖 Non-covered 🔖 Limited Coverage ⊞ Combination (See Appendix E) DRG Non-OR Non-OR 🔖 Hospital-Acquired Condition

SECTION: Ø MEDICAL AND SURGICAL
BODY SYSTEM: J SUBCUTANEOUS TISSUE AND FASCIA
OPERATION: J INSPECTION: Visually and/or manually exploring a body part

Body Part	Approach	Device	Qualifier
S Subcutaneous Tissue and Fascia, Head and Neck T Subcutaneous Tissue and Fascia, Trunk V Subcutaneous Tissue and Fascia, Upper Extremity W Subcutaneous Tissue and Fascia, Lower Extremity	Ø Open 3 Percutaneous X External	Z No Device	Z No Qualifier

Non-OR All Values

SECTION: Ø MEDICAL AND SURGICAL
BODY SYSTEM: J SUBCUTANEOUS TISSUE AND FASCIA
OPERATION: N RELEASE: Freeing a body part from an abnormal physical constraint by cutting or by the use of force

Body Part	Approach	Device	Qualifier
Ø Subcutaneous Tissue and Fascia, Scalp 1 Subcutaneous Tissue and Fascia, Face 4 Subcutaneous Tissue and Fascia, Right Neck 5 Subcutaneous Tissue and Fascia, Left Neck 6 Subcutaneous Tissue and Fascia, Chest 7 Subcutaneous Tissue and Fascia, Back 8 Subcutaneous Tissue and Fascia, Abdomen 9 Subcutaneous Tissue and Fascia, Buttock B Subcutaneous Tissue and Fascia, Perineum C Subcutaneous Tissue and Fascia, Pelvic Region D Subcutaneous Tissue and Fascia, Right Upper Arm F Subcutaneous Tissue and Fascia, Left Upper Arm G Subcutaneous Tissue and Fascia, Right Lower Arm H Subcutaneous Tissue and Fascia, Left Lower Arm J Subcutaneous Tissue and Fascia, Right Hand K Subcutaneous Tissue and Fascia, Left Hand L Subcutaneous Tissue and Fascia, Right Upper Leg M Subcutaneous Tissue and Fascia, Left Upper Leg N Subcutaneous Tissue and Fascia, Right Lower Leg P Subcutaneous Tissue and Fascia, Left Lower Leg Q Subcutaneous Tissue and Fascia, Right Foot R Subcutaneous Tissue and Fascia, Left Foot	Ø Open 3 Percutaneous X External	Z No Device	Z No Qualifier

Non-OR ØJN[1456789BCDFGHJKLMNPQR]XZZ

Coding Clinic: 2017, Q3, P12 – ØJN[LMNPQR]ØZZ

SECTION: Ø MEDICAL AND SURGICAL
BODY SYSTEM: J SUBCUTANEOUS TISSUE AND FASCIA
OPERATION: P REMOVAL: Taking out or off a device from a body part

Body Part	Approach	Device	Qualifier
S Subcutaneous Tissue and Fascia, Head and Neck	Ø Open 3 Percutaneous	Ø Drainage Device 1 Radioactive Element 3 Infusion Device 7 Autologous Tissue Substitute J Synthetic Substitute K Nonautologous Tissue Substitute N Tissue Expander Y Other Device	Z No Qualifier
S Subcutaneous Tissue and Fascia, Head and Neck	X External	Ø Drainage Device 1 Radioactive Element 3 Infusion Device	Z No Qualifier
T Subcutaneous Tissue and Fascia, Trunk 🔖	Ø Open 3 Percutaneous	Ø Drainage Device 1 Radioactive Element 2 Monitoring Device 3 Infusion Device 7 Autologous Tissue Substitute H Contraceptive Device J Synthetic Substitute K Nonautologous Tissue Substitute M Stimulator Generator N Tissue Expander P Cardiac Rhythm Related Device V Infusion Device, Pump W Vascular Access Device, Totally Implantable X Vascular Access Device, Tunneled Y Other Device	Z No Qualifier
T Subcutaneous Tissue and Fascia, Trunk	X External	Ø Drainage Device 1 Radioactive Element 2 Monitoring Device 3 Infusion Device H Contraceptive Device V Infusion Device, Pump X Vascular Access Device, Tunneled	Z No Qualifier
V Subcutaneous Tissue and Fascia, Upper Extremity W Subcutaneous Tissue and Fascia, Lower Extremity	Ø Open 3 Percutaneous	Ø Drainage Device 1 Radioactive Element 3 Infusion Device 7 Autologous Tissue Substitute H Contraceptive Device J Synthetic Substitute K Nonautologous Tissue Substitute N Tissue Expander V Infusion Device, Pump W Vascular Access Device, Totally Implantable X Vascular Access Device, Tunneled Y Other Device	Z No Qualifier
V Subcutaneous Tissue and Fascia, Upper Extremity W Subcutaneous Tissue and Fascia, Lower Extremity	X External	Ø Drainage Device 1 Radioactive Element 3 Infusion Device H Contraceptive Device V Infusion Pump X Vascular Access Device, Tunneled	Z No Qualifier

Non-OR ØJPS[Ø3][Ø137JKN]Z
Non-OR ØJPSX[Ø13]Z
Non-OR ØJPT[Ø3][Ø1237HJKMNVWX]Z
Non-OR ØJPTX[Ø123HVX]Z

Non-OR ØJP[VW][Ø3][Ø137HJKNVWX]Z
Non-OR ØJP[VW]X[Ø13HVX]Z
🔖 ØJPT[Ø3]PZ when reported with Secondary Diagnosis K68.11, T81.4XXA, T82.6XXA, or T82.7XXA

Coding Clinic: 2012, Q4, P105 – ØJPTØPZ
Coding Clinic: 2016, Q2, P15; 2015, Q4, P32 – ØJPTØXZ

SECTION: Ø MEDICAL AND SURGICAL

BODY SYSTEM: J   SUBCUTANEOUS TISSUE AND FASCIA

OPERATION: **Q REPAIR:** Restoring, to the extent possible, a body part to its normal anatomic structure and function

Body Part	Approach	Device	Qualifier
Ø Subcutaneous Tissue and Fascia, Scalp	Ø Open	Z No Device	Z No Qualifier
1 Subcutaneous Tissue and Fascia, Face	3 Percutaneous		
4 Subcutaneous Tissue and Fascia, Right Neck			
5 Subcutaneous Tissue and Fascia, Left Neck			
6 Subcutaneous Tissue and Fascia, Chest			
7 Subcutaneous Tissue and Fascia, Back			
8 Subcutaneous Tissue and Fascia, Abdomen			
9 Subcutaneous Tissue and Fascia, Buttock			
B Subcutaneous Tissue and Fascia, Perineum			
C Subcutaneous Tissue and Fascia, Pelvic Region			
D Subcutaneous Tissue and Fascia, Right Upper Arm			
F Subcutaneous Tissue and Fascia, Left Upper Arm			
G Subcutaneous Tissue and Fascia, Right Lower Arm			
H Subcutaneous Tissue and Fascia, Left Lower Arm			
J Subcutaneous Tissue and Fascia, Right Hand			
K Subcutaneous Tissue and Fascia, Left Hand			
L Subcutaneous Tissue and Fascia, Right Upper Leg			
M Subcutaneous Tissue and Fascia, Left Upper Leg			
N Subcutaneous Tissue and Fascia, Right Lower Leg			
P Subcutaneous Tissue and Fascia, Left Lower Leg			
Q Subcutaneous Tissue and Fascia, Right Foot			
R Subcutaneous Tissue and Fascia, Left Foot			

DRG Non-OR   ØJQ[Ø1456789BCDFGHJKLMNPQR][Ø3]ZZ

Non-OR   ØJQ[Ø1456789BCDFGHJKLMNPQR]3ZZ

Coding Clinic: 2Ø17, Q3, P19 – ØJQCØZZ

New/Revised Text in Green   ~~deleted~~ Deleted   ♀ Females Only   ♂ Males Only   **Coding Clinic**

Non-covered   Limited Coverage   ⊞ Combination (See Appendix E)   DRG Non-OR   Non-OR   Hospital-Acquired Condition

SECTION: Ø MEDICAL AND SURGICAL
BODY SYSTEM: J SUBCUTANEOUS TISSUE AND FASCIA
OPERATION: R REPLACEMENT: Putting in or on biological or synthetic material that physically takes the place and/or function of all or a portion of a body part

Body Part	Approach	Device	Qualifier
Ø Subcutaneous Tissue and Fascia, Scalp	Ø Open	7 Autologous Tissue Substitute	Z No Qualifier
1 Subcutaneous Tissue and Fascia, Face	3 Percutaneous	J Synthetic Substitute	
4 Subcutaneous Tissue and Fascia, Right Neck		K Nonautologous Tissue Substitute	
5 Subcutaneous Tissue and Fascia, Left Neck			
6 Subcutaneous Tissue and Fascia, Chest			
7 Subcutaneous Tissue and Fascia, Back			
8 Subcutaneous Tissue and Fascia, Abdomen			
9 Subcutaneous Tissue and Fascia, Buttock			
B Subcutaneous Tissue and Fascia, Perineum			
C Subcutaneous Tissue and Fascia, Pelvic Region			
D Subcutaneous Tissue and Fascia, Right Upper Arm			
F Subcutaneous Tissue and Fascia, Left Upper Arm			
G Subcutaneous Tissue and Fascia, Right Lower Arm			
H Subcutaneous Tissue and Fascia, Left Lower Arm			
J Subcutaneous Tissue and Fascia, Right Hand			
K Subcutaneous Tissue and Fascia, Left Hand			
L Subcutaneous Tissue and Fascia, Right Upper Leg			
M Subcutaneous Tissue and Fascia, Left Upper Leg			
N Subcutaneous Tissue and Fascia, Right Lower Leg			
P Subcutaneous Tissue and Fascia, Left Lower Leg			
Q Subcutaneous Tissue and Fascia, Right Foot			
R Subcutaneous Tissue and Fascia, Left Foot			

Coding Clinic: 2Ø15, Q2, P13 – ØJR1Ø7Z

Ø: M/S

J: SUBCUTANEOUS TISSUE AND FASCIA

R: REPLACEMENT

SECTION: Ø MEDICAL AND SURGICAL

BODY SYSTEM: J SUBCUTANEOUS TISSUE AND FASCIA

OPERATION: U SUPPLEMENT: Putting in or on biological or synthetic material that physically reinforces and/or augments the function of a portion of a body part

Body Part	Approach	Device	Qualifier
Ø Subcutaneous Tissue and Fascia, Scalp 1 Subcutaneous Tissue and Fascia, Face 4 Subcutaneous Tissue and Fascia, Right Neck 5 Subcutaneous Tissue and Fascia, Left Neck 6 Subcutaneous Tissue and Fascia, Chest 7 Subcutaneous Tissue and Fascia, Back 8 Subcutaneous Tissue and Fascia, Abdomen 9 Subcutaneous Tissue and Fascia, Buttock B Subcutaneous Tissue and Fascia, Perineum C Subcutaneous Tissue and Fascia, Pelvic Region D Subcutaneous Tissue and Fascia, Right Upper Arm F Subcutaneous Tissue and Fascia, Left Upper Arm G Subcutaneous Tissue and Fascia, Right Lower Arm H Subcutaneous Tissue and Fascia, Left Lower Arm J Subcutaneous Tissue and Fascia, Right Hand K Subcutaneous Tissue and Fascia, Left Hand L Subcutaneous Tissue and Fascia, Right Upper Leg M Subcutaneous Tissue and Fascia, Left Upper Leg N Subcutaneous Tissue and Fascia, Right Lower Leg P Subcutaneous Tissue and Fascia, Left Lower Leg Q Subcutaneous Tissue and Fascia, Right Foot R Subcutaneous Tissue and Fascia, Left Foot	Ø Open 3 Percutaneous	7 Autologous Tissue Substitute J Synthetic Substitute K Nonautologous Tissue Substitute	Z No Qualifier

Coding Clinic: 2Ø18, Q1, P7 – ØJU7Ø7Z
Coding Clinic: 2Ø18, Q2, P2Ø – ØJUHØKZ

SECTION: Ø MEDICAL AND SURGICAL

BODY SYSTEM: J SUBCUTANEOUS TISSUE AND FASCIA

OPERATION: W REVISION: *(on multiple pages)*
Correcting, to the extent possible, a portion of a malfunctioning device or the position of a displaced device

Body Part	Approach	Device	Qualifier
S Subcutaneous Tissue and Fascia, Head and Neck	Ø Open 3 Percutaneous	Ø Drainage Device 3 Infusion Device 7 Autologous Tissue Substitute J Synthetic Substitute K Nonautologous Tissue Substitute N Tissue Expander Y Other Device	Z No Qualifier
S Subcutaneous Tissue and Fascia, Head and Neck	X External	Ø Drainage Device 3 Infusion Device 7 Autologous Tissue Substitute J Synthetic Substitute K Nonautologous Tissue Substitute N Tissue Expander	Z No Qualifier
T Subcutaneous Tissue and Fascia, Trunk 🔖	Ø Open 3 Percutaneous	Ø Drainage Device 2 Monitoring Device 3 Infusion Device 7 Autologous Tissue Substitute H Contraceptive Device J Synthetic Substitute K Nonautologous Tissue Substitute M Stimulator Generator N Tissue Expander P Cardiac Rhythm Related Device V Infusion Device, Pump W Vascular Access Device, Totally Implantable X Vascular Access Device, Tunneled Y Other Device	Z No Qualifier
T Subcutaneous Tissue and Fascia, Trunk	X External	Ø Drainage Device 2 Monitoring Device 3 Infusion Device 7 Autologous Tissue Substitute H Contraceptive Device J Synthetic Substitute K Nonautologous Tissue Substitute M Stimulator Generator N Tissue Expander P Cardiac Rhythm Related Device V Infusion Device, Pump W Vascular Access Device, Totally Implantable X Vascular Access Device, Tunneled	Z No Qualifier

DRG Non-OR   ØJWS[Ø3][Ø37JKN]Z
DRG Non-OR   ØJWT[Ø3][Ø37HJKNVWX]Z
Non-OR   ØJWSX[Ø37JKN]Z
Non-OR   ØJWTX[Ø237HJKNPVWX]Z
🔖 ØJWT[Ø3]PZ when reported with Secondary Diagnosis K68.11, T81.4XXA, T82.6XXA, or T82.7XXA

Coding Clinic: 2012, Q4, P106 – ØJWTØPZ
Coding Clinic: 2015, Q2, P10 – ØJWSØJZ
Coding Clinic: 2015, Q4, P33 – ØJWT33Z
Coding Clinic: 2018, Q1, P9 – ØJWTØJZ

New/Revised Text in Green   ~~deleted~~ Deleted   ♀ Females Only   ♂ Males Only   **Coding Clinic**
🔖 Non-covered   🔖 Limited Coverage   ⊡ Combination (See Appendix E)   DRG Non-OR   Non-OR   🔖 Hospital-Acquired Condition

SECTION: Ø MEDICAL AND SURGICAL
BODY SYSTEM: J SUBCUTANEOUS TISSUE AND FASCIA
OPERATION: W REVISION: *(continued)*
Correcting, to the extent possible, a portion of a malfunctioning device or the position of a displaced device

Body Part	Approach	Device	Qualifier
V Subcutaneous Tissue and Fascia, Upper Extremity W Subcutaneous Tissue and Fascia, Lower Extremity	Ø Open 3 Percutaneous	Ø Drainage Device 3 Infusion Device 7 Autologous Tissue Substitute H Contraceptive Device J Synthetic Substitute K Nonautologous Tissue Substitute N Tissue Expander V Infusion Device, Pump W Vascular Access Device, Totally Implantable X Vascular Access Device, Tunneled Y Other Device	Z No Qualifier
V Subcutaneous Tissue and Fascia, Upper Extremity W Subcutaneous Tissue and Fascia, Lower Extremity	X External	Ø Drainage Device 3 Infusion Device 7 Autologous Tissue Substitute H Contraceptive Device J Synthetic Substitute K Nonautologous Tissue Substitute N Tissue Expander V Infusion Device, Pump W Vascular Access Device, Totally Implantable X Vascular Access Device, Tunneled	Z No Qualifier

DRG Non-OR ØJW[VW][Ø3][Ø37HJKNVWX]Z
Non-OR ØJW[VW]X[Ø37HJKNVWX]Z

New/Revised Text in Green   ~~deleted~~ Deleted   ♀ Females Only   ♂ Males Only   **Coding Clinic**
Non-covered   Limited Coverage   ⊞ Combination (See Appendix E)   DRG Non-OR   Non-OR   Hospital-Acquired Condition

SECTION: Ø MEDICAL AND SURGICAL
BODY SYSTEM: J SUBCUTANEOUS TISSUE AND FASCIA
OPERATION: X TRANSFER: Moving, without taking out, all or a portion of a body part to another location to take over the function of all or a portion of a body part

Body Part	Approach	Device	Qualifier
Ø Subcutaneous Tissue and Fascia, Scalp 1 Subcutaneous Tissue and Fascia, Face 4 Subcutaneous Tissue and Fascia, Right Neck 5 Subcutaneous Tissue and Fascia, Left Neck 6 Subcutaneous Tissue and Fascia, Chest 7 Subcutaneous Tissue and Fascia, Back 8 Subcutaneous Tissue and Fascia, Abdomen 9 Subcutaneous Tissue and Fascia, Buttock B Subcutaneous Tissue and Fascia, Perineum C Subcutaneous Tissue and Fascia, Pelvic Region D Subcutaneous Tissue and Fascia, Right Upper Arm F Subcutaneous Tissue and Fascia, Left Upper Arm G Subcutaneous Tissue and Fascia, Right Lower Arm H Subcutaneous Tissue and Fascia, Left Lower Arm J Subcutaneous Tissue and Fascia, Right Hand K Subcutaneous Tissue and Fascia, Left Hand L Subcutaneous Tissue and Fascia, Right Upper Leg M Subcutaneous Tissue and Fascia, Left Upper Leg N Subcutaneous Tissue and Fascia, Right Lower Leg P Subcutaneous Tissue and Fascia, Left Lower Leg Q Subcutaneous Tissue and Fascia, Right Foot R Subcutaneous Tissue and Fascia, Left Foot	Ø Open 3 Percutaneous	Z No Device	B Skin and Subcutaneous Tissue C Skin, Subcutaneous Tissue and Fascia Z No Qualifier

Coding Clinic: 2018, Q1, P10 – ØJX00ZC

SECTION: Ø MEDICAL AND SURGICAL

BODY SYSTEM: K MUSCLES

OPERATION: 2 **CHANGE:** Taking out or off a device from a body part and putting back an identical or similar device in or on the same body part without cutting or puncturing the skin or a mucous membrane

Body Part	Approach	Device	Qualifier
X Upper Muscle Y Lower Muscle	X External	Ø Drainage Device Y Other Device	Z No Qualifier

Non-OR All Values

SECTION: Ø MEDICAL AND SURGICAL

BODY SYSTEM: K MUSCLES

OPERATION: 5 **DESTRUCTION:** Physical eradication of all or a portion of a body part by the direct use of energy, force, or a destructive agent

Body Part	Approach	Device	Qualifier
Ø Head Muscle 1 Facial Muscle 2 Neck Muscle, Right 3 Neck Muscle, Left 4 Tongue, Palate, Pharynx Muscle 5 Shoulder Muscle, Right 6 Shoulder Muscle, Left 7 Upper Arm Muscle, Right 8 Upper Arm Muscle, Left 9 Lower Arm and Wrist Muscle, Right B Lower Arm and Wrist Muscle, Left C Hand Muscle, Right D Hand Muscle, Left F Trunk Muscle, Right G Trunk Muscle, Left H Thorax Muscle, Right J Thorax Muscle, Left K Abdomen Muscle, Right L Abdomen Muscle, Left M Perineum Muscle N Hip Muscle, Right P Hip Muscle, Left Q Upper Leg Muscle, Right R Upper Leg Muscle, Left S Lower Leg Muscle, Right T Lower Leg Muscle, Left V Foot Muscle, Right W Foot Muscle, Left	Ø Open 3 Percutaneous 4 Percutaneous Endoscopic	Z No Device	Z No Qualifier

SECTION: Ø MEDICAL AND SURGICAL
BODY SYSTEM: K MUSCLES
OPERATION: 8 DIVISION: Cutting into a body part, without draining fluids and/or gases from the body part, in order to separate or transect a body part

Body Part	Approach	Device	Qualifier
Ø Head Muscle 1 Facial Muscle 2 Neck Muscle, Right 3 Neck Muscle, Left 4 Tongue, Palate, Pharynx Muscle 5 Shoulder Muscle, Right 6 Shoulder Muscle, Left 7 Upper Arm Muscle, Right 8 Upper Arm Muscle, Left 9 Lower Arm and Wrist Muscle, Right B Lower Arm and Wrist Muscle, Left C Hand Muscle, Right D Hand Muscle, Left F Trunk Muscle, Right G Trunk Muscle, Left H Thorax Muscle, Right J Thorax Muscle, Left K Abdomen Muscle, Right L Abdomen Muscle, Left M Perineum Muscle N Hip Muscle, Right P Hip Muscle, Left Q Upper Leg Muscle, Right R Upper Leg Muscle, Left S Lower Leg Muscle, Right T Lower Leg Muscle, Left V Foot Muscle, Right W Foot Muscle, Left	Ø Open 3 Percutaneous 4 Percutaneous Endoscopic	Z No Device	Z No Qualifier

SECTION: Ø MEDICAL AND SURGICAL
BODY SYSTEM: K MUSCLES
OPERATION: 9 DRAINAGE: *(on multiple pages)*
Taking or letting out fluids and/or gases from a body part

Body Part	Approach	Device	Qualifier
Ø Head Muscle 1 Facial Muscle 2 Neck Muscle, Right 3 Neck Muscle, Left 4 Tongue, Palate, Pharynx Muscle 5 Shoulder Muscle, Right 6 Shoulder Muscle, Left 7 Upper Arm Muscle, Right 8 Upper Arm Muscle, Left 9 Lower Arm and Wrist Muscle, Right B Lower Arm and Wrist Muscle, Left C Hand Muscle, Right D Hand Muscle, Left F Trunk Muscle, Right G Trunk Muscle, Left H Thorax Muscle, Right J Thorax Muscle, Left K Abdomen Muscle, Right L Abdomen Muscle, Left M Perineum Muscle N Hip Muscle, Right P Hip Muscle, Left Q Upper Leg Muscle, Right R Upper Leg Muscle, Left S Lower Leg Muscle, Right T Lower Leg Muscle, Left V Foot Muscle, Right W Foot Muscle, Left	Ø Open 3 Percutaneous 4 Percutaneous Endoscopic	Ø Drainage Device	Z No Qualifier

Non-OR ØK9[Ø123456789BCDFGHJKLMNPQRSTVW]3ØZ

SECTION: Ø MEDICAL AND SURGICAL
BODY SYSTEM: K MUSCLES
OPERATION: 9 DRAINAGE: *(continued)*
Taking or letting out fluids and/or gases from a body part

Body Part	Approach	Device	Qualifier
Ø Head Muscle	Ø Open	Z No Device	X Diagnostic
1 Facial Muscle	3 Percutaneous		Z No Qualifier
2 Neck Muscle, Right	4 Percutaneous Endoscopic		
3 Neck Muscle, Left			
4 Tongue, Palate, Pharynx Muscle			
5 Shoulder Muscle, Right			
6 Shoulder Muscle, Left			
7 Upper Arm Muscle, Right			
8 Upper Arm Muscle, Left			
9 Lower Arm and Wrist Muscle, Right			
B Lower Arm and Wrist Muscle, Left			
C Hand Muscle, Right			
D Hand Muscle, Left			
F Trunk Muscle, Right			
G Trunk Muscle, Left			
H Thorax Muscle, Right			
J Thorax Muscle, Left			
K Abdomen Muscle, Right			
L Abdomen Muscle, Left			
M Perineum Muscle			
N Hip Muscle, Right			
P Hip Muscle, Left			
Q Upper Leg Muscle, Right			
R Upper Leg Muscle, Left			
S Lower Leg Muscle, Right			
T Lower Leg Muscle, Left			
V Foot Muscle, Right			
W Foot Muscle, Left			

Non-OR   ØK9[Ø123456789BFGHJKLMNPQRSTVW]3ZZ
Non-OR   ØK9[CD][34]ZZ

SECTION: Ø MEDICAL AND SURGICAL

BODY SYSTEM: K MUSCLES

OPERATION: B **EXCISION:** Cutting out or off, without replacement, a portion of a body part

Body Part	Approach	Device	Qualifier
Ø Head Muscle 1 Facial Muscle 2 Neck Muscle, Right 3 Neck Muscle, Left 4 Tongue, Palate, Pharynx Muscle 5 Shoulder Muscle, Right 6 Shoulder Muscle, Left 7 Upper Arm Muscle, Right 8 Upper Arm Muscle, Left 9 Lower Arm and Wrist Muscle, Right B Lower Arm and Wrist Muscle, Left C Hand Muscle, Right D Hand Muscle, Left F Trunk Muscle, Right G Trunk Muscle, Left H Thorax Muscle, Right J Thorax Muscle, Left K Abdomen Muscle, Right L Abdomen Muscle, Left M Perineum Muscle N Hip Muscle, Right P Hip Muscle, Left Q Upper Leg Muscle, Right R Upper Leg Muscle, Left S Lower Leg Muscle, Right T Lower Leg Muscle, Left V Foot Muscle, Right W Foot Muscle, Left	Ø Open 3 Percutaneous 4 Percutaneous Endoscopic	Z No Device	X Diagnostic Z No Qualifier

Coding Clinic: 2016, Q3, P20 – ØKB[NP]ØZZ

SECTION: Ø MEDICAL AND SURGICAL

BODY SYSTEM: K MUSCLES

OPERATION: C EXTIRPATION: Taking or cutting out solid matter from a body part

Body Part	Approach	Device	Qualifier
Ø Head Muscle	Ø Open	Z No Device	Z No Qualifier
1 Facial Muscle	3 Percutaneous		
2 Neck Muscle, Right	4 Percutaneous Endoscopic		
3 Neck Muscle, Left			
4 Tongue, Palate, Pharynx Muscle			
5 Shoulder Muscle, Right			
6 Shoulder Muscle, Left			
7 Upper Arm Muscle, Right			
8 Upper Arm Muscle, Left			
9 Lower Arm and Wrist Muscle, Right			
B Lower Arm and Wrist Muscle, Left			
C Hand Muscle, Right			
D Hand Muscle, Left			
F Trunk Muscle, Right			
G Trunk Muscle, Left			
H Thorax Muscle, Right			
J Thorax Muscle, Left			
K Abdomen Muscle, Right			
L Abdomen Muscle, Left			
M Perineum Muscle			
N Hip Muscle, Right			
P Hip Muscle, Left			
Q Upper Leg Muscle, Right			
R Upper Leg Muscle, Left			
S Lower Leg Muscle, Right			
T Lower Leg Muscle, Left			
V Foot Muscle, Right			
W Foot Muscle, Left			

C: EXTIRPATION

K: MUSCLES

Ø: M/S

SECTION: Ø MEDICAL AND SURGICAL
BODY SYSTEM: K MUSCLES
OPERATION: D EXTRACTION: Pulling or stripping out or off all or a portion of a body part by the use of force

Body Part	Approach	Device	Qualifier
Ø Head Muscle	Ø Open	Z No Device	Z No Qualifier
1 Facial Muscle			
2 Neck Muscle, Right			
3 Neck Muscle, Left			
4 Tongue, Palate, Pharynx Muscle			
5 Shoulder Muscle, Right			
6 Shoulder Muscle, Left			
7 Upper Arm Muscle, Right			
8 Upper Arm Muscle, Left			
9 Lower Arm and Wrist Muscle, Right			
B Lower Arm and Wrist Muscle, Left			
C Hand Muscle, Right			
D Hand Muscle, Left			
F Trunk Muscle, Right			
G Trunk Muscle, Left			
H Thorax Muscle, Right			
J Thorax Muscle, Left			
K Abdomen Muscle, Right			
L Abdomen Muscle, Left			
M Perineum Muscle			
N Hip Muscle, Right			
P Hip Muscle, Left			
Q Upper Leg Muscle, Right			
R Upper Leg Muscle, Left			
S Lower Leg Muscle, Right			
T Lower Leg Muscle, Left			
V Foot Muscle, Right			
W Foot Muscle, Left			

Coding Clinic: 2Ø17, Q4, P42 – ØKDSØZZ

SECTION: Ø MEDICAL AND SURGICAL
BODY SYSTEM: K MUSCLES
OPERATION: H INSERTION: Putting in a nonbiological appliance that monitors, assists, performs, or prevents a physiological function but does not physically take the place of a body part

Body Part	Approach	Device	Qualifier
X Upper Muscle	Ø Open	M Stimulator Lead	Z No Qualifier
Y Lower Muscle	3 Percutaneous	Y Other Device	
	4 Percutaneous Endoscopic		

SECTION: Ø MEDICAL AND SURGICAL

BODY SYSTEM: K MUSCLES
OPERATION: **J INSPECTION:** Visually and/or manually exploring a body part

Body Part	Approach	Device	Qualifier
X Upper Muscle Y Lower Muscle	Ø Open 3 Percutaneous 4 Percutaneous Endoscopic X External	Z No Device	Z No Qualifier

Non-OR ØKJ[XY][3X]ZZ

SECTION: Ø MEDICAL AND SURGICAL

BODY SYSTEM: K MUSCLES
OPERATION: **M REATTACHMENT:** Putting back in or on all or a portion of a separated body part to its normal location or other suitable location

Body Part	Approach	Device	Qualifier
Ø Head Muscle 1 Facial Muscle 2 Neck Muscle, Right 3 Neck Muscle, Left 4 Tongue, Palate, Pharynx Muscle 5 Shoulder Muscle, Right 6 Shoulder Muscle, Left 7 Upper Arm Muscle, Right 8 Upper Arm Muscle, Left 9 Lower Arm and Wrist Muscle, Right B Lower Arm and Wrist Muscle, Left C Hand Muscle, Right D Hand Muscle, Left F Trunk Muscle, Right G Trunk Muscle, Left H Thorax Muscle, Right J Thorax Muscle, Left K Abdomen Muscle, Right L Abdomen Muscle, Left M Perineum Muscle N Hip Muscle, Right P Hip Muscle, Left Q Upper Leg Muscle, Right R Upper Leg Muscle, Left S Lower Leg Muscle, Right T Lower Leg Muscle, Left V Foot Muscle, Right W Foot Muscle, Left	Ø Open 4 Percutaneous Endoscopic	Z No Device	Z No Qualifier

SECTION: Ø MEDICAL AND SURGICAL

BODY SYSTEM: K MUSCLES

OPERATION: N RELEASE: Freeing a body part from an abnormal physical constraint by cutting or by the use of force

Body Part	Approach	Device	Qualifier
Ø Head Muscle 1 Facial Muscle 2 Neck Muscle, Right 3 Neck Muscle, Left 4 Tongue, Palate, Pharynx Muscle 5 Shoulder Muscle, Right 6 Shoulder Muscle, Left 7 Upper Arm Muscle, Right 8 Upper Arm Muscle, Left 9 Lower Arm and Wrist Muscle, Right B Lower Arm and Wrist Muscle, Left C Hand Muscle, Right D Hand Muscle, Left F Trunk Muscle, Right G Trunk Muscle, Left H Thorax Muscle, Right J Thorax Muscle, Left K Abdomen Muscle, Right L Abdomen Muscle, Left M Perineum Muscle N Hip Muscle, Right P Hip Muscle, Left Q Upper Leg Muscle, Right R Upper Leg Muscle, Lefta S Lower Leg Muscle, Right T Lower Leg Muscle, Left V Foot Muscle, Right W Foot Muscle, Left	Ø Open 3 Percutaneous 4 Percutaneous Endoscopic X External	Z No Device	Z No Qualifier

Non-OR ØKN[Ø123456789BCDFGHJKLMNPQRSTVW]XZZ

Coding Clinic: 2Ø15, Q2, P22 – ØKN84ZZ
Coding Clinic: 2Ø17, Q2, P13 – ØKNVØZZ
Coding Clinic: 2Ø17, Q2, P14 – ØKNTØZZ

SECTION: Ø MEDICAL AND SURGICAL

BODY SYSTEM: K MUSCLES

OPERATION: P REMOVAL: Taking out or off a device from a body part

Body Part	Approach	Device	Qualifier
X Upper Muscle Y Lower Muscle	Ø Open 3 Percutaneous 4 Percutaneous Endoscopic	Ø Drainage Device 7 Autologous Tissue Substitute J Synthetic Substitute K Nonautologous Tissue Substitute M Stimulator Lead Y Other Device	Z No Qualifier
X Upper Muscle Y Lower Muscle	X External	Ø Drainage Device M Stimulator Lead	Z No Qualifier

Non-OR ØKP[XY]X[ØM]Z

New/Revised Text in Green   ~~deleted~~ Deleted   ♀ Females Only   ♂ Males Only   **Coding Clinic**

Non-covered   Limited Coverage   ⊞ Combination (See Appendix E)   DRG Non-OR   Non-OR   Hospital-Acquired Condition

SECTION: Ø MEDICAL AND SURGICAL

BODY SYSTEM: **K MUSCLES**

OPERATION: **Q REPAIR:** Restoring, to the extent possible, a body part to its normal anatomic structure and function

Body Part	Approach	Device	Qualifier
Ø Head Muscle	Ø Open	Z No Device	Z No Qualifier
1 Facial Muscle	3 Percutaneous		
2 Neck Muscle, Right	4 Percutaneous Endoscopic		
3 Neck Muscle, Left			
4 Tongue, Palate, Pharynx Muscle			
5 Shoulder Muscle, Right			
6 Shoulder Muscle, Left			
7 Upper Arm Muscle, Right			
8 Upper Arm Muscle, Left			
9 Lower Arm and Wrist Muscle, Right			
B Lower Arm and Wrist Muscle, Left			
C Hand Muscle, Right			
D Hand Muscle, Left			
F Trunk Muscle, Right			
G Trunk Muscle, Left			
H Thorax Muscle, Right			
J Thorax Muscle, Left			
K Abdomen Muscle, Right			
L Abdomen Muscle, Left			
M Perineum Muscle			
N Hip Muscle, Right			
P Hip Muscle, Left			
Q Upper Leg Muscle, Right			
R Upper Leg Muscle, Left			
S Lower Leg Muscle, Right			
T Lower Leg Muscle, Left			
V Foot Muscle, Right			
W Foot Muscle, Left			

Coding Clinic: 2016, Q2, P35, Q1, P7 – ØKQMØZZ

SECTION: Ø MEDICAL AND SURGICAL
BODY SYSTEM: K MUSCLES
OPERATION: R REPLACEMENT: Putting in or on biological or synthetic material that physically takes the place and/or function of all or a portion of a body part

Body Part	Approach	Device	Qualifier
Ø Head Muscle 1 Facial Muscle 2 Neck Muscle, Right 3 Neck Muscle, Left 4 Tongue, Palate, Pharynx Muscle 5 Shoulder Muscle, Right 6 Shoulder Muscle, Left 7 Upper Arm Muscle, Right 8 Upper Arm Muscle, Left 9 Lower Arm and Wrist Muscle, Right B Lower Arm and Wrist Muscle, Left C Hand Muscle, Right D Hand Muscle, Left F Trunk Muscle, Right G Trunk Muscle, Left H Thorax Muscle, Right J Thorax Muscle, Left K Abdomen Muscle, Right L Abdomen Muscle, Left M Perineum Muscle N Hip Muscle, Right P Hip Muscle, Left Q Upper Leg Muscle, Right R Upper Leg Muscle, Left S Lower Leg Muscle, Right T Lower Leg Muscle, Left V Foot Muscle, Right W Foot Muscle, Left	Ø Open 4 Percutaneous Endoscopic	7 Autologous Tissue Substitute J Synthetic Substitute K Nonautologous Tissue Substitute	Z No Qualifier

SECTION: Ø MEDICAL AND SURGICAL
BODY SYSTEM: K MUSCLES
OPERATION: S REPOSITION: Moving to its normal location, or other suitable location, all or a portion of a body part

Body Part	Approach	Device	Qualifier
Ø Head Muscle	Ø Open	Z No Device	Z No Qualifier
1 Facial Muscle	4 Percutaneous Endoscopic		
2 Neck Muscle, Right			
3 Neck Muscle, Left			
4 Tongue, Palate, Pharynx Muscle			
5 Shoulder Muscle, Right			
6 Shoulder Muscle, Left			
7 Upper Arm Muscle, Right			
8 Upper Arm Muscle, Left			
9 Lower Arm and Wrist Muscle, Right			
B Lower Arm and Wrist Muscle, Left			
C Hand Muscle, Right			
D Hand Muscle, Left			
F Trunk Muscle, Right			
G Trunk Muscle, Left			
H Thorax Muscle, Right			
J Thorax Muscle, Left			
K Abdomen Muscle, Right			
L Abdomen Muscle, Left			
M Perineum Muscle			
N Hip Muscle, Right			
P Hip Muscle, Left			
Q Upper Leg Muscle, Right			
R Upper Leg Muscle, Left			
S Lower Leg Muscle, Right			
T Lower Leg Muscle, Left			
V Foot Muscle, Right			
W Foot Muscle, Left			

S: REPOSITION

K: MUSCLES

Ø: M/S

New/Revised Text in Green   deleted Deleted   ♀ Females Only   ♂ Males Only   **Coding Clinic**
  Non-covered   Limited Coverage   ⊞ Combination (See Appendix E)   DRG Non-OR   Non-OR   Hospital-Acquired Condition

SECTION: Ø MEDICAL AND SURGICAL

BODY SYSTEM: K MUSCLES

OPERATION: T RESECTION: Cutting out or off, without replacement, all of a body part

Body Part	Approach	Device	Qualifier
Ø Head Muscle	Ø Open	Z No Device	Z No Qualifier
1 Facial Muscle	4 Percutaneous Endoscopic		
2 Neck Muscle, Right			
3 Neck Muscle, Left			
4 Tongue, Palate, Pharynx Muscle			
5 Shoulder Muscle, Right			
6 Shoulder Muscle, Left			
7 Upper Arm Muscle, Right			
8 Upper Arm Muscle, Left			
9 Lower Arm and Wrist Muscle, Right			
B Lower Arm and Wrist Muscle, Left			
C Hand Muscle, Right			
D Hand Muscle, Left			
F Trunk Muscle, Right			
G Trunk Muscle, Left			
H Thorax Muscle, Right ⊞			
J Thorax Muscle, Left ⊞			
K Abdomen Muscle, Right			
L Abdomen Muscle, Left			
M Perineum Muscle			
N Hip Muscle, Right			
P Hip Muscle, Left			
Q Upper Leg Muscle, Right			
R Upper Leg Muscle, Left			
S Lower Leg Muscle, Right			
T Lower Leg Muscle, Left			
V Foot Muscle, Right			
W Foot Muscle, Left			

⊞ ØKT[HJ]ØZZ

Coding Clinic: 2015, Q1, P38 – ØKTMØZZ
Coding Clinic: 2016, Q2, P13 – ØKT3ØZZ

Ø: M/S

K: MUSCLES

T: RESECTION

SECTION: Ø MEDICAL AND SURGICAL

BODY SYSTEM: K MUSCLES

OPERATION: **U SUPPLEMENT:** Putting in or on biological or synthetic material that physically reinforces and/or augments the function of a portion of a body part

Body Part	Approach	Device	Qualifier
Ø Head Muscle 1 Facial Muscle 2 Neck Muscle, Right 3 Neck Muscle, Left 4 Tongue, Palate, Pharynx Muscle 5 Shoulder Muscle, Right 6 Shoulder Muscle, Left 7 Upper Arm Muscle, Right 8 Upper Arm Muscle, Left 9 Lower Arm and Wrist Muscle, Right B Lower Arm and Wrist Muscle, Left C Hand Muscle, Right D Hand Muscle, Left F Trunk Muscle, Right G Trunk Muscle, Left H Thorax Muscle, Right J Thorax Muscle, Left K Abdomen Muscle, Right L Abdomen Muscle, Left M Perineum Muscle N Hip Muscle, Right P Hip Muscle, Left Q Upper Leg Muscle, Right R Upper Leg Muscle, Left S Lower Leg Muscle, Right T Lower Leg Muscle, Left V Foot Muscle, Right W Foot Muscle, Left	Ø Open 4 Percutaneous Endoscopic	7 Autologous Tissue Substitute J Synthetic Substitute K Nonautologous Tissue Substitute	Z No Qualifier

SECTION: Ø MEDICAL AND SURGICAL

BODY SYSTEM: K MUSCLES

OPERATION: **W REVISION:** Correcting, to the extent possible, a portion of a malfunctioning device or the position of a displaced device

Body Part	Approach	Device	Qualifier
X Upper Muscle Y Lower Muscle	Ø Open 3 Percutaneous 4 Percutaneous Endoscopic	Ø Drainage Device 7 Autologous Tissue Substitute J Synthetic Substitute K Nonautologous Tissue Substitute M Stimulator Lead Y Other device	Z No Qualifier
X Upper Muscle Y Lower Muscle	X External	Ø Drainage Device 7 Autologous Tissue Substitute J Synthetic Substitute K Nonautologous Tissue Substitute M Stimulator Lead	Z No Qualifier

Non-OR   ØKW[XY]X[Ø7JKM]Z

New/Revised Text in Green   ~~deleted~~ Deleted   ♀ Females Only   ♂ Males Only   **Coding Clinic**

⬡ Non-covered   ⬡ Limited Coverage   ⊡ Combination (See Appendix E)   DRG Non-OR   Non-OR   ⬡ Hospital-Acquired Condition

SECTION: Ø MEDICAL AND SURGICAL
BODY SYSTEM: K MUSCLES
OPERATION: X TRANSFER: Moving, without taking out, all or a portion of a body part to another location to take over the function of all or a portion of a body part

Body Part	Approach	Device	Qualifier
Ø Head Muscle 1 Facial Muscle 2 Neck Muscle, Right 3 Neck Muscle, Left 4 Tongue, Palate, Pharynx Muscle 5 Shoulder Muscle, Right 6 Shoulder Muscle, Left 7 Upper Arm Muscle, Right 8 Upper Arm Muscle, Left 9 Lower Arm and Wrist Muscle, Right B Lower Arm and Wrist Muscle, Left C Hand Muscle, Right D Hand Muscle, Left H Thorax Muscle, Right J Thorax Muscle, Left M Perineum Muscle N Hip Muscle, Right P Hip Muscle, Left Q Upper Leg Muscle, Right R Upper Leg Muscle, Left S Lower Leg Muscle, Right T Lower Leg Muscle, Left V Foot Muscle, Right W Foot Muscle, Left	Ø Open 4 Percutaneous Endoscopic	Z No Device	Ø Skin 1 Subcutaneous Tissue 2 Skin and Subcutaneous Tissue Z No Qualifier
F Trunk Muscle, Right G Trunk Muscle, Left	Ø Open 4 Percutaneous Endoscopic	Z No Device	Ø Skin 1 Subcutaneous Tissue 2 Skin and Subcutaneous Tissue 5 Latissimus Dorsi Myocutaneous Flap 7 Deep Inferior Epigastric Artery Perforator Flap 8 Superficial Inferior Epigastric Artery Flap 9 Gluteal Artery Perforator Flap Z No Qualifier
K Abdomen Muscle, Right L Abdomen Muscle, Left	Ø Open 4 Percutaneous Endoscopic	Z No Device	Ø Skin 1 Subcutaneous Tissue 2 Skin and Subcutaneous Tissue 6 Transverse Rectus Abdominis Myocutaneous Flap Z No Qualifier

Coding Clinic: 2015, Q2, P26 – ØKX4ØZ2
Coding Clinic: 2015, Q3, P33 – ØKX1ØZ2
Coding Clinic: 2016, Q3, P30-31 – ØKX[QR]ØZZ
Coding Clinic: 2017, Q4, P67 – ØKXFØZ5

Ø: M/S

K: MUSCLES

X: TRANSFER

New/Revised Text in Green   ~~deleted~~ Deleted   ♀ Females Only   ♂ Males Only   **Coding Clinic**

Non-covered   Limited Coverage   ⊞ Combination (See Appendix E)   DRG Non-OR   Non-OR   Hospital-Acquired Condition

SECTION: Ø MEDICAL AND SURGICAL

BODY SYSTEM: L TENDONS

OPERATION: 2 **CHANGE:** Taking out or off a device from a body part and putting back an identical or similar device in or on the same body part without cutting or puncturing the skin or a mucous membrane

Body Part	Approach	Device	Qualifier
X Upper Tendon Y Lower Tendon	X External	Ø Drainage Device Y Other Device	Z No Qualifier

Non-OR All Values

SECTION: Ø MEDICAL AND SURGICAL

BODY SYSTEM: L TENDONS

OPERATION: 5 **DESTRUCTION:** Physical eradication of all or a portion of a body part by the direct use of energy, force, or a destructive agent

Body Part	Approach	Device	Qualifier
Ø Head and Neck Tendon 1 Shoulder Tendon, Right 2 Shoulder Tendon, Left 3 Upper Arm Tendon, Right 4 Upper Arm Tendon, Left 5 Lower Arm and Wrist Tendon, Right 6 Lower Arm and Wrist Tendon, Left 7 Hand Tendon, Right 8 Hand Tendon, Left 9 Trunk Tendon, Right B Trunk Tendon, Left C Thorax Tendon, Right D Thorax Tendon, Left F Abdomen Tendon, Right G Abdomen Tendon, Left H Perineum Tendon J Hip Tendon, Right K Hip Tendon, Left L Upper Leg Tendon, Right M Upper Leg Tendon, Left N Lower Leg Tendon, Right P Lower Leg Tendon, Left Q Knee Tendon, Right R Knee Tendon, Left S Ankle Tendon, Right T Ankle Tendon, Left V Foot Tendon, Right W Foot Tendon, Left	Ø Open 3 Percutaneous 4 Percutaneous Endoscopic	Z No Device	Z No Qualifier

New/Revised Text in Green deleted Deleted ♀ Females Only ♂ Males Only **Coding Clinic**
⬚ Non-covered ⬚ Limited Coverage ⊞ Combination (See Appendix E) DRG Non-OR Non-OR ⬚ Hospital-Acquired Condition

341

SECTION: Ø MEDICAL AND SURGICAL
BODY SYSTEM: L TENDONS
OPERATION: 8 DIVISION: Cutting into a body part, without draining fluids and/or gases from the body part, in order to separate or transect a body part

Body Part	Approach	Device	Qualifier
Ø Head and Neck Tendon 1 Shoulder Tendon, Right 2 Shoulder Tendon, Left 3 Upper Arm Tendon, Right 4 Upper Arm Tendon, Left 5 Lower Arm and Wrist Tendon, Right 6 Lower Arm and Wrist Tendon, Left 7 Hand Tendon, Right 8 Hand Tendon, Left 9 Trunk Tendon, Right B Trunk Tendon, Left C Thorax Tendon, Right D Thorax Tendon, Left F Abdomen Tendon, Right G Abdomen Tendon, Left H Perineum Tendon J Hip Tendon, Right K Hip Tendon, Left L Upper Leg Tendon, Right M Upper Leg Tendon, Left N Lower Leg Tendon, Right P Lower Leg Tendon, Left Q Knee Tendon, Right R Knee Tendon, Left S Ankle Tendon, Right T Ankle Tendon, Left V Foot Tendon, Right W Foot Tendon, Left	Ø Open 3 Percutaneous 4 Percutaneous Endoscopic	Z No Device	Z No Qualifier

Coding Clinic: 2Ø16, Q3, P31 – ØL8JØZZ

New/Revised Text in Green deleted Deleted ♀ Females Only ♂ Males Only **Coding Clinic**
Non-covered Limited Coverage Combination (See Appendix E) DRG Non-OR Non-OR Hospital-Acquired Condition

SECTION: Ø MEDICAL AND SURGICAL

BODY SYSTEM: L TENDONS

OPERATION: 9 DRAINAGE: Taking or letting out fluids and/or gases from a body part

Body Part	Approach	Device	Qualifier
Ø Head and Neck Tendon 1 Shoulder Tendon, Right 2 Shoulder Tendon, Left 3 Upper Arm Tendon, Right 4 Upper Arm Tendon, Left 5 Lower Arm and Wrist Tendon, Right 6 Lower Arm and Wrist Tendon, Left 7 Hand Tendon, Right 8 Hand Tendon, Left 9 Trunk Tendon, Right B Trunk Tendon, Left C Thorax Tendon, Right D Thorax Tendon, Left F Abdomen Tendon, Right G Abdomen Tendon, Left H Perineum Tendon J Hip Tendon, Right K Hip Tendon, Left L Upper Leg Tendon, Right M Upper Leg Tendon, Left N Lower Leg Tendon, Right P Lower Leg Tendon, Left Q Knee Tendon, Right R Knee Tendon, Left S Ankle Tendon, Right T Ankle Tendon, Left V Foot Tendon, Right W Foot Tendon, Left	Ø Open 3 Percutaneous 4 Percutaneous Endoscopic	Ø Drainage Device	Z No Qualifier
Ø Head and Neck Tendon 1 Shoulder Tendon, Right 2 Shoulder Tendon, Left 3 Upper Arm Tendon, Right 4 Upper Arm Tendon, Left 5 Lower Arm and Wrist Tendon, Right 6 Lower Arm and Wrist Tendon, Left 7 Hand Tendon, Right 8 Hand Tendon, Left 9 Trunk Tendon, Right B Trunk Tendon, Left C Thorax Tendon, Right D Thorax Tendon, Left F Abdomen Tendon, Right G Abdomen Tendon, Left H Perineum Tendon J Hip Tendon, Right K Hip Tendon, Left L Upper Leg Tendon, Right M Upper Leg Tendon, Left N Lower Leg Tendon, Right P Lower Leg Tendon, Left Q Knee Tendon, Right R Knee Tendon, Left S Ankle Tendon, Right T Ankle Tendon, Left V Foot Tendon, Right W Foot Tendon, Left	Ø Open 3 Percutaneous 4 Percutaneous Endoscopic	Z No Device	X Diagnostic Z No Qualifier

Non-OR ØL9[Ø123456789BCDFGHJKLMNPQRSTVW]3ØZ   Non-OR ØL9[78][34]ZZ

Non-OR ØL9[Ø1234569BCDFGHJKLMNPQRSTVW]3ZZ

New/Revised Text in Green   ~~deleted~~ Deleted   ♀ Females Only   ♂ Males Only   **Coding Clinic**

⊘ Non-covered   ⊘ Limited Coverage   ⊞ Combination (See Appendix E)   DRG Non-OR   Non-OR   ⊘ Hospital-Acquired Condition

SECTION: Ø MEDICAL AND SURGICAL
BODY SYSTEM: L TENDONS
OPERATION: B EXCISION: Cutting out or off, without replacement, a portion of a body part

Body Part	Approach	Device	Qualifier
Ø Head and Neck Tendon	Ø Open	Z No Device	X Diagnostic
1 Shoulder Tendon, Right	3 Percutaneous		Z No Qualifier
2 Shoulder Tendon, Left	4 Percutaneous Endoscopic		
3 Upper Arm Tendon, Right			
4 Upper Arm Tendon, Left			
5 Lower Arm and Wrist Tendon, Right			
6 Lower Arm and Wrist Tendon, Left			
7 Hand Tendon, Right			
8 Hand Tendon, Left			
9 Trunk Tendon, Right			
B Trunk Tendon, Left			
C Thorax Tendon, Right			
D Thorax Tendon, Left			
F Abdomen Tendon, Right			
G Abdomen Tendon, Left			
H Perineum Tendon			
J Hip Tendon, Right			
K Hip Tendon, Left			
L Upper Leg Tendon, Right			
M Upper Leg Tendon, Left			
N Lower Leg Tendon, Right			
P Lower Leg Tendon, Left			
Q Knee Tendon, Right			
R Knee Tendon, Left			
S Ankle Tendon, Right			
T Ankle Tendon, Left			
V Foot Tendon, Right			
W Foot Tendon, Left			

Coding Clinic: 2015, Q3, P27 – ØLB60ZZ
Coding Clinic: 2017, Q2, P22 – ØLBLØZZ

B: EXCISION   L: TENDONS   Ø: M/S

SECTION: Ø MEDICAL AND SURGICAL

BODY SYSTEM: L TENDONS

OPERATION: C EXTIRPATION: Taking or cutting out solid matter from a body part

Body Part	Approach	Device	Qualifier
Ø Head and Neck Tendon	Ø Open	Z No Device	Z No Qualifier
1 Shoulder Tendon, Right	3 Percutaneous		
2 Shoulder Tendon, Left	4 Percutaneous Endoscopic		
3 Upper Arm Tendon, Right			
4 Upper Arm Tendon, Left			
5 Lower Arm and Wrist Tendon, Right			
6 Lower Arm and Wrist Tendon, Left			
7 Hand Tendon, Right			
8 Hand Tendon, Left			
9 Trunk Tendon, Right			
B Trunk Tendon, Left			
C Thorax Tendon, Right			
D Thorax Tendon, Left			
F Abdomen Tendon, Right			
G Abdomen Tendon, Left			
H Perineum Tendon			
J Hip Tendon, Right			
K Hip Tendon, Left			
L Upper Leg Tendon, Right			
M Upper Leg Tendon, Left			
N Lower Leg Tendon, Right			
P Lower Leg Tendon, Left			
Q Knee Tendon, Right			
R Knee Tendon, Left			
S Ankle Tendon, Right			
T Ankle Tendon, Left			
V Foot Tendon, Right			
W Foot Tendon, Left			

New/Revised Text in Green   deleted Deleted   ♀ Females Only   ♂ Males Only   **Coding Clinic**
🚫 Non-covered   🚫 Limited Coverage   ⊞ Combination (See Appendix E)   DRG Non-OR   Non-OR   🚫 Hospital-Acquired Condition

345

SECTION: Ø MEDICAL AND SURGICAL
BODY SYSTEM: L TENDONS

OPERATION: **D EXTRACTION:** Pulling or stripping out or off all or a portion of a body part by the use of force

Body Part	Approach	Device	Qualifier
Ø Head and Neck Tendon 1 Shoulder Tendon, Right 2 Shoulder Tendon, Left 3 Upper Arm Tendon, Right 4 Upper Arm Tendon, Left 5 Lower Arm and Wrist Tendon, Right 6 Lower Arm and Wrist Tendon, Left 7 Hand Tendon, Right 8 Hand Tendon, Left 9 Trunk Tendon, Right B Trunk Tendon, Left C Thorax Tendon, Right D Thorax Tendon, Left F Abdomen Tendon, Right G Abdomen Tendon, Left H Perineum Tendon J Hip Tendon, Right K Hip Tendon, Left L Upper Leg Tendon, Right M Upper Leg Tendon, Left N Lower Leg Tendon, Right P Lower Leg Tendon, Left Q Knee Tendon, Right R Knee Tendon, Left S Ankle Tendon, Right T Ankle Tendon, Left V Foot Tendon, Right W Foot Tendon, Left	Ø Open	Z No Device	Z No Qualifier

SECTION: Ø MEDICAL AND SURGICAL
BODY SYSTEM: L TENDONS

OPERATION: **H INSERTION:** Putting in a nonbiological appliance that monitors, assists, performs, or prevents a physiological function but does not physically take the place of a body part

Body Part	Approach	Device	Qualifier
X Upper Tendon Y Lower Tendon	Ø Open 3 Percutaneous 4 Percutaneous Endoscopic	Y Other Device	Z No Qualifier

D: EXTRACTION   H: INSERTION

L: TENDONS

Ø: M/S

SECTION: Ø MEDICAL AND SURGICAL

BODY SYSTEM: L TENDONS

OPERATION: J INSPECTION: Visually and/or manually exploring a body part

Body Part	Approach	Device	Qualifier
X Upper Tendon Y Lower Tendon	Ø Open 3 Percutaneous 4 Percutaneous Endoscopic X External	Z No Device	Z No Qualifier

Non-OR ØLJ[XY][3X]ZZ

SECTION: Ø MEDICAL AND SURGICAL

BODY SYSTEM: L TENDONS

OPERATION: M REATTACHMENT: Putting back in or on all or a portion of a separated body part to its normal location or other suitable location

Body Part	Approach	Device	Qualifier
Ø Head and Neck Tendon 1 Shoulder Tendon, Right 2 Shoulder Tendon, Left 3 Upper Arm Tendon, Right 4 Upper Arm Tendon, Left 5 Lower Arm and Wrist Tendon, Right 6 Lower Arm and Wrist Tendon, Left 7 Hand Tendon, Right 8 Hand Tendon, Left 9 Trunk Tendon, Right B Trunk Tendon, Left C Thorax Tendon, Right D Thorax Tendon, Left F Abdomen Tendon, Right G Abdomen Tendon, Left H Perineum Tendon J Hip Tendon, Right K Hip Tendon, Left L Upper Leg Tendon, Right M Upper Leg Tendon, Left N Lower Leg Tendon, Right P Lower Leg Tendon, Left Q Knee Tendon, Right R Knee Tendon, Left S Ankle Tendon, Right T Ankle Tendon, Left V Foot Tendon, Right W Foot Tendon, Left	Ø Open 4 Percutaneous Endoscopic	Z No Device	Z No Qualifier

SECTION: Ø MEDICAL AND SURGICAL

BODY SYSTEM: L TENDONS

OPERATION: N RELEASE: Freeing a body part from an abnormal physical constraint by cutting or by the use of force

Body Part	Approach	Device	Qualifier
Ø Head and Neck Tendon 1 Shoulder Tendon, Right 2 Shoulder Tendon, Left 3 Upper Arm Tendon, Right 4 Upper Arm Tendon, Left 5 Lower Arm and Wrist Tendon, Right 6 Lower Arm and Wrist Tendon, Left 7 Hand Tendon, Right 8 Hand Tendon, Left 9 Trunk Tendon, Right B Trunk Tendon, Left C Thorax Tendon, Right D Thorax Tendon, Left F Abdomen Tendon, Right G Abdomen Tendon, Left H Perineum Tendon J Hip Tendon, Right K Hip Tendon, Left L Upper Leg Tendon, Right M Upper Leg Tendon, Left N Lower Leg Tendon, Right P Lower Leg Tendon, Left Q Knee Tendon, Right R Knee Tendon, Left S Ankle Tendon, Right T Ankle Tendon, Left V Foot Tendon, Right W Foot Tendon, Left	Ø Open 3 Percutaneous 4 Percutaneous Endoscopic X External	Z No Device	Z No Qualifier

Non-OR ØLN[Ø123456789BCDFGHJKLMNPQRSTVW]XZZ

SECTION: Ø MEDICAL AND SURGICAL

BODY SYSTEM: L TENDONS

OPERATION: P REMOVAL: Taking out or off a device from a body part

Body Part	Approach	Device	Qualifier
X Upper Tendon Y Lower Tendon	Ø Open 3 Percutaneous 4 Percutaneous Endoscopic	Ø Drainage Device 7 Autologous Tissue Substitute J Synthetic Substitute K Nonautologous Tissue Substitute Y Other Device	Z No Qualifier
X Upper Tendon Y Lower Tendon	X External	Ø Drainage Device	Z No Qualifier

Non-OR ØLP[XY]3ØZ
Non-OR ØLP[XY]XØZ

New/Revised Text in Green   ~~deleted~~ Deleted   ♀ Females Only   ♂ Males Only   **Coding Clinic**

Non-covered   Limited Coverage   ⊞ Combination (See Appendix E)   DRG Non-OR   Non-OR   Hospital-Acquired Condition

SECTION: Ø MEDICAL AND SURGICAL

BODY SYSTEM: L TENDONS

OPERATION: Q REPAIR: Restoring, to the extent possible, a body part to its normal anatomic structure and function

Body Part	Approach	Device	Qualifier
Ø Head and Neck Tendon	Ø Open	Z No Device	Z No Qualifier
1 Shoulder Tendon, Right	3 Percutaneous		
2 Shoulder Tendon, Left	4 Percutaneous Endoscopic		
3 Upper Arm Tendon, Right			
4 Upper Arm Tendon, Left			
5 Lower Arm and Wrist Tendon, Right			
6 Lower Arm and Wrist Tendon, Left			
7 Hand Tendon, Right			
8 Hand Tendon, Left			
9 Trunk Tendon, Right			
B Trunk Tendon, Left			
C Thorax Tendon, Right			
D Thorax Tendon, Left			
F Abdomen Tendon, Right			
G Abdomen Tendon, Left			
H Perineum Tendon			
J Hip Tendon, Right			
K Hip Tendon, Left			
L Upper Leg Tendon, Right			
M Upper Leg Tendon, Left			
N Lower Leg Tendon, Right			
P Lower Leg Tendon, Left			
Q Knee Tendon, Right			
R Knee Tendon, Left			
S Ankle Tendon, Right			
T Ankle Tendon, Left			
V Foot Tendon, Right			
W Foot Tendon, Left			

Coding Clinic: 2013, Q3, P21 – ØLQ14ZZ
Coding Clinic: 2016, Q3, P33 – ØLQ14ZZ

Ø: M/S

L: TENDONS

Q: REPAIR

SECTION: Ø MEDICAL AND SURGICAL
BODY SYSTEM: L TENDONS
OPERATION: R **REPLACEMENT:** Putting in or on biological or synthetic material that physically takes the place and/or function of all or a portion of a body part

Body Part	Approach	Device	Qualifier
Ø Head and Neck Tendon	Ø Open	7 Autologous Tissue Substitute	Z No Qualifier
1 Shoulder Tendon, Right	4 Percutaneous Endoscopic	J Synthetic Substitute	
2 Shoulder Tendon, Left		K Nonautologous Tissue Substitute	
3 Upper Arm Tendon, Right			
4 Upper Arm Tendon, Left			
5 Lower Arm and Wrist Tendon, Right			
6 Lower Arm and Wrist Tendon, Left			
7 Hand Tendon, Right			
8 Hand Tendon, Left			
9 Trunk Tendon, Right			
B Trunk Tendon, Left			
C Thorax Tendon, Right			
D Thorax Tendon, Left			
F Abdomen Tendon, Right			
G Abdomen Tendon, Left			
H Perineum Tendon			
J Hip Tendon, Right			
K Hip Tendon, Left			
L Upper Leg Tendon, Right			
M Upper Leg Tendon, Left			
N Lower Leg Tendon, Right			
P Lower Leg Tendon, Left			
Q Knee Tendon, Right			
R Knee Tendon, Left			
S Ankle Tendon, Right			
T Ankle Tendon, Left			
V Foot Tendon, Right			
W Foot Tendon, Left			

New/Revised Text in Green ~~deleted~~ Deleted ♀ Females Only ♂ Males Only **Coding Clinic**
Non-covered Limited Coverage Combination (See Appendix E) DRG Non-OR Non-OR Hospital-Acquired Condition

SECTION: Ø MEDICAL AND SURGICAL

BODY SYSTEM: L TENDONS

OPERATION: S REPOSITION: Moving to its normal location, or other suitable location, all or a portion of a body part

Body Part	Approach	Device	Qualifier
Ø Head and Neck Tendon	Ø Open	Z No Device	Z No Qualifier
1 Shoulder Tendon, Right	4 Percutaneous Endoscopic		
2 Shoulder Tendon, Left			
3 Upper Arm Tendon, Right			
4 Upper Arm Tendon, Left			
5 Lower Arm and Wrist Tendon, Right			
6 Lower Arm and Wrist Tendon, Left			
7 Hand Tendon, Right			
8 Hand Tendon, Left			
9 Trunk Tendon, Right			
B Trunk Tendon, Left			
C Thorax Tendon, Right			
D Thorax Tendon, Left			
F Abdomen Tendon, Right			
G Abdomen Tendon, Left			
H Perineum Tendon			
J Hip Tendon, Right			
K Hip Tendon, Left			
L Upper Leg Tendon, Right			
M Upper Leg Tendon, Left			
N Lower Leg Tendon, Right			
P Lower Leg Tendon, Left			
Q Knee Tendon, Right			
R Knee Tendon, Left			
S Ankle Tendon, Right			
T Ankle Tendon, Left			
V Foot Tendon, Right			
W Foot Tendon, Left			

Coding Clinic: 2015, Q3, P15 – ØLS40ZZ
Coding Clinic: 2016, Q3, P33 – ØLS30ZZ

Ø: M/S

L: TENDONS

S: REPOSITION

SECTION: Ø MEDICAL AND SURGICAL
BODY SYSTEM: L TENDONS
OPERATION: T RESECTION: Cutting out or off, without replacement, all of a body part

Body Part	Approach	Device	Qualifier
Ø Head and Neck Tendon	Ø Open	Z No Device	Z No Qualifier
1 Shoulder Tendon, Right	4 Percutaneous Endoscopic		
2 Shoulder Tendon, Left			
3 Upper Arm Tendon, Right			
4 Upper Arm Tendon, Left			
5 Lower Arm and Wrist Tendon, Right			
6 Lower Arm and Wrist Tendon, Left			
7 Hand Tendon, Right			
8 Hand Tendon, Left			
9 Trunk Tendon, Right			
B Trunk Tendon, Left			
C Thorax Tendon, Right			
D Thorax Tendon, Left			
F Abdomen Tendon, Right			
G Abdomen Tendon, Left			
H Perineum Tendon			
J Hip Tendon, Right			
K Hip Tendon, Left			
L Upper Leg Tendon, Right			
M Upper Leg Tendon, Left			
N Lower Leg Tendon, Right			
P Lower Leg Tendon, Left			
Q Knee Tendon, Right			
R Knee Tendon, Left			
S Ankle Tendon, Right			
T Ankle Tendon, Left			
V Foot Tendon, Right			
W Foot Tendon, Left			

T: RESECTION

L: TENDONS

Ø: M/S

New/Revised Text in Green   ~~deleted~~ Deleted   ♀ Females Only   ♂ Males Only   **Coding Clinic**

Non-covered   Limited Coverage   ⊞ Combination (See Appendix E)   DRG Non-OR   Non-OR   Hospital-Acquired Condition

SECTION: Ø MEDICAL AND SURGICAL
BODY SYSTEM: L TENDONS
OPERATION: U SUPPLEMENT: Putting in or on biological or synthetic material that physically reinforces and/or augments the function of a portion of a body part

Body Part	Approach	Device	Qualifier
Ø Head and Neck Tendon 1 Shoulder Tendon, Right 2 Shoulder Tendon, Left 3 Upper Arm Tendon, Right 4 Upper Arm Tendon, Left 5 Lower Arm and Wrist Tendon, Right 6 Lower Arm and Wrist Tendon, Left 7 Hand Tendon, Right 8 Hand Tendon, Left 9 Trunk Tendon, Right B Trunk Tendon, Left C Thorax Tendon, Right D Thorax Tendon, Left F Abdomen Tendon, Right G Abdomen Tendon, Left H Perineum Tendon J Hip Tendon, Right K Hip Tendon, Left L Upper Leg Tendon, Right M Upper Leg Tendon, Left N Lower Leg Tendon, Right P Lower Leg Tendon, Left Q Knee Tendon, Right R Knee Tendon, Left S Ankle Tendon, Right T Ankle Tendon, Left V Foot Tendon, Right W Foot Tendon, Left	Ø Open 4 Percutaneous Endoscopic	7 Autologous Tissue Substitute J Synthetic Substitute K Nonautologous Tissue Substitute	Z No Qualifier

Coding Clinic: 2Ø15, Q2, P11 – ØLU[QM]ØKZ

SECTION: Ø MEDICAL AND SURGICAL
BODY SYSTEM: L TENDONS
OPERATION: W REVISION: Correcting, to the extent possible, a portion of a malfunctioning device or the position of a displaced device

Body Part	Approach	Device	Qualifier
X Upper Tendon Y Lower Tendon	Ø Open 3 Percutaneous 4 Percutaneous Endoscopic	Ø Drainage Device 7 Autologous Tissue Substitute J Synthetic Substitute K Nonautologous Tissue Substitute Y Other Device	Z No Qualifier
X Upper Tendon Y Lower Tendon	X External	Ø Drainage Device 7 Autologous Tissue Substitute J Synthetic Substitute K Nonautologous Tissue Substitute	Z No Qualifier

Non-OR ØLW[XY]X[Ø7JK]Z

SECTION: Ø MEDICAL AND SURGICAL

BODY SYSTEM: L TENDONS

OPERATION: X TRANSFER: Moving, without taking out, all or a portion of a body part to another location to take over the function of all or a portion of a body part

Body Part	Approach	Device	Qualifier
Ø Head and Neck Tendon	Ø Open	Z No Device	Z No Qualifier
1 Shoulder Tendon, Right	4 Percutaneous Endoscopic		
2 Shoulder Tendon, Left			
3 Upper Arm Tendon, Right			
4 Upper Arm Tendon, Left			
5 Lower Arm and Wrist Tendon, Right			
6 Lower Arm and Wrist Tendon, Left			
7 Hand Tendon, Right			
8 Hand Tendon, Left			
9 Trunk Tendon, Right			
B Trunk Tendon, Left			
C Thorax Tendon, Right			
D Thorax Tendon, Left			
F Abdomen Tendon, Right			
G Abdomen Tendon, Left			
H Perineum Tendon			
J Hip Tendon, Right			
K Hip Tendon, Left			
L Upper Leg Tendon, Right			
M Upper Leg Tendon, Left			
N Lower Leg Tendon, Right			
P Lower Leg Tendon, Left			
Q Knee Tendon, Right			
R Knee Tendon, Left			
S Ankle Tendon, Right			
T Ankle Tendon, Left			
V Foot Tendon, Right			
W Foot Tendon, Left			

X: TRANSFER

L: TENDONS

Ø: M/S

SECTION: Ø MEDICAL AND SURGICAL

BODY SYSTEM: M BURSAE AND LIGAMENTS

OPERATION: 2 **CHANGE:** Taking out or off a device from a body part and putting back an identical or similar device in or on the same body part without cutting or puncturing the skin or a mucous membrane

Body Part	Approach	Device	Qualifier
X Upper Bursa and Ligament Y Lower Bursa and Ligament	X External	Ø Drainage Device Y Other Device	Z No Qualifier

Non-OR   All Values

SECTION: Ø MEDICAL AND SURGICAL

BODY SYSTEM: M BURSAE AND LIGAMENTS

OPERATION: 5 **DESTRUCTION:** Physical eradication of all or a portion of a body part by the direct use of energy, force, or a destructive agent

Body Part	Approach	Device	Qualifier
Ø Head and Neck Bursa and Ligament 1 Shoulder Bursa and Ligament, Right 2 Shoulder Bursa and Ligament, Left 3 Elbow Bursa and Ligament, Right 4 Elbow Bursa and Ligament, Left 5 Wrist Bursa and Ligament, Right 6 Wrist Bursa and Ligament, Left 7 Hand Bursa and Ligament, Right 8 Hand Bursa and Ligament, Left 9 Upper Extremity Bursa and Ligament, Right B Upper Extremity Bursa and Ligament, Left C Upper Spine Bursa and Ligament D Lower Spine Bursa and Ligament F Sternum Bursa and Ligament G Rib(s) Bursa and Ligament H Abdomen Bursa and Ligament, Right J Abdomen Bursa and Ligament, Left K Perineum Bursa and Ligament L Hip Bursa and Ligament, Right M Hip Bursa and Ligament, Left N Knee Bursa and Ligament, Right P Knee Bursa and Ligament, Left Q Ankle Bursa and Ligament, Right R Ankle Bursa and Ligament, Left S Foot Bursa and Ligament, Right T Foot Bursa and Ligament, Left V Lower Extremity Bursa and Ligament, Right W Lower Extremity Bursa and Ligament, Left	Ø Open 3 Percutaneous 4 Percutaneous Endoscopic	Z No Device	Z No Qualifier

SECTION: Ø MEDICAL AND SURGICAL

BODY SYSTEM: M BURSAE AND LIGAMENTS

OPERATION: 8 DIVISION: Cutting into a body part, without draining fluids and/or gases from the body part, in order to separate or transect a body part

Body Part	Approach	Device	Qualifier
Ø Head and Neck Bursa and Ligament 1 Shoulder Bursa and Ligament, Right 2 Shoulder Bursa and Ligament, Left 3 Elbow Bursa and Ligament, Right 4 Elbow Bursa and Ligament, Left 5 Wrist Bursa and Ligament, Right 6 Wrist Bursa and Ligament, Left 7 Hand Bursa and Ligament, Right 8 Hand Bursa and Ligament, Left 9 Upper Extremity Bursa and Ligament, Right B Upper Extremity Bursa and Ligament, Left C Upper Spine Bursa and Ligament D Lower Spine Bursa and Ligament F Sternum Bursa and Ligament G Rib(s) Bursa and Ligament H Abdomen Bursa and Ligament, Right J Abdomen Bursa and Ligament, Left K Perineum Bursa and Ligament L Hip Bursa and Ligament, Right M Hip Bursa and Ligament, Left N Knee Bursa and Ligament, Right P Knee Bursa and Ligament, Left Q Ankle Bursa and Ligament, Right R Ankle Bursa and Ligament, Left S Foot Bursa and Ligament, Right T Foot Bursa and Ligament, Left V Lower Extremity Bursa and Ligament, Right W Lower Extremity Bursa and Ligament, Left	Ø Open 3 Percutaneous 4 Percutaneous Endoscopic	Z No Device	Z No Qualifier

SECTION: Ø MEDICAL AND SURGICAL

BODY SYSTEM: M BURSAE AND LIGAMENTS

OPERATION: 9 DRAINAGE: Taking or letting out fluids and/or gases from a body part

Body Part	Approach	Device	Qualifier
Ø Head and Neck Bursa and Ligament 1 Shoulder Bursa and Ligament, Right 2 Shoulder Bursa and Ligament, Left 3 Elbow Bursa and Ligament, Right 4 Elbow Bursa and Ligament, Left 5 Wrist Bursa and Ligament, Right 6 Wrist Bursa and Ligament, Left 7 Hand Bursa and Ligament, Right 8 Hand Bursa and Ligament, Left 9 Upper Extremity Bursa and Ligament, Right B Upper Extremity Bursa and Ligament, Left C Upper Spine Bursa and Ligament D Lower Spine Bursa and Ligament F Sternum Bursa and Ligament G Rib(s) Bursa and Ligament H Abdomen Bursa and Ligament, Right J Abdomen Bursa and Ligament, Left K Perineum Bursa and Ligament L Hip Bursa and Ligament, Right M Hip Bursa and Ligament, Left N Knee Bursa and Ligament, Right P Knee Bursa and Ligament, Left Q Ankle Bursa and Ligament, Right R Ankle Bursa and Ligament, Left S Foot Bursa and Ligament, Right T Foot Bursa and Ligament, Left V Lower Extremity Bursa and Ligament, Right W Lower Extremity Bursa and Ligament, Left	Ø Open 3 Percutaneous 4 Percutaneous Endoscopic	Ø Drainage Device	Z No Qualifier
Ø Head and Neck Bursa and Ligament 1 Shoulder Bursa and Ligament, Right 2 Shoulder Bursa and Ligament, Left 3 Elbow Bursa and Ligament, Right 4 Elbow Bursa and Ligament, Left 5 Wrist Bursa and Ligament, Right 6 Wrist Bursa and Ligament, Left 7 Hand Bursa and Ligament, Right 8 Hand Bursa and Ligament, Left 9 Upper Extremity Bursa and Ligament, Right B Upper Extremity Bursa and Ligament, Left C Upper Spine Bursa and Ligament D Lower Spine Bursa and Ligament F Sternum Bursa and Ligament G Rib(s) Bursa and Ligament H Abdomen Bursa and Ligament, Right J Abdomen Bursa and Ligament, Left K Perineum Bursa and Ligament L Hip Bursa and Ligament, Right M Hip Bursa and Ligament, Left N Knee Bursa and Ligament, Right P Knee Bursa and Ligament, Left Q Ankle Bursa and Ligament, Right R Ankle Bursa and Ligament, Left S Foot Bursa and Ligament, Right T Foot Bursa and Ligament, Left V Lower Extremity Bursa and Ligament, Right W Lower Extremity Bursa and Ligament, Left	Ø Open 3 Percutaneous 4 Percutaneous Endoscopic	Z No Device	X Diagnostic Z No Qualifier

Non-OR ØM9[1234789BCDFGHJKLMVW][34]ØZ

Non-OR ØM9[Ø56NPQRST]3ØZ

Non-OR ØM9[Ø12345678CDFGLMNPQRST][Ø34]ZX

Non-OR ØM9[Ø56789BCDFGHJKNPQRSTVW][34]ZZ

Non-OR ØM9[1234LM]3ZZ

New/Revised Text in Green ~~deleted~~ Deleted ♀ Females Only ♂ Males Only **Coding Clinic**

Non-covered Limited Coverage ⊞ Combination (See Appendix E) DRG Non-OR Non-OR Hospital-Acquired Condition

SECTION: Ø MEDICAL AND SURGICAL

BODY SYSTEM: M BURSAE AND LIGAMENTS

OPERATION: B EXCISION: Cutting out or off, without replacement, a portion of a body part

Body Part	Approach	Device	Qualifier
Ø Head and Neck Bursa and Ligament	Ø Open	Z No Device	X Diagnostic
1 Shoulder Bursa and Ligament, Right	3 Percutaneous		Z No Qualifier
2 Shoulder Bursa and Ligament, Left	4 Percutaneous Endoscopic		
3 Elbow Bursa and Ligament, Right			
4 Elbow Bursa and Ligament, Left			
5 Wrist Bursa and Ligament, Right			
6 Wrist Bursa and Ligament, Left			
7 Hand Bursa and Ligament, Right			
8 Hand Bursa and Ligament, Left			
9 Upper Extremity Bursa and Ligament, Right			
B Upper Extremity Bursa and Ligament, Left			
C Upper Spine Bursa and Ligament			
D Lower Spine Bursa and Ligament			
F Sternum Bursa and Ligament			
G Rib(s) Bursa and Ligament			
H Abdomen Bursa and Ligament, Right			
J Abdomen Bursa and Ligament, Left			
K Perineum Bursa and Ligament			
L Hip Bursa and Ligament, Right			
M Hip Bursa and Ligament, Left			
N Knee Bursa and Ligament, Right			
P Knee Bursa and Ligament, Left			
Q Ankle Bursa and Ligament, Right			
R Ankle Bursa and Ligament, Left			
S Foot Bursa and Ligament, Right			
T Foot Bursa and Ligament, Left			
V Lower Extremity Bursa and Ligament, Right			
W Lower Extremity Bursa and Ligament, Left			

Non-OR ØMB[Ø12345678BCDFGLMNPQRST][Ø34]ZX
Non-OR ØMB94ZX

SECTION: Ø MEDICAL AND SURGICAL
BODY SYSTEM: M BURSAE AND LIGAMENTS
OPERATION: C EXTIRPATION: Taking or cutting out solid matter from a body part

Body Part	Approach	Device	Qualifier
Ø Head and Neck Bursa and Ligament	Ø Open	Z No Device	Z No Qualifier
1 Shoulder Bursa and Ligament, Right	3 Percutaneous		
2 Shoulder Bursa and Ligament, Left	4 Percutaneous Endoscopic		
3 Elbow Bursa and Ligament, Right			
4 Elbow Bursa and Ligament, Left			
5 Wrist Bursa and Ligament, Right			
6 Wrist Bursa and Ligament, Left			
7 Hand Bursa and Ligament, Right			
8 Hand Bursa and Ligament, Left			
9 Upper Extremity Bursa and Ligament, Right			
B Upper Extremity Bursa and Ligament, Left			
C Upper Spine Bursa and Ligament			
D Lower Spine Bursa and Ligament			
F Sternum Bursa and Ligament			
G Rib(s) Bursa and Ligament			
H Abdomen Bursa and Ligament, Right			
J Abdomen Bursa and Ligament, Left			
K Perineum Bursa and Ligament			
L Hip Bursa and Ligament, Right			
M Hip Bursa and Ligament, Left			
N Knee Bursa and Ligament, Right			
P Knee Bursa and Ligament, Left			
Q Ankle Bursa and Ligament, Right			
R Ankle Bursa and Ligament, Left			
S Foot Bursa and Ligament, Right			
T Foot Bursa and Ligament, Left			
V Lower Extremity Bursa and Ligament, Right			
W Lower Extremity Bursa and Ligament, Left			

C: EXTIRPATION

M: BURSAE AND LIGAMENTS

Ø: M/S

SECTION:　Ø　MEDICAL AND SURGICAL

BODY SYSTEM: M　BURSAE AND LIGAMENTS

OPERATION:　　D　EXTRACTION: Pulling or stripping out or off all or a portion of a body part by the use of force

Body Part	Approach	Device	Qualifier
Ø Head and Neck Bursa and Ligament 1 Shoulder Bursa and Ligament, Right 2 Shoulder Bursa and Ligament, Left 3 Elbow Bursa and Ligament, Right 4 Elbow Bursa and Ligament, Left 5 Wrist Bursa and Ligament, Right 6 Wrist Bursa and Ligament, Left 7 Hand Bursa and Ligament, Right 8 Hand Bursa and Ligament, Left 9 Upper Extremity Bursa and Ligament, Right B Upper Extremity Bursa and Ligament, Left C Upper Spine Bursa and Ligament D Lower Spine Bursa and Ligament F Sternum Bursa and Ligament G Rib(s) Bursa and Ligament H Abdomen Bursa and Ligament, Right J Abdomen Bursa and Ligament, Left K Perineum Bursa and Ligament L Hip Bursa and Ligament, Right M Hip Bursa and Ligament, Left N Knee Bursa and Ligament, Right P Knee Bursa and Ligament, Left Q Ankle Bursa and Ligament, Right R Ankle Bursa and Ligament, Left S Foot Bursa and Ligament, Right T Foot Bursa and Ligament, Left V Lower Extremity Bursa and Ligament, Right W Lower Extremity Bursa and Ligament, Left	Ø Open 3 Percutaneous 4 Percutaneous Endoscopic	Z No Device	Z No Qualifier

SECTION:　Ø　MEDICAL AND SURGICAL

BODY SYSTEM: M　BURSAE AND LIGAMENTS

OPERATION:　　H　INSERTION: Putting in a nonbiological appliance that monitors, assists, performs, or prevents a physiological function but does not physically take the place of a body part

Body Part	Approach	Device	Qualifier
X Upper Bursa and Ligament Y Lower Bursa and Ligament	Ø Open 3 Percutaneous 4 Percutaneous Endoscopic	Y Other Device	Z No Qualifier

SECTION: Ø MEDICAL AND SURGICAL

BODY SYSTEM: M BURSAE AND LIGAMENTS
OPERATION: J INSPECTION: Visually and/or manually exploring a body part

Body Part	Approach	Device	Qualifier
X Upper Bursa and Ligament Y Lower Bursa and Ligament	Ø Open 3 Percutaneous 4 Percutaneous Endoscopic X External	Z No Device	Z No Qualifier

Non-OR ØMJ[XY][3X]ZZ

SECTION: Ø MEDICAL AND SURGICAL

BODY SYSTEM: M BURSAE AND LIGAMENTS
OPERATION: M REATTACHMENT: Putting back in or on all or a portion of a separated
                   body part to its normal location or other suitable location

Body Part	Approach	Device	Qualifier
Ø Head and Neck Bursa and Ligament 1 Shoulder Bursa and Ligament, Right 2 Shoulder Bursa and Ligament, Left 3 Elbow Bursa and Ligament, Right 4 Elbow Bursa and Ligament, Left 5 Wrist Bursa and Ligament, Right 6 Wrist Bursa and Ligament, Left 7 Hand Bursa and Ligament, Right 8 Hand Bursa and Ligament, Left 9 Upper Extremity Bursa and Ligament, Right B Upper Extremity Bursa and Ligament, Left C Upper Spine Bursa and Ligament D Lower Spine Bursa and Ligament F Sternum Bursa and Ligament G Rib(s) Bursa and Ligament H Abdomen Bursa and Ligament, Right J Abdomen Bursa and Ligament, Left K Perineum Bursa and Ligament L Hip Bursa and Ligament, Right M Hip Bursa and Ligament, Left N Knee Bursa and Ligament, Right P Knee Bursa and Ligament, Left Q Ankle Bursa and Ligament, Right R Ankle Bursa and Ligament, Left S Foot Bursa and Ligament, Right T Foot Bursa and Ligament, Left V Lower Extremity Bursa and Ligament, Right W Lower Extremity Bursa and Ligament, Left	Ø Open 4 Percutaneous Endoscopic	Z No Device	Z No Qualifier

Coding Clinic: 2013, Q3, P22 – ØMM14ZZ

SECTION: Ø MEDICAL AND SURGICAL

BODY SYSTEM: M BURSAE AND LIGAMENTS
OPERATION: N RELEASE: Freeing a body part from an abnormal physical constraint by cutting or by the use of force

Body Part	Approach	Device	Qualifier
Ø Head and Neck Bursa and Ligament	Ø Open	Z No Device	Z No Qualifier
1 Shoulder Bursa and Ligament, Right	3 Percutaneous		
2 Shoulder Bursa and Ligament, Left	4 Percutaneous Endoscopic		
3 Elbow Bursa and Ligament, Right	X External		
4 Elbow Bursa and Ligament, Left			
5 Wrist Bursa and Ligament, Right			
6 Wrist Bursa and Ligament, Left			
7 Hand Bursa and Ligament, Right			
8 Hand Bursa and Ligament, Left			
9 Upper Extremity Bursa and Ligament, Right			
B Upper Extremity Bursa and Ligament, Left			
C Upper Spine Bursa and Ligament			
D Lower Spine Bursa and Ligament			
F Sternum Bursa and Ligament			
G Rib(s) Bursa and Ligament			
H Abdomen Bursa and Ligament, Right			
J Abdomen Bursa and Ligament, Left			
K Perineum Bursa and Ligament			
L Hip Bursa and Ligament, Right			
M Hip Bursa and Ligament, Left			
N Knee Bursa and Ligament, Right			
P Knee Bursa and Ligament, Left			
Q Ankle Bursa and Ligament, Right			
R Ankle Bursa and Ligament, Left			
S Foot Bursa and Ligament, Right			
T Foot Bursa and Ligament, Left			
V Lower Extremity Bursa and Ligament, Right			
W Lower Extremity Bursa and Ligament, Left			

Non-OR ØMN[Ø123456789BCDFGHJKLMNPQRSTVW]XZZ

SECTION: Ø MEDICAL AND SURGICAL

BODY SYSTEM: M BURSAE AND LIGAMENTS
OPERATION: P REMOVAL: Taking out or off a device from a body part

Body Part	Approach	Device	Qualifier
X Upper Bursa and Ligament Y Lower Bursa and Ligament	Ø Open 3 Percutaneous 4 Percutaneous Endoscopic	Ø Drainage Device 7 Autologous Tissue Substitute J Synthetic Substitute K Nonautologous Tissue Substitute Y Other Device	Z No Qualifier
X Upper Bursa and Ligament Y Lower Bursa and Ligament	X External	Ø Drainage Device	Z No Qualifier

Non-OR ØMP[XY]3ØZ
Non-OR ØMP[XY]XØZ

New/Revised Text in Green ~~deleted~~ Deleted ♀ Females Only ♂ Males Only **Coding Clinic**
Non-covered Limited Coverage ⊞ Combination (See Appendix E) DRG Non-OR Non-OR Hospital-Acquired Condition

363

SECTION: Ø MEDICAL AND SURGICAL
BODY SYSTEM: M BURSAE AND LIGAMENTS
OPERATION: Q REPAIR: Restoring, to the extent possible, a body part to its normal anatomic structure and function

Body Part	Approach	Device	Qualifier
Ø Head and Neck Bursa and Ligament 1 Shoulder Bursa and Ligament, Right 2 Shoulder Bursa and Ligament, Left 3 Elbow Bursa and Ligament, Right 4 Elbow Bursa and Ligament, Left 5 Wrist Bursa and Ligament, Right 6 Wrist Bursa and Ligament, Left 7 Hand Bursa and Ligament, Right 8 Hand Bursa and Ligament, Left 9 Upper Extremity Bursa and Ligament, Right B Upper Extremity Bursa and Ligament, Left C Upper Spine Bursa and Ligament D Lower Spine Bursa and Ligament F Sternum Bursa and Ligament G Rib(s) Bursa and Ligament H Abdomen Bursa and Ligament, Right J Abdomen Bursa and Ligament, Left K Perineum Bursa and Ligament L Hip Bursa and Ligament, Right M Hip Bursa and Ligament, Left N Knee Bursa and Ligament, Right P Knee Bursa and Ligament, Left Q Ankle Bursa and Ligament, Right R Ankle Bursa and Ligament, Left S Foot Bursa and Ligament, Right T Foot Bursa and Ligament, Left V Lower Extremity Bursa and Ligament, Right W Lower Extremity Bursa and Ligament, Left	Ø Open 3 Percutaneous 4 Percutaneous Endoscopic	Z No Device	Z No Qualifier

Q: REPAIR

M: BURSAE AND LIGAMENTS

Ø: M/S

New/Revised Text in Green   ~~deleted~~ Deleted   ♀ Females Only   ♂ Males Only   **Coding Clinic**

🚫 Non-covered   🚫 Limited Coverage   ⊟ Combination (See Appendix E)   DRG Non-OR   Non-OR   🚫 Hospital-Acquired Condition

SECTION: Ø MEDICAL AND SURGICAL

BODY SYSTEM: M BURSAE AND LIGAMENTS

OPERATION: R REPLACEMENT: Putting in or on biological or synthetic material that physically takes the place and/or function of all or a portion of a body part

Body Part	Approach	Device	Qualifier
Ø Head and Neck Bursa and Ligament 1 Shoulder Bursa and Ligament, Right 2 Shoulder Bursa and Ligament, Left 3 Elbow Bursa and Ligament, Right 4 Elbow Bursa and Ligament, Left 5 Wrist Bursa and Ligament, Right 6 Wrist Bursa and Ligament, Left 7 Hand Bursa and Ligament, Right 8 Hand Bursa and Ligament, Left 9 Upper Extremity Bursa and Ligament, Right B Upper Extremity Bursa and Ligament, Left C Upper Spine Bursa and Ligament D Lower Spine Bursa and Ligament F Sternum Bursa and Ligament G Rib(s) Bursa and Ligament H Abdomen Bursa and Ligament, Right J Abdomen Bursa and Ligament, Left K Perineum Bursa and Ligament L Hip Bursa and Ligament, Right M Hip Bursa and Ligament, Left N Knee Bursa and Ligament, Right P Knee Bursa and Ligament, Left Q Ankle Bursa and Ligament, Right R Ankle Bursa and Ligament, Left S Foot Bursa and Ligament, Right T Foot Bursa and Ligament, Left V Lower Extremity Bursa and Ligament, Right W Lower Extremity Bursa and Ligament, Left	Ø Open 4 Percutaneous Endoscopic	7 Autologous Tissue Substitute J Synthetic Substitute K Nonautologous Tissue Substitute	Z No Qualifier

SECTION: Ø MEDICAL AND SURGICAL

BODY SYSTEM: M BURSAE AND LIGAMENTS

OPERATION: S REPOSITION: Moving to its normal location, or other suitable location, all or a portion of a body part

Body Part	Approach	Device	Qualifier
Ø Head and Neck Bursa and Ligament 1 Shoulder Bursa and Ligament, Right 2 Shoulder Bursa and Ligament, Left 3 Elbow Bursa and Ligament, Right 4 Elbow Bursa and Ligament, Left 5 Wrist Bursa and Ligament, Right 6 Wrist Bursa and Ligament, Left 7 Hand Bursa and Ligament, Right 8 Hand Bursa and Ligament, Left 9 Upper Extremity Bursa and Ligament, Right B Upper Extremity Bursa and Ligament, Left C Upper Spine Bursa and Ligament D Lower Spine Bursa and Ligament F Sternum Bursa and Ligament G Rib(s) Bursa and Ligament H Abdomen Bursa and Ligament, Right J Abdomen Bursa and Ligament, Left K Perineum Bursa and Ligament L Hip Bursa and Ligament, Right M Hip Bursa and Ligament, Left N Knee Bursa and Ligament, Right P Knee Bursa and Ligament, Left Q Ankle Bursa and Ligament, Right R Ankle Bursa and Ligament, Left S Foot Bursa and Ligament, Right T Foot Bursa and Ligament, Left V Lower Extremity Bursa and Ligament, Right W Lower Extremity Bursa and Ligament, Left	Ø Open 4 Percutaneous Endoscopic	Z No Device	Z No Qualifier

New/Revised Text in Green   ~~deleted~~ Deleted   ♀ Females Only   ♂ Males Only   **Coding Clinic**
🚫 Non-covered   🚫 Limited Coverage   ⊞ Combination (See Appendix E)   DRG Non-OR   Non-OR   🚫 Hospital-Acquired Condition

SECTION: Ø MEDICAL AND SURGICAL
BODY SYSTEM: M BURSAE AND LIGAMENTS
OPERATION: T RESECTION: Cutting out or off, without replacement, all of a body part

Body Part	Approach	Device	Qualifier
Ø Head and Neck Bursa and Ligament	Ø Open	Z No Device	Z No Qualifier
1 Shoulder Bursa and Ligament, Right	4 Percutaneous Endoscopic		
2 Shoulder Bursa and Ligament, Left			
3 Elbow Bursa and Ligament, Right			
4 Elbow Bursa and Ligament, Left			
5 Wrist Bursa and Ligament, Right			
6 Wrist Bursa and Ligament, Left			
7 Hand Bursa and Ligament, Right			
8 Hand Bursa and Ligament, Left			
9 Upper Extremity Bursa and Ligament, Right			
B Upper Extremity Bursa and Ligament, Left			
C Upper Spine Bursa and Ligament			
D Lower Spine Bursa and Ligament			
F Sternum Bursa and Ligament			
G Rib(s) Bursa and Ligament			
H Abdomen Bursa and Ligament, Right			
J Abdomen Bursa and Ligament, Left			
K Perineum Bursa and Ligament			
L Hip Bursa and Ligament, Right			
M Hip Bursa and Ligament, Left			
N Knee Bursa and Ligament, Right			
P Knee Bursa and Ligament, Left			
Q Ankle Bursa and Ligament, Right			
R Ankle Bursa and Ligament, Left			
S Foot Bursa and Ligament, Right			
T Foot Bursa and Ligament, Left			
V Lower Extremity Bursa and Ligament, Right			
W Lower Extremity Bursa and Ligament, Left			

Ø: M/S

M: BURSAE AND LIGAMENTS

T: RESECTION

SECTION: Ø MEDICAL AND SURGICAL
BODY SYSTEM: M BURSAE AND LIGAMENTS
OPERATION: U SUPPLEMENT: Putting in or on biological or synthetic material that physically reinforces and/or augments the function of a portion of a body part

Body Part	Approach	Device	Qualifier
Ø Head and Neck Bursa and Ligament 1 Shoulder Bursa and Ligament, Right 2 Shoulder Bursa and Ligament, Left 3 Elbow Bursa and Ligament, Right 4 Elbow Bursa and Ligament, Left 5 Wrist Bursa and Ligament, Right 6 Wrist Bursa and Ligament, Left 7 Hand Bursa and Ligament, Right 8 Hand Bursa and Ligament, Left 9 Upper Extremity Bursa and Ligament, Right B Upper Extremity Bursa and Ligament, Left C Upper Spine Bursa and Ligament D Lower Spine Bursa and Ligament F Sternum Bursa and Ligament G Rib(s) Bursa and Ligament H Abdomen Bursa and Ligament, Right J Abdomen Bursa and Ligament, Left K Perineum Bursa and Ligament L Hip Bursa and Ligament, Right M Hip Bursa and Ligament, Left N Knee Bursa and Ligament, Right P Knee Bursa and Ligament, Left Q Ankle Bursa and Ligament, Right R Ankle Bursa and Ligament, Left S Foot Bursa and Ligament, Right T Foot Bursa and Ligament, Left V Lower Extremity Bursa and Ligament, Right W Lower Extremity Bursa and Ligament, Left	Ø Open 4 Percutaneous Endoscopic	7 Autologous Tissue Substitute J Synthetic Substitute K Nonautologous Tissue Substitute	Z No Qualifier

Coding Clinic: 2017, Q2, P22 – ØMUN47Z

SECTION: Ø MEDICAL AND SURGICAL
BODY SYSTEM: M BURSAE AND LIGAMENTS
OPERATION: W REVISION: Correcting, to the extent possible, a portion of a malfunctioning device or the position of a displaced device

Body Part	Approach	Device	Qualifier
X Upper Bursa and Ligament Y Lower Bursa and Ligament	Ø Open 3 Percutaneous 4 Percutaneous Endoscopic	Ø Drainage Device 7 Autologous Tissue Substitute J Synthetic Substitute K Nonautologous Tissue Substitute Y Other Device	Z No Qualifier
X Upper Bursa and Ligament Y Lower Bursa and Ligament	X External	Ø Drainage Device 7 Autologous Tissue Substitute J Synthetic Substitute K Nonautologous Tissue Substitute	Z No Qualifier

Non-OR   ØMW[XY]X[Ø7JK]Z

SECTION: Ø MEDICAL AND SURGICAL
BODY SYSTEM: M BURSAE AND LIGAMENTS
OPERATION: X TRANSFER: Moving, without taking out, all or a portion of a body part to another location to take over the function of all or a portion of a body part

Body Part	Approach	Device	Qualifier
Ø Head and Neck Bursa and Ligament	Ø Open	Z No Device	Z No Qualifier
1 Shoulder Bursa and Ligament, Right	4 Percutaneous Endoscopic		
2 Shoulder Bursa and Ligament, Left			
3 Elbow Bursa and Ligament, Right			
4 Elbow Bursa and Ligament, Left			
5 Wrist Bursa and Ligament, Right			
6 Wrist Bursa and Ligament, Left			
7 Hand Bursa and Ligament, Right			
8 Hand Bursa and Ligament, Left			
9 Upper Extremity Bursa and Ligament, Right			
B Upper Extremity Bursa and Ligament, Left			
C Upper Spine Bursa and Ligament			
D Lower Spine Bursa and Ligament			
F Sternum Bursa and Ligament			
G Rib(s) Bursa and Ligament			
H Abdomen Bursa and Ligament, Right			
J Abdomen Bursa and Ligament, Left			
K Perineum Bursa and Ligament			
L Hip Bursa and Ligament, Right			
M Hip Bursa and Ligament, Left			
N Knee Bursa and Ligament, Right			
P Knee Bursa and Ligament, Left			
Q Ankle Bursa and Ligament, Right			
R Ankle Bursa and Ligament, Left			
S Foot Bursa and Ligament, Right			
T Foot Bursa and Ligament, Left			
V Lower Extremity Bursa and Ligament, Right			
W Lower Extremity Bursa and Ligament, Left			

Ø: M/S

M: BURSAE AND LIGAMENTS

X: TRANSFER

SECTION: Ø MEDICAL AND SURGICAL

BODY SYSTEM: N HEAD AND FACIAL BONES

OPERATION: 2 **CHANGE:** Taking out or off a device from a body part and putting back an identical or similar device in or on the same body part without cutting or puncturing the skin or a mucous membrane

Body Part	Approach	Device	Qualifier
Ø Skull B Nasal Bone W Facial Bone	X External	Ø Drainage Device Y Other Device	Z No Qualifier

Non-OR All Values

SECTION: Ø MEDICAL AND SURGICAL

BODY SYSTEM: N HEAD AND FACIAL BONES

OPERATION: 5 **DESTRUCTION:** Physical eradication of all or a portion of a body part by the direct use of energy, force, or a destructive agent

Body Part	Approach	Device	Qualifier
Ø Skull 1 Frontal Bone 3 Parietal Bone, Right 4 Parietal Bone, Left 5 Temporal Bone, Right 6 Temporal Bone, Left 7 Occipital Bone B Nasal Bone C Sphenoid Bone F Ethmoid Bone, Right G Ethmoid Bone, Left H Lacrimal Bone, Right J Lacrimal Bone, Left K Palatine Bone, Right L Palatine Bone, Left M Zygomatic Bone, Right N Zygomatic Bone, Left P Orbit, Right Q Orbit, Left R Maxilla T Mandible, Right V Mandible, Left X Hyoid Bone	Ø Open 3 Percutaneous 4 Percutaneous Endoscopic	Z No Device	Z No Qualifier

SECTION: 0   MEDICAL AND SURGICAL

BODY SYSTEM: N   HEAD AND FACIAL BONES

OPERATION: 8   **DIVISION:** Cutting into a body part, without draining fluids and/or gases from the body part, in order to separate or transect a body part

Body Part	Approach	Device	Qualifier
0 Skull	0 Open	Z No Device	Z No Qualifier
1 Frontal Bone	3 Percutaneous		
3 Parietal Bone, Right	4 Percutaneous Endoscopic		
4 Parietal Bone, Left			
5 Temporal Bone, Right			
6 Temporal Bone, Left			
7 Occipital Bonet			
B Nasal Bone			
C Sphenoid Bone			
F Ethmoid Bone, Right			
G Ethmoid Bone, Left			
H Lacrimal Bone, Right			
J Lacrimal Bone, Left			
K Palatine Bone, Right			
L Palatine Bone, Left			
M Zygomatic Bone, Right			
N Zygomatic Bone, Left			
P Orbit, Right			
Q Orbit, Left			
R Maxilla			
T Mandible, Right			
V Mandible, Left			
X Hyoid Bone			

Non-OR   0N8B[034]ZZ

SECTION: Ø MEDICAL AND SURGICAL

BODY SYSTEM: N HEAD AND FACIAL BONES

OPERATION: 9 DRAINAGE: Taking or letting out fluids and/or gases from a body part

Body Part	Approach	Device	Qualifier
Ø Skull 1 Frontal Bone 3 Parietal Bone, Right 4 Parietal Bone, Left 5 Temporal Bone, Right 6 Temporal Bone, Left 7 Occipital Bone B Nasal Bone C Sphenoid Bone F Ethmoid Bone, Right G Ethmoid Bone, Left H Lacrimal Bone, Right J Lacrimal Bone, Left K Palatine Bone, Right L Palatine Bone, Left M Zygomatic Bone, Right N Zygomatic Bone, Left P Orbit, Right Q Orbit, Left R Maxilla T Mandible, Right V Mandible, Left X Hyoid Bone	Ø Open 3 Percutaneous 4 Percutaneous Endoscopic	Ø Drainage Device	Z No Qualifier
Ø Skull 1 Frontal Bone 3 Parietal Bone, Right 4 Parietal Bone, Left 5 Temporal Bone, Right 6 Temporal Bone, Left 7 Occipital Bone B Nasal Bone C Sphenoid Bone F Ethmoid Bone, Right G Ethmoid Bone, Left H Lacrimal Bone, Right J Lacrimal Bone, Left K Palatine Bone, Right L Palatine Bone, Left M Zygomatic Bone, Right N Zygomatic Bone, Left P Orbit, Right Q Orbit, Left R Maxilla T Mandible, Right V Mandible, Left X Hyoid Bone	Ø Open 3 Percutaneous 4 Percutaneous Endoscopic	Z No Device	X Diagnostic Z No Qualifier

Non-OR ØN9[Ø134567CFGHJKLMNPQX]3ØZ
Non-OR ØN9[BRTV][Ø34]ØZ
Non-OR ØN9[Ø134567CFGHJKLMNPQX]3ZZ

Non-OR ØN9B[Ø34]ZX
Non-OR ØN9[BRTV][Ø34]ZZ

New/Revised Text in Green ~~deleted~~ Deleted ♀ Females Only ♂ Males Only **Coding Clinic**

Non-covered Limited Coverage ⊡ Combination (See Appendix E) DRG Non-OR Non-OR Hospital-Acquired Condition

SECTION: Ø MEDICAL AND SURGICAL
BODY SYSTEM: N HEAD AND FACIAL BONES
OPERATION: B EXCISION: Cutting out or off, without replacement, a portion of a body part

Body Part	Approach	Device	Qualifier
Ø Skull 1 Frontal Bone 3 Parietal Bone, Right 4 Parietal Bone, Left 5 Temporal Bone, Right 6 Temporal Bone, Left 7 Occipital Bone B Nasal Bone C Sphenoid Bone F Ethmoid Bone, Right G Ethmoid Bone, Left H Lacrimal Bone, Right J Lacrimal Bone, Left K Palatine Bone, Right L Palatine Bone, Left M Zygomatic Bone, Right N Zygomatic Bone, Left P Orbit, Right Q Orbit, Left R Maxilla T Mandible, Right V Mandible, Left X Hyoid Bone	Ø Open 3 Percutaneous 4 Percutaneous Endoscopic	Z No Device	X Diagnostic Z No Qualifier

Non-OR ØNB[BRTV][Ø34]ZX

Coding Clinic: 2Ø15, Q2, P13 – ØNBQØZZ
Coding Clinic: 2Ø17, Q1, P2Ø – ØNBBØZZ

New/Revised Text in Green   deleted Deleted   ♀ Females Only   ♂ Males Only   **Coding Clinic**
🦠 Non-covered   🦠 Limited Coverage   ⊞ Combination (See Appendix E)   DRG Non-OR   Non-OR   🦠 Hospital-Acquired Condition

SECTION: Ø MEDICAL AND SURGICAL
BODY SYSTEM: N HEAD AND FACIAL BONES
OPERATION: C EXTIRPATION: Taking or cutting out solid matter from a body part

Body Part	Approach	Device	Qualifier
1 Frontal Bone 3 Parietal Bone, Right 4 Parietal Bone, Left 5 Temporal Bone, Right 6 Temporal Bone, Left 7 Occipital Bone B Nasal Bone C Sphenoid Bone F Ethmoid Bone, Right G Ethmoid Bone, Left H Lacrimal Bone, Right J Lacrimal Bone, Left K Palatine Bone, Right L Palatine Bone, Left M Zygomatic Bone, Right N Zygomatic Bone, Left P Orbit, Right Q Orbit, Left R Maxilla T Mandible, Right V Mandible, Left X Hyoid Bone	Ø Open 3 Percutaneous 4 Percutaneous Endoscopic	Z No Device	Z No Qualifier

Non-OR   ØNC[BRTV][Ø34]ZZ

SECTION: Ø MEDICAL AND SURGICAL

BODY SYSTEM: N HEAD AND FACIAL BONES

OPERATION: D EXTRACTION: Pulling or stripping out or off all or a portion of a body part by the use of force

Body Part	Approach	Device	Qualifier
Ø Skull 1 Frontal Bone 3 Parietal Bone, Right 4 Parietal Bone, Left 5 Temporal Bone, Right 6 Temporal Bone, Left 7 Occipital Bone B Nasal Bone C Sphenoid Bone F Ethmoid Bone, Right G Ethmoid Bone, Left H Lacrimal Bone, Right J Lacrimal Bone, Left K Palatine Bone, Right L Palatine Bone, Left M Zygomatic Bone, Right N Zygomatic Bone, Left P Orbit, Right Q Orbit, Left R Maxilla T Mandible, Right V Mandible, Left X Hyoid Bone	Ø Open	Z No Device	Z No Qualifier

New/Revised Text in Green   deleted Deleted   ♀ Females Only   ♂ Males Only   **Coding Clinic**

🔖 Non-covered   🔖 Limited Coverage   ⊞ Combination (See Appendix E)   DRG Non-OR   Non-OR   🔖 Hospital-Acquired Condition

SECTION: Ø MEDICAL AND SURGICAL

BODY SYSTEM: N HEAD AND FACIAL BONES

OPERATION: H INSERTION: Putting in a nonbiological appliance that monitors, assists, performs, or prevents a physiological function but does not physically take the place of a body part

Body Part	Approach	Device	Qualifier
Ø Skull ⊞	Ø Open	4 Internal Fixation Device 5 External Fixation Device M Bone Growth Stimulator N Neurostimulator Generator	Z No Qualifier
Ø Skull	3 Percutaneous 4 Percutaneous Endoscopic	4 Internal Fixation Device 5 External Fixation Device M Bone Growth Stimulator	Z No Qualifier
1 Frontal Bone 3 Parietal Bone, Right 4 Parietal Bone, Left 7 Occipital Bone C Sphenoid Bone F Ethmoid Bone, Right G Ethmoid Bone, Left H Lacrimal Bone, Right J Lacrimal Bone, Left K Palatine Bone, Right L Palatine Bone, Left M Zygomatic Bone, Right N Zygomatic Bone, Left P Orbit, Right Q Orbit, Left X Hyoid Bone	Ø Open 3 Percutaneous 4 Percutaneous Endoscopic	4 Internal Fixation Device	Z No Qualifier
5 Temporal Bone, Right 6 Temporal Bone, Left	Ø Open 3 Percutaneous 4 Percutaneous Endoscopic	4 Internal Fixation Device S Hearing Device	Z No Qualifier
B Nasal Bone	Ø Open 3 Percutaneous 4 Percutaneous Endoscopic	4 Internal Fixation Device M Bone Growth Stimulator	Z No Qualifier
R Maxilla T Mandible, Right V Mandible, Left	Ø Open 3 Percutaneous 4 Percutaneous Endoscopic	4 Internal Fixation Device 5 External Fixation Device	Z No Qualifier
W Facial Bone	Ø Open 3 Percutaneous 4 Percutaneous Endoscopic	M Bone Growth Stimulator	Z No Qualifier

⊞ ØNHØØNZ
Non-OR ØNHØØ5Z
Non-OR ØNHØ[34]5Z
Non-OR ØNHB[Ø34][4M]Z

Coding Clinic: 2Ø15, Q3, P14 – ØNHØØ4Z

SECTION: Ø MEDICAL AND SURGICAL

BODY SYSTEM: N HEAD AND FACIAL BONES

OPERATION: J INSPECTION: Visually and/or manually exploring a body part

Body Part	Approach	Device	Qualifier
Ø Skull B Nasal Bone W Facial Bone	Ø Open 3 Percutaneous 4 Percutaneous Endoscopic X External	Z No Device	Z No Qualifier

Non-OR   ØNJ[ØBW][3X]ZZ

SECTION: Ø MEDICAL AND SURGICAL

BODY SYSTEM: N HEAD AND FACIAL BONES

OPERATION: N RELEASE: Freeing a body part from an abnormal physical constraint by cutting or by the use of force

Body Part	Approach	Device	Qualifier
1 Frontal Bone 3 Parietal Bone, Right 4 Parietal Bone, Left 5 Temporal Bone, Right 6 Temporal Bone, Left 7 Occipital Bone B Nasal Bone C Sphenoid Bone F Ethmoid Bone, Right G Ethmoid Bone, Left H Lacrimal Bone, Right J Lacrimal Bone, Left K Palatine Bone, Right L Palatine Bone, Left M Zygomatic Bone, Right N Zygomatic Bone, Left P Orbit, Right Q Orbit, Left R Maxilla T Mandible, Right V Mandible, Left X Hyoid Bone	Ø Open 3 Percutaneous 4 Percutaneous Endoscopic	Z No Device	Z No Qualifier

Non-OR   ØNNB[Ø34]ZZ

SECTION: Ø MEDICAL AND SURGICAL
BODY SYSTEM: N HEAD AND FACIAL BONES
OPERATION: P REMOVAL: Taking out or off a device from a body part

Body Part	Approach	Device	Qualifier
Ø Skull	Ø Open	Ø Drainage Device 4 Internal Fixation Device 5 External Fixation Device 7 Autologous Tissue Substitute J Synthetic Substitute K Nonautologous Tissue Substitute M Bone Growth Stimulator N Neurostimulator Generator S Hearing Device	Z No Qualifier
Ø Skull	3 Percutaneous 4 Percutaneous Endoscopic	Ø Drainage Device 4 Internal Fixation Device 5 External Fixation Device 7 Autologous Tissue Substitute J Synthetic Substitute K Nonautologous Tissue Substitute M Bone Growth Stimulator S Hearing Device	Z No Qualifier
Ø Skull	X External	Ø Drainage Device 4 Internal Fixation Device 5 External Fixation Device M Bone Growth Stimulator S Hearing Device	Z No Qualifier
B Nasal Bone W Facial Bone	Ø Open 3 Percutaneous 4 Percutaneous Endoscopic	Ø Drainage Device 4 Internal Fixation Device 7 Autologous Tissue Substitute J Synthetic Substitute K Nonautologous Tissue Substitute M Bone Growth Stimulator	Z No Qualifier
B Nasal Bone W Facial Bone	X External	Ø Drainage Device 4 Internal Fixation Device M Bone Growth Stimulator	Z No Qualifier

Non-OR ØNPØ[34]5Z
Non-OR ØNPØX[Ø5]Z
Non-OR ØNPB[Ø34][Ø47JKM]Z
Non-OR ØNPBX[Ø4M]Z
Non-OR ØNPWX[ØM]Z

Coding Clinic: 2Ø15, Q3, P14 – ØNPØØ4Z

New/Revised Text in Green ~~deleted~~ Deleted ♀ Females Only ♂ Males Only **Coding Clinic**
Non-covered Limited Coverage ⊕ Combination (See Appendix E) DRG Non-OR Non-OR Hospital-Acquired Condition

379

SECTION: Ø MEDICAL AND SURGICAL

BODY SYSTEM: N HEAD AND FACIAL BONES

OPERATION: Q REPAIR: Restoring, to the extent possible, a body part to its normal anatomic structure and function

Body Part	Approach	Device	Qualifier
Ø Skull	Ø Open	Z No Device	Z No Qualifier
1 Frontal Bone	3 Percutaneous		
3 Parietal Bone, Right	4 Percutaneous Endoscopic		
4 Parietal Bone, Left	X External		
5 Temporal Bone, Right			
6 Temporal Bone, Left			
7 Occipital Bone			
B Nasal Bone			
C Sphenoid Bone			
F Ethmoid Bone, Right			
G Ethmoid Bone, Left			
H Lacrimal Bone, Right			
J Lacrimal Bone, Left			
K Palatine Bone, Right			
L Palatine Bone, Left			
M Zygomatic Bone, Right			
N Zygomatic Bone, Left			
P Orbit, Right			
Q Orbit, Left			
R Maxilla			
T Mandible, Right			
V Mandible, Left			
X Hyoid Bone			

DRG Non-OR   ØNQ[Ø12345678BCDFGHJKLMNPQRSTVX]XZZ

Coding Clinic: 2Ø16, Q3, P29 – ØNQSØZZ

New/Revised Text in Green   ~~deleted~~ Deleted   ♀ Females Only   ♂ Males Only   **Coding Clinic**
Non-covered   Limited Coverage   ⊞ Combination (See Appendix E)   DRG Non-OR   Non-OR   Hospital-Acquired Condition

SECTION: Ø MEDICAL AND SURGICAL
BODY SYSTEM: N HEAD AND FACIAL BONES
OPERATION: R REPLACEMENT: Putting in or on biological or synthetic material that physically takes the place and/or function of all or a portion of a body part

Body Part	Approach	Device	Qualifier
Ø Skull 1 Frontal Bone 3 Parietal Bone, Right 4 Parietal Bone, Left 5 Temporal Bone, Right 6 Temporal Bone, Left 7 Occipital Bone B Nasal Bone C Sphenoid Bone F Ethmoid Bone, Right G Ethmoid Bone, Left H Lacrimal Bone, Right J Lacrimal Bone, Left K Palatine Bone, Right L Palatine Bone, Left M Zygomatic Bone, Right N Zygomatic Bone, Left P Orbit, Right Q Orbit, Left R Maxilla T Mandible, Right V Mandible, Left X Hyoid Bone	Ø Open 3 Percutaneous 4 Percutaneous Endoscopic	7 Autologous Tissue Substitute J Synthetic Substitute K Nonautologous Tissue Substitute	Z No Qualifier

Coding Clinic: 2017, Q1, P24 – ØNRVØ[7J]Z
Coding Clinic: 2017, Q3, P17 – ØNR8ØJZ

SECTION: Ø MEDICAL AND SURGICAL
BODY SYSTEM: N HEAD AND FACIAL BONES
OPERATION: S REPOSITION: *(on multiple pages)*
Moving to its normal location, or other suitable location, all or a portion of a body part

Body Part	Approach	Device	Qualifier
Ø Skull R Maxilla T Mandible, Right V Mandible, Left	Ø Open 3 Percutaneous 4 Percutaneous Endoscopic	4 Internal Fixation Device 5 External Fixation Device Z No Device	Z No Qualifier
Ø Skull R Maxilla T Mandible, Right V Mandible, Left	X External	Z No Device	Z No Qualifier

Non-OR ØNS[RTV][34][45Z]Z
Non-OR ØNS[RTV]XZZ

Coding Clinic: 2016, Q2, P30; 2015, Q3, P18 – ØNS00ZZ
Coding Clinic: 2017, Q1, P21 – ØNS[RS]0ZZ
Coding Clinic: 2017, Q3, P22 – ØNS004Z

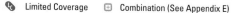

New/Revised Text in Green   ~~deleted~~ Deleted   ♀ Females Only   ♂ Males Only   **Coding Clinic**

Non-covered   Limited Coverage   ⊞ Combination (See Appendix E)   DRG Non-OR   Non-OR   Hospital-Acquired Condition

SECTION: Ø MEDICAL AND SURGICAL
BODY SYSTEM: N HEAD AND FACIAL BONES
OPERATION: S REPOSITION: *(continued)*

Moving to its normal location, or other suitable location, all or a portion of a body part

Body Part	Approach	Device	Qualifier
1 Frontal Bone 3 Parietal Bone, Right 4 Parietal Bone, Left 5 Temporal Bone, Right 6 Temporal Bone, Left 7 Occipital Bone B Nasal Bone C Sphenoid Bone F Ethmoid Bone, Right G Ethmoid Bone, Left H Lacrimal Bone, Right J Lacrimal Bone, Left K Palatine Bone, Right L Palatine Bone, Left M Zygomatic Bone, Right N Zygomatic Bone, Left P Orbit, Right Q Orbit, Left X Hyoid Bone	Ø Open 3 Percutaneous 4 Percutaneous Endoscopic	4 Internal Fixation Device Z No Device	Z No Qualifier
1 Frontal Bone 3 Parietal Bone, Right 4 Parietal Bone, Left 5 Temporal Bone, Right 6 Temporal Bone, Left 7 Occipital Bone B Nasal Bone C Sphenoid Bone F Ethmoid Bone, Right G Ethmoid Bone, Left H Lacrimal Bone, Right J Lacrimal Bone, Left K Palatine Bone, Right L Palatine Bone, Left M Zygomatic Bone, Right N Zygomatic Bone, Left P Orbit, Right Q Orbit, Left X Hyoid Bone	X External	Z No Device	Z No Qualifier

Non-OR ØNS[BCFGHJKLMNPQX][34][4Z]Z
Non-OR ØNS[BCFGHJKLMNPQX]XZZ

Coding Clinic: 2013, Q3, P25 – ØNSØØ5Z, ØNS1Ø4Z
Coding Clinic: 2015, Q3, P28 – ØNS5Ø4Z

S: REPOSITION

N: HEAD AND FACIAL BONES

Ø: M/S

New/Revised Text in Green   ~~deleted~~ Deleted   ♀ Females Only   ♂ Males Only   **Coding Clinic**

Non-covered   Limited Coverage   ⊞ Combination (See Appendix E)   DRG Non-OR   Non-OR   Hospital-Acquired Condition

SECTION: Ø MEDICAL AND SURGICAL

BODY SYSTEM: N HEAD AND FACIAL BONES

OPERATION: T RESECTION: Cutting out or off, without replacement, all of a body part

Body Part	Approach	Device	Qualifier
1 Frontal Bone	Ø Open	Z No Device	Z No Qualifier
3 Parietal Bone, Right			
4 Parietal Bone, Left			
5 Temporal Bone, Right			
6 Temporal Bone, Left			
7 Occipital Bone			
B Nasal Bone			
C Sphenoid Bone			
F Ethmoid Bone, Right			
G Ethmoid Bone, Left			
H Lacrimal Bone, Right			
J Lacrimal Bone, Left			
K Palatine Bone, Right			
L Palatine Bone, Left			
M Zygomatic Bone, Right			
N Zygomatic Bone, Left			
P Orbit, Right			
Q Orbit, Left			
R Maxilla			
T Mandible, Right			
V Mandible, Left			
X Hyoid Bone			

SECTION: Ø MEDICAL AND SURGICAL

BODY SYSTEM: N HEAD AND FACIAL BONES

OPERATION: U SUPPLEMENT: Putting in or on biological or synthetic material that physically reinforces and/or augments the function of a portion of a body part

Body Part	Approach	Device	Qualifier
Ø Skull	Ø Open	7 Autologous Tissue Substitute	Z No Qualifier
1 Frontal Bone	3 Percutaneous	J Synthetic Substitute	
3 Parietal Bone, Right	4 Percutaneous Endoscopic	K Nonautologous Tissue	
4 Parietal Bone, Left		Substitute	
5 Temporal Bone, Right			
6 Temporal Bone, Left			
7 Occipital Bone			
B Nasal Bone			
C Sphenoid Bone			
F Ethmoid Bone, Right			
G Ethmoid Bone, Left			
H Lacrimal Bone, Right			
J Lacrimal Bone, Left			
K Palatine Bone, Right			
L Palatine Bone, Left			
M Zygomatic Bone, Right			
N Zygomatic Bone, Left			
P Orbit, Right			
Q Orbit, Left			
R Maxilla			
T Mandible, Right			
V Mandible, Left			
X Hyoid Bone			

Coding Clinic: 2013, Q3, P25 – ØNUØØJZ
Coding Clinic: 2016, Q3, P29 – ØNURØ7Z

New/Revised Text in Green   deleted Deleted   ♀ Females Only   ♂ Males Only   **Coding Clinic**
Non-covered   Limited Coverage   ⊟ Combination (See Appendix E)   DRG Non-OR   Non-OR   Hospital-Acquired Condition

SECTION: Ø MEDICAL AND SURGICAL

BODY SYSTEM: N HEAD AND FACIAL BONES

OPERATION: W REVISION: Correcting, to the extent possible, a portion of a malfunctioning device or the position of a displaced device

Body Part	Approach	Device	Qualifier
Ø Skull	Ø Open	Ø Drainage Device 4 Internal Fixation Device 5 External Fixation Device 7 Autologous Tissue Substitute J Synthetic Substitute K Nonautologous Tissue Substitute M Bone Growth Stimulator N Neurostimulator Generator S Hearing Device	Z No Qualifier
Ø Skull	3 Percutaneous 4 Percutaneous Endoscopic X External	Ø Drainage Device 4 Internal Fixation Device 5 External Fixation Device 7 Autologous Tissue Substitute J Synthetic Substitute K Nonautologous Tissue Substitute M Bone Growth Stimulator S Hearing Device	Z No Qualifier
B Nasal Bone W Facial Bone	Ø Open 3 Percutaneous 4 Percutaneous Endoscopic X External	Ø Drainage Device 4 Internal Fixation Device 7 Autologous Tissue Substitute J Synthetic Substitute K Nonautologous Tissue Substitute M Bone Growth Stimulator	Z No Qualifier

Non-OR ØNWØX[Ø457JKMS]Z
Non-OR ØNWB[Ø34X][Ø47JKM]Z
Non-OR ØNWWX[Ø47JKM]Z

New/Revised Text in Green   ~~deleted~~ Deleted   ♀ Females Only   ♂ Males Only   **Coding Clinic**

🚫 Non-covered   🚫 Limited Coverage   ⊞ Combination (See Appendix E)   DRG Non-OR   Non-OR   🚫 Hospital-Acquired Condition

SECTION: Ø MEDICAL AND SURGICAL

BODY SYSTEM: P UPPER BONES

OPERATION: 2 **CHANGE:** Taking out or off a device from a body part and putting back an identical or similar device in or on the same body part without cutting or puncturing the skin or a mucous membrane

Body Part	Approach	Device	Qualifier
Y Upper Bone	X External	Ø Drainage Device Y Other Device	Z No Qualifier

Non-OR All Values

SECTION: Ø MEDICAL AND SURGICAL

BODY SYSTEM: P UPPER BONES

OPERATION: 5 **DESTRUCTION:** Physical eradication of all or a portion of a body part by the direct use of energy, force, or a destructive agent

Body Part	Approach	Device	Qualifier
Ø Sternum 1 Rib, 1 to 2 2 Rib, 3 or More 3 Cervical Vertebra 4 Thoracic Vertebra 5 Scapula, Right 6 Scapula, Left 7 Glenoid Cavity, Right 8 Glenoid Cavity, Left 9 Clavicle, Right B Clavicle, Left C Humeral Head, Right D Humeral Head, Left F Humeral Shaft, Right G Humeral Shaft, Left H Radius, Right J Radius, Left K Ulna, Right L Ulna, Left M Carpal, Right N Carpal, Left P Metacarpal, Right Q Metacarpal, Left R Thumb Phalanx, Right S Thumb Phalanx, Left T Finger Phalanx, Right V Finger Phalanx, Left	Ø Open 3 Percutaneous 4 Percutaneous Endoscopic	Z No Device	Z No Qualifier

SECTION: Ø MEDICAL AND SURGICAL

BODY SYSTEM: P UPPER BONES

OPERATION: 8 DIVISION: Cutting into a body part, without draining fluids and/or gases from the body part, in order to separate or transect a body part

Body Part	Approach	Device	Qualifier
Ø Sternum	Ø Open	Z No Device	Z No Qualifier
1 Rib, 1 to 2	3 Percutaneous		
2 Rib, 3 or More	4 Percutaneous Endoscopic		
3 Cervical Vertebra			
4 Thoracic Vertebra			
5 Scapula, Right			
6 Scapula, Left			
7 Glenoid Cavity, Right			
8 Glenoid Cavity, Left			
9 Clavicle, Right			
B Clavicle, Left			
C Humeral Head, Right			
D Humeral Head, Left			
F Humeral Shaft, Right			
G Humeral Shaft, Left			
H Radius, Right			
J Radius, Left			
K Ulna, Right			
L Ulna, Left			
M Carpal, Right			
N Carpal, Left			
P Metacarpal, Right			
Q Metacarpal, Left			
R Thumb Phalanx, Right			
S Thumb Phalanx, Left			
T Finger Phalanx, Right			
V Finger Phalanx, Left			

SECTION: Ø MEDICAL AND SURGICAL
BODY SYSTEM: P UPPER BONES
OPERATION: 9 DRAINAGE: Taking or letting out fluids and/or gases from a body part

Body Part	Approach	Device	Qualifier
Ø Sternum 1 Rib, 1 to 2 2 Rib, 3 or More 3 Cervical Vertebra 4 Thoracic Vertebra 5 Scapula, Right 6 Scapula, Left 7 Glenoid Cavity, Right 8 Glenoid Cavity, Left 9 Clavicle, Right B Clavicle, Left C Humeral Head, Right D Humeral Head, Left F Humeral Shaft, Right G Humeral Shaft, Left H Radius, Right J Radius, Left K Ulna, Right L Ulna, Left M Carpal, Right N Carpal, Left P Metacarpal, Right Q Metacarpal, Left R Thumb Phalanx, Right S Thumb Phalanx, Left T Finger Phalanx, Right V Finger Phalanx, Left	Ø Open 3 Percutaneous 4 Percutaneous Endoscopic	Ø Drainage Device	Z No Qualifier
Ø Sternum 1 Rib, 1 to 2 2 Rib, 3 or More 3 Cervical Vertebra 4 Thoracic Vertebra 5 Scapula, Right 6 Scapula, Left 7 Glenoid Cavity, Right 8 Glenoid Cavity, Left 9 Clavicle, Right B Clavicle, Left C Humeral Head, Right D Humeral Head, Left F Humeral Shaft, Right G Humeral Shaft, Left H Radius, Right J Radius, Left K Ulna, Right L Ulna, Left M Carpal, Right N Carpal, Left P Metacarpal, Right Q Metacarpal, Left R Thumb Phalanx, Right S Thumb Phalanx, Left T Finger Phalanx, Right V Finger Phalanx, Left	Ø Open 3 Percutaneous 4 Percutaneous Endoscopic	Z No Device	X Diagnostic Z No Qualifier

Non-OR ØP9[Ø123456789BCDFGHJKLMNPQRSTV]3ØZ
Non-OR ØP9[Ø123456789BCDFGHJKLMNPQRSTV]3ZZ

New/Revised Text in Green   ~~deleted~~ Deleted   ♀ Females Only   ♂ Males Only   **Coding Clinic**
 Non-covered   Limited Coverage   ⊞ Combination (See Appendix E)   DRG Non-OR   Non-OR   Hospital-Acquired Condition

SECTION: Ø MEDICAL AND SURGICAL
BODY SYSTEM: P UPPER BONES
OPERATION: B EXCISION: Cutting out or off, without replacement, a portion of a body part

Body Part	Approach	Device	Qualifier
Ø Sternum	Ø Open	Z No Device	X Diagnostic
1 Rib, 1 to 2	3 Percutaneous		Z No Qualifier
2 Rib, 3 or More	4 Percutaneous Endoscopic		
3 Cervical Vertebra			
4 Thoracic Vertebra			
5 Scapula, Right			
6 Scapula, Left			
7 Glenoid Cavity, Right			
8 Glenoid Cavity, Left			
9 Clavicle, Right			
B Clavicle, Left			
C Humeral Head, Right			
D Humeral Head, Left			
F Humeral Shaft, Right			
G Humeral Shaft, Left			
H Radius, Right			
J Radius, Left			
K Ulna, Right			
L Ulna, Left			
M Carpal, Right			
N Carpal, Left			
P Metacarpal, Right			
Q Metacarpal, Left			
R Thumb Phalanx, Right			
S Thumb Phalanx, Left			
T Finger Phalanx, Right			
V Finger Phalanx, Left			

Coding Clinic: 2012, Q4, P101 – ØPB1ØZZ
Coding Clinic: 2013, Q3, P22 – ØPB54ZZ

New/Revised Text in Green   deleted Deleted   ♀ Females Only   ♂ Males Only   **Coding Clinic**
🚫 Non-covered   🚫 Limited Coverage   ⊕ Combination (See Appendix E)   DRG Non-OR   Non-OR   🚫 Hospital-Acquired Condition

SECTION: Ø MEDICAL AND SURGICAL
BODY SYSTEM: P UPPER BONES
OPERATION: C EXTIRPATION: Taking or cutting out solid matter from a body part

Body Part	Approach	Device	Qualifier
Ø Sternum	Ø Open	Z No Device	Z No Qualifier
1 Rib, 1 to 2	3 Percutaneous		
2 Rib, 3 or More	4 Percutaneous Endoscopic		
3 Cervical Vertebra			
4 Thoracic Vertebra			
5 Scapula, Right			
6 Scapula, Left			
7 Glenoid Cavity, Right			
8 Glenoid Cavity, Left			
9 Clavicle, Right			
B Clavicle, Left			
C Humeral Head, Right			
D Humeral Head, Left			
F Humeral Shaft, Right			
G Humeral Shaft, Left			
H Radius, Right			
J Radius, Left			
K Ulna, Right			
L Ulna, Left			
M Carpal, Right			
N Carpal, Left			
P Metacarpal, Right			
Q Metacarpal, Left			
R Thumb Phalanx, Right			
S Thumb Phalanx, Left			
T Finger Phalanx, Right			
V Finger Phalanx, Left			

SECTION: Ø MEDICAL AND SURGICAL

BODY SYSTEM: P UPPER BONES

OPERATION: D **EXTRACTION:** Pulling or stripping out or off all or a portion of a body part by the use of force

Body Part	Approach	Device	Qualifier
Ø Sternum	Ø Open	Z No Device	Z No Qualifier
1 Rib, 1 to 2			
2 Rib, 3 or More			
3 Cervical Vertebra			
4 Thoracic Vertebra			
5 Scapula, Right			
6 Scapula, Left			
7 Glenoid Cavity, Right			
8 Glenoid Cavity, Left			
9 Clavicle, Right			
B Clavicle, Left			
C Humeral Head, Right			
D Humeral Head, Left			
F Humeral Shaft, Right			
G Humeral Shaft, Left			
H Radius, Right			
J Radius, Left			
K Ulna, Right			
L Ulna, Left			
M Carpal, Right			
N Carpal, Left			
P Metacarpal, Right			
Q Metacarpal, Left			
R Thumb Phalanx, Right			
S Thumb Phalanx, Left			
T Finger Phalanx, Right			
V Finger Phalanx, Left			

D: EXTRACTION

P: UPPER BONES

Ø: M/S

SECTION: Ø MEDICAL AND SURGICAL
BODY SYSTEM: P UPPER BONES
OPERATION: H INSERTION: Putting in a nonbiological appliance that monitors, assists, performs, or prevents a physiological function but does not physically take the place of a body part

Body Part	Approach	Device	Qualifier
Ø Sternum	Ø Open 3 Percutaneous 4 Percutaneous Endoscopic	Ø Internal Fixation Device, Rigid Plate 4 Internal Fixation Device	Z No Qualifier
1 Rib, 1 to 2 2 Rib, 3 or More 3 Cervical Vertebra 4 Thoracic Vertebra 5 Scapula, Right 6 Scapula, Left 7 Glenoid Cavity, Right 8 Glenoid Cavity, Left 9 Clavicle, Right B Clavicle, Left	Ø Open 3 Percutaneous 4 Percutaneous Endoscopic	4 Internal Fixation Device	Z No Qualifier
C Humeral Head, Right D Humeral Head, Left F Humeral Shaft, Right G Humeral Shaft, Left H Radius, Right J Radius, Left K Ulna, Right L Ulna, Left	Ø Open 3 Percutaneous 4 Percutaneous Endoscopic	4 Internal Fixation Device 5 External Fixation Device 6 Internal Fixation Device, Intramedullary 8 External Fixation Device, Limb Lengthening B External Fixation Device, Monoplanar C External Fixation Device, Ring D External Fixation Device, Hybrid	Z No Qualifier
M Carpal, Right N Carpal, Left P Metacarpal, Right Q Metacarpal, Left R Thumb Phalanx, Right S Thumb Phalanx, Left T Finger Phalanx, Right V Finger Phalanx, Left	Ø Open 3 Percutaneous 4 Percutaneous Endoscopic	4 Internal Fixation Device 5 External Fixation Device	Z No Qualifier
Y Upper Bone	Ø Open 3 Percutaneous 4 Percutaneous Endoscopic	M Bone Growth Stimulator	Z No Qualifier
Y Upper Bone	Ø Open 3 Percutaneous 4 Percutaneous Endoscopic X External	Z No Device	Z No Qualifier

Non-OR ØPH[CDFGHJKL][Ø34]8Z

New/Revised Text in Green   ~~deleted~~ Deleted   ♀ Females Only   ♂ Males Only   **Coding Clinic**
 Non-covered   Limited Coverage   ⊞ Combination (See Appendix E)   DRG Non-OR   Non-OR   Hospital-Acquired Condition

SECTION: Ø MEDICAL AND SURGICAL
BODY SYSTEM: P UPPER BONES
OPERATION: J INSPECTION: Visually and/or manually exploring a body part

Body Part	Approach	Device	Qualifier
Y Upper Bone	Ø Open 3 Percutaneous 4 Percutaneous Endoscopic X External	Z No Device	Z No Qualifier

Non-OR ØPJY[3X]ZZ

SECTION: Ø MEDICAL AND SURGICAL
BODY SYSTEM: P UPPER BONES
OPERATION: N RELEASE: Freeing a body part from an abnormal physical constraint by cutting or by the use of force

Body Part	Approach	Device	Qualifier
Ø Sternum 1 Rib, 1 to 2 2 Rib, 3 or More 3 Cervical Vertebra 4 Thoracic Vertebra 5 Scapula, Right 6 Scapula, Left 7 Glenoid Cavity, Right 8 Glenoid Cavity, Left 9 Clavicle, Right B Clavicle, Left C Humeral Head, Right D Humeral Head, Left F Humeral Shaft, Right G Humeral Shaft, Left H Radius, Right J Radius, Left K Ulna, Right L Ulna, Left M Carpal, Right N Carpal, Left P Metacarpal, Right Q Metacarpal, Left R Thumb Phalanx, Right S Thumb Phalanx, Left T Finger Phalanx, Right V Finger Phalanx, Left	Ø Open 3 Percutaneous 4 Percutaneous Endoscopic	Z No Device	Z No Qualifier

SECTION: Ø MEDICAL AND SURGICAL
BODY SYSTEM: P UPPER BONES
OPERATION: P REMOVAL: *(on multiple pages)*
Taking out or off a device from a body part

Body Part	Approach	Device	Qualifier
Ø Sternum 1 Rib, 1 to 2 2 Rib, 3 or More 3 Cervical Vertebra 4 Thoracic Vertebra 5 Scapula, Right 6 Scapula, Left 7 Glenoid Cavity, Right 8 Glenoid Cavity, Left 9 Clavicle, Right B Clavicle, Left	Ø Open 3 Percutaneous 4 Percutaneous Endoscopic	4 Internal Fixation Device 7 Autologous Tissue Substitute J Synthetic Substitute K Nonautologous Tissue Substitute	Z No Qualifier
Ø Sternum 1 Rib, 1 to 2 2 Rib, 3 or More 3 Cervical Vertebra 4 Thoracic Vertebra 5 Scapula, Right 6 Scapula, Left 7 Glenoid Cavity, Right 8 Glenoid Cavity, Left 9 Clavicle, Right B Clavicle, Left	X External	4 Internal Fixation Device	Z No Qualifier
C Humeral Head, Right D Humeral Head, Left F Humeral Shaft, Right G Humeral Shaft, Left H Radius, Right J Radius, Left K Ulna, Right L Ulna, Left M Carpal, Right N Carpal, Left P Metacarpal, Right Q Metacarpal, Left R Thumb Phalanx, Right S Thumb Phalanx, Left T Finger Phalanx, Right V Finger Phalanx, Left	Ø Open 3 Percutaneous 4 Percutaneous Endoscopic	4 Internal Fixation Device 5 External Fixation Device 7 Autologous Tissue Substitute J Synthetic Substitute K Nonautologous Tissue Substitute	Z No Qualifier

Non-OR ØPP[Ø123456789B]X4Z

New/Revised Text in Green ~~deleted~~ Deleted ♀ Females Only ♂ Males Only **Coding Clinic**
🚫 Non-covered 🚫 Limited Coverage ⊞ Combination (See Appendix E) DRG Non-OR Non-OR 🚫 Hospital-Acquired Condition

395

SECTION: Ø MEDICAL AND SURGICAL
BODY SYSTEM: P UPPER BONES
OPERATION: P REMOVAL: *(continued)*
              Taking out or off a device from a body part

Body Part	Approach	Device	Qualifier
C Humeral Head, Right D Humeral Head, Left F Humeral Shaft, Right G Humeral Shaft, Left H Radius, Right J Radius, Left K Ulna, Right L Ulna, Left M Carpal, Right N Carpal, Left P Metacarpal, Right Q Metacarpal, Left R Thumb Phalanx, Right S Thumb Phalanx, Left T Finger Phalanx, Right V Finger Phalanx, Left	X External	4 Internal Fixation Device 5 External Fixation Device	Z No Qualifier
Y Upper Bone	Ø Open 3 Percutaneous 4 Percutaneous Endoscopic X External	Ø Drainage Device M Bone Growth Stimulator	Z No Qualifier

Non-OR   ØPP[CDFGHJKLMNPQRSTV]X[45]Z
Non-OR   ØPPY3ØZ
Non-OR   ØPPYX[ØM]Z

SECTION: Ø MEDICAL AND SURGICAL
BODY SYSTEM: P UPPER BONES
OPERATION: Q REPAIR: Restoring, to the extent possible, a body part to its normal anatomic structure and function

Body Part	Approach	Device	Qualifier
Ø Sternum	Ø Open	Z No Device	Z No Qualifier
1 Rib, 1 to 2	3 Percutaneous		
2 Rib, 3 or More	4 Percutaneous Endoscopic		
3 Cervical Vertebra	X External		
4 Thoracic Vertebra			
5 Scapula, Right			
6 Scapula, Left			
7 Glenoid Cavity, Right			
8 Glenoid Cavity, Left			
9 Clavicle, Right			
B Clavicle, Left			
C Humeral Head, Right			
D Humeral Head, Left			
F Humeral Shaft, Right			
G Humeral Shaft, Left			
H Radius, Right			
J Radius, Left			
K Ulna, Right			
L Ulna, Left			
M Carpal, Right			
N Carpal, Left			
P Metacarpal, Right			
Q Metacarpal, Left			
R Thumb Phalanx, Right			
S Thumb Phalanx, Left			
T Finger Phalanx, Right			
V Finger Phalanx, Left			

DRG Non-OR   ØPQ[Ø123456789BCDFGHJKLMNPQRSTV]XZZ

Ø: M/S

P: UPPER BONES

Q: REPAIR

SECTION: Ø MEDICAL AND SURGICAL

BODY SYSTEM: P UPPER BONES

OPERATION: R REPLACEMENT: Putting in or on biological or synthetic material that physically takes the place and/or function of all or a portion of a body part

Body Part	Approach	Device	Qualifier
Ø Sternum 1 Rib, 1 to 2 2 Rib, 3 or More 3 Cervical Vertebra 4 Thoracic Vertebra 5 Scapula, Right 6 Scapula, Left 7 Glenoid Cavity, Right 8 Glenoid Cavity, Left 9 Clavicle, Right B Clavicle, Left C Humeral Head, Right D Humeral Head, Left F Humeral Shaft, Right G Humeral Shaft, Left H Radius, Right J Radius, Left K Ulna, Right L Ulna, Left M Carpal, Right N Carpal, Left P Metacarpal, Right Q Metacarpal, Left R Thumb Phalanx, Right S Thumb Phalanx, Left T Finger Phalanx, Right V Finger Phalanx, Left	Ø Open 3 Percutaneous 4 Percutaneous Endoscopic	7 Autologous Tissue Substitute J Synthetic Substitute K Nonautologous Tissue Substitute	Z No Qualifier

SECTION: Ø MEDICAL AND SURGICAL

BODY SYSTEM: P UPPER BONES

OPERATION: S REPOSITION: *(on multiple pages)*
Moving to its normal location, or other suitable location, all or a portion of a body part

Body Part	Approach	Device	Qualifier
Ø Sternum	Ø Open 3 Percutaneous 4 Percutaneous Endoscopic	Ø Internal Fixation Device, Rigid Plate 4 Internal Fixation Device Z No Device	Z No Qualifier
Ø Sternum	X External	Z No Device	Z No Qualifier
1 Rib, 1 to 2 2 Rib, 3 or More 3 Cervical Vertebra ⊞ 4 Thoracic Vertebra ⊞ 5 Scapula, Right 6 Scapula, Left 7 Glenoid Cavity, Right 8 Glenoid Cavity, Left 9 Clavicle, Right B Clavicle, Left	Ø Open 3 Percutaneous 4 Percutaneous Endoscopic	4 Internal Fixation Device Z No Device	Z No Qualifier

⊞ ØPS3[34]ZZ

Non-OR ØPSØ[34]ZZ
Non-OR ØPSØXZZ
Non-OR ØPS[1256789B][34]ZZ

Coding Clinic: 2015, Q4, P34 – ØPSØØZZ
Coding Clinic: 2016, Q1, P21 – ØPS4XZZ
Coding Clinic: 2017, Q4, P53 – ØPS2Ø4Z

New/Revised Text in Green   ~~deleted~~ Deleted   ♀ Females Only   ♂ Males Only   **Coding Clinic**
🗞 Non-covered   🗞 Limited Coverage   ⊞ Combination (See Appendix E)   DRG Non-OR   Non-OR   🗞 Hospital-Acquired Condition

SECTION: Ø MEDICAL AND SURGICAL
BODY SYSTEM: P UPPER BONES
OPERATION: S REPOSITION: *(continued)*

Moving to its normal location, or other suitable location, all or a portion of a body part

Body Part	Approach	Device	Qualifier
1 Rib, 1 to 2 2 Rib, 3 or More 3 Cervical Vertebra 4 Thoracic Vertebra 5 Scapula, Right 6 Scapula, Left 7 Glenoid Cavity, Right 8 Glenoid Cavity, Left 9 Clavicle, Right B Clavicle, Left	X External	Z No Device	Z No Qualifier
C Humeral Head, Right D Humeral Head, Left F Humeral Shaft, Right G Humeral Shaft, Left H Radius, Right J Radius, Left K Ulna, Right L Ulna, Left	Ø Open 3 Percutaneous 4 Percutaneous Endoscopic	4 Internal Fixation Device 5 External Fixation Device 6 Internal Fixation Device, Intramedullary B External Fixation Device, Monoplanar C External Fixation Device, Ring D External Fixation Device, Hybrid Z No Device	Z No Qualifier
C Humeral Head, Right D Humeral Head, Left F Humeral Shaft, Right G Humeral Shaft, Left H Radius, Right J Radius, Left K Ulna, Right L Ulna, Left	X External	Z No Device	Z No Qualifier
M Carpal, Right N Carpal, Left P Metacarpal, Right Q Metacarpal, Left R Thumb Phalanx, Right S Thumb Phalanx, Left T Finger Phalanx, Right V Finger Phalanx, Left	Ø Open 3 Percutaneous 4 Percutaneous Endoscopic	4 Internal Fixation Device 5 External Fixation Device Z No Device	Z No Qualifier
M Carpal, Right N Carpal, Left P Metacarpal, Right Q Metacarpal, Left R Thumb Phalanx, Right S Thumb Phalanx, Left T Finger Phalanx, Right V Finger Phalanx, Left	X External	Z No Device	Z No Qualifier

Non-OR ØPS[1256789B]XZZ
Non-OR ØPS[CDFGHJKL][34]ZZ
Non-OR ØPS[CDFGHJKL]XZZ
Non-OR ØPS[MNPQRSTV][34]ZZ
Non-OR ØPS[MNPQRSTV]XZZ

Coding Clinic: 2Ø15, Q2, P35 – ØPS3XZZ

New/Revised Text in Green ~~deleted~~ Deleted ♀ Females Only ♂ Males Only **Coding Clinic**
Non-covered Limited Coverage ⊞ Combination (See Appendix E) DRG Non-OR Non-OR Hospital-Acquired Condition

SECTION: Ø MEDICAL AND SURGICAL

BODY SYSTEM: P UPPER BONES
OPERATION: T RESECTION: Cutting out or off, without replacement, all of a body part

Body Part	Approach	Device	Qualifier
Ø Sternum	Ø Open	Z No Device	Z No Qualifier
1 Rib, 1 to 2			
2 Rib, 3 or More			
5 Scapula, Right			
6 Scapula, Left			
7 Glenoid Cavity, Right			
8 Glenoid Cavity, Left			
9 Clavicle, Right			
B Clavicle, Left			
C Humeral Head, Right			
D Humeral Head, Left			
F Humeral Shaft, Right			
G Humeral Shaft, Left			
H Radius, Right			
J Radius, Left			
K Ulna, Right			
L Ulna, Left			
M Carpal, Right			
N Carpal, Left			
P Metacarpal, Right			
Q Metacarpal, Left			
R Thumb Phalanx, Right			
S Thumb Phalanx, Left			
T Finger Phalanx, Right			
V Finger Phalanx, Left			

Coding Clinic: 2015, Q3, P27 – ØPTNØZZ

T: RESECTION

P: UPPER BONES

Ø: M/S

SECTION: Ø MEDICAL AND SURGICAL
BODY SYSTEM: P UPPER BONES
OPERATION: U SUPPLEMENT: Putting in or on biological or synthetic material that physically reinforces and/or augments the function of a portion of a body part

Body Part	Approach	Device	Qualifier
Ø Sternum	Ø Open	7 Autologous Tissue Substitute	Z No Qualifier
1 Rib, 1 to 2	3 Percutaneous	J Synthetic Substitute	
2 Rib, 3 or More	4 Percutaneous Endoscopic	K Nonautologous Tissue Substitute	
3 Cervical Vertebra ⊞			
4 Thoracic Vertebra ⊞			
5 Scapula, Right			
6 Scapula, Left			
7 Glenoid Cavity, Right			
8 Glenoid Cavity, Left			
9 Clavicle, Right			
B Clavicle, Left			
C Humeral Head, Right			
D Humeral Head, Left			
F Humeral Shaft, Right			
G Humeral Shaft, Left			
H Radius, Right			
J Radius, Left			
K Ulna, Right			
L Ulna, Left			
M Carpal, Right			
N Carpal, Left			
P Metacarpal, Right			
Q Metacarpal, Left			
R Thumb Phalanx, Right			
S Thumb Phalanx, Left			
T Finger Phalanx, Right			
V Finger Phalanx, Left			

⊞ ØPU[34]3JZ

Coding Clinic: 2015, Q2, P20 – ØPU30KZ

SECTION: Ø MEDICAL AND SURGICAL
BODY SYSTEM: P UPPER BONES
OPERATION: W REVISION: Correcting, to the extent possible, a portion of a malfunctioning device or the position of a displaced device

W: REVISION

P: UPPER BONES

Ø: M/S

Body Part	Approach	Device	Qualifier
Ø Sternum 1 Rib, 1 to 2 2 Rib, 3 or More 3 Cervical Vertebra 4 Thoracic Vertebra 5 Scapula, Right 6 Scapula, Left 7 Glenoid Cavity, Right 8 Glenoid Cavity, Left 9 Clavicle, Right B Clavicle, Left	Ø Open 3 Percutaneous 4 Percutaneous Endoscopic X External	4 Internal Fixation Device 7 Autologous Tissue Substitute J Synthetic Substitute K Nonautologous Tissue Substitute	Z No Qualifier
C Humeral Head, Right D Humeral Head, Left F Humeral Shaft, Right G Humeral Shaft, Left H Radius, Right J Radius, Left K Ulna, Right L Ulna, Left M Carpal, Right N Carpal, Left P Metacarpal, Right Q Metacarpal, Left R Thumb Phalanx, Right S Thumb Phalanx, Left T Finger Phalanx, Right V Finger Phalanx, Left	Ø Open 3 Percutaneous 4 Percutaneous Endoscopic X External	4 Internal Fixation Device 5 External Fixation Device 7 Autologous Tissue Substitute J Synthetic Substitute K Nonautologous Tissue Substitute	Z No Qualifier
Y Upper Bone	Ø Open 3 Percutaneous 4 Percutaneous Endoscopic X External	Ø Drainage Device M Bone Growth Stimulator	Z No Qualifier

Non-OR ØPW[Ø123456789B]X[47JK]Z
Non-OR ØPW[CDFGHJKLMNPQRSTV]X[457JK]Z
Non-OR ØPWYX[ØM]Z

SECTION: Ø MEDICAL AND SURGICAL
BODY SYSTEM: Q LOWER BONES
OPERATION: 2 **CHANGE:** Taking out or off a device from a body part and putting back an identical or similar device in or on the same body part without cutting or puncturing the skin or a mucous membrane

Body Part	Approach	Device	Qualifier
Y Lower Bone	X External	Ø Drainage Device Y Other Device	Z No Qualifier

Non-OR All Values

SECTION: Ø MEDICAL AND SURGICAL
BODY SYSTEM: Q LOWER BONES
OPERATION: 5 **DESTRUCTION:** Physical eradication of all or a portion of a body part by the direct use of energy, force, or a destructive agent

Body Part	Approach	Device	Qualifier
Ø Lumbar Vertebra 1 Sacrum 2 Pelvic Bone, Right 3 Pelvic Bone, Left 4 Acetabulum, Right 5 Acetabulum, Left 6 Upper Femur, Right 7 Upper Femur, Left 8 Femoral Shaft, Right 9 Femoral Shaft, Left B Lower Femur, Right C Lower Femur, Left D Patella, Right F Patella, Left G Tibia, Right H Tibia, Left J Fibula, Right K Fibula, Left L Tarsal, Right M Tarsal, Left N Metatarsal, Right P Metatarsal, Left Q Toe Phalanx, Right R Toe Phalanx, Left S Coccyx	Ø Open 3 Percutaneous 4 Percutaneous Endoscopic	Z No Device	Z No Qualifier

2: CHANGE 5: DESTRUCTION
Q: LOWER BONES
Ø: M/S

SECTION: 0 MEDICAL AND SURGICAL

BODY SYSTEM: Q LOWER BONES

OPERATION: 8 DIVISION: Cutting into a body part, without draining fluids and/or gases from the body part, in order to separate or transect a body part

Body Part	Approach	Device	Qualifier
0 Lumbar Vertebra 1 Sacrum 2 Pelvic Bone, Right 3 Pelvic Bone, Left 4 Acetabulum, Right 5 Acetabulum, Left 6 Upper Femur, Right 7 Upper Femur, Left 8 Femoral Shaft, Right 9 Femoral Shaft, Left B Lower Femur, Right C Lower Femur, Left D Patella, Right F Patella, Left G Tibia, Right H Tibia, Left J Fibula, Right K Fibula, Left L Tarsal, Right M Tarsal, Left N Metatarsal, Right P Metatarsal, Left Q Toe Phalanx, Right R Toe Phalanx, Left S Coccyx	0 Open 3 Percutaneous 4 Percutaneous Endoscopic	Z No Device	Z No Qualifier

Coding Clinic: 2016, Q2, P32 – 0Q830ZZ

SECTION: 0 MEDICAL AND SURGICAL

BODY SYSTEM: Q LOWER BONES

OPERATION: 9 DRAINAGE: Taking or letting out fluids and/or gases from a body part

Body Part	Approach	Device	Qualifier
0 Lumbar Vertebra 1 Sacrum 2 Pelvic Bone, Right 3 Pelvic Bone, Left 4 Acetabulum, Right 5 Acetabulum, Left 6 Upper Femur, Right 7 Upper Femur, Left 8 Femoral Shaft, Right 9 Femoral Shaft, Left B Lower Femur, Right C Lower Femur, Left D Patella, Right F Patella, Left G Tibia, Right H Tibia, Left J Fibula, Right K Fibula, Left L Tarsal, Right M Tarsal, Left N Metatarsal, Right P Metatarsal, Left Q Toe Phalanx, Right R Toe Phalanx, Left S Coccyx	0 Open 3 Percutaneous 4 Percutaneous Endoscopic	0 Drainage Device	Z No Qualifier
0 Lumbar Vertebra 1 Sacrum 2 Pelvic Bone, Right 3 Pelvic Bone, Left 4 Acetabulum, Right 5 Acetabulum, Left 6 Upper Femur, Right 7 Upper Femur, Left 8 Femoral Shaft, Right 9 Femoral Shaft, Left B Lower Femur, Right C Lower Femur, Left D Patella, Right F Patella, Left G Tibia, Right H Tibia, Left J Fibula, Right K Fibula, Left L Tarsal, Right M Tarsal, Left N Metatarsal, Right P Metatarsal, Left Q Toe Phalanx, Right R Toe Phalanx, Left S Coccyx	0 Open 3 Percutaneous 4 Percutaneous Endoscopic	Z No Device	X Diagnostic Z No Qualifier

Non-OR 0Q9[0123456789BCDFGHJKLMNPQRS]30Z
Non-OR 0Q9[0123456789BCDFGHJKLMNPQRS]3ZZ

9: DRAINAGE

Q: LOWER BONES

0: M/S

SECTION: Ø MEDICAL AND SURGICAL

BODY SYSTEM: Q LOWER BONES

OPERATION: B EXCISION: Cutting out or off, without replacement, a portion of a body part

Body Part	Approach	Device	Qualifier
Ø Lumbar Vertebra 1 Sacrum 2 Pelvic Bone, Right 3 Pelvic Bone, Left 4 Acetabulum, Right 5 Acetabulum, Left 6 Upper Femur, Right 7 Upper Femur, Left 8 Femoral Shaft, Right 9 Femoral Shaft, Left B Lower Femur, Right C Lower Femur, Left D Patella, Right F Patella, Left G Tibia, Right H Tibia, Left J Fibula, Right K Fibula, Left L Tarsal, Right M Tarsal, Left N Metatarsal, Right P Metatarsal, Left Q Toe Phalanx, Right R Toe Phalanx, Left S Coccyx	Ø Open 3 Percutaneous 4 Percutaneous Endoscopic	Z No Device	X Diagnostic Z No Qualifier

Coding Clinic: 2013, Q2, P40 – ØQBKØZZ
Coding Clinic: 2015, Q3, P4 – ØQBSØZZ
Coding Clinic: 2017, Q1, P24 – ØQBJØZZ

SECTION: Ø MEDICAL AND SURGICAL
BODY SYSTEM: Q LOWER BONES
OPERATION: C EXTIRPATION: Taking or cutting out solid matter from a body part

Body Part	Approach	Device	Qualifier
Ø Lumbar Vertebra 1 Sacrum 2 Pelvic Bone, Right 3 Pelvic Bone, Left 4 Acetabulum, Right 5 Acetabulum, Left 6 Upper Femur, Right 7 Upper Femur, Left 8 Femoral Shaft, Right 9 Femoral Shaft, Left B Lower Femur, Right C Lower Femur, Left D Patella, Right F Patella, Left G Tibia, Right H Tibia, Left J Fibula, Right K Fibula, Left L Tarsal, Right M Tarsal, Left N Metatarsal, Right P Metatarsal, Left Q Toe Phalanx, Right R Toe Phalanx, Left S Coccyx	Ø Open 3 Percutaneous 4 Percutaneous Endoscopic	Z No Device	Z No Qualifier

C: EXTIRPATION

Q: LOWER BONES

Ø: M/S

SECTION: 0 MEDICAL AND SURGICAL

BODY SYSTEM: Q LOWER BONES

OPERATION: D **EXTRACTION:** Pulling or stripping out or off all or a portion of a body part by the use of force

Body Part	Approach	Device	Qualifier
0 Lumbar Vertebra	0 Open	Z No Device	Z No Qualifier
1 Sacrum			
2 Pelvic Bone, Right			
3 Pelvic Bone, Left			
4 Acetabulum, Right			
5 Acetabulum, Left			
6 Upper Femur, Right			
7 Upper Femur, Left			
8 Femoral Shaft, Right			
9 Femoral Shaft, Left			
B Lower Femur, Right			
C Lower Femur, Left			
D Patella, Right			
F Patella, Left			
G Tibia, Right			
H Tibia, Left			
J Fibula, Right			
K Fibula, Left			
L Tarsal, Right			
M Tarsal, Left			
N Metatarsal, Right			
P Metatarsal, Left			
Q Toe Phalanx, Right			
R Toe Phalanx, Left			
S Coccyx			

SECTION: Ø MEDICAL AND SURGICAL

BODY SYSTEM: Q LOWER BONES

OPERATION: H INSERTION: Putting in a nonbiological appliance that monitors, assists, performs, or prevents a physiological function but does not physically take the place of a body part

Body Part	Approach	Device	Qualifier
Ø Lumbar Vertebra 1 Sacrum 2 Pelvic Bone, Right 3 Pelvic Bone, Left 4 Acetabulum, Right 5 Acetabulum, Left D Patella, Right F Patella, Left L Tarsal, Right M Tarsal, Left N Metatarsal, Right P Metatarsal, Left Q Toe Phalanx, Right R Toe Phalanx, Left S Coccyx	Ø Open 3 Percutaneous 4 Percutaneous Endoscopic	4 Internal Fixation Device 5 External Fixation Device	Z No Qualifier
6 Upper Femur, Right 7 Upper Femur, Left 8 Femoral Shaft, Right 9 Femoral Shaft, Left B Lower Femur, Right C Lower Femur, Left G Tibia, Right H Tibia, Left J Fibula, Right K Fibula, Left	Ø Open 3 Percutaneous 4 Percutaneous Endoscopic	4 Internal Fixation Device 5 External Fixation Device 6 Internal Fixation Device, Intramedullary 8 External Fixation Device, Limb Lengthening B External Fixation Device, Monoplanar C External Fixation Device, Ring D External Fixation Device, Hybrid	Z No Qualifier
Y Lower Bone	Ø Open 3 Percutaneous 4 Percutaneous Endoscopic	M Bone Growth Stimulator	Z No Qualifier

Non-OR ØQH[6789BCGHJK][Ø34]8Z

Coding Clinic: 2Ø16, Q3, P35 – ØQH[GJ]Ø4Z
Coding Clinic: 2Ø17, Q1, P22 – ØQH[23]Ø4Z

H: INSERTION

Q: LOWER BONES

Ø: M/S

SECTION: Ø MEDICAL AND SURGICAL

BODY SYSTEM: Q LOWER BONES

OPERATION: J INSPECTION: Visually and/or manually exploring a body part

Body Part	Approach	Device	Qualifier
Y Lower Bone	Ø Open 3 Percutaneous 4 Percutaneous Endoscopic X External	Z No Device	Z No Qualifier

Non-OR ØQJY[3X]ZZ

SECTION: Ø MEDICAL AND SURGICAL

BODY SYSTEM: Q LOWER BONES

OPERATION: N RELEASE: Freeing a body part from an abnormal physical constraint by cutting or by the use of force

Body Part	Approach	Device	Qualifier
Ø Lumbar Vertebra 1 Sacrum 2 Pelvic Bone, Right 3 Pelvic Bone, Left 4 Acetabulum, Right 5 Acetabulum, Left 6 Upper Femur, Right 7 Upper Femur, Left 8 Femoral Shaft, Right 9 Femoral Shaft, Left B Lower Femur, Right C Lower Femur, Left D Patella, Right F Patella, Left G Tibia, Right H Tibia, Left J Fibula, Right K Fibula, Left L Tarsal, Right M Tarsal, Left N Metatarsal, Right P Metatarsal, Left Q Toe Phalanx, Right R Toe Phalanx, Left S Coccyx	Ø Open 3 Percutaneous 4 Percutaneous Endoscopic	Z No Device	Z No Qualifier

Ø: M/S   Q: LOWER BONES   J: INSPECTION   N: RELEASE

SECTION: Ø MEDICAL AND SURGICAL

BODY SYSTEM: Q LOWER BONES

OPERATION: P REMOVAL: *(on multiple pages)*

Taking out or off a device from a body part

Body Part	Approach	Device	Qualifier
Ø Lumbar Vertebra 1 Sacrum 4 Acetabulum, Right 5 Acetabulum, Left S Coccyx	Ø Open 3 Percutaneous 4 Percutaneous Endoscopic	4 Internal Fixation Device 7 Autologous Tissue Substitute J Synthetic Substitute K Nonautologous Tissue Substitute	Z No Qualifier
Ø Lumbar Vertebra 1 Sacrum 4 Acetabulum, Right 5 Acetabulum, Left S Coccyx	X External	4 Internal Fixation Device	Z No Qualifier
2 Pelvic Bone, Right 3 Pelvic Bone, Left 6 Upper Femur, Right 7 Upper Femur, Left 8 Femoral Shaft, Right 9 Femoral Shaft, Left B Lower Femur, Right C Lower Femur, Left D Patella, Right F Patella, Left G Tibia, Right H Tibia, Left J Fibula, Right K Fibula, Left L Tarsal, Right M Tarsal, Left N Metatarsal, Right P Metatarsal, Left Q Toe Phalanx, Right R Toe Phalanx, Left	Ø Open 3 Percutaneous 4 Percutaneous Endoscopic	4 Internal Fixation Device 5 External Fixation Device 7 Autologous Tissue Substitute J Synthetic Substitute K Nonautologous Tissue Substitute	Z No Qualifier
2 Pelvic Bone, Right 3 Pelvic Bone, Left 6 Upper Femur, Right 7 Upper Femur, Left 8 Femoral Shaft, Right 9 Femoral Shaft, Left B Lower Femur, Right C Lower Femur, Left D Patella, Right F Patella, Left G Tibia, Right H Tibia, Left J Fibula, Right K Fibula, Left L Tarsal, Right M Tarsal, Left N Metatarsal, Right P Metatarsal, Left Q Toe Phalanx, Right R Toe Phalanx, Left	X External	4 Internal Fixation Device 5 External Fixation Device	Z No Qualifier

P: REMOVAL

Q: LOWER BONES

Ø: M/S

Non-OR ØQP[Ø145S]X4Z

Non-OR ØQP[236789BCDFGHJKLMNPQR]X[45]Z

Coding Clinic: 2Ø15, Q2, P6 – ØQPGØ4Z

Coding Clinic: 2Ø17, Q4, P75 – ØQPØØ4Z

New/Revised Text in Green   ~~deleted~~ Deleted   ♀ Females Only   ♂ Males Only   **Coding Clinic**

Non-covered   Limited Coverage   ⊞ Combination (See Appendix E)   DRG Non-OR   Non-OR   Hospital-Acquired Condition

SECTION: 0 MEDICAL AND SURGICAL

BODY SYSTEM: Q LOWER BONES

OPERATION: P REMOVAL: *(continued)*
Taking out or off a device from a body part

Body Part	Approach	Device	Qualifier
Y Lower Bone	0 Open 3 Percutaneous 4 Percutaneous Endoscopic X External	0 Drainage Device M Bone Growth Stimulator	Z No Qualifier

Non-OR 0QPY30Z
Non-OR 0QPYX[0M]Z

SECTION: 0 MEDICAL AND SURGICAL

BODY SYSTEM: Q LOWER BONES

OPERATION: Q REPAIR: Restoring, to the extent possible, a body part to its normal anatomic structure and function

Body Part	Approach	Device	Qualifier
0 Lumbar Vertebra 1 Sacrum 2 Pelvic Bone, Right 3 Pelvic Bone, Left 4 Acetabulum, Right 5 Acetabulum, Left 6 Upper Femur, Right 7 Upper Femur, Left 8 Femoral Shaft, Right 9 Femoral Shaft, Left B Lower Femur, Right C Lower Femur, Left D Patella, Right F Patella, Left G Tibia, Right H Tibia, Left J Fibula, Right K Fibula, Left L Tarsal, Right M Tarsal, Left N Metatarsal, Right P Metatarsal, Left Q Toe Phalanx, Right R Toe Phalanx, Left S Coccyx	0 Open 3 Percutaneous 4 Percutaneous Endoscopic X External	Z No Device	Z No Qualifier

DRG Non-OR 0QQ[0123456789BCDFGHJKLMNPQRS]XZZ

Coding Clinic: 2018, Q1, P15 – 0QQ[23]0ZZ

SECTION: Ø MEDICAL AND SURGICAL

BODY SYSTEM: Q LOWER BONES

OPERATION: R REPLACEMENT: Putting in or on biological or synthetic material that physically takes the place and/or function of all or a portion of a body part

Body Part	Approach	Device	Qualifier
Ø Lumbar Vertebra	Ø Open	7 Autologous Tissue Substitute	Z No Qualifier
1 Sacrum	3 Percutaneous	J Synthetic Substitute	
2 Pelvic Bone, Right	4 Percutaneous Endoscopic	K Nonautologous Tissue	
3 Pelvic Bone, Left		Substitute	
4 Acetabulum, Right			
5 Acetabulum, Left			
6 Upper Femur, Right			
7 Upper Femur, Left			
8 Femoral Shaft, Right			
9 Femoral Shaft, Left			
B Lower Femur, Right			
C Lower Femur, Left			
D Patella, Right			
F Patella, Left			
G Tibia, Right			
H Tibia, Left			
J Fibula, Right			
K Fibula, Left			
L Tarsal, Right			
M Tarsal, Left			
N Metatarsal, Right			
P Metatarsal, Left			
Q Toe Phalanx, Right			
R Toe Phalanx, Left			
S Coccyx			

R: REPLACEMENT

Q: LOWER BONES

Ø: M/S

SECTION: Ø MEDICAL AND SURGICAL

BODY SYSTEM: Q LOWER BONES
OPERATION: S REPOSITION: *(on multiple pages)*
Moving to its normal location, or other suitable location, all or a portion of a body part

Body Part	Approach	Device	Qualifier
Ø Lumbar Vertebra ⊞ 1 Sacrum ⊞ 4 Acetabulum, Right 5 Acetabulum, Left S Coccyx ⊞	Ø Open 3 Percutaneous 4 Percutaneous Endoscopic	4 Internal Fixation Device Z No Device	Z No Qualifier
Ø Lumbar Vertebra 1 Sacrum 4 Acetabulum, Right 5 Acetabulum, Left S Coccyx	X External	Z No Device	Z No Qualifier
2 Pelvic Bone, Right 3 Pelvic Bone, Left D Patella, Right F Patella, Left L Tarsal, Right M Tarsal, Left Q Toe Phalanx, Right R Toe Phalanx, Left	Ø Open 3 Percutaneous 4 Percutaneous Endoscopic	4 Internal Fixation Device 5 External Fixation Device Z No Device	Z No Qualifier
2 Pelvic Bone, Right 3 Pelvic Bone, Left D Patella, Right F Patella, Left L Tarsal, Right M Tarsal, Left Q Toe Phalanx, Right R Toe Phalanx, Left	X External	Z No Device	Z No Qualifier
6 Upper Femur, Right 7 Upper Femur, Left 8 Femoral Shaft, Right 9 Femoral Shaft, Left B Lower Femur, Right C Lower Femur, Left G Tibia, Right H Tibia, Left J Fibula, Right K Fibula, Left	Ø Open 3 Percutaneous 4 Percutaneous Endoscopic	4 Internal Fixation Device 5 External Fixation Device 6 Internal Fixation Device, Intramedullary B External Fixation Device, Monoplanar C External Fixation Device, Ring D External Fixation Device, Hybrid Z No Device	Z No Qualifier

⊞ ØQS[Ø1S]3ZZ

Non-OR ØQS[45][34]ZZ

Non-OR ØQS[45]XZZ

Non-OR ØQS[23DFLMQR][34]ZZ

Non-OR ØQS[23DFLMQR]XZZ

Non-OR ØQS[6789BCGHJK][34]ZZ

Coding Clinic: 2016, Q3, P35 – ØQS[FH]Ø4Z
Coding Clinic: 2016, Q3, P35 – ØQSKØZZ
Coding Clinic: 2018, Q1, P13 – ØQS[LM]Ø4Z

Ø: M/S   Q: LOWER BONES   S: REPOSITION

SECTION: **Ø   MEDICAL AND SURGICAL**

BODY SYSTEM: Q LOWER BONES

OPERATION: S   **REPOSITION:** *(continued)*
Moving to its normal location, or other suitable location, all or a portion of a body part

Body Part	Approach	Device	Qualifier
6 Upper Femur, Right 7 Upper Femur, Left 8 Femoral Shaft, Right 9 Femoral Shaft, Left B Lower Femur, Right C Lower Femur, Left G Tibia, Right H Tibia, Left J Fibula, Right K Fibula, Left	X External	Z No Device	Z No Qualifier
N Metatarsal, Right P Metatarsal, Left	Ø Open 3 Percutaneous 4 Percutaneous Endoscopic	4 Internal Fixation Device 5 External Fixation Device Z No Device	2 Sesamoid Bone(s) 1st Toe Z No Qualifier
N Metatarsal, Right P Metatarsal, Left	X External	Z No Device	2 Sesamoid Bone(s) 1st Toe Z No Qualifier

Non-OR   ØQS[6789BCGHJK]XZZ   Non-OR   ØQS[NP][34]ZZ   Non-OR   ØQS[NP]XZZ

SECTION: **Ø   MEDICAL AND SURGICAL**

BODY SYSTEM: Q LOWER BONES

OPERATION: T   **RESECTION:** Cutting out or off, without replacement, all of a body part

Body Part	Approach	Device	Qualifier
2 Pelvic Bone, Right 3 Pelvic Bone, Left 4 Acetabulum, Right 5 Acetabulum, Left 6 Upper Femur, Right 7 Upper Femur, Left 8 Femoral Shaft, Right 9 Femoral Shaft, Left B Lower Femur, Right C Lower Femur, Left D Patella, Right F Patella, Left G Tibia, Right H Tibia, Left J Fibula, Right K Fibula, Left L Tarsal, Right M Tarsal, Left N Metatarsal, Right P Metatarsal, Left Q Toe Phalanx, Right R Toe Phalanx, Left S Coccyx	Ø Open	Z No Device	Z No Qualifier

Coding Clinic: 2015, Q3, P26 – ØQT7ØZZ
Coding Clinic: 2016, Q3, P30 – ØQT[67]ØZZ

New/Revised Text in Green   ~~deleted~~ Deleted   ♀ Females Only   ♂ Males Only   **Coding Clinic**
🔷 Non-covered   🔷 Limited Coverage   ⊕ Combination (See Appendix E)   DRG Non-OR   Non-OR   🔷 Hospital-Acquired Condition

SECTION: Ø MEDICAL AND SURGICAL

BODY SYSTEM: Q LOWER BONES

OPERATION: U SUPPLEMENT: Putting in or on biological or synthetic material that physically reinforces and/or augments the function of a portion of a body part

Body Part	Approach	Device	Qualifier
Ø Lumbar Vertebra ⊞ 1 Sacrum ⊞ 2 Pelvic Bone, Right 3 Pelvic Bone, Left 4 Acetabulum, Right 5 Acetabulum, Left 6 Upper Femur, Right 7 Upper Femur, Left 8 Femoral Shaft, Right 9 Femoral Shaft, Left B Lower Femur, Right C Lower Femur, Left D Patella, Right F Patella, Left G Tibia, Right H Tibia, Left J Fibula, Right K Fibula, Left L Tarsal, Right M Tarsal, Left N Metatarsal, Right P Metatarsal, Left Q Toe Phalanx, Right R Toe Phalanx, Left S Coccyx	Ø Open 3 Percutaneous 4 Percutaneous Endoscopic	7 Autologous Tissue Substitute J Synthetic Substitute K Nonautologous Tissue Substitute	Z No Qualifier

⊞ ØQU[Ø1S]3JZ

Coding Clinic: 2013, Q2, P36 – ØQU2ØJZ
Coding Clinic: 2015, Q3, P19 – ØQU5ØJZ

SECTION: Ø MEDICAL AND SURGICAL
BODY SYSTEM: Q LOWER BONES
OPERATION: W REVISION: Correcting, to the extent possible, a portion of a malfunctioning device or the position of a displaced device

Body Part	Approach	Device	Qualifier
Ø Lumbar Vertebra 1 Sacrum 4 Acetabulum, Right 5 Acetabulum, Left S Coccyx	Ø Open 3 Percutaneous 4 Percutaneous Endoscopic X External	4 Internal Fixation Device 7 Autologous Tissue Substitute J Synthetic Substitute K Nonautologous Tissue Substitute	Z No Qualifier
2 Pelvic Bone, Right 3 Pelvic Bone, Left 6 Upper Femur, Right 7 Upper Femur, Left 8 Femoral Shaft, Right 9 Femoral Shaft, Left B Lower Femur, Right C Lower Femur, Left D Patella, Right F Patella, Left G Tibia, Right H Tibia, Left J Fibula, Right K Fibula, Left L Tarsal, Right M Tarsal, Left N Metatarsal, Right P Metatarsal, Left Q Toe Phalanx, Right R Toe Phalanx, Left	Ø Open 3 Percutaneous 4 Percutaneous Endoscopic X External	4 Internal Fixation Device 5 External Fixation Device 7 Autologous Tissue Substitute J Synthetic Substitute K Nonautologous Tissue Substitute	Z No Qualifier
Y Lower Bone	Ø Open 3 Percutaneous 4 Percutaneous Endoscopic X External	Ø Drainage Device M Bone Growth Stimulator	Z No Qualifier

Non-OR ØQW[0145S]X[47JK]Z
Non-OR ØQW[236789BCDFGHJKLMNPQR]X[457JK]Z
Non-OR ØQWYX[ØM]Z

Coding Clinic: 2Ø17, Q4, P75 – ØQWØ34Z

New/Revised Text in Green   ~~deleted~~ Deleted   ♀ Females Only   ♂ Males Only   **Coding Clinic**

Non-covered   Limited Coverage   Combination (See Appendix E)   DRG Non-OR   Non-OR   Hospital-Acquired Condition

SECTION: Ø MEDICAL AND SURGICAL

BODY SYSTEM: R UPPER JOINTS

OPERATION: 2 **CHANGE:** Taking out or off a device from a body part and putting back an identical or similar device in or on the same body part without cutting or puncturing the skin or a mucous membrane

Body Part	Approach	Device	Qualifier
Y Upper Joint	X External	Ø Drainage Device Y Other Device	Z No Qualifier

Non-OR   All Values

SECTION: Ø MEDICAL AND SURGICAL

BODY SYSTEM: R UPPER JOINTS

OPERATION: 5 **DESTRUCTION:** Physical eradication of all or a portion of a body part by the direct use of energy, force, or destructive agent

Body Part	Approach	Device	Qualifier
Ø Occipital-cervical Joint 1 Cervical Vertebral Joint 3 Cervical Vertebral Disc 4 Cervicothoracic Vertebral Joint 5 Cervicothoracic Vertebral Disc 6 Thoracic Vertebral Joint 9 Thoracic Vertebral Disc A Thoracolumbar Vertebral Joint B Thoracolumbar Vertebral Disc C Temporomandibular Joint, Right D Temporomandibular Joint, Left E Sternoclavicular Joint, Right F Sternoclavicular Joint, Left G Acromioclavicular Joint, Right H Acromioclavicular Joint, Left J Shoulder Joint, Right K Shoulder Joint, Left L Elbow Joint, Right M Elbow Joint, Left N Wrist Joint, Right P Wrist Joint, Left Q Carpal Joint, Right R Carpal Joint, Left S Carpometacarpal Joint, Right T Carpometacarpal Joint, Left U Metacarpophalangeal Joint, Right V Metacarpophalangeal Joint, Left W Finger Phalangeal Joint, Right X Finger Phalangeal Joint, Left	Ø Open 3 Percutaneous 4 Percutaneous Endoscopic	Z No Device	Z No Qualifier

Non-OR   ØR5[359B][34]ZZ

SECTION: Ø MEDICAL AND SURGICAL
BODY SYSTEM: R UPPER JOINTS
OPERATION: 9 DRAINAGE: *(on multiple pages)*
Taking or letting out fluids and/or gases from a body part

Body Part	Approach	Device	Qualifier
Ø Occipital-cervical Joint	Ø Open	Ø Drainage Device	Z No Qualifier
1 Cervical Vertebral Joint	3 Percutaneous		
3 Cervical Vertebral Disc	4 Percutaneous Endoscopic		
4 Cervicothoracic Vertebral Joint			
5 Cervicothoracic Vertebral Disc			
6 Thoracic Vertebral Joint			
9 Thoracic Vertebral Disc			
A Thoracolumbar Vertebral Joint			
B Thoracolumbar Vertebral Disc			
C Temporomandibular Joint, Right			
D Temporomandibular Joint, Left			
E Sternoclavicular Joint, Right			
F Sternoclavicular Joint, Left			
G Acromioclavicular Joint, Right			
H Acromioclavicular Joint, Left			
J Shoulder Joint, Right			
K Shoulder Joint, Left			
L Elbow Joint, Right			
M Elbow Joint, Left			
N Wrist Joint, Right			
P Wrist Joint, Left			
Q Carpal Joint, Right			
R Carpal Joint, Left			
S Carpometacarpal Joint, Right			
T Carpometacarpal Joint, Left			
U Metacarpophalangeal Joint, Right			
V Metacarpophalangeal Joint, Left			
W Finger Phalangeal Joint, Right			
X Finger Phalangeal Joint, Left			

Non-OR ØR9[CD]30Z
Non-OR ØR9[0134569ABEFGHJKLMNPQRSTUVWX][34]0Z

SECTION: Ø MEDICAL AND SURGICAL

BODY SYSTEM: R UPPER JOINTS

OPERATION: 9 DRAINAGE: *(continued)*
Taking or letting out fluids and/or gases from a body part

Body Part	Approach	Device	Qualifier
Ø Occipital-cervical Joint	Ø Open	Z No Device	X Diagnostic
1 Cervical Vertebral Joint	3 Percutaneous		Z No Qualifier
3 Cervical Vertebral Disc	4 Percutaneous Endoscopic		
4 Cervicothoracic Vertebral Joint			
5 Cervicothoracic Vertebral Disc			
6 Thoracic Vertebral Joint			
9 Thoracic Vertebral Disc			
A Thoracolumbar Vertebral Joint			
B Thoracolumbar Vertebral Disc			
C Temporomandibular Joint, Right			
D Temporomandibular Joint, Left			
E Sternoclavicular Joint, Right			
F Sternoclavicular Joint, Left			
G Acromioclavicular Joint, Right			
H Acromioclavicular Joint, Left			
J Shoulder Joint, Right			
K Shoulder Joint, Left			
L Elbow Joint, Right			
M Elbow Joint, Left			
N Wrist Joint, Right			
P Wrist Joint, Left			
Q Carpal Joint, Right			
R Carpal Joint, Left			
S Carpometacarpal Joint, Right			
T Carpometacarpal Joint, Left			
U Metacarpophalangeal Joint, Right			
V Metacarpophalangeal Joint, Left			
W Finger Phalangeal Joint, Right			
X Finger Phalangeal Joint, Left			

DRG Non-OR ØR9[CD]3ZZ
Non-OR ØR9[Ø134569ABEFGHJKLMNPQRSTUVWX][Ø34]ZX
Non-OR ØR9[Ø134569ABEFGHJKLMNPQRSTUVWX][34]ZZ

SECTION: Ø MEDICAL AND SURGICAL

BODY SYSTEM: R UPPER JOINTS

OPERATION: B EXCISION: Cutting out or off, without replacement, a portion of a body part

Body Part	Approach	Device	Qualifier
Ø Occipital-cervical Joint 1 Cervical Vertebral Joint 3 Cervical Vertebral Disc 4 Cervicothoracic Vertebral Joint 5 Cervicothoracic Vertebral Disc 6 Thoracic Vertebral Joint 9 Thoracic Vertebral Disc A Thoracolumbar Vertebral Joint B Thoracolumbar Vertebral Disc C Temporomandibular Joint, Right D Temporomandibular Joint, Left E Sternoclavicular Joint, Right F Sternoclavicular Joint, Left G Acromioclavicular Joint, Right H Acromioclavicular Joint, Left J Shoulder Joint, Right K Shoulder Joint, Left L Elbow Joint, Right M Elbow Joint, Left N Wrist Joint, Right P Wrist Joint, Left Q Carpal Joint, Right R Carpal Joint, Left S Carpometacarpal Joint, Right T Carpometacarpal Joint, Left U Metacarpophalangeal Joint, Right V Metacarpophalangeal Joint, Left W Finger Phalangeal Joint, Right X Finger Phalangeal Joint, Left	Ø Open 3 Percutaneous 4 Percutaneous Endoscopic	Z No Device	X Diagnostic Z No Qualifier

Non-OR   ØRB[Ø134569ABEFGHJKLMNPQRSTUVWX][Ø34]ZX

New/Revised Text in Green   deleted Deleted   ♀ Females Only   ♂ Males Only   Coding Clinic
Non-covered   Limited Coverage   ⊞ Combination (See Appendix E)   DRG Non-OR   Non-OR   Hospital-Acquired Condition

423

SECTION: Ø MEDICAL AND SURGICAL

BODY SYSTEM: R UPPER JOINTS

OPERATION: C EXTIRPATION: Taking or cutting out solid matter from a body part

Body Part	Approach	Device	Qualifier
Ø Occipital-cervical Joint 1 Cervical Vertebral Joint 3 Cervical Vertebral Disc 4 Cervicothoracic Vertebral Joint 5 Cervicothoracic Vertebral Disc 6 Thoracic Vertebral Joint 9 Thoracic Vertebral Disc A Thoracolumbar Vertebral Joint B Thoracolumbar Vertebral Disc C Temporomandibular Joint, Right D Temporomandibular Joint, Left E Sternoclavicular Joint, Right F Sternoclavicular Joint, Left G Acromioclavicular Joint, Right H Acromioclavicular Joint, Left J Shoulder Joint, Right K Shoulder Joint, Left L Elbow Joint, Right M Elbow Joint, Left N Wrist Joint, Right P Wrist Joint, Left Q Carpal Joint, Right R Carpal Joint, Left S Carpometacarpal Joint, Right T Carpometacarpal Joint, Left U Metacarpophalangeal Joint, Right V Metacarpophalangeal Joint, Left W Finger Phalangeal Joint, Right X Finger Phalangeal Joint, Left	Ø Open 3 Percutaneous 4 Percutaneous Endoscopic	Z No Device	Z No Qualifier

C: EXTIRPATION

R: UPPER JOINTS

Ø: M/S

New/Revised Text in Green   ~~deleted~~ Deleted   ♀ Females Only   ♂ Males Only   **Coding Clinic**

Non-covered   Limited Coverage   ⊟ Combination (See Appendix E)   DRG Non-OR   Non-OR   Hospital-Acquired Condition

SECTION: Ø MEDICAL AND SURGICAL
BODY SYSTEM: R UPPER JOINTS
OPERATION: **G FUSION:** Joining together portions of an articular body part, rendering the articular body part immobile

Body Part	Approach	Device	Qualifier
Ø Occipital-cervical Joint 🔖 1 Cervical Vertebral Joint 🔖 2 Cervical Vertebral Joints, 2 or more 🔖 4 Cervicothoracic Vertebral Joint 🔖 6 Thoracic Vertebral Joint 🔖 7 Thoracic Vertebral Joint, 2 to 7 ⊞ 🔖 8 Thoracic Vertebral Joint, 8 or more 🔖 A Thoracolumbar Vertebral Joint 🔖	Ø Open 3 Percutaneous 4 Percutaneous Endoscopic	7 Autologous Tissue Substitute J Synthetic Substitute K Nonautologous Tissue Substitute ~~Z No Device~~	Ø Anterior Approach, Anterior Column 1 Posterior Approach, Posterior Column J Posterior Approach, Anterior Column
Ø Occipital-cervical Joint 🔖 1 Cervical Vertebral Joint 🔖 2 Cervical Vertebral Joints, 2 or more 🔖 4 Cervicothoracic Vertebral Joint 🔖 6 Thoracic Vertebral Joint 🔖 7 Thoracic Vertebral Joints, 2 to 7 ⊞ 🔖 8 Thoracic Vertebral Joints, 8 or more 🔖 A Thoracolumbar Vertebral Joint 🔖	Ø Open 3 Percutaneous 4 Percutaneous Endoscopic	A Interbody Fusion Device	Ø Anterior Approach, Anterior Column J Posterior Approach, Anterior Column
C Temporomandibular Joint, Right D Temporomandibular Joint, Left E Sternoclavicular Joint, Right 🔖 F Sternoclavicular Joint, Left 🔖 G Acromioclavicular Joint, Right 🔖 H Acromioclavicular Joint, Left 🔖 J Shoulder Joint, Right 🔖 K Shoulder Joint, Left 🔖	Ø Open 3 Percutaneous 4 Percutaneous Endoscopic	4 Internal Fixation Device 7 Autologous Tissue Substitute J Synthetic Substitute K Nonautologous Tissue Substitute ~~Z No Device~~	Z No Qualifier
L Elbow Joint, Right 🔖 M Elbow Joint, Left 🔖 N Wrist Joint, Right P Wrist Joint, Left Q Carpal Joint, Right R Carpal Joint, Left S Carpometacarpal Joint, Right T Carpometacarpal Joint, Left U Metacarpophalangeal Joint, Right V Metacarpophalangeal Joint, Left W Finger Phalangeal Joint, Right X Finger Phalangeal Joint, Left	Ø Open 3 Percutaneous 4 Percutaneous Endoscopic	4 Internal Fixation Device 5 External Fixation Device 7 Autologous Tissue Substitute J Synthetic Substitute K Nonautologous Tissue Substitute ~~Z No Device~~	Z No Qualifier

⊞ ØRG7[Ø34][7JKZ][Ø1J]
⊞ ØRG7[Ø34]A[ØJ]
🔖 ØRG[Ø124678A][Ø34][7JKZ][Ø1J] when reported with Secondary Diagnosis K68.11, T81.4XXA, or T84.60XA-T84.7XXA
🔖 ØRG[Ø124678A][Ø34]A[ØJ] when reported with Secondary Diagnosis K68.11, T81.4XXA, or T84.60XA-T84.7XXA
🔖 ØRG[EFGHJK][Ø34][47JKZ]Z when reported with Secondary Diagnosis K68.11, T81.4XXA, or T84.60XA-T84.7XXA
🔖 ØRG[LM][Ø34][457JKZ]Z when reported with Secondary Diagnosis K68.11, T81.4XXA, or T84.60XA-T84.7XXA

Coding Clinic: 2013, Q1, P29 – ØRG40AØ
Coding Clinic: 2013, Q1, P22 – ØRG7071, ØRGAØ71
Coding Clinic: 2017, Q4, P62 – ØRGWØ4Z

New/Revised Text in Green   ~~deleted~~ Deleted   ♀ Females Only   ♂ Males Only   **Coding Clinic**
🔖 Non-covered   ⊞ Limited Coverage   ⊞ Combination (See Appendix E)   DRG Non-OR   Non-OR   🔖 Hospital-Acquired Condition

425

SECTION: Ø MEDICAL AND SURGICAL

BODY SYSTEM: R UPPER JOINTS

OPERATION: H INSERTION: Putting in a nonbiological appliance that monitors, assists, performs, or prevents a physiological function but does not physically take the place of a body part

H: INSERTION

R: UPPER JOINTS

Ø: M/S

Body Part	Approach	Device	Qualifier
Ø Occipital-cervical Joint 1 Cervical Vertebral Joint 4 Cervicothoracic Vertebral Joint 6 Thoracic Vertebral Joint A Thoracolumbar Vertebral Joint	Ø Open 3 Percutaneous 4 Percutaneous Endoscopic	3 Infusion Device 4 Internal Fixation Device 8 Spacer B Spinal Stabilization Device, Interspinous Process C Spinal Stabilization Device, Pedicle-Based D Spinal Stabilization Device, Facet Replacement	Z No Qualifier
3 Cervical Vertebral Disc 5 Cervicothoracic Vertebral Disc 9 Thoracic Vertebral Disc B Thoracolumbar Vertebral Disc	Ø Open 3 Percutaneous 4 Percutaneous Endoscopic	3 Infusion Device	Z No Qualifier
C Temporomandibular Joint, Right D Temporomandibular Joint, Left E Sternoclavicular Joint, Right F Sternoclavicular Joint, Left G Acromioclavicular Joint, Right H Acromioclavicular Joint, Left J Shoulder Joint, Right K Shoulder Joint, Left	Ø Open 3 Percutaneous 4 Percutaneous Endoscopic	3 Infusion Device 4 Internal Fixation Device 8 Spacer	Z No Qualifier
L Elbow Joint, Right M Elbow Joint, Left N Wrist Joint, Right P Wrist Joint, Left Q Carpal Joint, Right R Carpal Joint, Left S Carpometacarpal Joint, Right T Carpometacarpal Joint, Left U Metacarpophalangeal Joint, Right V Metacarpophalangeal Joint, Left W Finger Phalangeal Joint, Right X Finger Phalangeal Joint, Left	Ø Open 3 Percutaneous 4 Percutaneous Endoscopic	3 Infusion Device 4 Internal Fixation Device 5 External Fixation Device 8 Spacer	Z No Qualifier

DRG Non-OR   ØRH[Ø146A][34]3Z
DRG Non-OR   ØRH[359B][34]3Z
DRG Non-OR   ØRH[EFGHJK][34]3Z
DRG Non-OR   ØRH[LMNPQRSTUVWX][34]3Z
Non-OR   ØRH[Ø146A][Ø34][38]Z
Non-OR   ØRH[359B][Ø34]3Z
Non-OR   ØRH[CD]33Z
Non-OR   ØRH[CD][Ø34]8Z
Non-OR   ØRH[EFGHJK][Ø34][38]Z
Non-OR   ØRH[LMNPQRSTUVWX][Ø34][38]Z

Coding Clinic: 2016, Q3, P33 – ØRHJØ4ZZ
Coding Clinic: 2017, Q2, P24 – ØRH1Ø4Z

New/Revised Text in Green   ~~deleted~~ Deleted   ♀ Females Only   ♂ Males Only   **Coding Clinic**
Non-covered   Limited Coverage   ⊞ Combination (See Appendix E)   DRG Non-OR   Non-OR   Hospital-Acquired Condition

SECTION: Ø MEDICAL AND SURGICAL

BODY SYSTEM: R UPPER JOINTS

OPERATION: J INSPECTION: Visually and/or manually exploring a body part

Body Part	Approach	Device	Qualifier
Ø Occipital-cervical Joint	Ø Open	Z No Device	Z No Qualifier
1 Cervical Vertebral Joint	3 Percutaneous		
3 Cervical Vertebral Disc	4 Percutaneous Endoscopic		
4 Cervicothoracic Vertebral Joint	X External		
5 Cervicothoracic Vertebral Disc			
6 Thoracic Vertebral Joint			
9 Thoracic Vertebral Disc			
A Thoracolumbar Vertebral Joint			
B Thoracolumbar Vertebral Disc			
C Temporomandibular Joint, Right			
D Temporomandibular Joint, Left			
E Sternoclavicular Joint, Right			
F Sternoclavicular Joint, Left			
G Acromioclavicular Joint, Right			
H Acromioclavicular Joint, Left			
J Shoulder Joint, Right			
K Shoulder Joint, Left			
L Elbow Joint, Right			
M Elbow Joint, Left			
N Wrist Joint, Right			
P Wrist Joint, Left			
Q Carpal Joint, Right			
R Carpal Joint, Left			
S Carpometacarpal Joint, Right			
T Carpometacarpal Joint, Left			
U Metacarpophalangeal Joint, Right			
V Metacarpophalangeal Joint, Left			
W Finger Phalangeal Joint, Right			
X Finger Phalangeal Joint, Left			

Non-OR ØRJ[Ø134569ABCDEFGHJKLMNPQRSTUVWX][3X]ZZ

Ø: M/S

R: UPPER JOINTS

J: INSPECTION

SECTION: Ø MEDICAL AND SURGICAL

BODY SYSTEM: R UPPER JOINTS

OPERATION: N RELEASE: Freeing a body part from an abnormal physical constraint by cutting or by the use of force

Body Part	Approach	Device	Qualifier
Ø Occipital-cervical Joint	Ø Open	Z No Device	Z No Qualifier
1 Cervical Vertebral Joint	3 Percutaneous		
3 Cervical Vertebral Disc	4 Percutaneous Endoscopic		
4 Cervicothoracic Vertebral Joint	X External		
5 Cervicothoracic Vertebral Disc			
6 Thoracic Vertebral Joint			
9 Thoracic Vertebral Disc			
A Thoracolumbar Vertebral Joint			
B Thoracolumbar Vertebral Disc			
C Temporomandibular Joint, Right			
D Temporomandibular Joint, Left			
E Sternoclavicular Joint, Right			
F Sternoclavicular Joint, Left			
G Acromioclavicular Joint, Right			
H Acromioclavicular Joint, Left			
J Shoulder Joint, Right			
K Shoulder Joint, Left			
L Elbow Joint, Right			
M Elbow Joint, Left			
N Wrist Joint, Right			
P Wrist Joint, Left			
Q Carpal Joint, Right			
R Carpal Joint, Left			
S Carpometacarpal Joint, Right			
T Carpometacarpal Joint, Left			
U Metacarpophalangeal Joint, Right			
V Metacarpophalangeal Joint, Left			
W Finger Phalangeal Joint, Right			
X Finger Phalangeal Joint, Left			

Non-OR ØRN[Ø134569ABCDEFGHJKLMNPQRSTUVWX]XZZ

Coding Clinic: 2Ø15, Q2, P23 – ØRNK4ZZ
Coding Clinic: 2Ø16, Q3, P33 – ØRNJ4ZZ

SECTION: Ø MEDICAL AND SURGICAL

BODY SYSTEM: R UPPER JOINTS

OPERATION: P REMOVAL: *(on multiple pages)*
Taking out or off a device from a body part

Body Part	Approach	Device	Qualifier
Ø Occipital-cervical Joint	Ø Open	Ø Drainage Device	Z No Qualifier
1 Cervical Vertebral Joint	3 Percutaneous	3 Infusion Device	
4 Cervicothoracic Vertebral Joint	4 Percutaneous Endoscopic	4 Internal Fixation Device	
6 Thoracic Vertebral Joint		7 Autologous Tissue Substitute	
A Thoracolumbar Vertebral Joint		8 Spacer	
		A Interbody Fusion Device	
		J Synthetic Substitute	
		K Nonautologous Tissue Substitute	

DRG Non-OR ØRQ[Ø134569ABEFGHJKLMNPQRSTUVWX]XZZ
Non-OR ØRP[Ø146A]3[Ø3]Z
Non-OR ØRP[Ø146A][Ø34]8Z

New/Revised Text in Green   ~~deleted~~ Deleted   ♀ Females Only   ♂ Males Only   **Coding Clinic**
Non-covered   Limited Coverage   ⊞ Combination (See Appendix E)   DRG Non-OR   Non-OR   Hospital-Acquired Condition

SECTION: 0 MEDICAL AND SURGICAL
BODY SYSTEM: R UPPER JOINTS
OPERATION: P REMOVAL: *(continued)*
Taking out or off a device from a body part

Body Part	Approach	Device	Qualifier
0 Occipital-cervical Joint 1 Cervical Vertebral Joint 4 Cervicothoracic Vertebral Joint 6 Thoracic Vertebral Joint A Thoracolumbar Vertebral Joint	X External	0 Drainage Device 3 Infusion Device 4 Internal Fixation Device	Z No Qualifier
3 Cervical Vertebral Disc 5 Cervicothoracic Vertebral Disc 9 Thoracic Vertebral Disc B Thoracolumbar Vertebral Disc	0 Open 3 Percutaneous 4 Percutaneous Endoscopic	0 Drainage Device 3 Infusion Device 7 Autologous Tissue Substitute J Synthetic Substitute K Nonautologous Tissue Substitute	Z No Qualifier
3 Cervical Vertebral Disc 5 Cervicothoracic Vertebral Disc 9 Thoracic Vertebral Disc B Thoracolumbar Vertebral Disc	X External	0 Drainage Device 3 Infusion Device	Z No Qualifier
C Temporomandibular Joint, Right D Temporomandibular Joint, Left E Sternoclavicular Joint, Right F Sternoclavicular Joint, Left G Acromioclavicular Joint, Right H Acromioclavicular Joint, Left J Shoulder Joint, Right K Shoulder Joint, Left	0 Open 3 Percutaneous 4 Percutaneous Endoscopic	0 Drainage Device 3 Infusion Device 4 Internal Fixation Device 7 Autologous Tissue Substitute 8 Spacer J Synthetic Substitute K Nonautologous Tissue Substitute	Z No Qualifier
C Temporomandibular Joint, Right D Temporomandibular Joint, Left E Sternoclavicular Joint, Right F Sternoclavicular Joint, Left G Acromioclavicular Joint, Right H Acromioclavicular Joint, Left J Shoulder Joint, Right K Shoulder Joint, Left	X External	0 Drainage Device 3 Infusion Device 4 Internal Fixation Device	Z No Qualifier
L Elbow Joint, Right M Elbow Joint, Left N Wrist Joint, Right P Wrist Joint, Left Q Carpal Joint, Right R Carpal Joint, Left S Carpometacarpal Joint, Right T Carpometacarpal Joint, Left U Metacarpophalangeal Joint, Right V Metacarpophalangeal Joint, Left W Finger Phalangeal Joint, Right X Finger Phalangeal Joint, Left	0 Open 3 Percutaneous 4 Percutaneous Endoscopic	0 Drainage Device 3 Infusion Device 4 Internal Fixation Device 5 External Fixation Device 7 Autologous Tissue Substitute 8 Spacer J Synthetic Substitute K Nonautologous Tissue Substitute	Z No Qualifier

Non-OR 0RP[0146A]X[034]Z
Non-OR 0RP[359B]3[03]Z
Non-OR 0RP[359B]X[03]Z
Non-OR 0RP[CDEFGHJK][034]8Z
Non-OR 0RP[CDEFGHJK]3[03]Z
Non-OR 0RP[CD]X[03]Z
Non-OR 0RP[EFGHJK]X[034]Z
Non-OR 0RP[LMNPQRSTUVWX]3[03]Z
Non-OR 0RP[LMNPQRSTUVWX][034]8Z

0: M/S   R: UPPER JOINTS   P: REMOVAL

New/Revised Text in Green   deleted Deleted   ♀ Females Only   ♂ Males Only   **Coding Clinic**
Non-covered   Limited Coverage   Combination (See Appendix E)   DRG Non-OR   Non-OR   Hospital-Acquired Condition

429

SECTION: Ø MEDICAL AND SURGICAL

BODY SYSTEM: R UPPER JOINTS
OPERATION: P REMOVAL: *(continued)*
Taking out or off a device from a body part

Body Part	Approach	Device	Qualifier
L Elbow Joint, Right M Elbow Joint, Left N Wrist Joint, Right P Wrist Joint, Left Q Carpal Joint, Right R Carpal Joint, Left S Carpometacarpal Joint, Right T Carpometacarpal Joint, Left U Metacarpophalangeal Joint, Right V Metacarpophalangeal Joint, Left W Finger Phalangeal Joint, Right X Finger Phalangeal Joint, Left	X External	Ø Drainage Device 3 Infusion Device 4 Internal Fixation Device 5 External Fixation Device	Z No Qualifier

Non-OR ØRP[LMNPQRSTUVWX]X[Ø345]Z

SECTION: Ø MEDICAL AND SURGICAL

BODY SYSTEM: R UPPER JOINTS
OPERATION: Q REPAIR: Restoring, to the extent possible, a body part to its normal anatomic structure and function

Body Part	Approach	Device	Qualifier
Ø Occipital-cervical Joint 1 Cervical Vertebral Joint 3 Cervical Vertebral Disc 4 Cervicothoracic Vertebral Joint 5 Cervicothoracic Vertebral Disc 6 Thoracic Vertebral Joint 9 Thoracic Vertebral Disc A Thoracolumbar Vertebral Joint B Thoracolumbar Vertebral Disc C Temporomandibular Joint, Right D Temporomandibular Joint, Left E Sternoclavicular Joint, Right 🔖 F Sternoclavicular Joint, Left 🔖 G Acromioclavicular Joint, Right 🔖 H Acromioclavicular Joint, Left 🔖 J Shoulder Joint, Right 🔖 K Shoulder Joint, Left 🔖 L Elbow Joint, Right 🔖 M Elbow Joint, Left 🔖 N Wrist Joint, Right P Wrist Joint, Left Q Carpal Joint, Right R Carpal Joint, Left S Carpometacarpal Joint, Right T Carpometacarpal Joint, Left U Metacarpophalangeal Joint, Right V Metacarpophalangeal Joint, Left W Finger Phalangeal Joint, Right X Finger Phalangeal Joint, Left	Ø Open 3 Percutaneous 4 Percutaneous Endoscopic X External	Z No Device	Z No Qualifier

DRG Non-OR ØRQ[Ø134569ABEFGHJKLMNPQRSTUVWX]XZZ
Non-OR ØRQ[CD]XZZ

🔖 ØRQ[EFGHJKLM][Ø34X]ZZ when reported with Secondary Diagnosis K68.11, T81.4XXA, or T84.60XA-T84.7XXA

Coding Clinic: 2Ø16, Q1, P3Ø – ØRQJ4ZZ

New/Revised Text in Green ~~deleted~~ Deleted ♀ Females Only ♂ Males Only **Coding Clinic**
🔖 Non-covered 🔖 Limited Coverage ⊞ Combination (See Appendix E) DRG Non-OR Non-OR 🔖 Hospital-Acquired Condition

SECTION: Ø MEDICAL AND SURGICAL

BODY SYSTEM: R UPPER JOINTS

OPERATION: R **REPLACEMENT:** Putting in or on biological or synthetic material that physically takes the place and/or function of all or a portion of a body part

Body Part	Approach	Device	Qualifier
Ø Occipital-cervical Joint 1 Cervical Vertebral Joint 3 Cervical Vertebral Disc 4 Cervicothoracic Vertebral Joint 5 Cervicothoracic Vertebral Disc 6 Thoracic Vertebral Joint 9 Thoracic Vertebral Disc A Thoracolumbar Vertebral Joint B Thoracolumbar Vertebral Disc C Temporomandibular Joint, Right D Temporomandibular Joint, Left E Sternoclavicular Joint, Right F Sternoclavicular Joint, Left G Acromioclavicular Joint, Right H Acromioclavicular Joint, Left L Elbow Joint, Right M Elbow Joint, Left N Wrist Joint, Right P Wrist Joint, Left Q Carpal Joint, Right R Carpal Joint, Left S Carpometacarpal Joint, Right T Carpometacarpal Joint, Left U Metacarpophalangeal Joint, Right V Metacarpophalangeal Joint, Left W Finger Phalangeal Joint, Right X Finger Phalangeal Joint, Left	Ø Open	7 Autologous Tissue Substitute J Synthetic Substitute K Nonautologous Tissue Substitute	Z No Qualifier
J Shoulder Joint, Right K Shoulder Joint, Left	Ø Open	Ø Synthetic Substitute, Reverse Ball and Socket 7 Autologous Tissue Substitute K Nonautologous Tissue Substitute	Z No Qualifier
J Shoulder Joint, Right K Shoulder Joint, Left	Ø Open	J Synthetic Substitute	6 Humeral Surface 7 Glenoid Surface Z No Qualifier

Coding Clinic: 2015, Q1, P27 – ØRRJ00Z
Coding Clinic: 2015, Q3, P15 – ØRRKØJ6

Ø: M/S

R: UPPER JOINTS

R: REPLACEMENT

SECTION: Ø MEDICAL AND SURGICAL

BODY SYSTEM: R UPPER JOINTS

OPERATION: S REPOSITION: Moving to its normal location, or other suitable location, all or a portion of a body part

Body Part	Approach	Device	Qualifier
Ø Occipital-cervical Joint 1 Cervical Vertebral Joint 4 Cervicothoracic Vertebral Joint 6 Thoracic Vertebral Joint A Thoracolumbar Vertebral Joint C Temporomandibular Joint, Right D Temporomandibular Joint, Left E Sternoclavicular Joint, Right F Sternoclavicular Joint, Left G Acromioclavicular Joint, Right H Acromioclavicular Joint, Left J Shoulder Joint, Right K Shoulder Joint, Left	Ø Open 3 Percutaneous 4 Percutaneous Endoscopic X External	4 Internal Fixation Device Z No Device	Z No Qualifier
L Elbow Joint, Right M Elbow Joint, Left N Wrist Joint, Right P Wrist Joint, Left Q Carpal Joint, Right R Carpal Joint, Left S Carpometacarpal Joint, Right T Carpometacarpal Joint, Left U Metacarpophalangeal Joint, Right V Metacarpophalangeal Joint, Left W Finger Phalangeal Joint, Right X Finger Phalangeal Joint, Left	Ø Open 3 Percutaneous 4 Percutaneous Endoscopic X External	4 Internal Fixation Device 5 External Fixation Device Z No Device	Z No Qualifier

Non-OR   ØRS[Ø146ACDEFGHJK][34X][4Z]Z
Non-OR   ØRS[LMNPQRSTUVWX][34X][45Z]Z

Coding Clinic: 2015, Q2, P35; 2013, Q2, P39 – ØRS1XZZ

S: REPOSITION

R: UPPER JOINTS

Ø: M/S

New/Revised Text in Green   ~~deleted~~ Deleted   ♀ Females Only   ♂ Males Only   **Coding Clinic**

⬥ Non-covered   ⬥ Limited Coverage   ⊡ Combination (See Appendix E)   DRG Non-OR   Non-OR   ⬥ Hospital-Acquired Condition

SECTION: Ø MEDICAL AND SURGICAL

BODY SYSTEM: R UPPER JOINTS

OPERATION: T RESECTION: Cutting out or off, without replacement, all of a body part

Body Part	Approach	Device	Qualifier
3 Cervical Vertebral Disc	Ø Open	Z No Device	Z No Qualifier
4 Cervicothoracic Vertebral Joint			
5 Cervicothoracic Vertebral Disc			
9 Thoracic Vertebral Disc			
B Thoracolumbar Vertebral Disc			
C Temporomandibular Joint, Right			
D Temporomandibular Joint, Left			
E Sternoclavicular Joint, Right			
F Sternoclavicular Joint, Left			
G Acromioclavicular Joint, Right			
H Acromioclavicular Joint, Left			
J Shoulder Joint, Right			
K Shoulder Joint, Left			
L Elbow Joint, Right			
M Elbow Joint, Left			
N Wrist Joint, Right			
P Wrist Joint, Left			
Q Carpal Joint, Right			
R Carpal Joint, Left			
S Carpometacarpal Joint, Right			
T Carpometacarpal Joint, Left			
U Metacarpophalangeal Joint, Right			
V Metacarpophalangeal Joint, Left			
W Finger Phalangeal Joint, Right			
X Finger Phalangeal Joint, Left			

Ø: M/S

R: UPPER JOINTS

T: RESECTION

SECTION: Ø MEDICAL AND SURGICAL
BODY SYSTEM: R UPPER JOINTS
OPERATION: U SUPPLEMENT: Putting in or on biological or synthetic material that physically reinforces and/or augments the function of a portion of a body part

Body Part	Approach	Device	Qualifier
Ø Occipital-cervical Joint	Ø Open	7 Autologous Tissue Substitute	Z No Qualifier
1 Cervical Vertebral Joint	3 Percutaneous	J Synthetic Substitute	
3 Cervical Vertebral Disc	4 Percutaneous Endoscopic	K Nonautologous Tissue	
4 Cervicothoracic Vertebral Joint		Substitute	
5 Cervicothoracic Vertebral Disc			
6 Thoracic Vertebral Joint			
9 Thoracic Vertebral Disc			
A Thoracolumbar Vertebral Joint			
B Thoracolumbar Vertebral Disc			
C Temporomandibular Joint, Right			
D Temporomandibular Joint, Left			
E Sternoclavicular Joint, Right 🕮			
F Sternoclavicular Joint, Left 🕮			
G Acromioclavicular Joint, Right 🕮			
H Acromioclavicular Joint, Left 🕮			
J Shoulder Joint, Right 🕮			
K Shoulder Joint, Left 🕮			
L Elbow Joint, Right 🕮			
M Elbow Joint, Left 🕮			
N Wrist Joint, Right			
P Wrist Joint, Left			
Q Carpal Joint, Right			
R Carpal Joint, Left			
S Carpometacarpal Joint, Right			
T Carpometacarpal Joint, Left			
U Metacarpophalangeal Joint, Right			
V Metacarpophalangeal Joint, Left			
W Finger Phalangeal Joint, Right			
X Finger Phalangeal Joint, Left			

🕮 ØRU[EFGHJKLM][Ø34][7JK]Z when reported with Secondary Diagnosis K68.11, T81.4XXA, or T84.60XA-T84.7XXA

Coding Clinic: 2Ø15, Q3, P27 – ØRUTØ7Z

SECTION: Ø MEDICAL AND SURGICAL
BODY SYSTEM: R UPPER JOINTS
OPERATION: W REVISION: Correcting, to the extent possible, a portion of a malfunctioning device or the position of a displaced device

Body Part	Approach	Device	Qualifier
Ø Occipital-cervical Joint 1 Cervical Vertebral Joint 4 Cervicothoracic Vertebral Joint 6 Thoracic Vertebral Joint A Thoracolumbar Vertebral Joint	Ø Open 3 Percutaneous 4 Percutaneous Endoscopic X External	Ø Drainage Device 3 Infusion Device 4 Internal Fixation Device 7 Autologous Tissue Substitute 8 Spacer A Interbody Fusion Device J Synthetic Substitute K Nonautologous Tissue Substitute	Z No Qualifier
3 Cervical Vertebral Disc 5 Cervicothoracic Vertebral Disc 9 Thoracic Vertebral Disc B Thoracolumbar Vertebral Disc	Ø Open 3 Percutaneous 4 Percutaneous Endoscopic X External	Ø Drainage Device 3 Infusion Device 7 Autologous Tissue Substitute J Synthetic Substitute K Nonautologous Tissue Substitute	Z No Qualifier
C Temporomandibular Joint, Right D Temporomandibular Joint, Left E Sternoclavicular Joint, Right F Sternoclavicular Joint, Left G Acromioclavicular Joint, Right H Acromioclavicular Joint, Left J Shoulder Joint, Right K Shoulder Joint, Left	Ø Open 3 Percutaneous 4 Percutaneous Endoscopic X External	Ø Drainage Device 3 Infusion Device 4 Internal Fixation Device 7 Autologous Tissue Substitute 8 Spacer J Synthetic Substitute K Nonautologous Tissue Substitute	Z No Qualifier
L Elbow Joint, Right M Elbow Joint, Left N Wrist Joint, Right P Wrist Joint, Left Q Carpal Joint, Right R Carpal Joint, Left S Carpometacarpal Joint, Right T Carpometacarpal Joint, Left U Metacarpophalangeal Joint, Right V Metacarpophalangeal Joint, Left W Finger Phalangeal Joint, Right X Finger Phalangeal Joint, Left	Ø Open 3 Percutaneous 4 Percutaneous Endoscopic X External	Ø Drainage Device 3 Infusion Device 4 Internal Fixation Device 5 External Fixation Device 7 Autologous Tissue Substitute 8 Spacer J Synthetic Substitute K Nonautologous Tissue Substitute	Z No Qualifier

Non-OR ØRW[Ø146A]X[Ø3478AJK]Z
Non-OR ØRW[359B]X[Ø37JK]Z
Non-OR ØRW[CDEFGHJK]X[Ø3478JK]Z
Non-OR ØRW[LMNPQRSTUVWX]X[Ø34578JK]Z

SECTION: Ø MEDICAL AND SURGICAL

BODY SYSTEM: S LOWER JOINTS
OPERATION: 2 **CHANGE:** Taking out or off a device from a body part and putting back an identical or similar device in or on the same body part without cutting or puncturing the skin or a mucous membrane

Body Part	Approach	Device	Qualifier
Y Lower Joint	X External	Ø Drainage Device Y Other Device	Z No Qualifier

Non-OR All Values

SECTION: Ø MEDICAL AND SURGICAL

BODY SYSTEM: S LOWER JOINTS
OPERATION: 5 **DESTRUCTION:** Physical eradication of all or a portion of a body part by the direct use of energy, force, or destructive agent

Body Part	Approach	Device	Qualifier
Ø Lumbar Vertebral Joint 2 Lumbar Vertebral Disc 3 Lumbosacral Joint 4 Lumbosacral Disc 5 Sacrococcygeal Joint 6 Coccygeal Joint 7 Sacroiliac Joint, Right 8 Sacroiliac Joint, Left 9 Hip Joint, Right B Hip Joint, Left C Knee Joint, Right D Knee Joint, Left F Ankle Joint, Right G Ankle Joint, Left H Tarsal Joint, Right J Tarsal Joint, Left K Tarsometatarsal Joint, Right L Tarsometatarsal Joint, Left M Metatarsal-Phalangeal Joint, Right N Metatarsal-Phalangeal Joint, Left P Toe Phalangeal Joint, Right Q Toe Phalangeal Joint, Left	Ø Open 3 Percutaneous 4 Percutaneous Endoscopic	Z No Device	Z No Qualifier

0: M/S   **S: LOWER JOINTS**   **2: CHANGE**   **5: DESTRUCTION**

SECTION: Ø MEDICAL AND SURGICAL

BODY SYSTEM: S LOWER JOINTS

OPERATION: 9 DRAINAGE: Taking or letting out fluids and/or gases from a body part

Body Part	Approach	Device	Qualifier
Ø Lumbar Vertebral Joint 2 Lumbar Vertebral Disc 3 Lumbosacral Joint 4 Lumbosacral Disc 5 Sacrococcygeal Joint 6 Coccygeal Joint 7 Sacroiliac Joint, Right 8 Sacroiliac Joint, Left 9 Hip Joint, Right B Hip Joint, Left C Knee Joint, Right D Knee Joint, Left F Ankle Joint, Right G Ankle Joint, Left H Tarsal Joint, Right J Tarsal Joint, Left K Tarsometatarsal Joint, Right L Tarsometatarsal Joint, Left M Metatarsal-Phalangeal Joint, Right N Metatarsal-Phalangeal Joint, Left P Toe Phalangeal Joint, Right Q Toe Phalangeal Joint, Left	Ø Open 3 Percutaneous 4 Percutaneous Endoscopic	Ø Drainage Device	Z No Qualifier
Ø Lumbar Vertebral Joint 2 Lumbar Vertebral Disc 3 Lumbosacral Joint 4 Lumbosacral Disc 5 Sacrococcygeal Joint 6 Coccygeal Joint 7 Sacroiliac Joint, Right 8 Sacroiliac Joint, Left 9 Hip Joint, Right B Hip Joint, Left C Knee Joint, Right D Knee Joint, Left F Ankle Joint, Right G Ankle Joint, Left H Tarsal Joint, Right J Tarsal Joint, Left K Tarsometatarsal Joint, Right L Tarsometatarsal Joint, Left M Metatarsal-Phalangeal Joint, Right N Metatarsal-Phalangeal Joint, Left P Toe Phalangeal Joint, Right Q Toe Phalangeal Joint, Left	Ø Open 3 Percutaneous 4 Percutaneous Endoscopic	Z No Device	X Diagnostic Z No Qualifier

Non-OR ØS9[Ø23456789BCDFGHJKLMNPQ][34]ØZ
Non-OR ØS9[Ø23456789BCDFGHJKLMNPQ][Ø34]ZX
Non-OR ØS9[Ø23456789BCDFGHJKLMNPQ][34]ZZ

Coding Clinic: 2Ø18, Q2, P17 – ØS9D4ZZ

New/Revised Text in Green   ~~deleted~~ Deleted   ♀ Females Only   ♂ Males Only   **Coding Clinic**

Non-covered   Limited Coverage   ⊡ Combination (See Appendix E)   DRG Non-OR   Non-OR   Hospital-Acquired Condition

SECTION: Ø MEDICAL AND SURGICAL

BODY SYSTEM: S LOWER JOINTS

OPERATION: B EXCISION: Cutting out or off, without replacement, a portion of a body part

Body Part	Approach	Device	Qualifier
Ø Lumbar Vertebral Joint 2 Lumbar Vertebral Disc 3 Lumbosacral Joint 4 Lumbosacral Disc 5 Sacrococcygeal Joint 6 Coccygeal Joint 7 Sacroiliac Joint, Right 8 Sacroiliac Joint, Left 9 Hip Joint, Right B Hip Joint, Left C Knee Joint, Right D Knee Joint, Left F Ankle Joint, Right G Ankle Joint, Left H Tarsal Joint, Right J Tarsal Joint, Left K Tarsometatarsal Joint, Right L Tarsometatarsal Joint, Left M Metatarsal-Phalangeal Joint, Right N Metatarsal-Phalangeal Joint, Left P Toe Phalangeal Joint, Right Q Toe Phalangeal Joint, Left	Ø Open 3 Percutaneous 4 Percutaneous Endoscopic	Z No Device	X Diagnostic Z No Qualifier

Non-OR ØSB[Ø23456789BCDFGHJKLMNPQ][Ø34]ZX

Coding Clinic: 2015, Q1, P34 – ØSBD4ZZ
Coding Clinic: 2017, Q4, P76; 2016, Q2, P16 – ØSB2ØZZ
Coding Clinic: 2017, Q4, P76 – ØSB4ØZZ

SECTION: Ø MEDICAL AND SURGICAL

BODY SYSTEM: S LOWER JOINTS

OPERATION: C EXTIRPATION: Taking or cutting out solid matter from a body part

Body Part	Approach	Device	Qualifier
Ø Lumbar Vertebral Joint 2 Lumbar Vertebral Disc 3 Lumbosacral Joint 4 Lumbosacral Disc 5 Sacrococcygeal Joint 6 Coccygeal Joint 7 Sacroiliac Joint, Right 8 Sacroiliac Joint, Left 9 Hip Joint, Right B Hip Joint, Left C Knee Joint, Right D Knee Joint, Left F Ankle Joint, Right G Ankle Joint, Left H Tarsal Joint, Right J Tarsal Joint, Left K Tarsometatarsal Joint, Right L Tarsometatarsal Joint, Left M Metatarsal-Phalangeal Joint, Right N Metatarsal-Phalangeal Joint, Left P Toe Phalangeal Joint, Right Q Toe Phalangeal Joint, Left	Ø Open 3 Percutaneous 4 Percutaneous Endoscopic	Z No Device	Z No Qualifier

SECTION: Ø MEDICAL AND SURGICAL

BODY SYSTEM: S LOWER JOINTS

OPERATION: G FUSION: Joining together portions of an articular body part, rendering the articular body part immobile

Body Part	Approach	Device	Qualifier
Ø Lumbar Vertebral Joint 🦠 1 Lumbar Vertebral Joints, 2 or more ⊞ 🦠 3 Lumbosacral Joint 🦠	Ø Open 3 Percutaneous 4 Percutaneous Endoscopic	7 Autologous Tissue Substitute J Synthetic Substitute K Nonautologous Tissue Substitute ~~Z No Device~~	Ø Anterior Approach, Anterior Column 1 Posterior Approach, Posterior Column J Posterior Approach, Anterior Column
Ø Lumbar Vertebral Joint 🦠 1 Lumbar Vertebral Joints, 2 or more ⊞ 🦠 3 Lumbosacral Joint 🦠	Ø Open 3 Percutaneous 4 Percutaneous Endoscopic	A Interbody Fusion Device	Ø Anterior Approach, Anterior Column J Posterior Approach, Anterior Column
5 Sacrococcygeal Joint 6 Coccygeal Joint 7 Sacroiliac Joint, Right 🦠 8 Sacroiliac Joint, Left 🦠	Ø Open 3 Percutaneous 4 Percutaneous Endoscopic	4 Internal Fixation Device 7 Autologous Tissue Substitute J Synthetic Substitute K Nonautologous Tissue Substitute ~~Z No Device~~	Z No Qualifier
9 Hip Joint, Right B Hip Joint, Left C Knee Joint, Right D Knee Joint, Left F Ankle Joint, Right G Ankle Joint, Left H Tarsal Joint, Right J Tarsal Joint, Left K Tarsometatarsal Joint, Right L Tarsometatarsal Joint, Left M Metatarsal-Phalangeal Joint, Right N Metatarsal-Phalangeal Joint, Left P Toe Phalangeal Joint, Right Q Toe Phalangeal Joint, Left	Ø Open 3 Percutaneous 4 Percutaneous Endoscopic	4 Internal Fixation Device 5 External Fixation Device 7 Autologous Tissue Substitute J Synthetic Substitute K Nonautologous Tissue Substitute ~~Z No Device~~	Z No Qualifier

⊞ ØSG1[Ø34][7JKZ][Ø1J]

⊞ ØSG1[Ø34]A[ØJ]

🦠 ØSG[Ø13][Ø34][7JKZ][Ø1J] when reported with Secondary Diagnosis K68.11, T81.4XXA, or T84.6ØXA-T84.7XXA

🦠 ØSG[Ø13][Ø34]A[ØJ] when reported with Secondary Diagnosis K68.11, T81.4XXA, or T84.6ØXA-T84.7XXA

🦠 ØSG[78][Ø34][47JKZ]Z when reported with Secondary Diagnosis K68.11, T81.4XXA, or T84.6ØXA-T84.7XXA

Coding Clinic: 2Ø13, Q3, P26, Q1, P23 – ØSGØØ71
Coding Clinic: 2Ø13, Q3, P26 – ØSGØØAJ
Coding Clinic: 2Ø13, Q2, P4Ø – ØSGGØ4Z, ØSGGØ7Z

New/Revised Text in Green   ~~deleted~~ Deleted   ♀ Females Only   ♂ Males Only   **Coding Clinic**
🦠 Non-covered   🦠 Limited Coverage   ⊞ Combination (See Appendix E)   DRG Non-OR   Non-OR   🦠 Hospital-Acquired Condition

SECTION: Ø MEDICAL AND SURGICAL

BODY SYSTEM: S LOWER JOINTS

OPERATION: H **INSERTION:** Putting in a nonbiological appliance that monitors, assists, performs, or prevents a physiological function but does not physically take the place of a body part

Body Part	Approach	Device	Qualifier
Ø Lumbar Vertebral Joint 3 Lumbosacral Joint	Ø Open 3 Percutaneous 4 Percutaneous Endoscopic	3 Infusion Device 4 Internal Fixation Device 8 Spacer B Spinal Stabilization Device, Interspinous Process C Spinal Stabilization Device, Pedicle-Based D Spinal Stabilization Device, Facet Replacement	Z No Qualifier
2 Lumbar Vertebral Disc 4 Lumbosacral Disc	Ø Open 3 Percutaneous 4 Percutaneous Endoscopic	3 Infusion Device 8 Spacer	Z No Qualifier
5 Sacrococcygeal Joint 6 Coccygeal Joint 7 Sacroiliac Joint, Right 8 Sacroiliac Joint, Left	Ø Open 3 Percutaneous 4 Percutaneous Endoscopic	3 Infusion Device 4 Internal Fixation Device 8 Spacer	Z No Qualifier
9 Hip Joint, Right B Hip Joint, Left C Knee Joint, Right D Knee Joint, Left F Ankle Joint, Right G Ankle Joint, Left H Tarsal Joint, Right J Tarsal Joint, Left K Tarsometatarsal Joint, Right L Tarsometatarsal Joint, Left M Metatarsal-Phalangeal Joint, Right N Metatarsal-Phalangeal Joint, Left P Toe Phalangeal Joint, Right Q Toe Phalangeal Joint, Left	Ø Open 3 Percutaneous 4 Percutaneous Endoscopic	3 Infusion Device 4 Internal Fixation Device 5 External Fixation Device 8 Spacer	Z No Qualifier

DRG Non-OR ØSH[Ø3][34]3Z
DRG Non-OR ØSH[24][34]3Z
DRG Non-OR ØSH[5678][34]3Z
DRG Non-OR ØSH[9BCDFGHJKLMNPQ][34]3Z
Non-OR ØSH[Ø3]Ø3Z
Non-OR ØSH[Ø3][Ø34]8Z
Non-OR ØSH[24]Ø3Z
Non-OR ØSH[24][Ø34]8Z
Non-OR ØSH[5678]Ø3Z
Non-OR ØSH[5678][Ø34]8Z
Non-OR ØSH[9BCDFGHJKLMNPQ]Ø3Z
Non-OR ØSH[9BCDFGHJKLMNPQ][Ø34]8Z

New/Revised Text in Green   ~~deleted~~ Deleted   ♀ Females Only   ♂ Males Only   **Coding Clinic**

🔲 Non-covered   🔲 Limited Coverage   ⊞ Combination (See Appendix E)   DRG Non-OR   Non-OR   🔲 Hospital-Acquired Condition

J: INSPECTION   N: RELEASE

S: LOWER JOINTS   Ø: M/S

SECTION: Ø MEDICAL AND SURGICAL
BODY SYSTEM: S LOWER JOINTS
OPERATION: J INSPECTION: Visually and/or manually exploring a body part

Body Part	Approach	Device	Qualifier
Ø Lumbar Vertebral Joint	Ø Open	Z No Device	Z No Qualifier
2 Lumbar Vertebral Disc	3 Percutaneous		
3 Lumbosacral Joint	4 Percutaneous Endoscopic		
4 Lumbosacral Disc	X External		
5 Sacrococcygeal Joint			
6 Coccygeal Joint			
7 Sacroiliac Joint, Right			
8 Sacroiliac Joint, Left			
9 Hip Joint, Right			
B Hip Joint, Left			
C Knee Joint, Right			
D Knee Joint, Left			
F Ankle Joint, Right			
G Ankle Joint, Left			
H Tarsal Joint, Right			
J Tarsal Joint, Left			
K Tarsometatarsal Joint, Right			
L Tarsometatarsal Joint, Left			
M Metatarsal-Phalangeal Joint, Right			
N Metatarsal-Phalangeal Joint, Left			
P Toe Phalangeal Joint, Right			
Q Toe Phalangeal Joint, Left			

Non-OR   ØSJ[Ø23456789BCDFGHJKLMNPQ][3X]ZZ

Coding Clinic: 2017, Q1, P5Ø – ØSJG3ZZ

SECTION: Ø MEDICAL AND SURGICAL
BODY SYSTEM: S LOWER JOINTS
OPERATION: N RELEASE: Freeing a body part from an abnormal physical constraint by cutting or by the use of force

Body Part	Approach	Device	Qualifier
Ø Lumbar Vertebral Joint	Ø Open	Z No Device	Z No Qualifier
2 Lumbar Vertebral Disc	3 Percutaneous		
3 Lumbosacral Joint	4 Percutaneous Endoscopic		
4 Lumbosacral Disc	X External		
5 Sacrococcygeal Joint			
6 Coccygeal Joint			
7 Sacroiliac Joint, Right			
8 Sacroiliac Joint, Left			
9 Hip Joint, Right			
B Hip Joint, Left			
C Knee Joint, Right			
D Knee Joint, Left			
F Ankle Joint, Right			
G Ankle Joint, Left			
H Tarsal Joint, Right			
J Tarsal Joint, Left			
K Tarsometatarsal Joint, Right			
L Tarsometatarsal Joint, Left			
M Metatarsal-Phalangeal Joint, Right			
N Metatarsal-Phalangeal Joint, Left			
P Toe Phalangeal Joint, Right			
Q Toe Phalangeal Joint, Left			

Non-OR   ØSN[Ø23456789BCDFGHJKLMNPQ]XZZ

New/Revised Text in Green   ~~deleted~~ Deleted   ♀ Females Only   ♂ Males Only   **Coding Clinic**

🔖 Non-covered   🔖 Limited Coverage   ⊞ Combination (See Appendix E)   DRG Non-OR   Non-OR   🔖 Hospital-Acquired Condition

SECTION: Ø MEDICAL AND SURGICAL
BODY SYSTEM: S LOWER JOINTS
OPERATION: P REMOVAL: *(on multiple pages)*
Taking out or off a device from a body part

Body Part	Approach	Device	Qualifier
Ø Lumbar Vertebral Joint 3 Lumbosacral Joint	Ø Open 3 Percutaneous 4 Percutaneous Endoscopic	Ø Drainage Device 3 Infusion Device 4 Internal Fixation Device 7 Autologous Tissue Substitute 8 Spacer A Interbody Fusion Device J Synthetic Substitute K Nonautologous Tissue Substitute	Z No Qualifier
Ø Lumbar Vertebral Joint 3 Lumbosacral Joint	X External	Ø Drainage Device 3 Infusion Device 4 Internal Fixation Device	Z No Qualifier
2 Lumbar Vertebral Disc 4 Lumbosacral Disc	Ø Open 3 Percutaneous 4 Percutaneous Endoscopic	Ø Drainage Device 3 Infusion Device 7 Autologous Tissue Substitute J Synthetic Substitute K Nonautologous Tissue Substitute	Z No Qualifier
2 Lumbar Vertebral Disc 4 Lumbosacral Disc	X External	Ø Drainage Device 3 Infusion Device	Z No Qualifier
5 Sacrococcygeal Joint 6 Coccygeal Joint 7 Sacroiliac Joint, Right 8 Sacroiliac Joint, Left	Ø Open 3 Percutaneous 4 Percutaneous Endoscopic	Ø Drainage Device 3 Infusion Device 4 Internal Fixation Device 7 Autologous Tissue Substitute 8 Spacer J Synthetic Substitute K Nonautologous Tissue Substitute	Z No Qualifier
5 Sacrococcygeal Joint 6 Coccygeal Joint 7 Sacroiliac Joint, Right 8 Sacroiliac Joint, Left	X External	Ø Drainage Device 3 Infusion Device 4 Internal Fixation Device	Z No Qualifier
9 Hip Joint, Right ⊞ B Hip Joint, Left ⊞	Ø Open	Ø Drainage Device 3 Infusion Device 4 Internal Fixation Device 5 External Fixation Device 7 Autologous Tissue Substitute 8 Spacer 9 Liner B Resurfacing Device E Articulating Spacer J Synthetic Substitute K Nonautologous Tissue Substitute	Z No Qualifier
9 Hip Joint, Right ⊞ B Hip Joint, Left ⊞	3 Percutaneous 4 Percutaneous Endoscopic	Ø Drainage Device 3 Infusion Device 4 Internal Fixation Device 5 External Fixation Device 7 Autologous Tissue Substitute 8 Spacer J Synthetic Substitute K Nonautologous Tissue Substitute	Z No Qualifier

⊞ ØSP[9B]Ø[89BJ]Z
⊞ ØSP[9B]4[8J]Z
DRG Non-OR ØSP[9B]Ø8Z
DRG Non-OR ØSP[9B]48Z
Non-OR ØSP[Ø3][Ø34]8Z

Non-OR ØSP[Ø3]3[Ø3]Z
Non-OR ØSP[Ø3]X[Ø34]Z
Non-OR ØSP[24]3[Ø3]Z
Non-OR ØSP[24]X[Ø3]Z
Non-OR ØSP[5678][Ø34]8Z

Non-OR ØSP[5678]3[Ø3]Z
Non-OR ØSP[5678]X[Ø34]Z
Non-OR ØSP[9B]3[Ø38]Z

Coding Clinic: 2015, Q2, P20 – ØSP9Ø9Z
Coding Clinic: 2016, Q4, P112 – ØSP9Ø9Z

Ø: M/S

S: LOWER JOINTS

P: REMOVAL

SECTION: Ø MEDICAL AND SURGICAL
BODY SYSTEM: S LOWER JOINTS
OPERATION: P REMOVAL: *(continued)*
Taking out or off a device from a body part

Body Part	Approach	Device	Qualifier
9 Hip Joint, Right B Hip Joint, Left	X External	Ø Drainage Device 3 Infusion Device 4 Internal Fixation Device 5 External Fixation Device	Z No Qualifier
A Hip Joint, Acetabular Surface, Right ⊞ E Hip Joint, Acetabular Surface, Left ⊞ R Hip Joint, Femoral Surface, Right ⊞ S Hip Joint, Femoral Surface, Left ⊞ T Knee Joint, Femoral Surface, Right ⊞ U Knee Joint, Femoral Surface, Left ⊞ V Knee Joint, Tibial Surface, Right ⊞ W Knee Joint, Tibial Surface, Left ⊞	Ø Open 3 Percutaneous 4 Percutaneous Endoscopic	J Synthetic Substitute	Z No Qualifier
C Knee Joint, Right ⊞ D Knee Joint, Left ⊞	Ø Open	Ø Drainage Device 3 Infusion Device 4 Internal Fixation Device 5 External Fixation Device 7 Autologous Tissue Substitute 8 Spacer 9 Liner E Articulating Spacer K Nonautologous Tissue Substitute L Synthetic Substitute, Unicondylar Medial M Synthetic Substitute, Unicondylar Lateral N Synthetic Substitute, Patellofemoral	Z No Qualifier
C Knee Joint, Right ⊞ D Knee Joint, Left ⊞	Ø Open	J Synthetic Substitute	C Patellar Surface Z No Qualifier
C Knee Joint, Right ⊞ D Knee Joint, Left ⊞	3 Percutaneous 4 Percutaneous Endoscopic	Ø Drainage Device 3 Infusion Device 4 Internal Fixation Device 5 External Fixation Device 7 Autologous Tissue Substitute 8 Spacer K Nonautologous Tissue Substitute L Synthetic Substitute, Unicondylar Medial M Synthetic Substitute, Unicondylar Lateral N Synthetic Substitute, Patellofemoral	Z No Qualifier
C Knee Joint, Right ⊞ D Knee Joint, Left ⊞	3 Percutaneous 4 Percutaneous Endoscopic	J Synthetic Substitute	C Patellar Surface Z No Qualifier
C Knee Joint, Right D Knee Joint, Left	X External	Ø Drainage Device 3 Infusion Device 4 Internal Fixation Device 5 External Fixation Device	Z No Qualifier

⊞ ØSP[AERSTUVW][Ø4]JZ
⊞ ØSP[CD]Ø[89]Z
⊞ ØSP[CD]ØJ[CZ]
⊞ ØSP[CD][34]8Z
⊞ ØSP[CD]4J[CZ]

DRG Non-OR ØSP[CD]Ø8Z
DRG Non-OR ØSP[CD][34]8Z
Non-OR ØSP[9B]X[Ø345]Z
Non-OR ØSP[CD]3[Ø3]Z
Non-OR ØSP[CD]X[Ø345]Z

Coding Clinic: 2015, Q2, P18 – ØSPCØJZ
Coding Clinic: 2015, Q2, P2Ø – ØSP9ØJZ
Coding Clinic: 2016, Q4, P112 – ØSPRØJZ
Coding Clinic: 2018, Q2, P16 – ØSPWØJZ

New/Revised Text in Green ~~deleted~~ Deleted ♀ Females Only ♂ Males Only **Coding Clinic**
🚫 Non-covered 🚫 Limited Coverage ⊞ Combination (See Appendix E) DRG Non-OR Non-OR 🚫 Hospital-Acquired Condition

SECTION: Ø MEDICAL AND SURGICAL
BODY SYSTEM: S LOWER JOINTS
OPERATION: P REMOVAL: *(continued)*
Taking out or off a device from a body part

Body Part	Approach	Device	Qualifier
F Ankle Joint, Right G Ankle Joint, Left H Tarsal Joint, Right J Tarsal Joint, Left K Tarsometatarsal Joint, Right L Tarsometatarsal Joint, Left M Metatarsal-Phalangeal Joint, Right N Metatarsal-Phalangeal Joint, Left P Toe Phalangeal Joint, Right Q Toe Phalangeal Joint, Left	Ø Open 3 Percutaneous 4 Percutaneous Endoscopic	Ø Drainage Device 3 Infusion Device 4 Internal Fixation Device 5 External Fixation Device 7 Autologous Tissue Substitute 8 Spacer J Synthetic Substitute K Nonautologous Tissue Substitute	Z No Qualifier
F Ankle Joint, Right G Ankle Joint, Left H Tarsal Joint, Right J Tarsal Joint, Left K Tarsometatarsal Joint, Right L Tarsometatarsal Joint, Left M Metatarsal-Phalangeal Joint, Right N Metatarsal-Phalangeal Joint, Left P Toe Phalangeal Joint, Right Q Toe Phalangeal Joint, Left	X External	Ø Drainage Device 3 Infusion Device 4 Internal Fixation Device 5 External Fixation Device	Z No Qualifier

Non-OR ØSP[FGHJKLMNPQ]3[Ø3]Z
Non-OR ØSP[FGHJKLMNPQ][Ø34]8Z
Non-OR ØSP[FGHJKLMNPQ]X[Ø345]Z

Coding Clinic: 2013, Q2, P40 – ØSPG04Z
Coding Clinic: 2016, Q4, P111 – ØSP
Coding Clinic: 2017, Q4, P108 – ØSPFØJZ

SECTION: Ø MEDICAL AND SURGICAL
BODY SYSTEM: S LOWER JOINTS
OPERATION: Q REPAIR: Restoring, to the extent possible, a body part to its normal anatomic structure and function

Body Part	Approach	Device	Qualifier
Ø Lumbar Vertebral Joint 2 Lumbar Vertebral Disc 3 Lumbosacral Joint 4 Lumbosacral Disc 5 Sacrococcygeal Joint 6 Coccygeal Joint 7 Sacroiliac Joint, Right 8 Sacroiliac Joint, Left 9 Hip Joint, Right B Hip Joint, Left C Knee Joint, Right D Knee Joint, Left F Ankle Joint, Right G Ankle Joint, Left H Tarsal Joint, Right J Tarsal Joint, Left K Tarsometatarsal Joint, Right L Tarsometatarsal Joint, Left M Metatarsal-Phalangeal Joint, Right N Metatarsal-Phalangeal Joint, Left P Toe Phalangeal Joint, Right Q Toe Phalangeal Joint, Left	Ø Open 3 Percutaneous 4 Percutaneous Endoscopic X External	Z No Device	Z No Qualifier

DRG Non-OR ØSQ[Ø23456789BCDFGHJKLMNPQ]XZZ

New/Revised Text in Green ~~deleted~~ Deleted ♀ Females Only ♂ Males Only **Coding Clinic**
Non-covered Limited Coverage Combination (See Appendix E) DRG Non-OR Non-OR Hospital-Acquired Condition

Q: REPAIR

S: LOWER JOINTS

Ø: M/S

SECTION: Ø MEDICAL AND SURGICAL
BODY SYSTEM: S LOWER JOINTS
OPERATION: R REPLACEMENT: *(on multiple pages)*
Putting in or on biological or synthetic material that physically takes the place and/or function of all or a portion of a body part

Body Part	Approach	Device	Qualifier
Ø Lumbar Vertebral Joint 2 Lumbar Vertebral Disc 🗞 3 Lumbosacral Joint 4 Lumbosacral Disc 🗞 5 Sacrococcygeal Joint 6 Coccygeal Joint 7 Sacroiliac Joint, Right 8 Sacroiliac Joint, Left H Tarsal Joint, Right J Tarsal Joint, Left K Tarsometatarsal Joint, Right L Tarsometatarsal Joint, Left M Metatarsal-Phalangeal Joint, Right N Metatarsal-Phalangeal Joint, Left P Toe Phalangeal Joint, Right Q Toe Phalangeal Joint, Left	Ø Open	7 Autologous Tissue Substitute J Synthetic Substitute K Nonautologous Tissue Substitute	Z No Qualifier
9 Hip Joint, Right ⊞ 🗞 B Hip Joint, Left ⊞ 🗞	Ø Open	1 Synthetic Substitute, Metal 2 Synthetic Substitute, Metal on Polyethylene 3 Synthetic Substitute, Ceramic 4 Synthetic Substitute, Ceramic on Polyethylene 6 Synthetic Substitute, Oxidized Zirconium on Polyethylene J Synthetic Substitute	9 Cemented A Uncemented Z No Qualifier
9 Hip Joint, Right 🗞 B Hip Joint, Left 🗞	Ø Open	7 Autologous Tissue Substitute E Articulating Spacer K Nonautologous Tissue Substitute	Z No Qualifier
A Hip Joint, Acetabular Surface, Right ⊞ 🗞 E Hip Joint, Acetabular Surface, Left ⊞ 🗞	Ø Open	Ø Synthetic Substitute, Polyethylene 1 Synthetic Substitute, Metal 3 Synthetic Substitute, Ceramic J Synthetic Substitute	9 Cemented A Uncemented Z No Qualifier
A Hip Joint, Acetabular Surface, Right 🗞 E Hip Joint, Acetabular Surface, Left 🗞	Ø Open	7 Autologous Tissue Substitute K Nonautologous Tissue Substitute	Z No Qualifier

🗞 ØSR[24]Ø[7JK]Z when the beneficiary is over age 6Ø
🗞 ØSR[24]ØJZ when beneficiary is over age 6Ø
⊞ ØSR[9B]Ø[1234J][9AZ]
⊞ ØSR[AE]Ø[Ø13J][9AZ]
🗞 ØSR[9B]Ø[1234J][9AZ] when reported with Secondary Diagnosis from I26.Ø2-I26.Ø9, I26.92-I26.99, or I82.4Ø1-I82.4Z9
🗞 ØSR[9B]Ø[7K]Z when reported with Secondary Diagnosis from I26.Ø2-I26.Ø9, I26.92-I26.99, or I82.4Ø1-I82.4Z9

🗞 ØSR[AE]Ø[Ø13J][9AZ] when reported with Secondary Diagnosis from I26.Ø2-I26.Ø9, I26.92-I26.99, or I82.4Ø1-I82.4Z9
🗞 ØSR[AE]Ø[7K]Z when reported with Secondary Diagnosis from I26.Ø2-I26.Ø9, I26.92-I26.99, or I82.4Ø1-I82.4Z9

Coding Clinic: 2016, Q4, P109 – ØSR
Coding Clinic: 2017, Q4, P39 – ØSRBØ6Z

New/Revised Text in Green   ~~deleted~~ Deleted   ♀ Females Only   ♂ Males Only   **Coding Clinic**
🗞 Non-covered   🗞 Limited Coverage   ⊞ Combination (See Appendix E)   DRG Non-OR   Non-OR   🗞 Hospital-Acquired Condition

SECTION: Ø MEDICAL AND SURGICAL
BODY SYSTEM: S LOWER JOINTS
OPERATION: R REPLACEMENT: *(continued)*
Putting in or on biological or synthetic material that physically takes the place and/or function of all or a portion of a body part

Body Part	Approach	Device	Qualifier
C Knee Joint, Right ⊡ ✎ D Knee Joint, Left ⊡ ✎	Ø Open	6 Synthetic Substitute, Oxidized Zirconium on Polyethylene J Synthetic Substitute L Synthetic Substitute, Unicondylar Medial M Synthetic Substitute, Unicondylar Lateral N Synthetic Substitute, Patellofemoral	9 Cemented A Uncemented Z No Qualifier
C Knee Joint, Right ✎ D Knee Joint, Left ✎	Ø Open	7 Autologous Tissue Substitute E Articulating Spacer K Nonautologous Tissue Substitute	Z No Qualifier
F Ankle Joint, Right G Ankle Joint, Left T Knee Joint, Femoral Surface, Right ✎ U Knee Joint, Femoral Surface, Left ✎ V Knee Joint, Tibial Surface, Right ✎ W Knee Joint, Tibial Surface, Left ✎	Ø Open	7 Autologous Tissue Substitute K Nonautologous Tissue Substitute	Z No Qualifier
F Ankle Joint, Right G Ankle Joint, Left T Knee Joint, Femoral Surface, Right ⊡ ✎ U Knee Joint, Femoral Surface, Left ⊡ ✎ V Knee Joint, Tibial Surface, Right ⊡ ✎ W Knee Joint, Tibial Surface, Left ⊡ ✎	Ø Open	J Synthetic Substitute	9 Cemented A Uncemented Z No Qualifier
R Hip Joint, Femoral Surface, Right ⊡ ✎ S Hip Joint, Femoral Surface, Left ⊡ ✎	Ø Open	1 Synthetic Substitute, Metal 3 Synthetic Substitute, Ceramic J Synthetic Substitute	9 Cemented A Uncemented Z No Qualifier
R Hip Joint, Femoral Surface, Right ✎ S Hip Joint, Femoral Surface, Left ✎	Ø Open	7 Autologous Tissue Substitute K Nonautologous Tissue Substitute	Z No Qualifier

⊡ ØSR[CDTUVW]ØJ[9AZ]
⊡ ØSR[CD]ØL[9AZ]
⊡ ØSR[RS]Ø[13J][9AZ]
✎ ØSR[CD]Ø[7K]Z when reported with Secondary Diagnosis from I26.Ø2-I26.Ø9, I26.92-I26.99, or I82.4Ø1-I82.4Z9
✎ ØSR[CD]ØL[9AZ] when reported with Secondary Diagnosis from I26.Ø2-I26.Ø9, I26.92-I26.99, or I82.4Ø1-I82.4Z9
✎ ØSR[TUVW]Ø[7K]Z when reported with Secondary Diagnosis from I26.Ø2-I26.Ø9, I26.92-I26.99, or I82.4Ø1-I82.4Z9
✎ ØSR[CD]ØJ[9AZ] when reported with Secondary Diagnosis from I26.Ø2-I26.Ø9, I26.92-I26.99, or I82.4Ø1-I82.4Z9
✎ ØSR[TUVW]ØJ[9AZ] when reported with Secondary Diagnosis from I26.Ø2-I26.Ø9, I26.92-I26.99, or I82.4Ø1-I82.4Z9

✎ ØSR[RS]Ø[13J][9AZ] when reported with Secondary Diagnosis from I26.Ø2-I26.Ø9, I26.92-I26.99, or I82.4Ø1-I82.4Z9
✎ ØSR[RS]Ø[7K]Z when reported with Secondary Diagnosis from I26.Ø2-I26.Ø9, I26.92-I26.99, or I82.4Ø1-I82.4Z9

Coding Clinic: 2015, Q2, P18 – ØSRCØJ9
Coding Clinic: 2015, Q2, P20 – ØSRRØ3A
Coding Clinic: 2015, Q3, P19 – ØSRBØJ9
Coding Clinic: 2016, Q4, P110 – ØSRDØ[JL]Z
Coding Clinic: 2016, Q4, P111 – ØSRRØJ9
Coding Clinic: 2017, Q4, P108 – ØSRFØJA
Coding Clinic: 2018, Q2, P16 – ØSRWØJZ

SECTION: Ø MEDICAL AND SURGICAL

BODY SYSTEM: S LOWER JOINTS

OPERATION: S REPOSITION: Moving to its normal location, or other suitable location, all or a portion of a body part

Body Part	Approach	Device	Qualifier
Ø Lumbar Vertebral Joint 3 Lumbosacral Joint 5 Sacrococcygeal Joint 6 Coccygeal Joint 7 Sacroiliac Joint, Right 8 Sacroiliac Joint, Left	Ø Open 3 Percutaneous 4 Percutaneous Endoscopic X External	4 Internal Fixation Device Z No Device	Z No Qualifier
9 Hip Joint, Right B Hip Joint, Left C Knee Joint, Right D Knee Joint, Left F Ankle Joint, Right G Ankle Joint, Left H Tarsal Joint, Right J Tarsal Joint, Left K Tarsometatarsal Joint, Right L Tarsometatarsal Joint, Left M Metatarsal-Phalangeal Joint, Right N Metatarsal-Phalangeal Joint, Left P Toe Phalangeal Joint, Right Q Toe Phalangeal Joint, Left	Ø Open 3 Percutaneous 4 Percutaneous Endoscopic X External	4 Internal Fixation Device 5 External Fixation Device Z No Device	Z No Qualifier

Non-OR ØSS[Ø35678][34X][4Z]Z
Non-OR ØSS[9BCDFGHJKLMNPQ][34X][45Z]Z

Coding Clinic: 2Ø16, Q2, P32 – ØSSBØ4Z

SECTION: Ø MEDICAL AND SURGICAL

BODY SYSTEM: S LOWER JOINTS

OPERATION: T RESECTION: Cutting out or off, without replacement, all of a body part

Body Part	Approach	Device	Qualifier
2 Lumbar Vertebral Disc 4 Lumbosacral Disc 5 Sacrococcygeal Joint 6 Coccygeal Joint 7 Sacroiliac Joint, Right 8 Sacroiliac Joint, Left 9 Hip Joint, Right B Hip Joint, Left C Knee Joint, Right D Knee Joint, Left F Ankle Joint, Right G Ankle Joint, Left H Tarsal Joint, Right J Tarsal Joint, Left K Tarsometatarsal Joint, Right L Tarsometatarsal Joint, Left M Metatarsal-Phalangeal Joint, Right N Metatarsal-Phalangeal Joint, Left P Toe Phalangeal Joint, Right Q Toe Phalangeal Joint, Left	Ø Open	Z No Device	Z No Qualifier

Coding Clinic: 2Ø16, Q1, P2Ø – ØSTMØZZ

SECTION: Ø MEDICAL AND SURGICAL
BODY SYSTEM: S LOWER JOINTS
OPERATION: U SUPPLEMENT: Putting in or on biological or synthetic material that physically reinforces and/or augments the function of a portion of a body part

Body Part	Approach	Device	Qualifier
Ø Lumbar Vertebral Joint 2 Lumbar Vertebral Disc 3 Lumbosacral Joint 4 Lumbosacral Disc 5 Sacrococcygeal Joint 6 Coccygeal Joint 7 Sacroiliac Joint, Right 8 Sacroiliac Joint, Left F Ankle Joint, Right G Ankle Joint, Left H Tarsal Joint, Right J Tarsal Joint, Left K Tarsometatarsal Joint, Right L Tarsometatarsal Joint, Left M Metatarsal-Phalangeal Joint, Right N Metatarsal-Phalangeal Joint, Left P Toe Phalangeal Joint, Right Q Toe Phalangeal Joint, Left	Ø Open 3 Percutaneous 4 Percutaneous Endoscopic	7 Autologous Tissue Substitute J Synthetic Substitute K Nonautologous Tissue Substitute	Z No Qualifier
9 Hip Joint, Right ⊞ ⬥ B Hip Joint, Left ⊞ ⬥	Ø Open	7 Autologous Tissue Substitute 9 Liner B Resurfacing Device J Synthetic Substitute K Nonautologous Tissue Substitute	Z No Qualifier
9 Hip Joint, Right B Hip Joint, Left	3 Percutaneous 4 Percutaneous Endoscopic	7 Autologous Tissue Substitute J Synthetic Substitute K Nonautologous Tissue Substitute	Z No Qualifier
A Hip Joint, Acetabular Surface, Right ⊞ ⬥ E Hip Joint, Acetabular Surface, Left ⊞ ⬥ R Hip Joint, Femoral Surface, Right ⊞ ⬥ S Hip Joint, Femoral Surface, Left ⊞ ⬥	Ø Open	9 Liner B Resurfacing Device	Z No Qualifier
C Knee Joint, Right D Knee Joint, Left	Ø Open	7 Autologous Tissue Substitute J Synthetic Substitute K Nonautologous Tissue Substitute	Z No Qualifier
C Knee Joint, Right D Knee Joint, Left	Ø Open	9 Liner	C Patellar Surface Z No Qualifier
C Knee Joint, Right D Knee Joint, Left	3 Percutaneous 4 Percutaneous Endoscopic	7 Autologous Tissue Substitute J Synthetic Substitute K Nonautologous Tissue Substitute	Z No Qualifier
T Knee Joint, Femoral Surface, Right ⊞ U Knee Joint, Femoral Surface, Left ⊞ V Knee Joint, Tibial Surface, Right ⊞ W Knee Joint, Tibial Surface, Left ⊞	Ø Open	9 Liner	Z No Qualifier

⊞ ØSU[9B]Ø9Z
⊞ ØSU[AERS]Ø9Z
⊞ ØSU[VW]Ø9Z

⬥ ØSU[9B]ØBZ when reported with Secondary Diagnosis from I26.02-I26.09, I26.92-I26.99, or I82.401-I82.4Z9
⬥ ØSU[AERS]ØBZ when reported with Secondary Diagnosis from I26.02-I26.09, I26.92-I26.99, or I82.401-I82.4Z9

Coding Clinic: 2015, Q2, P20 – ØSUAØ9Z
Coding Clinic: 2016, Q4, P112 – ØSUAØ9Z

New/Revised Text in Green ~~deleted~~ Deleted ♀ Females Only ♂ Males Only **Coding Clinic**
⬥ Non-covered ⬥ Limited Coverage ⊞ Combination (See Appendix E) DRG Non-OR Non-OR ⬥ Hospital-Acquired Condition

SECTION: Ø MEDICAL AND SURGICAL

BODY SYSTEM: S LOWER JOINTS

OPERATION: W REVISION: *(on multiple pages)*

Correcting, to the extent possible, a portion of a malfunctioning device or the position of a displaced device

Body Part	Approach	Device	Qualifier
Ø Lumbar Vertebral Joint 3 Lumbosacral Joint	Ø Open 3 Percutaneous 4 Percutaneous Endoscopic X External	Ø Drainage Device 3 Infusion Device 4 Internal Fixation Device 7 Autologous Tissue Substitute 8 Spacer A Interbody Fusion Device J Synthetic Substitute K Nonautologous Tissue Substitute	Z No Qualifier
2 Lumbar Vertebral Disc 4 Lumbosacral Disc	Ø Open 3 Percutaneous 4 Percutaneous Endoscopic X External	Ø Drainage Device 3 Infusion Device 7 Autologous Tissue Substitute J Synthetic Substitute K Nonautologous Tissue Substitute	Z No Qualifier
5 Sacrococcygeal Joint 6 Coccygeal Joint 7 Sacroiliac Joint, Right 8 Sacroiliac Joint, Left	Ø Open 3 Percutaneous 4 Percutaneous Endoscopic X External	Ø Drainage Device 3 Infusion Device 4 Internal Fixation Device 7 Autologous Tissue Substitute 8 Spacer J Synthetic Substitute K Nonautologous Tissue Substitute	Z No Qualifier
9 Hip Joint, Right B Hip Joint, Left	Ø Open	Ø Drainage Device 3 Infusion Device 4 Internal Fixation Device 5 External Fixation Device 7 Autologous Tissue Substitute 8 Spacer 9 Liner B Resurfacing Device J Synthetic Substitute K Nonautologous Tissue Substitute	Z No Qualifier
9 Hip Joint, Right B Hip Joint, Left	3 Percutaneous 4 Percutaneous Endoscopic X External	Ø Drainage Device 3 Infusion Device 4 Internal Fixation Device 5 External Fixation Device 7 Autologous Tissue Substitute 8 Spacer J Synthetic Substitute K Nonautologous Tissue Substitute	Z No Qualifier

Non-OR ØSW[Ø3]X[Ø3478AJK]Z
Non-OR ØSW[24]X[Ø37JK]Z
Non-OR ØSW[5678]X[Ø3478JK]Z
Non-OR ØSW[9B]X[Ø34578JK]Z

Coding Clinic: 2Ø16, Q4, P111 – ØSW

New/Revised Text in Green   deleted Deleted   ♀ Females Only   ♂ Males Only   Coding Clinic
Non-covered   Limited Coverage   Combination (See Appendix E)   DRG Non-OR   Non-OR   Hospital-Acquired Condition

Ø: M/S

S: LOWER JOINTS

W: REVISION

SECTION: Ø MEDICAL AND SURGICAL

BODY SYSTEM: S LOWER JOINTS

OPERATION: W REVISION: *(continued)*

Correcting, to the extent possible, a portion of a malfunctioning device or the position of a displaced device

Body Part	Approach	Device	Qualifier
A Hip Joint, Acetabular Surface, Right E Hip Joint, Acetabular Surface, Left R Hip Joint, Femoral Surface, Right S Hip Joint, Femoral Surface, Left T Knee Joint, Femoral Surface, Right U Knee Joint, Femoral Surface, Left V Knee Joint, Tibial Surface, Right W Knee Joint, Tibial Surface, Left	Ø Open 3 Percutaneous 4 Percutaneous Endoscopic X External	J Synthetic Substitute	Z No Qualifier
C Knee Joint, Right D Knee Joint, Left	Ø Open	Ø Drainage Device 3 Infusion Device 4 Internal Fixation Device 5 External Fixation Device 7 Autologous Tissue Substitute 8 Spacer 9 Liner K Nonautologous Tissue Substitute	Z No Qualifier
C Knee Joint, Right D Knee Joint, Left	Ø Open	J Synthetic Substitute	C Patellar Surface Z No Qualifier
C Knee Joint, Right D Knee Joint, Left	3 Percutaneous 4 Percutaneous Endoscopic X External	Ø Drainage Device 3 Infusion Device 4 Internal Fixation Device 5 External Fixation Device 7 Autologous Tissue Substitute 8 Spacer K Nonautologous Tissue Substitute	Z No Qualifier
C Knee Joint, Right D Knee Joint, Left	3 Percutaneous 4 Percutaneous Endoscopic X External	J Synthetic Substitute	C Patellar Surface Z No Qualifier
F Ankle Joint, Right G Ankle Joint, Left H Tarsal Joint, Right J Tarsal Joint, Left K Tarsometatarsal Joint, Right L Tarsometatarsal Joint, Left M Metatarsal-Phalangeal Joint, Right N Metatarsal-Phalangeal Joint, Left P Toe Phalangeal Joint, Right Q Toe Phalangeal Joint, Left	Ø Open 3 Percutaneous 4 Percutaneous Endoscopic X External	Ø Drainage Device 3 Infusion Device 4 Internal Fixation Device 5 External Fixation Device 7 Autologous Tissue Substitute 8 Spacer J Synthetic Substitute K Nonautologous Tissue Substitute	Z No Qualifier

Non-OR ØSW[AERSTUVW]XJZ
Non-OR ØSW[CD]X[Ø34578K]Z
Non-OR ØSW[CD]XJZ
Non-OR ØSW[FGHJKLMNPQ]X[Ø34578JK]Z

Coding Clinic: 2016, Q4, P112 – ØSWWØJZ
Coding Clinic: 2017, Q4, P107 – ØSWFØJZ

SECTION: Ø MEDICAL AND SURGICAL

BODY SYSTEM: T URINARY SYSTEM

OPERATION: 1 BYPASS: Altering the route of passage of the contents of a tubular body part

Body Part	Approach	Device	Qualifier
3 Kidney Pelvis, Right 4 Kidney Pelvis, Left	Ø Open 4 Percutaneous Endoscopic	7 Autologous Tissue Substitute J Synthetic Substitute K Nonautologous Tissue Substitute Z No Device	3 Kidney Pelvis, Right 4 Kidney Pelvis, Left 6 Ureter, Right 7 Ureter, Left 8 Colon 9 Colocutaneous A Ileum B Bladder C Ileocutaneous D Cutaneous
3 Kidney Pelvis, Right 4 Kidney Pelvis, Left	3 Percutaneous	J Synthetic Substitute	D Cutaneous
6 Ureter, Right 7 Ureter, Left 8 Ureters, Bilateral	Ø Open 4 Percutaneous Endoscopic	7 Autologous Tissue Substitute J Synthetic Substitute K Nonautologous Tissue Substitute Z No Device	6 Ureter, Right 7 Ureter, Left 8 Colon 9 Colocutaneous A Ileum B Bladder C Ileocutaneous D Cutaneous
6 Ureter, Right 7 Ureter, Left 8 Ureters, Bilateral	3 Percutaneous	J Synthetic Substitute	D Cutaneous
B Bladder	Ø Open 4 Percutaneous Endoscopic	7 Autologous Tissue Substitute J Synthetic Substitute K Nonautologous Tissue Substitute Z No Device	9 Colocutaneous C Ileocutaneous D Cutaneous
B Bladder	3 Percutaneous	J Synthetic Substitute	D Cutaneous

Coding Clinic: 2015, Q3, P35 – ØT17ØZB
Coding Clinic: 2017, Q3, P21-22 – ØT1[8B]ØZ[9C]

SECTION: Ø MEDICAL AND SURGICAL

BODY SYSTEM: T URINARY SYSTEM

OPERATION: 2 CHANGE: Taking out or off a device from a body part and putting back an identical or similar device in or on the same body part without cutting or puncturing the skin or a mucous membrane

Body Part	Approach	Device	Qualifier
5 Kidney 9 Ureter B Bladder D Urethra	X External	Ø Drainage Device Y Other Device	Z No Qualifier

Non-OR **All Values**

Ø: M/S   1: BYPASS   2: CHANGE   T: URINARY SYSTEM

SECTION: Ø MEDICAL AND SURGICAL

BODY SYSTEM: T URINARY SYSTEM

OPERATION: 5 DESTRUCTION: Physical eradication of all or a portion of a body part by the direct use of energy, force, or a destructive agent

Body Part	Approach	Device	Qualifier
Ø Kidney, Right 1 Kidney, Left 3 Kidney Pelvis, Right 4 Kidney Pelvis, Left 6 Ureter, Right 7 Ureter, Left B Bladder C Bladder Neck	Ø Open 3 Percutaneous 4 Percutaneous Endoscopic 7 Via Natural or Artificial Opening 8 Via Natural or Artificial Opening Endoscopic	Z No Device	Z No Qualifier
D Urethra	Ø Open 3 Percutaneous 4 Percutaneous Endoscopic 7 Via Natural or Artificial Opening 8 Via Natural or Artificial Opening Endoscopic X External	Z No Device	Z No Qualifier

Non-OR ØT5D[Ø3478X]ZZ

SECTION: Ø MEDICAL AND SURGICAL

BODY SYSTEM: T URINARY SYSTEM

OPERATION: 7 DILATION: Expanding an orifice or the lumen of a tubular body part

Body Part	Approach	Device	Qualifier
3 Kidney Pelvis, Right 4 Kidney Pelvis, Left 6 Ureter, Right 7 Ureter, Left 8 Ureters, Bilateral B Bladder C Bladder Neck D Urethra	Ø Open 3 Percutaneous 4 Percutaneous Endoscopic 7 Via Natural or Artificial Opening 8 Via Natural or Artificial Opening Endoscopic	D Intraluminal Device Z No Device	Z No Qualifier

Non-OR ØT7[67][Ø3478]DZ
Non-OR ØT7[8D][Ø34]DZ
Non-OR ØT7[8D][78][DZ]Z
Non-OR ØT7C[Ø3478][DZ]Z

Coding Clinic: 2Ø16, Q2, P28 – ØT767DZ

SECTION: Ø MEDICAL AND SURGICAL

BODY SYSTEM: T URINARY SYSTEM

OPERATION: 8 DIVISION: Cutting into a body part, without draining fluids and/or gases from the body part, in order to separate or transect a body part

Body Part	Approach	Device	Qualifier
2 Kidneys, Bilateral C Bladder Neck	Ø Open 3 Percutaneous 4 Percutaneous Endoscopic	Z No Device	Z No Qualifier

New/Revised Text in Green   ~~deleted~~ Deleted   ♀ Females Only   ♂ Males Only   **Coding Clinic**

Non-covered   Limited Coverage   ⊞ Combination (See Appendix E)   DRG Non-OR   Non-OR   Hospital-Acquired Condition

SECTION: Ø MEDICAL AND SURGICAL

BODY SYSTEM: T URINARY SYSTEM

OPERATION: 9 **DRAINAGE:** Taking or letting out fluids and/or gases from a body part

Body Part	Approach	Device	Qualifier
Ø Kidney, Right 1 Kidney, Left 3 Kidney Pelvis, Right 4 Kidney Pelvis, Left 6 Ureter, Right 7 Ureter, Left 8 Ureters, Bilateral B Bladder C Bladder Neck	Ø Open 3 Percutaneous 4 Percutaneous Endoscopic 7 Via Natural or Artificial Opening 8 Via Natural or Artificial Opening Endoscopic	Ø Drainage Device	Z No Qualifier
Ø Kidney, Right 1 Kidney, Left 3 Kidney Pelvis, Right 4 Kidney Pelvis, Left 6 Ureter, Right 7 Ureter, Left 8 Ureters, Bilateral B Bladder C Bladder Neck	Ø Open 3 Percutaneous 4 Percutaneous Endoscopic 7 Via Natural or Artificial Opening 8 Via Natural or Artificial Opening Endoscopic	Z No Device	X Diagnostic Z No Qualifier
D Urethra	Ø Open 3 Percutaneous 4 Percutaneous Endoscopic 7 Via Natural or Artificial Opening 8 Via Natural or Artificial Opening Endoscopic X External	Ø Drainage Device	Z No Qualifier
D Urethrav	Ø Open 3 Percutaneous 4 Percutaneous Endoscopic 7 Via Natural or Artificial Opening 8 Via Natural or Artificial Opening Endoscopic X External	Z No Device	X Diagnostic Z No Qualifier

DRG Non-OR ØT9[34]3ØZ
Non-OR ØT9[678][Ø3478]ØZ
Non-OR ØT9[678]3ZZ
Non-OR ØT9[BC][3478]ØZ

Non-OR ØT9[Ø134678][3478]ZX
Non-OR ØT9[Ø134][34]ZZ
Non-OR ØT9[BC][3478]ZZ
Non-OR ØT9D[Ø3478X]ZX

Non-OR ØT9D3ØZ
Non-OR ØT9D3ZZ

Coding Clinic: 2Ø17, Q3, P2Ø – ØT968ØZ

9: DRAINAGE

T: URINARY SYSTEM

Ø: M/S

New/Revised Text in Green   ~~deleted~~ Deleted   ♀ Females Only   ♂ Males Only   **Coding Clinic**
Non-covered   Limited Coverage   Combination (See Appendix E)   DRG Non-OR   Non-OR   Hospital-Acquired Condition

SECTION: Ø MEDICAL AND SURGICAL

BODY SYSTEM: T URINARY SYSTEM

OPERATION: B EXCISION: Cutting out or off, without replacement, a portion of a body part

Body Part	Approach	Device	Qualifier
Ø Kidney, Right 1 Kidney, Left 3 Kidney Pelvis, Right 4 Kidney Pelvis, Left 6 Ureter, Right 7 Ureter, Left B Bladder C Bladder Neck	Ø Open 3 Percutaneous 4 Percutaneous Endoscopic 7 Via Natural or Artificial Opening 8 Via Natural or Artificial Opening Endoscopic	Z No Device	X Diagnostic Z No Qualifier
D Urethra	Ø Open 3 Percutaneous 4 Percutaneous Endoscopic 7 Via Natural or Artificial Opening 8 Via Natural or Artificial Opening Endoscopic X External	Z No Device	X Diagnostic Z No Qualifier

Non-OR ØTB[013467][3478]ZX
Non-OR ØTBD[03478X]ZX

Coding Clinic: 2015, Q3, P34 – ØTBD8ZZ
Coding Clinic: 2016, Q1, P19 – ØTBB8ZX

SECTION: Ø MEDICAL AND SURGICAL

BODY SYSTEM: T URINARY SYSTEM

OPERATION: C EXTIRPATION: Taking or cutting out solid matter from a body part

Body Part	Approach	Device	Qualifier
Ø Kidney, Right 1 Kidney, Left 3 Kidney Pelvis, Right 4 Kidney Pelvis, Left 6 Ureter, Right 7 Ureter, Left B Bladder C Bladder Neck	Ø Open 3 Percutaneous 4 Percutaneous Endoscopic 7 Via Natural or Artificial Opening 8 Via Natural or Artificial Opening Endoscopic	Z No Device	Z No Qualifier
D Urethra	Ø Open 3 Percutaneous 4 Percutaneous Endoscopic 7 Via Natural or Artificial Opening 8 Via Natural or Artificial Opening Endoscopic X External	Z No Device	Z No Qualifier

Non-OR ØTC[BC][78]ZZ
Non-OR ØTCD[78X]ZZ

Coding Clinic: 2015, Q2, P8 – ØTC48ZZ
Coding Clinic: 2015, Q2, P9 – ØTC18ZZ, ØTC78ZZ, ØTCB8ZZ, ØTC78DZ
Coding Clinic: 2016, Q3, P24 – ØTCB8ZZ

SECTION: Ø MEDICAL AND SURGICAL

BODY SYSTEM: T URINARY SYSTEM

OPERATION: D EXTRACTION: Pulling or stripping out or off all or a portion of a body part by the use of force

Body Part	Approach	Device	Qualifier
Ø Kidney, Right 1 Kidney, Left	Ø Open 3 Percutaneous 4 Percutaneous Endoscopic	Z No Device	Z No Qualifier

New/Revised Text in Green   deleted Deleted   ♀ Females Only   ♂ Males Only   **Coding Clinic**
🔹 Non-covered   🔹 Limited Coverage   ⊞ Combination (See Appendix E)   DRG Non-OR   Non-OR   🔹 Hospital-Acquired Condition

457

SECTION: Ø MEDICAL AND SURGICAL

BODY SYSTEM: T URINARY SYSTEM

OPERATION: F FRAGMENTATION: Breaking solid matter in a body part into pieces

Body Part	Approach	Device	Qualifier
3 Kidney Pelvis, Right 4 Kidney Pelvis, Left 6 Ureter, Right 7 Ureter, Left B Bladder C Bladder Neck D Urethra	0 Open 3 Percutaneous 4 Percutaneous Endoscopic 7 Via Natural or Artificial Opening 8 Via Natural or Artificial Opening Endoscopic X External	Z No Device	Z No Qualifier

ØTFDXZZ

DRG Non-OR ØTF[3467BC]XZZ

Non-OR ØTF[34][078]ZZ

Non-OR ØTF[67BC][03478]ZZ

Non-OR ØTFD[03478X]ZZ

SECTION: Ø MEDICAL AND SURGICAL

BODY SYSTEM: T URINARY SYSTEM

OPERATION: H INSERTION: Putting in a nonbiological appliance that monitors, assists, performs, or prevents a physiological function but does not physically take the place of a body part

Body Part	Approach	Device	Qualifier
5 Kidney	0 Open 3 Percutaneous 4 Percutaneous Endoscopic 7 Via Natural or Artificial Opening 8 Via Natural or Artificial Opening Endoscopic	2 Monitoring Device 3 Infusion Device Y Other Device	Z No Qualifier
9 Ureter	0 Open 3 Percutaneous 4 Percutaneous Endoscopic 7 Via Natural or Artificial Opening 8 Via Natural or Artificial Opening Endoscopic	2 Monitoring Device 3 Infusion Device M Stimulator Lead Y Other Device	Z No Qualifier
B Bladder	0 Open 3 Percutaneous 4 Percutaneous Endoscopic 7 Via Natural or Artificial Opening 8 Via Natural or Artificial Opening Endoscopic	2 Monitoring Device 3 Infusion Device L Artificial Sphincter M Stimulator Lead Y Other Device	Z No Qualifier
C Bladder Neck	0 Open 3 Percutaneous 4 Percutaneous Endoscopic 7 Via Natural or Artificial Opening 8 Via Natural or Artificial Opening Endoscopic	L Artificial Sphincter	Z No Qualifier
D Urethra	0 Open 3 Percutaneous 4 Percutaneous Endoscopic 7 Via Natural or Artificial Opening 8 Via Natural or Artificial Opening Endoscopic	2 Monitoring Device 3 Infusion Device L Artificial Sphincter Y Other Device	Z No Qualifier
D Urethra	X External	2 Monitoring Device 3 Infusion Device L Artificial Sphincter	Z No Qualifier

ØTHB[03478]MZ

Non-OR ØTH5[03478]3Z

Non-OR ØTH5[78]2Z

Non-OR ØTH9[03478]3Z

Non-OR ØTH9[78]2Z

Non-OR ØTHB[03478]3Z

Non-OR ØTHB[78]2Z

Non-OR ØTHD[03478]3Z

Non-OR ØTHD[78]2Z

Non-OR ØTHDX3Z

New/Revised Text in Green ~~deleted~~ Deleted ♀ Females Only ♂ Males Only **Coding Clinic**

Non-covered Limited Coverage ⊞ Combination (See Appendix E) DRG Non-OR Non-OR Hospital-Acquired Condition

Left margin: F: FRAGMENTATION H: INSERTION | T: URINARY SYSTEM | Ø: M/S

SECTION: Ø MEDICAL AND SURGICAL

BODY SYSTEM: T URINARY SYSTEM
OPERATION: J INSPECTION: Visually and/or manually exploring a body part

Body Part	Approach	Device	Qualifier
5 Kidney 9 Ureter B Bladder D Urethra	Ø Open 3 Percutaneous 4 Percutaneous Endoscopic 7 Via Natural or Artificial Opening 8 Via Natural or Artificial Opening Endoscopic X External	Z No Device	Z No Qualifier

DRG Non-OR ØTJ[5B][37]ZZ
Non-OR ØTJ9[37]ZZ
Non-OR ØTJ[59][48X]ZZ
Non-OR ØTJB[8X]ZZ
Non-OR ØTJD[3478X]ZZ

SECTION: Ø MEDICAL AND SURGICAL

BODY SYSTEM: T URINARY SYSTEM
OPERATION: L OCCLUSION: Completely closing an orifice or the lumen of a tubular body part

Body Part	Approach	Device	Qualifier
3 Kidney Pelvis, Right 4 Kidney Pelvis, Left 6 Ureter, Right 7 Ureter, Left B Bladder C Bladder Neck	Ø Open 3 Percutaneous 4 Percutaneous Endoscopic	C Extraluminal Device D Intraluminal Device Z No Device	Z No Qualifier
3 Kidney Pelvis, Right 4 Kidney Pelvis, Left 6 Ureter, Right 7 Ureter, Left B Bladder C Bladder Neck	7 Via Natural or Artificial Opening 8 Via Natural or Artificial Opening Endoscopic	D Intraluminal Device Z No Device	Z No Qualifier
D Urethra	Ø Open 3 Percutaneous 4 Percutaneous Endoscopic X External	C Extraluminal Device D Intraluminal Device Z No Device	Z No Qualifier
D Urethra	7 Via Natural or Artificial Opening 8 Via Natural or Artificial Opening Endoscopic	D Intraluminal Device Z No Device	Z No Qualifier

SECTION: Ø MEDICAL AND SURGICAL

BODY SYSTEM: T URINARY SYSTEM

OPERATION: M **REATTACHMENT:** Putting back in or on all or a portion of a separated body part to its normal location or other suitable location

Body Part	Approach	Device	Qualifier
Ø Kidney, Right 1 Kidney, Left 2 Kidneys, Bilateral 3 Kidney Pelvis, Right 4 Kidney Pelvis, Left 6 Ureter, Right 7 Ureter, Left 8 Ureters, Bilateral B Bladder C Bladder Neck D Urethra	Ø Open 4 Percutaneous Endoscopic	Z No Device	Z No Qualifier

SECTION: Ø MEDICAL AND SURGICAL

BODY SYSTEM: T URINARY SYSTEM

OPERATION: N **RELEASE:** Freeing a body part from an abnormal physical constraint by cutting or by the use of force

Body Part	Approach	Device	Qualifier
Ø Kidney, Right 1 Kidney, Left 3 Kidney Pelvis, Right 4 Kidney Pelvis, Left 6 Ureter, Right 7 Ureter, Left B Bladder C Bladder Neck	Ø Open 3 Percutaneous 4 Percutaneous Endoscopic 7 Via Natural or Artificial Opening 8 Via Natural or Artificial Opening Endoscopic	Z No Device	Z No Qualifier
D Urethra	Ø Open 3 Percutaneous 4 Percutaneous Endoscopic 7 Via Natural or Artificial Opening 8 Via Natural or Artificial Opening Endoscopic X External	Z No Device	Z No Qualifier

M: REATTACHMENT N: RELEASE

T: URINARY SYSTEM

Ø: M/S

New/Revised Text in Green   ~~deleted~~ Deleted   ♀ Females Only   ♂ Males Only   **Coding Clinic**
Non-covered   Limited Coverage   ⊞ Combination (See Appendix E)   DRG Non-OR   Non-OR   Hospital-Acquired Condition

SECTION: Ø MEDICAL AND SURGICAL
BODY SYSTEM: T URINARY SYSTEM
OPERATION: P REMOVAL: *(on multiple pages)*
Taking out or off a device from a body part

Body Part	Approach	Device	Qualifier
5 Kidney	Ø Open 3 Percutaneous 4 Percutaneous Endoscopic 7 Via Natural or Artificial Opening 8 Via Natural or Artificial Opening Endoscopic	Ø Drainage Device 2 Monitoring Device 3 Infusion Device 7 Autologous Tissue Substitute C Extraluminal Device D Intraluminal Device J Synthetic Substitute K Nonautologous Tissue Substitute Y Other Device	Z No Qualifier
5 Kidney	X External	Ø Drainage Device 2 Monitoring Device 3 Infusion Device D Intraluminal Device	Z No Qualifier
9 Ureter	Ø Open 3 Percutaneous 4 Percutaneous Endoscopic 7 Via Natural or Artificial Opening 8 Via Natural or Artificial Opening Endoscopic	Ø Drainage Device 2 Monitoring Device 3 Infusion Device 7 Autologous Tissue Substitute C Extraluminal Device D Intraluminal Device J Synthetic Substitute K Nonautologous Tissue Substitute M Stimulator Lead Y Other Device	Z No Qualifier
9 Ureter	X External	Ø Drainage Device 2 Monitoring Device 3 Infusion Device D Intraluminal Device M Stimulator Lead	Z No Qualifier
B Bladder 🕲	Ø Open 3 Percutaneous 4 Percutaneous Endoscopic 7 Via Natural or Artificial Opening 8 Via Natural or Artificial Opening Endoscopic	Ø Drainage Device 2 Monitoring Device 3 Infusion Device 7 Autologous Tissue Substitute C Extraluminal Device D Intraluminal Device J Synthetic Substitute K Nonautologous Tissue Substitute L Artificial Sphincter M Stimulator Lead Y Other Device	Z No Qualifier
B Bladder	X External	Ø Drainage Device 2 Monitoring Device 3 Infusion Device D Intraluminal Device L Artificial Sphincter M Stimulator Lead	Z No Qualifier

🕲 ØTPB[Ø3478]MZ
Non-OR ØTP5[78][Ø23D]Z
Non-OR ØTP5X[Ø23D]Z

Non-OR ØTP9[78][Ø23D]Z
Non-OR ØTP9X[Ø23D]Z
Non-OR ØTPB[78][Ø23D]Z

Non-OR ØTPBX[Ø23DL]Z

Coding Clinic: 2Ø16, Q2, P28 – Ø2P98DZ

Ø: M/S

T: URINARY SYSTEM

P: REMOVAL

SECTION: Ø MEDICAL AND SURGICAL

BODY SYSTEM: T URINARY SYSTEM
OPERATION: P REMOVAL: *(continued)*
Taking out or off a device from a body part

Body Part	Approach	Device	Qualifier
D Urethra	Ø Open 3 Percutaneous 4 Percutaneous Endoscopic 7 Via Natural or Artificial Opening 8 Via Natural or Artificial Opening Endoscopic	Ø Drainage Device 2 Monitoring Device 3 Infusion Device 7 Autologous Tissue Substitute C Extraluminal Device D Intraluminal Device J Synthetic Substitute K Nonautologous Tissue Substitute L Artificial Sphincter Y Other Device	Z No Qualifier
D Urethra	X External	Ø Drainage Device 2 Monitoring Device 3 Infusion Device D Intraluminal Device L Artificial Sphincter	Z No Qualifier

Non-OR ØTPD[78][Ø23D]Z
Non-OR ØTPDX[Ø23D]Z

SECTION: Ø MEDICAL AND SURGICAL

BODY SYSTEM: T URINARY SYSTEM
OPERATION: Q REPAIR: Restoring, to the extent possible, a body part to its normal anatomic structure and function

Body Part	Approach	Device	Qualifier
Ø Kidney, Right 1 Kidney, Left 3 Kidney Pelvis, Right 4 Kidney Pelvis, Left 6 Ureter, Right 7 Ureter, Left B Bladder C Bladder Neck	Ø Open 3 Percutaneous 4 Percutaneous Endoscopic 7 Via Natural or Artificial Opening 8 Via Natural or Artificial Opening Endoscopic	Z No Device	Z No Qualifier
D Urethra	Ø Open 3 Percutaneous 4 Percutaneous Endoscopic 7 Via Natural or Artificial Opening 8 Via Natural or Artificial Opening Endoscopic X External	Z No Device	Z No Qualifier

Coding Clinic: 2017, Q1, P38 – ØTQDØZZ

New/Revised Text in Green ~~deleted~~ Deleted ♀ Females Only ♂ Males Only **Coding Clinic**
🐾 Non-covered 🐾 Limited Coverage ⊞ Combination (See Appendix E) DRG Non-OR Non-OR 🐾 Hospital-Acquired Condition

SECTION: Ø MEDICAL AND SURGICAL

BODY SYSTEM: T URINARY SYSTEM
OPERATION: R REPLACEMENT: Putting in or on biological or synthetic material that physically takes the place and/or function of all or a portion of a body part

Body Part	Approach	Device	Qualifier
3 Kidney Pelvis, Right 4 Kidney Pelvis, Left 6 Ureter, Right 7 Ureter, Left B Bladder C Bladder Neck	Ø Open 4 Percutaneous Endoscopic 7 Via Natural or Artificial Opening 8 Via Natural or Artificial Opening Endoscopic	7 Autologous Tissue Substitute J Synthetic Substitute K Nonautologous Tissue Substitute	Z No Qualifier
D Urethra	Ø Open 4 Percutaneous Endoscopic 7 Via Natural or Artificial Opening 8 Via Natural or Artificial Opening Endoscopic X External	7 Autologous Tissue Substitute J Synthetic Substitute K Nonautologous Tissue Substitute	Z No Qualifier

Coding Clinic: 2017, Q3, P20 – ØTRBØ7Z

SECTION: Ø MEDICAL AND SURGICAL

BODY SYSTEM: T URINARY SYSTEM
OPERATION: S REPOSITION: Moving to its normal location, or other suitable location, all or a portion of a body part

Body Part	Approach	Device	Qualifier
Ø Kidney, Right 1 Kidney, Left 2 Kidneys, Bilateral 3 Kidney Pelvis, Right 4 Kidney Pelvis, Left 6 Ureter, Right 7 Ureter, Left 8 Ureters, Bilateral B Bladder C Bladder Neck D Urethra	Ø Open 4 Percutaneous Endoscopic	Z No Device	Z No Qualifier

Coding Clinic: 2016, Q1, P15 – ØTSDØZZ
Coding Clinic: 2017, Q1, P37 – ØTS6ØZZ

SECTION: Ø MEDICAL AND SURGICAL

BODY SYSTEM: T URINARY SYSTEM

OPERATION: T RESECTION: Cutting out or off, without replacement, all of a body part

Body Part	Approach	Device	Qualifier
Ø Kidney, Right 1 Kidney, Left 2 Kidneys, Bilateral	Ø Open 4 Percutaneous Endoscopic	Z No Device	Z No Qualifier
3 Kidney Pelvis, Right 4 Kidney Pelvis, Left 6 Ureter, Right 7 Ureter, Left B Bladder C Bladder Neck D Urethra	Ø Open 4 Percutaneous Endoscopic 7 Via Natural or Artificial Opening 8 Via Natural or Artificial Opening Endoscopic	Z No Device	Z No Qualifier

Non-OR ØTTD[0478]ZZ

SECTION: Ø MEDICAL AND SURGICAL

BODY SYSTEM: T URINARY SYSTEM

OPERATION: U SUPPLEMENT: Putting in or on biological or synthetic material that physically reinforces and/or augments the function of a portion of a body part

Body Part	Approach	Device	Qualifier
3 Kidney Pelvis, Right 4 Kidney Pelvis, Left 6 Ureter, Right 7 Ureter, Left B Bladder C Bladder Neck	Ø Open 4 Percutaneous Endoscopic 7 Via Natural or Artificial Opening 8 Via Natural or Artificial Opening Endoscopic	7 Autologous Tissue Substitute J Synthetic Substitute K Nonautologous Tissue Substitute	Z No Qualifier
D Urethra	Ø Open 4 Percutaneous Endoscopic 7 Via Natural or Artificial Opening 8 Via Natural or Artificial Opening Endoscopic X External	7 Autologous Tissue Substitute J Synthetic Substitute K Nonautologous Tissue Substitute	Z No Qualifier

Coding Clinic: 2017, Q3, P21 – ØTUBØ7Z

SECTION: Ø MEDICAL AND SURGICAL

BODY SYSTEM: T URINARY SYSTEM

OPERATION: V RESTRICTION: Partially closing an orifice or the lumen of a tubular body part

Body Part	Approach	Device	Qualifier
3 Kidney Pelvis, Right 4 Kidney Pelvis, Left 6 Ureter, Right 7 Ureter, Left B Bladder C Bladder Neck	Ø Open 3 Percutaneous 4 Percutaneous Endoscopic	C Extraluminal Device D Intraluminal Device Z No Device	Z No Qualifier
3 Kidney Pelvis, Right 4 Kidney Pelvis, Left 6 Ureter, Right 7 Ureter, Left B Bladder C Bladder Neck	7 Via Natural or Artificial Opening 8 Via Natural or Artificial Opening Endoscopic	D Intraluminal Device Z No Device	Z No Qualifier
D Urethra	Ø Open 3 Percutaneous 4 Percutaneous Endoscopic	C Extraluminal Device D Intraluminal Device Z No Device	Z No Qualifier
D Urethra	7 Via Natural or Artificial Opening 8 Via Natural or Artificial Opening Endoscopic	D Intraluminal Device Z No Device	Z No Qualifier
D Urethra	X External	Z No Device	Z No Qualifier

Coding Clinic: 2015, Q2, P12 – ØTV[67]8ZZ

SECTION: Ø MEDICAL AND SURGICAL
BODY SYSTEM: T URINARY SYSTEM
OPERATION: W REVISION: *(on multiple pages)*
Correcting, to the extent possible, a portion of a malfunctioning device or the position of a displaced device

Body Part	Approach	Device	Qualifier
5 Kidney	Ø Open 3 Percutaneous 4 Percutaneous Endoscopic 7 Via Natural or Artificial Opening 8 Via Natural or Artificial Opening Endoscopic	Ø Drainage Device 2 Monitoring Device 3 Infusion Device 7 Autologous Tissue Substitute C Extraluminal Device D Intraluminal Device J Synthetic Substitute K Nonautologous Tissue Substitute Y Other Device	Z No Qualifier
5 Kidney	X External	Ø Drainage Device 2 Monitoring Device 3 Infusion Device 7 Autologous Tissue Substitute C Extraluminal Device D Intraluminal Device J Synthetic Substitute K Nonautologous Tissue Substitute	Z No Qualifier
9 Ureter	Ø Open 3 Percutaneous 4 Percutaneous Endoscopic 7 Via Natural or Artificial Opening 8 Via Natural or Artificial Opening Endoscopic	Ø Drainage Device 2 Monitoring Device 3 Infusion Device 7 Autologous Tissue Substitute C Extraluminal Device D Intraluminal Device J Synthetic Substitute K Nonautologous Tissue Substitute M Stimulator Lead Y Other Device	Z No Qualifier
9 Ureter	X External	Ø Drainage Device 2 Monitoring Device 3 Infusion Device 7 Autologous Tissue Substitute C Extraluminal Device D Intraluminal Device J Synthetic Substitute K Nonautologous Tissue Substitute M Stimulator Lead	Z No Qualifier

Non-OR   ØTW5X[Ø237CDJK]Z

SECTION: Ø MEDICAL AND SURGICAL
BODY SYSTEM: T URINARY SYSTEM
OPERATION: W REVISION: *(continued)*

Correcting, to the extent possible, a portion of a malfunctioning device or the position of a displaced device

Body Part	Approach	Device	Qualifier
B Bladder	Ø Open 3 Percutaneous 4 Percutaneous Endoscopic 7 Via Natural or Artificial Opening 8 Via Natural or Artificial Opening Endoscopic	Ø Drainage Device 2 Monitoring Device 3 Infusion Device 7 Autologous Tissue Substitute C Extraluminal Device D Intraluminal Device J Synthetic Substitute K Nonautologous Tissue Substitute L Artificial Sphincter M Stimulator Lead Y Other Device	Z No Qualifier
B Bladder	X External	Ø Drainage Device 2 Monitoring Device 3 Infusion Device 7 Autologous Tissue Substitute C Extraluminal Device D Intraluminal Device J Synthetic Substitute K Nonautologous Tissue Substitute L Artificial Sphincter M Stimulator Lead	Z No Qualifier
D Urethra	Ø Open 3 Percutaneous 4 Percutaneous Endoscopic 7 Via Natural or Artificial Opening 8 Via Natural or Artificial Opening Endoscopic	Ø Drainage Device 2 Monitoring Device 3 Infusion Device 7 Autologous Tissue Substitute C Extraluminal Device D Intraluminal Device J Synthetic Substitute K Nonautologous Tissue Substitute L Artificial Sphincter Y Other Device	Z No Qualifier
D Urethra	X External	Ø Drainage Device 2 Monitoring Device 3 Infusion Device 7 Autologous Tissue Substitute C Extraluminal Device D Intraluminal Device J Synthetic Substitute K Nonautologous Tissue Substitute L Artificial Sphincter	Z No Qualifier

Non-OR ØTW9X[0237CDJKM]Z
Non-OR ØTWBX[0237CDJKLM]Z
Non-OR ØTWDX[0237CDJKL]Z

Ø: M/S

T: URINARY SYSTEM

W: REVISION

SECTION: Ø MEDICAL AND SURGICAL
BODY SYSTEM: T URINARY SYSTEM
OPERATION: Y TRANSPLANTATION: Putting in or on all or a portion of a living body part taken from another individual or animal to physically take the place and/or function of all or a portion of a similar body part

Body Part	Approach	Device	Qualifier
Ø Kidney, Right 🅟 ⊞ 1 Kidney, Left 🅟 ⊞	Ø Open	Z No Device	Ø Allogeneic 1 Syngeneic 2 Zooplastic

🅟 ØTY[Ø1]ØZ[Ø12]
⊞ ØTY[Ø1]ØZ[Ø12]

Y: TRANSPLANTATION

T: URINARY SYSTEM

Ø: M/S

SECTION: Ø **MEDICAL AND SURGICAL**

BODY SYSTEM: U FEMALE REPRODUCTIVE SYSTEM

OPERATION: 1 **BYPASS:** Altering the route of passage of the contents of a tubular body part

Body Part	Approach	Device	Qualifier
5 Fallopian Tube, Right ♀ 6 Fallopian Tube, Left ♀	Ø Open 4 Percutaneous Endoscopic	7 Autologous Tissue Substitute J Synthetic Substitute K Nonautologous Tissue Substitute Z No Device	5 Fallopian Tube, Right 6 Fallopian Tube, Left 9 Uterus

SECTION: Ø **MEDICAL AND SURGICAL**

BODY SYSTEM: U FEMALE REPRODUCTIVE SYSTEM

OPERATION: 2 **CHANGE:** Taking out or off a device from a body part and putting back an identical or similar device in or on the same body part without cutting or puncturing the skin or a mucous membrane

Body Part	Approach	Device	Qualifier
3 Ovary ♀ 8 Fallopian Tube ♀ M Vulva ♀	X External	Ø Drainage Device Y Other Device	Z No Qualifier
D Uterus and Cervix ♀	X External	Ø Drainage Device H Contraceptive Device Y Other Device	Z No Qualifier
H Vagina and Cul-de-sac ♀	X External	Ø Drainage Device G Intraluminal Device, Pessary Y Other Device	Z No Qualifier

Non-OR All Values

1: BYPASS 2: CHANGE
U: FEMALE REPRODUCTIVE SYSTEM
Ø: M/S

SECTION: Ø MEDICAL AND SURGICAL

BODY SYSTEM: U FEMALE REPRODUCTIVE SYSTEM

OPERATION: 5 DESTRUCTION: Physical eradication of all or a portion of a body part by the direct use of energy, force, or a destructive agent

Body Part	Approach	Device	Qualifier
Ø Ovary, Right ♀ 1 Ovary, Left ♀ 2 Ovaries, Bilateral ♀ 4 Uterine Supporting Structure ♀	Ø Open 3 Percutaneous 4 Percutaneous Endoscopic 8 Via Natural or Artificial Opening Endoscopic	Z No Device	Z No Qualifier
5 Fallopian Tube, Right ♀ 6 Fallopian Tube, Left ♀ 7 Fallopian Tubes, Bilateral ♀ 🕸 9 Uterus ♀ B Endometrium ♀ C Cervix ♀ F Cul-de-sac ♀	Ø Open 3 Percutaneous 4 Percutaneous Endoscopic 7 Via Natural or Artificial Opening 8 Via Natural or Artificial Opening Endoscopic	Z No Device	Z No Qualifier
G Vagina ♀ K Hymen ♀	Ø Open 3 Percutaneous 4 Percutaneous Endoscopic 7 Via Natural or Artificial Opening 8 Via Natural or Artificial Opening Endoscopic X External	Z No Device	Z No Qualifier
J Clitoris ♀ L Vestibular Gland ♀ M Vulva ♀	Ø Open X External	Z No Device	Z No Qualifier

🕸 ØU57[Ø3478]ZZ when Z3Ø.2 is listed as the principal diagnosis

SECTION: 0 MEDICAL AND SURGICAL
BODY SYSTEM: U FEMALE REPRODUCTIVE SYSTEM
OPERATION: 7 DILATION: Expanding an orifice or the lumen of a tubular body part

Body Part	Approach	Device	Qualifier
5 Fallopian Tube, Right ♀ 6 Fallopian Tube, Left ♀ 7 Fallopian Tubes, Bilateral ♀ 9 Uterus ♀ C Cervix ♀ G Vagina ♀	0 Open 3 Percutaneous 4 Percutaneous Endoscopic 7 Via Natural or Artificial Opening 8 Via Natural or Artificial Opening Endoscopic	D Intraluminal Device Z No Device	Z No Qualifier
K Hymen ♀	0 Open 3 Percutaneous 4 Percutaneous Endoscopic 7 Via Natural or Artificial Opening 8 Via Natural or Artificial Opening Endoscopic X External	D Intraluminal Device Z No Device	Z No Qualifier

Non-OR 0U7C[03478][DZ]Z
Non-OR 0U7G[78][DZ]Z

SECTION: 0 MEDICAL AND SURGICAL
BODY SYSTEM: U FEMALE REPRODUCTIVE SYSTEM
OPERATION: 8 DIVISION: Cutting into a body part, without draining fluids and/or gases from the body part, in order to separate or transect a body part

Body Part	Approach	Device	Qualifier
0 Ovary, Right ♀ 1 Ovary, Left ♀ 2 Ovaries, Bilateral ♀ 4 Uterine Supporting Structure ♀	0 Open 3 Percutaneous 4 Percutaneous Endoscopic	Z No Device	Z No Qualifier
K Hymen ♀	7 Via Natural or Artificial Opening 8 Via Natural or Artificial Opening Endoscopic X External	Z No Device	Z No Qualifier

Non-OR 0U8K[78X]ZZ

SECTION: Ø MEDICAL AND SURGICAL

BODY SYSTEM: U FEMALE REPRODUCTIVE SYSTEM
OPERATION: 9 DRAINAGE: *(on multiple pages)*
Taking or letting out fluids and/or gases from a body part

Body Part	Approach	Device	Qualifier
Ø Ovary, Right ♀ 1 Ovary, Left ♀ 2 Ovaries, Bilateral ♀	Ø Open 3 Percutaneous 4 Percutaneous Endoscopic 8 Via Natural or Artificial Opening Endoscopic	Ø Drainage Device	Z No Qualifier
Ø Ovary, Right ♀ 1 Ovary, Left ♀ 2 Ovaries, Bilateral ♀	Ø Open 3 Percutaneous 4 Percutaneous Endoscopic 8 Via Natural or Artificial Opening Endoscopic	Z No Device	X Diagnostic Z No Qualifier
Ø Ovary, Right ♀ 1 Ovary, Left ♀ 2 Ovaries, Bilateral ♀	X External	Z No Device	Z No Qualifier
4 Uterine Supporting Structure ♀	Ø Open 3 Percutaneous 4 Percutaneous Endoscopic 8 Via Natural or Artificial Opening Endoscopic	Ø Drainage Device	Z No Qualifier
4 Uterine Supporting Structure ♀	Ø Open 3 Percutaneous 4 Percutaneous Endoscopic 8 Via Natural or Artificial Opening Endoscopic	Z No Device	X Diagnostic Z No Qualifier
5 Fallopian Tube, Right ♀ 6 Fallopian Tube, Left ♀ 7 Fallopian Tubes, Bilateral ♀ 9 Uterus ♀ C Cervix ♀ F Cul-de-sac ♀	Ø Open 3 Percutaneous 4 Percutaneous Endoscopic 7 Via Natural or Artificial Opening 8 Via Natural or Artificial Opening Endoscopic	Ø Drainage Device	Z No Qualifier
5 Fallopian Tube, Right ♀ 6 Fallopian Tube, Left ♀ 7 Fallopian Tubes, Bilateral ♀ 9 Uterus ♀ C Cervix ♀ F Cul-de-sac ♀	Ø Open 3 Percutaneous 4 Percutaneous Endoscopic 7 Via Natural or Artificial Opening 8 Via Natural or Artificial Opening Endoscopic	Z No Device	X Diagnostic Z No Qualifier
G Vagina ♀ K Hymen ♀	Ø Open 3 Percutaneous 4 Percutaneous Endoscopic 7 Via Natural or Artificial Opening 8 Via Natural or Artificial Opening Endoscopic X External	Ø Drainage Device	Z No Qualifier

Non-OR ØU9[Ø12]3ØZ	Non-OR ØU9F[34]ØZ	Non-OR ØU9K[Ø3478X]ZZ
Non-OR ØU9[Ø12]3ZZ	Non-OR ØU9[567][3478]ZZ	Non-OR ØU9[9C]3ZZ
Non-OR ØU943ØZ	Non-OR ØU9F[34]ZZ	Non-OR ØU9G3ØZ
Non-OR ØU943ZZ	Non-OR ØU9K[Ø3478X]ØZ	Non-OR ØU9G3ZZ
Non-OR ØU9[5679C]3ØZ		

New/Revised Text in Green   deleted Deleted   ♀ Females Only   ♂ Males Only   **Coding Clinic**
🝫 Non-covered   🝫 Limited Coverage   ⊞ Combination (See Appendix E)   DRG Non-OR   Non-OR   🝫 Hospital-Acquired Condition

SECTION: 0 MEDICAL AND SURGICAL
BODY SYSTEM: U FEMALE REPRODUCTIVE SYSTEM
OPERATION: 9 DRAINAGE: *(continued)*
Taking or letting out fluids and/or gases from a body part

Body Part	Approach	Device	Qualifier
G Vagina ♀ K Hymen ♀	0 Open 3 Percutaneous 4 Percutaneous Endoscopic 7 Via Natural or Artificial Opening 8 Via Natural or Artificial Opening Endoscopic X External	Z No Device	X Diagnostic Z No Qualifier
J Clitoris ♀ L Vestibular Gland ♀ M Vulva ♀	0 Open X External	0 Drainage Device	Z No Qualifier
J Clitoris ♀ L Vestibular Gland ♀ M Vulva ♀	0 Open X External	Z No Device	X Diagnostic Z No Qualifier

Non-OR 0U9L[0X]0Z
Non-OR 0U9L[0X]ZZ

SECTION: 0 MEDICAL AND SURGICAL
BODY SYSTEM: U FEMALE REPRODUCTIVE SYSTEM
OPERATION: B EXCISION: Cutting out or off, without replacement, a portion of a body part

Body Part	Approach	Device	Qualifier
0 Ovary, Right ♀ 1 Ovary, Left ♀ 2 Ovaries, Bilateral ♀ 4 Uterine Supporting Structure ♀ 5 Fallopian Tube, Right ♀ 6 Fallopian Tube, Left ♀ 7 Fallopian Tubes, Bilateral ♀ 9 Uterus ♀ C Cervix ♀ F Cul-de-sac ♀	0 Open 3 Percutaneous 4 Percutaneous Endoscopic 7 Via Natural or Artificial Opening 8 Via Natural or Artificial Opening Endoscopic	Z No Device	X Diagnostic Z No Qualifier
G Vagina ♀ K Hymen ♀	0 Open 3 Percutaneous 4 Percutaneous Endoscopic 7 Via Natural or Artificial Opening 8 Via Natural or Artificial Opening Endoscopic X External	Z No Device	X Diagnostic Z No Qualifier
J Clitoris ♀ L Vestibular Gland ♀ M Vulva ♀	0 Open X External	Z No Device	X Diagnostic Z No Qualifier

Coding Clinic: 2015, Q3, P31 – 0UB70ZZ
Coding Clinic: 2015, Q3, P32 – 0UB64ZZ

New/Revised Text in Green   ~~deleted~~ Deleted   ♀ Females Only   ♂ Males Only   **Coding Clinic**
🚫 Non-covered   🚫 Limited Coverage   ⊞ Combination (See Appendix E)   DRG Non-OR   Non-OR   🚫 Hospital-Acquired Condition

SECTION: Ø MEDICAL AND SURGICAL

BODY SYSTEM: U FEMALE REPRODUCTIVE SYSTEM

OPERATION: C EXTIRPATION: Taking or cutting out solid matter from a body part

Body Part	Approach	Device	Qualifier
Ø Ovary, Right ♀ 1 Ovary, Left ♀ 2 Ovaries, Bilateral ♀ 4 Uterine Supporting Structure ♀	Ø Open 3 Percutaneous 4 Percutaneous Endoscopic 8 Via Natural or Artificial Opening Endoscopic	Z No Device	Z No Qualifier
5 Fallopian Tube, Right ♀ 6 Fallopian Tube, Left ♀ 7 Fallopian Tubes, Bilateral ♀ 9 Uterus ♀ B Endometrium ♀ C Cervix ♀ F Cul-de-sac ♀	Ø Open 3 Percutaneous 4 Percutaneous Endoscopic 7 Via Natural or Artificial Opening 8 Via Natural or Artificial Opening Endoscopic	Z No Device	Z No Qualifier
G Vagina ♀ K Hymen ♀	Ø Open 3 Percutaneous 4 Percutaneous Endoscopic 7 Via Natural or Artificial Opening 8 Via Natural or Artificial Opening Endoscopic X External	Z No Device	Z No Qualifier
J Clitoris ♀ L Vestibular Gland ♀ M Vulva ♀	Ø Open X External	Z No Device	Z No Qualifier

Non-OR   ØUC9[78]ZZ
Non-OR   ØUCG[78X]ZZ
Non-OR   ØUCK[Ø3478X]ZZ
Non-OR   ØUCMXZZ

Coding Clinic: 2Ø13, Q2, P38 – ØUC97ZZ
Coding Clinic: 2Ø15, Q3, P3Ø-31 – ØUCC[78]ZZ

New/Revised Text in Green   ~~deleted~~ Deleted   ♀ Females Only   ♂ Males Only   **Coding Clinic**
Non-covered   Limited Coverage   ⊞ Combination (See Appendix E)   DRG Non-OR   Non-OR   Hospital-Acquired Condition

475

SECTION: Ø MEDICAL AND SURGICAL

BODY SYSTEM: U FEMALE REPRODUCTIVE SYSTEM

OPERATION: D **EXTRACTION:** Pulling or stripping out or off all or a portion of a body part by the use of force

Body Part	Approach	Device	Qualifier
B Endometrium ♀	7 Via Natural or Artificial Opening 8 Via Natural or Artificial Opening Endoscopic	Z No Device	X Diagnostic Z No Qualifier
N Ova ♀	Ø Open 3 Percutaneous 4 Percutaneous Endoscopic	Z No Device	Z No Qualifier

SECTION: Ø MEDICAL AND SURGICAL

BODY SYSTEM: U FEMALE REPRODUCTIVE SYSTEM

OPERATION: F **FRAGMENTATION:** Breaking solid matter in a body part into pieces

Body Part	Approach	Device	Qualifier
5 Fallopian Tube, Right ♀ 🦠 6 Fallopian Tube, Left ♀ 🦠 7 Fallopian Tubes, Bilateral ♀ 🦠 9 Uterus ♀ 🦠	Ø Open 3 Percutaneous 4 Percutaneous Endoscopic 7 Via Natural or Artificial Opening 8 Via Natural or Artificial Opening Endoscopic X External	Z No Device	Z No Qualifier

🦠 ØUF[5679]XZZ
Non-OR   ØUF[5679]XZZ

SECTION: Ø MEDICAL AND SURGICAL

BODY SYSTEM: U FEMALE REPRODUCTIVE SYSTEM

OPERATION: H **INSERTION:** Putting in a nonbiological appliance that monitors, assists, performs, or prevents a physiological function but does not physically take the place of a body part

Body Part	Approach	Device	Qualifier
3 Ovary ♀	Ø Open 3 Percutaneous 4 Percutaneous Endoscopic	3 Infusion Device Y Other Device	Z No Qualifier
3 Ovary ♀	7 Via Natural or Artificial Opening 8 Via Natural or Artificial Opening Endoscopic	Y Other Device	Z No Qualifier
8 Fallopian Tube ♀ D Uterus and Cervix ♀ H Vagina and Cul-de-sac ♀	Ø Open 3 Percutaneous 4 Percutaneous Endoscopic 7 Via Natural or Artificial Opening 8 Via Natural or Artificial Opening Endoscopic	3 Infusion Device Y Other Device	Z No Qualifier
9 Uterus ♀	Ø Open 7 Via Natural or Artificial Opening 8 Via Natural or Artificial Opening Endoscopic	H Contraceptive Device	Z No Qualifier
C Cervix ♀	Ø Open 3 Percutaneous 4 Percutaneous Endoscopic	1 Radioactive Element	Z No Qualifier
C Cervix ♀	7 Via Natural or Artificial Opening 8 Via Natural or Artificial Opening Endoscopic	1 Radioactive Element H Contraceptive Device	Z No Qualifier
F Cul-de-sac ♀	7 Via Natural or Artificial Opening 8 Via Natural or Artificial Opening Endoscopic	G Intraluminal Device, Pessary	Z No Qualifier
G Vagina ♀	Ø Open 3 Percutaneous 4 Percutaneous Endoscopic X External	1 Radioactive Element	Z No Qualifier
G Vagina ♀	7 Via Natural or Artificial Opening 8 Via Natural or Artificial Opening Endoscopic	1 Radioactive Element G Intraluminal Device, Pessary	Z No Qualifier

Non-OR ØUH3[Ø34]3Z
Non-OR ØUH[8D][Ø3478]3Z
Non-OR ØUHH[78]3Z
Non-OR ØUH9[78]HZ
Non-OR ØUHC[78]HZ
Non-OR ØUHF[78]GZ
Non-OR ØUHG[78]GZ

Coding Clinic: 2013, Q2, P34 – ØUH97HZ

SECTION: Ø MEDICAL AND SURGICAL

BODY SYSTEM: U FEMALE REPRODUCTIVE SYSTEM

OPERATION: **J** INSPECTION: Visually and/or manually exploring a body part

Body Part	Approach	Device	Qualifier
3 Ovary ♀	Ø Open 3 Percutaneous 4 Percutaneous Endoscopic 8 Via Natural or Artificial Opening Endoscopic X External	Z No Device	Z No Qualifier
8 Fallopian Tube ♀ D Uterus and Cervix ♀ H Vagina and Cul-de-sac ♀	Ø Open 3 Percutaneous 4 Percutaneous Endoscopic 7 Via Natural or Artificial Opening 8 Via Natural or Artificial Opening Endoscopic X External	Z No Device	Z No Qualifier
M Vulva ♀	Ø Open X External	Z No Device	Z No Qualifier

Non-OR ØUJ8[378]ZZ
Non-OR ØUJD3ZZ
Non-OR ØUJ3[3X]ZZ
Non-OR ØUJ8XZZ
Non-OR ØUJD[78X]ZZ
Non-OR ØUJH[378X]ZZ
Non-OR ØUJMXZZ

Coding Clinic: 2015, Q1, P34 – ØUJD4ZZ

SECTION: Ø MEDICAL AND SURGICAL

BODY SYSTEM: U FEMALE REPRODUCTIVE SYSTEM

OPERATION: **L** OCCLUSION: Completely closing an orifice or the lumen of a tubular body part

Body Part	Approach	Device	Qualifier
5 Fallopian Tube, Right ♀ 6 Fallopian Tube, Left ♀ 7 Fallopian Tubes, Bilateral ♀ 🚫	Ø Open 3 Percutaneous 4 Percutaneous Endoscopic	C Extraluminal Device D Intraluminal Device Z No Device	Z No Qualifier
5 Fallopian Tube, Right ♀ 6 Fallopian Tube, Left ♀ 7 Fallopian Tubes, Bilateral ♀ 🚫	7 Via Natural or Artificial Opening 8 Via Natural or Artificial Opening Endoscopic	D Intraluminal Device Z No Device	Z No Qualifier
F Cul-de-sac ♀ G Vagina ♀	7 Via Natural or Artificial Opening 8 Via Natural or Artificial Opening Endoscopic	D Intraluminal Device Z No Device	Z No Qualifier

🚫 ØUL7[Ø34][CDZ]Z when Z30.2 is listed as the principal diagnosis
🚫 ØUL7[78][DZ]Z when Z30.2 is listed as the principal diagnosis

Side tab labels: J: INSPECTION   L: OCCLUSION   U: FEMALE REPRODUCTIVE SYSTEM   Ø: M/S

SECTION: Ø MEDICAL AND SURGICAL
BODY SYSTEM: U FEMALE REPRODUCTIVE SYSTEM
OPERATION: M REATTACHMENT: Putting back in or on all or a portion of a separated body part to its normal location or other suitable location

Body Part	Approach	Device	Qualifier
Ø Ovary, Right ♀ 1 Ovary, Left ♀ 2 Ovaries, Bilateral ♀ 4 Uterine Supporting Structure ♀ 5 Fallopian Tube, Right ♀ 6 Fallopian Tube, Left ♀ 7 Fallopian Tubes, Bilateral ♀ 9 Uterus ♀ C Cervix ♀ F Cul-de-sac ♀ G Vagina ♀	Ø Open 4 Percutaneous Endoscopic	Z No Device	Z No Qualifier
J Clitoris ♀ M Vulva ♀	X External	Z No Device	Z No Qualifier
K Hymen ♀	Ø Open 4 Percutaneous Endoscopic X External	Z No Device	Z No Qualifier

SECTION: Ø MEDICAL AND SURGICAL
BODY SYSTEM: U FEMALE REPRODUCTIVE SYSTEM
OPERATION: N RELEASE: Freeing a body part from an abnormal physical constraint by cutting or by the use of force

Body Part	Approach	Device	Qualifier
Ø Ovary, Right ♀ 1 Ovary, Left ♀ 2 Ovaries, Bilateral ♀ 4 Uterine Supporting Structure ♀	Ø Open 3 Percutaneous 4 Percutaneous Endoscopic 8 Via Natural or Artificial Opening Endoscopic	Z No Device	Z No Qualifier
5 Fallopian Tube, Right ♀ 6 Fallopian Tube, Left ♀ 7 Fallopian Tubes, Bilateral ♀ 9 Uterus ♀ C Cervix ♀ F Cul-de-sac ♀	Ø Open 3 Percutaneous 4 Percutaneous Endoscopic 7 Via Natural or Artificial Opening 8 Via Natural or Artificial Opening Endoscopic	Z No Device	Z No Qualifier
G Vagina ♀ K Hymen ♀	Ø Open 3 Percutaneous 4 Percutaneous Endoscopic 7 Via Natural or Artificial Opening 8 Via Natural or Artificial Opening Endoscopic X External	Z No Device	Z No Qualifier
J Clitoris ♀ L Vestibular Gland ♀ M Vulva ♀	Ø Open X External	Z No Device	Z No Qualifier

SECTION: Ø MEDICAL AND SURGICAL

BODY SYSTEM: U FEMALE REPRODUCTIVE SYSTEM
OPERATION: P REMOVAL: *(on multiple pages)*
Taking out or off a device from a body part

P: REMOVAL

U: FEMALE REPRODUCTIVE SYSTEM

Ø: M/S

Body Part	Approach	Device	Qualifier
3 Ovary ♀	Ø Open 3 Percutaneous 4 Percutaneous Endoscopic	Ø Drainage Device 3 Infusion Device Y Other Device	Z No Qualifier
3 Ovary ♀	7 Via Natural or Artificial Opening 8 Via Natural or Artificial Opening Endoscopic	Y Other Device	Z No Qualifier
3 Ovary ♀	X External	Ø Drainage Device 3 Infusion Device	Z No Qualifier
8 Fallopian Tube ♀	Ø Open 3 Percutaneous 4 Percutaneous Endoscopic 7 Via Natural or Artificial Opening 8 Via Natural or Artificial Opening Endoscopic	Ø Drainage Device 3 Infusion Device 7 Autologous Tissue Substitute C Extraluminal Device D Intraluminal Device J Synthetic Substitute K Nonautologous Tissue Substitute Y Other Device	Z No Qualifier
8 Fallopian Tube ♀	X External	Ø Drainage Device 3 Infusion Device D Intraluminal Device	Z No Qualifier
D Uterus and Cervix ♀	Ø Open 3 Percutaneous 4 Percutaneous Endoscopic 7 Via Natural or Artificial Opening 8 Via Natural or Artificial Opening Endoscopic	Ø Drainage Device 1 Radioactive Element 3 Infusion Device 7 Autologous Tissue Substitute C Extraluminal Device D Intraluminal Device H Contraceptive Device J Synthetic Substitute K Nonautologous Tissue Substitute Y Other Device	Z No Qualifier
D Uterus and Cervix ♀	X External	Ø Drainage Device 3 Infusion Device D Intraluminal Device H Contraceptive Device	Z No Qualifier
H Vagina and Cul-de-sac ♀	Ø Open 3 Percutaneous 4 Percutaneous Endoscopic 7 Via Natural or Artificial Opening 8 Via Natural or Artificial Opening Endoscopic	Ø Drainage Device 1 Radioactive Element 3 Infusion Device 7 Autologous Tissue Substitute D Intraluminal Device J Synthetic Substitute K Nonautologous Tissue Substitute Y Other Device	Z No Qualifier

Non-OR ØUP3X[Ø3]Z
Non-OR ØUP8[78][Ø3D]Z
Non-OR ØUP8X[Ø3D]Z

Non-OR ØUPD[34]CZ
Non-OR ØUPD[78][Ø3CDH]Z

Non-OR ØUPDX[Ø3DH]Z
Non-OR ØUPH[78][Ø3D]Z

New/Revised Text in Green   ~~deleted~~ Deleted   ♀ Females Only   ♂ Males Only   **Coding Clinic**
🚫 Non-covered   🚫 Limited Coverage   ⊞ Combination (See Appendix E)   DRG Non-OR   Non-OR   🚫 Hospital-Acquired Condition

SECTION: Ø MEDICAL AND SURGICAL

BODY SYSTEM: U FEMALE REPRODUCTIVE SYSTEM

OPERATION: P REMOVAL: *(continued)*
Taking out or off a device from a body part

Body Part	Approach	Device	Qualifier
H Vagina and Cul-de-sac ♀	X External	Ø Drainage Device 1 Radioactive Element 3 Infusion Device D Intraluminal Device	Z No Qualifier
M Vulva ♀	Ø Open	Ø Drainage Device 7 Autologous Tissue Substitute J Synthetic Substitute K Nonautologous Tissue Substitute	Z No Qualifier
M Vulva ♀	X External	Ø Drainage Device	Z No Qualifier

Non-OR ØUPHX[Ø13D]Z
Non-OR ØUPMXØZ

SECTION: Ø MEDICAL AND SURGICAL

BODY SYSTEM: U FEMALE REPRODUCTIVE SYSTEM

OPERATION: Q REPAIR: Restoring, to the extent possible, a body part to its normal anatomic structure and function

Body Part	Approach	Device	Qualifier
Ø Ovary, Right ♀ 1 Ovary, Left ♀ 2 Ovaries, Bilateral ♀ 4 Uterine Supporting Structure ♀	Ø Open 3 Percutaneous 4 Percutaneous Endoscopic 8 Via Natural or Artificial Opening Endoscopic	Z No Device	Z No Qualifier
5 Fallopian Tube, Right ♀ 6 Fallopian Tube, Left ♀ 7 Fallopian Tubes, Bilateral ♀ 9 Uterus ♀ C Cervix ♀ F Cul-de-sac ♀	Ø Open 3 Percutaneous 4 Percutaneous Endoscopic 7 Via Natural or Artificial Opening 8 Via Natural or Artificial Opening Endoscopic	Z No Device	Z No Qualifier
G Vagina ♀ K Hymen ♀	Ø Open 3 Percutaneous 4 Percutaneous Endoscopic 7 Via Natural or Artificial Opening 8 Via Natural or Artificial Opening Endoscopic X External	Z No Device	Z No Qualifier
J Clitoris ♀ L Vestibular Gland ♀ M Vulva ♀	Ø Open X External	Z No Device	Z No Qualifier

U: FEMALE REPRODUCTIVE SYSTEM

S: REPOSITION   T: RESECTION

SECTION: Ø **MEDICAL AND SURGICAL**

BODY SYSTEM: U FEMALE REPRODUCTIVE SYSTEM

OPERATION: S **REPOSITION:** Moving to its normal location, or other suitable location, all or a portion of a body part

Body Part	Approach	Device	Qualifier
Ø Ovary, Right ♀ 1 Ovary, Left ♀ 2 Ovaries, Bilateral ♀ 4 Uterine Supporting Structure ♀ 5 Fallopian Tube, Right ♀ 6 Fallopian Tube, Left ♀ 7 Fallopian Tubes, Bilateral ♀ C Cervix ♀ F Cul-de-sac ♀	Ø Open 4 Percutaneous Endoscopic 8 Via Natural or Artificial Opening Endoscopic	Z No Device	Z No Qualifier
9 Uterus ♀ G Vagina ♀	Ø Open 4 Percutaneous Endoscopic 7 Via Natural or Artificial Opening 8 Via Natural or Artificial Opening Endoscopic X External	Z No Device	Z No Qualifier

Non-OR ØUS9XZZ

Coding Clinic: 2016, Q1, P9 – ØUS9XZZ
Coding Clinic: 2017, Q4, P68 – ØUT9[Ø7]Z[LZ]

SECTION: Ø **MEDICAL AND SURGICAL**

BODY SYSTEM: U FEMALE REPRODUCTIVE SYSTEM

OPERATION: T **RESECTION:** Cutting out or off, without replacement, all of a body part

Body Part	Approach	Device	Qualifier
Ø Ovary, Right ♀ 1 Ovary, Left ♀ 2 Ovaries, Bilateral ♀ 5 Fallopian Tube, Right ♀ 6 Fallopian Tube, Left ♀ 7 Fallopian Tubes, Bilateral ♀	Ø Open 4 Percutaneous Endoscopic 7 Via Natural or Artificial Opening 8 Via Natural or Artificial Opening Endoscopic F Via Natural or Artificial Opening With Percutaneous Endoscopic Assistance	Z No Device	Z No Qualifier
4 Uterine Supporting Structure ♀ ⊞ C Cervix ♀ ⊞ F Cul-de-sac ♀ G Vagina ♀	Ø Open 4 Percutaneous Endoscopic 7 Via Natural or Artificial Opening 8 Via Natural or Artificial Opening Endoscopic	Z No Device	Z No Qualifier
9 Uterus ♀ ⊞	Ø Open 4 Percutaneous Endoscopic 7 Via Natural or Artificial Opening 8 Via Natural or Artificial Opening Endoscopic F Via Natural or Artificial Opening With Percutaneous Endoscopic Assistance	Z No Device	L Supracervical Z No Qualifier
J Clitoris ♀ L Vestibular Gland ♀ M Vulva ♀ ⊞	Ø Open X External	Z No Device	Z No Qualifier
K Hymen ♀	Ø Open 4 Percutaneous Endoscopic 7 Via Natural or Artificial Opening 8 Via Natural or Artificial Opening Endoscopic X External	Z No Device	Z No Qualifier

⊞ ØUT9[Ø478F]ZZ
⊞ ØUT[4C][Ø478]ZZ
⊞ ØUTM[ØX]ZZ

Coding Clinic: 2013, Q1, P24 – ØUTØØZZ
Coding Clinic: 2015, Q1, P33-34; 2013, Q3, P28 – ØUT9ØZZ, ØUTCØZZ
Coding Clinic: 2015, Q1, P34 – ØUT2ØZZ, ØUT7ØZZ

Ø: M/S

New/Revised Text in Green   ~~deleted~~ Deleted   ♀ Females Only   ♂ Males Only   **Coding Clinic**
🚫 Non-covered   🚫 Limited Coverage   ⊞ Combination (See Appendix E)   DRG Non-OR   Non-OR   🚫 Hospital-Acquired Condition

SECTION: Ø MEDICAL AND SURGICAL

BODY SYSTEM: U FEMALE REPRODUCTIVE SYSTEM

OPERATION: U SUPPLEMENT: Putting in or on biological or synthetic material that physically reinforces and/or augments the function of a portion of a body part

Body Part	Approach	Device	Qualifier
4 Uterine Supporting Structure ♀	Ø Open 4 Percutaneous Endoscopic	7 Autologous Tissue Substitute J Synthetic Substitute K Nonautologous Tissue Substitute	Z No Qualifier
5 Fallopian Tube Right ♀ 6 Fallopian Tube, Left ♀ 7 Fallopian Tubes, Bilateral ♀ F Cul-de-sac ♀	Ø Open 4 Percutaneous Endoscopic 7 Via Natural or Artificial Opening 8 Via Natural or Artificial Opening Endoscopic	7 Autologous Tissue Substitute J Synthetic Substitute K Nonautologous Tissue Substitute	Z No Qualifier
G Vagina ♀ K Hymen ♀	Ø Open 4 Percutaneous Endoscopic 7 Via Natural or Artificial Opening 8 Via Natural or Artificial Opening Endoscopic X External	7 Autologous Tissue Substitute J Synthetic Substitute K Nonautologous Tissue Substitute	Z No Qualifier
J Clitoris ♀ M Vulva ♀	Ø Open X External	7 Autologous Tissue Substitute J Synthetic Substitute K Nonautologous Tissue Substitute	Z No Qualifier

SECTION: Ø MEDICAL AND SURGICAL

BODY SYSTEM: U FEMALE REPRODUCTIVE SYSTEM

OPERATION: V RESTRICTION: Partially closing an orifice or the lumen of a tubular body part

Body Part	Approach	Device	Qualifier
C Cervix ♀	Ø Open 3 Percutaneous 4 Percutaneous Endoscopic	C Extraluminal Device D Intraluminal Device Z No Device	Z No Qualifier
C Cervix ♀	7 Via Natural or Artificial Opening 8 Via Natural or Artificial Opening Endoscopic	D Intraluminal Device Z No Device	Z No Qualifier

Coding Clinic: 2015, Q3, P3Ø – ØUVC7ZZ

SECTION: Ø   MEDICAL AND SURGICAL

BODY SYSTEM: U   FEMALE REPRODUCTIVE SYSTEM

OPERATION: W   REVISION: *(on multiple pages)*

                  Correcting, to the extent possible, a portion of a malfunctioning device or the position of a displaced device

Body Part	Approach	Device	Qualifier
3 Ovary ♀	Ø Open 3 Percutaneous 4 Percutaneous Endoscopic	Ø Drainage Device 3 Infusion Device Y Other Device	Z No Qualifier
3 Ovary ♀	7 Via Natural or Artificial Opening 8 Via Natural or Artificial Opening Endoscopic	Y Other Device	Z No Qualifier
3 Ovary ♀	X External	Ø Drainage Device 3 Infusion Device	Z No Qualifier
8 Fallopian Tube ♀	Ø Open 3 Percutaneous 4 Percutaneous Endoscopic 7 Via Natural or Artificial Opening 8 Via Natural or Artificial Opening Endoscopic	Ø Drainage Device 3 Infusion Device 7 Autologous Tissue Substitute C Extraluminal Device D Intraluminal Device J Synthetic Substitute K Nonautologous Tissue Substitute Y Other Device	Z No Qualifier
8 Fallopian Tube ♀	X External	Ø Drainage Device 3 Infusion Device 7 Autologous Tissue Substitute C Extraluminal Device D Intraluminal Device J Synthetic Substitute K Nonautologous Tissue Substitute	Z No Qualifier
D Uterus and Cervix ♀	Ø Open 3 Percutaneous 4 Percutaneous Endoscopic 7 Via Natural or Artificial Opening 8 Via Natural or Artificial Opening Endoscopic	Ø Drainage Device 1 Radioactive Element 3 Infusion Device 7 Autologous Tissue Substitute C Extraluminal Device D Intraluminal Device H Contraceptive Device J Synthetic Substitute K Nonautologous Tissue Substitute Y Other Device	Z No Qualifier
D Uterus and Cervix ♀	X External	Ø Drainage Device 3 Infusion Device 7 Autologous Tissue Substitute C Extraluminal Device D Intraluminal Device H Contraceptive Device J Synthetic Substitute K Nonautologous Tissue Substitute	Z No Qualifier
H Vagina and Cul-de-sac ♀	Ø Open 3 Percutaneous 4 Percutaneous Endoscopic 7 Via Natural or Artificial Opening 8 Via Natural or Artificial Opening Endoscopic	Ø Drainage Device 1 Radioactive Element 3 Infusion Device 7 Autologous Tissue Substitute D Intraluminal Device J Synthetic Substitute K Nonautologous Tissue Substitute Y Other Device	Z No Qualifier

Non-OR   ØUW3X[Ø3]Z   Non-OR   ØUW8X[Ø37CDJK]Z   Non-OR   ØUWDX[Ø37CDHJK]Z

New/Revised Text in Green   ~~deleted~~ Deleted   ♀ Females Only   ♂ Males Only   **Coding Clinic**

🖫 Non-covered   🖫 Limited Coverage   ⊞ Combination (See Appendix E)   DRG Non-OR   Non-OR   🖫 Hospital-Acquired Condition

SECTION: Ø MEDICAL AND SURGICAL

BODY SYSTEM: U FEMALE REPRODUCTIVE SYSTEM

OPERATION: W REVISION: *(continued)*
Correcting, to the extent possible, a portion of a malfunctioning device or the position of a displaced device

Body Part	Approach	Device	Qualifier
H Vagina and Cul-de-sac ♀	X External	Ø Drainage Device 3 Infusion Device 7 Autologous Tissue Substitute D Intraluminal Device J Synthetic Substitute K Nonautologous Tissue Substitute	Z No Qualifier
M Vulva ♀	Ø Open X External	Ø Drainage Device 7 Autologous Tissue Substitute J Synthetic Substitute K Nonautologous Tissue Substitute	Z No Qualifier

Non-OR   ØUWHX[Ø37DJK]Z
Non-OR   ØUWMX[Ø7JK]Z

SECTION: Ø MEDICAL AND SURGICAL

BODY SYSTEM: U FEMALE REPRODUCTIVE SYSTEM

OPERATION: Y TRANSPLANTATION: Putting in or on all or a portion of a living body part taken from another individual or animal to physically take the place and/or function of all or a portion of a similar body part

Body Part	Approach	Device	Qualifier
Ø Ovary, Right ♀ 1 Ovary, Left ♀ 9 Uterus ♀	Ø Open	Z No Device	Ø Allogeneic 1 Syngeneic 2 Zooplastic

New/Revised Text in Green   ~~deleted~~ Deleted   ♀ Females Only   ♂ Males Only   **Coding Clinic**
Non-covered   Limited Coverage   ⊞ Combination (See Appendix E)   DRG Non-OR   Non-OR   Hospital-Acquired Condition

SECTION: Ø MEDICAL AND SURGICAL

BODY SYSTEM: V MALE REPRODUCTIVE SYSTEM

OPERATION: 1 BYPASS: Altering the route of passage of the contents of a tubular body part

Body Part	Approach	Device	Qualifier
N Vas Deferens, Right ♂ P Vas Deferens, Left ♂ Q Vas Deferens, Bilateral ♂	Ø Open 4 Percutaneous Endoscopic	7 Autologous Tissue Substitute J Synthetic Substitute K Nonautologous Tissue Substitute Z No Device	J Epididymis, Right K Epididymis, Left N Vas Deferens, Right P Vas Deferens, Left

SECTION: Ø MEDICAL AND SURGICAL

BODY SYSTEM: V MALE REPRODUCTIVE SYSTEM

OPERATION: 2 CHANGE: Taking out or off a device from a body part and putting back an identical or similar device in or on the same body part without cutting or puncturing the skin or a mucous membrane

Body Part	Approach	Device	Qualifier
4 Prostate and Seminal Vesicles ♂ 8 Scrotum and Tunica Vaginalis ♂ D Testis ♂ M Epididymis and Spermatic Cord ♂ R Vas Deferens ♂ S Penis ♂	X External	Ø Drainage Device Y Other Device	Z No Qualifier

Non-OR **All Values**

SECTION: Ø MEDICAL AND SURGICAL
BODY SYSTEM: V MALE REPRODUCTIVE SYSTEM
OPERATION: 5 DESTRUCTION: Physical eradication of all or a portion of a body part by the direct use of energy, force, or a destructive agent

Body Part	Approach	Device	Qualifier
Ø Prostate ♂	Ø Open 3 Percutaneous 4 Percutaneous Endoscopic 7 Via Natural or Artificial Opening 8 Via Natural or Artificial Opening Endoscopic	Z No Device	Z No Qualifier
1 Seminal Vesicle, Right ♂ 2 Seminal Vesicle, Left ♂ 3 Seminal Vesicles, Bilateral ♂ 6 Tunica Vaginalis, Right ♂ 7 Tunica Vaginalis, Left ♂ 9 Testis, Right ♂ B Testis, Left ♂ C Testes, Bilateral ♂	Ø Open 3 Percutaneous 4 Percutaneous Endoscopic	Z No Device	Z No Qualifier
5 Scrotum ♂ S Penis ♂ T Prepuce ♂	Ø Open 3 Percutaneous 4 Percutaneous Endoscopic X External	Z No Device	Z No Qualifier
F Spermatic Cord, Right ♂ G Spermatic Cord, Left ♂ H Spermatic Cords, Bilateral ♂ J Epididymis, Right ♂ K Epididymis, Left ♂ L Epididymis, Bilateral ♂ N Vas Deferens, Right ♂ 🔒 P Vas Deferens, Left ♂ 🔒 Q Vas Deferens, Bilateral ♂ 🔒	Ø Open 3 Percutaneous 4 Percutaneous Endoscopic 8 Via Natural or Artificial Opening Endoscopic	Z No Device	Z No Qualifier

🔒 ØV5[NPQ][Ø34]ZZ when Z30.2 is listed as the principal diagnosis
Non-OR ØV5[NPQ][Ø34]ZZ
Non-OR ØV55[Ø34X]ZZ

SECTION: Ø MEDICAL AND SURGICAL
BODY SYSTEM: V MALE REPRODUCTIVE SYSTEM
OPERATION: 7 DILATION: Expanding an orifice or the lumen of a tubular body part

Body Part	Approach	Device	Qualifier
N Vas Deferens, Right ♂ P Vas Deferens, Left ♂ Q Vas Deferens, Bilateral ♂	Ø Open 3 Percutaneous 4 Percutaneous Endoscopic	D Intraluminal Device Z No Device	Z No Qualifier

5: DESTRUCTION   7: DILATION

V: MALE REPRODUCTIVE SYSTEM

Ø: M/S

New/Revised Text in Green   ~~deleted~~ Deleted   ♀ Females Only   ♂ Males Only   **Coding Clinic**
🔒 Non-covered   🔒 Limited Coverage   ⊞ Combination (See Appendix E)   DRG Non-OR   Non-OR   🔒 Hospital-Acquired Condition

SECTION: 0 MEDICAL AND SURGICAL
BODY SYSTEM: V MALE REPRODUCTIVE SYSTEM
OPERATION: 9 DRAINAGE: *(on multiple pages)*
Taking or letting out fluids and/or gases from a body part

Body Part	Approach	Device	Qualifier
0 Prostate ♂	0 Open 3 Percutaneous 4 Percutaneous Endoscopic 7 Via Natural or Artificial Opening 8 Via Natural or Artificial Opening Endoscopic	0 Drainage Device	Z No Qualifier
0 Prostate ♂	0 Open 3 Percutaneous 4 Percutaneous Endoscopic 7 Via Natural or Artificial Opening 8 Via Natural or Artificial Opening Endoscopic	Z No Device	X Diagnostic Z No Qualifier
1 Seminal Vesicle, Right ♂ 2 Seminal Vesicle, Left ♂ 3 Seminal Vesicles, Bilateral ♂ 6 Tunica Vaginalis, Right ♂ 7 Tunica Vaginalis, Left ♂ 9 Testis, Right ♂ B Testis, Left ♂ C Testes, Bilateral ♂ F Spermatic Cord, Right ♂ G Spermatic Cord, Left ♂ H Spermatic Cords, Bilateral ♂ J Epididymis, Right ♂ K Epididymis, Left ♂ L Epididymis, Bilateral ♂ N Vas Deferens, Right ♂ P Vas Deferens, Left ♂ Q Vas Deferens, Bilateral ♂	0 Open 3 Percutaneous 4 Percutaneous Endoscopic	0 Drainage Device	Z No Qualifier
1 Seminal Vesicle, Right ♂ 2 Seminal Vesicle, Left ♂ 3 Seminal Vesicles, Bilateral ♂ 6 Tunica Vaginalis, Right ♂ 7 Tunica Vaginalis, Left ♂ 9 Testis, Right ♂ B Testis, Left ♂ C Testes, Bilateral ♂ F Spermatic Cord, Right ♂ G Spermatic Cord, Left ♂ H Spermatic Cords, Bilateral ♂ J Epididymis, Right ♂ K Epididymis, Left ♂ L Epididymis, Bilateral ♂ N Vas Deferens, Right ♂ P Vas Deferens, Left ♂ Q Vas Deferens, Bilateral ♂	0 Open 3 Percutaneous 4 Percutaneous Endoscopic	Z No Device	X Diagnostic Z No Qualifier

Non-OR 0V90[34]0Z
Non-OR 0V90[34]ZZ
Non-OR 0V90[3478]ZX
Non-OR 0V9[1239BC][34]0Z
Non-OR 0V9[67FGHNPQ][034]0Z

Non-OR 0V9[JKL]30Z
Non-OR 0V9[1239BC][34]Z[XZ]
Non-OR 0V9[67FGHJKLNPQ][034]ZX
Non-OR 0V9[67FGHNPQ][034]ZZ
Non-OR 0V9[JKL]3ZZ

0: M/S

V: MALE REPRODUCTIVE SYSTEM

9: DRAINAGE

SECTION: Ø MEDICAL AND SURGICAL
BODY SYSTEM: V MALE REPRODUCTIVE SYSTEM
OPERATION: 9 DRAINAGE: *(continued)*
Taking or letting out fluids and/or gases from a body part

Body Part	Approach	Device	Qualifier
5 Scrotum ♂ S Penis ♂ T Prepuce ♂	Ø Open 3 Percutaneous 4 Percutaneous Endoscopic X External	Ø Drainage Device	Z No Qualifier
5 Scrotum ♂ S Penis ♂ T Prepuce ♂	Ø Open 3 Percutaneous 4 Percutaneous Endoscopic X External	Z No Device	X Diagnostic Z No Qualifier

Non-OR ØV9[ST]3ØZ
Non-OR ØV9[ST]3ZZ

Non-OR ØV95[Ø34X]Z[XZ]

SECTION: Ø MEDICAL AND SURGICAL
BODY SYSTEM: V MALE REPRODUCTIVE SYSTEM
OPERATION: B EXCISION: *(on multiple pages)*
Cutting out or off, without replacement, a portion of a body part

Body Part	Approach	Device	Qualifier
Ø Prostate ♂	Ø Open 3 Percutaneous 4 Percutaneous Endoscopic 7 Via Natural or Artificial Opening 8 Via Natural or Artificial Opening Endoscopic	Z No Device	X Diagnostic Z No Qualifier
1 Seminal Vesicle, Right ♂ 2 Seminal Vesicle, Left ♂ 3 Seminal Vesicles, Bilateral ♂ 6 Tunica Vaginalis, Right ♂ 7 Tunica Vaginalis, Left ♂ 9 Testis, Right ♂ B Testis, Left ♂ C Testes, Bilateral ♂	Ø Open 3 Percutaneous 4 Percutaneous Endoscopic	Z No Device	X Diagnostic Z No Qualifier
5 Scrotum ♂ S Penis ♂ T Prepuce ♂	Ø Open 3 Percutaneous 4 Percutaneous Endoscopic X External	Z No Device	X Diagnostic Z No Qualifier

ØVB[NPQ][Ø34]ZZ when Z30.2 is listed as the principal diagnosis
Non-OR ØVBØ[3478]ZX
Non-OR ØVB[1239BC][34]ZX
Non-OR ØVB[67F][Ø34]ZX
Non-OR ØVB5[Ø34X]Z[XZ]

Coding Clinic: 2016, Q1, P23 – ØVBQ4ZZ

SECTION: Ø MEDICAL AND SURGICAL
BODY SYSTEM: V MALE REPRODUCTIVE SYSTEM
OPERATION: B EXCISION: *(continued)*
Cutting out or off, without replacement, a portion of a body part

Body Part	Approach	Device	Qualifier
F Spermatic Cord, Right ♂ G Spermatic Cord, Left ♂ H Spermatic Cords, Bilateral ♂ J Epididymis, Right ♂ K Epididymis, Left ♂ L Epididymis, Bilateral ♂ N Vas Deferens, Right ♂ 🗣 P Vas Deferens, Left ♂ 🗣 Q Vas Deferens, Bilateral ♂ 🗣	Ø Open 3 Percutaneous 4 Percutaneous Endoscopic 8 Via Natural or Artificial Opening Endoscopic	Z No Device	X Diagnostic Z No Qualifier

Non-OR ØVB[GHJKL][Ø34]ZX
Non-OR ØVB[NPQ][Ø34]Z[XZ]

SECTION: Ø MEDICAL AND SURGICAL
BODY SYSTEM: V MALE REPRODUCTIVE SYSTEM
OPERATION: C EXTIRPATION: Taking or cutting out solid matter from a body part

Body Part	Approach	Device	Qualifier
Ø Prostate ♂	Ø Open 3 Percutaneous 4 Percutaneous Endoscopic 7 Via Natural or Artificial Opening 8 Via Natural or Artificial Opening Endoscopic	Z No Device	Z No Qualifier
1 Seminal Vesicle, Right ♂ 2 Seminal Vesicle, Left ♂ 3 Seminal Vesicles, Bilateral ♂ 6 Tunica Vaginalis, Right ♂ 7 Tunica Vaginalis, Left ♂ 9 Testis, Right ♂ B Testis, Left ♂ C Testes, Bilateral ♂ F Spermatic Cord, Right ♂ G Spermatic Cord, Left ♂ H Spermatic Cords, Bilateral ♂ J Epididymis, Right ♂ K Epididymis, Left ♂ L Epididymis, Bilateral ♂ N Vas Deferens, Right ♂ P Vas Deferens, Left ♂ Q Vas Deferens, Bilateral ♂	Ø Open 3 Percutaneous 4 Percutaneous Endoscopic	Z No Device	Z No Qualifier
5 Scrotum ♂ S Penis ♂ T Prepuce ♂	Ø Open 3 Percutaneous 4 Percutaneous Endoscopic X External	Z No Device	Z No Qualifier

Non-OR ØVC[67NPQ][Ø34]ZZ
Non-OR ØVC5[Ø34X]ZZ
Non-OR ØVCSXZZ

SECTION: Ø MEDICAL AND SURGICAL
BODY SYSTEM: V MALE REPRODUCTIVE SYSTEM
OPERATION: H **INSERTION:** Putting in a nonbiological appliance that monitors, assists, performs, or prevents a physiological function but does not physically take the place of a body part

Body Part	Approach	Device	Qualifier
Ø Prostate ♂	Ø Open 3 Percutaneous 4 Percutaneous Endoscopic 7 Via Natural or Artificial Opening 8 Via Natural or Artificial Opening Endoscopic	1 Radioactive Element	Z No Qualifier
4 Prostate and Seminal Vesicles ♂ 8 Scrotum and Tunica Vaginalis ♂ D Testis ♂ M Epididymis and Spermatic Cord ♂ R Vas Deferens ♂	Ø Open 3 Percutaneous 4 Percutaneous Endoscopic 7 Via Natural or Artificial Opening 8 Via Natural or Artificial Opening Endoscopic	3 Infusion Device Y Other Device	Z No Qualifier
S Penis ♂	Ø Open 3 Percutaneous 4 Percutaneous Endoscopic	3 Infusion Device Y Other Device	Z No Qualifier
S Penis ♂	7 Via Natural or Artificial Opening 8 Via Natural or Artificial Opening Endoscopic	Y Other Device	Z No Qualifier
S Penis ♂	X External	3 Infusion Device	Z No Qualifier

DRG Non-OR ØVH[48DMR][Ø3478]3Z
DRG Non-OR ØVHS[Ø34]3Z
DRG Non-OR ØVHSX3Z

SECTION: Ø MEDICAL AND SURGICAL
BODY SYSTEM: V MALE REPRODUCTIVE SYSTEM
OPERATION: J **INSPECTION:** Visually and/or manually exploring a body part

Body Part	Approach	Device	Qualifier
4 Prostate and Seminal Vesicles ♂ 8 Scrotum and Tunica Vaginalis ♂ D Testis ♂ M Epididymis and Spermatic Cord ♂ R Vas Deferens ♂ S Penis ♂	Ø Open 3 Percutaneous 4 Percutaneous Endoscopic X External	Z No Device	Z No Qualifier

Non-OR ØVJ[4DMR][3X]ZZ
Non-OR ØVJ[8S][Ø34X]ZZ

SECTION: Ø MEDICAL AND SURGICAL

BODY SYSTEM: V MALE REPRODUCTIVE SYSTEM

OPERATION: L OCCLUSION: Completely closing an orifice or the lumen of a tubular body part

Body Part	Approach	Device	Qualifier
F Spermatic Cord, Right ♂ 🔖 G Spermatic Cord, Left ♂ 🔖 H Spermatic Cords, Bilateral ♂ 🔖 N Vas Deferens, Right ♂ 🔖 P Vas Deferens, Left ♂ 🔖 Q Vas Deferens, Bilateral ♂ 🔖	Ø Open 3 Percutaneous 4 Percutaneous Endoscopic 8 Via Natural or Artificial Opening Endoscopic	C Extraluminal Device D Intraluminal Device Z No Device	Z No Qualifier

🔖 ØVL[FGH][Ø34][CDZ]Z when Z30.2 is listed as the principal diagnosis
🔖 ØVL[NPQ][Ø34][CZ]Z when Z30.2 is listed as the principal diagnosis
Non-OR ØVL[FGH][Ø34][CDZ]Z
Non-OR ØVL[NPQ][Ø34][CZ]Z

SECTION: Ø MEDICAL AND SURGICAL

BODY SYSTEM: V MALE REPRODUCTIVE SYSTEM

OPERATION: M REATTACHMENT: Putting back in or on all or a portion of a separated body part to its normal location or other suitable location

Body Part	Approach	Device	Qualifier
5 Scrotum ♂ S Penis ♂	X External	Z No Device	Z No Qualifier
6 Tunica Vaginalis, Right ♂ 7 Tunica Vaginalis, Left ♂ 9 Testis, Right ♂ B Testis, Left ♂ C Testes, Bilateral ♂ F Spermatic Cord, Right ♂ G Spermatic Cord, Left ♂ H Spermatic Cords, Bilateral ♂	Ø Open 4 Percutaneous Endoscopic	Z No Device	Z No Qualifier

SECTION: Ø MEDICAL AND SURGICAL
BODY SYSTEM: V MALE REPRODUCTIVE SYSTEM
OPERATION: N RELEASE: Freeing a body part from an abnormal physical restraint by cutting or by the use of force

Body Part	Approach	Device	Qualifier
Ø Prostate ♂	Ø Open 3 Percutaneous 4 Percutaneous Endoscopic 7 Via Natural or Artificial Opening 8 Via Natural or Artificial Opening Endoscopic	Z No Device	Z No Qualifier
1 Seminal Vesicle, Right ♂ 2 Seminal Vesicle, Left ♂ 3 Seminal Vesicles, Bilateral ♂ 6 Tunica Vaginalis, Right ♂ 7 Tunica Vaginalis, Left ♂ 9 Testis, Right ♂ B Testis, Left ♂ C Testes, Bilateral ♂	Ø Open 3 Percutaneous 4 Percutaneous Endoscopic	Z No Device	Z No Qualifier
5 Scrotum ♂ S Penis ♂ T Prepuce ♂	Ø Open 3 Percutaneous 4 Percutaneous Endoscopic X External	Z No Device	Z No Qualifier
F Spermatic Cord, Right ♂ G Spermatic Cord, Left ♂ H Spermatic Cords, Bilateral ♂ J Epididymis, Right ♂ K Epididymis, Left ♂ L Epididymis, Bilateral ♂ N Vas Deferens, Right ♂ P Vas Deferens, Left ♂ Q Vas Deferens, Bilateral ♂	Ø Open 3 Percutaneous 4 Percutaneous Endoscopic 8 Via Natural or Artificial Opening Endoscopic	Z No Device	Z No Qualifier

Non-OR   ØVN[9BC][Ø34]ZZ
Non-OR   ØVNT[Ø34X]ZZ

New/Revised Text in Green   ~~deleted~~ Deleted   ♀ Females Only   ♂ Males Only   **Coding Clinic**

Non-covered   Limited Coverage   ⊞ Combination (See Appendix E)   DRG Non-OR   Non-OR   Hospital-Acquired Condition

SECTION: 0 MEDICAL AND SURGICAL
BODY SYSTEM: V MALE REPRODUCTIVE SYSTEM
OPERATION: P REMOVAL: Taking out or off a device from a body part

Body Part	Approach	Device	Qualifier
4 Prostate and Seminal Vesicles ♂	0 Open 3 Percutaneous 4 Percutaneous Endoscopic 7 Via Natural or Artificial Opening 8 Via Natural or Artificial Opening Endoscopic	0 Drainage Device 1 Radioactive Element 3 Infusion Device 7 Autologous Tissue Substitute J Synthetic Substitute K Nonautologous Tissue Substitute Y Other Device	Z No Qualifier
4 Prostate and Seminal Vesicles ♂	X External	0 Drainage Device 1 Radioactive Element 3 Infusion Device	Z No Qualifier
8 Scrotum and Tunica Vaginalis ♂ D Testis ♂ S Penis ♂	0 Open 3 Percutaneous 4 Percutaneous Endoscopic 7 Via Natural or Artificial Opening 8 Via Natural or Artificial Opening Endoscopic	0 Drainage Device 3 Infusion Device 7 Autologous Tissue Substitute J Synthetic Substitute K Nonautologous Tissue Substitute Y Other Device	Z No Qualifier
8 Scrotum and Tunica Vaginalis ♂ D Testis ♂ S Penis ♂	X External	0 Drainage Device 3 Infusion Device	Z No Qualifier
M Epididymis and Spermatic Cord ♂	0 Open 3 Percutaneous 4 Percutaneous Endoscopic 7 Via Natural or Artificial Opening 8 Via Natural or Artificial Opening Endoscopic	0 Drainage Device 3 Infusion Device 7 Autologous Tissue Substitute C Extraluminal Device J Synthetic Substitute K Nonautologous Tissue Substitute Y Other Device	Z No Qualifier
M Epididymis and Spermatic Cord ♂	X External	0 Drainage Device 3 Infusion Device	Z No Qualifier
R Vas Deferens ♂	0 Open 3 Percutaneous 4 Percutaneous Endoscopic 7 Via Natural or Artificial Opening 8 Via Natural or Artificial Opening Endoscopic	0 Drainage Device 3 Infusion Device 7 Autologous Tissue Substitute C Extraluminal Device D Intraluminal Device J Synthetic Substitute K Nonautologous Tissue Substitute Y Other Device	Z No Qualifier
R Vas Deferens ♂	X External	0 Drainage Device 3 Infusion Device D Intraluminal Device	Z No Qualifier

Non-OR 0VP4[78][03]Z
Non-OR 0VP4X[013]Z
Non-OR 0VP8[03478][037JK]Z
Non-OR 0VPD[78][03]Z
Non-OR 0VPS[78][03]Z
Non-OR 0VP[8DS]X[03]Z
Non-OR 0VPM[78][03]Z

Non-OR 0VPMX[03]Z
Non-OR 0VPR[03478][037CDJK]Z
Non-OR 0VPR[78]DZ
Non-OR 0VPRX[03D]Z
Coding Clinic: 2016, Q2, P28 – 0VPS0JZ

SECTION: Ø MEDICAL AND SURGICAL
BODY SYSTEM: V MALE REPRODUCTIVE SYSTEM
OPERATION: Q REPAIR: Restoring, to the extent possible, a body part to its normal anatomic structure and function

Body Part	Approach	Device	Qualifier
Ø Prostate ♂	Ø Open 3 Percutaneous 4 Percutaneous Endoscopic 7 Via Natural or Artificial Opening 8 Via Natural or Artificial Opening Endoscopic	Z No Device	Z No Qualifier
1 Seminal Vesicle, Right ♂ 2 Seminal Vesicle, Left ♂ 3 Seminal Vesicles, Bilateral ♂ 6 Tunica Vaginalis, Right ♂ 7 Tunica Vaginalis, Left ♂ 9 Testis, Right ♂ B Testis, Left ♂ C Testes, Bilateral ♂	Ø Open 3 Percutaneous 4 Percutaneous Endoscopic	Z No Device	Z No Qualifier
5 Scrotum ♂ S Penis ♂ T Prepuce ♂	Ø Open 3 Percutaneous 4 Percutaneous Endoscopic X External	Z No Device	Z No Qualifier
F Spermatic Cord, Right ♂ G Spermatic Cord, Left ♂ H Spermatic Cords, Bilateral ♂ J Epididymis, Right ♂ K Epididymis, Left ♂ L Epididymis, Bilateral ♂ N Vas Deferens, Right ♂ P Vas Deferens, Left ♂ Q Vas Deferens, Bilateral ♂	Ø Open 3 Percutaneous 4 Percutaneous Endoscopic 8 Via Natural or Artificial Opening Endoscopic	Z No Device	Z No Qualifier

Non-OR   ØVQ[67][Ø34]ZZ
Non-OR   ØVQ5[Ø34X]ZZ

SECTION: Ø MEDICAL AND SURGICAL
BODY SYSTEM: V MALE REPRODUCTIVE SYSTEM
OPERATION: R REPLACEMENT: Putting in or on biological or synthetic material that physically takes the place and/or function of all or a portion of a body part

Body Part	Approach	Device	Qualifier
9 Testis, Right ♂ B Testis, Left ♂ C Testis, Bilateral ♂	Ø Open	J Synthetic Substitute	Z No Qualifier

New/Revised Text in Green   ~~deleted~~ Deleted   ♀ Females Only   ♂ Males Only   **Coding Clinic**
🚫 Non-covered   🚫 Limited Coverage   ⊡ Combination (See Appendix E)   DRG Non-OR   Non-OR   🚫 Hospital-Acquired Condition

Q: REPAIR   R: REPLACEMENT

V: MALE REPRODUCTIVE SYSTEM

Ø: M/S

SECTION: Ø MEDICAL AND SURGICAL
BODY SYSTEM: V MALE REPRODUCTIVE SYSTEM
OPERATION: S REPOSITION: Moving to its normal location or other suitable location all or a portion of a body part

Body Part	Approach	Device	Qualifier
9 Testis, Right ♂ B Testis, Left ♂ C Testes, Bilateral ♂ F Spermatic Cord, Right ♂ G Spermatic Cord, Left ♂ H Spermatic Cords, Bilateral ♂	Ø Open 3 Percutaneous 4 Percutaneous Endoscopic 8 Via Natural or Artificial Opening Endoscopic	Z No Device	Z No Qualifier

SECTION: Ø MEDICAL AND SURGICAL
BODY SYSTEM: V MALE REPRODUCTIVE SYSTEM
OPERATION: T RESECTION: Cutting out or off, without replacement, all of a body part

Body Part	Approach	Device	Qualifier
Ø Prostate ♂ ⊞	Ø Open 4 Percutaneous Endoscopic 7 Via Natural or Artificial Opening 8 Via Natural or Artificial Opening Endoscopic	Z No Device	Z No Qualifier
1 Seminal Vesicle, Right ♂ 2 Seminal Vesicle, Left ♂ 3 Seminal Vesicles, Bilateral ♂ ⊞ 6 Tunica Vaginalis, Right ♂ 7 Tunica Vaginalis, Left ♂ 9 Testis, Right ♂ B Testis, Left ♂ C Testes, Bilateral ♂ F Spermatic Cord, Right ♂ G Spermatic Cord, Left ♂ H Spermatic Cords, Bilateral ♂ J Epididymis, Right ♂ K Epididymis, Left ♂ L Epididymis, Bilateral ♂ N Vas Deferens, Right ♂ 🚫 P Vas Deferens, Left ♂ 🚫 Q Vas Deferens, Bilateral ♂ 🚫	Ø Open 4 Percutaneous Endoscopic	Z No Device	Z No Qualifier
5 Scrotum ♂ S Penis ♂ T Prepuce ♂	Ø Open 4 Percutaneous Endoscopic X External	Z No Device	Z No Qualifier

🚫 ØVT[NPQ][04]ZZ when Z30.2 is listed as the principal diagnosis
⊞ ØVTØ[0478]ZZ
⊞ ØVT3[04]ZZ
Non-OR ØVT[NPQ][04]ZZ
Non-OR ØVT[5T][04X]ZZ

SECTION: Ø MEDICAL AND SURGICAL
BODY SYSTEM: V MALE REPRODUCTIVE SYSTEM
OPERATION: U SUPPLEMENT: Putting in or on biological or synthetic material that physically reinforces and/or augments the function of a portion of a body part

Body Part	Approach	Device	Qualifier
1 Seminal Vesicle, Right ♂ 2 Seminal Vesicle, Left ♂ 3 Seminal Vesicles, Bilateral ♂ 6 Tunica Vaginalis, Right ♂ 7 Tunica Vaginalis, Left ♂ F Spermatic Cord, Right ♂ G Spermatic Cord, Left ♂ H Spermatic Cords, Bilateral ♂ J Epididymis, Right ♂ K Epididymis, Left ♂ L Epididymis, Bilateral ♂ N Vas Deferens, Right ♂ P Vas Deferens, Left ♂ Q Vas Deferens, Bilateral ♂	Ø Open 4 Percutaneous Endoscopic 8 Via Natural or Artificial Opening Endoscopic	7 Autologous Tissue Substitute J Synthetic Substitute K Nonautologous Tissue Substitute	Z No Qualifier
5 Scrotum ♂ S Penis ♂ T Prepuce ♂	Ø Open 4 Percutaneous Endoscopic X External	7 Autologous Tissue Substitute J Synthetic Substitute K Nonautologous Tissue Substitute	Z No Qualifier
9 Testis, Right ♂ B Testis, Left ♂ C Testis, Bilateral ♂	Ø Open	7 Autologous Tissue Substitute J Synthetic Substitute K Nonautologous Tissue Substitute	Z No Qualifier

Non-OR ØVUSX[7JK]Z

Coding Clinic: 2016, Q2, P29; 2015, Q3, P25 – ØVUSØJZ

New/Revised Text in Green ~~deleted~~ Deleted ♀ Females Only ♂ Males Only **Coding Clinic**
Non-covered Limited Coverage ⊞ Combination (See Appendix E) DRG Non-OR Non-OR Hospital-Acquired Condition

SECTION: Ø MEDICAL AND SURGICAL
BODY SYSTEM: V MALE REPRODUCTIVE SYSTEM
OPERATION: W REVISION: Correcting, to the extent possible, a portion of a malfunctioning device or the position of a displaced device

Body Part	Approach	Device	Qualifier
4 Prostate and Seminal Vesicles ♂ 8 Scrotum and Tunica Vaginalis ♂ D Testis A ♂ S Penis A ♂	Ø Open 3 Percutaneous 4 Percutaneous Endoscopic 7 Via Natural or Artificial Opening 8 Via Natural or Artificial Opening Endoscopic	Ø Drainage Device 3 Infusion Device 7 Autologous Tissue Substitute J Synthetic Substitute K Nonautologous Tissue Substitute Y Other Device	Z No Qualifier
4 Prostate and Seminal Vesicles ♂ 8 Scrotum and Tunica Vaginalis ♂ D Testis ♂ S Penis ♂	X External	Ø Drainage Device 3 Infusion Device 7 Autologous Tissue Substitute J Synthetic Substitute K Nonautologous Tissue Substitute	Z No Qualifier
M Epididymis and Spermatic Cord ♂	Ø Open 3 Percutaneous 4 Percutaneous Endoscopic 7 Via Natural or Artificial Opening 8 Via Natural or Artificial Opening Endoscopic	Ø Drainage Device 3 Infusion Device 7 Autologous Tissue Substitute C Extraluminal Device J Synthetic Substitute K Nonautologous Tissue Substitute Y Other Device	Z No Qualifier
M Epididymis and Spermatic Cord ♂	X External	Ø Drainage Device 3 Infusion Device 7 Autologous Tissue Substitute C Extraluminal Device J Synthetic Substitute K Nonautologous Tissue Substitute	Z No Qualifier
R Vas Deferens ♂	Ø Open 3 Percutaneous 4 Percutaneous Endoscopic 7 Via Natural or Artificial Opening 8 Via Natural or Artificial Opening Endoscopic	Ø Drainage Device 3 Infusion Device 7 Autologous Tissue Substitute C Extraluminal Device D Intraluminal Device J Synthetic Substitute K Nonautologous Tissue Substitute Y Other Device	Z No Qualifier
R Vas Deferens ♂	X External	Ø Drainage Device 3 Infusion Device 7 Autologous Tissue Substitute C Extraluminal Device D Intraluminal Device J Synthetic Substitute K Nonautologous Tissue Substitute	Z No Qualifier

Non-OR ØVW[4DS]X[Ø37JK]Z
Non-OR ØVW8[Ø3478][Ø37JK]Z
Non-OR ØVW8X[Ø37]Z
Non-OR ØVWMX[Ø37CJK]Z
Non-OR ØVWR[Ø3478][Ø37CDJK]Z
Non-OR ØVWRX[Ø37CDJK]Z

SECTION: Ø MEDICAL AND SURGICAL
BODY SYSTEM: V MALE REPRODUCTIVE SYSTEM
OPERATION: X TRANSFER: Moving, without taking out, all or a portion of a body part to another location to take over the function of all or a portion of a body part

Body Part	Approach	Device	Qualifier
T Prepuce ♂	Ø Open X External	Z No Device	D Urethra S Penis

New/Revised Text in Green   ~~deleted~~ Deleted   ♀ Females Only   ♂ Males Only   **Coding Clinic**
Non-covered   Limited Coverage   ⊞ Combination (See Appendix E)   DRG Non-OR   Non-OR   Hospital-Acquired Condition

SECTION: Ø MEDICAL AND SURGICAL
BODY SYSTEM: W ANATOMICAL REGIONS, GENERAL
OPERATION: Ø ALTERATION: Modifying the anatomic structure of a body part without affecting the function of the body part

Body Part	Approach	Device	Qualifier
Ø Head 2 Face 4 Upper Jaw 5 Lower Jaw 6 Neck 8 Chest Wall F Abdominal Wall K Upper Back L Lower Back M Perineum, Male ♂ N Perineum, Female ♀	Ø Open 3 Percutaneous 4 Percutaneous Endoscopic	7 Autologous Tissue Substitute J Synthetic Substitute K Nonautologous Tissue Substitute Z No Device	Z No Qualifier

Coding Clinic: 2Ø15, Q1, P31 – ØWØ2ØZZ

SECTION: Ø MEDICAL AND SURGICAL
BODY SYSTEM: W ANATOMICAL REGIONS, GENERAL
OPERATION: 1 BYPASS: Altering the route of passage of the contents of a tubular body part

Body Part	Approach	Device	Qualifier
1 Cranial Cavity	Ø Open	J Synthetic Substitute	9 Pleural Cavity, Right B Pleural Cavity, Left G Peritoneal Cavity J Pelvic Cavity
9 Pleural Cavity, Right B Pleural Cavity, Left G Peritoneal Cavity J Pelvic Cavity	Ø Open 3 Percutaneous 4 Percutaneous Endoscopic	J Synthetic Substitute	4 Cutaneous 9 Pleural Cavity, Right B Pleural Cavity, Left G Peritoneal Cavity J Pelvic Cavity W Upper Vein Y Lower Vein
9 Pleural Cavity, Right B Pleural Cavity, Left G Peritoneal Cavity J Pelvic Cavity	3 Percutaneous	J Synthetic Substitute	4 Cutaneous

Non-OR   ØW1[9B][Ø4]J[4GY]
Non-OR   ØW1G[Ø4]J[9BGJ]
Non-OR   ØW1J[Ø4]J[4Y]
Non-OR   ØW1[9BJ]3J4

SECTION: Ø MEDICAL AND SURGICAL

BODY SYSTEM: W ANATOMICAL REGIONS, GENERAL

OPERATION: 2 CHANGE: Taking out or off a device from a body part and putting back an identical or similar device in or on the same body part without cutting or puncturing the skin or a mucous membrane

Body Part	Approach	Device	Qualifier
Ø Head	X External	Ø Drainage Device	Z No Qualifier
1 Cranial Cavity		Y Other Device	
2 Face			
4 Upper Jaw			
5 Lower Jaw			
6 Neck			
8 Chest Wall			
9 Pleural Cavity, Right			
B Pleural Cavity, Left			
C Mediastinum			
D Pericardial Cavity			
F Abdominal Wall			
G Peritoneal Cavity			
H Retroperitoneum			
J Pelvic Cavity			
K Upper Back			
L Lower Back			
M Perineum, Male ♂			
N Perineum, Female ♀			

Non-OR All Values

SECTION: Ø MEDICAL AND SURGICAL

BODY SYSTEM: W ANATOMICAL REGIONS, GENERAL

OPERATION: 3 CONTROL: *(on multiple pages)*
Stopping, or attempting to stop, postprocedure or other acute bleeding

Body Part	Approach	Device	Qualifier
Ø Head	Ø Open	Z No Device	Z No Qualifier
1 Cranial Cavity	3 Percutaneous		
2 Face	4 Percutaneous Endoscopic		
3 Oral Cavity and Throat			
4 Upper Jaw			
5 Lower Jaw			
6 Neck			
8 Chest Wall			
9 Pleural Cavity, Right			
B Pleural Cavity, Left			
C Mediastinum			
D Pericardial Cavity			
F Abdominal Wall			
G Peritoneal Cavity			
H Retroperitoneum			
J Pelvic Cavity			
K Upper Back			
L Lower Back			
M Perineum, Male ♂			
N Perineum, Female ♀			

Non-OR ØW3GØZZ

Coding Clinic: 2016, Q4, P99 – ØW3

Coding Clinic: 2016, Q4, P100 – ØW3P8ZZ
Coding Clinic: 2016, Q4, P101 – ØW3FØZZ
Coding Clinic: 2017, Q4, P105-106 – ØW3[PQ][78]ZZ

New/Revised Text in Green   ~~deleted~~ Deleted   ♀ Females Only   ♂ Males Only   **Coding Clinic**

🔖 Non-covered   🔖 Limited Coverage   ⊞ Combination (See Appendix E)   DRG Non-OR   Non-OR   🔖 Hospital-Acquired Condition

SECTION: Ø MEDICAL AND SURGICAL

BODY SYSTEM: W ANATOMICAL REGIONS, GENERAL

OPERATION: 3 CONTROL: *(continued)*
Stopping, or attempting to stop, postprocedure or other acute bleeding

Body Part	Approach	Device	Qualifier
3 Oral Cavity and Throat	Ø Open 3 Percutaneous 4 Percutaneous Endoscopic 7 Via Natural or Artificial Opening 8 Via Natural or Artificial Opening Endoscopic X External	Z No Device	Z No Qualifier
P Gastrointestinal Tract Q Respiratory Tract R Genitourinary Tract	Ø Open 3 Percutaneous 4 Percutaneous Endoscopic 7 Via Natural or Artificial Opening 8 Via Natural or Artificial Opening Endoscopic	Z No Device	Z No Qualifier

Non-OR ØW3P8ZZ

Coding Clinic: 2018, Q1, P19-20 – ØW3[PQ]8ZZ

SECTION: Ø MEDICAL AND SURGICAL

BODY SYSTEM: W ANATOMICAL REGIONS, GENERAL

OPERATION: 4 CREATION: Putting in or on biological or synthetic material to form a new body part that to the extent possible replicates the anatomic structure or function of an absent body part

Body Part	Approach	Device	Qualifier
M Perineum, Male ♂	Ø Open	7 Autologous Tissue Substitute J Synthetic Substitute K Nonautologous Tissue Substitute Z No Device	Ø Vagina
N Perineum, Female ♀	Ø Open	7 Autologous Tissue Substitute J Synthetic Substitute K Nonautologous Tissue Substitute Z No Device	1 Penis

Coding Clinic: 2016, Q4, P1Ø1 – ØW4

SECTION: Ø MEDICAL AND SURGICAL

BODY SYSTEM: W ANATOMICAL REGIONS, GENERAL

OPERATION: 8 DIVISION: Cutting into a body part, without draining fluids and/or gases from the body part, in order to separate or transect a body part

Body Part	Approach	Device	Qualifier
N Perineum, Female ♀	X External	Z No Device	Z No Qualifier

Non-OR ØW8NXZZ

New/Revised Text in Green   ~~deleted~~ Deleted   ♀ Females Only   ♂ Males Only   **Coding Clinic**

🝆 Non-covered   🝆 Limited Coverage   ⊞ Combination (See Appendix E)   DRG Non-OR   Non-OR   🝆 Hospital-Acquired Condition

SECTION: Ø MEDICAL AND SURGICAL
BODY SYSTEM: W ANATOMICAL REGIONS, GENERAL
OPERATION: 9 DRAINAGE: Taking or letting out fluids and/or gases from a body part

Body Part	Approach	Device	Qualifier
Ø Head 1 Cranial Cavity 2 Face 3 Oral Cavity and Throat 4 Upper Jaw 5 Lower Jaw 6 Neck 8 Chest Wall 9 Pleural Cavity, Right B Pleural Cavity, Left C Mediastinum D Pericardial Cavity F Abdominal Wall G Peritoneal Cavity H Retroperitoneum J Pelvic Cavity K Upper Back L Lower Back M Perineum, Male ♂ N Perineum, Female ♀	Ø Open 3 Percutaneous 4 Percutaneous Endoscopic	Ø Drainage Device	Z No Qualifier
Ø Head 1 Cranial Cavity 2 Face 3 Oral Cavity and Throat 4 Upper Jaw 5 Lower Jaw 6 Neck 8 Chest Wall 9 Pleural Cavity, Right B Pleural Cavity, Left C Mediastinum D Pericardial Cavity F Abdominal Wall G Peritoneal Cavity H Retroperitoneum J Pelvic Cavity K Upper Back L Lower Back M Perineum, Male ♂ N Perineum, Female ♀	Ø Open 3 Percutaneous 4 Percutaneous Endoscopic	Z No Device	X Diagnostic Z No Qualifier

DRG Non-OR ØW9H3ØZ
DRG Non-OR ØW9H3ZZ
Non-OR ØW9[Ø8KLM][Ø34]ØZ
Non-OR ØW9[9B][Ø3]ØZ
Non-OR ØW9[1DFG][34]ØZ
Non-OR ØW9J3ØZ
Non-OR ØW9[Ø234568KLMN][Ø34]ZX
Non-OR ØW9G3ZX

Non-OR ØW9[9B][Ø3]ZZ
Non-OR ØW9[Ø8KLM][Ø34]ZZ
Non-OR ØW9[9B][Ø3]ZZ
Non-OR ØW9[1CD][34]ZX
Non-OR ØW9[1DFG][34]ZZ
Non-OR ØW9J3ZZ

Coding Clinic: 2017, Q2, P17 – ØW93ØZZ
Coding Clinic: 2017, Q3, P13 – ØW9G3ZZ

0: M/S   W: ANATOMICAL REGIONS, GENERAL   9: DRAINAGE

New/Revised Text in Green   deleted Deleted   ♀ Females Only   ♂ Males Only   Coding Clinic
Non-covered   Limited Coverage   Combination (See Appendix E)   DRG Non-OR   Non-OR   Hospital-Acquired Condition   505

SECTION: Ø MEDICAL AND SURGICAL
BODY SYSTEM: W ANATOMICAL REGIONS, GENERAL
OPERATION: B EXCISION: Cutting out or off, without replacement, a portion of a body part

Body Part	Approach	Device	Qualifier
Ø Head 2 Face 3 Oral Cavity and Throat 4 Upper Jaw 5 Lower Jaw 8 Chest Wall K Upper Back L Lower Back M Perineum, Male ♂ N Perineum, Female ♀	Ø Open 3 Percutaneous 4 Percutaneous Endoscopic X External	Z No Device	X Diagnostic Z No Qualifier
6 Neck F Abdominal Wall	Ø Open 3 Percutaneous 4 Percutaneous Endoscopic	Z No Device	X Diagnostic Z No Qualifier
6 Neck F Abdominal Wall	X External	Z No Device	2 Stoma X Diagnostic Z No Qualifier
C Mediastinum H Retroperitoneum	Ø Open 3 Percutaneous 4 Percutaneous Endoscopic	Z No Device	X Diagnostic Z No Qualifier

Non-OR ØWB[02458KLM][034X]ZX
Non-OR ØWB6[034]ZX
Non-OR ØWB6XZX

Non-OR ØWB[CH][34]ZX

Coding Clinic: 2016, Q1, P22 – ØWBF4ZZ

SECTION: Ø MEDICAL AND SURGICAL
BODY SYSTEM: W ANATOMICAL REGIONS, GENERAL
OPERATION: C EXTIRPATION: Taking or cutting out solid matter from a body part

Body Part	Approach	Device	Qualifier
1 Cranial Cavity 3 Oral Cavity and Throat 9 Pleural Cavity, Right B Pleural Cavity, Left C Mediastinum D Pericardial Cavity G Peritoneal Cavity H Retroperitoneum J Pelvic Cavity	Ø Open 3 Percutaneous 4 Percutaneous Endoscopic X External	Z No Device	Z No Qualifier
P Gastrointestinal Tract Q Respiratory Tract R Genitourinary Tract	Ø Open 3 Percutaneous 4 Percutaneous Endoscopic 7 Via Natural or Artificial Opening 8 Via Natural or Artificial Opening Endoscopic X External	Z No Device	Z No Qualifier

Non-OR ØWC[13]XZZ
Non-OR ØWC[9B][034X]ZZ
Non-OR ØWC[CDGJ]XZZ
Non-OR ØWCP[78X]ZZ

Non-OR ØWCQ[034X]ZZ
Non-OR ØWCR[78X]ZZ

Coding Clinic: 2017, Q2, P16 – ØWC3ØZZ

New/Revised Text in Green ~~deleted~~ Deleted ♀ Females Only ♂ Males Only **Coding Clinic**
Non-covered Limited Coverage ⊞ Combination (See Appendix E) DRG Non-OR Non-OR Hospital-Acquired Condition

B: EXCISION   C: EXTIRPATION
W: ANATOMICAL REGIONS, GENERAL
Ø: M/S

SECTION: Ø MEDICAL AND SURGICAL
BODY SYSTEM: W ANATOMICAL REGIONS, GENERAL
OPERATION: **F FRAGMENTATION:** Breaking solid matter in a body part into pieces

Body Part	Approach	Device	Qualifier
1 Cranial Cavity 🔖 3 Oral Cavity and Throat 🔖 9 Pleural Cavity, Right 🔖 B Pleural Cavity, Left 🔖 C Mediastinum 🔖 D Pericardial Cavity G Peritoneal Cavity 🔖 J Pelvic Cavity 🔖	Ø Open 3 Percutaneous 4 Percutaneous Endoscopic X External	Z No Device	Z No Qualifier
P Gastrointestinal Tract 🔖 Q Respiratory Tract 🔖 R Genitourinary Tract	Ø Open 3 Percutaneous 4 Percutaneous Endoscopic 7 Via Natural or Artificial Opening 8 Via Natural or Artificial Opening Endoscopic X External	Z No Device	Z No Qualifier

🔖 ØWF[139BCGJ]XZZ
🔖 ØWF[PQ]XZZ
DRG Non-OR ØWFRXZZ
Non-OR ØWF[139BCG]XZZ
Non-OR ØWFJ[Ø34X]ZZ
Non-OR ØWFP[Ø3478X]ZZ
Non-OR ØWFQXZZ
Non-OR ØWFR[Ø3478]ZZ

New/Revised Text in Green   deleted Deleted   ♀ Females Only   ♂ Males Only   **Coding Clinic**
🔖 Non-covered   🔖 Limited Coverage   ⊞ Combination (See Appendix E)   DRG Non-OR   Non-OR   🔖 Hospital-Acquired Condition

507

Ø: M/S

W: ANATOMICAL REGIONS, GENERAL

F: FRAGMENTATION

SECTION: Ø MEDICAL AND SURGICAL
BODY SYSTEM: W ANATOMICAL REGIONS, GENERAL
OPERATION: H INSERTION: Putting in a nonbiological appliance that monitors, assists, performs, or prevents a physiological function but does not physically take the place of a body part

Body Part	Approach	Device	Qualifier
Ø Head 1 Cranial Cavity 2 Face 3 Oral Cavity and Throat 4 Upper Jaw 5 Lower Jaw 6 Neck 8 Chest Wall 9 Pleural Cavity, Right B Pleural Cavity, Left C Mediastinum D Pericardial Cavity F Abdominal Wall G Peritoneal Cavity H Retroperitoneum J Pelvic Cavity K Upper Back L Lower Back M Perineum, Male ♂ N Perineum, Female ♀	Ø Open 3 Percutaneous 4 Percutaneous Endoscopic	1 Radioactive Element 3 Infusion Device Y Other Device	Z No Qualifier
P Gastrointestinal Tract Q Respiratory Tract R Genitourinary Tract	Ø Open 3 Percutaneous 4 Percutaneous Endoscopic 7 Via Natural or Artificial Opening 8 Via Natural or Artificial Opening Endoscopic	1 Radioactive Element 3 Infusion Device Y Other Device	Z No Qualifier

DRG Non-OR ØWH[Ø2456KLM][Ø34][3Y]Z
Non-OR ØWH1[Ø34]3Z
Non-OR ØWH[89B][Ø34][3Y]Z
Non-OR ØWHPØYZ
Non-OR ØWHP[3478][3Y]Z
Non-OR ØWHQ[Ø78][3Y]Z
Non-OR ØWHR[Ø3478][3Y]Z

Coding Clinic: 2Ø16, Q2, P14 – ØWHG33Z
Coding Clinic: 2Ø17, Q4, P1Ø4 – ØUHD7YZ

SECTION: Ø MEDICAL AND SURGICAL
BODY SYSTEM: W ANATOMICAL REGIONS, GENERAL
OPERATION: J INSPECTION: Visually and/or manually exploring a body part

Body Part	Approach	Device	Qualifier
Ø Head 2 Face 3 Oral Cavity and Throat 4 Upper Jaw 5 Lower Jaw 6 Neck 8 Chest Wall F Abdominal Wall K Upper Back L Lower Back M Perineum, Male ♂ N Perineum, Female ♀	Ø Open 3 Percutaneous 4 Percutaneous Endoscopic X External	Z No Device	Z No Qualifier
1 Cranial Cavity 9 Pleural Cavity, Right B Pleural Cavity, Left C Mediastinum D Pericardial Cavity G Peritoneal Cavity H Retroperitoneum J Pelvic Cavity	Ø Open 3 Percutaneous 4 Percutaneous Endoscopic	Z No Device	Z No Qualifier
P Gastrointestinal Tract Q Respiratory Tract R Genitourinary Tract	Ø Open 3 Percutaneous 4 Percutaneous Endoscopic 7 Via Natural or Artificial Opening 8 Via Natural or Artificial Opening Endoscopic	Z No Device	Z No Qualifier

DRG Non-OR ØWJ[Ø245KL]ØZZ
DRG Non-OR ØWJF3ZZ
DRG Non-OR ØWJM[Ø4]ZZ
DRG Non-OR ØWJ[1GHJ]3ZZ
DRG Non-OR ØWJ[PR][378]ZZ

Non-OR ØWJ[Ø245KL][34X]ZZ
Non-OR ØWJ[68]3ZZ
Non-OR ØWJ3[Ø34X]ZZ
Non-OR ØWJ[68FN]XZZ
Non-OR OWJM[3X]ZZ

Non-OR ØWJ[9BC]3ZZ
Non-OR ØWJD[Ø3]ZZ
Non-OR ØWJQ[378]ZZ

Coding Clinic: 2013, Q2, P37 – ØWJG4ZZ

SECTION: Ø MEDICAL AND SURGICAL
BODY SYSTEM: W ANATOMICAL REGIONS, GENERAL
OPERATION: M REATTACHMENT: Putting back in or on all or a portion of a separated body part to its normal location or other suitable location

Body Part	Approach	Device	Qualifier
2 Face 4 Upper Jaw 5 Lower Jaw 6 Neck 8 Chest Wall F Abdominal Wall K Upper Back L Lower Back M Perineum, Male ♂ N Perineum, Female ♀	Ø Open	Z No Device	Z No Qualifier

New/Revised Text in Green ~~deleted~~ Deleted ♀ Females Only ♂ Males Only **Coding Clinic**
☙ Non-covered ☙ Limited Coverage ⊞ Combination (See Appendix E) DRG Non-OR Non-OR ☙ Hospital-Acquired Condition

SECTION: Ø MEDICAL AND SURGICAL
BODY SYSTEM: W ANATOMICAL REGIONS, GENERAL
OPERATION: P REMOVAL: Taking out or off a device from a body part

Body Part	Approach	Device	Qualifier
Ø Head 2 Face 4 Upper Jaw 5 Lower Jaw 6 Neck 8 Chest Wall C Mediastinum F Abdominal Wall K Upper Back L Lower Back M Perineum, Male ♂ N Perineum, Female ♀	Ø Open 3 Percutaneous 4 Percutaneous Endoscopic X External	Ø Drainage Device 1 Radioactive Element 3 Infusion Device 7 Autologous Tissue Substitute J Synthetic Substitute K Nonautologous Tissue Substitute Y Other Device	Z No Qualifier
1 Cranial Cavity 9 Pleural Cavity, Right B Pleural Cavity, Left G Peritoneal Cavity J Pelvic Cavity	Ø Open 3 Percutaneous 4 Percutaneous Endoscopic	Ø Drainage Device 1 Radioactive Element 3 Infusion Device J Synthetic Substitute Y Other Device	Z No Qualifier
1 Cranial Cavity 9 Pleural Cavity, Right B Pleural Cavity, Left G Peritoneal Cavity J Pelvic Cavity	X External	Ø Drainage Device 1 Radioactive Element 3 Infusion Device	Z No Qualifier
D Pericardial Cavity H Retroperitoneum	Ø Open 3 Percutaneous 4 Percutaneous Endoscopic	Ø Drainage Device 1 Radioactive Element 3 Infusion Device Y Other Device	Z No Qualifier
D Pericardial Cavity H Retroperitoneum	X External	Ø Drainage Device 1 Radioactive Element 3 Infusion Device	Z No Qualifier
P Gastrointestinal Tract Q Respiratory Tract R Genitourinary Tract	Ø Open 3 Percutaneous 4 Percutaneous Endoscopic 7 Via Natural or Artificial Opening 8 Via Natural or Artificial Opening Endoscopic X External	1 Radioactive Element 3 Infusion Device Y Other Device	Z No Qualifier

Non-OR	ØWP[Ø24568KL][Ø34X][Ø137JKY]Z
Non-OR	ØWPM[Ø34][Ø13JY]Z
Non-OR	ØWPMX[Ø13Y]Z
Non-OR	ØWP[CFN]X[Ø137JKY]Z
Non-OR	ØWP1[Ø34]3Z
Non-OR	ØWP[9BJ][Ø34][Ø13JY]Z
Non-OR	ØWP[19BGJ]X[Ø13]Z
Non-OR	ØWP[DH]X[Ø13]Z
Non-OR	ØWPP[3478X][13Y]Z
Non-OR	ØWPQ73Z
Non-OR	ØWPQ8[3Y]Z
Non-OR	ØWPQ[ØX][13Y]Z
Non-OR	ØWPR[Ø3478X][13Y]Z

New/Revised Text in Green   ~~deleted~~ Deleted   ♀ Females Only   ♂ Males Only   **Coding Clinic**
Non-covered   Limited Coverage   ⊞ Combination (See Appendix E)   DRG Non-OR   Non-OR   Hospital-Acquired Condition

SECTION: Ø MEDICAL AND SURGICAL

BODY SYSTEM: W ANATOMICAL REGIONS, GENERAL

OPERATION: Q REPAIR: Restoring, to the extent possible, a body part to its normal anatomic structure and function

Body Part	Approach	Device	Qualifier
Ø Head 2 Face 3 Oral Cavity and Throat 4 Upper Jaw 5 Lower Jaw 8 Chest Wall K Upper Back L Lower Back M Perineum, Male ♂ N Perineum, Female ♀	Ø Open 3 Percutaneous 4 Percutaneous Endoscopic X External	Z No Device	Z No Qualifier
6 Neck F Abdominal Wall	Ø Open 3 Percutaneous 4 Percutaneous Endoscopic	Z No Device	Z No Qualifier
6 Neck F Abdominal Wall ⊞	X External	Z No Device	2 Stoma Z No Qualifier
C Mediastinum	Ø Open 3 Percutaneous 4 Percutaneous Endoscopic	Z No Device	Z No Qualifier

⊞ ØWQFXZ[2Z]

Non-OR ØWQNXZZ

Coding Clinic: 2Ø16, Q3, P6 – ØWQFØZZ
Coding Clinic: 2Ø17, Q3, P9 – ØWQFØZZ

SECTION: Ø MEDICAL AND SURGICAL

BODY SYSTEM: W ANATOMICAL REGIONS, GENERAL

OPERATION: U SUPPLEMENT: Putting in or on biological or synthetic material that physically reinforces and/or augments the function of a portion of a body part

Body Part	Approach	Device	Qualifier
Ø Head 2 Face 4 Upper Jaw 5 Lower Jaw 6 Neck 8 Chest Wall C Mediastinum F Abdominal Wall K Upper Back L Lower Back M Perineum, Male ♂ N Perineum, Female ♀	Ø Open 4 Percutaneous Endoscopic	7 Autologous Tissue Substitute J Synthetic Substitute K Nonautologous Tissue Substitute	Z No Qualifier

Coding Clinic: 2Ø12, Q4, P1Ø1 – ØWU8ØJZ
Coding Clinic: 2Ø16, Q3, P41 – ØWUFØ7Z
Coding Clinic: 2Ø17, Q3, P8 – ØWUFØJZ

New/Revised Text in Green   deleted Deleted   ♀ Females Only   ♂ Males Only   **Coding Clinic**

⬡ Non-covered   ⬡ Limited Coverage   ⊞ Combination (See Appendix E)   DRG Non-OR   Non-OR   ⬡ Hospital-Acquired Condition

511

0: M/S   W: ANATOMICAL REGIONS, GENERAL   Q: REPAIR   U: SUPPLEMENT

SECTION: Ø MEDICAL AND SURGICAL

BODY SYSTEM: W ANATOMICAL REGIONS, GENERAL

OPERATION: W REVISION: Correcting, to the extent possible, a portion of a malfunctioning device or the position of a displaced device

Body Part	Approach	Device	Qualifier
Ø Head 2 Face 4 Upper Jaw 5 Lower Jaw 6 Neck 8 Chest Wall C Mediastinum F Abdominal Wall K Upper Back L Lower Back M Perineum, Male ♂ N Perineum, Female ♀	Ø Open 3 Percutaneous 4 Percutaneous Endoscopic X External	Ø Drainage Device 1 Radioactive Element 3 Infusion Device 7 Autologous Tissue Substitute J Synthetic Substitute K Nonautologous Tissue Substitute Y Other Device	Z No Qualifier
1 Cranial Cavity 9 Pleural Cavity, Right B Pleural Cavity, Left G Peritoneal Cavity J Pelvic Cavity	Ø Open 3 Percutaneous 4 Percutaneous Endoscopic X External	Ø Drainage Device 1 Radioactive Element 3 Infusion Device J Synthetic Substitute Y Other Device	Z No Qualifier
D Pericardial Cavity H Retroperitoneum	Ø Open 3 Percutaneous 4 Percutaneous Endoscopic X External	Ø Drainage Device 1 Radioactive Element 3 Infusion Device Y Other Device	Z No Qualifier
P Gastrointestinal Tract Q Respiratory Tract R Genitourinary Tract	Ø Open 3 Percutaneous 4 Percutaneous Endoscopic 7 Via Natural or Artificial Opening 8 Via Natural or Artificial Opening Endoscopic X External	1 Radioactive Element 3 Infusion Device Y Other Device	Z No Qualifier

DRG Non-OR   ØWW[Ø2456KL][Ø34][Ø137JKY]Z
DRG Non-OR   ØWWM[Ø34][Ø13JY]Z
Non-OR   ØWW[Ø2456CFKLMN]X[Ø137JKY]Z
Non-OR   ØWW8[Ø34X][Ø137JKY]Z
Non-OR   ØWW[1GJ]X[Ø13JY]Z
Non-OR   ØWW[9B][Ø34X][Ø13JY]Z

Non-OR   ØWW[DH]X[Ø13Y]Z
Non-OR   ØWWP[3478X][13Y]Z
Non-OR   ØWWQ[ØX][13Y]Z
Non-OR   ØWWR[Ø3478X][13Y]Z

Coding Clinic: 2015, Q2, P10 – ØWWG4JZ
Coding Clinic: 2016, Q4, P112 – ØWY

SECTION: Ø MEDICAL AND SURGICAL

BODY SYSTEM: W ANATOMICAL REGIONS, GENERAL

OPERATION: Y TRANSPLANTATION: Putting in or on all or a portion of a living body part taken from another individual or animal to physically take the place and/or function of all or a portion of a similar body part

Body Part	Approach	Device	Qualifier
2 Face	Ø Open	Z No Device	Ø Allogeneic 1 Syngeneic

New/Revised Text in Green   ~~deleted~~ Deleted   ♀ Females Only   ♂ Males Only   **Coding Clinic**
Non-covered   Limited Coverage   ⊞ Combination (See Appendix E)   DRG Non-OR   Non-OR   Hospital-Acquired Condition

Side tab text: Y: TRANSPLANTATION   W: REVISION   W: ANATOMICAL REGIONS, GENERAL   Ø: M/S

SECTION: Ø MEDICAL AND SURGICAL
BODY SYSTEM: X ANATOMICAL REGIONS, UPPER EXTREMITIES
OPERATION: Ø ALTERATION: Modifying the anatomic structure of a body part without affecting the function of the body part

Body Part	Approach	Device	Qualifier
2 Shoulder Region, Right 3 Shoulder Region, Left 4 Axilla, Right 5 Axilla, Left 6 Upper Extremity, Right 7 Upper Extremity, Left 8 Upper Arm, Right 9 Upper Arm, Left B Elbow Region, Right C Elbow Region, Left D Lower Arm, Right F Lower Arm, Left G Wrist Region, Right H Wrist Region, Left	Ø Open 3 Percutaneous 4 Percutaneous Endoscopic	7 Autologous Tissue Substitute J Synthetic Substitute K Nonautologous Tissue Substitute Z No Device	Z No Qualifier

SECTION: Ø MEDICAL AND SURGICAL
BODY SYSTEM: X ANATOMICAL REGIONS, UPPER EXTREMITIES
OPERATION: 2 CHANGE: Taking out or off a device from a body part and putting back an identical or similar device in or on the same body part without cutting or puncturing the skin or a mucous membrane

Body Part	Approach	Device	Qualifier
6 Upper Extremity, Right 7 Upper Extremity, Left	X External	Ø Drainage Device Y Other Device	Z No Qualifier

Non-OR All Values

SECTION: Ø MEDICAL AND SURGICAL
BODY SYSTEM: X ANATOMICAL REGIONS, UPPER EXTREMITIES
OPERATION: 3 CONTROL: Stopping, or attempting to stop, postprocedure or other acute bleeding

Body Part	Approach	Device	Qualifier
2 Shoulder Region, Right 3 Shoulder Region, Left 4 Axilla, Right 5 Axilla, Left 6 Upper Extremity, Right 7 Upper Extremity, Left 8 Upper Arm, Right 9 Upper Arm, Left B Elbow Region, Right C Elbow Region, Left D Lower Arm, Right F Lower Arm, Left G Wrist Region, Right H Wrist Region, Left J Hand, Right K Hand, Left	Ø Open 3 Percutaneous 4 Percutaneous Endoscopic	Z No Device	Z No Qualifier

Coding Clinic: 2015, Q1, P35 – ØX37ØZZ   Coding Clinic: 2016, Q4, P99 – ØX3

New/Revised Text in Green   deleted Deleted   ♀ Females Only   ♂ Males Only   Coding Clinic
Non-covered   Limited Coverage   Combination (See Appendix E)   DRG Non-OR   Non-OR   Hospital-Acquired Condition

SECTION: Ø MEDICAL AND SURGICAL
BODY SYSTEM: X ANATOMICAL REGIONS, UPPER EXTREMITIES
OPERATION: 6 **DETACHMENT:** Cutting off all or a portion of the upper or lower extremities

Body Part	Approach	Device	Qualifier
Ø Forequarter, Right 1 Forequarter, Left 2 Shoulder Region, Right 3 Shoulder Region, Left B Elbow Region, Right C Elbow Region, Left	Ø Open	Z No Device	Z No Qualifier
8 Upper Arm, Right 9 Upper Arm, Left D Lower Arm, Right F Lower Arm, Left	Ø Open	Z No Device	1 High 2 Mid 3 Low
J Hand, Right K Hand, Left	Ø Open	Z No Device	Ø Complete 4 Complete 1st Ray 5 Complete 2nd Ray 6 Complete 3rd Ray 7 Complete 4th Ray 8 Complete 5th Ray 9 Partial 1st Ray B Partial 2nd Ray C Partial 3rd Ray D Partial 4th Ray F Partial 5th Ray
L Thumb, Right M Thumb, Left N Index Finger, Right P Index Finger, Left Q Middle Finger, Right R Middle Finger, Left S Ring Finger, Right T Ring Finger, Left V Little Finger, Right W Little Finger, Left	Ø Open	Z No Device	Ø Complete 1 High 2 Mid 3 Low

Coding Clinic: 2016, Q3, P34 – ØX6[MTW]ØZ1
Coding Clinic: 2017, Q1, P52 – ØX6[MTW]ØZ3
Coding Clinic: 2017, Q2, P19 – ØX6VØZØ

Ø: M/S

X: ANATOMICAL REGIONS, UPPER EXTREMITIES

6: DETACHMENT

SECTION: Ø MEDICAL AND SURGICAL

BODY SYSTEM: X ANATOMICAL REGIONS, UPPER EXTREMITIES
OPERATION: 9 DRAINAGE: Taking or letting out fluids and/or gases from a body part

Body Part	Approach	Device	Qualifier
2 Shoulder Region, Right 3 Shoulder Region, Left 4 Axilla, Right 5 Axilla, Left 6 Upper Extremity, Right 7 Upper Extremity, Left 8 Upper Arm, Right 9 Upper Arm, Left B Elbow Region, Right C Elbow Region, Left D Lower Arm, Right F Lower Arm, Left G Wrist Region, Right H Wrist Region, Left J Hand, Right K Hand, Left	Ø Open 3 Percutaneous 4 Percutaneous Endoscopic	Ø Drainage Device	Z No Qualifier
2 Shoulder Region, Right 3 Shoulder Region, Left 4 Axilla, Right 5 Axilla, Left 6 Upper Extremity, Right 7 Upper Extremity, Left 8 Upper Arm, Right 9 Upper Arm, Left B Elbow Region, Right C Elbow Region, Left D Lower Arm, Right F Lower Arm, Left G Wrist Region, Right H Wrist Region, Left J Hand, Right K Hand, Left	Ø Open 3 Percutaneous 4 Percutaneous Endoscopic	Z No Device	X Diagnostic Z No Qualifier

Non-OR All Values

9: DRAINAGE

X: ANATOMICAL REGIONS, UPPER EXTREMITIES

Ø: M/S

SECTION: Ø MEDICAL AND SURGICAL
BODY SYSTEM: X ANATOMICAL REGIONS, UPPER EXTREMITIES
OPERATION: B EXCISION: Cutting out or off, without replacement, a portion of a body part

Body Part	Approach	Device	Qualifier
2 Shoulder Region, Right 3 Shoulder Region, Left 4 Axilla, Right 5 Axilla, Left 6 Upper Extremity, Right 7 Upper Extremity, Left 8 Upper Arm, Right 9 Upper Arm, Left B Elbow Region, Right C Elbow Region, Left D Lower Arm, Right F Lower Arm, Left G Wrist Region, Right H Wrist Region, Left J Hand, Right K Hand, Left	Ø Open 3 Percutaneous 4 Percutaneous Endoscopic	Z No Device	X Diagnostic Z No Qualifier

Non-OR ØXB[23456789BCDFGHJK][Ø34]ZX

SECTION: Ø MEDICAL AND SURGICAL
BODY SYSTEM: X ANATOMICAL REGIONS, UPPER EXTREMITIES
OPERATION: H INSERTION: Putting in a nonbiological appliance that monitors, assists, performs, or prevents a physiological function but does not physically take the place of a body part

Body Part	Approach	Device	Qualifier
2 Shoulder Region, Right 3 Shoulder Region, Left 4 Axilla, Right 5 Axilla, Left 6 Upper Extremity, Right 7 Upper Extremity, Left 8 Upper Arm, Right 9 Upper Arm, Left B Elbow Region, Right C Elbow Region, Left D Lower Arm, Right F Lower Arm, Left G Wrist Region, Right H Wrist Region, Left J Hand, Right K Hand, Left	Ø Open 3 Percutaneous 4 Percutaneous Endoscopic	1 Radioactive Element 3 Infusion Device Y Other Device	Z No Qualifier

DRG Non-OR ØXH[23456789BCDFGHJK][Ø34][3Y]Z
Coding Clinic: 2017, Q2, P21 – ØXH9ØYZ

New/Revised Text in Green deleted Deleted ♀ Females Only ♂ Males Only Coding Clinic
Non-covered Limited Coverage ⊕ Combination (See Appendix E) DRG Non-OR Non-OR Hospital-Acquired Condition

SECTION: Ø MEDICAL AND SURGICAL

BODY SYSTEM: X ANATOMICAL REGIONS, UPPER EXTREMITIES

OPERATION: J INSPECTION: Visually and/or manually exploring a body part

Body Part	Approach	Device	Qualifier
2 Shoulder Region, Right 3 Shoulder Region, Left 4 Axilla, Right 5 Axilla, Left 6 Upper Extremity, Right 7 Upper Extremity, Left 8 Upper Arm, Right 9 Upper Arm, Left B Elbow Region, Right C Elbow Region, Left D Lower Arm, Right F Lower Arm, Left G Wrist Region, Right H Wrist Region, Left J Hand, Right K Hand, Left	Ø Open 3 Percutaneous 4 Percutaneous Endoscopic X External	Z No Device	Z No Qualifier

DRG Non-OR ØXJ[23456789BCDFGHJK]ØZZ   Non-OR ØXJ[JK]3ZZ
Non-OR ØXJ[23456789BCDFGH][34X]ZZ   Non-OR ØXJ[JK]XZZ

SECTION: Ø MEDICAL AND SURGICAL

BODY SYSTEM: X ANATOMICAL REGIONS, UPPER EXTREMITIES

OPERATION: M REATTACHMENT: Putting back in or on all or a portion of a separated body part to its normal location or other suitable location

Body Part	Approach	Device	Qualifier
Ø Forequarter, Right 1 Forequarter, Left 2 Shoulder Region, Right 3 Shoulder Region, Left 4 Axilla, Right 5 Axilla, Left 6 Upper Extremity, Right 7 Upper Extremity, Left 8 Upper Arm, Right 9 Upper Arm, Left B Elbow Region, Right C Elbow Region, Left D Lower Arm, Right F Lower Arm, Left G Wrist Region, Right H Wrist Region, Left J Hand, Right K Hand, Left L Thumb, Right M Thumb, Left N Index Finger, Right P Index Finger, Left Q Middle Finger, Right R Middle Finger, Left S Ring Finger, Right T Ring Finger, Left V Little Finger, Right W Little Finger, Left	Ø Open	Z No Device	Z No Qualifier

New/Revised Text in Green   ~~deleted~~ Deleted   ♀ Females Only   ♂ Males Only   **Coding Clinic**
🚫 Non-covered   🚫 Limited Coverage   ⊟ Combination (See Appendix E)   DRG Non-OR   Non-OR   🚫 Hospital-Acquired Condition

SECTION: Ø MEDICAL AND SURGICAL
BODY SYSTEM: X ANATOMICAL REGIONS, UPPER EXTREMITIES
OPERATION: P REMOVAL: Taking out or off a device from a body part

Body Part	Approach	Device	Qualifier
6 Upper Extremity, Right 7 Upper Extremity, Left	Ø Open 3 Percutaneous 4 Percutaneous Endoscopic X External	Ø Drainage Device 1 Radioactive Element 3 Infusion Device 7 Autologous Tissue Substitute J Synthetic Substitute K Nonautologous Tissue Substitute Y Other Device	Z No Qualifier

Non-OR All Values

Coding Clinic: 2017, Q2, P21 – ØXP70YZ

SECTION: Ø MEDICAL AND SURGICAL
BODY SYSTEM: X ANATOMICAL REGIONS, UPPER EXTREMITIES
OPERATION: Q REPAIR: Restoring, to the extent possible, a body part to its normal anatomic structure and function

Body Part	Approach	Device	Qualifier
2 Shoulder Region, Right 3 Shoulder Region, Left 4 Axilla, Right 5 Axilla, Left 6 Upper Extremity, Right 7 Upper Extremity, Left 8 Upper Arm, Right 9 Upper Arm, Left B Elbow Region, Right C Elbow Region, Left D Lower Arm, Right F Lower Arm, Left G Wrist Region, Right H Wrist Region, Left J Hand, Right K Hand, Left L Thumb, Right M Thumb, Left N Index Finger, Right P Index Finger, Left Q Middle Finger, Right R Middle Finger, Left S Ring Finger, Right T Ring Finger, Left V Little Finger, Right W Little Finger, Left	Ø Open 3 Percutaneous 4 Percutaneous Endoscopic X External	Z No Device	Z No Qualifier

SECTION: Ø MEDICAL AND SURGICAL

BODY SYSTEM: X ANATOMICAL REGIONS, UPPER EXTREMITIES
OPERATION: R **REPLACEMENT:** Putting in or on biological or synthetic material that physically takes the place and/or function of all or a portion of a body part

Body Part	Approach	Device	Qualifier
L Thumb, Right M Thumb, Left	Ø Open 4 Percutaneous Endoscopic	7 Autologous Tissue Substitute	N Toe, Right P Toe, Left

SECTION: Ø MEDICAL AND SURGICAL

BODY SYSTEM: X ANATOMICAL REGIONS, UPPER EXTREMITIES
OPERATION: U **SUPPLEMENT:** Putting in or on biological or synthetic material that physically reinforces and/or augments the function of a portion of a body part

Body Part	Approach	Device	Qualifier
2 Shoulder Region, Right 3 Shoulder Region, Left 4 Axilla, Right 5 Axilla, Left 6 Upper Extremity, Right 7 Upper Extremity, Left 8 Upper Arm, Right 9 Upper Arm, Left B Elbow Region, Right C Elbow Region, Left D Lower Arm, Right F Lower Arm, Left G Wrist Region, Right H Wrist Region, Left J Hand, Right K Hand, Left L Thumb, Right M Thumb, Left N Index Finger, Right P Index Finger, Left Q Middle Finger, Right R Middle Finger, Left S Ring Finger, Right T Ring Finger, Left V Little Finger, Right W Little Finger, Left	Ø Open 4 Percutaneous Endoscopic	7 Autologous Tissue Substitute J Synthetic Substitute K Nonautologous Tissue Substitute	Z No Qualifier

SECTION: Ø MEDICAL AND SURGICAL
BODY SYSTEM: X ANATOMICAL REGIONS, UPPER EXTREMITIES
OPERATION: **W REVISION:** Correcting, to the extent possible, a portion of a malfunctioning device or the position of displaced device

Body Part	Approach	Device	Qualifier
6 Upper Extremity, Right 7 Upper Extremity, Left	Ø Open 3 Percutaneous 4 Percutaneous Endoscopic X External	Ø Drainage Device 3 Infusion Device 7 Autologous Tissue Substitute J Synthetic Substitute K Nonautologous Tissue Substitute Y Other Device	Z No Qualifier

DRG Non-OR   ØXW[67][Ø34][Ø37JKY]Z
Non-OR   ØXW[67]X[Ø37JKY]Z

SECTION: Ø MEDICAL AND SURGICAL
BODY SYSTEM: X ANATOMICAL REGIONS, UPPER EXTREMITIES
OPERATION: **X TRANSFER:** Moving, without taking out, all or a portion of a body part to another location to take over the function of all or a portion of a body part

Body Part	Approach	Device	Qualifier
N Index Finger, Right	Ø Open	Z No Device	L Thumb, Right
P Index Finger, Left	Ø Open	Z No Device	M Thumb, Left

SECTION: Ø MEDICAL AND SURGICAL
BODY SYSTEM: X ANATOMICAL REGIONS, UPPER EXTREMITIES
OPERATION: **Y TRANSPLANTATION:** Putting in or on all or a portion of a living body part taken from another individual or animal to physically take the place and/or function of all or a portion of a similar body part

Body Part	Approach	Device	Qualifier
J Hand, Right K Hand, Left	Ø Open	Z No Device	Ø Allogeneic 1 Syngeneic

Coding Clinic: 2016, Q4, P112 – ØXY

New/Revised Text in Green   ~~deleted~~ Deleted   ♀ Females Only   ♂ Males Only   **Coding Clinic**

Non-covered   Limited Coverage   Combination (See Appendix E)   DRG Non-OR   Non-OR   Hospital-Acquired Condition

SECTION: Ø MEDICAL AND SURGICAL
BODY SYSTEM: Y ANATOMICAL REGIONS, LOWER EXTREMITIES
OPERATION: Ø ALTERATION: Modifying the anatomic structure of a body part without affecting the function of the body part

Body Part	Approach	Device	Qualifier
Ø Buttock, Right 1 Buttock, Left 9 Lower Extremity, Right B Lower Extremity, Left C Upper Leg, Right D Upper Leg, Left F Knee Region, Right G Knee Region, Left H Lower Leg, Right J Lower Leg, Left K Ankle Region, Right L Ankle Region, Left	Ø Open 3 Percutaneous 4 Percutaneous Endoscopic	7 Autologous Tissue Substitute J Synthetic Substitute K Nonautologous Tissue Substitute Z No Device	Z No Qualifier

SECTION: Ø MEDICAL AND SURGICAL
BODY SYSTEM: Y ANATOMICAL REGIONS, LOWER EXTREMITIES
OPERATION: 2 CHANGE: Taking out or off a device from a body part and putting back an identical or similar device in or on the same body part without cutting or puncturing the skin or a mucous membrane

Body Part	Approach	Device	Qualifier
9 Lower Extremity, Right B Lower Extremity, Left	X External	Ø Drainage Device Y Other Device	Z No Qualifier

Non-OR All Values

SECTION: Ø MEDICAL AND SURGICAL
BODY SYSTEM: Y ANATOMICAL REGIONS, LOWER EXTREMITIES
OPERATION: 3 CONTROL: Stopping, or attempting to stop, postprocedure or other acute bleeding

Body Part	Approach	Device	Qualifier
Ø Buttock, Right 1 Buttock, Left 5 Inguinal Region, Right 6 Inguinal Region, Left 7 Femoral Region, Right 8 Femoral Region, Left 9 Lower Extremity, Right B Lower Extremity, Left C Upper Leg, Right D Upper Leg, Left F Knee Region, Right G Knee Region, Left H Lower Leg, Right J Lower Leg, Left K Ankle Region, Right L Ankle Region, Left M Foot, Right N Foot, Left	Ø Open 3 Percutaneous 4 Percutaneous Endoscopic	Z No Device	Z No Qualifier

Coding Clinic: 2Ø16, Q4, P99 – ØY3

SECTION: Ø MEDICAL AND SURGICAL

BODY SYSTEM: Y ANATOMICAL REGIONS, LOWER EXTREMITIES

OPERATION: 6 DETACHMENT: Cutting off all or a portion of the upper or lower extremities

6: DETACHMENT

Y: ANATOMICAL REGIONS, LOWER EXTREMITIES

Ø: M/S

Body Part	Approach	Device	Qualifier
2 Hindquarter, Right 3 Hindquarter, Left 4 Hindquarter, Bilateral 7 Femoral Region, Right 8 Femoral Region, Left F Knee Region, Right G Knee Region, Left	Ø Open	Z No Device	Z No Qualifier
C Upper Leg, Right D Upper Leg, Left H Lower Leg, Right J Lower Leg, Left	Ø Open	Z No Device	1 High 2 Mid 3 Low
M Foot, Right N Foot, Left	Ø Open	Z No Device	Ø Complete 4 Complete 1st Ray 5 Complete 2nd Ray 6 Complete 3rd Ray 7 Complete 4th Ray 8 Complete 5th Ray 9 Partial 1st Ray B Partial 2nd Ray C Partial 3rd Ray D Partial 4th Ray F Partial 5th Ray
P 1st Toe, Right Q 1st Toe, Left R 2nd Toe, Right S 2nd Toe, Left T 3rd Toe, Right U 3rd Toe, Left V 4th Toe, Right W 4th Toe, Left X 5th Toe, Right Y 5th Toe, Left	Ø Open	Z No Device	Ø Complete 1 High 2 Mid 3 Low

Coding Clinic: 2015, Q1, P28 – ØY6NØZØ
Coding Clinic: 2015, Q2, P29 – ØY6[PQ]ØZ3
Coding Clinic: 2017, Q1, P23 – ØY6NØZØ

New/Revised Text in Green   ~~deleted~~ Deleted   ♀ Females Only   ♂ Males Only   **Coding Clinic**

Non-covered   Limited Coverage   ⊞ Combination (See Appendix E)   DRG Non-OR   Non-OR   Hospital-Acquired Condition

SECTION: Ø MEDICAL AND SURGICAL

BODY SYSTEM: Y ANATOMICAL REGIONS, LOWER EXTREMITIES

OPERATION: 9 DRAINAGE: Taking or letting out fluids and/or gases from a body part

Body Part	Approach	Device	Qualifier
Ø Buttock, Right 1 Buttock, Left 5 Inguinal Region, Right 6 Inguinal Region, Left 7 Femoral Region, Right 8 Femoral Region, Left 9 Lower Extremity, Right B Lower Extremity, Left C Upper Leg, Right D Upper Leg, Left F Knee Region, Right G Knee Region, Left H Lower Leg, Right J Lower Leg, Left K Ankle Region, Right L Ankle Region, Left M Foot, Right N Foot, Left	Ø Open 3 Percutaneous 4 Percutaneous Endoscopic	Ø Drainage Device	Z No Qualifier
Ø Buttock, Right 1 Buttock, Left 5 Inguinal Region, Right 6 Inguinal Region, Left 7 Femoral Region, Right 8 Femoral Region, Left 9 Lower Extremity, Right B Lower Extremity, Left C Upper Leg, Right D Upper Leg, Left F Knee Region, Right G Knee Region, Left H Lower Leg, Right J Lower Leg, Left K Ankle Region, Right L Ankle Region, Left M Foot, Right N Foot, Left	Ø Open 3 Percutaneous 4 Percutaneous Endoscopic	Z No Device	X Diagnostic Z No Qualifier

DRG Non-OR ØY9[56]3ØZ
DRG Non-OR ØY9[56]3ZZ
Non-OR ØY9[Ø1789BCDFGHJKLMN][Ø34]ØZ
Non-OR ØY9[Ø1789BCDFGHJKLMN][Ø34]Z[XZ]

Coding Clinic: 2Ø15, Q1, P22-23 – ØY98ØZZ

New/Revised Text in Green   deleted Deleted   ♀ Females Only   ♂ Males Only   **Coding Clinic**
🦚 Non-covered   🦚 Limited Coverage   ⊞ Combination (See Appendix E)   DRG Non-OR   Non-OR   🦚 Hospital-Acquired Condition

525

SECTION: Ø MEDICAL AND SURGICAL

BODY SYSTEM: Y ANATOMICAL REGIONS, LOWER EXTREMITIES
OPERATION: B EXCISION: Cutting out or off, without replacement, a portion of a body part

Body Part	Approach	Device	Qualifier
Ø Buttock, Right 1 Buttock, Left 5 Inguinal Region, Right 6 Inguinal Region, Left 7 Femoral Region, Right 8 Femoral Region, Left 9 Lower Extremity, Right B Lower Extremity, Left C Upper Leg, Right D Upper Leg, Left F Knee Region, Right G Knee Region, Left H Lower Leg, Right J Lower Leg, Left K Ankle Region, Right L Ankle Region, Left M Foot, Right N Foot, Left	Ø Open 3 Percutaneous 4 Percutaneous Endoscopic	Z No Device	X Diagnostic Z No Qualifier

Non-OR ØYB[Ø19BCDFGHJKLMN][Ø34]ZX

SECTION: Ø MEDICAL AND SURGICAL

BODY SYSTEM: Y ANATOMICAL REGIONS, LOWER EXTREMITIES
OPERATION: H INSERTION: Putting in a nonbiological appliance that monitors, assists, performs, or prevents a physiological function but does not physically take the place of a body part

Body Part	Approach	Device	Qualifier
Ø Buttock, Right 1 Buttock, Left 5 Inguinal Region, Right 6 Inguinal Region, Left 7 Femoral Region, Right 8 Femoral Region, Left 9 Lower Extremity, Right B Lower Extremity, Left C Upper Leg, Right D Upper Leg, Left F Knee Region, Right G Knee Region, Left H Lower Leg, Right J Lower Leg, Left K Ankle Region, Right L Ankle Region, Left M Foot, Right N Foot, Left	Ø Open 3 Percutaneous 4 Percutaneous Endoscopic	1 Radioactive Element 3 Infusion Device Y Other Device	Z No Qualifier

DRG Non-OR ØYH[Ø156789BCDFGHJKLMN][Ø34][3Y]Z

SECTION: Ø MEDICAL AND SURGICAL

BODY SYSTEM: Y ANATOMICAL REGIONS, LOWER EXTREMITIES

OPERATION: J INSPECTION: Visually and/or manually exploring a body part

Body Part	Approach	Device	Qualifier
Ø Buttock, Right	Ø Open	Z No Device	Z No Qualifier
1 Buttock, Left	3 Percutaneous		
5 Inguinal Region, Right	4 Percutaneous Endoscopic		
6 Inguinal Region, Left	X External		
7 Femoral Region, Right			
8 Femoral Region, Left			
9 Lower Extremity, Right			
A Inguinal Region, Bilateral			
B Lower Extremity, Left			
C Upper Leg, Right			
D Upper Leg, Left			
E Femoral Region, Bilateral			
F Knee Region, Right			
G Knee Region, Left			
H Lower Leg, Right			
J Lower Leg, Left			
K Ankle Region, Right			
L Ankle Region, Left			
M Foot, Right			
N Foot, Left			

DRG Non-OR ØYJ[Ø19BCDFGHJKLMN]ØZZ
DRG Non-OR ØYJ[567A]3ZZ
DRG Non-OR ØYJ[8E][Ø3]ZZ
Non-OR ØYJ[Ø19BCDFGHJKLMN][34X]ZZ
Non-OR ØYJ[5678AE]XZZ

SECTION: Ø MEDICAL AND SURGICAL
BODY SYSTEM: Y ANATOMICAL REGIONS, LOWER EXTREMITIES
OPERATION: M REATTACHMENT: Putting back in or on all or a portion of a separated body part to its normal location or other suitable location

Body Part	Approach	Device	Qualifier
Ø Buttock, Right	Ø Open	Z No Device	Z No Qualifier
1 Buttock, Left			
2 Hindquarter, Right			
3 Hindquarter, Left			
4 Hindquarter, Bilateral			
5 Inguinal Region, Right			
6 Inguinal Region, Left			
7 Femoral Region, Right			
8 Femoral Region, Left			
9 Lower Extremity, Right			
B Lower Extremity, Left			
C Upper Leg, Right			
D Upper Leg, Left			
F Knee Region, Right			
G Knee Region, Left			
H Lower Leg, Right			
J Lower Leg, Left			
K Ankle Region, Right			
L Ankle Region, Left			
M Foot, Right			
N Foot, Left			
P 1st Toe, Right			
Q 1st Toe, Left			
R 2nd Toe, Right			
S 2nd Toe, Left			
T 3rd Toe, Right			
U 3rd Toe, Left			
V 4th Toe, Right			
W 4th Toe, Left			
X 5th Toe, Right			
Y 5th Toe, Left			

SECTION: Ø MEDICAL AND SURGICAL
BODY SYSTEM: Y ANATOMICAL REGIONS, LOWER EXTREMITIES
OPERATION: P REMOVAL: Taking out or off a device from a body part

Body Part	Approach	Device	Qualifier
9 Lower Extremity, Right	Ø Open	Ø Drainage Device	Z No Qualifier
B Lower Extremity, Left	3 Percutaneous	1 Radioactive Element	
	4 Percutaneous Endoscopic	3 Infusion Device	
	X External	7 Autologous Tissue Substitute	
		J Synthetic Substitute	
		K Nonautologous Tissue Substitute	
		Y Other Device	

Non-OR **All Values**

SECTION: Ø MEDICAL AND SURGICAL

BODY SYSTEM: Y ANATOMICAL REGIONS, LOWER EXTREMITIES

OPERATION: Q REPAIR: Restoring, to the extent possible, a body part to its normal anatomic structure and function

Body Part	Approach	Device	Qualifier
Ø Buttock, Right 1 Buttock, Left 5 Inguinal Region, Right 6 Inguinal Region, Left 7 Femoral Region, Right 8 Femoral Region, Left 9 Lower Extremity, Right A Inguinal Region, Bilateral B Lower Extremity, Left C Upper Leg, Right D Upper Leg, Left E Femoral Region, Bilateral F Knee Region, Right G Knee Region, Left H Lower Leg, Right J Lower Leg, Left K Ankle Region, Right L Ankle Region, Left M Foot, Right N Foot, Left P 1st Toe, Right Q 1st Toe, Left R 2nd Toe, Right S 2nd Toe, Left T 3rd Toe, Right U 3rd Toe, Left V 4th Toe, Right W 4th Toe, Left X 5th Toe, Right Y 5th Toe, Left	Ø Open 3 Percutaneous 4 Percutaneous Endoscopic X External	Z No Device	Z No Qualifier

Non-OR ØYQ[5678AE]XZZ

SECTION: Ø MEDICAL AND SURGICAL

BODY SYSTEM: Y ANATOMICAL REGIONS, LOWER EXTREMITIES

OPERATION: U SUPPLEMENT: Putting in or on biological or synthetic material that physically reinforces and/or augments the function of a portion of a body part

Body Part	Approach	Device	Qualifier
Ø Buttock, Right 1 Buttock, Left 5 Inguinal Region, Right 6 Inguinal Region, Left 7 Femoral Region, Right 8 Femoral Region, Left 9 Lower Extremity, Right A Inguinal Region, Bilateral B Lower Extremity, Left C Upper Leg, Right D Upper Leg, Left E Femoral Region, Bilateral F Knee Region, Right G Knee Region, Left H Lower Leg, Right J Lower Leg, Left K Ankle Region, Right L Ankle Region, Left M Foot, Right N Foot, Left P 1st Toe, Right Q 1st Toe, Left R 2nd Toe, Right S 2nd Toe, Left T 3rd Toe, Right U 3rd Toe, Left V 4th Toe, Right W 4th Toe, Left X 5th Toe, Right Y 5th Toe, Left	Ø Open 4 Percutaneous Endoscopic	7 Autologous Tissue Substitute J Synthetic Substitute K Nonautologous Tissue Substitute	Z No Qualifier

SECTION: Ø MEDICAL AND SURGICAL

BODY SYSTEM: Y ANATOMICAL REGIONS, LOWER EXTREMITIES

OPERATION: W REVISION: Correcting, to the extent possible, a portion of a malfunctioning device or the position of a displaced device

Body Part	Approach	Device	Qualifier
9 Lower Extremity, Right B Lower Extremity, Left	Ø Open 3 Percutaneous 4 Percutaneous Endoscopic X External	Ø Drainage Device 3 Infusion Device 7 Autologous Tissue Substitute J Synthetic Substitute K Nonautologous Tissue Substitute Y Other Device	Z No Qualifier

DRG Non-OR ØYW[9B][Ø34][Ø37JKY]Z

Non-OR ØYW[9B]X[Ø37JKY]Z

New/Revised Text in Green   deleted Deleted   ♀ Females Only   ♂ Males Only   **Coding Clinic**
Non-covered   Limited Coverage   Combination (See Appendix E)   DRG Non-OR   Non-OR   Hospital-Acquired Condition

1 Obstetrics

ICD-10-PCS Coding Guidelines

Obstetric Section Guidelines (section 1)

C. Obstetrics Section

Products of conception

C1

Procedures performed on the products of conception are coded to the Obstetrics section. Procedures performed on the pregnant female other than the products of conception are coded to the appropriate root operation in the Medical and Surgical section.

Example: Amniocentesis is coded to the products of conception body part in the Obstetrics section. Repair of obstetric urethral laceration is coded to the urethra body part in the Medical and Surgical section.

Procedures following delivery or abortion

C2

Procedures performed following a delivery or abortion for curettage of the endometrium or evacuation of retained products of conception are all coded in the Obstetrics section, to the root operation Extraction and the body part Products of Conception, Retained. Diagnostic or therapeutic dilation and curettage performed during times other than the postpartum or post-abortion period are all coded in the Medical and Surgical section, to the root operation Extraction and the body part Endometrium.

SECTION: 1 OBSTETRICS
BODY SYSTEM: Ø PREGNANCY
OPERATION: 2 **CHANGE:** Taking out or off a device from a body part and putting back an identical or similar device in or on the same body part without cutting or puncturing the skin or a mucous membrane

Body Part	Approach	Device	Qualifier
Ø Products of Conception ♀	7 Via Natural or Artificial Opening	3 Monitoring Electrode Y Other Device	Z No Qualifier

Non-OR All Values

SECTION: 1 OBSTETRICS
BODY SYSTEM: Ø PREGNANCY
OPERATION: 9 **DRAINAGE:** Taking or letting out fluids and/or gases from a body part

Body Part	Approach	Device	Qualifier
Ø Products of Conception ♀	Ø Open 3 Percutaneous 4 Percutaneous Endoscopic 7 Via Natural or Artificial Opening 8 Via Natural or Artificial Opening Endoscopic	Z No Device	9 Fetal Blood A Fetal Cerebrospinal Fluid B Fetal Fluid, Other C Amniotic Fluid, Therapeutic D Fluid, Other U Amniotic Fluid, Diagnostic

Non-OR All Values

SECTION: 1 OBSTETRICS
BODY SYSTEM: Ø PREGNANCY
OPERATION: A **ABORTION:** Artificially terminating a pregnancy

Body Part	Approach	Device	Qualifier
Ø Products of Conception ♀	Ø Open 3 Percutaneous 4 Percutaneous Endoscopic 8 Via Natural or Artificial Opening Endoscopic	Z No Device	Z No Qualifier
Ø Products of Conception ♀	7 Via Natural or Artificial Opening	Z No Device	6 Vacuum W Laminaria X Abortifacient Z No Qualifier

DRG Non-OR 10AØ7Z6
Non-OR 10AØ7Z[WX]

Vertical side tab: 1: OBSTETRICS   Ø: PREGNANCY   2: CHANGE   9: DRAINAGE   A: ABORTION

SECTION: 1 OBSTETRICS
BODY SYSTEM: Ø PREGNANCY
OPERATION: D **EXTRACTION:** Pulling or stripping out or off all or a portion of a body part by the use of force

Body Part	Approach	Device	Qualifier
Ø Products of Conception ♀	Ø Open	Z No Device	Ø High 1 Low Ø Classical 1 Low Cervical 2 Extraperitoneal
Ø Products of Conception ♀	7 Via Natural or Artificial Opening	Z No Device	3 Low Forceps 4 Mid Forceps 5 High Forceps 6 Vacuum 7 Internal Version 8 Other
1 Products of Conception, Retained ♀	7 Via Natural or Artificial Opening 8 Via Natural or Artificial Opening Endoscopic	Z No Device	9 Manual Z No Qualifier
2 Products of Conception, Ectopic ♀	7 Via Natural or Artificial Opening 8 Via Natural or Artificial Opening Endoscopic	Z No Device	Z No Qualifier

DRG Non-OR 1ØDØ7Z[345678]

Coding Clinic: 2016, Q1, P10 – 1ØDØ7Z3
Coding Clinic: 2018, Q2, P18 – 1ØDØØZØ

SECTION: 1 OBSTETRICS
BODY SYSTEM: Ø PREGNANCY
OPERATION: E **DELIVERY:** Assisting the passage of the products of conception from the genital canal

Body Part	Approach	Device	Qualifier
Ø Products of Conception ♀	X External	Z No Device	Z No Qualifier

DRG Non-OR 1ØEØXZZ

Coding Clinic: 2016, Q2, P34-35 – 1ØEØXZZ
Coding Clinic: 2017, Q3, P5 – 1ØEØXZZ

SECTION: 1 OBSTETRICS
BODY SYSTEM: Ø PREGNANCY
OPERATION: H **INSERTION:** Putting in a nonbiological appliance that monitors, assists, performs, or prevents a physiological function but does not physically take the place of a body part

Body Part	Approach	Device	Qualifier
Ø Products of Conception ♀	Ø Open 7 Via Natural or Artificial Opening	3 Monitoring Electrode Y Other Device	Z No Qualifier

Non-OR 1ØHØ7[3Y]Z

Coding Clinic: 2013, Q2, P36 – 1ØHØ7YZ

New/Revised Text in Green   deleted Deleted   ♀ Females Only   ♂ Males Only   **Coding Clinic**
Non-covered   Limited Coverage   ⊞ Combination (See Appendix E)   DRG Non-OR   Non-OR   Hospital-Acquired Condition

SECTION: 1 OBSTETRICS

BODY SYSTEM: Ø PREGNANCY

OPERATION: J INSPECTION: Visually and/or manually exploring a body part

Body Part	Approach	Device	Qualifier
Ø Products of Conception ♀ 1 Products of Conception, Retained ♀ 2 Products of Conception, Ectopic ♀	Ø Open 3 Percutaneous 4 Percutaneous Endoscopic 7 Via Natural or Artificial Opening 8 Via Natural or Artificial Opening Endoscopic X External	Z No Device	Z No Qualifier

Non-OR   All Values

SECTION: 1 OBSTETRICS

BODY SYSTEM: Ø PREGNANCY

OPERATION: P REMOVAL: Taking out or off a device from a body part, region or orifice

Body Part	Approach	Device	Qualifier
Ø Products of Conception ♀	Ø Open 7 Via Natural or Artificial Opening	3 Monitoring Electrode Y Other Device	Z No Qualifier

Non-OR   1ØP7[3Y]Z

SECTION: 1 OBSTETRICS

BODY SYSTEM: Ø PREGNANCY

OPERATION: Q REPAIR: Restoring, to the extent possible, a body part to its normal anatomic structure and function

Body Part	Approach	Device	Qualifier
Ø Products of Conception ♀	Ø Open 3 Percutaneous 4 Percutaneous Endoscopic 7 Via Natural or Artificial Opening 8 Via Natural or Artificial Opening Endoscopic	Y Other Device Z No Device	E Nervous System F Cardiovascular System G Lymphatics and Hemic H Eye J Ear, Nose, and Sinus K Respiratory System L Mouth and Throat M Gastrointestinal System N Hepatobiliary and Pancreas P Endocrine System Q Skin R Musculoskeletal System S Urinary System T Female Reproductive System V Male Reproductive System Y Other Body System

Left margin: Q: REPAIR   P: REMOVAL   J: INSPECTION   Ø: PREGNANCY   1: OBSTETRICS

SECTION: 1 OBSTETRICS

BODY SYSTEM: Ø PREGNANCY
OPERATION: **S REPOSITION:** Moving to its normal location or other suitable location all or a portion of a body part

Body Part	Approach	Device	Qualifier
Ø Products of Conception ♀	7 Via Natural or Artificial Opening X External	Z No Device	Z No Qualifier
2 Products of Conception, Ectopic ♀	Ø Open 3 Percutaneous 4 Percutaneous Endoscopic 7 Via Natural or Artificial Opening 8 Via Natural or Artificial Opening Endoscopic	Z No Device	Z No Qualifier

DRG Non-OR 10S07ZZ
Non-OR 10S0XZZ

SECTION: 1 OBSTETRICS

BODY SYSTEM: Ø PREGNANCY
OPERATION: **T RESECTION:** Cutting out or off, without replacement, all of a body part

Body Part	Approach	Device	Qualifier
2 Products of Conception, Ectopic ♀	Ø Open 3 Percutaneous 4 Percutaneous Endoscopic 7 Via Natural or Artificial Opening 8 Via Natural or Artificial Opening Endoscopic	Z No Device	Z No Qualifier

Coding Clinic: 2015, Q3, P32 – 10T24ZZ

SECTION: 1 OBSTETRICS

BODY SYSTEM: Ø PREGNANCY
OPERATION: **Y TRANSPLANTATION:** Putting in or on all or a portion of a living body part taken from another individual or animal to physically take the place and/or function of all or a portion of a similar body part

Body Part	Approach	Device	Qualifier
Ø Products of Conception ♀	3 Percutaneous 4 Percutaneous Endoscopic 7 Via Natural or Artificial Opening	Z No Device	E Nervous System F Cardiovascular System G Lymphatics and Hemic H Eye J Ear, Nose, and Sinus K Respiratory System L Mouth and Throat M Gastrointestinal System N Hepatobiliary and Pancreas P Endocrine System Q Skin R Musculoskeletal System S Urinary System T Female Reproductive System V Male Reproductive System Y Other Body System

New/Revised Text in Green   ~~deleted~~ Deleted   ♀ Females Only   ♂ Males Only   **Coding Clinic**

Non-covered   Limited Coverage   ⊞ Combination (See Appendix E)   DRG Non-OR   Non-OR   Hospital-Acquired Condition

SECTION: 2 PLACEMENT

BODY SYSTEM: W ANATOMICAL REGIONS

OPERATION: 0 **CHANGE:** Taking out or off a device from a body part and putting back an identical or similar device in or on the same body part without cutting or puncturing the skin or a mucous membrane

Body Region	Approach	Device	Qualifier
0 Head 2 Neck 3 Abdominal Wall 4 Chest Wall 5 Back 6 Inguinal Region, Right 7 Inguinal Region, Left 8 Upper Extremity, Right 9 Upper Extremity, Left A Upper Arm, Right B Upper Arm, Left C Lower Arm, Right D Lower Arm, Left E Hand, Right F Hand, Left G Thumb, Right H Thumb, Left J Finger, Right K Finger, Left L Lower Extremity, Right M Lower Extremity, Left N Upper Leg, Right P Upper Leg, Left Q Lower Leg, Right R Lower Leg, Left S Foot, Right T Foot, Left U Toe, Right V Toe, Left	X External	0 Traction Apparatus 1 Splint 2 Cast 3 Brace 4 Bandage 5 Packing Material 6 Pressure Dressing 7 Intermittent Pressure Device Y Other Device	Z No Qualifier
1 Face	X External	0 Traction Apparatus 1 Splint 2 Cast 3 Brace 4 Bandage 5 Packing Material 6 Pressure Dressing 7 Intermittent Pressure Device 9 Wire Y Other Device	Z No Qualifier

SECTION: 2 PLACEMENT
BODY SYSTEM: W ANATOMICAL REGIONS
OPERATION: 1 COMPRESSION: Putting pressure on a body region

Body Region	Approach	Device	Qualifier
0 Head	X External	6 Pressure Dressing	Z No Qualifier
1 Face		7 Intermittent Pressure Device	
2 Neck			
3 Abdominal Wall			
4 Chest Wall			
5 Back			
6 Inguinal Region, Right			
7 Inguinal Region, Left			
8 Upper Extremity, Right			
9 Upper Extremity, Left			
A Upper Arm, Right			
B Upper Arm, Left			
C Lower Arm, Right			
D Lower Arm, Left			
E Hand, Right			
F Hand, Left			
G Thumb, Right			
H Thumb, Left			
J Finger, Right			
K Finger, Left			
L Lower Extremity, Right			
M Lower Extremity, Left			
N Upper Leg, Right			
P Upper Leg, Left			
Q Lower Leg, Right			
R Lower Leg, Left			
S Foot, Right			
T Foot, Left			
U Toe, Right			
V Toe, Left			

New/Revised Text in Green   ~~deleted~~ Deleted   ♀ Females Only   ♂ Males Only   **Coding Clinic**
Non-covered   Limited Coverage   ⊞ Combination (See Appendix E)   DRG Non-OR   Non-OR   Hospital-Acquired Condition

SECTION: 2 PLACEMENT

BODY SYSTEM: W ANATOMICAL REGIONS
OPERATION: 2 DRESSING: Putting material on a body region for protection

Body Region	Approach	Device	Qualifier
0 Head	X External	4 Bandage	Z No Qualifier
1 Face			
2 Neck			
3 Abdominal Wall			
4 Chest Wall			
5 Back			
6 Inguinal Region, Right			
7 Inguinal Region, Left			
8 Upper Extremity, Right			
9 Upper Extremity, Left			
A Upper Arm, Right			
B Upper Arm, Left			
C Lower Arm, Right			
D Lower Arm, Left			
E Hand, Right			
F Hand, Left			
G Thumb, Right			
H Thumb, Left			
J Finger, Right			
K Finger, Left			
L Lower Extremity, Right			
M Lower Extremity, Left			
N Upper Leg, Right			
P Upper Leg, Left			
Q Lower Leg, Right			
R Lower Leg, Left			
S Foot, Right			
T Foot, Left			
U Toe, Right			
V Toe, Left			

SECTION: 2 PLACEMENT

BODY SYSTEM: W ANATOMICAL REGIONS

OPERATION: 3 IMMOBILIZATION: Limiting or preventing motion of a body region

Body Region	Approach	Device	Qualifier
Ø Head 2 Neck 3 Abdominal Wall 4 Chest Wall 5 Back 6 Inguinal Region, Right 7 Inguinal Region, Left 8 Upper Extremity, Right 9 Upper Extremity, Left A Upper Arm, Right B Upper Arm, Left C Lower Arm, Right D Lower Arm, Left E Hand, Right F Hand, Left G Thumb, Right H Thumb, Left J Finger, Right K Finger, Left L Lower Extremity, Right M Lower Extremity, Left N Upper Leg, Right P Upper Leg, Left Q Lower Leg, Right R Lower Leg, Left S Foot, Right T Foot, Left U Toe, Right V Toe, Left	X External	1 Splint 2 Cast 3 Brace Y Other Device	Z No Qualifier
1 Face	X External	1 Splint 2 Cast 3 Brace 9 Wire Y Other Device	Z No Qualifier

Sidebar: 3: IMMOBILIZATION　W: ANATOMICAL REGIONS　2: PLACEMENT

SECTION: 2 PLACEMENT

BODY SYSTEM: W ANATOMICAL REGIONS

OPERATION: 4 PACKING: Putting material in a body region or orifice

Body Region	Approach	Device	Qualifier
Ø Head	X External	5 Packing Material	Z No Qualifier
1 Face			
2 Neck			
3 Abdominal Wall			
4 Chest Wall			
5 Back			
6 Inguinal Region, Right			
7 Inguinal Region, Left			
8 Upper Extremity, Right			
9 Upper Extremity, Left			
A Upper Arm, Right			
B Upper Arm, Left			
C Lower Arm, Right			
D Lower Arm, Left			
E Hand, Right			
F Hand, Left			
G Thumb, Right			
H Thumb, Left			
J Finger, Right			
K Finger, Left			
L Lower Extremity, Right			
M Lower Extremity, Left			
N Upper Leg, Right			
P Upper Leg, Left			
Q Lower Leg, Right			
R Lower Leg, Left			
S Foot, Right			
T Foot, Left			
U Toe, Right			
V Toe, Left			

2: PLACEMENT

W: ANATOMICAL REGIONS

4: PACKING

SECTION: 2 PLACEMENT

BODY SYSTEM: W ANATOMICAL REGIONS

OPERATION: 5 REMOVAL: Taking out or off a device from a body part

Body Region	Approach	Device	Qualifier
Ø Head 2 Neck 3 Abdominal Wall 4 Chest Wall 5 Back 6 Inguinal Region, Right 7 Inguinal Region, Left 8 Upper Extremity, Right 9 Upper Extremity, Left A Upper Arm, Right B Upper Arm, Left C Lower Arm, Right D Lower Arm, Left E Hand, Right F Hand, Left G Thumb, Right H Thumb, Left J Finger, Right K Finger, Left L Lower Extremity, Right M Lower Extremity, Left N Upper Leg, Right P Upper Leg, Left Q Lower Leg, Right R Lower Leg, Left S Foot, Right T Foot, Left U Toe, Right V Toe, Left	X External	Ø Traction Apparatus 1 Splint 2 Cast 3 Brace 4 Bandage 5 Packing Material 6 Pressure Dressing 7 Intermittent Pressure Device Y Other Device	Z No Qualifier
1 Face	X External	Ø Traction Apparatus 1 Splint 2 Cast 3 Brace 4 Bandage 5 Packing Material 6 Pressure Dressing 7 Intermittent Pressure Device 9 Wire Y Other Device	Z No Qualifier

SECTION: 2 PLACEMENT

BODY SYSTEM: W ANATOMICAL REGIONS

OPERATION: 6 **TRACTION:** Exerting a pulling force on a body region in a distal direction

Body Region	Approach	Device	Qualifier
Ø Head	X External	Ø Traction Apparatus	Z No Qualifier
1 Face		Z No Device	
2 Neck			
3 Abdominal Wall			
4 Chest Wall			
5 Back			
6 Inguinal Region, Right			
7 Inguinal Region, Left			
8 Upper Extremity, Right			
9 Upper Extremity, Left			
A Upper Arm, Right			
B Upper Arm, Left			
C Lower Arm, Right			
D Lower Arm, Left			
E Hand, Right			
F Hand, Left			
G Thumb, Right			
H Thumb, Left			
J Finger, Right			
K Finger, Left			
L Lower Extremity, Right			
M Lower Extremity, Left			
N Upper Leg, Right			
P Upper Leg, Left			
Q Lower Leg, Right			
R Lower Leg, Left			
S Foot, Right			
T Foot, Left			
U Toe, Right			
V Toe, Left			

Coding Clinic: 2015, Q2, P35; 2013, Q2, P39 – 2W60XØZ
Coding Clinic: 2015, Q2, P35 – 2W62XØZ

SECTION: 2 PLACEMENT

BODY SYSTEM: Y ANATOMICAL ORIFICES

OPERATION: Ø **CHANGE:** Taking out or off a device from a body part and putting back an identical or similar device in or on the same body part without cutting or puncturing the skin or a mucous membrane

Body Region	Approach	Device	Qualifier
Ø Mouth and Pharynx 1 Nasal 2 Ear 3 Anorectal 4 Female Genital Tract ♀ 5 Urethra	X External	5 Packing Material	Z No Qualifier

SECTION: 2 PLACEMENT

BODY SYSTEM: Y ANATOMICAL ORIFICES

OPERATION: 4 **PACKING:** Putting material in a body region or orifice

Body Region	Approach	Device	Qualifier
Ø Mouth and Pharynx 1 Nasal 2 Ear 3 Anorectal 4 Female Genital Tract ♀ 5 Urethra	X External	5 Packing Material	Z No Qualifier

Coding Clinic: 2017, Q4, P106 – 2Y41X5Z

SECTION: 2 PLACEMENT

BODY SYSTEM: Y ANATOMICAL ORIFICES

OPERATION: 5 **REMOVAL:** Taking out or off a device from a body part

Body Region	Approach	Device	Qualifier
Ø Mouth and Pharynx 1 Nasal 2 Ear 3 Anorectal 4 Female Genital Tract ♀ 5 Urethra	X External	5 Packing Material	Z No Qualifier

SECTION: 3 ADMINISTRATION
BODY SYSTEM: Ø CIRCULATORY
OPERATION: 2 TRANSFUSION: *(on multiple pages)*
Putting in blood or blood products

2: TRANSFUSION

Ø: CIRCULATORY

3: ADMINISTRATION

Body System / Region	Approach	Substance	Qualifier
3 Peripheral Vein 🔒 4 Central Vein 🔒	Ø Open 3 Percutaneous	A Stem Cells, Embryonic	Z No Qualifier
3 Peripheral Vein 🔒 4 Central Vein 🔒	Ø Open 3 Percutaneous	G Bone Marrow X Stem Cells, Cord Blood Y Stem Cells, Hematopoietic	Ø Autologous 2 Allogeneic, Related 3 Allogeneic, Unrelated 4 Allogeneic, Unspecified
3 Peripheral Vein 4 Central Vein	Ø Open 3 Percutaneous	H Whole Blood J Serum Albumin K Frozen Plasma L Fresh Plasma M Plasma Cryoprecipitate N Red Blood Cells P Frozen Red Cells Q White Cells R Platelets S Globulin T Fibrinogen V Antihemophilic Factors W Factor IX	Ø Autologous 1 Nonautologous
5 Peripheral Artery 🔒 6 Central Artery 🔒	Ø Open 3 Percutaneous	G Bone Marrow H Whole Blood J Serum Albumin K Frozen Plasma L Fresh Plasma M Plasma Cryoprecipitate N Red Blood Cells P Frozen Red Cells Q White Cells R Platelets S Globulin T Fibrinogen V Antihemophilic Factors W Factor IX X Stem Cells, Cord Blood Y Stem Cells, Hematopoietic	Ø Autologous 1 Nonautologous

🔒 302[34][Ø3]AZ and 302[56][Ø3][GY]1 are identified as non-covered when a code from the diagnosis list below is present as a principal or secondary diagnosis

C91ØØ	C924Ø	C93ØØ
C92ØØ	C925Ø	C94ØØ
C921Ø	C926Ø	C95ØØ
C9211	C92AØ	

🔒 302[34][Ø3][GY][234] and 302[56][Ø3][GY]1 are identified as non-covered when C90.00 or C90.01 are present as a principal or secondary diagnosis

`DRG Non-OR` 302[34]3AZ *(proposed)*
`DRG Non-OR` 302[34]3[GXY]Z *(proposed)*
`DRG Non-OR` 302[56]3[GXY]ZZ *(proposed)*
`Non-OR` 302[34][Ø3][HJKLMNPQRSTVW][Ø1]
`Non-OR` 302[56][Ø3][HJKLMNPQRSTVW][Ø1]

New/Revised Text in Green   ~~deleted~~ Deleted   ♀ Females Only   ♂ Males Only   **Coding Clinic**
🔒 Non-covered   🔒 Limited Coverage   ⊞ Combination (See Appendix E)   `DRG Non-OR`   `Non-OR`   🔒 Hospital-Acquired Condition

SECTION: 3 ADMINISTRATION
BODY SYSTEM: Ø CIRCULATORY
OPERATION: 2 TRANSFUSION: *(continued)*

Putting in blood or blood products

Body System / Region	Approach	Substance	Qualifier
7 Products of Conception, Circulatory ♀	3 Percutaneous 7 Via Natural or Artificial Opening	H Whole Blood J Serum Albumin K Frozen Plasma L Fresh Plasma M Plasma Cryoprecipitate N Red Blood Cells P Frozen Red Cells Q White Cells R Platelets S Globulin T Fibrinogen V Antihemophilic Factors W Factor IX	1 Nonautologous
8 Vein	Ø Open 3 Percutaneous	B 4-Factor Prothrombin Complex Concentrate	1 Nonautologous

Non-OR 3027[37][HJKLMNPQRSTVW]1
Non-OR 3028[Ø3]B1

SECTION: 3 ADMINISTRATION
BODY SYSTEM: C INDWELLING DEVICE
OPERATION: 1 IRRIGATION: Putting in or on a cleansing substance

Body System / Region	Approach	Substance	Qualifier
Z None	X External	8 Irrigating Substance	Z No Qualifier

SECTION: 3 ADMINISTRATION
BODY SYSTEM: E PHYSIOLOGICAL SYSTEMS AND ANATOMICAL REGIONS
OPERATION: Ø INTRODUCTION: *(on multiple pages)*
Putting in or on a therapeutic, diagnostic, nutritional, physiological, or prophylactic substance except blood or blood products

Body System / Region	Approach	Substance	Qualifier
Ø Skin and Mucous Membranes	X External	Ø Antineoplastic	5 Other Antineoplastic M Monoclonal Antibody
Ø Skin and Mucous Membranes	X External	2 Anti-infective	8 Oxazolidinones 9 Other Anti-infective
Ø Skin and Mucous Membranes	X External	3 Anti-inflammatory 4 Serum, Toxoid and Vaccine B Anesthetic Agent K Other Diagnostic Substance M Pigment N Analgesics, Hypnotics, Sedatives T Destructive Agent	Z No Qualifier
Ø Skin and Mucous Membranes	X External	G Other Therapeutic Substance	C Other Substance
1 Subcutaneous Tissue	Ø Open	2 Anti-infective	A Anti-Infective Envelope
1 Subcutaneous Tissue	3 Percutaneous	Ø Antineoplastic	5 Other Antineoplastic M Monoclonal Antibody
1 Subcutaneous Tissue	3 Percutaneous	2 Anti-infective	8 Oxazolidinones 9 Other Anti-infective A Anti-Infective Envelope
1 Subcutaneous Tissue	3 Percutaneous	3 Anti-inflammatory 6 Nutritional Substance 7 Electrolytic and Water Balance Substance B Anesthetic Agent H Radioactive Substance K Other Diagnostic Substance N Analgesics, Hypnotics, Sedatives T Destructive Agent	Z No Qualifier
1 Subcutaneous Tissue	3 Percutaneous	4 Serum, Toxoid and Vaccine	Ø Influenza Vaccine Z No Qualifier
1 Subcutaneous Tissue	3 Percutaneous	G Other Therapeutic Substance	C Other Substance
1 Subcutaneous Tissue	3 Percutaneous	V Hormone	G Insulin J Other Hormone
2 Muscle	3 Percutaneous	Ø Antineoplastic	5 Other Antineoplastic M Monoclonal Antibody

SECTION: 3 ADMINISTRATION
BODY SYSTEM: E PHYSIOLOGICAL SYSTEMS AND ANATOMICAL REGIONS
OPERATION: Ø INTRODUCTION: *(continued)*

Putting in or on a therapeutic, diagnostic, nutritional, physiological, or prophylactic substance except blood or blood products

Body System / Region	Approach	Substance	Qualifier
2 Muscle	3 Percutaneous	2 Anti-infective	8 Oxazolidinones 9 Other Anti-infective
2 Muscle	3 Percutaneous	3 Anti-inflammatory 4 ~~Serum, Toxoid and Vaccine~~ 6 Nutritional Substance 7 Electrolytic and Water Balance Substance B Anesthetic Agent H Radioactive Substance K Other Diagnostic Substance N Analgesics, Hypnotics, Sedatives T Destructive Agent	Z No Qualifier
2 Muscle	3 Percutaneous	4 Serum, Toxoid and Vaccine	Ø Influenza Vaccine Z No Qualifier
2 Muscle	3 Percutaneous	G Other Therapeutic Substance	C Other Substance
3 Peripheral Vein	Ø Open	Ø Antineoplastic	2 High-dose Interleukin-2 3 Low-dose Interleukin-2 5 Other Antineoplastic M Monoclonal Antibody P Clofarabine
3 Peripheral Vein	Ø Open	1 Thrombolytic	6 Recombinant Human-activated Protein C 7 Other Thrombolytic
3 Peripheral Vein	Ø Open	2 Anti-infective	8 Oxazolidinones 9 Other Anti-infective
3 Peripheral Vein	Ø Open	3 Anti-inflammatory 4 Serum, Toxoid and Vaccine 6 Nutritional Substance 7 Electrolytic and Water Balance Substance F Intracirculatory Anesthetic H Radioactive Substance K Other Diagnostic Substance N Analgesics, Hypnotics, Sedatives P Platelet Inhibitor R Antiarrhythmic T Destructive Agent X Vasopressor	Z No Qualifier
3 Peripheral Vein	Ø Open	G Other Therapeutic Substance	C Other Substance N Blood Brain Barrier Disruption
3 Peripheral Vein	Ø Open	U Pancreatic Islet Cells	Ø Autologous 1 Nonautologous
3 Peripheral Vein	Ø Open	V Hormone	G Insulin H Human B-type Natriuretic Peptide J Other Hormone
3 Peripheral Vein	Ø Open	W Immunotherapeutic	K Immunostimulator L Immunosuppressive

DRG Non-OR 3E03002
DRG Non-OR 3E03017
DRG Non-OR 3E030U[01]

SECTION: 3 ADMINISTRATION
BODY SYSTEM: E PHYSIOLOGICAL SYSTEMS AND ANATOMICAL REGIONS
OPERATION: Ø INTRODUCTION: *(continued)*

Putting in or on a therapeutic, diagnostic, nutritional, physiological, or prophylactic substance except blood or blood products

Body System / Region	Approach	Substance	Qualifier
3 Peripheral Vein	3 Percutaneous	Ø Antineoplastic	2 High-dose Interleukin-2 3 Low-dose Interleukin-2 5 Other Antineoplastic M Monoclonal Antibody P Clofarabine
3 Peripheral Vein	3 Percutaneous	1 Thrombolytic	6 Recombinant Human-activated Protein C 7 Other Thrombolytic
3 Peripheral Vein	3 Percutaneous	2 Anti-infective	8 Oxazolidinones 9 Other Anti-infective
3 Peripheral Vein	3 Percutaneous	3 Anti-inflammatory 4 Serum, Toxoid and Vaccine 6 Nutritional Substance 7 Electrolytic and Water Balance Substance F Intracirculatory Anesthetic H Radioactive Substance K Other Diagnostic Substance N Analgesics, Hypnotics, Sedatives P Platelet Inhibitor R Antiarrhythmic T Destructive Agent X Vasopressor	Z No Qualifier
3 Peripheral Vein	3 Percutaneous	G Other Therapeutic Substance	C Other Substance N Blood Brain Barrier Disruption Q Glucarpidase
3 Peripheral Vein	3 Percutaneous	U Pancreatic Islet Cells	Ø Autologous 1 Nonautologous
3 Peripheral Vein	3 Percutaneous	V Hormone	G Insulin H Human B-type Natriuretic Peptide J Other Hormone
3 Peripheral Vein	3 Percutaneous	W Immunotherapeutic	K Immunostimulator L Immunosuppressive
4 Central Vein	Ø Open	Ø Antineoplastic	2 High-dose Interleukin-2 3 Low-dose Interleukin-2 5 Other Antineoplastic M Monoclonal Antibody P Clofarabine
4 Central Vein	Ø Open	1 Thrombolytic	6 Recombinant Human-activated Protein C 7 Other Thrombolytic
4 Central Vein	Ø Open	2 Anti-infective	8 Oxazolidinones 9 Other Anti-infective

DRG Non-OR 3E03302
DRG Non-OR 3E03317
DRG Non-OR 3E033U[Ø1]
DRG Non-OR 3E04002
DRG Non-OR 3E0417
DRG Non-OR 3E033TZ *(proposed)*

New/Revised Text in Green ~~deleted~~ Deleted ♀ Females Only ♂ Males Only **Coding Clinic**
Non-covered Limited Coverage ⊡ Combination (See Appendix E) DRG Non-OR Non-OR Hospital-Acquired Condition

SECTION: 3 ADMINISTRATION
BODY SYSTEM: E PHYSIOLOGICAL SYSTEMS AND ANATOMICAL REGIONS
OPERATION: 0 INTRODUCTION: *(continued)*
Putting in or on a therapeutic, diagnostic, nutritional, physiological, or prophylactic substance except blood or blood products

Body System / Region	Approach	Substance	Qualifier
4 Central Vein	0 Open	3 Anti-inflammatory 4 Serum, Toxoid and Vaccine 6 Nutritional Substance 7 Electrolytic and Water Balance Substance F Intracirculatory Anesthetic H Radioactive Substance K Other Diagnostic Substance N Analgesics, Hypnotics, Sedatives P Platelet Inhibitor R Antiarrhythmic T Destructive Agent X Vasopressor	Z No Qualifier
4 Central Vein	0 Open	G Other Therapeutic Substance	C Other Substance N Blood Brain Barrier Disruption
4 Central Vein	0 Open	V Hormone	G Insulin H Human B-type Natriuretic Peptide J Other Hormone
4 Central Vein	0 Open	W Immunotherapeutic	K Immunostimulator L Immunosuppressive
4 Central Vein	3 Percutaneous	0 Antineoplastic	2 High-dose Interleukin-2 3 Low-dose Interleukin-2 5 Other Antineoplastic M Monoclonal Antibody P Clofarabine
4 Central Vein	3 Percutaneous	1 Thrombolytic	6 Recombinant Human-activated Protein C 7 Other Thrombolytic
4 Central Vein	3 Percutaneous	2 Anti-infective	8 Oxazolidinones 9 Other Anti-infective
4 Central Vein	3 Percutaneous	3 Anti-inflammatory 4 Serum, Toxoid and Vaccine 6 Nutritional Substance 7 Electrolytic and Water Balance Substance F Intracirculatory Anesthetic H Radioactive Substance K Other Diagnostic Substance N Analgesics, Hypnotics, Sedatives P Platelet Inhibitor R Antiarrhythmic T Destructive Agent X Vasopressor	Z No Qualifier
4 Central Vein	3 Percutaneous	G Other Therapeutic Substance	C Other Substance N Blood Brain Barrier Disruption Q Glucarpidase
4 Central Vein	3 Percutaneous	V Hormone	G Insulin H Human B-type Natriuretic Peptide J Other Hormone

DRG Non-OR 3E04302
DRG Non-OR 3E04317
DRG Non-OR 3E043TZ *(proposed)*

SECTION: 3 ADMINISTRATION
BODY SYSTEM: E PHYSIOLOGICAL SYSTEMS AND ANATOMICAL REGIONS
OPERATION: Ø INTRODUCTION: *(continued)*

Putting in or on a therapeutic, diagnostic, nutritional, physiological, or prophylactic substance except blood or blood products

Body System / Region	Approach	Substance	Qualifier
4 Central Vein	3 Percutaneous	W Immunotherapeutic	K Immunostimulator L Immunosuppressive
5 Peripheral Artery 6 Central Artery	Ø Open 3 Percutaneous	Ø Antineoplastic	2 High-dose Interleukin-2 3 Low-dose Interleukin-2 5 Other Antineoplastic M Monoclonal Antibody P Clofarabine
5 Peripheral Artery 6 Central Artery	Ø Open 3 Percutaneous	1 Thrombolytic	6 Recombinant Human-activated Protein C 7 Other Thrombolytic
5 Peripheral Artery 6 Central Artery	Ø Open 3 Percutaneous	2 Anti-infective	8 Oxazolidinones 9 Other Anti-infective
5 Peripheral Artery 6 Central Artery	Ø Open 3 Percutaneous	3 Anti-inflammatory 4 Serum, Toxoid and Vaccine 6 Nutritional Substance 7 Electrolytic and Water Balance Substance F Intracirculatory Anesthetic H Radioactive Substance K Other Diagnostic Substance N Analgesics, Hypnotics, Sedatives P Platelet Inhibitor R Antiarrhythmic T Destructive Agent X Vasopressor	Z No Qualifier
5 Peripheral Artery 6 Central Artery	Ø Open 3 Percutaneous	G Other Therapeutic Substance	C Other Substance N Blood Brain Barrier Disruption
5 Peripheral Artery 6 Central Artery	Ø Open 3 Percutaneous	V Hormone	G Insulin H Human B-type Natriuretic Peptide J Other Hormone
5 Peripheral Artery 6 Central Artery	Ø Open 3 Percutaneous	W Immunotherapeutic	K Immunostimulator L Immunosuppressive
7 Coronary Artery 8 Heart	Ø Open 3 Percutaneous	1 Thrombolytic	6 Recombinant Human-activated Protein C 7 Other Thrombolytic
7 Coronary Artery 8 Heart	Ø Open 3 Percutaneous	G Other Therapeutic Substance	C Other Substance
7 Coronary Artery 8 Heart	Ø Open 3 Percutaneous	K Other Diagnostic Substance P Platelet Inhibitor	Z No Qualifier
7 Coronary Artery 8 Heart	4 Percutaneous Endoscopic	G Other Therapeutic Substance	C Other Substance
9 Nose	3 Percutaneous 7 Via Natural or Artificial Opening X External	Ø Antineoplastic	5 Other Antineoplastic M Monoclonal Antibody
9 Nose	3 Percutaneous 7 Via Natural or Artificial Opening X External	2 Anti-infective	8 Oxazolidinones 9 Other Anti-infective

DRG Non-OR 3EØ[56][Ø3]Ø2
DRG Non-OR 3EØ[56][Ø3]17
DRG Non-OR 3EØ8[Ø3]17

New/Revised Text in Green   ~~deleted~~ Deleted   ♀ Females Only   ♂ Males Only   **Coding Clinic**

🐾 Non-covered   🐾 Limited Coverage   ⊞ Combination (See Appendix E)   DRG Non-OR   Non-OR   🐾 Hospital-Acquired Condition

0: INTRODUCTION

E: PHYSIOLOGICAL SYSTEMS AND ANATOMICAL REGIONS

3: ADMINISTRATION

SECTION: 3 ADMINISTRATION
BODY SYSTEM: E PHYSIOLOGICAL SYSTEMS AND ANATOMICAL REGIONS
OPERATION: 0 INTRODUCTION: *(continued)*

Putting in or on a therapeutic, diagnostic, nutritional, physiological, or prophylactic substance except blood or blood products

Body System / Region	Approach	Substance	Qualifier
9 Nose	3 Percutaneous 7 Via Natural or Artificial Opening X External	3 Anti-inflammatory 4 Serum, Toxoid and Vaccine B Anesthetic Agent H Radioactive Substance K Other Diagnostic Substance N Analgesics, Hypnotics, Sedatives T Destructive Agent	Z No Qualifier
9 Nose	3 Percutaneous 7 Via Natural or Artificial Opening X External	G Other Therapeutic Substance	C Other Substance
A Bone Marrow	3 Percutaneous	0 Antineoplastic	5 Other Antineoplastic M Monoclonal Antibody
A Bone Marrow	3 Percutaneous	G Other Therapeutic Substance	C Other Substance
B Ear	3 Percutaneous 7 Via Natural or Artificial Opening X External	0 Antineoplastic	4 Liquid Brachytherapy Radioisotope 5 Other Antineoplastic M Monoclonal Antibody
B Ear	3 Percutaneous 7 Via Natural or Artificial Opening X External	2 Anti-infective	8 Oxazolidinones 9 Other Anti-infective
B Ear	3 Percutaneous 7 Via Natural or Artificial Opening X External	3 Anti-inflammatory B Anesthetic Agent H Radioactive Substance K Other Diagnostic Substance N Analgesics, Hypnotics, Sedatives T Destructive Agent	Z No Qualifier
B Ear	3 Percutaneous 7 Via Natural or Artificial Opening X External	G Other Therapeutic Substance	C Other Substance
C Eye	3 Percutaneous 7 Via Natural or Artificial Opening X External	0 Antineoplastic	4 Liquid Brachytherapy Radioisotope 5 Other Antineoplastic M Monoclonal Antibody
C Eye	3 Percutaneous 7 Via Natural or Artificial Opening X External	2 Anti-infective	8 Oxazolidinones 9 Other Anti-infective
C Eye	3 Percutaneous 7 Via Natural or Artificial Opening X External	3 Anti-inflammatory B Anesthetic Agent H Radioactive Substance K Other Diagnostic Substance M Pigment N Analgesics, Hypnotics, Sedatives T Destructive Agent	Z No Qualifier
C Eye	3 Percutaneous 7 Via Natural or Artificial Opening X External	G Other Therapeutic Substance	C Other Substance

DRG Non-OR 3E0B329 *(proposed)*
DRG Non-OR 3E0B33Z *(proposed)*
DRG Non-OR 3E0B3[GHKT]C *(proposed)*
DRG Non-OR 3E0B[7X]29 *(proposed)*
DRG Non-OR 3E0B[7X][3BHKT]Z *(proposed)*
DRG Non-OR 3E0B[7X]GC *(proposed)*

DRG Non-OR 3E0C[37X][3BHKMT]Z *(proposed)*
DRG Non-OR 3E0C[37X]GC *(proposed)*
DRG Non-OR 3E0C[37X]SF *(proposed)*
DRG Non-OR 3E0C[7X]29 *(proposed)*

New/Revised Text in Green   deleted Deleted   ♀ Females Only   ♂ Males Only   **Coding Clinic**
🚫 Non-covered   🚫 Limited Coverage   ⊞ Combination (See Appendix E)   DRG Non-OR   Non-OR   🚫 Hospital-Acquired Condition

SECTION: 3 ADMINISTRATION
BODY SYSTEM: E PHYSIOLOGICAL SYSTEMS AND ANATOMICAL REGIONS
OPERATION: Ø INTRODUCTION: *(continued)*
Putting in or on a therapeutic, diagnostic, nutritional, physiological, or prophylactic substance except blood or blood products

Body System / Region	Approach	Substance	Qualifier
C Eye	3 Percutaneous 7 Via Natural or Artificial Opening X External	S Gas	F Other Gas
D Mouth and Pharynx	3 Percutaneous 7 Via Natural or Artificial Opening X External	Ø Antineoplastic	4 Liquid Brachytherapy Radioisotope 5 Other Antineoplastic M Monoclonal Antibody
D Mouth and Pharynx	3 Percutaneous 7 Via Natural or Artificial Opening X External	2 Anti-infective	8 Oxazolidinones 9 Other Anti-infective
D Mouth and Pharynx	3 Percutaneous 7 Via Natural or Artificial Opening X External	3 Anti-inflammatory 4 Serum, Toxoid and Vaccine 6 Nutritional Substance 7 Electrolytic and Water Balance Substance B Anesthetic Agent H Radioactive Substance K Other Diagnostic Substance N Analgesics, Hypnotics, Sedatives R Antiarrhythmic T Destructive Agent	Z No Qualifier
D Mouth and Pharynx	3 Percutaneous 7 Via Natural or Artificial Opening X External	G Other Therapeutic Substance	C Other Substance
E Products of Conception ♀ G Upper GI H Lower GI K Genitourinary Tract N Male Reproductive ♂	3 Percutaneous 7 Via Natural or Artificial Opening 8 Via Natural or Artificial Opening Endoscopic	Ø Antineoplastic	4 Liquid Brachytherapy Radioisotope 5 Other Antineoplastic M Monoclonal Antibody
E Products of Conception ♀ G Upper GI H Lower GI K Genitourinary Tract N Male Reproductive ♂	3 Percutaneous 7 Via Natural or Artificial Opening 8 Via Natural or Artificial Opening Endoscopic	2 Anti-infective	8 Oxazolidinones 9 Other Anti-infective
E Products of Conception ♀ G Upper GI H Lower GI K Genitourinary Tract N Male Reproductive ♂	3 Percutaneous 7 Via Natural or Artificial Opening 8 Via Natural or Artificial Opening Endoscopic	3 Anti-inflammatory 6 Nutritional Substance 7 Electrolytic and Water Balance Substance B Anesthetic Agent H Radioactive Substance K Other Diagnostic Substance N Analgesics, Hypnotics, Sedatives T Destructive Agent	Z No Qualifier
E Products of Conception ♀ G Upper GI H Lower GI K Genitourinary Tract N Male Reproductive ♂	3 Percutaneous 7 Via Natural or Artificial Opening 8 Via Natural or Artificial Opening Endoscopic	G Other Therapeutic Substance	C Other Substance

DRG Non-OR 3EØG3GC *(proposed)*
Coding Clinic: 2Ø15, Q2, P29 – 3EØG76Z

Coding Clinic: 2Ø15, Q3, P25 – 3EØG8GC
Coding Clinic: 2Ø17, Q1, P37 – 3EØH3GC

SECTION: 3 ADMINISTRATION

BODY SYSTEM: E **PHYSIOLOGICAL SYSTEMS AND ANATOMICAL REGIONS**
OPERATION: Ø **INTRODUCTION:** *(continued)*

Putting in or on a therapeutic, diagnostic, nutritional, physiological, or prophylactic substance except blood or blood products

Body System / Region	Approach	Substance	Qualifier
E Products of Conception ♀ G Upper GI H Lower GI K Genitourinary Tract N Male Reproductive ♂	3 Percutaneous 7 Via Natural or Artificial Opening 8 Via Natural or Artificial Opening Endoscopic	S Gas	F Other Gas
E Products of Conception ♀ G Upper GI H Lower GI K Genitourinary Tract N Male Reproductive ♂	4 Percutaneous Endoscopic	G Other Therapeutic Substance	C Other Substance
F Respiratory Tract	3 Percutaneous 7 Via Natural or Artificial Opening 8 Via Natural or Artificial Opening Endoscopic	Ø Antineoplastic	4 Liquid Brachytherapy Radioisotope 5 Other Antineoplastic M Monoclonal Antibody
F Respiratory Tract	3 Percutaneous 7 Via Natural or Artificial Opening 8 Via Natural or Artificial Opening Endoscopic	2 Anti-infective	8 Oxazolidinones 9 Other Anti-infective
F Respiratory Tract	3 Percutaneous 7 Via Natural or Artificial Opening 8 Via Natural or Artificial Opening Endoscopic	3 Anti-inflammatory 6 Nutritional Substance 7 Electrolytic and Water Balance Substance B Anesthetic Agent H Radioactive Substance K Other Diagnostic Substance N Analgesics, Hypnotics, Sedatives T Destructive Agent	Z No Qualifier
F Respiratory Tract	3 Percutaneous 7 Via Natural or Artificial Opening 8 Via Natural or Artificial Opening Endoscopic	G Other Therapeutic Substance	C Other Substance
F Respiratory Tract	3 Percutaneous 7 Via Natural or Artificial Opening 8 Via Natural or Artificial Opening Endoscopic	S Gas	D Nitric Oxide F Other Gas
F Respiratory Tract	4 Percutaneous Endoscopic	G Other Therapeutic Substance	C Other Substance

SECTION: 3 ADMINISTRATION
BODY SYSTEM: E PHYSIOLOGICAL SYSTEMS AND ANATOMICAL REGIONS
OPERATION: Ø INTRODUCTION: *(continued)*

Putting in or on a therapeutic, diagnostic, nutritional, physiological, or prophylactic substance except blood or blood products

Body System / Region	Approach	Substance	Qualifier
J Biliary and Pancreatic Tract	3 Percutaneous 7 Via Natural or Artificial Opening 8 Via Natural or Artificial Opening Endoscopic	Ø Antineoplastic	4 Liquid Brachytherapy Radioisotope 5 Other Antineoplastic M Monoclonal Antibody
J Biliary and Pancreatic Tract	3 Percutaneous 7 Via Natural or Artificial Opening 8 Via Natural or Artificial Opening Endoscopic	2 Anti-infective	8 Oxazolidinones 9 Other Anti-infective
J Biliary and Pancreatic Tract	3 Percutaneous 7 Via Natural or Artificial Opening 8 Via Natural or Artificial Opening Endoscopic	3 Anti-inflammatory 6 Nutritional Substance 7 Electrolytic and Water Balance Substance B Anesthetic Agent H Radioactive Substance K Other Diagnostic Substance N Analgesics, Hypnotics, Sedatives T Destructive Agent	Z No Qualifier
J Biliary and Pancreatic Tract	3 Percutaneous 7 Via Natural or Artificial Opening 8 Via Natural or Artificial Opening Endoscopic	G Other Therapeutic Substance	C Other Substance
J Biliary and Pancreatic Tract	3 Percutaneous 7 Via Natural or Artificial Opening 8 Via Natural or Artificial Opening Endoscopic	S Gas	F Other Gas
J Biliary and Pancreatic Tract	3 Percutaneous 7 Via Natural or Artificial Opening 8 Via Natural or Artificial Opening Endoscopic	U Pancreatic Islet Cells	Ø Autologous 1 Nonautologous
J Biliary and Pancreatic Tract	4 Percutaneous Endoscopic	G Other Therapeutic Substance	C Other Substance
L Pleural Cavity M Peritoneal Cavity	Ø Open	5 Adhesion Barrier	Z No Qualifier
L Pleural Cavity M Peritoneal Cavity	3 Percutaneous	Ø Antineoplastic	4 Liquid Brachytherapy Radioisotope 5 Other Antineoplastic M Monoclonal Antibody
L Pleural Cavity M Peritoneal Cavity	3 Percutaneous	2 Anti-infective	8 Oxazolidinones 9 Other Anti-infective
L Pleural Cavity M Peritoneal Cavity	3 Percutaneous	3 Anti-inflammatory 5 Adhesion Barrier 6 Nutritional Substance 7 Electrolytic and Water Balance Substance B Anesthetic Agent H Radioactive Substance K Other Diagnostic Substance N Analgesics, Hypnotics, Sedatives T Destructive Agent	Z No Qualifier

DRG Non-OR 3EØJ[378]U[Ø1]

SECTION:　3 ADMINISTRATION
BODY SYSTEM: E PHYSIOLOGICAL SYSTEMS AND ANATOMICAL REGIONS
OPERATION:　Ø INTRODUCTION: *(continued)*

Putting in or on a therapeutic, diagnostic, nutritional, physiological, or prophylactic substance except blood or blood products

Body System / Region	Approach	Substance	Qualifier
L Pleural Cavity M Peritoneal Cavity	3 Percutaneous	G Other Therapeutic Substance	C Other Substance
L Pleural Cavity M Peritoneal Cavity	3 Percutaneous	S Gas	F Other Gas
L Pleural Cavity M Peritoneal Cavity	4 Percutaneous Endoscopic	5 Adhesion Barrier	Z No Qualifier
L Pleural Cavity M Peritoneal Cavity	4 Percutaneous Endoscopic	G Other Therapeutic Substance	C Other Substance
L Pleural Cavity M Peritoneal Cavity	7 Via Natural or Artificial Opening	Ø Antineoplastic	4 Liquid Brachytherapy Radioisotope 5 Other Antineoplastic M Monoclonal Antibody
L Pleural Cavity M Peritoneal Cavity	7 Via Natural or Artificial Opening	S Gas	F Other Gas
P Female Reproductive ♀	Ø Open	5 Adhesion Barrier	Z No Qualifier
P Female Reproductive ♀	3 Percutaneous	Ø Antineoplastic	4 Liquid Brachytherapy Radioisotope 5 Other Antineoplastic M Monoclonal Antibody
P Female Reproductive ♀	3 Percutaneous	2 Anti-infective	8 Oxazolidinones 9 Other Anti-infective
P Female Reproductive ♀	3 Percutaneous	3 Anti-inflammatory 5 Adhesion Barrier 6 Nutritional Substance 7 Electrolytic and Water Balance Substance B Anesthetic Agent H Radioactive Substance K Other Diagnostic Substance L Sperm N Analgesics, Hypnotics, Sedatives T Destructive Agent V Hormone	Z No Qualifier
P Female Reproductive ♀	3 Percutaneous	G Other Therapeutic Substance	C Other Substance
P Female Reproductive ♀	3 Percutaneous	Q Fertilized Ovum	Ø Autologous 1 Nonautologous
P Female Reproductive ♀	3 Percutaneous	S Gas	F Other Gas
P Female Reproductive ♀	4 Percutaneous Endoscopic	5 Adhesion Barrier	Z No Qualifier
P Female Reproductive ♀	4 Percutaneous Endoscopic	G Other Therapeutic Substance	C Other Substance
P Female Reproductive ♀	7 Via Natural or Artificial Opening	Ø Antineoplastic	4 Liquid Brachytherapy Radioisotope 5 Other Antineoplastic M Monoclonal Antibody
P Female Reproductive ♀	7 Via Natural or Artificial Opening	2 Anti-infective	8 Oxazolidinones 9 Other Anti-infective

Coding Clinic: 2017, Q2, P15; 2015, Q2, P31 – 3E0L3GC

SECTION: 3 ADMINISTRATION
BODY SYSTEM: E PHYSIOLOGICAL SYSTEMS AND ANATOMICAL REGIONS
OPERATION: 0 INTRODUCTION: *(continued)*

Putting in or on a therapeutic, diagnostic, nutritional, physiological, or prophylactic substance except blood or blood products

0: INTRODUCTION

E: PHYSIOLOGICAL SYSTEMS AND ANATOMICAL REGIONS

3: ADMINISTRATION

Body System / Region	Approach	Substance	Qualifier
P Female Reproductive ♀	7 Via Natural or Artificial Opening	3 Anti-inflammatory 6 Nutritional Substance 7 Electrolytic and Water Balance Substance B Anesthetic Agent H Radioactive Substance K Other Diagnostic Substance L Sperm N Analgesics, Hypnotics, Sedatives T Destructive Agent V Hormone	Z No Qualifier
P Female Reproductive ♀	7 Via Natural or Artificial Opening	G Other Therapeutic Substance	C Other Substance
P Female Reproductive ♀	7 Via Natural or Artificial Opening	Q Fertilized Ovum	0 Autologous 1 Nonautologous
P Female Reproductive ♀	7 Via Natural or Artificial Opening	S Gas	F Other Gas
P Female Reproductive ♀	8 Via Natural or Artificial Opening Endoscopic	0 Antineoplastic	4 Liquid Brachytherapy Radioisotope 5 Other Antineoplastic M Monoclonal Antibody
P Female Reproductive ♀	8 Via Natural or Artificial Opening Endoscopic	2 Anti-infective	8 Oxazolidinones 9 Other Anti-infective
P Female Reproductive ♀	8 Via Natural or Artificial Opening Endoscopic	3 Anti-inflammatory 6 Nutritional Substance 7 Electrolytic and Water Balance Substance B Anesthetic Agent H Radioactive Substance K Other Diagnostic Substance N Analgesics, Hypnotics, Sedatives T Destructive Agent	Z No Qualifier
P Female Reproductive ♀	8 Via Natural or Artificial Opening Endoscopic	G Other Therapeutic Substance	C Other Substance
P Female Reproductive ♀	8 Via Natural or Artificial Opening Endoscopic	S Gas	F Other Gas
Q Cranial Cavity and Brain	0 Open 3 Percutaneous	0 Antineoplastic	4 Liquid Brachytherapy Radioisotope 5 Other Antineoplastic M Monoclonal Antibody
Q Cranial Cavity and Brain	0 Open 3 Percutaneous	2 Anti-infective	8 Oxazolidinones 9 Other Anti-infective
Q Cranial Cavity and Brain	0 Open 3 Percutaneous	3 Anti-inflammatory 6 Nutritional Substance 7 Electrolytic and Water Balance Substance A Stem Cells, Embryonic B Anesthetic Agent H Radioactive Substance K Other Diagnostic Substance N Analgesics, Hypnotics, Sedatives T Destructive Agent	Z No Qualifier

DRG Non-OR 3E0Q[03]05
DRG Non-OR 3E0P73Z *(proposed)*

Coding Clinic: 2016, Q4, P114 – 3E0Q005

New/Revised Text in Green   ~~deleted~~ Deleted   ♀ Females Only   ♂ Males Only   **Coding Clinic**
🖢 Non-covered   🖢 Limited Coverage   ⊞ Combination (See Appendix E)   DRG Non-OR   Non-OR   🖢 Hospital-Acquired Condition

SECTION: 3 ADMINISTRATION

BODY SYSTEM: E PHYSIOLOGICAL SYSTEMS AND ANATOMICAL REGIONS
OPERATION: 0 INTRODUCTION: *(continued)*

Putting in or on a therapeutic, diagnostic, nutritional, physiological, or prophylactic substance except blood or blood products

Body System / Region	Approach	Substance	Qualifier
Q Cranial Cavity and Brain	0 Open 3 Percutaneous	E Stem Cells, Somatic	0 Autologous 1 Nonautologous
Q Cranial Cavity and Brain	0 Open 3 Percutaneous	G Other Therapeutic Substance	C Other Substance
Q Cranial Cavity and Brain	0 Open 3 Percutaneous	S Gas	F Other Gas
Q Cranial Cavity and Brain	7 Via Natural or Artificial Opening	0 Antineoplastic	4 Liquid Brachytherapy Radioisotope 5 Other Antineoplastic M Monoclonal Antibody
Q Cranial Cavity and Brain	7 Via Natural or Artificial Opening	S Gas	F Other Gas
R Spinal Canal	0 Open	A Stem Cells, Embryonic	Z No Qualifier
R Spinal Canal	0 Open	A Stem Cells, Somatic	0 Autologous 1 Nonautologous
R Spinal Canal	3 Percutaneous	0 Antineoplastic	2 High-dose Interleukin-2 3 Low-dose Interleukin-2 4 Liquid Brachytherapy Radioisotope 5 Other Antineoplastic M Monoclonal Antibody
R Spinal Canal	3 Percutaneous	2 Anti-infective	8 Oxazolidinones 9 Other Anti-infective
R Spinal Canal	3 Percutaneous	3 Anti-inflammatory 6 Nutritional Substance 7 Electrolytic and Water Balance Substance A Stem Cells, Embryonic B Anesthetic Agent H Radioactive Substance K Other Diagnostic Substance N Analgesics, Hypnotics, Sedatives T Destructive Agent	Z No Qualifier
R Spinal Canal	3 Percutaneous	E Stem Cells, Somatic	0 Autologous 1 Nonautologous
R Spinal Canal	3 Percutaneous	G Other Therapeutic Substance	C Other Substance
R Spinal Canal	3 Percutaneous	S Gas	F Other Gas
R Spinal Canal	7 Via Natural or Artificial Opening	S Gas	F Other Gas
S Epidural Space	3 Percutaneous	0 Antineoplastic	2 High-dose Interleukin-2 3 Low-dose Interleukin-2 4 Liquid Brachytherapy Radioisotope 5 Other Antineoplastic M Monoclonal Antibody
S Epidural Space	3 Percutaneous	2 Anti-infective	8 Oxazolidinones 9 Other Anti-infective

DRG Non-OR 3E0Q705
DRG Non-OR 3E0R302

Ø: INTRODUCTION

E: PHYSIOLOGICAL SYSTEMS AND ANATOMICAL REGIONS

3: ADMINISTRATION

SECTION: 3 ADMINISTRATION

BODY SYSTEM: E PHYSIOLOGICAL SYSTEMS AND ANATOMICAL REGIONS

OPERATION: Ø INTRODUCTION: *(continued)*
Putting in or on a therapeutic, diagnostic, nutritional, physiological, or prophylactic substance except blood or blood products

Body System / Region	Approach	Substance	Qualifier
S Epidural Space	3 Percutaneous	3 Anti-inflammatory 6 Nutritional Substance 7 Electrolytic and Water Balance Substance B Anesthetic Agent H Radioactive Substance K Other Diagnostic Substance N Analgesics, Hypnotics, Sedatives T Destructive Agent	Z No Qualifier
S Epidural Space	3 Percutaneous	G Other Therapeutic Substance	C Other Substance
S Epidural Space	3 Percutaneous	S Gas	F Other Gas
S Epidural Space	7 Via Natural or Artificial Opening	S Gas	F Other Gas
T Peripheral Nerves and Plexi X Cranial Nerves	3 Percutaneous	3 Anti-inflammatory B Anesthetic Agent T Destructive Agent	Z No Qualifier
T Peripheral Nerves and Plexi X Cranial Nerves	3 Percutaneous	G Other Therapeutic Substance	C Other Substance
U Joints	Ø Open	2 Anti-infective	8 Oxazolidinones 9 Other Anti-infective
U Joints	Ø Open	G Other Therapeutic Substance	B Recombinant Bone Morphogenetic Protein
U Joints	3 Percutaneous	Ø Antineoplastic	4 Liquid Brachytherapy Radioisotope 5 Other Antineoplastic M Monoclonal Antibody
U Joints	3 Percutaneous	2 Anti-infective	8 Oxazolidinones 9 Other Anti-infective
U Joints	3 Percutaneous	3 Anti-inflammatory 6 Nutritional Substance 7 Electrolytic and Water Balance Substance B Anesthetic Agent H Radioactive Substance K Other Diagnostic Substance N Analgesics, Hypnotics, Sedatives T Destructive Agent	Z No Qualifier
U Joints	3 Percutaneous	G Other Therapeutic Substance	B Recombinant Bone Morphogenetic Protein C Other Substance
U Joints	3 Percutaneous	S Gas	F Other Gas
U Joints	3 Percutaneous Endoscopic	G Other Therapeutic Substance	C Other Substance

DRG Non-OR 3EØS3Ø2

Coding Clinic: 2Ø18, Q1, P8 – 3EØUØGB

SECTION: 3 ADMINISTRATION
BODY SYSTEM: E PHYSIOLOGICAL SYSTEMS AND ANATOMICAL REGIONS
OPERATION: Ø INTRODUCTION: *(continued)*
Putting in or on a therapeutic, diagnostic, nutritional, physiological, or prophylactic substance except blood or blood products

Body System / Region	Approach	Substance	Qualifier
V Bones	Ø Open	G Other Therapeutic Substance	B Recombinant Bone Morphogenetic Protein
V Bones	3 Percutaneous	Ø Antineoplastic	5 Other Antineoplastic M Monoclonal Antibody
V Bones	3 Percutaneous	2 Anti-infective	8 Oxazolidinones 9 Other Anti-infective
V Bones	3 Percutaneous	3 Anti-inflammatory 6 Nutritional Substance 7 Electrolytic and Water Balance Substance B Anesthetic Agent H Radioactive Substance K Other Diagnostic Substance N Analgesics, Hypnotics, Sedatives T Destructive Agent	Z No Qualifier
V Bones	3 Percutaneous	G Other Therapeutic Substance	B Recombinant Bone Morphogenetic Protein C Other Substance
W Lymphatics	3 Percutaneous	Ø Antineoplastic	5 Other Antineoplastic M Monoclonal Antibody
W Lymphatics	3 Percutaneous	2 Anti-infective	8 Oxazolidinones 9 Other Anti-infective
W Lymphatics	3 Percutaneous	3 Anti-inflammatory 6 Nutritional Substance 7 Electrolytic and Water Balance Substance B Anesthetic Agent H Radioactive Substance K Other Diagnostic Substance N Analgesics, Hypnotics, Sedatives T Destructive Agent	Z No Qualifier
W Lymphatics	3 Percutaneous	G Other Therapeutic Substance	C Other Substance
Y Pericardial Cavity	3 Percutaneous	Ø Antineoplastic	4 Liquid Brachytherapy Radioisotope 5 Other Antineoplastic M Monoclonal Antibody
Y Pericardial Cavity	3 Percutaneous	2 Anti-infective	8 Oxazolidinones 9 Other Anti-infective
Y Pericardial Cavity	3 Percutaneous	3 Anti-inflammatory 6 Nutritional Substance 7 Electrolytic and Water Balance Substance B Anesthetic Agent H Radioactive Substance K Other Diagnostic Substance N Analgesics, Hypnotics, Sedatives T Destructive Agent	Z No Qualifier

Coding Clinic: 2Ø16, Q3, P3Ø – 3EØVØGB

SECTION: 3 ADMINISTRATION
BODY SYSTEM: E PHYSIOLOGICAL SYSTEMS AND ANATOMICAL REGIONS
OPERATION: Ø INTRODUCTION: *(continued)*
Putting in or on a therapeutic, diagnostic, nutritional, physiological, or prophylactic substance except blood or blood products

Body System / Region	Approach	Substance	Qualifier
Y Pericardial Cavity	3 Percutaneous	G Other Therapeutic Substance	C Other Substance
Y Pericardial Cavity	3 Percutaneous	S Gas	F Other Gas
Y Pericardial Cavity	3 Percutaneous Endoscopic	G Other Therapeutic Substance	C Other Substance
Y Pericardial Cavity	7 Via Natural or Artificial Opening	Ø Antineoplastic	4 Liquid Brachytherapy Radioisotope 5 Other Antineoplastic M Monoclonal Antibody
Y Pericardial Cavity	7 Via Natural or Artificial Opening	S Gas	F Other Gas

Coding Clinic: 2013, Q1, P27 – 3EØG8TZ
Coding Clinic: 2015, Q1, P31 – 3EØR3Ø5
Coding Clinic: 2015, Q1, P38 – 3EØ53Ø5

SECTION: 3 ADMINISTRATION
BODY SYSTEM: E PHYSIOLOGICAL SYSTEMS AND ANATOMICAL REGIONS
OPERATION: 1 IRRIGATION: Putting in or on a cleansing substance

Body System / Region	Approach	Substance	Qualifier
Ø Skin and Mucous Membranes C Eye	3 Percutaneous X External	8 Irrigating Substance	X Diagnostic Z No Qualifier
9 Nose B Ear F Respiratory Tract G Upper GI H Lower GI J Biliary and Pancreatic Tract K Genitourinary Tract N Male Reproductive ♂ P Female Reproductive ♀	3 Percutaneous 7 Via Natural or Artificial Opening 8 Via Natural or Artificial Opening Endoscopic	8 Irrigating Substance	X Diagnostic Z No Qualifier
L Pleural Cavity Q Cranial Cavity and Brain R Spinal Canal S Epidural Space U Joints Y Pericardial Cavity	3 Percutaneous	8 Irrigating Substance	X Diagnostic Z No Qualifier
M Peritoneal Cavity	3 Percutaneous	8 Irrigating Substance	X Diagnostic Z No Qualifier
M Peritoneal Cavity	3 Percutaneous	9 Dialysate	Z No Qualifier

New/Revised Text in Green ~~deleted~~ Deleted ♀ Females Only ♂ Males Only **Coding Clinic**
Non-covered Limited Coverage ⊞ Combination (See Appendix E) DRG Non-OR Non-OR Hospital-Acquired Condition

SECTION: 4 MEASUREMENT AND MONITORING
BODY SYSTEM: A PHYSIOLOGICAL SYSTEMS
OPERATION: 0 MEASUREMENT: *(on multiple pages)*
Determining the level of a physiological or physical function at a point in time

0: MEASUREMENT

A: PHYSIOLOGICAL SYSTEMS

4: MEASUREMENT AND MONITORING

Body System	Approach	Function / Device	Qualifier
0 Central Nervous	0 Open	2 Conductivity 4 Electrical Activity B Pressure	Z No Qualifier
0 Central Nervous	3 Percutaneous 7 Via Natural or Artificial Opening 8 Via Natural or Artificial Opening Endoscopic	4 Electrical Activity	Z No Qualifier
0 Central Nervous	3 Percutaneous 7 Via Natural or Artificial Opening 8 Via Natural or Artificial Opening Endoscopic	B Pressure K Temperature R Saturation	D Intracranial
0 Central Nervous	X External	2 Conductivity 4 Electrical Activity	Z No Qualifier
1 Peripheral Nervous	0 Open 3 Percutaneous 7 Via Natural or Artificial Opening 8 Via Natural or Artificial Opening Endoscopic X External	2 Conductivity	9 Sensory B Motor
1 Peripheral Nervous	0 Open 3 Percutaneous 7 Via Natural or Artificial Opening 8 Via Natural or Artificial Opening Endoscopic X External	4 Electrical Activity	Z No Qualifier
2 Cardiac	0 Open 3 Percutaneous 7 Via Natural or Artificial Opening 8 Via Natural or Artificial Opening Endoscopic	4 Electrical Activity 9 Output C Rate F Rhythm H Sound P Action Currents	Z No Qualifier
2 Cardiac	0 Open 3 Percutaneous 7 Via Natural or Artificial Opening 8 Via Natural or Artificial Opening Endoscopic	N Sampling and Pressure	6 Right Heart 7 Left Heart 8 Bilateral
2 Cardiac	X External	4 Electrical Activity	A Guidance Z No Qualifier
2 Cardiac	X External	9 Output C Rate F Rhythm H Sound P Action Currents	Z No Qualifier
2 Cardiac	X External	M Total Activity	4 Stress
3 Arterial	0 Open 3 Percutaneous	5 Flow J Pulse	1 Peripheral 3 Pulmonary C Coronary
3 Arterial	0 Open 3 Percutaneous	B Pressure	1 Peripheral 3 Pulmonary C Coronary F Other Thoracic

DRG Non-OR 4A023FZ
DRG Non-OR 4A02[03]N[678]
Non-OR 4A02X4A

Coding Clinic: 2015, Q3, P29 – 4A02X4Z
Coding Clinic: 2016, Q3, P37 – 4A033BC
Coding Clinic: 2018, Q1, P13 – 4A023N8

New/Revised Text in Green   ~~deleted~~ Deleted   ♀ Females Only   ♂ Males Only   **Coding Clinic**
Non-covered   Limited Coverage   ⊕ Combination (See Appendix E)   DRG Non-OR   Non-OR   Hospital-Acquired Condition

SECTION: 4 MEASUREMENT AND MONITORING
BODY SYSTEM: A PHYSIOLOGICAL SYSTEMS
OPERATION: Ø MEASUREMENT: *(continued)*
Determining the level of a physiological or physical function at a point in time

Body System	Approach	Function / Device	Qualifier
3 Arterial	Ø Open 3 Percutaneous	H Sound R Saturation	1 Peripheral
3 Arterial	X External	5 Flow B Pressure H Sound J Pulse R Saturation	1 Peripheral
4 Venous	Ø Open 3 Percutaneous	5 Flow B Pressure J Pulse	Ø Central 1 Peripheral 2 Portal 3 Pulmonary
4 Venous	Ø Open 3 Percutaneous	R Saturation	1 Peripheral
4 Venous	X External	5 Flow B Pressure J Pulse R Saturation	1 Peripheral
5 Circulatory	X External	L Volume	Z No Qualifier
6 Lymphatic	Ø Open 3 Percutaneous 7 Via Natural or Artificial Opening 8 Via Natural or Artificial Opening Endoscopic	5 Flow B Pressure	Z No Qualifier
7 Visual	X External	Ø Acuity 7 Mobility B Pressure	Z No Qualifier
8 Olfactory	X External	Ø Acuity	Z No Qualifier
9 Respiratory	7 Via Natural or Artificial Opening 8 Via Natural or Artificial Opening Endoscopic X External	1 Capacity 5 Flow C Rate D Resistance L Volume M Total Activity	Z No Qualifier
B Gastrointestinal	7 Via Natural or Artificial Opening 8 Via Natural or Artificial Opening Endoscopic	8 Motility B Pressure G Secretion	Z No Qualifier
C Biliary	3 Percutaneous 4 Percutaneous Endoscopic 7 Via Natural or Artificial Opening 8 Via Natural or Artificial Opening Endoscopic	5 Flow B Pressure	Z No Qualifier
D Urinary	7 Via Natural or Artificial Opening 8 Via Natural or Artificial Opening Endoscopic	3 Contractility 5 Flow B Pressure D Resistance L Volume	Z No Qualifier
F Musculoskeletal	3 Percutaneous X External	3 Contractility	Z No Qualifier
H Products of Conception, Cardiac ♀	7 Via Natural or Artificial Opening 8 Via Natural or Artificial Opening Endoscopic X External	4 Electrical Activity C Rate F Rhythm H Sound	Z No Qualifier

SECTION: 4 MEASUREMENT AND MONITORING
BODY SYSTEM: A PHYSIOLOGICAL SYSTEMS
OPERATION: 0 MEASUREMENT: *(continued)*
Determining the level of a physiological or physical function at a point in time

Body System	Approach	Function / Device	Qualifier
J Products of Conception, Nervous ♀	7 Via Natural or Artificial Opening 8 Via Natural or Artificial Opening Endoscopic X External	2 Conductivity 4 Electrical Activity B Pressure	Z No Qualifier
Z None	7 Via Natural or Artificial Opening	6 Metabolism K Temperature	Z No Qualifier
Z None	X External	6 Metabolism K Temperature Q Sleep	Z No Qualifier

SECTION: 4 MEASUREMENT AND MONITORING
BODY SYSTEM: A PHYSIOLOGICAL SYSTEMS
OPERATION: 1 MONITORING: *(on multiple pages)*
Determining the level of a physiological or physical function repetitively over a period of time

Body System	Approach	Function / Device	Qualifier
0 Central Nervous	0 Open	2 Conductivity B Pressure	Z No Qualifier
0 Central Nervous	0 Open	4 Electrical Activity	G Intraoperative Z No Qualifier
0 Central Nervous	3 Percutaneous 7 Via Natural or Artificial Opening 8 Via Natural or Artificial Opening Endoscopic	4 Electrical Activity	G Intraoperative Z No Qualifier
0 Central Nervous	3 Percutaneous 7 Via Natural or Artificial Opening 8 Via Natural or Artificial Opening Endoscopic	B Pressure K Temperature R Saturation	D Intracranial
0 Central Nervous	X External	2 Conductivity	Z No Qualifier
0 Central Nervous	X External	4 Electrical Activity	G Intraoperative Z No Qualifier
1 Peripheral Nervous	0 Open 3 Percutaneous 7 Via Natural or Artificial Opening 8 Via Natural or Artificial Opening Endoscopic X External	2 Conductivity	9 Sensory B Motor
1 Peripheral Nervous	0 Open 3 Percutaneous 7 Via Natural or Artificial Opening 8 Via Natural or Artificial Opening Endoscopic X External	4 Electrical Activity	G Intraoperative Z No Qualifier

Coding Clinic: 2015, Q2, P14 – 4A11X4G
Coding Clinic: 2016, Q2, P29 – 4A103BD

New/Revised Text in Green   ~~deleted~~ Deleted   ♀ Females Only   ♂ Males Only   **Coding Clinic**
Non-covered   Limited Coverage   ⊞ Combination (See Appendix E)   DRG Non-OR   Non-OR   Hospital-Acquired Condition

SECTION: 4 MEASUREMENT AND MONITORING
BODY SYSTEM: A PHYSIOLOGICAL SYSTEMS
OPERATION: 1 MONITORING: *(continued)*
Determining the level of a physiological or physical function repetitively over a period of time

Body System	Approach	Function / Device	Qualifier
2 Cardiac	Ø Open 3 Percutaneous 7 Via Natural or Artificial Opening 8 Via Natural or Artificial Opening Endoscopic	4 Electrical Activity 9 Output C Rate F Rhythm H Sound	Z No Qualifier
2 Cardiac	X External	4 Electrical Activity	5 Ambulatory Z No Qualifier
2 Cardiac	X External	9 Output C Rate F Rhythm H Sound	Z No Qualifier
2 Cardiac	X External	M Total Activity	4 Stress
2 Cardiac	X External	S Vascular Perfusion	H Indocyanine Green Dye
3 Arterial	Ø Open 3 Percutaneous	5 Flow B Pressure J Pulse	1 Peripheral 3 Pulmonary C Coronary
3 Arterial	Ø Open 3 Percutaneous	H Sound R Saturation	1 Peripheral
3 Arterial	X External	5 Flow B Pressure H Sound J Pulse R Saturation	1 Peripheral
4 Venous	Ø Open 3 Percutaneous	5 Flow B Pressure J Pulse	Ø Central 1 Peripheral 2 Portal 3 Pulmonary
4 Venous	Ø Open 3 Percutaneous	R Saturation	Ø Central 2 Portal 3 Pulmonary
4 Venous	X External	5 Flow B Pressure J Pulse	1 Peripheral
6 Lymphatic	Ø Open 3 Percutaneous 7 Via Natural or Artificial Opening 8 Via Natural or Artificial Opening Endoscopic	5 Flow B Pressure	Z No Qualifier
9 Respiratory	7 Via Natural or Artificial Opening X External	1 Capacity 5 Flow C Rate D Resistance L Volume	Z No Qualifier
B Gastrointestinal	7 Via Natural or Artificial Opening 8 Via Natural or Artificial Opening Endoscopic	8 Motility B Pressure G Secretion	Z No Qualifier

Coding Clinic: 2015, Q3, P35 – 4A1239Z, 4A133B3
Coding Clinic: 2016, Q2, P33 – 4A133[BJ]1

SECTION: 4 MEASUREMENT AND MONITORING

BODY SYSTEM: A PHYSIOLOGICAL SYSTEMS

OPERATION: 1 MONITORING: *(continued)*
Determining the level of a physiological or physical function repetitively over a period of time

Body System	Approach	Function / Device	Qualifier
B Gastrointestinal	X External	S Vascular Perfusion	H Indocyanine Green Dye
D Urinary	7 Via Natural or Artificial Opening 8 Via Natural or Artificial Opening Endoscopic	3 Contractility 5 Flow B Pressure D Resistance L Volume	Z No Qualifier
G Skin and Breast	X External	S Vascular Perfusion	H Indocyanine Green Dye
H Products of Conception, Cardiac ♀	7 Via Natural or Artificial Opening 8 Via Natural or Artificial Opening Endoscopic X External	4 Electrical Activity C Rate F Rhythm H Sound	Z No Qualifier
J Products of Conception, Nervous ♀	7 Via Natural or Artificial Opening 8 Via Natural or Artificial Opening Endoscopic X External	2 Conductivity 4 Electrical Activity B Pressure	Z No Qualifier
Z None	7 Via Natural or Artificial Opening	K Temperature	Z No Qualifier
Z None	X External	K Temperature Q Sleep	Z No Qualifier

Coding Clinic: 2015, Q1, P26 – 4A11X4G

SECTION: 4 MEASUREMENT AND MONITORING

BODY SYSTEM: B PHYSIOLOGICAL DEVICES

OPERATION: Ø MEASUREMENT: Determining the level of a physiological or physical function at a point in time

Body System	Approach	Function / Device	Qualifier
Ø Central Nervous 1 Peripheral Nervous F Musculoskeletal	X External	V Stimulator	Z No Qualifier
2 Cardiac	X External	S Pacemaker T Defibrillator	Z No Qualifier
9 Respiratory	X External	S Pacemaker	Z No Qualifier

SECTION: 5 EXTRACORPOREAL OR SYSTEMIC ASSISTANCE AND PERFORMANCE

BODY SYSTEM: A PHYSIOLOGICAL SYSTEMS

OPERATION: Ø ASSISTANCE: Taking over a portion of a physiological function by extracorporeal means

Body System	Duration	Function	Qualifier
2 Cardiac	1 Intermittent 2 Continuous	1 Output	Ø Balloon Pump 5 Pulsatile Compression 6 Pump D Impeller Pump
5 Circulatory	1 Intermittent 2 Continuous	2 Oxygenation	1 Hyperbaric C Supersaturated
9 Respiratory	2 Continuous	Ø Filtration	Z No Qualifier
9 Respiratory	3 Less than 24 Consecutive Hours 4 24-96 Consecutive Hours 5 Greater than 96 Consecutive Hours	5 Ventilation	7 Continuous Positive Airway Pressure 8 Intermittent Positive Airway Pressure 9 Continuous Negative Airway Pressure B Intermittent Negative Airway Pressure Z No Qualifier

Coding Clinic: 2013, Q3, P19 – 5AØ221Ø
Coding Clinic: 2017, Q1, P10-11, 29; 2016, Q4, P137 – 5AØ
Coding Clinic: 2017, Q1, P11-12; 2016, Q4, P139 – 5AØ221D
Coding Clinic: 2017, Q4, P44-45 – 5AØ221D
Coding Clinic: 2018, Q2, P4-5 – 5AØ221Ø

New/Revised Text in Green   ~~deleted~~ Deleted   ♀ Females Only   ♂ Males Only   **Coding Clinic**
Non-covered   Limited Coverage   ⊞ Combination (See Appendix E)   DRG Non-OR   Non-OR   Hospital-Acquired Condition

SECTION: 5 EXTRACORPOREAL OR SYSTEMIC ASSISTANCE AND PERFORMANCE

BODY SYSTEM: A PHYSIOLOGICAL SYSTEMS

OPERATION: 1 PERFORMANCE: Completely taking over a physiological function by extracorporeal means

Body System	Duration	Function	Qualifier
2 Cardiac	Ø Single	1 Output	2 Manual
2 Cardiac	1 Intermittent	3 Pacing	Z No Qualifier
2 Cardiac	2 Continuous	1 Output 3 Pacing	Z No Qualifier
5 Circulatory	2 Continuous	2 Oxygenation	3 Membrane F Membrane, Central G Membrane, Peripheral Veno-arterial H Membrane, Peripheral Veno-venous
9 Respiratory	Ø Single	5 Ventilation	4 Nonmechanical
9 Respiratory	3 Less than 24 Consecutive Hours 4 24-96 Consecutive Hours 5 Greater than 96 Consecutive Hours	5 Ventilation	Z No Qualifier
C Biliary	Ø Single 6 Multiple	Ø Filtration	Z No Qualifier
D Urinary	7 Intermittent, Less than 6 Hours Per Day 8 Prolonged Intermittent, 6-18 Hours Per Day 9 Continuous, Greater than 18 Hours Per Day	Ø Filtration	Z No Qualifier

DRG Non-OR 5A19[345]5Z

NOTE: 5A1955Z should only be coded on claims when the respiratory ventilation is provided for greater than four consecutive days during the length of stay.

Coding Clinic: 2013, Q3, P19 – 5A1223Z
Coding Clinic: 2015, Q4, P23-25; 2013, Q3, P19 – 5A1221Z
Coding Clinic: 2016, Q1, P28 – 5A1221Z
Coding Clinic: 2016, Q1, P29 – 5A1C00Z, 5A1D60Z

Coding Clinic: 2017, Q1, P20 – 5A1221Z
Coding Clinic: 2017, Q3, P7 – 5A1221Z
Coding Clinic: 2017, Q4, P72-73 – 51AD[789]0Z
Coding Clinic: 2018, Q1, P14 – 5A1935Z

SECTION: 5 EXTRACORPOREAL OR SYSTEMIC ASSISTANCE AND PERFORMANCE

BODY SYSTEM: A PHYSIOLOGICAL SYSTEMS

OPERATION: 2 RESTORATION: Returning, or attempting to return, a physiological function to its original state by extracorporeal means

Body System	Duration	Function	Qualifier
2 Cardiac	Ø Single	4 Rhythm	Z No Qualifier

New/Revised Text in Green   deleted Deleted   ♀ Females Only   ♂ Males Only   **Coding Clinic**

Non-covered   Limited Coverage   Combination (See Appendix E)   DRG Non-OR   Non-OR   Hospital-Acquired Condition

New/Revised Text in Green   ~~deleted~~ Deleted   ♀ Females Only   ♂ Males Only   **Coding Clinic**

Non-covered   Limited Coverage   ⊞ Combination (See Appendix E)   DRG Non-OR   Non-OR   Hospital-Acquired Condition

SECTION: 6 EXTRACORPOREAL OR SYSTEMIC THERAPIES
BODY SYSTEM: A PHYSIOLOGICAL SYSTEMS
OPERATION: Ø **ATMOSPHERIC CONTROL:** Extracorporeal control of atmospheric pressure and composition

Body System	Duration	Qualifier	Qualifier
Z None	Ø Single 1 Multiple	Z No Qualifier	Z No Qualifier

SECTION: 6 EXTRACORPOREAL OR SYSTEMIC THERAPIES
BODY SYSTEM: A PHYSIOLOGICAL SYSTEMS
OPERATION: 1 **DECOMPRESSION:** Extracorporeal elimination of undissolved gas from body fluids

Body System	Duration	Qualifier	Qualifier
5 Circulatory	Ø Single 1 Multiple	Z No Qualifier	Z No Qualifier

SECTION: 6 EXTRACORPOREAL OR SYSTEMIC THERAPIES
BODY SYSTEM: A PHYSIOLOGICAL SYSTEMS
OPERATION: 2 **ELECTROMAGNETIC THERAPY:** Extracorporeal treatment by electromagnetic rays

Body System	Duration	Qualifier	Qualifier
1 Urinary 2 Central Nervous	Ø Single 1 Multiple	Z No Qualifier	Z No Qualifier

SECTION: 6 EXTRACORPOREAL OR SYSTEMIC THERAPIES
BODY SYSTEM: A PHYSIOLOGICAL SYSTEMS
OPERATION: 3 **HYPERTHERMIA:** Extracorporeal raising of body temperature

Body System	Duration	Qualifier	Qualifier
Z None	Ø Single 1 Multiple	Z No Qualifier	Z No Qualifier

SECTION: 6 EXTRACORPOREAL OR SYSTEMIC THERAPIES
BODY SYSTEM: A PHYSIOLOGICAL SYSTEMS
OPERATION: 4 **HYPOTHERMIA:** Extracorporeal lowering of body temperature

Body System	Duration	Qualifier	Qualifier
Z None	Ø Single 1 Multiple	Z No Qualifier	Z No Qualifier

6: EXTRACORPOREAL OR SYSTEMIC THERAPIES   A: PHYSIOLOGICAL SYSTEMS   Ø; 1; 2; 3; 4

SECTION: 6 EXTRACORPOREAL OR SYSTEMIC THERAPIES

BODY SYSTEM: A PHYSIOLOGICAL SYSTEMS

OPERATION: 5 PHERESIS: Extracorporeal separation of blood products

Body System	Duration	Qualifier	Qualifier
5 Circulatory	Ø Single 1 Multiple	Z No Qualifier	Ø Erythrocytes 1 Leukocytes 2 Platelets 3 Plasma T Stem Cells, Cord Blood V Stem Cells, Hematopoietic

SECTION: 6 EXTRACORPOREAL OR SYSTEMIC THERAPIES

BODY SYSTEM: A PHYSIOLOGICAL SYSTEMS

OPERATION: 6 PHOTOTHERAPY: Extracorporeal treatment by light rays

Body System	Duration	Qualifier	Qualifier
Ø Skin 5 Circulatory	Ø Single 1 Multiple	Z No Qualifier	Z No Qualifier

SECTION: 6 EXTRACORPOREAL OR SYSTEMIC THERAPIES

BODY SYSTEM: A PHYSIOLOGICAL SYSTEMS

OPERATION: 7 ULTRASOUND THERAPY: Extracorporeal treatment by ultrasound

Body System	Duration	Qualifier	Qualifier
5 Circulatory	Ø Single 1 Multiple	Z No Qualifier	4 Head and Neck Vessels 5 Heart 6 Peripheral Vessels 7 Other Vessels Z No Qualifier

SECTION: 6 EXTRACORPOREAL OR SYSTEMIC THERAPIES

BODY SYSTEM: A PHYSIOLOGICAL SYSTEMS

OPERATION: 8 ULTRAVIOLET LIGHT THERAPY: Extracorporeal treatment by ultraviolet light

Body System	Duration	Qualifier	Qualifier
Ø Skin	Ø Single 1 Multiple	Z No Qualifier	Z No Qualifier

New/Revised Text in Green   ~~deleted~~ Deleted   ♀ Females Only   ♂ Males Only   **Coding Clinic**

Non-covered   Limited Coverage   Combination (See Appendix E)   DRG Non-OR   Non-OR   Hospital-Acquired Condition

SECTION: 6 EXTRACORPOREAL OR SYSTEMIC THERAPIES
BODY SYSTEM: A PHYSIOLOGICAL SYSTEMS
OPERATION: 9 SHOCK WAVE THERAPY: Extracorporeal treatment by shock waves

Body System	Duration	Qualifier	Qualifier
3 Musculoskeletal	Ø Single 1 Multiple	Z No Qualifier	Z No Qualifier

SECTION: 6 EXTRACORPOREAL OR SYSTEMIC THERAPIES
BODY SYSTEM: A PHYSIOLOGICAL SYSTEMS
OPERATION: B PERFUSION: Extracorporeal treatment by diffusion of therapeutic fluid

Body System	Duration	Qualifier	Qualifier
5 Circulatory B Respiratory System F Hepatobiliary System and Pancreas T Urinary System	Ø Single	B Donor Organ	Z No Qualifier

SECTION: 7 OSTEOPATHIC
BODY SYSTEM: W ANATOMICAL REGIONS
OPERATION: Ø TREATMENT: Manual treatment to eliminate or alleviate somatic dysfunction and related disorders

Body Region	Approach	Method	Qualifier
Ø Head 1 Cervical 2 Thoracic 3 Lumbar 4 Sacrum 5 Pelvis 6 Lower Extremities 7 Upper Extremities 8 Rib Cage 9 Abdomen	X External	Ø Articulatory-Raising 1 Fascial Release 2 General Mobilization 3 High Velocity-Low Amplitude 4 Indirect 5 Low Velocity-High Amplitude 6 Lymphatic Pump 7 Muscle Energy-Isometric 8 Muscle Energy-Isotonic 9 Other Method	Z None

SECTION: 8 OTHER PROCEDURES

BODY SYSTEM: C INDWELLING DEVICE

OPERATION: Ø OTHER PROCEDURES: Methodologies which attempt to remediate or cure a disorder or disease

Body Region	Approach	Method	Qualifier
1 Nervous System	X External	6 Collection	J Cerebrospinal Fluid L Other Fluid
2 Circulatory System	X External	6 Collection	K Blood L Other Fluid

SECTION: 8 OTHER PROCEDURES

BODY SYSTEM: E PHYSIOLOGICAL SYSTEMS AND ANATOMICAL REGIONS

OPERATION: Ø OTHER PROCEDURES: Methodologies which attempt to remediate or cure a disorder or disease

Body Region	Approach	Method	Qualifier
1 Nervous System U Female Reproductive System ♀	X External	Y Other Method	7 Examination
2 Circulatory System	3 Percutaneous	D Near Infrared Spectroscopy	Z No Qualifier
9 Head and Neck Region W Trunk Region	Ø Open 3 Percutaneous 4 Percutaneous Endoscopic 7 Via Natural or Artificial Opening 8 Via Natural or Artificial Opening Endoscopic	C Robotic Assisted Procedure	Z No Qualifier
9 Head and Neck Region W Trunk Region	X External	B Computer Assisted Procedure	F With Fluoroscopy G With Computerized Tomography H With Magnetic Resonance Imaging Z No Qualifier
9 Head and Neck Region W Trunk Region	X External	C Robotic Assisted Procedure	Z No Qualifier
9 Head and Neck Region W Trunk Region	X External	Y Other Method	8 Suture Removal
H Integumentary System and Breast	3 Percutaneous	Ø Acupuncture	Ø Anesthesia Z No Qualifier
H Integumentary System and Breast	X External	6 Collection	2 Breast Milk ♀
H Integumentary System and Breast	X External	Y Other Method	9 Piercing
K Musculoskeletal System	X External	1 Therapeutic Massage	Z No Qualifier
K Musculoskeletal System	X External	Y Other Method	7 Examination
V Male Reproductive System ♂	X External	1 Therapeutic Massage	C Prostate D Rectum
V Male Reproductive System ♂	X External	6 Collection	3 Sperm
X Upper Extremity Y Lower Extremity	Ø Open 3 Percutaneous 4 Percutaneous Endoscopic	C Robotic Assisted Procedure	Z No Qualifier
X Upper Extremity Y Lower Extremity	X External	B Computer Assisted Procedure	F With Fluoroscopy G With Computerized Tomography H With Magnetic Resonance Imaging Z No Qualifier
X Upper Extremity Y Lower Extremity	X External	C Robotic Assisted Procedure	Z No Qualifier
X Upper Extremity Y Lower Extremity	X External	Y Other Method	8 Suture Removal
Z None	X External	Y Other Method	1 In Vitro Fertilization 4 Yoga Therapy 5 Meditation 6 Isolation

Coding Clinic: 2015, Q1, P34 – 8EØW4CZ

New/Revised Text in Green   ~~deleted~~ Deleted   ♀ Females Only   ♂ Males Only   **Coding Clinic**
Non-covered   Limited Coverage   ⊞ Combination (See Appendix E)   DRG Non-OR   Non-OR   Hospital-Acquired Condition

SECTION: 9 CHIROPRACTIC
BODY SYSTEM: W ANATOMICAL REGIONS
OPERATION: **B MANIPULATION:** Manual procedure that involves a directed thrust to move a joint past the physiological range of motion, without exceeding the anatomical limit

Body Region	Approach	Method	Qualifier
Ø Head	X External	B Non-Manual	Z None
1 Cervical		C Indirect Visceral	
2 Thoracic		D Extra-Articular	
3 Lumbar		F Direct Visceral	
4 Sacrum		G Long Lever Specific Contact	
5 Pelvis		H Short Lever Specific Contact	
6 Lower Extremities		J Long and Short Lever Specific Contact	
7 Upper Extremities			
8 Rib Cage		K Mechanically Assisted	
9 Abdomen		L Other Method	

B: MANIPULATION

W: ANATOMICAL REGIONS

9: CHIROPRACTIC

B Imaging

New/Revised Text in Green   ~~deleted~~ Deleted   ♀ Females Only   ♂ Males Only   **Coding Clinic**

🐾 Non-covered   🐾 Limited Coverage   ⊞ Combination (See Appendix E)   DRG Non-OR   Non-OR   🐾 Hospital-Acquired Condition

New/Revised Text in Green   ~~deleted~~ Deleted   ♀ Females Only   ♂ Males Only   **Coding Clinic**

🐾 Non-covered   🐾 Limited Coverage   ⊞ Combination (See Appendix E)   DRG Non-OR   Non-OR   🐾 Hospital-Acquired Condition

SECTION: B IMAGING
BODY SYSTEM: Ø CENTRAL NERVOUS SYSTEM
TYPE: Ø PLAIN RADIOGRAPHY: Planar display of an image developed from the capture of external ionizing radiation on photographic or photoconductive plate

Body Part	Contrast	Qualifier	Qualifier
B Spinal Cord	Ø High Osmolar 1 Low Osmolar Y Other Contrast Z None	Z None	Z None

SECTION: B IMAGING
BODY SYSTEM: Ø CENTRAL NERVOUS SYSTEM
TYPE: 1 FLUOROSCOPY: Single plane or bi-plane real time display of an image developed from the capture of external ionizing radiation on a fluorescent screen. The image may also be stored by either digital or analog means.

Body Part	Contrast	Qualifier	Qualifier
B Spinal Cord	Ø High Osmolar 1 Low Osmolar Y Other Contrast Z None	Z None	Z None

SECTION: B IMAGING
BODY SYSTEM: Ø CENTRAL NERVOUS SYSTEM
TYPE: 2 COMPUTERIZED TOMOGRAPHY (CT SCAN): Computer reformatted digital display of multiplanar images developed from the capture of multiple exposures of external ionizing radiation

Body Part	Contrast	Qualifier	Qualifier
Ø Brain 7 Cisterna 8 Cerebral Ventricle(s) 9 Sella Turcica/Pituitary Gland B Spinal Cord	Ø High Osmolar 1 Low Osmolar Y Other Contrast	Ø Unenhanced and Enhanced Z None	Z None
Ø Brain 7 Cisterna 8 Cerebral Ventricle(s) 9 Sella Turcica/Pituitary Gland B Spinal Cord	Z None	Z None	Z None

SECTION: B IMAGING

BODY SYSTEM: Ø CENTRAL NERVOUS SYSTEM

TYPE: 3 **MAGNETIC RESONANCE IMAGING (MRI):** Computer reformatted digital display of multiplanar images developed from the capture of radiofrequency signals emitted by nuclei in a body site excited within a magnetic field

Body Part	Contrast	Qualifier	Qualifier
Ø Brain 9 Sella Turcica/Pituitary Gland B Spinal Cord C Acoustic Nerves	Y Other Contrast	Ø Unenhanced and Enhanced Z None	Z None
Ø Brain 9 Sella Turcica/Pituitary Gland B Spinal Cord C Acoustic Nerves	Z None	Z None	Z None

SECTION: B IMAGING

BODY SYSTEM: Ø CENTRAL NERVOUS SYSTEM

TYPE: 4 **ULTRASONOGRAPHY:** Real time display of images of anatomy or flow information developed from the capture of reflected and attenuated high frequency sound waves

Body Part	Contrast	Qualifier	Qualifier
Ø Brain B Spinal Cord	Z None	Z None	Z None

SECTION: **B IMAGING**

BODY SYSTEM: 2 HEART

TYPE: Ø **PLAIN RADIOGRAPHY:** Planar display of an image developed from the capture of external ionizing radiation on photographic or photoconductive plate

Body Part	Contrast	Qualifier	Qualifier
Ø Coronary Artery, Single 1 Coronary Arteries, Multiple 2 Coronary Artery Bypass Graft, Single 3 Coronary Artery Bypass Grafts, Multiple 4 Heart, Right 5 Heart, Left 6 Heart, Right and Left 7 Internal Mammary Bypass Graft, Right 8 Internal Mammary Bypass Graft, Left F Bypass Graft, Other	Ø High Osmolar 1 Low Osmolar Y Other Contrast	Z None	Z None

`DRG Non-OR` All Values

Coding Clinic: 2Ø18, Q1, P13 – B2151ZZ

SECTION: **B IMAGING**

BODY SYSTEM: 2 HEART

TYPE: 1 **FLUOROSCOPY:** Single plane or bi-plane real time display of an image developed from the capture of external ionizing radiation on a fluorescent screen. The image may also be stored by either digital or analog means.

Body Part	Contrast	Qualifier	Qualifier
Ø Coronary Artery, Single 1 Coronary Arteries, Multiple 2 Coronary Artery Bypass Graft, Single 3 Coronary Artery Bypass Grafts, Multiple	Ø High Osmolar 1 Low Osmolar Y Other Contrast	1 Laser	Ø Intraoperative
Ø Coronary Artery, Single 1 Coronary Arteries, Multiple 2 Coronary Artery Bypass Graft, Single 3 Coronary Artery Bypass Grafts, Multiple	Ø High Osmolar 1 Low Osmolar Y Other Contrast	Z None	Z None
4 Heart, Right 5 Heart, Left 6 Heart, Right and Left 7 Internal Mammary Bypass Graft, Right 8 Internal Mammary Bypass Graft, Left F Bypass Graft, Other	Ø High Osmolar 1 Low Osmolar Y Other Contrast	Z None	Z None

`DRG Non-OR` B21[Ø123][Ø1Y]ZZ
`DRG Non-OR` B21[45678F][Ø1Y]ZZ

Coding Clinic: 2Ø16, Q3, P36 – B21

New/Revised Text in Green   deleted Deleted   ♀ Females Only   ♂ Males Only   **Coding Clinic**

 Non-covered   Limited Coverage   ⊞ Combination (See Appendix E)   `DRG Non-OR`   Non-OR   Hospital-Acquired Condition

SECTION: B IMAGING

BODY SYSTEM: 2 HEART

TYPE: 2 **COMPUTERIZED TOMOGRAPHY (CT SCAN):** Computer reformatted digital display of multiplanar images developed from the capture of multiple exposures of external ionizing radiation

Body Part	Contrast	Qualifier	Qualifier
1 Coronary Arteries, Multiple 3 Coronary Artery Bypass Grafts, Multiple 6 Heart, Right and Left	Ø High Osmolar 1 Low Osmolar Y Other Contrast	Ø Unenhanced and Enhanced Z None	Z None
1 Coronary Arteries, Multiple 3 Coronary Artery Bypass Grafts, Multiple 6 Heart, Right and Left	Z None	2 Intravascular Optical Coherence Z None	Z None

SECTION: B IMAGING

BODY SYSTEM: 2 HEART

TYPE: 3 **MAGNETIC RESONANCE IMAGING (MRI):** Computer reformatted digital display of multiplanar images developed from the capture of radiofrequency signals emitted by nuclei in a body site excited within a magnetic field

Body Part	Contrast	Qualifier	Qualifier
1 Coronary Arteries, Multiple 3 Coronary Artery Bypass Grafts, Multiple 6 Heart, Right and Left	Y Other Contrast	Ø Unenhanced and Enhanced Z None	Z None
1 Coronary Arteries, Multiple 3 Coronary Artery Bypass Grafts, Multiple 6 Heart, Right and Left	Z None	Z None	Z None

2: COMPUTERIZED TOMOGRAPHY (CT SCAN)   3: MAGNETIC RESONANCE IMAGING (MRI)

2: HEART

B: IMAGING

New/Revised Text in Green   ~~deleted~~ Deleted   ♀ Females Only   ♂ Males Only   **Coding Clinic**
🔖 Non-covered   🔖 Limited Coverage   ⊟ Combination (See Appendix E)   DRG Non-OR   Non-OR   🔖 Hospital-Acquired Condition

SECTION: B IMAGING
BODY SYSTEM: 2 HEART
TYPE: 4 **ULTRASONOGRAPHY:** Real time display of images of anatomy or flow information developed from the capture of reflected and attenuated high frequency sound waves

Body Part	Contrast	Qualifier	Qualifier
Ø Coronary Artery, Single 1 Coronary Arteries, Multiple 4 Heart, Right 5 Heart, Left 6 Heart, Right and Left B Heart with Aorta C Pericardium D Pediatric Heart	Y Other Contrast	Z None	Z None
Ø Coronary Artery, Single 1 Coronary Arteries, Multiple 4 Heart, Right 5 Heart, Left 6 Heart, Right and Left B Heart with Aorta C Pericardium D Pediatric Heart	Z None	Z None	3 Intravascular 4 Transesophageal Z None

New/Revised Text in Green ~~deleted~~ Deleted ♀ Females Only ♂ Males Only **Coding Clinic**
Non-covered Limited Coverage Combination (See Appendix E) DRG Non-OR Non-OR Hospital-Acquired Condition

589

SECTION: B IMAGING

BODY SYSTEM: 3 UPPER ARTERIES

TYPE: Ø **PLAIN RADIOGRAPHY:** Planar display of an image developed from the capture of external ionizing radiation on photographic or photoconductive plate

0: PLAIN RADIOGRAPHY

3: UPPER ARTERIES

B: IMAGING

Body Part	Contrast	Qualifier	Qualifier
Ø Thoracic Aorta	Ø High Osmolar	Z None	Z None
1 Brachiocephalic-Subclavian Artery, Right	1 Low Osmolar		
2 Subclavian Artery, Left	Y Other Contrast		
3 Common Carotid Artery, Right	Z None		
4 Common Carotid Artery, Left			
5 Common Carotid Arteries, Bilateral			
6 Internal Carotid Artery, Right			
7 Internal Carotid Artery, Left			
8 Internal Carotid Arteries, Bilateral			
9 External Carotid Artery, Right			
B External Carotid Artery, Left			
C External Carotid Arteries, Bilateral			
D Vertebral Artery, Right			
F Vertebral Artery, Left			
G Vertebral Arteries, Bilateral			
H Upper Extremity Arteries, Right			
J Upper Extremity Arteries, Left			
K Upper Extremity Arteries, Bilateral			
L Intercostal and Bronchial Arteries			
M Spinal Arteries			
N Upper Arteries, Other			
P Thoraco-Abdominal Aorta			
Q Cervico-Cerebral Arch			
R Intracranial Arteries			
S Pulmonary Artery, Right			
T Pulmonary Artery, Left			

SECTION: B IMAGING
BODY SYSTEM: 3 UPPER ARTERIES
TYPE: 1 FLUOROSCOPY: *(on multiple pages)*

Single plane or bi-plane real time display of an image developed from the capture of external ionizing radiation on a fluorescent screen. The image may also be stored by either digital or analog means.

Body Part	Contrast	Qualifier	Qualifier
Ø Thoracic Aorta	Ø High Osmolar	1 Laser	Ø Intraoperative
1 Brachiocephalic-Subclavian Artery, Right	1 Low Osmolar		
2 Subclavian Artery, Left	Y Other Contrast		
3 Common Carotid Artery, Right			
4 Common Carotid Artery, Left			
5 Common Carotid Arteries, Bilateral			
6 Internal Carotid Artery, Right			
7 Internal Carotid Artery, Left			
8 Internal Carotid Arteries, Bilateral			
9 External Carotid Artery, Right			
B External Carotid Artery, Left			
C External Carotid Arteries, Bilateral			
D Vertebral Artery, Right			
F Vertebral Artery, Left			
G Vertebral Arteries, Bilateral			
H Upper Extremity Arteries, Right			
J Upper Extremity Arteries, Left			
K Upper Extremity Arteries, Bilateral			
L Intercostal and Bronchial Arteries			
M Spinal Arteries			
N Upper Arteries, Other			
P Thoraco-Abdominal Aorta			
Q Cervico-Cerebral Arch			
R Intracranial Arteries			
S Pulmonary Artery, Right			
T Pulmonary Artery, Left			
U Pulmonary Trunk			

SECTION: B IMAGING
BODY SYSTEM: 3 UPPER ARTERIES
TYPE: 1 **FLUOROSCOPY:** *(continued)*

Single plane or bi-plane real time display of an image developed from the capture of external ionizing radiation on a fluorescent screen. The image may also be stored by either digital or analog means.

Body Part	Contrast	Qualifier	Qualifier
Ø Thoracic Aorta 1 Brachiocephalic-Subclavian Artery, Right 2 Subclavian Artery, Left 3 Common Carotid Artery, Right 4 Common Carotid Artery, Left 5 Common Carotid Arteries, Bilateral 6 Internal Carotid Artery, Right 7 Internal Carotid Artery, Left 8 Internal Carotid Arteries, Bilateral 9 External Carotid Artery, Right B External Carotid Artery, Left C External Carotid Arteries, Bilateral D Vertebral Artery, Right F Vertebral Artery, Left G Vertebral Arteries, Bilateral H Upper Extremity Arteries, Right J Upper Extremity Arteries, Left K Upper Extremity Arteries, Bilateral L Intercostal and Bronchial Arteries M Spinal Arteries N Upper Arteries, Other P Thoraco-Abdominal Aorta Q Cervico-Cerebral Arch R Intracranial Arteries S Pulmonary Artery, Right T Pulmonary Artery, Left U Pulmonary Trunk	Ø High Osmolar 1 Low Osmolar Y Other Contrast	Z None	Z None

1: FLUOROSCOPY

3: UPPER ARTERIES

B: IMAGING

New/Revised Text in Green — deleted Deleted ♀ Females Only ♂ Males Only **Coding Clinic**
Non-covered — Limited Coverage — ⊕ Combination (See Appendix E) — DRG Non-OR — Non-OR — Hospital-Acquired Condition

SECTION: B IMAGING

BODY SYSTEM: 3 UPPER ARTERIES

TYPE: 1 **FLUOROSCOPY:** *(continued)*
Single plane or bi-plane real time display of an image developed from the capture of external ionizing radiation on a fluorescent screen. The image may also be stored by either digital or analog means.

Body Part	Contrast	Qualifier	Qualifier
0 Thoracic Aorta 1 Brachiocephalic-Subclavian Artery, Right 2 Subclavian Artery, Left 3 Common Carotid Artery, Right 4 Common Carotid Artery, Left 5 Common Carotid Arteries, Bilateral 6 Internal Carotid Artery, Right 7 Internal Carotid Artery, Left 8 Internal Carotid Arteries, Bilateral 9 External Carotid Artery, Right B External Carotid Artery, Left C External Carotid Arteries, Bilateral D Vertebral Artery, Right F Vertebral Artery, Left G Vertebral Arteries, Bilateral H Upper Extremity Arteries, Right J Upper Extremity Arteries, Left K Upper Extremity Arteries, Bilateral L Intercostal and Bronchial Arteries M Spinal Arteries N Upper Arteries, Other P Thoraco-Abdominal Aorta Q Cervico-Cerebral Arch R Intracranial Arteries S Pulmonary Artery, Right T Pulmonary Artery, Left U Pulmonary Trunk	Z None	Z None	Z None

SECTION: B IMAGING

BODY SYSTEM: 3 UPPER ARTERIES

TYPE: 2 **COMPUTERIZED TOMOGRAPHY (CT SCAN):** Computer reformatted digital display of multiplanar images developed from the capture of multiple exposures of external ionizing radiation

Body Part	Contrast	Qualifier	Qualifier
0 Thoracic Aorta 5 Common Carotid Arteries, Bilateral 8 Internal Carotid Arteries, Bilateral G Vertebral Arteries, Bilateral R Intracranial Arteries S Pulmonary Artery, Right T Pulmonary Artery, Left	0 High Osmolar 1 Low Osmolar Y Other Contrast	Z None	Z None
0 Thoracic Aorta 5 Common Carotid Arteries, Bilateral 8 Internal Carotid Arteries, Bilateral G Vertebral Arteries, Bilateral R Intracranial Arteries S Pulmonary Artery, Right T Pulmonary Artery, Left	Z None	2 Intravascular Optical Coherence Z None	Z None

New/Revised Text in Green   ~~deleted~~ Deleted   ♀ Females Only   ♂ Males Only   **Coding Clinic**
Non-covered   Limited Coverage   ⊞ Combination (See Appendix E)   DRG Non-OR   Non-OR   Hospital-Acquired Condition

B: IMAGING   3: UPPER ARTERIES   1: FLUOROSCOPY   2: COMPUTERIZED TOMOGRAPHY (CT SCAN)

SECTION: B IMAGING

BODY SYSTEM: 3 UPPER ARTERIES

TYPE: 3 **MAGNETIC RESONANCE IMAGING (MRI):** Computer reformatted digital display of multiplanar images developed from the capture of radiofrequency signals emitted by nuclei in a body site excited within a magnetic field

Body Part	Contrast	Qualifier	Qualifier
Ø Thoracic Aorta 5 Common Carotid Arteries, Bilateral 8 Internal Carotid Arteries, Bilateral G Vertebral Arteries, Bilateral H Upper Extremity Arteries, Right J Upper Extremity Arteries, Left K Upper Extremity Arteries, Bilateral M Spinal Arteries Q Cervico-Cerebral Arch R Intracranial Arteries	Y Other Contrast	Ø Unenhanced and Enhanced Z None	Z None
Ø Thoracic Aorta 5 Common Carotid Arteries, Bilateral 8 Internal Carotid Arteries, Bilateral G Vertebral Arteries, Bilateral H Upper Extremity Arteries, Right J Upper Extremity Arteries, Left K Upper Extremity Arteries, Bilateral M Spinal Arteries Q Cervico-Cerebral Arch R Intracranial Arteries	Z None	Z None	Z None

SECTION: B IMAGING

BODY SYSTEM: 3 UPPER ARTERIES

TYPE: 4 **ULTRASONOGRAPHY:** Real time display of images of anatomy or flow information developed from the capture of reflected and attenuated high frequency sound waves

Body Part	Contrast	Qualifier	Qualifier
Ø Thoracic Aorta 1 Brachiocephalic-Subclavian Artery, Right 2 Subclavian Artery, Left 3 Common Carotid Artery, Right 4 Common Carotid Artery, Left 5 Common Carotid Arteries, Bilateral 6 Internal Carotid Artery, Right 7 Internal Carotid Artery, Left 8 Internal Carotid Arteries, Bilateral H Upper Extremity Arteries, Right J Upper Extremity Arteries, Left K Upper Extremity Arteries, Bilateral R Intracranial Arteries S Pulmonary Artery, Right T Pulmonary Artery, Left V Ophthalmic Arteries	Z None	Z None	3 Intravascular Z None

SECTION: B IMAGING
BODY SYSTEM: 4 LOWER ARTERIES
TYPE:

Ø **PLAIN RADIOGRAPHY:** Planar display of an image developed from the capture of external ionizing radiation on photographic or photoconductive plate

Body Part	Contrast	Qualifier	Qualifier
Ø Abdominal Aorta	Ø High Osmolar	Z None	Z None
2 Hepatic Artery	1 Low Osmolar		
3 Splenic Arteries	Y Other Contrast		
4 Superior Mesenteric Artery			
5 Inferior Mesenteric Artery			
6 Renal Artery, Right			
7 Renal Artery, Left			
8 Renal Arteries, Bilateral			
9 Lumbar Arteries			
B Intra-Abdominal Arteries, Other			
C Pelvic Arteries			
D Aorta and Bilateral Lower Extremity Arteries			
F Lower Extremity Arteries, Right			
G Lower Extremity Arteries, Left			
J Lower Arteries, Other			
M Renal Artery Transplant			

SECTION: B IMAGING

BODY SYSTEM: 4 LOWER ARTERIES

TYPE: 1 **FLUOROSCOPY:** Single plane or bi-plane real time display of an image developed from the capture of external ionizing radiation on a fluorescent screen. The image may also be stored by either digital or analog means.

Body Part	Contrast	Qualifier	Qualifier
0 Abdominal Aorta 2 Hepatic Artery 3 Splenic Arteries 4 Superior Mesenteric Artery 5 Inferior Mesenteric Artery 6 Renal Artery, Right 7 Renal Artery, Left 8 Renal Arteries, Bilateral 9 Lumbar Arteries B Intra-Abdominal Arteries, Other C Pelvic Arteries D Aorta and Bilateral Lower Extremity Arteries F Lower Extremity Arteries, Right G Lower Extremity Arteries, Left J Lower Arteries, Other	0 High Osmolar 1 Low Osmolar Y Other Contrast	1 Laser	0 Intraoperative
0 Abdominal Aorta 2 Hepatic Artery 3 Splenic Arteries 4 Superior Mesenteric Artery 5 Inferior Mesenteric Artery 6 Renal Artery, Right 7 Renal Artery, Left 8 Renal Arteries, Bilateral 9 Lumbar Arteries B Intra-Abdominal Arteries, Other C Pelvic Arteries D Aorta and Bilateral Lower Extremity Arteries F Lower Extremity Arteries, Right G Lower Extremity Arteries, Left J Lower Arteries, Other	0 High Osmolar 1 Low Osmolar Y Other Contrast	Z None	Z None
0 Abdominal Aorta 2 Hepatic Artery 3 Splenic Arteries 4 Superior Mesenteric Artery 5 Inferior Mesenteric Artery 6 Renal Artery, Right 7 Renal Artery, Left 8 Renal Arteries, Bilateral 9 Lumbar Arteries B Intra-Abdominal Arteries, Other C Pelvic Arteries D Aorta and Bilateral Lower Extremity Arteries F Lower Extremity Arteries, Right G Lower Extremity Arteries, Left J Lower Arteries, Other	Z None	Z None	Z None

1: FLUOROSCOPY

4: LOWER ARTERIES

B: IMAGING

SECTION: B IMAGING

BODY SYSTEM: 4 LOWER ARTERIES

TYPE: 2 **COMPUTERIZED TOMOGRAPHY (CT SCAN):** Computer reformatted digital display of multiplanar images developed from the capture of multiple exposures of external ionizing radiation

Body Part	Contrast	Qualifier	Qualifier
Ø Abdominal Aorta 1 Celiac Artery 4 Superior Mesenteric Artery 8 Renal Arteries, Bilateral C Pelvic Arteries F Lower Extremity Arteries, Right G Lower Extremity Arteries, Left H Lower Extremity Arteries, Bilateral M Renal Artery Transplant	Ø High Osmolar 1 Low Osmolar Y Other Contrast	Z None	Z None
Ø Abdominal Aorta 1 Celiac Artery 4 Superior Mesenteric Artery 8 Renal Arteries, Bilateral C Pelvic Arteries F Lower Extremity Arteries, Right G Lower Extremity Arteries, Left H Lower Extremity Arteries, Bilateral M Renal Artery Transplant	Z None	2 Intravascular Optical Coherence Z None	Z None

SECTION: B IMAGING

BODY SYSTEM: 4 LOWER ARTERIES

TYPE: 3 **MAGNETIC RESONANCE IMAGING (MRI):** Computer reformatted digital display of multiplanar images developed from the capture of radiofrequency signals emitted by nuclei in a body site excited within a magnetic field

Body Part	Contrast	Qualifier	Qualifier
Ø Abdominal Aorta 1 Celiac Artery 4 Superior Mesenteric Artery 8 Renal Arteries, Bilateral C Pelvic Arteries F Lower Extremity Arteries, Right G Lower Extremity Arteries, Left H Lower Extremity Arteries, Bilateral	Y Other Contrast	Ø Unenhanced and Enhanced Z None	Z None
Ø Abdominal Aorta 1 Celiac Artery 4 Superior Mesenteric Artery 8 Renal Arteries, Bilateral C Pelvic Arteries F Lower Extremity Arteries, Right G Lower Extremity Arteries, Left H Lower Extremity Arteries, Bilateral	Z None	Z None	Z None

SECTION: B IMAGING

BODY SYSTEM: 4 LOWER ARTERIES

TYPE: 4 **ULTRASONOGRAPHY:** Real time display of images of anatomy or flow information developed from the capture of reflected and attenuated high frequency sound waves

Body Part	Contrast	Qualifier	Qualifier
Ø Abdominal Aorta 4 Superior Mesenteric Artery 5 Inferior Mesenteric Artery 6 Renal Artery, Right 7 Renal Artery, Left 8 Renal Arteries, Bilateral B Intra-Abdominal Arteries, Other F Lower Extremity Arteries, Right G Lower Extremity Arteries, Left H Lower Extremity Arteries, Bilateral K Celiac and Mesenteric Arteries L Femoral Artery N Penile Arteries	Z None	Z None	3 Intravascular Z None

SECTION: B IMAGING

BODY SYSTEM: 5 VEINS
TYPE: Ø **PLAIN RADIOGRAPHY:** Planar display of an image developed from the capture of external ionizing radiation on photographic or photoconductive plate

Body Part	Contrast	Qualifier	Qualifier
Ø Epidural Veins 1 Cerebral and Cerebellar Veins 2 Intracranial Sinuses 3 Jugular Veins, Right 4 Jugular Veins, Left 5 Jugular Veins, Bilateral 6 Subclavian Vein, Right 7 Subclavian Vein, Left 8 Superior Vena Cava 9 Inferior Vena Cava B Lower Extremity Veins, Right C Lower Extremity Veins, Left D Lower Extremity Veins, Bilateral F Pelvic (Iliac) Veins, Right G Pelvic (Iliac) Veins, Left H Pelvic (Iliac) Veins, Bilateral J Renal Vein, Right K Renal Vein, Left L Renal Veins, Bilateral M Upper Extremity Veins, Right N Upper Extremity Veins, Left P Upper Extremity Veins, Bilateral Q Pulmonary Vein, Right R Pulmonary Vein, Left S Pulmonary Veins, Bilateral T Portal and Splanchnic Veins V Veins, Other W Dialysis Shunt/Fistula	Ø High Osmolar 1 Low Osmolar Y Other Contrast	Z None	Z None

SECTION: B IMAGING

BODY SYSTEM: 5 VEINS

TYPE: 1 **FLUOROSCOPY:** Single plane or bi-plane real time display of an image developed from the capture of external ionizing radiation on a fluorescent screen. The image may also be stored by either digital or analog means.

Body Part	Contrast	Qualifier	Qualifier
Ø Epidural Veins	Ø High Osmolar	Z None	A Guidance
1 Cerebral and Cerebellar Veins	1 Low Osmolar		Z None
2 Intracranial Sinuses	Y Other Contrast		
3 Jugular Veins, Right	Z None		
4 Jugular Veins, Left			
5 Jugular Veins, Bilateral			
6 Subclavian Vein, Right			
7 Subclavian Vein, Left			
8 Superior Vena Cava			
9 Inferior Vena Cava			
B Lower Extremity Veins, Right			
C Lower Extremity Veins, Left			
D Lower Extremity Veins, Bilateral			
F Pelvic (Iliac) Veins, Right			
G Pelvic (Iliac) Veins, Left			
H Pelvic (Iliac) Veins, Bilateral			
J Renal Vein, Right			
K Renal Vein, Left			
L Renal Veins, Bilateral			
M Upper Extremity Veins, Right			
N Upper Extremity Veins, Left			
P Upper Extremity Veins, Bilateral			
Q Pulmonary Vein, Right			
R Pulmonary Vein, Left			
S Pulmonary Veins, Bilateral			
T Portal and Splanchnic Veins			
V Veins, Other			
W Dialysis Shunt/Fistula			

Coding Clinic: 2015, Q4, P30 – B518ZZA

1: FLUOROSCOPY

5: VEINS

B: IMAGING

New/Revised Text in Green   ~~deleted~~ Deleted   ♀ Females Only   ♂ Males Only   **Coding Clinic**
 Non-covered   Limited Coverage   Combination (See Appendix E)   DRG Non-OR   Non-OR   Hospital-Acquired Condition

SECTION: B IMAGING
BODY SYSTEM: 5 VEINS
TYPE: 2 **COMPUTERIZED TOMOGRAPHY (CT SCAN):** Computer reformatted digital display of multiplanar images developed from the capture of multiple exposures of external ionizing radiation

Body Part	Contrast	Qualifier	Qualifier
2 Intracranial Sinuses 8 Superior Vena Cava 9 Inferior Vena Cava F Pelvic (Iliac) Veins, Right G Pelvic (Iliac) Veins, Left H Pelvic (Iliac) Veins, Bilateral J Renal Vein, Right K Renal Vein, Left L Renal Veins, Bilateral Q Pulmonary Vein, Right R Pulmonary Vein, Left S Pulmonary Veins, Bilateral T Portal and Splanchnic Veins	Ø High Osmolar 1 Low Osmolar Y Other Contrast	Ø Unenhanced and Enhanced Z None	Z None
2 Intracranial Sinuses 8 Superior Vena Cava 9 Inferior Vena Cava F Pelvic (Iliac) Veins, Right G Pelvic (Iliac) Veins, Left H Pelvic (Iliac) Veins, Bilateral J Renal Vein, Right K Renal Vein, Left L Renal Veins, Bilateral Q Pulmonary Vein, Right R Pulmonary Vein, Left S Pulmonary Veins, Bilateral T Portal and Splanchnic Veins	Z None	2 Intravascular Optical Coherence Z None	Z None

SECTION: B IMAGING
BODY SYSTEM: 5 VEINS
TYPE: 3 **MAGNETIC RESONANCE IMAGING (MRI):** Computer reformatted digital display of multiplanar images developed from the capture of radiofrequency signals emitted by nuclei in a body site excited within a magnetic field

Body Part	Contrast	Qualifier	Qualifier
1 Cerebral and Cerebellar Veins 2 Intracranial Sinuses 5 Jugular Veins, Bilateral 8 Superior Vena Cava 9 Inferior Vena Cava B Lower Extremity Veins, Right C Lower Extremity Veins, Left D Lower Extremity Veins, Bilateral H Pelvic (Iliac) Veins, Bilateral L Renal Veins, Bilateral M Upper Extremity Veins, Right N Upper Extremity Veins, Left P Upper Extremity Veins, Bilateral S Pulmonary Veins, Bilateral T Portal and Splanchnic Veins V Veins, Other	Y Other Contrast	Ø Unenhanced and Enhanced Z None	Z None
1 Cerebral and Cerebellar Veins 2 Intracranial Sinuses 5 Jugular Veins, Bilateral 8 Superior Vena Cava 9 Inferior Vena Cava B Lower Extremity Veins, Right C Lower Extremity Veins, Left D Lower Extremity Veins, Bilateral H Pelvic (Iliac) Veins, Bilateral L Renal Veins, Bilateral M Upper Extremity Veins, Right N Upper Extremity Veins, Left P Upper Extremity Veins, Bilateral S Pulmonary Veins, Bilateral T Portal and Splanchnic Veins V Veins, Other	Z None	Z None	Z None

3: MAGNETIC RESONANCE IMAGING (MRI)

5: VEINS

B: IMAGING

New/Revised Text in Green ~~deleted~~ Deleted ♀ Females Only ♂ Males Only **Coding Clinic**
⊘ Non-covered ⊘ Limited Coverage ⊞ Combination (See Appendix E) DRG Non-OR Non-OR ⊘ Hospital-Acquired Condition

SECTION: B IMAGING

BODY SYSTEM: 5 VEINS

TYPE: 4 **ULTRASONOGRAPHY:** Real time display of images of anatomy or flow information developed from the capture of reflected and attenuated high frequency sound waves

Body Part	Contrast	Qualifier	Qualifier
3 Jugular Veins, Right 4 Jugular Veins, Left 6 Subclavian Vein, Right 7 Subclavian Vein, Left 9 Inferior Vena Cava B Lower Extremity Veins, Right C Lower Extremity Veins, Left D Lower Extremity Veins, Bilateral J Renal Vein, Right K Renal Vein, Left L Renal Veins, Bilateral M Upper Extremity Veins, Right N Upper Extremity Veins, Left P Upper Extremity Veins, Bilateral T Portal and Splanchnic Veins	Z None	Z None	3 Intravascular A Guidance Z None

SECTION: B IMAGING
BODY SYSTEM: 7 LYMPHATIC SYSTEM
TYPE: Ø PLAIN RADIOGRAPHY: Planar display of an image developed from the capture of external ionizing radiation on photographic or photoconductive plate

Body Part	Contrast	Qualifier	Qualifier
Ø Abdominal/Retroperitoneal Lymphatics, Unilateral 1 Abdominal/Retroperitoneal Lymphatics, Bilateral 4 Lymphatics, Head and Neck 5 Upper Extremity Lymphatics, Right 6 Upper Extremity Lymphatics, Left 7 Upper Extremity Lymphatics, Bilateral 8 Lower Extremity Lymphatics, Right 9 Lower Extremity Lymphatics, Left B Lower Extremity Lymphatics, Bilateral C Lymphatics, Pelvic	Ø High Osmolar 1 Low Osmolar Y Other Contrast	Z None	Z None

Ø: PLAIN RADIOGRAPHY

7: LYMPHATIC SYSTEM

B: IMAGING

New/Revised Text in Green   deleted Deleted   ♀ Females Only   ♂ Males Only   **Coding Clinic**

Non-covered   Limited Coverage   Combination (See Appendix E)   DRG Non-OR   Non-OR   Hospital-Acquired Condition

SECTION: B IMAGING
BODY SYSTEM: 8 EYE
TYPE: Ø **PLAIN RADIOGRAPHY:** Planar display of an image developed from the capture of external ionizing radiation on photographic or photoconductive plate

Body Part	Contrast	Qualifier	Qualifier
Ø Lacrimal Duct, Right 1 Lacrimal Duct, Left 2 Lacrimal Ducts, Bilateral	Ø High Osmolar 1 Low Osmolar Y Other Contrast	Z None	Z None
3 Optic Foramina, Right 4 Optic Foramina, Left 5 Eye, Right 6 Eye, Left 7 Eyes, Bilateral	Z None	Z None	Z None

SECTION: B IMAGING
BODY SYSTEM: 8 EYE
TYPE: 2 **COMPUTERIZED TOMOGRAPHY (CT SCAN):** Computer reformatted digital display of multiplanar images developed from the capture of multiple exposures of external ionizing radiation

Body Part	Contrast	Qualifier	Qualifier
5 Eye, Right 6 Eye, Left 7 Eyes, Bilateral	Ø High Osmolar 1 Low Osmolar Y Other Contrast	Ø Unenhanced and Enhanced Z None	Z None
5 Eye, Right 6 Eye, Left 7 Eyes, Bilateral	Z None	Z None	Z None

SECTION: B IMAGING

BODY SYSTEM: 8 EYE

TYPE: 3 **MAGNETIC RESONANCE IMAGING (MRI):** Computer reformatted digital display of multiplanar images developed from the capture of radiofrequency signals emitted by nuclei in a body site excited within a magnetic field

Body Part	Contrast	Qualifier	Qualifier
5 Eye, Right 6 Eye, Left 7 Eyes, Bilateral	Y Other Contrast	Ø Unenhanced and Enhanced Z None	Z None
5 Eye, Right 6 Eye, Left 7 Eyes, Bilateral	Z None	Z None	Z None

SECTION: B IMAGING

BODY SYSTEM: 8 EYE

TYPE: 4 **ULTRASONOGRAPHY:** Real time display of images of anatomy or flow information developed from the capture of reflected and attenuated high frequency sound waves

Body Part	Contrast	Qualifier	Qualifier
5 Eye, Right 6 Eye, Left 7 Eyes, Bilateral	Z None	Z None	Z None

SECTION: **B IMAGING**

BODY SYSTEM: 9 **EAR, NOSE, MOUTH, AND THROAT**

TYPE: Ø **PLAIN RADIOGRAPHY:** Planar display of an image developed from the capture of external ionizing radiation on photographic or photoconductive plate

Body Part	Contrast	Qualifier	Qualifier
2 Paranasal Sinuses F Nasopharynx/Oropharynx H Mastoids	Z None	Z None	Z None
4 Parotid Gland, Right 5 Parotid Gland, Left 6 Parotid Glands, Bilateral 7 Submandibular Gland, Right 8 Submandibular Gland, Left 9 Submandibular Glands, Bilateral B Salivary Gland, Right C Salivary Gland, Left D Salivary Glands, Bilateral	Ø High Osmolar 1 Low Osmolar Y Other Contrast	Z None	Z None

SECTION: **B IMAGING**

BODY SYSTEM: 9 **EAR, NOSE, MOUTH, AND THROAT**

TYPE: 1 **FLUOROSCOPY:** Single plane or bi-plane real time display of an image developed from the capture of external ionizing radiation on a fluorescent screen. The image may also be stored by either digital or analog means.

Body Part	Contrast	Qualifier	Qualifier
G Pharynx and Epiglottis J Larynx	Y Other Contrast Z None	Z None	Z None

SECTION: B IMAGING

BODY SYSTEM: 9 EAR, NOSE, MOUTH, AND THROAT

TYPE: 2 **COMPUTERIZED TOMOGRAPHY (CT SCAN):** Computer reformatted digital display of multiplanar images developed from the capture of multiple exposures of external ionizing radiation

Body Part	Contrast	Qualifier	Qualifier
Ø Ear 2 Paranasal Sinuses 6 Parotid Glands, Bilateral 9 Submandibular Glands, Bilateral D Salivary Glands, Bilateral F Nasopharynx/Oropharynx J Larynx	Ø High Osmolar 1 Low Osmolar Y Other Contrast	Ø Unenhanced and Enhanced Z None	Z None
Ø Ear 2 Paranasal Sinuses 6 Parotid Glands, Bilateral 9 Submandibular Glands, Bilateral D Salivary Glands, Bilateral F Nasopharynx/Oropharynx J Larynx	Z None	Z None	Z None

SECTION: B IMAGING

BODY SYSTEM: 9 EAR, NOSE, MOUTH, AND THROAT

TYPE: 3 **MAGNETIC RESONANCE IMAGING (MRI):** Computer reformatted digital display of multiplanar images developed from the capture of radiofrequency signals emitted by nuclei in a body site excited within a magnetic field

Body Part	Contrast	Qualifier	Qualifier
Ø Ear 2 Paranasal Sinuses 6 Parotid Glands, Bilateral 9 Submandibular Glands, Bilateral D Salivary Glands, Bilateral F Nasopharynx/Oropharynx J Larynx	Y Other Contrast	Ø Unenhanced and Enhanced Z None	Z None
Ø Ear 2 Paranasal Sinuses 6 Parotid Glands, Bilateral 9 Submandibular Glands, Bilateral D Salivary Glands, Bilateral F Nasopharynx/Oropharynx J Larynx	Z None	Z None	Z None

2: CT SCAN 3: MRI

9: EAR, NOSE, MOUTH, AND THROAT

B: IMAGING

New/Revised Text in Green ~~deleted~~ Deleted ♀ Females Only ♂ Males Only **Coding Clinic**

 Non-covered   Limited Coverage ⊞ Combination (See Appendix E) DRG Non-OR Non-OR   Hospital-Acquired Condition

SECTION: B IMAGING
BODY SYSTEM: B RESPIRATORY SYSTEM
TYPE: Ø PLAIN RADIOGRAPHY: Planar display of an image developed from the capture of external ionizing radiation on photographic or photoconductive plate

Body Part	Contrast	Qualifier	Qualifier
7 Tracheobronchial Tree, Right 8 Tracheobronchial Tree, Left 9 Tracheobronchial Trees, Bilateral	Y Other Contrast	Z None	Z None
D Upper Airways	Z None	Z None	Z None

SECTION: B IMAGING
BODY SYSTEM: B RESPIRATORY SYSTEM
TYPE: 1 FLUOROSCOPY: Single plane or bi-plane real time display of an image developed from the capture of external ionizing radiation on a fluorescent screen. The image may also be stored by either digital or analog means.

Body Part	Contrast	Qualifier	Qualifier
2 Lung, Right 3 Lung, Left 4 Lungs, Bilateral 6 Diaphragm C Mediastinum D Upper Airways	Z None	Z None	Z None
7 Tracheobronchial Tree, Right 8 Tracheobronchial Tree, Left 9 Tracheobronchial Trees, Bilateral	Y Other Contrast	Z None	Z None

SECTION: B IMAGING
BODY SYSTEM: B RESPIRATORY SYSTEM
TYPE: 2 COMPUTERIZED TOMOGRAPHY (CT SCAN): Computer reformatted digital display of multiplanar images developed from the capture of multiple exposures of external ionizing radiation

Body Part	Contrast	Qualifier	Qualifier
4 Lungs, Bilateral 7 Tracheobronchial Tree, Right 8 Tracheobronchial Tree, Left 9 Tracheobronchial Trees, Bilateral F Trachea/Airways	Ø High Osmolar 1 Low Osmolar Y Other Contrast	Ø Unenhanced and Enhanced Z None	Z None
4 Lungs, Bilateral 7 Tracheobronchial Tree, Right 8 Tracheobronchial Tree, Left 9 Tracheobronchial Trees, Bilateral F Trachea/Airways	Z None	Z None	Z None

New/Revised Text in Green   ~~deleted~~ Deleted   ♀ Females Only   ♂ Males Only   **Coding Clinic**
Non-covered   Limited Coverage   ⊕ Combination (See Appendix E)   DRG Non-OR   Non-OR   Hospital-Acquired Condition

SECTION: B IMAGING

BODY SYSTEM: B RESPIRATORY SYSTEM

TYPE: 3 **MAGNETIC RESONANCE IMAGING (MRI):** Computer reformatted digital display of multiplanar images developed from the capture of radiofrequency signals emitted by nuclei in a body site excited within a magnetic field

Body Part	Contrast	Qualifier	Qualifier
G Lung Apices	Y Other Contrast	Ø Unenhanced and Enhanced Z None	Z None
G Lung Apices	Z None	Z None	Z None

SECTION: B IMAGING

BODY SYSTEM: B RESPIRATORY SYSTEM

TYPE: 4 **ULTRASONOGRAPHY:** Real time display of images of anatomy or flow information developed from the capture of reflected and attenuated high frequency sound waves

Body Part	Contrast	Qualifier	Qualifier
B Pleura C Mediastinum	Z None	Z None	Z None

New/Revised Text in Green   ~~deleted~~ Deleted   ♀ Females Only   ♂ Males Only   **Coding Clinic**

🔊 Non-covered   🔊 Limited Coverage   ⊞ Combination (See Appendix E)   DRG Non-OR   Non-OR   🔊 Hospital-Acquired Condition

SECTION: B IMAGING

BODY SYSTEM: D GASTROINTESTINAL SYSTEM

TYPE: 1 **FLUOROSCOPY:** Single plane or bi-plane real time display of an image developed from the capture of external ionizing radiation on a fluorescent screen. The image may also be stored by either digital or analog means.

Body Part	Contrast	Qualifier	Qualifier
1 Esophagus 2 Stomach 3 Small Bowel 4 Colon 5 Upper GI 6 Upper GI and Small Bowel 9 Duodenum B Mouth/Oropharynx	Y Other Contrast Z None	Z None	Z None

SECTION: B IMAGING

BODY SYSTEM: D GASTROINTESTINAL SYSTEM

TYPE: 2 **COMPUTERIZED TOMOGRAPHY (CT SCAN):** Computer reformatted digital display of multiplanar images developed from the capture of multiple exposures of external ionizing radiation

Body Part	Contrast	Qualifier	Qualifier
4 Colon	Ø High Osmolar 1 Low Osmolar Y Other Contrast	Ø Unenhanced and Enhanced Z None	Z None
4 Colon	Z None	Z None	Z None

SECTION: B IMAGING

BODY SYSTEM: D GASTROINTESTINAL SYSTEM

TYPE: 4 **ULTRASONOGRAPHY:** Real time display of images of anatomy or flow information developed from the capture of reflected and attenuated high frequency sound waves

Body Part	Contrast	Qualifier	Qualifier
1 Esophagus 2 Stomach 7 Gastrointestinal Tract 8 Appendix 9 Duodenum C Rectum	Z None	Z None	Z None

SECTION: B IMAGING

BODY SYSTEM: F HEPATOBILIARY SYSTEM AND PANCREAS

TYPE: 0 **PLAIN RADIOGRAPHY:** Planar display of an image developed from the capture of external ionizing radiation on photographic or photoconductive plate

Body Part	Contrast	Qualifier	Qualifier
0 Bile Ducts 3 Gallbladder and Bile Ducts C Hepatobiliary System, All	0 High Osmolar 1 Low Osmolar Y Other Contrast	Z None	Z None

Non-OR   BF0[3C][01Y]ZZ

SECTION: B IMAGING

BODY SYSTEM: F HEPATOBILIARY SYSTEM AND PANCREAS

TYPE: 1 **FLUOROSCOPY:** Single plane or bi-plane real time display of an image developed from the capture of external ionizing radiation on a fluorescent screen. The image may also be stored by either digital or analog means.

Body Part	Contrast	Qualifier	Qualifier
0 Bile Ducts 1 Biliary and Pancreatic Ducts 2 Gallbladder 3 Gallbladder and Bile Ducts 4 Gallbladder, Bile Ducts, and Pancreatic Ducts 8 Pancreatic Ducts	0 High Osmolar 1 Low Osmolar Y Other Contrast	Z None	Z None

SECTION: B IMAGING

BODY SYSTEM: F HEPATOBILIARY SYSTEM AND PANCREAS

TYPE: 2 **COMPUTERIZED TOMOGRAPHY (CT SCAN):** Computer reformatted digital display of multiplanar images developed from the capture of multiple exposures of external ionizing radiation

Body Part	Contrast	Qualifier	Qualifier
5 Liver 6 Liver and Spleen 7 Pancreas C Hepatobiliary System, All	Ø High Osmolar 1 Low Osmolar Y Other Contrast	Ø Unenhanced and Enhanced Z None	Z None
5 Liver 6 Liver and Spleen 7 Pancreas C Hepatobiliary System, All	Z None	Z None	Z None

SECTION: B IMAGING

BODY SYSTEM: F HEPATOBILIARY SYSTEM AND PANCREAS

TYPE: 3 **MAGNETIC RESONANCE IMAGING (MRI):** Computer reformatted digital display of multiplanar images developed from the capture of radiofrequency signals emitted by nuclei in a body site excited within a magnetic field

Body Part	Contrast	Qualifier	Qualifier
5 Liver 6 Liver and Spleen 7 Pancreas	Y Other Contrast	Ø Unenhanced and Enhanced Z None	Z None
5 Liver 6 Liver and Spleen 7 Pancreas	Z None	Z None	Z None

SECTION: B IMAGING

BODY SYSTEM: F HEPATOBILIARY SYSTEM AND PANCREAS

TYPE: 4 **ULTRASONOGRAPHY:** Real time display of images of anatomy or flow information developed from the capture of reflected and attenuated high frequency sound waves

Body Part	Contrast	Qualifier	Qualifier
Ø Bile Ducts 2 Gallbladder 3 Gallbladder and Bile Ducts 5 Liver 6 Liver and Spleen 7 Pancreas C Hepatobiliary System, All	Z None	Z None	Z None

New/Revised Text in Green   ~~deleted~~ Deleted   ♀ Females Only   ♂ Males Only   **Coding Clinic**

Non-covered   Limited Coverage   ⊕ Combination (See Appendix E)   DRG Non-OR   Non-OR   Hospital-Acquired Condition

SECTION: B IMAGING

BODY SYSTEM: G ENDOCRINE SYSTEM

TYPE: **2 COMPUTERIZED TOMOGRAPHY (CT SCAN):** Computer reformatted digital display of multiplanar images developed from the capture of multiple exposures of external ionizing radiation

Body Part	Contrast	Qualifier	Qualifier
2 Adrenal Glands, Bilateral 3 Parathyroid Glands 4 Thyroid Gland	Ø High Osmolar 1 Low Osmolar Y Other Contrast	Ø Unenhanced and Enhanced Z None	Z None
2 Adrenal Glands, Bilateral 3 Parathyroid Glands 4 Thyroid Gland	Z None	Z None	Z None

SECTION: B IMAGING

BODY SYSTEM: G ENDOCRINE SYSTEM

TYPE: **3 MAGNETIC RESONANCE IMAGING (MRI):** Computer reformatted digital display of multiplanar images developed from the capture of radiofrequency signals emitted by nuclei in a body site excited within a magnetic field

Body Part	Contrast	Qualifier	Qualifier
2 Adrenal Glands, Bilateral 3 Parathyroid Glands 4 Thyroid Gland	Y Other Contrast	Ø Unenhanced and Enhanced Z None	Z None
2 Adrenal Glands, Bilateral 3 Parathyroid Glands 4 Thyroid Gland	Z None	Z None	Z None

SECTION: B IMAGING

BODY SYSTEM: G ENDOCRINE SYSTEM

TYPE: **4 ULTRASONOGRAPHY:** Real time display of images of anatomy or flow information developed from the capture of reflected and attenuated high frequency sound waves

Body Part	Contrast	Qualifier	Qualifier
Ø Adrenal Gland, Right 1 Adrenal Gland, Left 2 Adrenal Glands, Bilateral 3 Parathyroid Glands 4 Thyroid Gland	Z None	Z None	Z None

SECTION: B IMAGING

BODY SYSTEM: H SKIN, SUBCUTANEOUS TISSUE AND BREAST

TYPE: Ø **PLAIN RADIOGRAPHY:** Planar display of an image developed from the capture of external ionizing radiation on photographic or photoconductive plate

Body Part	Contrast	Qualifier	Qualifier
Ø Breast, Right 1 Breast, Left 2 Breasts, Bilateral	Z None	Z None	Z None
3 Single Mammary Duct, Right 4 Single Mammary Duct, Left 5 Multiple Mammary Ducts, Right 6 Multiple Mammary Ducts, Left	Ø High Osmolar 1 Low Osmolar Y Other Contrast Z None	Z None	Z None

SECTION: B IMAGING

BODY SYSTEM: H SKIN, SUBCUTANEOUS TISSUE AND BREAST

TYPE: 3 **MAGNETIC RESONANCE IMAGING (MRI):** Computer reformatted digital display of multiplanar images developed from the capture of radiofrequency signals emitted by nuclei in a body site excited within a magnetic field

Body Part	Contrast	Qualifier	Qualifier
Ø Breast, Right 1 Breast, Left 2 Breasts, Bilateral D Subcutaneous Tissue, Head/Neck F Subcutaneous Tissue, Upper Extremity G Subcutaneous Tissue, Thorax H Subcutaneous Tissue, Abdomen and Pelvis J Subcutaneous Tissue, Lower Extremity	Y Other Contrast	Ø Unenhanced and Enhanced Z None	Z None
Ø Breast, Right 1 Breast, Left 2 Breasts, Bilateral D Subcutaneous Tissue, Head/Neck F Subcutaneous Tissue, Upper Extremity G Subcutaneous Tissue, Thorax H Subcutaneous Tissue, Abdomen and Pelvis J Subcutaneous Tissue, Lower Extremity	Z None	Z None	Z None

SECTION: B IMAGING

BODY SYSTEM: H SKIN, SUBCUTANEOUS TISSUE AND BREAST

TYPE: 4 **ULTRASONOGRAPHY:** Real time display of images of anatomy or flow information developed from the capture of reflected and attenuated high frequency sound waves

Body Part	Contrast	Qualifier	Qualifier
Ø Breast, Right 1 Breast, Left 2 Breasts, Bilateral 7 Extremity, Upper 8 Extremity, Lower 9 Abdominal Wall B Chest Wall C Head and Neck	Z None	Z None	Z None

SECTION: B IMAGING

BODY SYSTEM: L CONNECTIVE TISSUE

TYPE: 3 **MAGNETIC RESONANCE IMAGING (MRI):** Computer reformatted digital display of multiplanar images developed from the capture of radiofrequency signals emitted by nuclei in a body site excited within a magnetic field

Body Part	Contrast	Qualifier	Qualifier
Ø Connective Tissue, Upper Extremity 1 Connective Tissue, Lower Extremity 2 Tendons, Upper Extremity 3 Tendons, Lower Extremity	Y Other Contrast	Ø Unenhanced and Enhanced Z None	Z None
Ø Connective Tissue, Upper Extremity 1 Connective Tissue, Lower Extremity 2 Tendons, Upper Extremity 3 Tendons, Lower Extremity	Z None	Z None	Z None

SECTION: B IMAGING

BODY SYSTEM: L CONNECTIVE TISSUE

TYPE: 4 **ULTRASONOGRAPHY:** Real time display of images of anatomy or flow information developed from the capture of reflected and attenuated high frequency sound waves

Body Part	Contrast	Qualifier	Qualifier
Ø Connective Tissue, Upper Extremity 1 Connective Tissue, Lower Extremity 2 Tendons, Upper Extremity 3 Tendons, Lower Extremity	Z None	Z None	Z None

SECTION: **B IMAGING**

BODY SYSTEM: N SKULL AND FACIAL BONES

TYPE: Ø **PLAIN RADIOGRAPHY:** Planar display of an image developed from the capture of external ionizing radiation on photographic or photoconductive plate

Body Part	Contrast	Qualifier	Qualifier
Ø Skull 1 Orbit, Right 2 Orbit, Left 3 Orbits, Bilateral 4 Nasal Bones 5 Facial Bones 6 Mandible B Zygomatic Arch, Right C Zygomatic Arch, Left D Zygomatic Arches, Bilateral G Tooth, Single H Teeth, Multiple J Teeth, All	Z None	Z None	Z None
7 Temporomandibular Joint, Right 8 Temporomandibular Joint, Left 9 Temporomandibular Joints, Bilateral	Ø High Osmolar 1 Low Osmolar Y Other Contrast Z None	Z None	Z None

SECTION: **B IMAGING**

BODY SYSTEM: N SKULL AND FACIAL BONES

TYPE: 1 **FLUOROSCOPY:** Single plane or bi-plane real time display of an image developed from the capture of external ionizing radiation on a fluorescent screen. The image may also be stored by either digital or analog means.

Body Part	Contrast	Qualifier	Qualifier
7 Temporomandibular Joint, Right 8 Temporomandibular Joint, Left 9 Temporomandibular Joints, Bilateral	Ø High Osmolar 1 Low Osmolar Y Other Contrast Z None	Z None	Z None

Side tab: Ø: PLAIN RADIOGRAPHY   1: FLUOROSCOPY   N: SKULL AND FACIAL BONES   B: IMAGING

SECTION: B IMAGING

BODY SYSTEM: N SKULL AND FACIAL BONES

TYPE: 2 **COMPUTERIZED TOMOGRAPHY (CT SCAN):** Computer reformatted digital display of multiplanar images developed from the capture of multiple exposures of external ionizing radiation

Body Part	Contrast	Qualifier	Qualifier
Ø Skull 3 Orbits, Bilateral 5 Facial Bones 6 Mandible 9 Temporomandibular Joints, Bilateral F Temporal Bones	Ø High Osmolar 1 Low Osmolar Y Other Contrast Z None	Z None	Z None

SECTION: B IMAGING

BODY SYSTEM: N SKULL AND FACIAL BONES

TYPE: 3 **MAGNETIC RESONANCE IMAGING (MRI):** Computer reformatted digital display of multiplanar images developed from the capture of radiofrequency signals emitted by nuclei in a body site excited within a magnetic field

Body Part	Contrast	Qualifier	Qualifier
9 Temporomandibular Joints, Bilateral	Y Other Contrast Z None	Z None	Z None

B: IMAGING   N: SKULL AND FACIAL BONES   2: CT SCAN   3: MRI

SECTION: B IMAGING
BODY SYSTEM: P NON-AXIAL UPPER BONES
TYPE: Ø PLAIN RADIOGRAPHY: Planar display of an image developed from the capture of external ionizing radiation on photographic or photoconductive plate

Body Part	Contrast	Qualifier	Qualifier
Ø Sternoclavicular Joint, Right 1 Sternoclavicular Joint, Left 2 Sternoclavicular Joints, Bilateral 3 Acromioclavicular Joints, Bilateral 4 Clavicle, Right 5 Clavicle, Left 6 Scapula, Right 7 Scapula, Left A Humerus, Right B Humerus, Left E Upper Arm, Right F Upper Arm, Left J Forearm, Right K Forearm, Left N Hand, Right P Hand, Left R Finger(s), Right S Finger(s), Left X Ribs, Right Y Ribs, Left	Z None	Z None	Z None
8 Shoulder, Right 9 Shoulder, Left C Hand/Finger Joint, Right D Hand/Finger Joint, Left G Elbow, Right H Elbow, Left L Wrist, Right M Wrist, Left	Ø High Osmolar 1 Low Osmolar Y Other Contrast Z None	Z None	Z None

SECTION: B IMAGING
BODY SYSTEM: P NON-AXIAL UPPER BONES

TYPE: 1 FLUOROSCOPY: Single plane or bi-plane real time display of an image developed from the capture of external ionizing radiation on a fluorescent screen. The image may also be stored by either digital or analog means.

Body Part	Contrast	Qualifier	Qualifier
0 Sternoclavicular Joint, Right 1 Sternoclavicular Joint, Left 2 Sternoclavicular Joints, Bilateral 3 Acromioclavicular Joints, Bilateral 4 Clavicle, Right 5 Clavicle, Left 6 Scapula, Right 7 Scapula, Left A Humerus, Right B Humerus, Left E Upper Arm, Right F Upper Arm, Left J Forearm, Right K Forearm, Left N Hand, Right P Hand, Left R Finger(s), Right S Finger(s), Left X Ribs, Right Y Ribs, Left	Z None	Z None	Z None
8 Shoulder, Right 9 Shoulder, Left L Wrist, Right M Wrist, Left	0 High Osmolar 1 Low Osmolar Y Other Contrast Z None	Z None	Z None
C Hand/Finger Joint, Right D Hand/Finger Joint, Left G Elbow, Right H Elbow, Left	0 High Osmolar 1 Low Osmolar Y Other Contrast	Z None	Z None

B: IMAGING

P: NON-AXIAL UPPER BONES

1: FLUOROSCOPY

SECTION: B IMAGING

BODY SYSTEM: P NON-AXIAL UPPER BONES

TYPE: 2 **COMPUTERIZED TOMOGRAPHY (CT SCAN):** Computer reformatted digital display of multiplanar images developed from the capture of multiple exposures of external ionizing radiation

Body Part	Contrast	Qualifier	Qualifier
Ø Sternoclavicular Joint, Right 1 Sternoclavicular Joint, Left W Thorax	Ø High Osmolar 1 Low Osmolar Y Other Contrast	Z None	Z None
2 Sternoclavicular Joints, Bilateral 3 Acromioclavicular Joints, Bilateral 4 Clavicle, Right 5 Clavicle, Left 6 Scapula, Right 7 Scapula, Left 8 Shoulder, Right 9 Shoulder, Left A Humerus, Right B Humerus, Left E Upper Arm, Right F Upper Arm, Left G Elbow, Right H Elbow, Left J Forearm, Right K Forearm, Left L Wrist, Right M Wrist, Left N Hand, Right P Hand, Left Q Hands and Wrists, Bilateral R Finger(s), Right S Finger(s), Left T Upper Extremity, Right U Upper Extremity, Left V Upper Extremities, Bilateral X Ribs, Right Y Ribs, Left	Ø High Osmolar 1 Low Osmolar Y Other Contrast Z None	Z None	Z None
C Hand/Finger Joint, Right D Hand/Finger Joint, Left	Z None	Z None	Z None

SECTION: B IMAGING
BODY SYSTEM: P NON-AXIAL UPPER BONES

TYPE: 3 MAGNETIC RESONANCE IMAGING (MRI): Computer reformatted digital display of multiplanar images developed from the capture of radiofrequency signals emitted by nuclei in a body site excited within a magnetic field

Body Part	Contrast	Qualifier	Qualifier
8 Shoulder, Right 9 Shoulder, Left C Hand/Finger Joint, Right D Hand/Finger Joint, Left E Upper Arm, Right F Upper Arm, Left G Elbow, Right H Elbow, Left J Forearm, Right K Forearm, Left L Wrist, Right M Wrist, Left	Y Other Contrast	Ø Unenhanced and Enhanced Z None	Z None
8 Shoulder, Right 9 Shoulder, Left C Hand/Finger Joint, Right D Hand/Finger Joint, Left E Upper Arm, Right F Upper Arm, Left G Elbow, Right H Elbow, Left J Forearm, Right K Forearm, Left L Wrist, Right M Wrist, Left	Z None	Z None	Z None

SECTION: B IMAGING
BODY SYSTEM: P NON-AXIAL UPPER BONES

TYPE: 4 ULTRASONOGRAPHY: Real time display of images of anatomy or flow information developed from the capture of reflected and attenuated high frequency sound waves

Body Part	Contrast	Qualifier	Qualifier
8 Shoulder, Right 9 Shoulder, Left G Elbow, Right H Elbow, Left L Wrist, Right M Wrist, Left N Hand, Right P Hand, Left	Z None	Z None	1 Densitometry Z None

SECTION: B IMAGING

BODY SYSTEM: Q NON-AXIAL LOWER BONES

TYPE: Ø PLAIN RADIOGRAPHY: Planar display of an image developed from the capture of external ionizing radiation on photographic or photoconductive plate

Body Part	Contrast	Qualifier	Qualifier
Ø Hip, Right 1 Hip, Left	Ø High Osmolar 1 Low Osmolar Y Other Contrast	Z None	Z None
Ø Hip, Right 1 Hip, Left	Z None	Z None	1 Densitometry Z None
3 Femur, Right 4 Femur, Left	Z None	Z None	1 Densitometry Z None
7 Knee, Right 8 Knee, Left G Ankle, Right H Ankle, Left	Ø High Osmolar 1 Low Osmolar Y Other Contrast Z None	Z None	Z None
D Lower Leg, Right F Lower Leg, Left J Calcaneus, Right K Calcaneus, Left L Foot, Right M Foot, Left P Toe(s), Right Q Toe(s), Left V Patella, Right W Patella, Left	Z None	Z None	Z None
X Foot/Toe Joint, Right Y Foot/Toe Joint, Left	Ø High Osmolar 1 Low Osmolar Y Other Contrast	Z None	Z None

Ø: PLAIN RADIOGRAPHY

Q: NON-AXIAL LOWER BONES

B: IMAGING

SECTION: B IMAGING

BODY SYSTEM: Q NON-AXIAL LOWER BONES

TYPE: 1 **FLUOROSCOPY:** Single plane or bi-plane real time display of an image developed from the capture of external ionizing radiation on a fluorescent screen. The image may also be stored by either digital or analog means.

Body Part	Contrast	Qualifier	Qualifier
Ø Hip, Right 1 Hip, Left 7 Knee, Right 8 Knee, Left G Ankle, Right H Ankle, Left X Foot/Toe Joint, Right Y Foot/Toe Joint, Left	Ø High Osmolar 1 Low Osmolar Y Other Contrast Z None	Z None	Z None
3 Femur, Right 4 Femur, Left D Lower Leg, Right F Lower Leg, Left J Calcaneus, Right K Calcaneus, Left L Foot, Right M Foot, Left P Toe(s), Right Q Toe(s), Left V Patella, Right W Patella, Left	Z None	Z None	Z None

SECTION: B IMAGING

BODY SYSTEM: Q NON-AXIAL LOWER BONES

TYPE: 2 COMPUTERIZED TOMOGRAPHY (CT SCAN): Computer reformatted digital display of multiplanar images developed from the capture of multiple exposures of external ionizing radiation

Body Part	Contrast	Qualifier	Qualifier
Ø Hip, Right 1 Hip, Left 3 Femur, Right 4 Femur, Left 7 Knee, Right 8 Knee, Left D Lower Leg, Right F Lower Leg, Left G Ankle, Right H Ankle, Left J Calcaneus, Right K Calcaneus, Left L Foot, Right M Foot, Left P Toe(s), Right Q Toe(s), Left R Lower Extremity, Right S Lower Extremity, Left V Patella, Right W Patella, Left X Foot/Toe Joint, Right Y Foot/Toe Joint, Left	Ø High Osmolar 1 Low Osmolar Y Other Contrast Z None	Z None	Z None
B Tibia/Fibula, Right C Tibia/Fibula, Left	Ø High Osmolar 1 Low Osmolar Y Other Contrast	Z None	Z None

SECTION: B IMAGING

BODY SYSTEM: Q NON-AXIAL LOWER BONES

TYPE: 3 **MAGNETIC RESONANCE IMAGING (MRI):** Computer reformatted digital display of multiplanar images developed from the capture of radiofrequency signals emitted by nuclei in a body site excited within a magnetic field

Body Part	Contrast	Qualifier	Qualifier
Ø Hip, Right 1 Hip, Left 3 Femur, Right 4 Femur, Left 7 Knee, Right 8 Knee, Left D Lower Leg, Right F Lower Leg, Left G Ankle, Right H Ankle, Left J Calcaneus, Right K Calcaneus, Left L Foot, Right M Foot, Left P Toe(s), Right Q Toe(s), Left V Patella, Right W Patella, Left	Y Other Contrast	Ø Unenhanced and Enhanced Z None	Z None
Ø Hip, Right 1 Hip, Left 3 Femur, Right 4 Femur, Left 7 Knee, Right 8 Knee, Left D Lower Leg, Right F Lower Leg, Left G Ankle, Right H Ankle, Left J Calcaneus, Right K Calcaneus, Left L Foot, Right M Foot, Left P Toe(s), Right Q Toe(s), Left V Patella, Right W Patella, Left	Z None	Z None	Z None

SECTION: B IMAGING
BODY SYSTEM: Q NON-AXIAL LOWER BONES
TYPE: 4 **ULTRASONOGRAPHY:** Real time display of images of anatomy or flow information developed from the capture of reflected and attenuated high frequency sound waves

Body Part	Contrast	Qualifier	Qualifier
Ø Hip, Right 1 Hip, Left 2 Hips, Bilateral 7 Knee, Right 8 Knee, Left 9 Knees, Bilateral	Z None	Z None	Z None

SECTION: B IMAGING

BODY SYSTEM: R AXIAL SKELETON, EXCEPT SKULL AND FACIAL BONES

TYPE: Ø **PLAIN RADIOGRAPHY:** Planar display of an image developed from the capture of external ionizing radiation on photographic or photoconductive plate

Body Part	Contrast	Qualifier	Qualifier
Ø Cervical Spine 7 Thoracic Spine 9 Lumbar Spine G Whole Spine	Z None	Z None	1 Densitometry Z None
1 Cervical Disc(s) 2 Thoracic Disc(s) 3 Lumbar Disc(s) 4 Cervical Facet Joint(s) 5 Thoracic Facet Joint(s) 6 Lumbar Facet Joint(s) D Sacroiliac Joints	Ø High Osmolar 1 Low Osmolar Y Other Contrast Z None	Z None	Z None
8 Thoracolumbar Joint B Lumbosacral Joint C Pelvis F Sacrum and Coccyx H Sternum	Z None	Z None	Z None

SECTION: B IMAGING

BODY SYSTEM: R AXIAL SKELETON, EXCEPT SKULL AND FACIAL BONES

TYPE: 1 **FLUOROSCOPY:** Single plane or bi-plane real time display of an image developed from the capture of external ionizing radiation on a fluorescent screen. The image may also be stored by either digital or analog means.

Body Part	Contrast	Qualifier	Qualifier
Ø Cervical Spine 1 Cervical Disc(s) 2 Thoracic Disc(s) 3 Lumbar Disc(s) 4 Cervical Facet Joint(s) 5 Thoracic Facet Joint(s) 6 Lumbar Facet Joint(s) 7 Thoracic Spine 8 Thoracolumbar Joint 9 Lumbar Spine B Lumbosacral Joint C Pelvis D Sacroiliac Joints F Sacrum and Coccyx G Whole Spine H Sternum	Ø High Osmolar 1 Low Osmolar Y Other Contrast Z None	Z None	Z None

SECTION: **B IMAGING**

BODY SYSTEM: R AXIAL SKELETON, EXCEPT SKULL AND FACIAL BONES

TYPE: 2 **COMPUTERIZED TOMOGRAPHY (CT SCAN):** Computer reformatted digital display of multiplanar images developed from the capture of multiple exposures of external ionizing radiation

Body Part	Contrast	Qualifier	Qualifier
Ø Cervical Spine 7 Thoracic Spine 9 Lumbar Spine C Pelvis D Sacroiliac Joints F Sacrum and Coccyx	Ø High Osmolar 1 Low Osmolar Y Other Contrast Z None	Z None	Z None

SECTION: **B IMAGING**

BODY SYSTEM: R AXIAL SKELETON, EXCEPT SKULL AND FACIAL BONES

TYPE: 3 **MAGNETIC RESONANCE IMAGING (MRI):** Computer reformatted digital display of multiplanar images developed from the capture of radiofrequency signals emitted by nuclei in a body site excited within a magnetic field

Body Part	Contrast	Qualifier	Qualifier
Ø Cervical Spine 1 Cervical Disc(s) 2 Thoracic Disc(s) 3 Lumbar Disc(s) 7 Thoracic Spine 9 Lumbar Spine C Pelvis F Sacrum and Coccyx	Y Other Contrast	Ø Unenhanced and Enhanced Z None	Z None
Ø Cervical Spine 1 Cervical Disc(s) 2 Thoracic Disc(s) 3 Lumbar Disc(s) 7 Thoracic Spine 9 Lumbar Spine C Pelvis F Sacrum and Coccyx	Z None	Z None	Z None

SECTION: **B IMAGING**

BODY SYSTEM: R AXIAL SKELETON, EXCEPT SKULL AND FACIAL BONES

TYPE: 4 **ULTRASONOGRAPHY:** Real time display of images of anatomy or flow information developed from the capture of reflected and attenuated high frequency sound waves

Body Part	Contrast	Qualifier	Qualifier
Ø Cervical Spine 7 Thoracic Spine 9 Lumbar Spine F Sacrum and Coccyx	Z None	Z None	Z None

New/Revised Text in Green   ~~deleted~~ Deleted   ♀ Females Only   ♂ Males Only   **Coding Clinic**

🐾 Non-covered   🐾 Limited Coverage   ⊡ Combination (See Appendix E)   DRG Non-OR   Non-OR   🐾 Hospital-Acquired Condition

SECTION: B IMAGING
BODY SYSTEM: T URINARY SYSTEM
TYPE: Ø **PLAIN RADIOGRAPHY:** Planar display of an image developed from the capture of external ionizing radiation on photographic or photoconductive plate

Body Part	Contrast	Qualifier	Qualifier
Ø Bladder	Ø High Osmolar	Z None	Z None
1 Kidney, Right	1 Low Osmolar		
2 Kidney, Left	Y Other Contrast		
3 Kidneys, Bilateral	Z None		
4 Kidneys, Ureters, and Bladder			
5 Urethra			
6 Ureter, Right			
7 Ureter, Left			
8 Ureters, Bilateral			
B Bladder and Urethra			
C Ileal Diversion Loop			

SECTION: B IMAGING
BODY SYSTEM: T URINARY SYSTEM
TYPE: 1 **FLUOROSCOPY:** Single plane or bi-plane real time display of an image developed from the capture of external ionizing radiation on a fluorescent screen. The image may also be stored by either digital or analog means.

Body Part	Contrast	Qualifier	Qualifier
Ø Bladder	Ø High Osmolar	Z None	Z None
1 Kidney, Right	1 Low Osmolar		
2 Kidney, Left	Y Other Contrast		
3 Kidneys, Bilateral	Z None		
4 Kidneys, Ureters, and Bladder			
5 Urethra			
6 Ureter, Right			
7 Ureter, Left			
B Bladder and Urethra			
C Ileal Diversion Loop			
D Kidney, Ureter, and Bladder, Right			
F Kidney, Ureter, and Bladder, Left			
G Ileal Loop, Ureters, and Kidneys			

B: IMAGING

T: URINARY SYSTEM

Ø: PLAIN RADIOGRAPHY   1: FLUOROSCOPY

New/Revised Text in Green   ~~deleted~~ Deleted   ♀ Females Only   ♂ Males Only   **Coding Clinic**
🚫 Non-covered   🚫 Limited Coverage   ⊞ Combination (See Appendix E)   DRG Non-OR   Non-OR   🚫 Hospital-Acquired Condition

631

SECTION: B IMAGING

BODY SYSTEM: T URINARY SYSTEM

TYPE: 2 **COMPUTERIZED TOMOGRAPHY (CT SCAN):** Computer reformatted digital display of multiplanar images developed from the capture of multiple exposures of external ionizing radiation

Body Part	Contrast	Qualifier	Qualifier
Ø Bladder 1 Kidney, Right 2 Kidney, Left 3 Kidneys, Bilateral 9 Kidney Transplant	Ø High Osmolar 1 Low Osmolar Y Other Contrast	Ø Unenhanced and Enhanced Z None	Z None
Ø Bladder 1 Kidney, Right 2 Kidney, Left 3 Kidneys, Bilateral 9 Kidney Transplant	Z None	Z None	Z None

SECTION: B IMAGING

BODY SYSTEM: T URINARY SYSTEM

TYPE: 3 **MAGNETIC RESONANCE IMAGING (MRI):** Computer reformatted digital display of multiplanar images developed from the capture of radiofrequency signals emitted by nuclei in a body site excited within a magnetic field

Body Part	Contrast	Qualifier	Qualifier
Ø Bladder 1 Kidney, Right 2 Kidney, Left 3 Kidneys, Bilateral 9 Kidney Transplant	Y Other Contrast	Ø Unenhanced and Enhanced Z None	Z None
Ø Bladder 1 Kidney, Right 2 Kidney, Left 3 Kidneys, Bilateral 9 Kidney Transplant	Z None	Z None	Z None

2:CT SCAN 3:MRI

T: URINARY SYSTEM

B: IMAGING

New/Revised Text in Green ~~deleted~~ Deleted ♀ Females Only ♂ Males Only **Coding Clinic**

🞠 Non-covered 🞠 Limited Coverage ⊡ Combination (See Appendix E) DRG Non-OR Non-OR 🞠 Hospital-Acquired Condition

SECTION: B IMAGING

BODY SYSTEM: T URINARY SYSTEM

TYPE: 4 **ULTRASONOGRAPHY:** Real time display of images of anatomy or flow information developed from the capture of reflected and attenuated high frequency sound waves

Body Part	Contrast	Qualifier	Qualifier
Ø Bladder 1 Kidney, Right 2 Kidney, Left 3 Kidneys, Bilateral 5 Urethra 6 Ureter, Right 7 Ureter, Left 8 Ureters, Bilateral 9 Kidney Transplant J Kidneys and Bladder	Z None	Z None	Z None

B: IMAGING

T: URINARY SYSTEM

4: ULTRASONOGRAPHY

SECTION: B IMAGING

BODY SYSTEM: U FEMALE REPRODUCTIVE SYSTEM

TYPE: Ø PLAIN RADIOGRAPHY: Planar display of an image developed from the capture of external ionizing radiation on photographic or photoconductive plate

Body Part	Contrast	Qualifier	Qualifier
Ø Fallopian Tube, Right ♀ 1 Fallopian Tube, Left ♀ 2 Fallopian Tubes, Bilateral ♀ 6 Uterus ♀ 8 Uterus and Fallopian Tubes ♀ 9 Vagina ♀	Ø High Osmolar 1 Low Osmolar Y Other Contrast	Z None	Z None

SECTION: B IMAGING

BODY SYSTEM: U FEMALE REPRODUCTIVE SYSTEM

TYPE: 1 FLUOROSCOPY: Single plane or bi-plane real time display of an image developed from the capture of external ionizing radiation on a fluorescent screen. The image may also be stored by either digital or analog means.

Body Part	Contrast	Qualifier	Qualifier
Ø Fallopian Tube, Right ♀ 1 Fallopian Tube, Left ♀ 2 Fallopian Tubes, Bilateral ♀ 6 Uterus ♀ 8 Uterus and Fallopian Tubes ♀ 9 Vagina ♀	Ø High Osmolar 1 Low Osmolar Y Other Contrast Z None	Z None	Z None

SECTION:　B IMAGING

BODY SYSTEM: U　FEMALE REPRODUCTIVE SYSTEM

TYPE:　　　　3　**MAGNETIC RESONANCE IMAGING (MRI):** Computer reformatted digital display of multiplanar images developed from the capture of radiofrequency signals emitted by nuclei in a body site excited within a magnetic field

Body Part	Contrast	Qualifier	Qualifier
3　Ovary, Right ♀ 4　Ovary, Left ♀ 5　Ovaries, Bilateral ♀ 6　Uterus ♀ 9　Vagina ♀ B　Pregnant Uterus ♀ C　Uterus and Ovaries ♀	Y　Other Contrast	Ø　Unenhanced and Enhanced Z　None	Z　None
3　Ovary, Right ♀ 4　Ovary, Left ♀ 5　Ovaries, Bilateral ♀ 6　Uterus ♀ 9　Vagina ♀ B　Pregnant Uterus ♀ C　Uterus and Ovaries ♀	Z　None	Z　None	Z　None

SECTION:　B IMAGING

BODY SYSTEM: U　FEMALE REPRODUCTIVE SYSTEM

TYPE:　　　　4　**ULTRASONOGRAPHY:** Real time display of images of anatomy or flow information developed from the capture of reflected and attenuated high frequency sound waves

Body Part	Contrast	Qualifier	Qualifier
Ø　Fallopian Tube, Right ♀ 1　Fallopian Tube, Left ♀ 2　Fallopian Tubes, Bilateral ♀ 3　Ovary, Right ♀ 4　Ovary, Left ♀ 5　Ovaries, Bilateral ♀ 6　Uterus ♀ C　Uterus and Ovaries ♀	Y　Other Contrast Z　None	Z　None	Z　None

SECTION: **B IMAGING**
BODY SYSTEM: V MALE REPRODUCTIVE SYSTEM
TYPE: Ø **PLAIN RADIOGRAPHY:** Planar display of an image developed from the capture of external ionizing radiation on photographic or photoconductive plate

Body Part	Contrast	Qualifier	Qualifier
Ø Corpora Cavernosa ♂ 1 Epididymis, Right ♂ 2 Epididymis, Left ♂ 3 Prostate ♂ 5 Testicle, Right ♂ 6 Testicle, Left ♂ 8 Vasa Vasorum ♂	Ø High Osmolar 1 Low Osmolar Y Other Contrast	Z None	Z None

SECTION: **B IMAGING**
BODY SYSTEM: V MALE REPRODUCTIVE SYSTEM
TYPE: 1 **FLUOROSCOPY:** Single plane or bi-plane real time display of an image developed from the capture of external ionizing radiation on a fluorescent screen. The image may also be stored by either digital or analog means.

Body Part	Contrast	Qualifier	Qualifier
Ø Corpora Cavernosa ♂ 8 Vasa Vasorum ♂	Ø High Osmolar 1 Low Osmolar Y Other Contrast Z None	Z None	Z None

Ø: PLAIN RADIOGRAPHY   1: FLUOROSCOPY
V: MALE REPRODUCTIVE SYSTEM
B: IMAGING

SECTION: B IMAGING

BODY SYSTEM: V MALE REPRODUCTIVE SYSTEM

TYPE: 2 **COMPUTERIZED TOMOGRAPHY (CT SCAN):** Computer reformatted digital display of multiplanar images developed from the capture of multiple exposures of external ionizing radiation

Body Part	Contrast	Qualifier	Qualifier
3 Prostate ♂	Ø High Osmolar 1 Low Osmolar Y Other Contrast	Ø Unenhanced and Enhanced Z None	Z None
3 Prostate ♂	Z None	Z None	Z None

SECTION: B IMAGING

BODY SYSTEM: V MALE REPRODUCTIVE SYSTEM

TYPE: 3 **MAGNETIC RESONANCE IMAGING (MRI):** Computer reformatted digital display of multiplanar images developed from the capture of radiofrequency signals emitted by nuclei in a body site excited within a magnetic field

Body Part	Contrast	Qualifier	Qualifier
Ø Corpora Cavernosa ♂ 3 Prostate ♂ 4 Scrotum ♂ 5 Testicle, Right ♂ 6 Testicle, Left ♂ 7 Testicles, Bilateral ♂	Y Other Contrast	Ø Unenhanced and Enhanced Z None	Z None
Ø Corpora Cavernosa ♂ 3 Prostate ♂ 4 Scrotum ♂ 5 Testicle, Right ♂ 6 Testicle, Left ♂ 7 Testicles, Bilateral ♂	Z None	Z None	Z None

SECTION: B IMAGING

BODY SYSTEM: V MALE REPRODUCTIVE SYSTEM

TYPE: 4 **ULTRASONOGRAPHY:** Real time display of images of anatomy or flow information developed from the capture of reflected and attenuated high frequency sound waves

Body Part	Contrast	Qualifier	Qualifier
4 Scrotum ♂ 9 Prostate and Seminal Vesicles ♂ B Penis ♂	Z None	Z None	Z None

0: PLAIN RADIOGRAPHY   1: FLUOROSCOPY   2: CT SCAN

W: ANATOMICAL REGIONS

B: IMAGING

SECTION: B IMAGING
BODY SYSTEM: W ANATOMICAL REGIONS
TYPE: 0 PLAIN RADIOGRAPHY: Planar display of an image developed from the capture of external ionizing radiation on photographic or photoconductive plate

Body Part	Contrast	Qualifier	Qualifier
0 Abdomen 1 Abdomen and Pelvis 3 Chest B Long Bones, All C Lower Extremity J Upper Extremity K Whole Body L Whole Skeleton M Whole Body, Infant	Z None	Z None	Z None

SECTION: B IMAGING
BODY SYSTEM: W ANATOMICAL REGIONS
TYPE: 1 FLUOROSCOPY: Single plane or bi-plane real time display of an image developed from the capture of external ionizing radiation on a fluorescent screen. The image may also be stored by either digital or analog means.

Body Part	Contrast	Qualifier	Qualifier
1 Abdomen and Pelvis 9 Head and Neck C Lower Extremity J Upper Extremity	0 High Osmolar 1 Low Osmolar Y Other Contrast Z None	Z None	Z None

SECTION: B IMAGING
BODY SYSTEM: W ANATOMICAL REGIONS
TYPE: 2 COMPUTERIZED TOMOGRAPHY (CT SCAN): Computer reformatted digital display of multiplanar images developed from the capture of multiple exposures of external ionizing radiation

Body Part	Contrast	Qualifier	Qualifier
0 Abdomen 1 Abdomen and Pelvis 4 Chest and Abdomen 5 Chest, Abdomen, and Pelvis 8 Head 9 Head and Neck F Neck G Pelvic Region	0 High Osmolar 1 Low Osmolar Y Other Contrast	0 Unenhanced and Enhanced Z None	Z None
0 Abdomen 1 Abdomen and Pelvis 4 Chest and Abdomen 5 Chest, Abdomen, and Pelvis 8 Head 9 Head and Neck F Neck G Pelvic Region	Z None	Z None	Z None

SECTION: B IMAGING

BODY SYSTEM: W ANATOMICAL REGIONS

TYPE: 3 **MAGNETIC RESONANCE IMAGING (MRI):** Computer reformatted digital display of multiplanar images developed from the capture of radiofrequency signals emitted by nuclei in a body site excited within a magnetic field

Body Part	Contrast	Qualifier	Qualifier
Ø Abdomen 8 Head F Neck G Pelvic Region H Retroperitoneum P Brachial Plexus	Y Other Contrast	Ø Unenhanced and Enhanced Z None	Z None
Ø Abdomen 8 Head F Neck G Pelvic Region H Retroperitoneum P Brachial Plexus	Z None	Z None	Z None
3 Chest	Y Other Contrast	Ø Unenhanced and Enhanced Z None	Z None

SECTION: B IMAGING

BODY SYSTEM: W ANATOMICAL REGIONS

TYPE: 4 **ULTRASONOGRAPHY:** Real time display of images of anatomy or flow information developed from the capture of reflected and attenuated high frequency sound waves

Body Part	Contrast	Qualifier	Qualifier
Ø Abdomen 1 Abdomen and Pelvis F Neck G Pelvic Region	Z None	Z None	Z None

SECTION:　B IMAGING

BODY SYSTEM: Y　FETUS AND OBSTETRICAL

TYPE:　　　　　　3　**MAGNETIC RESONANCE IMAGING (MRI):** Computer reformatted digital display of multiplanar images developed from the capture of radiofrequency signals emitted by nuclei in a body site excited within a magnetic field

Body Part	Contrast	Qualifier	Qualifier
Ø Fetal Head ♀ 1 Fetal Heart ♀ 2 Fetal Thorax ♀ 3 Fetal Abdomen ♀ 4 Fetal Spine ♀ 5 Fetal Extremities ♀ 6 Whole Fetus ♀	Y Other Contrast	Ø Unenhanced and Enhanced Z None	Z None
Ø Fetal Head ♀ 1 Fetal Heart ♀ 2 Fetal Thorax ♀ 3 Fetal Abdomen ♀ 4 Fetal Spine ♀ 5 Fetal Extremities ♀ 6 Whole Fetus ♀	Z None	Z None	Z None

SECTION:　B IMAGING

BODY SYSTEM: Y　FETUS AND OBSTETRICAL

TYPE:　　　　　　4　**ULTRASONOGRAPHY:** Real time display of images of anatomy or flow information developed from the capture of reflected and attenuated high frequency sound waves

Body Part	Contrast	Qualifier	Qualifier
7 Fetal Umbilical Cord ♀ 8 Placenta ♀ 9 First Trimester, Single Fetus ♀ B First Trimester, Multiple Gestation ♀ C Second Trimester, Single Fetus ♀ D Second Trimester, Multiple Gestation ♀ F Third Trimester, Single Fetus ♀ G Third Trimester, Multiple Gestation ♀	Z None	Z None	Z None

0: CENTRAL NERVOUS SYSTEM

C: NUCLEAR MEDICINE

1; 2

SECTION: C NUCLEAR MEDICINE

BODY SYSTEM: Ø CENTRAL NERVOUS SYSTEM

TYPE: 1 **PLANAR NUCLEAR MEDICINE IMAGING:** Introduction of radioactive materials into the body for single plane display of images developed from the capture of radioactive emissions

Body Part	Radionuclide	Qualifier	Qualifier
Ø Brain	1 Technetium 99m (Tc-99m) Y Other Radionuclide	Z None	Z None
5 Cerebrospinal Fluid	D Indium 111 (In-111) Y Other Radionuclide	Z None	Z None
Y Central Nervous System	Y Other Radionuclide	Z None	Z None

SECTION: C NUCLEAR MEDICINE

BODY SYSTEM: Ø CENTRAL NERVOUS SYSTEM

TYPE: 2 **TOMOGRAPHIC (TOMO) NUCLEAR MEDICINE IMAGING:** Introduction of radioactive materials into the body for three dimensional display of images developed from the capture of radioactive emissions

Body Part	Radionuclide	Qualifier	Qualifier
Ø Brain	1 Technetium 99m (Tc-99m) F Iodine 123 (I-123) S Thallium 201 (Tl-201) Y Other Radionuclide	Z None	Z None
5 Cerebrospinal Fluid	D Indium 111 (In-111) Y Other Radionuclide	Z None	Z None
Y Central Nervous System	Y Other Radionuclide	Z None	Z None

SECTION: C NUCLEAR MEDICINE

BODY SYSTEM: Ø   CENTRAL NERVOUS SYSTEM

TYPE: **3 POSITRON EMISSION TOMOGRAPHIC (PET) IMAGING:** Introduction of radioactive materials into the body for three dimensional display of images developed from the simultaneous capture, 18Ø degrees apart, of radioactive emissions

Body Part	Radionuclide	Qualifier	Qualifier
Ø Brain	B Carbon 11 (C-11) K Fluorine 18 (F-18) M Oxygen 15 (O-15) Y Other Radionuclide	Z None	Z None
Y Central Nervous System	Y Other Radionuclide	Z None	Z None

SECTION: C NUCLEAR MEDICINE

BODY SYSTEM: Ø   CENTRAL NERVOUS SYSTEM

TYPE: **5 NONIMAGING NUCLEAR MEDICINE PROBE:** Introduction of radioactive materials into the body for the study of distribution and fate of certain substances by the detection of radioactive emissions; or, alternatively, measurement of absorption of radioactive emissions from an external source

Body Part	Radionuclide	Qualifier	Qualifier
Ø Brain	V Xenon 133 (Xe-133) Y Other Radionuclide	Z None	Z None
Y Central Nervous System	Y Other Radionuclide	Z None	Z None

SECTION: C NUCLEAR MEDICINE
BODY SYSTEM: 2 HEART
TYPE: **1 PLANAR NUCLEAR MEDICINE IMAGING:** Introduction of radioactive materials into the body for single plane display of images developed from the capture of radioactive emissions

Body Part	Radionuclide	Qualifier	Qualifier
6 Heart, Right and Left	1 Technetium 99m (Tc-99m) Y Other Radionuclide	Z None	Z None
G Myocardium	1 Technetium 99m (Tc-99m) D Indium 111 (In-111) S Thallium 201 (Tl-201) Y Other Radionuclide Z None	Z None	Z None
Y Heart	Y Other Radionuclide	Z None	Z None

SECTION: C NUCLEAR MEDICINE
BODY SYSTEM: 2 HEART
TYPE: **2 TOMOGRAPHIC (TOMO) NUCLEAR MEDICINE IMAGING:** Introduction of radioactive materials into the body for three dimensional display of images developed from the capture of radioactive emissions

Body Part	Radionuclide	Qualifier	Qualifier
6 Heart, Right and Left	1 Technetium 99m (Tc-99m) Y Other Radionuclide	Z None	Z None
G Myocardium	1 Technetium 99m (Tc-99m) D Indium 111 (In-111) K Fluorine 18 (F-18) S Thallium 201 (Tl-201) Y Other Radionuclide Z None	Z None	Z None
Y Heart	Y Other Radionuclide	Z None	Z None

1; 2

2: HEART

C: NUCLEAR MEDICINE

New/Revised Text in Green   ~~deleted~~ Deleted   ♀ Females Only   ♂ Males Only   **Coding Clinic**
   Non-covered   Limited Coverage   ⊞ Combination (See Appendix E)   DRG Non-OR   Non-OR   Hospital-Acquired Condition

SECTION: C NUCLEAR MEDICINE

BODY SYSTEM: 2 HEART

TYPE: 3 **POSITRON EMISSION TOMOGRAPHIC (PET) IMAGING:** Introduction of radioactive materials into the body for three dimensional display of images developed from the simultaneous capture, 18Ø degrees apart, of radioactive emissions

Body Part	Radionuclide	Qualifier	Qualifier
G Myocardium	K Fluorine 18 (F-18) M Oxygen 15 (O-15) Q Rubidium 82 (Rb-82) R Nitrogen 13 (N-13) Y Other Radionuclide	Z None	Z None
Y Heart	Y Other Radionuclide	Z None	Z None

SECTION: C NUCLEAR MEDICINE

BODY SYSTEM: 2 HEART

TYPE: 5 **NONIMAGING NUCLEAR MEDICINE PROBE:** Introduction of radioactive materials into the body for the study of distribution and fate of certain substances by the detection of radioactive emissions; or, alternatively, measurement of absorption of radioactive emissions from an external source

Body Part	Radionuclide	Qualifier	Qualifier
6 Heart, Right and Left	1 Technetium 99m (Tc-99m) Y Other Radionuclide	Z None	Z None
Y Heart	Y Other Radionuclide	Z None	Z None

C: NUCLEAR MEDICINE   2: HEART   3; 5

SECTION: C NUCLEAR MEDICINE
BODY SYSTEM: 5   VEINS

TYPE: 1   **PLANAR NUCLEAR MEDICINE IMAGING:** Introduction of radioactive materials into the body for single plane display of images developed from the capture of radioactive emissions

Body Part	Radionuclide	Qualifier	Qualifier
B Lower Extremity Veins, Right C Lower Extremity Veins, Left D Lower Extremity Veins, Bilateral N Upper Extremity Veins, Right P Upper Extremity Veins, Left Q Upper Extremity Veins, Bilateral R Central Veins	1 Technetium 99m (Tc-99m) Y Other Radionuclide	Z None	Z None
Y Veins	Y Other Radionuclide	Z None	Z None

New/Revised Text in Green   ~~deleted~~ Deleted   ♀ Females Only   ♂ Males Only   **Coding Clinic**

🚫 Non-covered   🚫 Limited Coverage   ⊞ Combination (See Appendix E)   DRG Non-OR   Non-OR   🚫 Hospital-Acquired Condition

SECTION: C NUCLEAR MEDICINE

BODY SYSTEM: 7 LYMPHATIC AND HEMATOLOGIC SYSTEM

TYPE: 1 **PLANAR NUCLEAR MEDICINE IMAGING:** Introduction of radioactive materials into the body for single plane display of images developed from the capture of radioactive emissions

Body Part	Radionuclide	Qualifier	Qualifier
Ø Bone Marrow	1 Technetium 99m (Tc-99m) D Indium 111 (In-111) Y Other Radionuclide	Z None	Z None
2 Spleen 5 Lymphatics, Head and Neck D Lymphatics, Pelvic J Lymphatics, Head K Lymphatics, Neck L Lymphatics, Upper Chest M Lymphatics, Trunk N Lymphatics, Upper Extremity P Lymphatics, Lower Extremity	1 Technetium 99m (Tc-99m) Y Other Radionuclide	Z None	Z None
3 Blood	D Indium 111 (In-111) Y Other Radionuclide	Z None	Z None
Y Lymphatic and Hematologic System	Y Other Radionuclide	Z None	Z None

SECTION: C NUCLEAR MEDICINE

BODY SYSTEM: 7 LYMPHATIC AND HEMATOLOGIC SYSTEM

TYPE: 2 **TOMOGRAPHIC (TOMO) NUCLEAR MEDICINE IMAGING:** Introduction of radioactive materials into the body for three dimensional display of images developed from the capture of radioactive emissions

Body Part	Radionuclide	Qualifier	Qualifier
2 Spleen	1 Technetium 99m (Tc-99m) Y Other Radionuclide	Z None	Z None
Y Lymphatic and Hematologic System	Y Other Radionuclide	Z None	Z None

SECTION: C NUCLEAR MEDICINE

BODY SYSTEM: 7 LYMPHATIC AND HEMATOLOGIC SYSTEM

TYPE: 5 **NONIMAGING NUCLEAR MEDICINE PROBE:** Introduction of radioactive materials into the body for the study of distribution and fate of certain substances by the detection of radioactive emissions; or, alternatively, measurement of absorption of radioactive emissions from an external source

Body Part	Radionuclide	Qualifier	Qualifier
5 Lymphatics, Head and Neck D Lymphatics, Pelvic J Lymphatics, Head K Lymphatics, Neck L Lymphatics, Upper Chest M Lymphatics, Trunk N Lymphatics, Upper Extremity P Lymphatics, Lower Extremity	1 Technetium 99m (Tc-99m) Y Other Radionuclide	Z None	Z None
Y Lymphatic and Hematologic System	Y Other Radionuclide	Z None	Z None

SECTION: C NUCLEAR MEDICINE

BODY SYSTEM: 7 LYMPHATIC AND HEMATOLOGIC SYSTEM

TYPE: 6 **NONIMAGING NUCLEAR MEDICINE ASSAY:** Introduction of radioactive materials into the body for the study of body fluids and blood elements, by the detection of radioactive emissions

Body Part	Radionuclide	Qualifier	Qualifier
3 Blood	1 Technetium 99m (Tc-99m) 7 Cobalt 58 (Co-58) C Cobalt 57 (Co-57) D Indium 111 (In-111) H Iodine 125 (I-125) W Chromium (Cr-51) Y Other Radionuclide	Z None	Z None
Y Lymphatic and Hematologic System	Y Other Radionuclide	Z None	Z None

5; 6

7: LYMPHATIC AND HEMATOLOGIC SYSTEM

C: NUCLEAR MEDICINE

SECTION: C NUCLEAR MEDICINE
BODY SYSTEM: 8 EYE
TYPE: 1 PLANAR NUCLEAR MEDICINE IMAGING: Introduction of radioactive materials into the body for single plane display of images developed from the capture of radioactive emissions

Body Part	Radionuclide	Qualifier	Qualifier
9 Lacrimal Ducts, Bilateral	1 Technetium 99m (Tc-99m) Y Other Radionuclide	Z None	Z None
Y Eye	Y Other Radionuclide	Z None	Z None

New/Revised Text in Green ~~deleted~~ Deleted ♀ Females Only ♂ Males Only Coding Clinic
Non-covered Limited Coverage Combination (See Appendix E) DRG Non-OR Non-OR Hospital-Acquired Condition

649

SECTION: **C NUCLEAR MEDICINE**

BODY SYSTEM: 9 **EAR, NOSE, MOUTH, AND THROAT**

TYPE: 1 **PLANAR NUCLEAR MEDICINE IMAGING:** Introduction of radioactive materials into the body for single plane display of images developed from the capture of radioactive emissions

Body Part	Radionuclide	Qualifier	Qualifier
B Salivary Glands, Bilateral	1 Technetium 99m (Tc-99m) Y Other Radionuclide	Z None	Z None
Y Ear, Nose, Mouth and Throat	Y Other Radionuclide	Z None	Z None

SECTION: C NUCLEAR MEDICINE
BODY SYSTEM: B RESPIRATORY SYSTEM
TYPE: **1 PLANAR NUCLEAR MEDICINE IMAGING:** Introduction of radioactive materials into the body for single plane display of images developed from the capture of radioactive emissions

Body Part	Radionuclide	Qualifier	Qualifier
2 Lungs and Bronchi	1 Technetium 99m (Tc-99m) 9 Krypton (Kr-81m) T Xenon 127 (Xe-127) V Xenon 133 (Xe-133) Y Other Radionuclide	Z None	Z None
Y Respiratory System	Y Other Radionuclide	Z None	Z None

SECTION: C NUCLEAR MEDICINE
BODY SYSTEM: B RESPIRATORY SYSTEM
TYPE: **2 TOMOGRAPHIC (TOMO) NUCLEAR MEDICINE IMAGING:** Introduction of radioactive materials into the body for three dimensional display of images developed from the capture of radioactive emissions

Body Part	Radionuclide	Qualifier	Qualifier
2 Lungs and Bronchi	1 Technetium 99m (Tc-99m) 9 Krypton (Kr-81m) Y Other Radionuclide	Z None	Z None
Y Respiratory System	Y Other Radionuclide	Z None	Z None

SECTION: C NUCLEAR MEDICINE
BODY SYSTEM: B RESPIRATORY SYSTEM
TYPE: **3 POSITRON EMISSION TOMOGRAPHIC (PET) IMAGING:** Introduction of radioactive materials into the body for three dimensional display of images developed from the simultaneous capture, 18Ø degrees apart, of radioactive emissions

Body Part	Radionuclide	Qualifier	Qualifier
2 Lungs and Bronchi	K Fluorine 18 (F-18) Y Other Radionuclide	Z None	Z None
Y Respiratory System	Y Other Radionuclide	Z None	Z None

New/Revised Text in Green   ~~deleted~~ Deleted   ♀ Females Only   ♂ Males Only   **Coding Clinic**
🐾 Non-covered   🐾 Limited Coverage   ⊞ Combination (See Appendix E)   DRG Non-OR   Non-OR   🐾 Hospital-Acquired Condition

SECTION: C NUCLEAR MEDICINE
BODY SYSTEM: D GASTROINTESTINAL SYSTEM
TYPE: **1 PLANAR NUCLEAR MEDICINE IMAGING:** Introduction of radioactive materials into the body for single plane display of images developed from the capture of radioactive emissions

Body Part	Radionuclide	Qualifier	Qualifier
5 Upper Gastrointestinal Tract 7 Gastrointestinal Tract	1 Technetium 99m (Tc-99m) D Indium 111 (In-111) Y Other Radionuclide	Z None	Z None
Y Digestive System	Y Other Radionuclide	Z None	Z None

SECTION: C NUCLEAR MEDICINE
BODY SYSTEM: D GASTROINTESTINAL SYSTEM
TYPE: **2 TOMOGRAPHIC (TOMO) NUCLEAR MEDICINE IMAGING:** Introduction of radioactive materials into the body for three dimensional display of images developed from the capture of radioactive emissions

Body Part	Radionuclide	Qualifier	Qualifier
7 Gastrointestinal Tract	1 Technetium 99m (Tc-99m) D Indium 111 (In-111) Y Other Radionuclide	Z None	Z None
Y Digestive System	Y Other Radionuclide	Z None	Z None

SECTION: C NUCLEAR MEDICINE
BODY SYSTEM: F HEPATOBILIARY SYSTEM AND PANCREAS
TYPE: **1 PLANAR NUCLEAR MEDICINE IMAGING:** Introduction of radioactive materials into the body for single plane display of images developed from the capture of radioactive emissions

Body Part	Radionuclide	Qualifier	Qualifier
4 Gallbladder 5 Liver 6 Liver and Spleen C Hepatobiliary System, All	1 Technetium 99m (Tc-99m) Y Other Radionuclide	Z None	Z None
Y Hepatobiliary System and Pancreas	Y Other Radionuclide	Z None	Z None

SECTION: C NUCLEAR MEDICINE
BODY SYSTEM: F HEPATOBILIARY SYSTEM AND PANCREAS
TYPE: **2 TOMOGRAPHIC (TOMO) NUCLEAR MEDICINE IMAGING:** Introduction of radioactive materials into the body for three dimensional display of images developed from the capture of radioactive emissions

Body Part	Radionuclide	Qualifier	Qualifier
4 Gallbladder 5 Liver 6 Liver and Spleen	1 Technetium 99m (Tc-99m) Y Other Radionuclide	Z None	Z None
Y Hepatobiliary System and Pancreas	Y Other Radionuclide	Z None	Z None

C: NUCLEAR MEDICINE

F: HEPATOBILIARY SYSTEM AND PANCREAS

1; 2

New/Revised Text in Green   ~~deleted~~ Deleted   ♀ Females Only   ♂ Males Only   **Coding Clinic**
🔖 Non-covered   🔖 Limited Coverage   ⊞ Combination (See Appendix E)   DRG Non-OR   Non-OR   🔖 Hospital-Acquired Condition

653

SECTION: C NUCLEAR MEDICINE
BODY SYSTEM: G ENDOCRINE SYSTEM
TYPE: 1 PLANAR NUCLEAR MEDICINE IMAGING: Introduction of radioactive materials into the body for single plane display of images developed from the capture of radioactive emissions

Body Part	Radionuclide	Qualifier	Qualifier
1 Parathyroid Glands	1 Technetium 99m (Tc-99m) S Thallium 201 (Tl-201) Y Other Radionuclide	Z None	Z None
2 Thyroid Gland	1 Technetium 99m (Tc-99m) F Iodine 123 (I-123) G Iodine 131 (I-131) Y Other Radionuclide	Z None	Z None
4 Adrenal Glands, Bilateral	G Iodine 131 (I-131) Y Other Radionuclide	Z None	Z None
Y Endocrine System	Y Other Radionuclide	Z None	Z None

SECTION: C NUCLEAR MEDICINE
BODY SYSTEM: G ENDOCRINE SYSTEM
TYPE: 2 TOMOGRAPHIC (TOMO) NUCLEAR MEDICINE IMAGING: Introduction of radioactive materials into the body for three dimensional display of images developed from the capture of radioactive emissions

Body Part	Radionuclide	Qualifier	Qualifier
1 Parathyroid Glands	1 Technetium 99m (Tc-99m) S Thallium 201 (Tl-201) Y Other Radionuclide	Z None	Z None
Y Endocrine System	Y Other Radionuclide	Z None	Z None

SECTION: C NUCLEAR MEDICINE
BODY SYSTEM: G ENDOCRINE SYSTEM
TYPE: 4 NONIMAGING NUCLEAR MEDICINE UPTAKE: Introduction of radioactive materials into the body for measurements of organ function, from the detection of radioactive emissions

Body Part	Radionuclide	Qualifier	Qualifier
2 Thyroid Gland	1 Technetium 99m (Tc-99m) F Iodine 123 (I-123) G Iodine 131 (I-131) Y Other Radionuclide	Z None	Z None
Y Endocrine System	Y Other Radionuclide	Z None	Z None

New/Revised Text in Green — deleted Deleted — ♀ Females Only — ♂ Males Only — **Coding Clinic**

🔻 Non-covered — 🔻 Limited Coverage — ⊞ Combination (See Appendix E) — DRG Non-OR — Non-OR — 🔻 Hospital-Acquired Condition

SECTION: C NUCLEAR MEDICINE

BODY SYSTEM: H SKIN, SUBCUTANEOUS TISSUE AND BREAST

TYPE: 1 **PLANAR NUCLEAR MEDICINE IMAGING:** Introduction of radioactive materials into the body for single plane display of images developed from the capture of radioactive emissions

Body Part	Radionuclide	Qualifier	Qualifier
Ø Breast, Right 1 Breast, Left 2 Breasts, Bilateral	1 Technetium 99m (Tc-99m) S Thallium 201 (Tl-201) Y Other Radionuclide	Z None	Z None
Y Skin, Subcutaneous Tissue, and Breast	Y Other Radionuclide	Z None	Z None

SECTION: C NUCLEAR MEDICINE

BODY SYSTEM: H SKIN, SUBCUTANEOUS TISSUE AND BREAST

TYPE: 2 **TOMOGRAPHIC (TOMO) NUCLEAR MEDICINE IMAGING:** Introduction of radioactive materials into the body for three dimensional display of images developed from the capture of radioactive emissions

Body Part	Radionuclide	Qualifier	Qualifier
Ø Breast, Right 1 Breast, Left 2 Breasts, Bilateral	1 Technetium 99m (Tc-99m) S Thallium 201 (Tl-201) Y Other Radionuclide	Z None	Z None
Y Skin, Subcutaneous Tissue, and Breast	Y Other Radionuclide	Z None	Z None

SECTION: **C NUCLEAR MEDICINE**
BODY SYSTEM: P MUSCULOSKELETAL SYSTEM
TYPE: 1 **PLANAR NUCLEAR MEDICINE IMAGING:** Introduction of radioactive materials into the body for single plane display of images developed from the capture of radioactive emissions

Body Part	Radionuclide	Qualifier	Qualifier
1 Skull 4 Thorax 5 Spine 6 Pelvis 7 Spine and Pelvis 8 Upper Extremity, Right 9 Upper Extremity, Left B Upper Extremities, Bilateral C Lower Extremity, Right D Lower Extremity, Left F Lower Extremities, Bilateral Z Musculoskeletal System, All	1 Technetium 99m (Tc-99m) Y Other Radionuclide	Z None	Z None
Y Musculoskeletal System, Other	Y Other Radionuclide	Z None	Z None

SECTION: **C NUCLEAR MEDICINE**
BODY SYSTEM: P MUSCULOSKELETAL SYSTEM
TYPE: 2 **TOMOGRAPHIC (TOMO) NUCLEAR MEDICINE IMAGING:** Introduction of radioactive materials into the body for three dimensional display of images developed from the capture of radioactive emissions

Body Part	Radionuclide	Qualifier	Qualifier
1 Skull 2 Cervical Spine 3 Skull and Cervical Spine 4 Thorax 6 Pelvis 7 Spine and Pelvis 8 Upper Extremity, Right 9 Upper Extremity, Left B Upper Extremities, Bilateral C Lower Extremity, Right D Lower Extremity, Left F Lower Extremities, Bilateral G Thoracic Spine H Lumbar Spine J Thoracolumbar Spine	1 Technetium 99m (Tc-99m) Y Other Radionuclide	Z None	Z None
Y Musculoskeletal System, Other	Y Other Radionuclide	Z None	Z None

P: MUSCULOSKELETAL SYSTEM   1; 2

C: NUCLEAR MEDICINE

SECTION: C NUCLEAR MEDICINE

BODY SYSTEM: P MUSCULOSKELETAL SYSTEM

TYPE: 5 **NONIMAGING NUCLEAR MEDICINE PROBE:** Introduction of radioactive materials into the body for the study of distribution and fate of certain substances by the detection of radioactive emissions; or, alternatively, measurement of absorption of radioactive emissions from an external source

Body Part	Radionuclide	Qualifier	Qualifier
5 Spine N Upper Extremities P Lower Extremities	Z None	Z None	Z None
Y Musculoskeletal System, Other	Y Other Radionuclide	Z None	Z None

New/Revised Text in Green   ~~deleted~~ Deleted   ♀ Females Only   ♂ Males Only   **Coding Clinic**
🜂 Non-covered   🜂 Limited Coverage   ⊞ Combination (See Appendix E)   DRG Non-OR   Non-OR   🜂 Hospital-Acquired Condition

657

SECTION: C NUCLEAR MEDICINE
BODY SYSTEM: T URINARY SYSTEM
TYPE: 1 PLANAR NUCLEAR MEDICINE IMAGING: Introduction of radioactive
                     materials into the body for single plane display of images developed from
                     the capture of radioactive emissions

Body Part	Radionuclide	Qualifier	Qualifier
3 Kidneys, Ureters, and Bladder	1 Technetium 99m (Tc-99m) F Iodine 123 (I-123) G Iodine 131 (I-131) Y Other Radionuclide	Z None	Z None
H Bladder and Ureters	1 Technetium 99m (Tc-99m) Y Other Radionuclide	Z None	Z None
Y Urinary System	Y Other Radionuclide	Z None	Z None

SECTION: C NUCLEAR MEDICINE
BODY SYSTEM: T URINARY SYSTEM
TYPE: 2 TOMOGRAPHIC (TOMO) NUCLEAR MEDICINE IMAGING: Introduction
                     of radioactive materials into the body for three dimensional display of
                     images developed from the capture of radioactive emissions

Body Part	Radionuclide	Qualifier	Qualifier
3 Kidneys, Ureters, and Bladder	1 Technetium 99m (Tc-99m) Y Other Radionuclide	Z None	Z None
Y Urinary System	Y Other Radionuclide	Z None	Z None

SECTION: C NUCLEAR MEDICINE
BODY SYSTEM: T URINARY SYSTEM
TYPE: 6 NONIMAGING NUCLEAR MEDICINE ASSAY: Introduction of
                     radioactive materials into the body for the study of body fluids and blood
                     elements, by the detection of radioactive emissions

Body Part	Radionuclide	Qualifier	Qualifier
3 Kidneys, Ureters, and Bladder	1 Technetium 99m (Tc-99m) F Iodine 123 (I-123) G Iodine 131 (I-131) H Iodine 125 (I-125) Y Other Radionuclide	Z None	Z None
Y Urinary System	Y Other Radionuclide	Z None	Z None

Side tab: 1; 2; 6 — T: URINARY SYSTEM — C: NUCLEAR MEDICINE

New/Revised Text in Green   ~~deleted~~ Deleted   ♀ Females Only   ♂ Males Only   **Coding Clinic**
⬡ Non-covered   ⬡ Limited Coverage   ⊞ Combination (See Appendix E)   DRG Non-OR   Non-OR   ⬡ Hospital-Acquired Condition

SECTION: C NUCLEAR MEDICINE
BODY SYSTEM: V MALE REPRODUCTIVE SYSTEM
TYPE: 1 **PLANAR NUCLEAR MEDICINE IMAGING:** Introduction of radioactive materials into the body for single plane display of images developed from the capture of radioactive emissions

Body Part	Radionuclide	Qualifier	Qualifier
9 Testicles, Bilateral ♂	1 Technetium 99m (Tc-99m) Y Other Radionuclide	Z None	Z None
Y Male Reproductive System ♂	Y Other Radionuclide	Z None	Z None

SECTION: C NUCLEAR MEDICINE
BODY SYSTEM: W ANATOMICAL REGIONS
TYPE: **1 PLANAR NUCLEAR MEDICINE IMAGING:** Introduction of radioactive materials into the body for single plane display of images developed from the capture of radioactive emissions

Body Part	Radionuclide	Qualifier	Qualifier
Ø Abdomen 1 Abdomen and Pelvis 4 Chest and Abdomen 6 Chest and Neck B Head and Neck D Lower Extremity J Pelvic Region M Upper Extremity N Whole Body	1 Technetium 99m (Tc-99m) D Indium 111 (In-111) F Iodine 123 (I-123) G Iodine 131 (I-131) L Gallium 67 (Ga-67) S Thallium 201 (Tl-201) Y Other Radionuclide	Z None	Z None
3 Chest	1 Technetium 99m (Tc-99m) D Indium 111 (In-111) F Iodine 123 (I-123) G Iodine 131 (I-131) K Fluorine 18 (F-18) L Gallium 67 (Ga-67) S Thallium 201 (Tl-201) Y Other Radionuclide	Z None	Z None
Y Anatomical Regions, Multiple	Y Other Radionuclide	Z None	Z None
Z Anatomical Region, Other	Z None	Z None	Z None

SECTION: C NUCLEAR MEDICINE
BODY SYSTEM: W ANATOMICAL REGIONS
TYPE: **2 TOMOGRAPHIC (TOMO) NUCLEAR MEDICINE IMAGING:** Introduction of radioactive materials into the body for three dimensional display of images developed from the capture of radioactive emissions

Body Part	Radionuclide	Qualifier	Qualifier
Ø Abdomen 1 Abdomen and Pelvis 3 Chest 4 Chest and Abdomen 6 Chest and Neck B Head and Neck D Lower Extremity J Pelvic Region M Upper Extremity	1 Technetium 99m (Tc-99m) D Indium 111 (In-111) F Iodine 123 (I-123) G Iodine 131 (I-131) K Fluorine 18 (F-18) L Gallium 67 (Ga-67) S Thallium 201 (Tl-201) Y Other Radionuclide	Z None	Z None
Y Anatomical Regions, Multiple	Y Other Radionuclide	Z None	Z None

C: NUCLEAR MEDICINE W: ANATOMICAL REGIONS 1; 2

New/Revised Text in Green ~~deleted~~ Deleted ♀ Females Only ♂ Males Only **Coding Clinic**
Non-covered Limited Coverage ⊞ Combination (See Appendix E) DRG Non-OR Non-OR Hospital-Acquired Condition

SECTION: C NUCLEAR MEDICINE
BODY SYSTEM: W ANATOMICAL REGIONS

TYPE: **3 POSITRON EMISSION TOMOGRAPHIC (PET) IMAGING:** Introduction of radioactive materials into the body for three dimensional display of images developed from the simultaneous capture, 18Ø degrees apart, of radioactive emissions

Body Part	Radionuclide	Qualifier	Qualifier
N Whole Body	Y Other Radionuclide	Z None	Z None

SECTION: C NUCLEAR MEDICINE
BODY SYSTEM: W ANATOMICAL REGIONS

TYPE: **5 NONIMAGING NUCLEAR MEDICINE PROBE:** Introduction of radioactive materials into the body for the study of distribution and fate of certain substances by the detection of radioactive emissions; or, alternatively, measurement of absorption of radioactive emissions from an external source

Body Part	Radionuclide	Qualifier	Qualifier
Ø Abdomen 1 Abdomen and Pelvis 3 Chest 4 Chest and Abdomen 6 Chest and Neck B Head and Neck D Lower Extremity J Pelvic Region M Upper Extremity	1 Technetium 99m (Tc-99m) D Indium 111 (In-111) Y Other Radionuclide	Z None	Z None

SECTION: C NUCLEAR MEDICINE
BODY SYSTEM: W ANATOMICAL REGIONS

TYPE: **7 SYSTEMIC NUCLEAR MEDICINE THERAPY:** Introduction of unsealed radioactive materials into the body for treatment

Body Part	Radionuclide	Qualifier	Qualifier
Ø Abdomen 3 Chest	N Phosphorus 32 (P-32) Y Other Radionuclide	Z None	Z None
G Thyroid	G Iodine 131 (I-131) Y Other Radionuclide	Z None	Z None
N Whole Body	8 Samarium 153 (Sm-153) G Iodine 131 (I-131) N Phosphorus 32 (P-32) P Strontium 89 (Sr-89) Y Other Radionuclide	Z None	Z None
Y Anatomical Regions, Multiple	Y Other Radionuclide	Z None	Z None

New/Revised Text in Green   ~~deleted~~ Deleted   ♀ Females Only   ♂ Males Only   **Coding Clinic**

🏷 Non-covered   🏷 Limited Coverage   ⊞ Combination (See Appendix E)   DRG Non-OR   Non-OR   🏷 Hospital-Acquired Condition

SECTION: D RADIATION THERAPY

BODY SYSTEM: Ø CENTRAL AND PERIPHERAL NERVOUS SYSTEM

MODALITY: Ø BEAM RADIATION

Treatment Site	Modality Qualifier	Isotope	Qualifier
Ø Brain 1 Brain Stem 6 Spinal Cord 7 Peripheral Nerve	Ø Photons <1 MeV 1 Photons 1 - 1Ø MeV 2 Photons >1Ø MeV 4 Heavy Particles (Protons,Ions) 5 Neutrons 6 Neutron Capture	Z None	Z None
Ø Brain 1 Brain Stem 6 Spinal Cord 7 Peripheral Nerve	3 Electrons	Z None	Ø Intraoperative Z None

SECTION: D RADIATION THERAPY

BODY SYSTEM: Ø CENTRAL AND PERIPHERAL NERVOUS SYSTEM

MODALITY: 1 BRACHYTHERAPY

Treatment Site	Modality Qualifier	Isotope	Qualifier
Ø Brain 1 Brain Stem 6 Spinal Cord 7 Peripheral Nerve	9 High Dose Rate (HDR) B Low Dose Rate (LDR)	7 Cesium 137 (Cs-137) 8 Iridium 192 (Ir-192) 9 Iodine 125 (I-125) B Palladium 1Ø3 (Pd-1Ø3) C Californium 252 (Cf-252) Y Other Isotope	Z None

SECTION: D RADIATION THERAPY

BODY SYSTEM: Ø CENTRAL AND PERIPHERAL NERVOUS SYSTEM

MODALITY: 2 STEREOTACTIC RADIOSURGERY

Treatment Site	Modality Qualifier	Isotope	Qualifier

Ø Brain
1 Brain Stem
6 Spinal Cord
7 Peripheral Nerve
	D Stereotactic Other Photon
	  Radiosurgery
	H Stereotactic Particulate
	  Radiosurgery
	J Stereotactic Gamma Beam
	  Radiosurgery
		Z None	Z None

DRG Non-OR   All Values

SECTION: D RADIATION THERAPY

BODY SYSTEM: Ø CENTRAL AND PERIPHERAL NERVOUS SYSTEM

MODALITY: Y OTHER RADIATION

Treatment Site	Modality Qualifier	Isotope	Qualifier
Ø Brain 1 Brain Stem 6 Spinal Cord 7 Peripheral Nerve	7 Contact Radiation 8 Hyperthermia F Plaque Radiation K Laser Interstitial Thermal Therapy	Z None	Z None

New/Revised Text in Green   ~~deleted~~ Deleted   ♀ Females Only   ♂ Males Only   **Coding Clinic**

🔖 Non-covered   🔖 Limited Coverage   ⊡ Combination (See Appendix E)   DRG Non-OR   Non-OR   🔖 Hospital-Acquired Condition

SECTION: D RADIATION THERAPY

BODY SYSTEM: 7 LYMPHATIC AND HEMATOLOGIC SYSTEM
MODALITY: Ø BEAM RADIATION

Treatment Site	Modality Qualifier	Isotope	Qualifier
Ø Bone Marrow 1 Thymus 2 Spleen 3 Lymphatics, Neck 4 Lymphatics, Axillary 5 Lymphatics, Thorax 6 Lymphatics, Abdomen 7 Lymphatics, Pelvis 8 Lymphatics, Inguinal	Ø Photons <1 MeV 1 Photons 1 - 1Ø MeV 2 Photons >1Ø MeV 4 Heavy Particles (Protons, Ions) 5 Neutrons 6 Neutron Capture	Z None	Z None
Ø Bone Marrow 1 Thymus 2 Spleen 3 Lymphatics, Neck 4 Lymphatics, Axillary 5 Lymphatics, Thorax 6 Lymphatics, Abdomen 7 Lymphatics, Pelvis 8 Lymphatics, Inguinal	3 Electrons	Z None	Ø Intraoperative Z None

SECTION: D RADIATION THERAPY

BODY SYSTEM: 7 LYMPHATIC AND HEMATOLOGIC SYSTEM
MODALITY: 1 BRACHYTHERAPY

Treatment Site	Modality Qualifier	Isotope	Qualifier
Ø Bone Marrow 1 Thymus 2 Spleen 3 Lymphatics, Neck 4 Lymphatics, Axillary 5 Lymphatics, Thorax 6 Lymphatics, Abdomen 7 Lymphatics, Pelvis 8 Lymphatics, Inguinal	9 High Dose Rate (HDR) B Low Dose Rate (LDR)	7 Cesium 137 (Cs-137) 8 Iridium 192 (Ir-192) 9 Iodine 125 (I-125) B Palladium 1Ø3 (Pd-1Ø3) C Californium 252 (Cf-252) Y Other Isotope	Z None

New/Revised Text in Green   ~~deleted~~ Deleted   ♀ Females Only   ♂ Males Only   **Coding Clinic**

Non-covered   Limited Coverage   ⊞ Combination (See Appendix E)   DRG Non-OR   Non-OR   Hospital-Acquired Condition

2; Y

SECTION: **D RADIATION THERAPY**
BODY SYSTEM: 7 **LYMPHATIC AND HEMATOLOGIC SYSTEM**
MODALITY: 2 **STEREOTACTIC RADIOSURGERY**

Treatment Site	Modality Qualifier	Isotope	Qualifier

Ø Bone Marrow
1 Thymus
2 Spleen
3 Lymphatics, Neck
4 Lymphatics, Axillary
5 Lymphatics, Thorax
6 Lymphatics, Abdomen
7 Lymphatics, Pelvis
8 Lymphatics, Inguinal
	D Stereotactic Other Photon
	   Radiosurgery
	H Stereotactic Particulate
	   Radiosurgery
	J Stereotactic Gamma Beam
	   Radiosurgery
		Z None	Z None

DRG Non-OR All Values

SECTION: **D RADIATION THERAPY**
BODY SYSTEM: 7 **LYMPHATIC AND HEMATOLOGIC SYSTEM**
MODALITY: Y **OTHER RADIATION**

Treatment Site	Modality Qualifier	Isotope	Qualifier
Ø Bone Marrow 1 Thymus 2 Spleen 3 Lymphatics, Neck 4 Lymphatics, Axillary 5 Lymphatics, Thorax 6 Lymphatics, Abdomen 7 Lymphatics, Pelvis 8 Lymphatics, Inguinal	8 Hyperthermia F Plaque Radiation	Z None	Z None

7: LYMPHATIC AND HEMATOLOGIC SYSTEM

D: RADIATION THERAPY

SECTION: D RADIATION THERAPY
BODY SYSTEM: 8 EYE
MODALITY: Ø BEAM RADIATION

Treatment Site	Modality Qualifier	Isotope	Qualifier
Ø Eye	Ø Photons <1 MeV 1 Photons 1 - 1Ø MeV 2 Photons >1Ø MeV 4 Heavy Particles (Protons, Ions) 5 Neutrons 6 Neutron Capture	Z None	Z None
Ø Eye	3 Electrons	Z None	Ø Intraoperative Z None

SECTION: D RADIATION THERAPY
BODY SYSTEM: 8 EYE
MODALITY: 1 BRACHYTHERAPY

Treatment Site	Modality Qualifier	Isotope	Qualifier
Ø Eye	9 High Dose Rate (HDR) B Low Dose Rate (LDR)	7 Cesium 137 (Cs-137) 8 Iridium 192 (Ir-192) 9 Iodine 125 (I-125) B Palladium 1Ø3 (Pd-1Ø3) C Californium 252 (Cf-252) Y Other Isotope	Z None

SECTION: D RADIATION THERAPY
BODY SYSTEM: 8 EYE
MODALITY: 2 STEREOTACTIC RADIOSURGERY

Treatment Site	Modality Qualifier	Isotope	Qualifier
Ø Eye	D Stereotactic Other Photon Radiosurgery H Stereotactic Particulate Radiosurgery J Stereotactic Gamma Beam Radiosurgery	Z None	Z None

DRG Non-OR All Values

SECTION: D RADIATION THERAPY
BODY SYSTEM: 8 EYE
MODALITY: Y OTHER RADIATION

Treatment Site	Modality Qualifier	Isotope	Qualifier
Ø Eye	7 Contact Radiation 8 Hyperthermia F Plaque Radiation	Z None	Z None

SECTION: D RADIATION THERAPY
BODY SYSTEM: 9 EAR, NOSE, MOUTH, AND THROAT
MODALITY: Ø BEAM RADIATION

Treatment Site	Modality Qualifier	Isotope	Qualifier
Ø Ear 1 Nose 3 Hypopharynx 4 Mouth 5 Tongue 6 Salivary Glands 7 Sinuses 8 Hard Palate 9 Soft Palate B Larynx D Nasopharynx F Oropharynx	Ø Photons <1 MeV 1 Photons 1 - 1Ø MeV 2 Photons >1Ø MeV 4 Heavy Particles (Protons, Ions) 5 Neutrons 6 Neutron Capture	Z None	Z None
Ø Ear 1 Nose 3 Hypopharynx 4 Mouth 5 Tongue 6 Salivary Glands 7 Sinuses 8 Hard Palate 9 Soft Palate B Larynx D Nasopharynx F Oropharynx	3 Electrons	Z None	Ø Intraoperative Z None

SECTION: D RADIATION THERAPY
BODY SYSTEM: 9 EAR, NOSE, MOUTH, AND THROAT
MODALITY: 1 BRACHYTHERAPY

Treatment Site	Modality Qualifier	Isotope	Qualifier
Ø Ear 1 Nose 3 Hypopharynx 4 Mouth 5 Tongue 6 Salivary Glands 7 Sinuses 8 Hard Palate 9 Soft Palate B Larynx D Nasopharynx F Oropharynx	9 High Dose Rate (HDR) B Low Dose Rate (LDR)	7 Cesium 137 (Cs-137) 8 Iridium 192 (Ir-192) 9 Iodine 125 (I-125) B Palladium 1Ø3 (Pd-1Ø3) C Californium 252 (Cf-252) Y Other Isotope	Z None

SECTION:　D RADIATION THERAPY
BODY SYSTEM: 9 EAR, NOSE, MOUTH, AND THROAT
MODALITY:　2 STEREOTACTIC RADIOSURGERY

Treatment Site	Modality Qualifier	Isotope	Qualifier
Ø Ear 1 Nose 4 Mouth 5 Tongue 6 Salivary Glands 7 Sinuses 8 Hard Palate 9 Soft Palate B Larynx C Pharynx D Nasopharynx	D Stereotactic Other Photon 　 Radiosurgery H Stereotactic Particulate 　 Radiosurgery J Stereotactic Gamma Beam 　 Radiosurgery	Z None	Z None

`DRG Non-OR`　All Values

SECTION:　D RADIATION THERAPY
BODY SYSTEM: 9 EAR, NOSE, MOUTH, AND THROAT
MODALITY:　Y OTHER RADIATION

Treatment Site	Modality Qualifier	Isotope	Qualifier
Ø Ear 1 Nose 5 Tongue 6 Salivary Glands 7 Sinuses 8 Hard Palate 9 Soft Palate	7 Contact Radiation 8 Hyperthermia F Plaque Radiation	Z None	Z None
3 Hypopharynx F Oropharynx	7 Contact Radiation 8 Hyperthermia	Z None	Z None
4 Mouth B Larynx D Nasopharynx	7 Contact Radiation 8 Hyperthermia C Intraoperative Radiation 　 Therapy (IORT) F Plaque Radiation	Z None	Z None
C Pharynx	C Intraoperative Radiation 　 Therapy (IORT) F Plaque Radiation	Z None	Z None

SECTION: D RADIATION THERAPY
BODY SYSTEM: B RESPIRATORY SYSTEM
MODALITY: Ø BEAM RADIATION

Treatment Site	Modality Qualifier	Isotope	Qualifier
Ø Trachea 1 Bronchus 2 Lung 5 Pleura 6 Mediastinum 7 Chest Wall 8 Diaphragm	Ø Photons <1 MeV 1 Photons 1 - 1Ø MeV 2 Photons >1Ø MeV 4 Heavy Particles (Protons, Ions) 5 Neutrons 6 Neutron Capture	Z None	Z None
Ø Trachea 1 Bronchus 2 Lung 5 Pleura 6 Mediastinum 7 Chest Wall 8 Diaphragm	3 Electrons	Z None	Ø Intraoperative Z None

SECTION: D RADIATION THERAPY
BODY SYSTEM: B RESPIRATORY SYSTEM
MODALITY: 1 BRACHYTHERAPY

Treatment Site	Modality Qualifier	Isotope	Qualifier
Ø Trachea 1 Bronchus 2 Lung 5 Pleura 6 Mediastinum 7 Chest Wall 8 Diaphragm	9 High Dose Rate (HDR) B Low Dose Rate (LDR)	7 Cesium 137 (Cs-137) 8 Iridium 192 (Ir-192) 9 Iodine 125 (I-125) B Palladium 1Ø3 (Pd-1Ø3) C Californium 252 (Cf-252) Y Other Isotope	Z None

B: RESPIRATORY SYSTEM   *Ø; 1*

D: RADIATION THERAPY

SECTION: D RADIATION THERAPY
BODY SYSTEM: B RESPIRATORY SYSTEM
MODALITY: 2 STEREOTACTIC RADIOSURGERY

Treatment Site	Modality Qualifier	Isotope	Qualifier

Ø Trachea
1 Bronchus
2 Lung
5 Pleura
6 Mediastinum
7 Chest Wall
8 Diaphragm
	D Stereotactic Other Photon
	   Radiosurgery
	H Stereotactic Particulate
	   Radiosurgery
	J Stereotactic Gamma Beam
	   Radiosurgery
		Z None	Z None

`DRG Non-OR` All Values

SECTION: D RADIATION THERAPY
BODY SYSTEM: B RESPIRATORY SYSTEM
MODALITY: Y OTHER RADIATION

Treatment Site	Modality Qualifier	Isotope	Qualifier
Ø Trachea 1 Bronchus 2 Lung 5 Pleura 6 Mediastinum 7 Chest Wall 8 Diaphragm	7 Contact Radiation 8 Hyperthermia F Plaque Radiation K Laser Interstitial Thermal Therapy	Z None	Z None

D: RADIATION THERAPY

B: RESPIRATORY SYSTEM

2;   Y

SECTION: **D RADIATION THERAPY**
BODY SYSTEM: D GASTROINTESTINAL SYSTEM
MODALITY: Ø BEAM RADIATION

Treatment Site	Modality Qualifier	Isotope	Qualifier
Ø Esophagus 1 Stomach 2 Duodenum 3 Jejunum 4 Ileum 5 Colon 7 Rectum	Ø Photons <1 MeV 1 Photons 1 - 1Ø MeV 2 Photons >1Ø MeV 4 Heavy Particles (Protons, Ions) 5 Neutrons 6 Neutron Capture	Z None	Z None
Ø Esophagus 1 Stomach 2 Duodenum 3 Jejunum 4 Ileum 5 Colon 7 Rectum	3 Electrons	Z None	Ø Intraoperative Z None

SECTION: **D RADIATION THERAPY**
BODY SYSTEM: D GASTROINTESTINAL SYSTEM
MODALITY: 1 BRACHYTHERAPY

Treatment Site	Modality Qualifier	Isotope	Qualifier
Ø Esophagus 1 Stomach 2 Duodenum 3 Jejunum 4 Ileum 5 Colon 7 Rectum	9 High Dose Rate (HDR) B Low Dose Rate (LDR)	7 Cesium 137 (Cs-137) 8 Iridium 192 (Ir-192) 9 Iodine 125 (I-125) B Palladium 1Ø3 (Pd-1Ø3) C Californium 252 (Cf-252) Y Other Isotope	Z None

SECTION: D RADIATION THERAPY
BODY SYSTEM: D GASTROINTESTINAL SYSTEM
MODALITY: 2 STEREOTACTIC RADIOSURGERY

Treatment Site	Modality Qualifier	Isotope	Qualifier
Ø Esophagus 1 Stomach 2 Duodenum 3 Jejunum 4 Ileum 5 Colon 7 Rectum	D Stereotactic Other Photon Radiosurgery H Stereotactic Particulate Radiosurgery J Stereotactic Gamma Beam Radiosurgery	Z None	Z None

`DRG Non-OR` All Values

SECTION: D RADIATION THERAPY
BODY SYSTEM: D GASTROINTESTINAL SYSTEM
MODALITY: Y OTHER RADIATION

Treatment Site	Modality Qualifier	Isotope	Qualifier
Ø Esophagus	7 Contact Radiation 8 Hyperthermia F Plaque Radiation K Laser Interstitial Thermal Therapy	Z None	Z None
1 Stomach 2 Duodenum 3 Jejunum 4 Ileum 5 Colon 7 Rectum	7 Contact Radiation 8 Hyperthermia C Intraoperative Radiation Therapy (IORT) F Plaque Radiation K Laser Interstitial Thermal Therapy	Z None	Z None
8 Anus	C Intraoperative Radiation Therapy (IORT) F Plaque Radiation K Laser Interstitial Thermal Therapy	Z None	Z None

Ø; 1; 2; Y

F: HEPATOBILIARY SYSTEM AND PANCREAS

D: RADIATION THERAPY

SECTION: D RADIATION THERAPY
BODY SYSTEM: F HEPATOBILIARY SYSTEM AND PANCREAS
MODALITY: Ø BEAM RADIATION

Treatment Site	Modality Qualifier	Isotope	Qualifier
Ø Liver 1 Gallbladder 2 Bile Ducts 3 Pancreas	Ø Photons <1 MeV 1 Photons 1 - 1Ø MeV 2 Photons >1Ø MeV 4 Heavy Particles (Protons, Ions) 5 Neutrons 6 Neutron Capture	Z None	Z None
Ø Liver 1 Gallbladder 2 Bile Ducts 3 Pancreas	3 Electrons	Z None	Ø Intraoperative Z None

SECTION: D RADIATION THERAPY
BODY SYSTEM: F HEPATOBILIARY SYSTEM AND PANCREAS
MODALITY: 1 BRACHYTHERAPY

Treatment Site	Modality Qualifier	Isotope	Qualifier
Ø Liver 1 Gallbladder 2 Bile Ducts 3 Pancreas	9 High Dose Rate (HDR) B Low Dose Rate (LDR)	7 Cesium 137 (Cs-137) 8 Iridium 192 (Ir-192) 9 Iodine 125 (I-125) B Palladium 1Ø3 (Pd-1Ø3) C Californium 252 (Cf-252) Y Other Isotope	Z None

SECTION: D RADIATION THERAPY
BODY SYSTEM: F HEPATOBILIARY SYSTEM AND PANCREAS
MODALITY: 2 STEREOTACTIC RADIOSURGERY

Treatment Site	Modality Qualifier	Isotope	Qualifier
Ø Liver 1 Gallbladder 2 Bile Ducts 3 Pancreas	D Stereotactic Other Photon Radiosurgery H Stereotactic Particulate Radiosurgery J Stereotactic Gamma Beam Radiosurgery	Z None	Z None

DRG Non-OR All Values

SECTION: D RADIATION THERAPY
BODY SYSTEM: F HEPATOBILIARY SYSTEM AND PANCREAS
MODALITY: Y OTHER RADIATION

Treatment Site	Modality Qualifier	Isotope	Qualifier
Ø Liver 1 Gallbladder 2 Bile Ducts 3 Pancreas	7 Contact Radiation 8 Hyperthermia C Intraoperative Radiation Therapy (IORT) F Plaque Radiation K Laser Interstitial Thermal Therapy	Z None	Z None

New/Revised Text in Green   deleted Deleted   ♀ Females Only   ♂ Males Only   **Coding Clinic**
Non-covered   Limited Coverage   ⊞ Combination (See Appendix E)   DRG Non-OR   Non-OR   Hospital-Acquired Condition

SECTION: D RADIATION THERAPY
BODY SYSTEM: G ENDOCRINE SYSTEM
MODALITY: Ø BEAM RADIATION

Treatment Site	Modality Qualifier	Isotope	Qualifier
Ø Pituitary Gland 1 Pineal Body 2 Adrenal Glands 4 Parathyroid Glands 5 Thyroid	Ø Photons <1 MeV 1 Photons 1 - 1Ø MeV 2 Photons >1Ø MeV 5 Neutrons 6 Neutron Capture	Z None	Z None
Ø Pituitary Gland 1 Pineal Body 2 Adrenal Glands 4 Parathyroid Glands 5 Thyroid	3 Electrons	Z None	Ø Intraoperative Z None

SECTION: D RADIATION THERAPY
BODY SYSTEM: G ENDOCRINE SYSTEM
MODALITY: 1 BRACHYTHERAPY

Treatment Site	Modality Qualifier	Isotope	Qualifier
Ø Pituitary Gland 1 Pineal Body 2 Adrenal Glands 4 Parathyroid Glands 5 Thyroid	9 High Dose Rate (HDR) B Low Dose Rate (LDR)	7 Cesium 137 (Cs-137) 8 Iridium 192 (Ir-192) 9 Iodine 125 (I-125) B Palladium 1Ø3 (Pd-1Ø3) C Californium 252 (Cf-252) Y Other Isotope	Z None

SECTION: D RADIATION THERAPY
BODY SYSTEM: G ENDOCRINE SYSTEM
MODALITY: 2 STEREOTACTIC RADIOSURGERY

Treatment Site	Modality Qualifier	Isotope	Qualifier

Ø Pituitary Gland
1 Pineal Body
2 Adrenal Glands
4 Parathyroid Glands
5 Thyroid
	D Stereotactic Other Photon
	   Radiosurgery
	H Stereotactic Particulate
	   Radiosurgery
	J Stereotactic Gamma Beam
	   Radiosurgery
		Z None	Z None

DRG Non-OR All Values

SECTION: D RADIATION THERAPY
BODY SYSTEM: G ENDOCRINE SYSTEM
MODALITY: Y OTHER RADIATION

Treatment Site	Modality Qualifier	Isotope	Qualifier
Ø Pituitary Gland 1 Pineal Body 2 Adrenal Glands 4 Parathyroid Glands 5 Thyroid	7 Contact Radiation 8 Hyperthermia F Plaque Radiation K Laser Interstitial Thermal Therapy	Z None	Z None

New/Revised Text in Green   ~~deleted~~ Deleted   ♀ Females Only   ♂ Males Only   **Coding Clinic**

Non-covered   Limited Coverage   Combination (See Appendix E)   DRG Non-OR   Non-OR   Hospital-Acquired Condition

SECTION: **D RADIATION THERAPY**
BODY SYSTEM: H SKIN
MODALITY: Ø BEAM RADIATION

Treatment Site	Modality Qualifier	Isotope	Qualifier
2 Skin, Face 3 Skin, Neck 4 Skin, Arm 6 Skin, Chest 7 Skin, Back 8 Skin, Abdomen 9 Skin, Buttock B Skin, Leg	Ø Photons <1 MeV 1 Photons 1 - 1Ø MeV 2 Photons >1Ø MeV 4 Heavy Particles (Protons, Ions) 5 Neutrons 6 Neutron Capture	Z None	Z None
2 Skin, Face 3 Skin, Neck 4 Skin, Arm 6 Skin, Chest 7 Skin, Back 8 Skin, Abdomen 9 Skin, Buttock B Skin, Leg	3 Electrons	Z None	Ø Intraoperative Z None

SECTION: **D RADIATION THERAPY**
BODY SYSTEM: H SKIN
MODALITY: Y OTHER RADIATION

Treatment Site	Modality Qualifier	Isotope	Qualifier
2 Skin, Face 3 Skin, Neck 4 Skin, Arm 6 Skin, Chest 7 Skin, Back 8 Skin, Abdomen 9 Skin, Buttock B Skin, Leg	7 Contact Radiation 8 Hyperthermia F Plaque Radiation	Z None	Z None
5 Skin, Hand C Skin, Foot	F Plaque Radiation	Z None	Z None

SECTION: D RADIATION THERAPY
BODY SYSTEM: M BREAST
MODALITY: Ø BEAM RADIATION

Treatment Site	Modality Qualifier	Isotope	Qualifier
Ø Breast, Left 1 Breast, Right	Ø Photons <1 MeV 1 Photons 1 - 1Ø MeV 2 Photons >1Ø MeV 4 Heavy Particles (Protons, Ions) 5 Neutrons 6 Neutron Capture	Z None	Z None
Ø Breast, Left 1 Breast, Right	3 Electrons	Z None	Ø Intraoperative Z None

SECTION: D RADIATION THERAPY
BODY SYSTEM: M BREAST
MODALITY: 1 BRACHYTHERAPY

Treatment Site	Modality Qualifier	Isotope	Qualifier
Ø Breast, Left 1 Breast, Right	9 High Dose Rate (HDR) B Low Dose Rate (LDR)	7 Cesium 137 (Cs-137) 8 Iridium 192 (Ir-192) 9 Iodine 125 (I-125) B Palladium 1Ø3 (Pd-1Ø3) C Californium 252 (Cf-252) Y Other Isotope	Z None

SECTION: D RADIATION THERAPY
BODY SYSTEM: M BREAST
MODALITY: 2 STEREOTACTIC RADIOSURGERY

Treatment Site	Modality Qualifier	Isotope	Qualifier
Ø Breast, Left 1 Breast, Right	D Stereotactic Other Photon Radiosurgery H Stereotactic Particulate Radiosurgery J Stereotactic Gamma Beam Radiosurgery	Z None	Z None

DRG Non-OR All Values

SECTION: D RADIATION THERAPY
BODY SYSTEM: M BREAST
MODALITY: Y OTHER RADIATION

Treatment Site	Modality Qualifier	Isotope	Qualifier
Ø Breast, Left 1 Breast, Right	7 Contact Radiation 8 Hyperthermia F Plaque Radiation K Laser Interstitial Thermal Therapy	Z None	Z None

D: RADIATION THERAPY   M: BREAST   Ø;   1;   2;   Y

SECTION: D RADIATION THERAPY
BODY SYSTEM: P MUSCULOSKELETAL SYSTEM
MODALITY: Ø BEAM RADIATION

Treatment Site	Modality Qualifier	Isotope	Qualifier
Ø Skull 2 Maxilla 3 Mandible 4 Sternum 5 Rib(s) 6 Humerus 7 Radius/Ulna 8 Pelvic Bones 9 Femur B Tibia/Fibula C Other Bone	Ø Photons <1 MeV 1 Photons 1 - 1Ø MeV 2 Photons >1Ø MeV 4 Heavy Particles (Protons, Ions) 5 Neutrons 6 Neutron Capture	Z None	Z None
Ø Skull 2 Maxilla 3 Mandible 4 Sternum 5 Rib(s) 6 Humerus 7 Radius/Ulna 8 Pelvic Bones 9 Femur B Tibia/Fibula C Other Bone	3 Electrons	Z None	Ø Intraoperative Z None

SECTION: D RADIATION THERAPY
BODY SYSTEM: P MUSCULOSKELETAL SYSTEM
MODALITY: Y OTHER RADIATION

Treatment Site	Modality Qualifier	Isotope	Qualifier
Ø Skull 2 Maxilla 3 Mandible 4 Sternum 5 Rib(s) 6 Humerus 7 Radius/Ulna 8 Pelvic Bones 9 Femur B Tibia/Fibula C Other Bone	7 Contact Radiation 8 Hyperthermia F Plaque Radiation	Z None	Z None

New/Revised Text in Green   ~~deleted~~ Deleted   ♀ Females Only   ♂ Males Only   **Coding Clinic**

Non-covered   Limited Coverage   ⊡ Combination (See Appendix E)   DRG Non-OR   Non-OR   Hospital-Acquired Condition

SECTION: D RADIATION THERAPY
BODY SYSTEM: T URINARY SYSTEM
MODALITY: Ø BEAM RADIATION

Treatment Site	Modality Qualifier	Isotope	Qualifier
Ø Kidney 1 Ureter 2 Bladder 3 Urethra	Ø Photons <1 MeV 1 Photons 1 - 1Ø MeV 2 Photons >1Ø MeV 4 Heavy Particles (Protons, Ions) 5 Neutrons 6 Neutron Capture	Z None	Z None
Ø Kidney 1 Ureter 2 Bladder 3 Urethra	3 Electrons	Z None	Ø Intraoperative Z None

SECTION: D RADIATION THERAPY
BODY SYSTEM: T URINARY SYSTEM
MODALITY: 1 BRACHYTHERAPY

Treatment Site	Modality Qualifier	Isotope	Qualifier
Ø Kidney 1 Ureter 2 Bladder 3 Urethra	9 High Dose Rate (HDR) B Low Dose Rate (LDR)	7 Cesium 137 (Cs-137) 8 Iridium 192 (Ir-192) 9 Iodine 125 (I-125) B Palladium 1Ø3 (Pd-1Ø3) C Californium 252 (Cf-252) Y Other Isotope	Z None

SECTION: D RADIATION THERAPY
BODY SYSTEM: T URINARY SYSTEM
MODALITY: 2 STEREOTACTIC RADIOSURGERY

Treatment Site	Modality Qualifier	Isotope	Qualifier
Ø Kidney 1 Ureter 2 Bladder 3 Urethra	D Stereotactic Other Photon Radiosurgery H Stereotactic Particulate Radiosurgery J Stereotactic Gamma Beam Radiosurgery	Z None	Z None

DRG Non-OR All Values

SECTION: D RADIATION THERAPY
BODY SYSTEM: T URINARY SYSTEM
MODALITY: Y OTHER RADIATION

Treatment Site	Modality Qualifier	Isotope	Qualifier
Ø Kidney 1 Ureter 2 Bladder 3 Urethra	7 Contact Radiation 8 Hyperthermia C Intraoperative Radiation Therapy (IORT) F Plaque Radiation	Z None	Z None

New/Revised Text in Green   deleted Deleted   ♀ Females Only   ♂ Males Only   **Coding Clinic**
🚫 Non-covered   🚫 Limited Coverage   ⊞ Combination (See Appendix E)   DRG Non-OR   Non-OR   🚫 Hospital-Acquired Condition

SECTION: D RADIATION THERAPY
BODY SYSTEM: U FEMALE REPRODUCTIVE SYSTEM
MODALITY: Ø BEAM RADIATION

Treatment Site	Modality Qualifier	Isotope	Qualifier
Ø Ovary ♀ 1 Cervix ♀ 2 Uterus ♀	Ø Photons <1 MeV 1 Photons 1 - 1Ø MeV 2 Photons >1Ø MeV 4 Heavy Particles (Protons, Ions) 5 Neutrons 6 Neutron Capture	Z None	Z None
Ø Ovary ♀ 1 Cervix ♀ 2 Uterus ♀	3 Electrons	Z None	Ø Intraoperative Z None

SECTION: D RADIATION THERAPY
BODY SYSTEM: U FEMALE REPRODUCTIVE SYSTEM
MODALITY: 1 BRACHYTHERAPY

Treatment Site	Modality Qualifier	Isotope	Qualifier
Ø Ovary ♀ 1 Cervix ♀ 2 Uterus ♀	9 High Dose Rate (HDR) B Low Dose Rate (LDR)	7 Cesium 137 (Cs-137) 8 Iridium 192 (Ir-192) 9 Iodine 125 (I-125) B Palladium 1Ø3 (Pd-1Ø3) C Californium 252 (Cf-252) Y Other Isotope	Z None

Coding Clinic: 2Ø17, Q4, P1Ø4 – DU11B7Z

SECTION: D RADIATION THERAPY
BODY SYSTEM: U FEMALE REPRODUCTIVE SYSTEM
MODALITY: 2 STEREOTACTIC RADIOSURGERY

Treatment Site	Modality Qualifier	Isotope	Qualifier
Ø Ovary ♀ 1 Cervix ♀ 2 Uterus ♀	D Stereotactic Other Photon Radiosurgery H Stereotactic Particulate Radiosurgery J Stereotactic Gamma Beam Radiosurgery	Z None	Z None

DRG Non-OR   All Values

SECTION: D RADIATION THERAPY
BODY SYSTEM: U FEMALE REPRODUCTIVE SYSTEM
MODALITY: Y OTHER RADIATION

Treatment Site	Modality Qualifier	Isotope	Qualifier
Ø Ovary ♀ 1 Cervix ♀ 2 Uterus ♀	7 Contact Radiation 8 Hyperthermia C Intraoperative Radiation Therapy (IORT) F Plaque Radiation	Z None	Z None

SECTION: D RADIATION THERAPY

BODY SYSTEM: V MALE REPRODUCTIVE SYSTEM
MODALITY: Ø BEAM RADIATION

Treatment Site	Modality Qualifier	Isotope	Qualifier
Ø Prostate ♂ 1 Testis ♂	Ø Photons <1 MeV 1 Photons 1 - 1Ø MeV 2 Photons >1Ø MeV 4 Heavy Particles (Protons, Ions) 5 Neutrons 6 Neutron Capture	Z None	Z None
Ø Prostate ♂ 1 Testis ♂	3 Electrons	Z None	Ø Intraoperative Z None

SECTION: D RADIATION THERAPY

BODY SYSTEM: V MALE REPRODUCTIVE SYSTEM
MODALITY: 1 BRACHYTHERAPY

Treatment Site	Modality Qualifier	Isotope	Qualifier
Ø Prostate ♂ 1 Testis ♂	9 High Dose Rate (HDR) B Low Dose Rate (LDR)	7 Cesium 137 (Cs-137) 8 Iridium 192 (Ir-192) 9 Iodine 125 (I-125) B Palladium 1Ø3 (Pd-1Ø3) C Californium 252 (Cf-252) Y Other Isotope	Z None

New/Revised Text in Green   ~~deleted~~ Deleted   ♀ Females Only   ♂ Males Only   **Coding Clinic**
🞫 Non-covered   🞫 Limited Coverage   ⊞ Combination (See Appendix E)   DRG Non-OR   Non-OR   🞫 Hospital-Acquired Condition

SECTION: D RADIATION THERAPY
BODY SYSTEM: V MALE REPRODUCTIVE SYSTEM
MODALITY: 2 STEREOTACTIC RADIOSURGERY

Treatment Site	Modality Qualifier	Isotope	Qualifier
Ø Prostate ♂ 1 Testis ♂	D Stereotactic Other Photon Radiosurgery H Stereotactic Particulate Radiosurgery J Stereotactic Gamma Beam Radiosurgery	Z None	Z None

DRG Non-OR All Values

SECTION: D RADIATION THERAPY
BODY SYSTEM: V MALE REPRODUCTIVE SYSTEM
MODALITY: Y OTHER RADIATION

Treatment Site	Modality Qualifier	Isotope	Qualifier
Ø Prostate ♂	7 Contact Radiation 8 Hyperthermia C Intraoperative Radiation Therapy (IORT) F Plaque Radiation K Laser Interstitial Thermal Therapy	Z None	Z None
1 Testis ♂	7 Contact Radiation 8 Hyperthermia F Plaque Radiation	Z None	Z None

SECTION: **D RADIATION THERAPY**

BODY SYSTEM: W ANATOMICAL REGIONS

MODALITY: Ø BEAM RADIATION

Treatment Site	Modality Qualifier	Isotope	Qualifier
1 Head and Neck 2 Chest 3 Abdomen 4 Hemibody 5 Whole Body 6 Pelvic Region	Ø Photons <1 MeV 1 Photons 1 - 1Ø MeV 2 Photons >1Ø MeV 4 Heavy Particles (Protons, Ions) 5 Neutrons 6 Neutron Capture	Z None	Z None
1 Head and Neck 2 Chest 3 Abdomen 4 Hemibody 5 Whole Body 6 Pelvic Region	3 Electrons	Z None	Ø Intraoperative Z None

SECTION: **D RADIATION THERAPY**

BODY SYSTEM: W ANATOMICAL REGIONS

MODALITY: 1 BRACHYTHERAPY

Treatment Site	Modality Qualifier	Isotope	Qualifier
1 Head and Neck 2 Chest 3 Abdomen 6 Pelvic Region	9 High Dose Rate (HDR) B Low Dose Rate (LDR)	7 Cesium 137 (Cs-137) 8 Iridium 192 (Ir-192) 9 Iodine 125 (I-125) B Palladium 1Ø3 (Pd-1Ø3) C Californium 252 (Cf-252) Y Other Isotope	Z None

SECTION: D RADIATION THERAPY
BODY SYSTEM: W ANATOMICAL REGIONS
MODALITY: 2 STEREOTACTIC RADIOSURGERY

Treatment Site	Modality Qualifier	Isotope	Qualifier
1 Head and Neck 2 Chest 3 Abdomen 6 Pelvic Region	D Stereotactic Other Photon Radiosurgery H Stereotactic Particulate Radiosurgery J Stereotactic Gamma Beam Radiosurgery	Z None	Z None

`DRG Non-OR` All Values

SECTION: D RADIATION THERAPY
BODY SYSTEM: W ANATOMICAL REGIONS
MODALITY: Y OTHER RADIATION

Treatment Site	Modality Qualifier	Isotope	Qualifier
1 Head and Neck 2 Chest 3 Abdomen 4 Hemibody 6 Pelvic Region	7 Contact Radiation 8 Hyperthermia F Plaque Radiation	Z None	Z None
5 Whole Body	7 Contact Radiation 8 Hyperthermia F Plaque Radiation	Z None	Z None
5 Whole Body	G Isotope Administration	D Iodine 131 (I-131) F Phosphorus 32 (P-32) G Strontium 89 (Sr-89) H Strontium 90 (Sr-90) Y Other Isotope	Z None

New/Revised Text in Green   ~~deleted~~ Deleted   ♀ Females Only   ♂ Males Only   **Coding Clinic**
🕭 Non-covered   🕭 Limited Coverage   ⊞ Combination (See Appendix E)   `DRG Non-OR`   Non-OR   🕭 Hospital-Acquired Condition

F Physical Rehabilitation and Diagnostic Audiology

SECTION: F PHYSICAL REHABILITATION AND DIAGNOSTIC AUDIOLOGY

SECTION QUALIFIER: 0 REHABILITATION

TYPE: **0** **SPEECH ASSESSMENT:** *(on multiple pages)*
Measurement of speech and related functions

Body System – Body Region	Type Qualifier	Equipment	Qualifier
3 Neurological System - Whole Body	G Communicative/Cognitive Integration Skills	K Audiovisual M Augmentative/Alternative Communication P Computer Y Other Equipment Z None	Z None
Z None	0 Filtered Speech 3 Staggered Spondaic Word Q Performance Intensity Phonetically Balanced Speech Discrimination R Brief Tone Stimuli S Distorted Speech T Dichotic Stimuli V Temporal Ordering of Stimuli W Masking Patterns	1 Audiometer 2 Sound Field/Booth K Audiovisual Z None	Z None
Z None	1 Speech Threshold 2 Speech/Word Recognition	1 Audiometer 2 Sound Field/Booth 9 Cochlear Implant K Audiovisual Z None	Z None
Z None	4 Sensorineural Acuity Level	1 Audiometer 2 Sound Field/Booth Z None	Z None
Z None	5 Synthetic Sentence Identification	1 Audiometer 2 Sound Field/Booth 9 Cochlear Implant K Audiovisual	Z None
Z None	6 Speech and/or Language Screening 7 Nonspoken Language 8 Receptive/Expressive Language C Aphasia G Communicative/Cognitive Integration Skills L Augmentative/Alternative Communication System	K Audiovisual M Augmentative/Alternative Communication P Computer Y Other Equipment Z None	Z None
Z None	9 Articulation/Phonology	K Audiovisual P Computer Q Speech Analysis Y Other Equipment Z None	Z None
Z None	B Motor Speech	K Audiovisual N Biosensory Feedback P Computer Q Speech Analysis T Aerodynamic Function Y Other Equipment Z None	Z None

DRG Non-OR   All Values

SECTION: F PHYSICAL REHABILITATION AND DIAGNOSTIC AUDIOLOGY

SECTION QUALIFIER: Ø REHABILITATION
TYPE: Ø SPEECH ASSESSMENT: *(continued)*
Measurement of speech and related functions

Body System – Body Region	Type Qualifier	Equipment	Qualifier
Z None	D Fluency	K Audiovisual N Biosensory Feedback P Computer Q Speech Analysis S Voice Analysis T Aerodynamic Function Y Other Equipment Z None	Z None
Z None	F Voice	K Audiovisual N Biosensory Feedback P Computer S Voice Analysis T Aerodynamic Function Y Other Equipment Z None	Z None
Z None	H Bedside Swallowing and Oral Function P Oral Peripheral Mechanism	Y Other Equipment Z None	Z None
Z None	J Instrumental Swallowing and Oral Function	T Aerodynamic Function W Swallowing Y Other Equipment	Z None
Z None	K Orofacial Myofunctional	K Audiovisual P Computer Y Other Equipment Z None	Z None
Z None	M Voice Prosthetic	K Audiovisual P Computer S Voice Analysis V Speech Prosthesis Y Other Equipment Z None	Z None
Z None	N Non-invasive Instrumental Status	N Biosensory Feedback P Computer Q Speech Analysis S Voice Analysis T Aerodynamic Function Y Other Equipment	Z None
Z None	X Other Specified Central Auditory Processing	Z None	Z None

DRG Non-OR All Values

SECTION: F PHYSICAL REHABILITATION AND DIAGNOSTIC AUDIOLOGY

SECTION QUALIFIER: Ø **REHABILITATION**

TYPE: 1 **MOTOR AND/OR NERVE FUNCTION ASSESSMENT:** *(on multiple pages)*
Measurement of motor, nerve, and related functions

Body System – Body Region	Type Qualifier	Equipment	Qualifier
Ø Neurological System - Head and Neck 1 Neurological System - Upper Back/Upper Extremity 2 Neurological System - Lower Back/Lower Extremity 3 Neurological System - Whole Body	Ø Muscle Performance	E Orthosis F Assistive, Adaptive, Supportive or Protective U Prosthesis Y Other Equipment Z None	Z None
Ø Neurological System - Head and Neck 1 Neurological System - Upper Back/Upper Extremity 2 Neurological System - Lower Back/Lower Extremity 3 Neurological System - Whole Body	1 Integumentary Integrity 3 Coordination/Dexterity 4 Motor Function G Reflex Integrity	Z None	Z None
Ø Neurological System - Head and Neck 1 Neurological System - Upper Back/Upper Extremity 2 Neurological System - Lower Back/Lower Extremity 3 Neurological System - Whole Body	5 Range of Motion and Joint Integrity 6 Sensory Awareness/Processing/Integrity	Y Other Equipment Z None	Z None
D Integumentary System - Head and Neck F Integumentary System - Upper Back/Upper Extremity G Integumentary System - Lower Back/Lower Extremity H Integumentary System - Whole Body J Musculoskeletal System - Head and Neck K Musculoskeletal System - Upper Back/Upper Extremity L Musculoskeletal System - Lower Back/Lower Extremity M Musculoskeletal System - Whole Body	Ø Muscle Performance	E Orthosis F Assistive, Adaptive, Supportive or Protective U Prosthesis Y Other Equipment Z None	Z None
D Integumentary System - Head and Neck F Integumentary System - Upper Back/Upper Extremity G Integumentary System - Lower Back/Lower Extremity H Integumentary System - Whole Body J Musculoskeletal System - Head and Neck K Musculoskeletal System - Upper Back/Upper Extremity L Musculoskeletal System - Lower Back/Lower Extremity M Musculoskeletal System - Whole Body	1 Integumentary Integrity	Z None	Z None
D Integumentary System - Head and Neck F Integumentary System - Upper Back/Upper Extremity G Integumentary System - Lower Back/Lower Extremity H Integumentary System - Whole Body J Musculoskeletal System - Head and Neck K Musculoskeletal System - Upper Back/Upper Extremity L Musculoskeletal System - Lower Back/Lower Extremity M Musculoskeletal System - Whole Body	5 Range of Motion and Joint Integrity 6 Sensory Awareness/Processing/Integrity	Y Other Equipment Z None	Z None

DRG Non-OR All Values

SECTION: F PHYSICAL REHABILITATION AND DIAGNOSTIC AUDIOLOGY

SECTION QUALIFIER: Ø   REHABILITATION

TYPE: 1   MOTOR AND/OR NERVE FUNCTION ASSESSMENT: *(continued)*

Measurement of motor, nerve, and related functions

Body System – Body Region	Type Qualifier	Equipment	Qualifier
N Genitourinary System	Ø Muscle Performance	E Orthosis F Assistive, Adaptive, Supportive or Protective U Prosthesis Y Other Equipment Z None	Z None
Z None	2 Visual Motor Integration	K Audiovisual M Augmentative/Alternative Communication N Biosensory Feedback P Computer Q Speech Analysis S Voice Analysis Y Other Equipment Z None	Z None
Z None	7 Facial Nerve Function	7 Electrophysiologic	Z None
Z None	9 Somatosensory Evoked Potentials	J Somatosensory	Z None
Z None	B Bed Mobility C Transfer F Wheelchair Mobility	E Orthosis F Assistive, Adaptive, Supportive or Protective U Prosthesis Z None	Z None
Z None	D Gait and/or Balance	E Orthosis F Assistive, Adaptive, Supportive or Protective U Prosthesis Y Other Equipment Z None	Z None

DRG Non-OR   All Values

Side tab: 1 · Ø: REHABILITATION · F: PHYSICAL REHABILITATION AND DIAGNOSTIC AUDIOLOGY

SECTION: F PHYSICAL REHABILITATION AND
                              DIAGNOSTIC AUDIOLOGY

SECTION QUALIFIER: Ø **REHABILITATION**

TYPE: 2 **ACTIVITIES OF DAILY LIVING ASSESSMENT:** *(on multiple pages)*
Measurement of functional level for activities of daily living

Body System – Body Region	Type Qualifier	Equipment	Qualifier
Ø Neurological System - Head and Neck	9 Cranial Nerve Integrity D Neuromotor Development	Y Other Equipment Z None	Z None
1 Neurological System - Upper Back/Upper Extremity 2 Neurological System - Lower Back/Lower Extremity 3 Neurological System - Whole Body	D Neuromotor Development	Y Other Equipment Z None	Z None
4 Circulatory System - Head and Neck 5 Circulatory System - Upper Back/Upper Extremity 6 Circulatory System - Lower Back/Lower Extremity 8 Respiratory System - Head and Neck 9 Respiratory System - Upper Back/Upper Extremity B Respiratory System - Lower Back/Lower Extremity	G Ventilation, Respiration and Circulation	C Mechanical G Aerobic Endurance and Conditioning Y Other Equipment Z None	Z None
7 Circulatory System - Whole Body C Respiratory System - Whole Body	7 Aerobic Capacity and Endurance	E Orthosis G Aerobic Endurance and Conditioning U Prosthesis Y Other Equipment Z None	Z None
7 Circulatory System - Whole Body C Respiratory System - Whole Body	G Ventilation, Respiration and Circulation	C Mechanical G Aerobic Endurance and Conditioning Y Other Equipment Z None	Z None

DRG Non-OR All Values

SECTION: F PHYSICAL REHABILITATION AND DIAGNOSTIC AUDIOLOGY

SECTION QUALIFIER: Ø REHABILITATION

TYPE: 2 ACTIVITIES OF DAILY LIVING ASSESSMENT: *(continued)*

Measurement of functional level for activities of daily living

Body System – Body Region	Type Qualifier	Equipment	Qualifier
Z None	Ø Bathing/Showering 1 Dressing 3 Grooming/Personal Hygiene 4 Home Management	E Orthosis F Assistive, Adaptive, Supportive or Protective U Prosthesis Z None	Z None
Z None	2 Feeding/Eating 8 Anthropometric Characteristics F Pain	Y Other Equipment Z None	Z None
Z None	5 Perceptual Processing	K Audiovisual M Augmentative/Alternative Communication N Biosensory Feedback P Computer Q Speech Analysis S Voice Analysis Y Other Equipment Z None	Z None
Z None	6 Psychosocial Skills	Z None	Z None
Z None	B Environmental, Home and Work Barriers C Ergonomics and Body Mechanics	E Orthosis F Assistive, Adaptive, Supportive or Protective U Prosthesis Y Other Equipment Z None	Z None
Z None	H Vocational Activities and Functional Community or Work Reintegration Skills	E Orthosis F Assistive, Adaptive, Supportive or Protective G Aerobic Endurance and Conditioning U Prosthesis Y Other Equipment Z None	Z None

DRG Non-OR   All Values

SECTION: F PHYSICAL REHABILITATION AND DIAGNOSTIC AUDIOLOGY

SECTION QUALIFIER: Ø REHABILITATION

TYPE: 6 SPEECH TREATMENT: *(on multiple pages)*

Application of techniques to improve, augment, or compensate for speech and related functional impairment

Body System – Body Region	Type Qualifier	Equipment	Qualifier
3 Neurological System - Whole Body	6 Communicative/Cognitive Integration Skills	K Audiovisual M Augmentative/Alternative Communication P Computer Y Other Equipment Z None	Z None
Z None	Ø Nonspoken Language 3 Aphasia 6 Communicative/Cognitive Integration Skills	K Audiovisual M Augmentative/Alternative Communication P Computer Y Other Equipment Z None	Z None
Z None	1 Speech-Language Pathology and Related Disorders Counseling 2 Speech-Language Pathology and Related Disorders Prevention	K Audiovisual Z None	Z None
Z None	4 Articulation/Phonology	K Audiovisual P Computer Q Speech Analysis T Aerodynamic Function Y Other Equipment Z None	Z None
Z None	5 Aural Rehabilitation	K Audiovisual L Assistive Listening M Augmentative/Alternative Communication N Biosensory Feedback P Computer Q Speech Analysis S Voice Analysis Y Other Equipment Z None	Z None
Z None	7 Fluency	4 Electroacoustic Immitance/ Acoustic Reflex K Audiovisual N Biosensory Feedback Q Speech Analysis S Voice Analysis T Aerodynamic Function Y Other Equipment Z None	Z None

`DRG Non-OR` All Values

New/Revised Text in Green   ~~deleted~~ Deleted   ♀ Females Only   ♂ Males Only   **Coding Clinic**

🔹 Non-covered   🔹 Limited Coverage   ⊡ Combination (See Appendix E)   `DRG Non-OR`   Non-OR   🔹 Hospital-Acquired Condition

6: SPEECH TREATMENT

0: REHABILITATION

F: PHYSICAL REHABILITATION AND DIAGNOSTIC AUDIOLOGY

SECTION: F PHYSICAL REHABILITATION AND DIAGNOSTIC AUDIOLOGY

SECTION QUALIFIER: 0 REHABILITATION
TYPE: 6 SPEECH TREATMENT: *(continued)*
Application of techniques to improve, augment, or compensate for speech and related functional impairment

Body System – Body Region	Type Qualifier	Equipment	Qualifier
Z None	8 Motor Speech	K Audiovisual N Biosensory Feedback P Computer Q Speech Analysis S Voice Analysis T Aerodynamic Function Y Other Equipment Z None	Z None
Z None	9 Orofacial Myofunctional	K Audiovisual P Computer Y Other Equipment Z None	Z None
Z None	B Receptive/Expressive Language	K Audiovisual L Assistive Listening M Augmentative/Alternative Communication P Computer Y Other Equipment Z None	Z None
Z None	C Voice	K Audiovisual N Biosensory Feedback P Computer S Voice Analysis T Aerodynamic Function V Speech Prosthesis Y Other Equipment Z None	Z None
Z None	D Swallowing Dysfunction	M Augmentative/Alternative Communication T Aerodynamic Function V Speech Prosthesis Y Other Equipment Z None	Z None

DRG Non-OR   All Values

SECTION: F PHYSICAL REHABILITATION AND DIAGNOSTIC AUDIOLOGY

SECTION QUALIFIER: Ø REHABILITATION

TYPE: 7 MOTOR TREATMENT: *(on multiple pages)*

Exercise or activities to increase or facilitate motor function

Body System – Body Region	Type Qualifier	Equipment	Qualifier
Ø Neurological System - Head and Neck 1 Neurological System - Upper Back/Upper Extremity 2 Neurological System - Lower Back/Lower Extremity 3 Neurological System - Whole Body D Integumentary System - Head and Neck F Integumentary System - Upper Back/Upper Extremity G Integumentary System - Lower Back/Lower Extremity H Integumentary System - Whole Body J Musculoskeletal System - Head and Neck K Musculoskeletal System - Upper Back/Upper Extremity L Musculoskeletal System - Lower Back/Lower Extremity M Musculoskeletal System - Whole Body	Ø Range of Motion and Joint Mobility 1 Muscle Performance 2 Coordination/Dexterity 3 Motor Function	E Orthosis F Assistive, Adaptive, Supportive or Protective U Prosthesis Y Other Equipment Z None	Z None
Ø Neurological System - Head and Neck 1 Neurological System - Upper Back/Upper Extremity 2 Neurological System - Lower Back/Lower Extremity 3 Neurological System - Whole Body D Integumentary System - Head and Neck F Integumentary System - Upper Back/Upper Extremity G Integumentary System - Lower Back/Lower Extremity H Integumentary System - Whole Body J Musculoskeletal System - Head and Neck K Musculoskeletal System - Upper Back/Upper Extremity L Musculoskeletal System - Lower Back/Lower Extremity M Musculoskeletal System - Whole Body	6 Therapeutic Exercise	B Physical Agents C Mechanical D Electrotherapeutic E Orthosis F Assistive, Adaptive, Supportive or Protective G Aerobic Endurance and Conditioning H Mechanical or Electromechanical U Prosthesis Y Other Equipment Z None	Z None
Ø Neurological System - Head and Neck 1 Neurological System - Upper Back/Upper Extremity 2 Neurological System - Lower Back/Lower Extremity 3 Neurological System - Whole Body D Integumentary System - Head and Neck F Integumentary System - Upper Back/Upper Extremity G Integumentary System - Lower Back/Lower Extremity H Integumentary System - Whole Body J Musculoskeletal System - Head and Neck K Musculoskeletal System - Upper Back/Upper Extremity L Musculoskeletal System - Lower Back/Lower Extremity M Musculoskeletal System - Whole Body	7 Manual Therapy Techniques	Z None	Z None

DRG Non-OR **All Values**

7: MOTOR TREATMENT

Ø: REHABILITATION

F: PHYSICAL REHABILITATION AND DIAGNOSTIC AUDIOLOGY

SECTION: F PHYSICAL REHABILITATION AND DIAGNOSTIC AUDIOLOGY

SECTION QUALIFIER: Ø REHABILITATION

TYPE: 7 MOTOR TREATMENT: *(continued)*
Exercise or activities to increase or facilitate motor function

Body System – Body Region	Type Qualifier	Equipment	Qualifier
4 Circulatory System - Head and Neck 5 Circulatory System - Upper Back/Upper Extremity 6 Circulatory System - Lower Back/Lower Extremity 7 Circulatory System - Whole Body 8 Respiratory System - Head and Neck 9 Respiratory System - Upper Back/Upper Extremity B Respiratory System - Lower Back/Lower Extremity C Respiratory System - Whole Body	6 Therapeutic Exercise	B Physical Agents C Mechanical D Electrotherapeutic E Orthosis F Assistive, Adaptive, Supportive or Protective G Aerobic Endurance and Conditioning H Mechanical or Electromechanical U Prosthesis Y Other Equipment Z None	Z None
N Genitourinary System	1 Muscle Performance	E Orthosis F Assistive, Adaptive, Supportive or Protective U Prosthesis Y Other Equipment Z None	Z None
N Genitourinary System	6 Therapeutic Exercise	B Physical Agents C Mechanical D Electrotherapeutic E Orthosis F Assistive, Adaptive, Supportive or Protective G Aerobic Endurance and Conditioning H Mechanical or Electromechanical U Prosthesis Y Other Equipment Z None	Z None
Z None	4 Wheelchair Mobility	D Electrotherapeutic E Orthosis F Assistive, Adaptive, Supportive or Protective U Prosthesis Y Other Equipment Z None	Z None
Z None	5 Bed Mobility	C Mechanical E Orthosis F Assistive, Adaptive, Supportive or Protective U Prosthesis Y Other Equipment Z None	Z None
Z None	8 Transfer Training	C Mechanical D Electrotherapeutic E Orthosis F Assistive, Adaptive, Supportive or Protective U Prosthesis Y Other Equipment Z None	Z None
Z None	9 Gait Training/Functional Ambulation	C Mechanical D Electrotherapeutic E Orthosis F Assistive, Adaptive, Supportive or Protective G Aerobic Endurance and Conditioning U Prosthesis Y Other Equipment Z None	Z None

New/Revised Text in Green ~~deleted~~ Deleted ♀ Females Only ♂ Males Only **Coding Clinic**
🔖 Non-covered 🔖 Limited Coverage ⊞ Combination (See Appendix E) DRG Non-OR Non-OR 🔖 Hospital-Acquired Condition

SECTION: F PHYSICAL REHABILITATION AND DIAGNOSTIC AUDIOLOGY

SECTION QUALIFIER: Ø REHABILITATION

TYPE: 8 ACTIVITIES OF DAILY LIVING TREATMENT: Exercise or activities to facilitate functional competence for activities of daily living

Body System – Body Region	Type Qualifier	Equipment	Qualifier
D Integumentary System - Head and Neck F Integumentary System - Upper Back/Upper Extremity G Integumentary System - Lower Back/Lower Extremity H Integumentary System - Whole Body J Musculoskeletal System - Head and Neck K Musculoskeletal System - Upper Back/Upper Extremity L Musculoskeletal System - Lower Back/Lower Extremity M Musculoskeletal System - Whole Body	5 Wound Management	B Physical Agents C Mechanical D Electrotherapeutic E Orthosis F Assistive, Adaptive, Supportive or Protective U Prosthesis Y Other Equipment Z None	Z None
Z None	Ø Bathing/Showering Techniques 1 Dressing Techniques 2 Grooming/Personal Hygiene	E Orthosis F Assistive, Adaptive, Supportive or Protective U Prosthesis Y Other Equipment Z None	Z None
Z None	3 Feeding/Eating	C Mechanical D Electrotherapeutic E Orthosis F Assistive, Adaptive, Supportive or Protective U Prosthesis Y Other Equipment Z None	Z None
Z None	4 Home Management	D Electrotherapeutic E Orthosis F Assistive, Adaptive, Supportive or Protective U Prosthesis Y Other Equipment Z None	Z None
Z None	6 Psychosocial Skills	Z None	Z None
Z None	7 Vocational Activities and Functional Community or Work Reintegration Skills	B Physical Agents C Mechanical D Electrotherapeutic E Orthosis F Assistive, Adaptive, Supportive or Protective G Aerobic Endurance and Conditioning U Prosthesis Y Other Equipment Z None	Z None

DRG Non-OR All Values

SECTION: F PHYSICAL REHABILITATION AND DIAGNOSTIC AUDIOLOGY

SECTION QUALIFIER: Ø REHABILITATION

TYPE: 9 **HEARING TREATMENT:** Application of techniques to improve, augment, or compensate for hearing and related functional impairment

Body System – Body Region	Type Qualifier	Equipment	Qualifier
Z None	Ø Hearing and Related Disorders Counseling 1 Hearing and Related Disorders Prevention	K Audiovisual Z None	Z None
Z None	2 Auditory Processing	K Audiovisual L Assistive Listening P Computer Y Other Equipment Z None	Z None
Z None	3 Cerumen Management	X Cerumen Management Z None	Z None

DRG Non-OR All Values

SECTION: F PHYSICAL REHABILITATION AND DIAGNOSTIC AUDIOLOGY

SECTION QUALIFIER: Ø REHABILITATION

TYPE: B **COCHLEAR IMPLANT TREATMENT:** Application of techniques to improve the communication abilities of individuals with cochlear implant

Body System – Body Region	Type Qualifier	Equipment	Qualifier
Z None	Ø Cochlear Implant Rehabilitation	1 Audiometer 2 Sound Field/Booth 9 Cochlear Implant K Audiovisual P Computer Y Other Equipment	Z None

DRG Non-OR All Values

SECTION: F PHYSICAL REHABILITATION AND DIAGNOSTIC AUDIOLOGY

SECTION QUALIFIER: Ø REHABILITATION
TYPE: **C** **VESTIBULAR TREATMENT:** Application of techniques to improve, augment, or compensate for vestibular and related functional impairment

Body System – Body Region	Type Qualifier	Equipment	Qualifier
3 Neurological System - Whole Body H Integumentary System - Whole Body M Musculoskeletal System - Whole Body	3 Postural Control	E Orthosis F Assistive, Adaptive, Supportive or Protective U Prosthesis Y Other Equipment Z None	Z None
Z None	Ø Vestibular	8 Vestibular/Balance Z None	Z None
Z None	1 Perceptual Processing 2 Visual Motor Integration	K Audiovisual L Assistive Listening N Biosensory Feedback P Computer Q Speech Analysis S Voice Analysis T Aerodynamic Function Y Other Equipment Z None	Z None

DRG Non-OR   All Values

SECTION: F PHYSICAL REHABILITATION AND DIAGNOSTIC AUDIOLOGY

SECTION QUALIFIER: Ø REHABILITATION
TYPE: **D** **DEVICE FITTING:** Fitting of a device designed to facilitate or support achievement of a higher level of function

Body System – Body Region	Type Qualifier	Equipment	Qualifier
Z None	Ø Tinnitus Masker	5 Hearing Aid Selection/Fitting/Test Z None	Z None
Z None	1 Monaural Hearing Aid 2 Binaural Hearing Aid 5 Assistive Listening Device	1 Audiometer 2 Sound Field/Booth 5 Hearing Aid Selection/Fitting/Test K Audiovisual L Assistive Listening Z None	Z None
Z None	3 Augmentative/Alternative Communication System	M Augmentative/Alternative Communication	Z None
Z None	4 Voice Prosthetic	S Voice Analysis V Speech Prosthesis	Z None
Z None	6 Dynamic Orthosis 7 Static Orthosis 8 Prosthesis 9 Assistive, Adaptive, Supportive or Protective Devices	E Orthosis F Assistive, Adaptive, Supportive or Protective U Prosthesis Z None	Z None

DRG Non-OR   FØDZØ[5Z]Z
DRG Non-OR   FØDZ[125][125KLZ]Z
DRG Non-OR   FØDZ3MZ

DRG Non-OR   FØDZ4[SV]Z
DRG Non-OR   FØDZ[67][EFUZ]Z
DRG Non-OR   FØDZ8[EFU]Z

New/Revised Text in Green   ~~deleted~~ Deleted   ♀ Females Only   ♂ Males Only   **Coding Clinic**
⟲ Non-covered   ⟲ Limited Coverage   ⊞ Combination (See Appendix E)   DRG Non-OR   Non-OR   ⟲ Hospital-Acquired Condition

SECTION: F PHYSICAL REHABILITATION AND DIAGNOSTIC AUDIOLOGY

SECTION QUALIFIER: Ø REHABILITATION

TYPE: F **CAREGIVER TRAINING:** Training in activities to support patient's optimal level of function

Body System – Body Region	Type Qualifier	Equipment	Qualifier
Z None	Ø Bathing/Showering Technique 1 Dressing 2 Feeding and Eating 3 Grooming/Personal Hygiene 4 Bed Mobility 5 Transfer 6 Wheelchair Mobility 7 Therapeutic Exercise 8 Airway Clearance Techniques 9 Wound Management B Vocational Activities and Functional Community or Work Reintegration Skills C Gait Training/Functional Ambulation D Application, Proper Use and Care Devices F Application, Proper Use and Care of Orthoses G Application, Proper Use and Care of Prosthesis H Home Management	E Orthosis F Assistive, Adaptive, Supportive or Protective U Prosthesis Z None	Z None
Z None	J Communication Skills	K Audiovisual L Assistive Listening M Augmentative/Alternative Communication P Computer Z None	Z None

DRG Non-OR **All Values**

SECTION: F PHYSICAL REHABILITATION AND DIAGNOSTIC AUDIOLOGY

SECTION QUALIFIER: 1 DIAGNOSTIC AUDIOLOGY

TYPE: 3 **HEARING ASSESSMENT:** Measurement of hearing and related functions

Body System – Body Region	Type Qualifier	Equipment	Qualifier
Z None	Ø Hearing Screening	Ø Occupational Hearing 1 Audiometer 2 Sound Field/Booth 3 Tympanometer 8 Vestibular/Balance 9 Cochlear Implant Z None	Z None
Z None	1 Pure Tone Audiometry, Air 2 Pure Tone Audiometry, Air and Bone	Ø Occupational Hearing 1 Audiometer 2 Sound Field/Booth Z None	Z None
Z None	3 Bekesy Audiometry 6 Visual Reinforcement Audiometry 9 Short Increment Sensitivity Index B Stenger C Pure Tone Stenger	1 Audiometer 2 Sound Field/Booth Z None	Z None
Z None	4 Conditioned Play Audiometry 5 Select Picture Audiometry	1 Audiometer 2 Sound Field/Booth K Audiovisual Z None	Z None
Z None	7 Alternate Binaural or Monaural Loudness Balance	1 Audiometer K Audiovisual Z None	Z None
Z None	8 Tone Decay D Tympanometry F Eustachian Tube Function G Acoustic Reflex Patterns H Acoustic Reflex Threshold J Acoustic Reflex Decay	3 Tympanometer 4 Electroacoustic Immitance/Acoustic Reflex Z None	Z None
Z None	K Electrocochleography L Auditory Evoked Potentials	7 Electrophysiologic Z None	Z None
Z None	M Evoked Otoacoustic Emissions, Screening N Evoked Otoacoustic Emissions, Diagnostic	6 Otoacoustic Emission (OAE) Z None	Z None
Z None	P Aural Rehabilitation Status	1 Audiometer 2 Sound Field/Booth 4 Electroacoustic Immitance/Acoustic Reflex 9 Cochlear Implant K Audiovisual L Assistive Listening P Computer Z None	Z None
Z None	Q Auditory Processing	K Audiovisual P Computer Y Other Equipment Z None	Z None

New/Revised Text in Green   ~~deleted~~ Deleted   ♀ Females Only   ♂ Males Only   **Coding Clinic**

Non-covered   Limited Coverage   Combination (See Appendix E)   DRG Non-OR   Non-OR   Hospital-Acquired Condition

SECTION: F PHYSICAL REHABILITATION AND
DIAGNOSTIC AUDIOLOGY

SECTION QUALIFIER: 1 DIAGNOSTIC AUDIOLOGY

TYPE: 4 **HEARING AID ASSESSMENT:** Measurement of the
appropriateness and/or effectiveness of a hearing device

Body System – Body Region	Type Qualifier	Equipment	Qualifier

Z None	Ø Cochlear Implant	1 Audiometer
		2 Sound Field/Booth
		3 Tympanometer
		4 Electroacoustic Immitance/
		  Acoustic Reflex
		5 Hearing Aid Selection/
		  Fitting/Test
		7 Electrophysiologic
		9 Cochlear Implant
		K Audiovisual
		L Assistive Listening
		P Computer
		Y Other Equipment
		Z None
			Z None

Z None	1 Ear Canal Probe Microphone
	6 Binaural Electroacoustic
	  Hearing Aid Check
	8 Monaural Electroacoustic
	  Hearing Aid Check
		5 Hearing Aid Selection/
		  Fitting/Test
		Z None
			Z None

Z None	2 Monaural Hearing Aid
	3 Binaural Hearing Aid
		1 Audiometer
		2 Sound Field/Booth
		3 Tympanometer
		4 Electroacoustic Immitance/
		  Acoustic Reflex
		5 Hearing Aid Selection/
		  Fitting/Test
		K Audiovisual
		L Assistive Listening
		P Computer
		Z None
			Z None

Z None	4 Assistive Listening System/
	  Device Selection
		1 Audiometer
		2 Sound Field/Booth
		3 Tympanometer
		4 Electroacoustic Immitance/
		  Acoustic Reflex
		K Audiovisual
		L Assistive Listening
		Z None
			Z None

Z None	5 Sensory Aids	1 Audiometer
		2 Sound Field/Booth
		3 Tympanometer
		4 Electroacoustic Immitance/
		  Acoustic Reflex
		5 Hearing Aid Selection/
		  Fitting/Test
		K Audiovisual
		L Assistive Listening
		Z None
			Z None

Z None	7 Ear Protector Attentuation	Ø Occupational Hearing Z None	Z None

F: PHYSICAL REHABILITATION AND DIAGNOSTIC AUDIOLOGY

1: DIAGNOSTIC AUDIOLOGY

4

SECTION: F PHYSICAL REHABILITATION AND DIAGNOSTIC AUDIOLOGY

SECTION QUALIFIER: 1 DIAGNOSTIC AUDIOLOGY

TYPE: 5 VESTIBULAR ASSESSMENT: Measurement of the vestibular system and related functions

Body System – Body Region	Type Qualifier	Equipment	Qualifier
Z None	Ø Bithermal, Binaural Caloric Irrigation 1 Bithermal, Monaural Caloric Irrigation 2 Unithermal Binaural Screen 3 Oscillating Tracking 4 Sinusoidal Vertical Axis Rotational 5 Dix-Hallpike Dynamic 6 Computerized Dynamic Posturography	8 Vestibular/Balance Z None	Z None
Z None	7 Tinnitus Masker	5 Hearing Aid Selection/ Fitting/Test Z None	Z None

New/Revised Text in Green   deleted Deleted   ♀ Females Only   ♂ Males Only   **Coding Clinic**
🚫 Non-covered   🚫 Limited Coverage   ⊞ Combination (See Appendix E)   DRG Non-OR   Non-OR   🚫 Hospital-Acquired Condition

SECTION: **G MENTAL HEALTH**
SECTION QUALIFIER: Z NONE
TYPE: 1 **PSYCHOLOGICAL TESTS:** The administration and interpretation of standardized psychological tests and measurement instruments for the assessment of psychological function

Qualifier	Qualifier	Qualifier	Qualifier
Ø Developmental 1 Personality and Behavioral 2 Intellectual and Psychoeducational 3 Neuropsychological 4 Neurobehavioral and Cognitive Status	Z None	Z None	Z None

SECTION: **G MENTAL HEALTH**
SECTION QUALIFIER: Z NONE
TYPE: 2 **CRISIS INTERVENTION:** Treatment of a traumatized, acutely disturbed or distressed individual for the purpose of short-term stabilization

Qualifier	Qualifier	Qualifier	Qualifier
Z None	Z None	Z None	Z None

SECTION: **G MENTAL HEALTH**
SECTION QUALIFIER: Z NONE
TYPE: 3 **MEDICATION MANAGEMENT:** Monitoring and adjusting the use of medications for the treatment of a mental health disorder

Qualifier	Qualifier	Qualifier	Qualifier
Z None	Z None	Z None	Z None

SECTION: **G MENTAL HEALTH**
SECTION QUALIFIER: Z NONE
TYPE: 5 **INDIVIDUAL PSYCHOTHERAPY:** Treatment of an individual with a mental health disorder by behavioral, cognitive, psychoanalytic, psychodynamic or psychophysiological means to improve functioning or well-being

Qualifier	Qualifier	Qualifier	Qualifier
Ø Interactive 1 Behavioral 2 Cognitive 3 Interpersonal 4 Psychoanalysis 5 Psychodynamic 6 Supportive 8 Cognitive-Behavioral 9 Psychophysiological	Z None	Z None	Z None

G: MENTAL HEALTH   Z: NONE   1; 2; 3; 5

New/Revised Text in Green   ~~deleted~~ Deleted   ♀ Females Only   ♂ Males Only   **Coding Clinic**
Non-covered   Limited Coverage   ⊞ Combination (See Appendix E)   DRG Non-OR   Non-OR   Hospital-Acquired Condition

SECTION: G MENTAL HEALTH

SECTION QUALIFIER: Z NONE

TYPE: 6 **COUNSELING:** The application of psychological methods to treat an individual with normal developmental issues and psychological problems in order to increase function, improve well-being, alleviate distress, maladjustment or resolve crises

Qualifier	Qualifier	Qualifier	Qualifier
Ø Educational 1 Vocational 3 Other Counseling	Z None	Z None	Z None

SECTION: G MENTAL HEALTH

SECTION QUALIFIER: Z NONE

TYPE: 7 **FAMILY PSYCHOTHERAPY:** Treatment that includes one or more family members of an individual with a mental health disorder by behavioral, cognitive, psychoanalytic, psychodynamic or psychophysiological means to improve functioning or well-being

Qualifier	Qualifier	Qualifier	Qualifier
2 Other Family Psychotherapy	Z None	Z None	Z None

SECTION: G MENTAL HEALTH

SECTION QUALIFIER: Z NONE

TYPE: B **ELECTROCONVULSIVE THERAPY:** The application of controlled electrical voltages to treat a mental health disorder

Qualifier	Qualifier	Qualifier	Qualifier
Ø Unilateral-Single Seizure 1 Unilateral-Multiple Seizure 2 Bilateral-Single Seizure 3 Bilateral-Multiple Seizure 4 Other Electroconvulsive Therapy	Z None	Z None	Z None

SECTION: G MENTAL HEALTH

SECTION QUALIFIER: Z NONE

TYPE: C **BIOFEEDBACK:** Provision of information from the monitoring and regulating of physiological processes in conjunction with cognitive-behavioral techniques to improve patient functioning or well-being

Qualifier	Qualifier	Qualifier	Qualifier
9 Other Biofeedback	Z None	Z None	Z None

G: MENTAL HEALTH

Z: NONE

6; 7; B; C

New/Revised Text in Green   ~~deleted~~ Deleted   ♀ Females Only   ♂ Males Only   **Coding Clinic**
🔖 Non-covered   🔖 Limited Coverage   ⊞ Combination (See Appendix E)   DRG Non-OR   Non-OR   🔖 Hospital-Acquired Condition

SECTION: G MENTAL HEALTH
SECTION QUALIFIER: Z NONE
TYPE: **F HYPNOSIS:** Induction of a state of heightened suggestibility by auditory, visual, and tactile techniques to elicit an emotional or behavioral response

Qualifier	Qualifier	Qualifier	Qualifier
Z None	Z None	Z None	Z None

SECTION: G MENTAL HEALTH
SECTION QUALIFIER: Z NONE
TYPE: **G NARCOSYNTHESIS:** Administration of intravenous barbiturates in order to release suppressed or repressed thoughts

Qualifier	Qualifier	Qualifier	Qualifier
Z None	Z None	Z None	Z None

SECTION: G MENTAL HEALTH
SECTION QUALIFIER: Z NONE
TYPE: **H GROUP PSYCHOTHERAPY:** Treatment of two or more individuals with a mental health disorder by behavioral, cognitive, psychoanalytic, psychodynamic, or psychophysiological means to improve functioning or well-being

Qualifier	Qualifier	Qualifier	Qualifier
Z None	Z None	Z None	Z None

SECTION: G MENTAL HEALTH
SECTION QUALIFIER: Z NONE
TYPE: **J LIGHT THERAPY:** Application of specialized light treatments to improve functioning or well-being

Qualifier	Qualifier	Qualifier	Qualifier
Z None	Z None	Z None	Z None

New/Revised Text in Green   ~~deleted~~ Deleted   ♀ Females Only   ♂ Males Only   **Coding Clinic**
🐧 Non-covered   🐧 Limited Coverage   ⊕ Combination (See Appendix E)   DRG Non-OR   Non-OR   🐧 Hospital-Acquired Condition

707

New/Revised Text in Green   ~~deleted~~ Deleted   ♀ Females Only   ♂ Males Only   **Coding Clinic**
Non-covered   Limited Coverage   Combination (See Appendix E)   DRG Non-OR   Non-OR   Hospital-Acquired Condition

SECTION: H SUBSTANCE ABUSE TREATMENT
SECTION QUALIFIER: Z NONE
TYPE: 2 **DETOXIFICATION SERVICES:** Detoxification from alcohol and/or drugs

Qualifier	Qualifier	Qualifier	Qualifier
Z None	Z None	Z None	Z None

SECTION: H SUBSTANCE ABUSE TREATMENT
SECTION QUALIFIER: Z NONE
TYPE: 3 **INDIVIDUAL COUNSELING:** The application of psychological methods to treat an individual with addictive behavior

Qualifier	Qualifier	Qualifier	Qualifier
Ø Cognitive 1 Behavioral 2 Cognitive-Behavioral 3 12-Step 4 Interpersonal 5 Vocational 6 Psychoeducation 7 Motivational Enhancement 8 Confrontational 9 Continuing Care B Spiritual C Pre/Post-Test Infectious Disease	Z None	Z None	Z None

DRG Non-OR HZ3[Ø123456789B]ZZZ

SECTION: H SUBSTANCE ABUSE TREATMENT
SECTION QUALIFIER: Z NONE
TYPE: 4 **GROUP COUNSELING:** The application of psychological methods to treat two or more individuals with addictive behavior

Qualifier	Qualifier	Qualifier	Qualifier
Ø Cognitive 1 Behavioral 2 Cognitive-Behavioral 3 12-Step 4 Interpersonal 5 Vocational 6 Psychoeducation 7 Motivational Enhancement 8 Confrontational 9 Continuing Care B Spiritual C Pre/Post-Test Infectious Disease	Z None	Z None	Z None

DRG Non-OR HZ4[Ø123456789B]ZZZ

H: SUBSTANCE ABUSE TREATMENT Z: NONE 2; 3; 4

SECTION: **H SUBSTANCE ABUSE TREATMENT**
SECTION QUALIFIER: **Z   NONE**
TYPE: **5   INDIVIDUAL PSYCHOTHERAPY:** Treatment of an individual with addictive behavior by behavioral, cognitive, psychoanalytic, psychodynamic, or psychophysiological means

Qualifier	Qualifier	Qualifier	Qualifier
Ø Cognitive 1 Behavioral 2 Cognitive-Behavioral 3 12-Step 4 Interpersonal 5 Interactive 6 Psychoeducation 7 Motivational Enhancement 8 Confrontational 9 Supportive B Psychoanalysis C Psychodynamic D Psychophysiological	Z None	Z None	Z None

`DRG Non-OR` All Values

SECTION: **H SUBSTANCE ABUSE TREATMENT**
SECTION QUALIFIER: **Z   NONE**
TYPE: **6   FAMILY COUNSELING:** The application of psychological methods that includes one or more family members to treat an individual with addictive behavior

Qualifier	Qualifier	Qualifier	Qualifier
3 Other Family Counseling	Z None	Z None	Z None

SECTION: **H SUBSTANCE ABUSE TREATMENT**
SECTION QUALIFIER: **Z   NONE**
TYPE: **8   MEDICATION MANAGEMENT:** Monitoring and adjusting the use of replacement medications for the treatment of addiction

Qualifier	Qualifier	Qualifier	Qualifier
Ø Nicotine Replacement 1 Methadone Maintenance 2 Levo-alpha-acetyl-methadol (LAAM) 3 Antabuse 4 Naltrexone 5 Naloxone 6 Clonidine 7 Bupropion 8 Psychiatric Medication 9 Other Replacement Medication	Z None	Z None	Z None

Side tab: 5; 6; 8   Z: NONE   H: SUBSTANCE ABUSE TREATMENT

SECTION: H SUBSTANCE ABUSE TREATMENT
SECTION QUALIFIER: Z NONE
TYPE: 9 **PHARMACOTHERAPY:** The use of replacement medications for the treatment of addiction

Qualifier	Qualifier	Qualifier	Qualifier
Ø Nicotine Replacement 1 Methadone Maintenance 2 Levo-alpha-acetyl-methadol (LAAM) 3 Antabuse 4 Naltrexone 5 Naloxone 6 Clonidine 7 Bupropion 8 Psychiatric Medication 9 Other Replacement Medication	Z None	Z None	Z None

H: SUBSTANCE ABUSE TREATMENT   Z: NONE   9: PHARMACOTHERAPY

ICD-10-PCS Coding Guidelines

New Technology Section Guidelines (section X)

D. New Technology Section

General guidelines

D1

Section X codes are standalone codes. They are not supplemental codes. Section X codes fully represent the specific procedure described in the code title, and do not require any additional codes from other sections of ICD-10-PCS. When section X contains a code title which describes a specific new technology procedure, only that X code is reported for the procedure. There is no need to report a broader, non-specific code in another section of ICD-10-PCS.

Example: XWØ4321 Introduction of Ceftazidime-Avibactam Anti-infective into Central Vein, Percutaneous Approach, New Technology Group 1, can be coded to indicate that Ceftazidime-Avibactam Anti-infective was administered via a central vein. A separate code from table 3EØ in the Administration section of ICD-10-PCS is not coded in addition to this code.

Selection of Principal Procedure

The following instructions should be applied in the selection of principal procedure and clarification on the importance of the relation to the principal diagnosis when more than one procedure is performed:

1. Procedure performed for definitive treatment of both principal diagnosis and secondary diagnosis

    a. Sequence procedure performed for definitive treatment most related to principal diagnosis as principal procedure.

2. Procedure performed for definitive treatment and diagnostic procedures performed for both principal diagnosis and secondary diagnosis

    a. Sequence procedure performed for definitive treatment most related to principal diagnosis as principal procedure

3. A diagnostic procedure was performed for the principal diagnosis and a procedure is performed for definitive treatment of a secondary diagnosis.

    a. Sequence diagnostic procedure as principal procedure, since the procedure most related to the principal diagnosis takes precedence.

4. No procedures performed that are related to principal diagnosis; procedures performed for definitive treatment and diagnostic procedures were performed for secondary diagnosis

    a. Sequence procedure performed for definitive treatment of secondary diagnosis as principal procedure, since there are no procedures (definitive or nondefinitive treatment) related to principal diagnosis.

New/Revised Text in Green   ~~deleted~~ Deleted   ♀ Females Only   ♂ Males Only   **Coding Clinic**

Non-covered   Limited Coverage   ⊕ Combination (See Appendix E)   DRG Non-OR   Non-OR   Hospital-Acquired Condition

SECTION: X NEW TECHNOLOGY
BODY SYSTEM: 2 CARDIOVASCULAR SYSTEM
OPERATION: A ASSISTANCE: Taking over a portion of a physiological function by extracorporeal means

Body Part	Approach	Device / Substance / Technology	Qualifier
5 Innominate Artery and Left Common Carotid Artery	3 Percutaneous	1 Cerebral Embolic Filtration, Dual Filter	2 New Technology Group 2

Coding Clinic: 2016, Q4, P115 – X2A

SECTION: X NEW TECHNOLOGY
BODY SYSTEM: 2 CARDIOVASCULAR SYSTEM
OPERATION: C EXTIRPATION: Taking or cutting out solid matter from a body part

Body Part	Approach	Device / Substance / Technology	Qualifier
0 Coronary Artery, One Artery 1 Coronary Artery, Two Arteries 2 Coronary Artery, Three Arteries 3 Coronary Artery, Four or More Arteries	3 Percutaneous	6 Orbital Atherectomy Technology	1 New Technology Group 1

Coding Clinic: 2015, Q4, P14 – X2C0361
Coding Clinic: 2016, Q4, P83 – X2C

SECTION: X NEW TECHNOLOGY
BODY SYSTEM: 2 CARDIOVASCULAR SYSTEM
OPERATION: R REPLACEMENT: Putting in or on biological or synthetic material that physically takes the place and/or function of all or a portion of a body part

Body Part	Approach	Device / Substance / Technology	Qualifier
F Aortic Valve	0 Open 3 Percutaneous 4 Percutaneous Endoscopic	3 Zooplastic Tissue, Rapid Deployment Technique	2 New Technology Group 2

Coding Clinic: 2016, Q4, P116 – X2R

New/Revised Text in Green ~~deleted~~ Deleted ♀ Females Only ♂ Males Only **Coding Clinic**
🐾 Non-covered 🐾 Limited Coverage ⊞ Combination (See Appendix E) DRG Non-OR Non-OR 🐾 Hospital-Acquired Condition

713

SECTION: **X NEW TECHNOLOGY**

BODY SYSTEM: **H SKIN, SUBCUTANEOUS TISSUE, FASCIA AND BREAST**

OPERATION: **R REPLACEMENT:** Putting in or on biological or synthetic material that physically takes the place and/or function of all or a portion of a body part

Body Part	Approach	Device / Substance / Technology	Qualifier
P Skin	X External	L Skin Substitute, Porcine Liver Derived	2 New Technology Group 2

SECTION: **X NEW TECHNOLOGY**

BODY SYSTEM: **K MUSCLES, TENDONS, BURSAE AND LIGAMENTS**

OPERATION: **Ø INTRODUCTION:** Putting in or on a therapeutic, diagnostic, nutritional, physiological, or prophylactic substance except blood or blood products

Body Part	Approach	Device / Substance / Technology	Qualifier
2 Muscle	3 Percutaneous	Ø Concentrated Bone Marrow Aspirate	3 New Technology Group 3

SECTION: **X NEW TECHNOLOGY**

BODY SYSTEM: **N BONES**

OPERATION: **S REPOSITION:** Moving to its normal location, or other suitable location, all or a portion of a body part

Body Part	Approach	Device / Substance / Technology	Qualifier
Ø Lumbar Vertebra 3 Cervical Vertebra 4 Thoracic Vertebra	Ø Open 3 Percutaneous	3 Magnetically Controlled Growth Rod(s)	2 New Technology Group 2

Coding Clinic: 2016, Q4, P117 – XNS
Coding Clinic: 2017, Q4, P75 – XNS0032

R: REPLACEMENT Ø: INTRODUCTION S: REPOSITION

H; K; N X: NEW TECHNOLOGY

New/Revised Text in Green ~~deleted~~ Deleted ♀ Females Only ♂ Males Only **Coding Clinic**
Non-covered Limited Coverage Combination (See Appendix E) DRG Non-OR Non-OR Hospital-Acquired Condition

SECTION: X NEW TECHNOLOGY
BODY SYSTEM: R JOINTS
OPERATION: 2 **MONITORING:** Determining the level of a physiological or physical function repetitively over a period of time

Body Part	Approach	Device / Substance / Technology	Qualifier
G Knee Joint, Right H Knee Joint, Left	Ø Open	2 Intraoperative Knee Replacement Sensor	1 New Technology Group 1

SECTION: X NEW TECHNOLOGY
BODY SYSTEM: R JOINTS *(on multiple pages)*
OPERATION: G **FUSION:** Joining together portions of an articular body part rendering the articular body part immobile

Body Part	Approach	Device / Substance / Technology	Qualifier
Ø Occipital-cervical Joint 🔖	Ø Open	9 Interbody Fusion Device, Nanotextured Surface	2 New Technology Group 2
Ø Occipital-cervical Joint	Ø Open	F Interbody Fusion Device, Radiolucent Porous	3 New Technology Group 3
1 Cervical Vertebral Joint 🔖	Ø Open	9 Interbody Fusion Device, Nanotextured Surface	2 New Technology Group 2
1 Cervical Vertebral Joint	Ø Open	F Interbody Fusion Device, Radiolucent Porous	3 New Technology Group 3
2 Cervical Vertebral Joints, 2 or more 🔖	Ø Open	9 Interbody Fusion Device, Nanotextured Surface	2 New Technology Group 2
2 Cervical Vertebral Joints, 2 or more	Ø Open	F Interbody Fusion Device, Radiolucent Porous	3 New Technology Group 3
4 Cervicothoracic Vertebral Joint 🔖	Ø Open	9 Interbody Fusion Device, Nanotextured Surface	2 New Technology Group 2
4 Cervicothoracic Vertebral Joint	Ø Open	F Interbody Fusion Device, Radiolucent Porous	3 New Technology Group 3
6 Thoracic Vertebral Joint 🔖	Ø Open	9 Interbody Fusion Device, Nanotextured Surface	2 New Technology Group 2
6 Thoracic Vertebral Joint	Ø Open	F Interbody Fusion Device, Radiolucent Porous	3 New Technology Group 3

🔖 XRG0092 when reported with Secondary Diagnosis K68.11, T81.4XXA, or T84.60XA-T84.7XXA
🔖 XRG1092 when reported with Secondary Diagnosis K68.11, T81.4XXA, or T84.60XA-T84.7XXA
🔖 XRG2092 when reported with Secondary Diagnosis K68.11, T81.4XXA, or T84.60XA-T84.7XXA
🔖 XRG4092 when reported with Secondary Diagnosis K68.11, T81.4XXA, or T84.60XA-T84.7XXA
🔖 XRG6092 when reported with Secondary Diagnosis K68.11, T81.4XXA, or T84.60XA-T84.7XXA

X: NEW TECHNOLOGY   R: JOINTS   2: MONITORING   G: FUSION

SECTION:

X NEW TECHNOLOGY

BODY SYSTEM: **R JOINTS** *(continued)*

OPERATION: **G FUSION:** Joining together portions of an articular body part rendering the articular body part immobile

Body Part	Approach	Device / Substance / Technology	Qualifier
7 Thoracic Vertebral Joints, 2 to 7 ⊞ ⬡	Ø Open	9 Interbody Fusion Device, Nanotextured Surface	2 New Technology Group 2
7 Thoracic Vertebral Joints, 2 to 7	Ø Open	F Interbody Fusion Device, Radiolucent Porous	3 New Technology Group 3
8 Thoracic Vertebral Joints, 8 or more ⬡	Ø Open	9 Interbody Fusion Device, Nanotextured Surface	2 New Technology Group 2
8 Thoracic Vertebral Joints, 8 or more	Ø Open	F Interbody Fusion Device, Radiolucent Porous	3 New Technology Group 3
A Thoracolumbar Vertebral Joint ⬡	Ø Open	9 Interbody Fusion Device, Nanotextured Surface	2 New Technology Group 2
A Thoracolumbar Vertebral Joint	Ø Open	F Interbody Fusion Device, Radiolucent Porous	3 New Technology Group 3
B Lumbar Vertebral Joint ⬡	Ø Open	9 Interbody Fusion Device, Nanotextured Surface	2 New Technology Group 2
B Lumbar Vertebral Joint	Ø Open	F Interbody Fusion Device, Radiolucent Porous	3 New Technology Group 3
C Lumbar Vertebral, Joints, 2 or more ⊞ ⬡	Ø Open	9 Interbody Fusion Device, Nanotextured Surface	2 New Technology Group 2
C Lumbar Vertebral Joints, 2 or more	Ø Open	F Interbody Fusion Device, Radiolucent Porous	3 New Technology Group 3
D Lumbosacral Joint ⬡	Ø Open	9 Interbody Fusion Device, Nanotextured Surface	2 New Technology Group 2
D Lumbosacral Joint	Ø Open	F Interbody Fusion Device, Radiolucent Porous	3 New Technology Group 3

⊞ XRG[7C]Ø92
⬡ XRG7Ø92 when reported with Secondary Diagnosis K68.11, T81.4XXA, or T84.6ØXA-T84.7XXA
⬡ XRG8Ø92 when reported with Secondary Diagnosis K68.11, T81.4XXA, or T84.6ØXA-T84.7XXA
⬡ XRGAØ92 when reported with Secondary Diagnosis K68.11, T81.4XXA, or T84.6ØXA-T84.7XXA
⬡ XRGBØ92 when reported with Secondary Diagnosis K68.11, T81.4XXA, or T84.6ØXA-T84.7XXA
⬡ XRGCØ92 when reported with Secondary Diagnosis K68.11, T81.4XXA, or T84.6ØXA-T84.7XXA
⬡ XRGDØ92 when reported with Secondary Diagnosis K68.11, T81.4XXA, or T84.6ØXA-T84.7XXA

Coding Clinic: 2Ø17, Q4, P76 – XRG[BD]F3

SECTION:

X NEW TECHNOLOGY

BODY SYSTEM: **V MALE REPRODUCTIVE SYSTEM**

OPERATION: **5 DESTRUCTION:** Physical eradication of all or a portion of a body part by the direct use of energy, force, or a destructive agent

Body Part	Approach	Device / Substance / Technology	Qualifier
Ø Prostate ♂	8 Via Natural or Artificial Opening Endoscopic	A Robotic Waterjet Ablation	4 New Technology Group 4

New/Revised Text in Green   ~~deleted~~ Deleted   ♀ Females Only   ♂ Males Only   **Coding Clinic**
⬡ Non-covered   ⬢ Limited Coverage   ⊞ Combination (See Appendix E)   DRG Non-OR   Non-OR   ⬡ Hospital-Acquired Condition

SECTION: X NEW TECHNOLOGY
BODY SYSTEM: W ANATOMICAL REGIONS
OPERATION: Ø **INTRODUCTION:** Putting in or on a therapeutic, diagnostic, nutritional, physiological, or prophylactic substance except blood or blood products

Body Part	Approach	Device / Substance / Technology	Qualifier
3 Peripheral Vein	3 Percutaneous	2 Ceftazidime-Avibactam Anti-infective 3 Idarucizumab, Dabigatran Reversal Agent 4 Isavuconazole Anti-infective 5 Blinatumomab Antineoplastic Immunotherapy	1 New Technology Group 1
3 Peripheral Vein	3 Percutaneous	7 Andexanet Alfa, Factor Xa Inhibitor Reversal Agent 9 Defibrotide Sodium Anticoagulant	2 New Technology Group 2
3 Peripheral Vein	3 Percutaneous	7 Andexanet Alfa, Factor Xa Inhibitor Reversal Agent 9 Defibrotide Sodium Anticoagulant	2 New Technology Group 2
3 Peripheral Vein	3 Percutaneous	A Bezlotoxumab Monoclonal Antibody B Cytarabine and Daunorubicin Liposome Antineoplastic C Engineered Autologous Chimeric Antigen Receptor T-cell Immunotherapy F Other New Technology Therapeutic Substance	3 New Technology Group 3
4 Central Vein	3 Percutaneous	G Plazomicin Anti-infective H Synthetic Human Angiotensin II	4 New Technology Group 4
4 Central Vein	3 Percutaneous	2 Ceftazidime-Avibactam Anti-infective 3 Idarucizumab, Dabigatran Reversal Agent 4 Isavuconazole Antiinfective 5 Blinatumomab Antineoplastic Immunotherapy	1 New Technology Group 1
4 Central Vein	3 Percutaneous	7 Andexanet Alfa, Factor Xa Inhibitor Reversal Agent 9 Defibrotide Sodium Anticoagulant	2 New Technology Group 2
4 Central Vein	3 Percutaneous	A Bezlotoxumab Monoclonal Antibody B Cytarabine and Daunorubicin Liposome Antineoplastic C Engineered Autologous Chimeric Antigen Receptor T-cell Immunotherapy F Other New Technology Therapeutic Substance	3 New Technology Group 3
D Mouth and Pharynx	X External	8 Uridine Triacetate	2 New Technology Group 2

Coding Clinic: 2Ø15, Q4, P13, P15 – XWØ4331, XWØ4351

New/Revised Text in Green ~~deleted~~ Deleted ♀ Females Only ♂ Males Only **Coding Clinic**
🔲 Non-covered 🔲 Limited Coverage ⊡ Combination (See Appendix E) DRG Non-OR Non-OR 🔲 Hospital-Acquired Condition

SECTION:

SECTION: **X NEW TECHNOLOGY**
BODY SYSTEM: Y EXTRACORPOREAL
OPERATION: Ø **INTRODUCTION:** Putting in or on a therapeutic, diagnostic, nutritional, physiological, or prophylactic substance except blood or blood products

Body Part	Approach	Device / Substance / Technology	Qualifier
V Vein Graft	X External	8 Endothelial Damage Inhibitor	3 New Technology Group 3

Ø: INTRODUCTION

Y: EXTRACORPOREAL

X: NEW TECHNOLOGY

3

3f (Aortic) Bioprosthesis valve *use* Zooplastic Tissue in Heart and Great Vessels

A

Abdominal aortic plexus *use* Abdominal Sympathetic Nerve
Abdominal esophagus *use* Esophagus, Lower
➡ Abdominohysterectomy *see* Resection, Uterus 0UT9
Abdominoplasty
  see Alteration, Abdominal Wall, 0W0F
  see Repair, Abdominal Wall, 0WQF
  see Supplement, Abdominal Wall, 0WUF
Abductor hallucis muscle
  use Foot Muscle, Right
  use Foot Muscle, Left
AbioCor® Total Replacement Heart *use* Synthetic Substitute
Ablation *see* Destruction
Abortion
  Products of Conception 10A0
  Abortifacient 10A07ZX
  Laminaria 10A07ZW
  Vacuum 10A07Z6
Abrasion *see* Extraction
Absolute Pro Vascular (OTW) Self-Expanding Stent System *use* Intraluminal Device
Accessory cephalic vein
  use Cephalic Vein, Right
  use Cephalic Vein, Left
Accessory obturator nerve *use* Lumbar Plexus
Accessory phrenic nerve *use* Phrenic Nerve
Accessory spleen *use* Spleen
Acculink (RX) Carotid Stent System *use* Intraluminal Device
Acellular Hydrated Dermis *use* Nonautologous Tissue Substitute
Acetabular cup *use* Liner in Lower Joints
Acetabulectomy
  see Excision, Lower Bones 0QB
  see Resection, Lower Bones 0QT
Acetabulofemoral joint
  use Hip Joint, Right
  use Hip Joint, Left
Acetabuloplasty
  see Repair, Lower Bones 0QQ
  see Replacement, Lower Bones 0QR
  see Supplement, Lower Bones 0QU
Achilles tendon
  use Lower Leg Tendon, Right
  use Lower Leg Tendon, Left
Achillorrhaphy *use* Repair, Tendons 0LQ
Achillotenotomy, achillotomy
  see Division, Tendons 0L8
  see Drainage, Tendons 0L9
Acromioclavicular ligament
  use Shoulder Bursa and Ligament, Right
  use Shoulder Bursa and Ligament, Left
Acromion (process)
  use Scapula, Right
  use Scapula, Left
Acromionectomy
  see Excision, Upper Joints 0RB
  see Resection, Upper Joints 0RT
Acromioplasty
  see Repair, Upper Joints 0RQ
  see Replacement, Upper Joints 0RR
  see Supplement, Upper Joints 0RU
Activa PC neurostimulator *use* Stimulator Generator, Multiple Array in 0JH
Activa RC neurostimulator *use* Stimulator Generator, Multiple Array Rechargeable in 0JH
Activa SC neurostimulator *use* Stimulator Generator, Single Array in 0JH
Activities of Daily Living Assessment F02
Activities of Daily Living Treatment F08

ACUITY™ Steerable Lead
  use Cardiac Lead, Pacemaker in 02H
  use Cardiac Lead, Defibrillator in O2H
Acupuncture
  Breast
    Anesthesia 8E0H300
    No Qualifier 8E0H30Z
  Integumentary System
    Anesthesia 8E0H300
    No Qualifier 8E0H30Z
Adductor brevis muscle
  use Upper Leg Muscle, Right
  use Upper Leg Muscle, Left
Adductor hallucis muscle
  use Foot Muscle, Right
  use Foot Muscle, Left
Adductor longus muscle
  use Upper Leg Muscle, Right
  use Upper Leg Muscle, Left
Adductor magnus muscle
  use Upper Leg Muscle, Right
  use Upper Leg Muscle, Left
Adenohypophysis *use* Pituitary Gland
Adenoidectomy
  see Excision, Adenoids 0CBQ
  see Resection, Adenoids 0CTQ
Adenoidotomy *see* Drainage, Adenoids 0C9Q
Adhesiolysis *see* Release
Administration
  Blood products *see* Transfusion
  Other substance *see* Introduction of substance in or on
Adrenalectomy
  see Excision, Endocrine System 0GB
  see Resection, Endocrine System 0GT
Adrenalorrhaphy *see* Repair, Endocrine System 0GQ
Adrenalotomy *see* Drainage, Endocrine System 0G9
Advancement
  see Reposition
  see Transfer
Advisa (MRI) *use* Pacemaker, Dual Chamber in 0JH
AFX® Endovascular AAA System *use* Intraluminal Device
AIGISRx Antibacterial Envelope *use* Anti-Infective Envelope
Alar ligament of axis *use* Head and Neck Bursa and Ligament
Alimentation *see* Introduction of substance in or on
Alteration
  Abdominal Wall 0W0F
  Ankle Region
    Left 0Y0L
    Right 0Y0K
  Arm
    Lower
      Left 0X0F
      Right 0X0D
    Upper
      Left 0X09
      Right 0X08
  Axilla
    Left 0X05
    Right 0X04
  Back
    Lower 0W0L
    Upper 0W0K
  Breast
    Bilateral 0H0V
    Left 0H0U
    Right 0H0T
  Buttock
    Left 0Y01
    Right 0Y00
  Chest Wall 0W08
  Ear
    Bilateral 0902
    Left 0901
    Right 0900

Alteration *(Continued)*
  Elbow Region
    Left 0X0C
    Right 0X0B
  Extremity
    Lower
      Left 0Y0B
      Right 0Y09
    Upper
      Left 0X07
      Right 0X06
  Eyelid
    Lower
      Left 080R
      Right 080Q
    Upper
      Left 080P
      Right 080N
  Face 0W02
  Head 0W00
  Jaw
    Lower 0W05
    Upper 0W04
  Knee Region
    Left 0Y0G
    Right 0Y0F
  Leg
    Lower
      Left 0Y0J
      Right 0Y0H
    Upper
      Left 0Y0D
      Right 0Y0C
  Lip
    Lower 0C01X
    Upper 0C00X
  Nasal Mucosa and Soft Tissue 090K
  Neck 0W06
  Perineum
    Female 0W0N
    Male 0W0M
  Shoulder Region
    Left 0X03
    Right 0X02
  Subcutaneous Tissue and Fascia
    Abdomen 0J08
    Back 0J07
    Buttock 0J09
    Chest 0J06
    Face 0J01
    Lower Arm
      Left 0J0H
      Right 0J0G
    Lower Leg
      Left 0J0P
      Right 0J0N
    Neck
      Left 0J05
      Right 0J04
    Upper Arm
      Left 0J0F
      Right 0J0D
    Upper Leg
      Left 0J0M
      Right 0J0L
  Wrist Region
    Left 0X0H
    Right 0X0G
Alveolar process of mandible *use* Maxilla
Alveolar process of maxilla
  use Maxilla, Right
  use Maxilla, Left
Alveolectomy
  see Excision, Head and Facial Bones 0NB
  see Resection, Head and Facial Bones 0NT
Alveoloplasty
  see Repair, Head and Facial Bones 0NQ
  see Replacement, Head and Facial Bones 0NR
  see Supplement, Head and Facial Bones 0NU

▶ New   ➡ Revised   ~~deleted~~ Deleted

Alveolotomy
  see Division, Head and Facial Bones 0N8
  see Drainage, Head and Facial Bones 0N9
Ambulatory cardiac monitoring 4A12X45
Amniocentesis *see* Drainage, Products of
  Conception 1090
Amnioinfusion *see* Introduction of substance in
  or on, Products of Conception 3E0E
Amnioscopy 10J08ZZ
Amniotomy *see* Drainage, Products of
  Conception 1090
AMPLATZER® Muscular VSD Occluder *use*
  Synthetic Substitute
Amputation *see* Detachment
AMS 800® Urinary Control System *use*
  Artificial Sphincter in Urinary System
Anal orifice *use* Anus
Analog radiography *see* Plain Radiography
Analog radiology *see* Plain Radiography
Anastomosis *see* Bypass
Anatomical snuffbox
  use Lower Arm and Wrist Muscle, Right
  use Lower Arm and Wrist Muscle, Left
Andexanet Alfa, Factor Xa Inhibitor Reversal
  Agent XW0
AneuRx® AAA Advantage® *use* Intraluminal
  Device
Angiectomy
  see Excision, Heart and Great Vessels 02B
  see Excision, Upper Arteries 03B
  see Excision, Lower Arteries 04B
  see Excision, Upper Veins 05B
  see Excision, Lower Veins 06B
Angiocardiography
  Combined right and left heart *see*
    Fluoroscopy, Heart, Right and Left B216
  Left Heart *see* Fluoroscopy, Heart, Left B215
  Right Heart *see* Fluoroscopy, Heart, Right B214
  SPY system intravascular fluorescence *see*
    Monitoring, Physiological Systems 4A1
Angiography
  see Plain Radiography, Heart B20
  see Fluoroscopy, Heart B21
Angioplasty
  see Dilation, Heart and Great Vessels 027
  see Repair, Heart and Great Vessels 02Q
  see Replacement, Heart and Great Vessels 02R
  see Supplement, Heart and Great Vessels 02U
  see Dilation, Upper Arteries 037
  see Repair, Upper Arteries 03Q
  see Replacement, Upper Arteries 03R
  see Supplement, Upper Arteries 03U
  see Dilation, Lower Arteries 047
  see Repair, Lower Arteries 04Q
  see Replacement, Lower Arteries 04R
  see Supplement, Lower Arteries 04U
Angiorrhaphy
  see Repair, Heart and Great Vessels 02Q
  see Repair, Upper Arteries 03Q
  see Repair, Lower Arteries 04Q
Angioscopy
  02JY4ZZ
  03JY4ZZ
  04JY4ZZ
▶**Angiotensin II** *use* Synthetic Human
  Angiotensin II
Angiotripsy
  see Occlusion, Upper Arteries 03L
  see Occlusion, Lower Arteries 04L
Angular artery *use* Face Artery
Angular vein
  use Face Vein, Right
  use Face Vein, Left
Annular ligament
  use Elbow Bursa and Ligament, Right
  use Elbow Bursa and Ligament, Left
Annuloplasty
  see Repair, Heart and Great Vessels 02Q
  see Supplement, Heart and Great Vessels
    02U
Annuloplasty ring *use* Synthetic Substitute

Anoplasty
  see Repair, Anus 0DQQ
  see Supplement, Anus 0DUQ
Anorectal junction *use* Rectum
Anoscopy 0DJD8ZZ
Ansa cervicalis *use* Cervical Plexus
Antabuse therapy HZ93ZZZ
Antebrachial fascia
  use Subcutaneous Tissue and Fascia, Right
    Lower Arm
  use Subcutaneous Tissue and Fascia, Left
    Lower Arm
Anterior (pectoral) lymph node
  use Lymphatic, Right Axillary
  use Lymphatic, Left Axillary
Anterior cerebral artery *use* Intracranial Artery
Anterior cerebral vein *use* Intracranial Vein
Anterior choroidal artery *use* Intracranial
  Artery
Anterior circumflex humeral artery
  use Axillary Artery, Right
  use Axillary Artery, Left
Anterior communicating artery *use* Intracranial
  Artery
Anterior cruciate ligament (ACL)
  use Knee Bursa and Ligament, Right
  use Knee Bursa and Ligament, Left
Anterior crural nerve *use* Femoral Nerve
Anterior facial vein
  use Face Vein, Right
  use Face Vein, Left
Anterior intercostal artery
  use Internal Mammary Artery, Right
  use Internal Mammary Artery, Left
Anterior interosseous nerve *use* Median Nerve
Anterior lateral malleolar artery
  use Anterior Tibial Artery, Right
  use Anterior Tibial Artery, Left
Anterior lingual gland *use* Minor Salivary
  Gland
Anterior medial malleolar artery
  use Anterior Tibial Artery, Right
  use Anterior Tibial Artery, Left
Anterior spinal artery
  use Vertebral Artery, Right
  use Vertebral Artery, Left
Anterior tibial recurrent artery
  use Anterior Tibial Artery, Right
  use Anterior Tibial Artery, Left
Anterior ulnar recurrent artery
  use Ulnar Artery, Right
  use Ulnar Artery, Left
Anterior vagal trunk *use* Vagus Nerve
Anterior vertebral muscle
  use Neck Muscle, Right
  use Neck Muscle, Left
Antigen-free air conditioning *see* Atmospheric
  Control, Physiological Systems 6A0
Antihelix
  use External Ear, Right
  use External Ear, Left
  use External Ear, Bilateral
Antimicrobial envelope *use* Anti-Infective
  Envelope
Antitragus
  use External Ear, Right
  use External Ear, Left
  use External Ear, Bilateral
Antrostomy *see* Drainage, Ear, Nose, Sinus 099
Antrotomy *see* Drainage, Ear, Nose, Sinus 099
Antrum of Highmore
  use Maxillary Sinus, Right
  use Maxillary Sinus, Left
Aortic annulus *use* Aortic Valve
Aortic arch *use* Thoracic Aorta, Ascending/Arch
Aortic intercostal artery *use* Upper Artery
Aortography
  see Plain Radiography, Upper Arteries B30
  see Fluoroscopy, Upper Arteries B31
  see Plain Radiography, Lower Arteries B40
  see Fluoroscopy, Lower Arteries B41

Aortoplasty
  see Repair, Aorta, Thoracic, Descending
    02QW
  see Repair, Aorta, Thoracic, Ascending/Arch
    02QX
  see Replacement, Aorta, Thoracic, Descending
    02RW
  see Replacement, Aorta, Thoracic, Ascending/
    Arch 02RX
  see Supplement, Aorta, Thoracic, Descending
    02UW
  see Supplement, Aorta, Thoracic, Ascending/
    Arch 02UX
  see Repair, Aorta, Abdominal 04Q0
  see Replacement, Aorta, Abdominal 04R0
  see Supplement, Aorta, Abdominal 04U0
Apical (subclavicular) lymph node
  use Lymphatic, Axillary, Right
  use Lymphatic, Axillary, Left
Apneustic center *use* Pons
Appendectomy
  see Excision, Appendix 0DBJ
  see Resection, Appendix 0DTJ
Appendicolysis *see* Release, Appendix 0DNJ
Appendicotomy *see* Drainage, Appendix 0D9J
Application *see* Introduction of substance in
  or on
▶**Aquablation therapy, prostate** XV508A4
Aquapheresis 6A550Z3
Aqueduct of Sylvius *use* Cerebral Ventricle
Aqueous humour
  use Anterior Chamber, Right
  use Anterior Chamber, Left
Arachnoid mater, intracranial *use* Cerebral
  Meninges
Arachnoid mater, spinal *use* Spinal Meninges
Arcuate artery
  use Foot Artery, Right
  use Foot Artery, Left
Areola
  use Nipple, Right
  use Nipple, Left
AROM (artificial rupture of membranes)
  10907ZC
Arterial canal (duct) *use* Pulmonary Artery, Left
Arterial pulse tracing *see* Measurement,
  Arterial 4A03
Arteriectomy
  see Excision, Heart and Great Vessels 02B
  see Excision, Upper Arteries 03B
  see Excision, Lower Arteries 04B
Arteriography
  see Plain Radiography, Heart B20
  see Fluoroscopy, Heart B21
  see Plain Radiography, Upper Arteries B30
  see Fluoroscopy, Upper Arteries B31
  see Plain Radiography, Lower Arteries B40
  see Fluoroscopy, Lower Arteries B41
Arterioplasty
  see Repair, Heart and Great Vessels 02Q
  see Replacement, Heart and Great Vessels 02R
  see Supplement, Heart and Great Vessels 02U
  see Repair, Upper Arteries 03Q
  see Replacement, Upper Arteries 03R
  see Supplement, Upper Arteries 03U
  see Repair, Lower Arteries 04Q
  see Replacement, Lower Arteries 04R
  see Supplement, Lower Arteries 04U
Arteriorrhaphy
  see Repair, Heart and Great Vessels 02Q
  see Repair, Upper Arteries 03Q
  see Repair, Lower Arteries 04Q
Arterioscopy
  see Inspection, Great Vessel 02JY
  see Inspection, Artery, Upper 03JY
  see Inspection, Artery, Lower 04JY
Arthrectomy
  see Excision, Upper Joints 0RB
  see Resection, Upper Joints 0RT
  see Excision, Lower Joints 0SB
  see Resection, Lower Joints 0ST

▶ New   ⇒ Revised   ~~deleted~~ Deleted

Arthrocentesis
 see Drainage, Upper Joints ØR9
 see Drainage, Lower Joints ØS9
Arthrodesis
 see Fusion, Upper Joints ØRG
 see Fusion, Lower Joints ØSG
Arthrography
 see Plain Radiography, Skull and Facial Bones BNØ
 see Plain Radiography, Non-Axial Upper Bones BPØ
 see Plain Radiography, Non-Axial Lower Bones BQØ
Arthrolysis
 see Release, Upper Joints ØRN
 see Release, Lower Joints ØSN
Arthropexy
 see Repair, Upper Joints ØRQ
 see Reposition, Upper Joints ØRS
 see Repair, Lower Joints ØSQ
 see Reposition, Lower Joints ØSS
Arthroplasty
 see Repair, Upper Joints ØRQ
 see Replacement, Upper Joints ØRR
 see Supplement, Upper Joints ØRU
 see Repair, Lower Joints ØSQ
 see Replacement, Lower Joints ØSR
 see Supplement, Lower Joints ØSU
▶Arthroplasty, radial head
 ▶see Replacement, Radius, Right ØPRH
 ▶see Replacement, Radius, Left ØPRJ
Arthroscopy
 see Inspection, Upper Joints ØRJ
 see Inspection, Lower Joints ØSJ
Arthrotomy
 see Drainage, Upper Joints ØR9
 see Drainage, Lower Joints ØS9
▶Articulating Spacer (Antibiotic) use
 Articulating Spacer in Lower Joints
Artificial anal sphincter (AAS) use Artificial Sphincter in Gastrointestinal System
Artificial bowel sphincter (neosphincter) use Artificial Sphincter in Gastrointestinal System
Artificial Sphincter
 Insertion of device in
  Anus ØDHQ
  Bladder ØTHB
  Bladder Neck ØTHC
  Urethra ØTHD
 Removal of device from
  Anus ØDPQ
  Bladder ØTPB
  Urethra ØTPD
 Revision of device in
  Anus ØDWQ
  Bladder ØTWB
  Urethra ØTWD
Artificial urinary sphincter (AUS) use Artificial Sphincter in Urinary System
Aryepiglottic fold use Larynx
Arytenoid cartilage use Larynx
Arytenoid muscle
 use Neck Muscle, Right
 use Neck Muscle, Left
Arytenoidectomy see Excision, Larynx ØCBS
Arytenoidopexy see Repair, Larynx ØCQS
Ascenda Intrathecal Catheter use Infusion Device
Ascending aorta use Thoracic Aorta, Ascending/Arch
Ascending palatine artery use Face Artery
Ascending pharyngeal artery
 use External Carotid Artery, Right
 use External Carotid Artery, Left
Aspiration, fine needle
 ⟩Fluid or gas see Drainage
 ▶Tissue biopsy
  ▶see Extraction
  ▶see Excision

Assessment
 Activities of daily living see Activities of Daily Living Assessment, Rehabilitation FØ2
 Hearing see Hearing Assessment, Diagnostic Audiology F13
 Hearing aid see Hearing Aid Assessment, Diagnostic Audiology F14
 Intravascular perfusion, using indocyanine green (ICG) dye see Monitoring, Physiological Systems 4A1
 Motor function see Motor Function Assessment, Rehabilitation FØ1
 Nerve function see Motor Function Assessment, Rehabilitation FØ1
 Speech see Speech Assessment, Rehabilitation FØØ
 Vestibular see Vestibular Assessment, Diagnostic Audiology F15
 Vocational see Activities of Daily Living Treatment, Rehabilitation FØ8
Assistance
 Cardiac
  Continuous
   Balloon Pump 5AØ221Ø
   Impeller Pump 5AØ221D
   Other Pump 5AØ2216
   Pulsatile Compression 5AØ2215
  Intermittent
   Balloon Pump 5AØ211Ø
   Impeller Pump 5AØ211D
   Other Pump 5AØ2116
   Pulsatile Compression 5AØ2115
 Circulatory
  Continuous
   Hyperbaric 5AØ5221
   Supersaturated 5AØ522C
  Intermittent
   Hyperbaric 5AØ5121
   Supersaturated 5AØ512C
 Respiratory
  24-96 Consecutive Hours
   Continuous Negative Airway Pressure 5AØ9459
   Continuous Positive Airway Pressure 5AØ9457
   Intermittent Negative Airway Pressure 5AØ945B
   Intermittent Positive Airway Pressure 5AØ9458
   No Qualifier 5AØ945Z
   Continuous, Filtration 5AØ92ØZ
  Greater than 96 Consecutive Hours
   Continuous Negative Airway Pressure 5AØ9559
   Continuous Positive Airway Pressure 5AØ9557
   Intermittent Negative Airway Pressure 5AØ955B
   Intermittent Positive Airway Pressure 5AØ9558
   No Qualifier 5AØ955Z
  Less than 24 Consecutive Hours
   Continuous Negative Airway Pressure 5AØ9359
   Continuous Positive Airway Pressure 5AØ9357
   Intermittent Negative Airway Pressure 5AØ935B
   Intermittent Positive Airway Pressure 5AØ9358
   No Qualifier 5AØ935Z
Assurant (Cobalt) stent use Intraluminal Device
Atherectomy
 see Extirpation, Heart and Great Vessels Ø2C
 see Extirpation, Upper Arteries Ø3C
 see Extirpation, Lower Arteries Ø4C
Atlantoaxial joint use Cervical Vertebral Joint
Atmospheric Control 6AØZ
AtriClip LAA Exclusion System use Extraluminal Device Atrioseptoplasty

 see Repair, Heart and Great Vessels Ø2Q
 see Replacement, Heart and Great Vessels Ø2R
 see Supplement, Heart and Great Vessels Ø2U
Atrioventricular node use Conduction Mechanism
Atrium dextrum cordis use Atrium, Right
Atrium pulmonale use Atrium, Left
Attain Ability® lead
 use Cardiac Lead, Pacemaker in Ø2H
 use Cardiac Lead, Defibrillator in Ø2H
Attain StarFix® (OTW) lead
 use Cardiac Lead, Pacemaker in Ø2H
 use Cardiac Lead, Defibrillator in O2H
Audiology, diagnostic
 see Hearing Assessment, Diagnostic Audiology F13
 see Hearing Aid Assessment, Diagnostic Audiology F14
 see Vestibular Assessment, Diagnostic Audiology F15
Audiometry see Hearing Assessment, Diagnostic Audiology F13
Auditory tube
 use Eustachian Tube, Right
 use Eustachian Tube, Left
Auerbach's (myenteric) plexus use Nerve, Abdominal Sympathetic
Auricle
 use External Ear, Right
 use External Ear, Left
 use External Ear, Bilateral
Auricularis muscle use Head Muscle
Autograft use Autologous Tissue Substitute
Autologous artery graft
 use Autologous Arterial Tissue in Heart and Great Vessels
 use Autologous Arterial Tissue in Upper Arteries
 use Autologous Arterial Tissue in Lower Arteries
 use Autologous Arterial Tissue in Upper Veins
 use Autologous Arterial Tissue in Lower Veins
Autologous vein graft
 use Autologous Venous Tissue in Heart and Great Vessels
 use Autologous Venous Tissue in Upper Arteries
 use Autologous Venous Tissue in Lower Arteries
 use Autologous Venous Tissue in Upper Veins
 use Autologous Venous Tissue in Lower Veins
Autotransfusion see Transfusion
Autotransplant
 Adrenal tissue see Reposition, Endocrine System ØGS
 Kidney
  see Reposition, Urinary System ØTS
 Pancreatic tissue see Reposition, Pancreas ØFSG
 Parathyroid tissue see Reposition, Endocrine System ØGS
 Thyroid tissue see Reposition, Endocrine System ØGS
 Tooth see Reattachment, Mouth and Throat ØCM
Avulsion see Extraction
Axial Lumbar Interbody Fusion System use Interbody Fusion Device in Lower Joints
AxiaLIF® System use Interbody Fusion Device in Lower Joints
Axicabtagene Ciloeucel use Engineered Autologous Chimeric Antigen Receptor T-cell Immunotherapy
Axillary fascia
 use Subcutaneous Tissue and Fascia, Right Upper Arm
 use Subcutaneous Tissue and Fascia, Left Upper Arm
Axillary nerve use Brachial Plexus

B

BAK/C® Interbody Cervical Fusion System
  use Interbody Fusion Device in Upper Joints
BAL (bronchial alveolar lavage), diagnostic *see* Drainage, Respiratory System 0B9
Balanoplasty
  see Repair, Penis 0VQS
  see Supplement, Penis 0VUS
Balloon atrial septostomy (BAS) 02163Z7
Balloon Pump
  Continuous, Output 5A02210
  Intermittent, Output 5A02110
Bandage, Elastic *see* Compression
Banding
  see Occlusion
  see Restriction
Banding, esophageal varices *see* Occlusion, Vein, Esophageal 06L3
Banding, laparoscopic (adjustable) gastric
  ▶ Surgical correction *see* Revision of device in, Stomach 0DW6
  Initial procedure 0DV64CZ
Bard® Composix® (E/X) (LP) mesh *use* Synthetic Substitute
Bard® Composix® Kugel® patch *use* Synthetic Substitute
Bard® Dulex™ mesh *use* Synthetic Substitute
Bard® Ventralex™ hernia patch *use* Synthetic Substitute
Barium swallow *see* Fluoroscopy, Gastrointestinal System BD1
Baroreflex Activation Therapy® (BAT®)
  use Stimulator Generator in Subcutaneous Tissue and Fascia
  use Stimulator Lead in Upper Arteries
Bartholin's (greater vestibular) gland *use* Vestibular Gland
Basal (internal) cerebral vein *use* Intracranial Vein
Basal metabolic rate (BMR) *see* Measurement, Physiological Systems 4A0Z
Basal nuclei *use* Basal Ganglia
Base of Tongue *use* Pharynx
Basilar artery *use* Intracranial Artery
Basis pontis *use* Pons
Beam Radiation
  Abdomen DW03
    Intraoperative DW033Z0
  Adrenal Gland DG02
    Intraoperative DG023Z0
  Bile Ducts DF02
    Intraoperative DF023Z0
  Bladder DT02
    Intraoperative DT023Z0
  Bone
    Other DP0C
    Intraoperative DP0C3Z0
  Bone Marrow D700
    Intraoperative D7003Z0
  Brain D000
    Intraoperative D0003Z0
  Brain Stem D001
    Intraoperative D0013Z0
  Breast
    Left DM00
      Intraoperative DM003Z0
    Right DM01
      Intraoperative DM013Z0
  Bronchus DB01
    Intraoperative DB013Z0
  Cervix DU01
    Intraoperative DU013Z0
  Chest DW02
    Intraoperative DW023Z0
  Chest Wall DB07
    Intraoperative DB073Z0
  Colon DD05
    Intraoperative DD053Z0

Beam Radiation *(Continued)*
  Diaphragm DB08
    Intraoperative DB083Z0
  Duodenum DD02
    Intraoperative DD023Z0
  Ear D900
    Intraoperative D9003Z0
  Esophagus DD00
    Intraoperative DD003Z0
  Eye D800
    Intraoperative D8003Z0
  Femur DP09
    Intraoperative DP093Z0
  Fibula DP0B
    Intraoperative DP0B3Z0
  Gallbladder DF01
    Intraoperative DF013Z0
  Gland
    Adrenal DG02
      Intraoperative DG023Z0
    Parathyroid DG04
      Intraoperative DG043Z0
    Pituitary DG00
      Intraoperative DG003Z0
    Thyroid DG05
      Intraoperative DG053Z0
  Glands
    Salivary D906
    Intraoperative D9063Z0
  Head and Neck DW01
    Intraoperative DW013Z0
  Hemibody DW04
    Intraoperative DW043Z0
  Humerus DP06
    Intraoperative DP063Z0
  Hypopharynx D903
    Intraoperative D9033Z0
  Ileum DD04
    Intraoperative DD043Z0
  Jejunum DD03
    Intraoperative DD033Z0
  Kidney DT00
    Intraoperative DT003Z0
  Larynx D90B
    Intraoperative D90B3Z0
  Liver DF00
    Intraoperative DF003Z0
  Lung DB02
    Intraoperative DB023Z0
  Lymphatics
    Abdomen D706
      Intraoperative D7063Z0
    Axillary D704
      Intraoperative D7043Z0
    Inguinal D708
      Intraoperative D7083Z0
    Neck D703
      Intraoperative D7033Z0
    Pelvis D707
      Intraoperative D7073Z0
    Thorax D705
      Intraoperative D7053Z0
  Mandible DP03
    Intraoperative DP033Z0
  Maxilla DP02
    Intraoperative DP023Z0
  Mediastinum DB06
    Intraoperative DB063Z0
  Mouth D904
    Intraoperative D9043Z0
  Nasopharynx D90D
    Intraoperative D90D3Z0
  Neck and Head DW01
    Intraoperative DW013Z0
  Nerve
    Peripheral D007
    Intraoperative D0073Z0
  Nose D901
    Intraoperative D9013Z0
  Oropharynx D90F
    Intraoperative D90F3Z0

Beam Radiation *(Continued)*
  Ovary DU00
    Intraoperative DU003Z0
  Palate
    Hard D908
      Intraoperative D9083Z0
    Soft D909
      Intraoperative D9093Z0
  Pancreas DF03
    Intraoperative DF033Z0
  Parathyroid Gland DG04
    Intraoperative DG043Z0
  Pelvic Bones DP08
    Intraoperative DP083Z0
  Pelvic Region DW06
    Intraoperative DW063Z0
  Pineal Body DG01
    Intraoperative DG013Z0
  Pituitary Gland DG00
    Intraoperative DG003Z0
  Pleura DB05
    Intraoperative DB053Z0
  Prostate DV00
    Intraoperative DV003Z0
  Radius DP07
    Intraoperative DP073Z0
  Rectum DD07
    Intraoperative DD073Z0
  Rib DP05
    Intraoperative DP053Z0
  Sinuses D907
    Intraoperative D9073Z0
  Skin
    Abdomen DH08
      Intraoperative DH083Z0
    Arm DH04
      Intraoperative DH043Z0
    Back DH07
      Intraoperative DH073Z0
    Buttock DH09
      Intraoperative DH093Z0
    Chest DH06
      Intraoperative DH063Z0
    Face DH02
      Intraoperative DH023Z0
    Leg DH0B
      Intraoperative DH0B3Z0
    Neck DH03
      Intraoperative DH033Z0
  Skull DP00
    Intraoperative DP003Z0
  Spinal Cord D006
    Intraoperative D0063Z0
  Spleen D702
    Intraoperative D7023Z0
  Sternum DP04
    Intraoperative DP043Z0
  Stomach DD01
    Intraoperative DD013Z0
  Testis DV01
    Intraoperative DV013Z0
  Thymus D701
    Intraoperative D7013Z0
  Thyroid Gland DG05
    Intraoperative DG053Z0
  Tibia DP0B
    Intraoperative DP0B3Z0
  Tongue D905
    Intraoperative D9053Z0
  Trachea DB00
    Intraoperative DB003Z0
  Ulna DP07
    Intraoperative DP073Z0
  Ureter DT01
    Intraoperative DT013Z0
  Urethra DT03
    Intraoperative DT033Z0
  Uterus DU02
    Intraoperative DU023Z0
  Whole Body DW05
    Intraoperative DW053Z0

▶ New   ⇒ Revised   ~~deleted~~ Deleted

Bedside swallow F00ZJWZ
Berlin Heart Ventricular Assist Device *use* Implantable Heart Assist System in Heart and Great Vessels
Bezlotoxumab Monoclonal Antibody XW0
Biceps brachii muscle
   use Upper Arm Muscle, Right
   use Upper Arm Muscle, Left
Biceps femoris muscle
   use Upper Leg Muscle, Right
   use Upper Leg Muscle, Left
Bicipital aponeurosis
   use Subcutaneous Tissue and Fascia, Right Lower Arm
   use Subcutaneous Tissue and Fascia, Left Lower Arm
Bicuspid valve *use* Mitral Valve
▶ Bill light therapy *see* Phototherapy, Skin 6A60
Bioactive embolization coil(s) *use* Intraluminal Device, Bioactive in Upper Arteries
Biofeedback GZC9ZZZ
Biopsy
   see Drainage with qualifier Diagnostic
   see Excision with qualifier Diagnostic
▶ *see* Extraction with qualifier Diagnostic
   ~~Bone Marrow see Extraction with qualifier Diagnostic~~
BiPAP *see* Assistance, Respiratory 5A09
Bisection *see* Division
Biventricular external heart assist system
   use Short-term External Heart Assist System in Heart and Great Vessels
Blepharectomy
   see Excision, Eye 08B
   see Resection, Eye 08T
Blepharoplasty
   see Repair, Eye 08Q
   see Replacement, Eye 08R
   see Reposition, Eye 08S
   see Supplement, Eye 08U
Blepharorrhaphy *see* Repair, Eye 08Q
Blepharotomy *see* Drainage, Eye 089
Blinatumomab Antineoplastic Immunotherapy XW0
Block, Nerve, anesthetic injection 3E0T3CZ
Blood glucose monitoring system *use* Monitoring Device
Blood pressure *see* Measurement, Arterial 4A03
BMR (basal metabolic rate) *see* Measurement, Physiological Systems 4A0Z
Body of femur
   use Femoral Shaft, Right
   use Femoral Shaft, Left
Body of fibula
   use Fibula, Right
   use Fibula, Left
Bone anchored hearing device
   use Hearing Device, Bone Conduction in 09H
   use Hearing Device, in Head and Facial Bones
Bone bank bone graft *use* Nonautologous Tissue Substitute
Bone Growth Stimulator
   Insertion of device in
      Bone
         Facial 0NHW
         Lower 0QHY
         Nasal 0NHB
         Upper 0PHY
         Skull 0NH0
   Removal of device from
      Bone
         Facial 0NPW
         Lower 0QPY
         Nasal 0NPB
         Upper 0PPY
         Skull 0NP0

Bone Growth Stimulator *(Continued)*
   Revision of device in
      Bone
         Facial 0NWW
         Lower 0QWY
         Nasal 0NWB
         Upper 0PWY
      Skull 0NW0
Bone marrow transplant *see* Transfusion, Circulatory 302
Bone morphogenetic protein 2 (BMP 2) *use* Recombinant Bone Morphogenetic Protein
Bone screw (interlocking) (lag) (pedicle) (recessed)
   use Internal Fixation Device in Head and Facial Bones
   use Internal Fixation Device in Upper Bones
   use Internal Fixation Device in Lower Bones
Bony labyrinth
   use Inner Ear, Right
   use Inner Ear, Left
Bony orbit
   use Orbit, Right
   use Orbit, Left
Bony vestibule
   use Inner Ear, Right
   use Inner Ear, Left
Botallo's duct *use* Pulmonary Artery, Left
Bovine pericardial valve *use* Zooplastic Tissue in Heart and Great Vessels
Bovine pericardium graft *use* Zooplastic Tissue in Heart and Great Vessels
BP (blood pressure) *see* Measurement, Arterial 4A03
Brachial (lateral) lymph node
   use Lymphatic, Axillary Right
   use Lymphatic, Axillary Left
Brachialis muscle
   use Upper Arm Muscle, Right
   use Upper Arm Muscle, Left
Brachiocephalic artery *use* Innominate Artery
Brachiocephalic trunk *use* Innominate Artery
Brachiocephalic vein
   use Innominate Vein, Right
   use Innominate Vein, Left
Brachioradialis muscle
   use Lower Arm and Wrist Muscle, Right
   use Lower Arm and Wrist Muscle, Left
Brachytherapy
   Abdomen DW13
   Adrenal Gland DG12
   Bile Ducts DF12
   Bladder DT12
   Bone Marrow D710
   Brain D010
   Brain Stem D011
   Breast
      Left DM10
      Right DM11
   Bronchus DB11
   Cervix DU11
   Chest DW12
   Chest Wall DB17
   Colon DD15
   Diaphragm DB18
   Duodenum DD12
   Ear D910
   Esophagus DD10
   Eye D810
   Gallbladder DF11
   Gland
      Adrenal DG12
      Parathyroid DG14
      Pituitary DG10
      Thyroid DG15
   Glands, Salivary D916
   Head and Neck DW11
   Hypopharynx D913
   Ileum DD14

Brachytherapy *(Continued)*
   Jejunum DD13
   Kidney DT10
   Larynx D91B
   Liver DF10
   Lung DB12
   Lymphatics
      Abdomen D716
      Axillary D714
      Inguinal D718
      Neck D713
      Pelvis D717
      Thorax D715
   Mediastinum DB16
   Mouth D914
   Nasopharynx D91D
   Neck and Head DW11
   Nerve, Peripheral D017
   Nose D911
   Oropharynx D91F
   Ovary DU10
   Palate
      Hard D918
      Soft D919
   Pancreas DF13
   Parathyroid Gland DG14
   Pelvic Region DW16
   Pineal Body DG11
   Pituitary Gland DG10
   Pleura DB15
   Prostate DV10
   Rectum DD17
   Sinuses D917
   Spinal Cord D016
   Spleen D712
   Stomach DD11
   Testis DV11
   Thymus D711
   Thyroid Gland DG15
   Tongue D915
   Trachea DB10
   Ureter DT11
   Urethra DT13
   Uterus DU12
Brachytherapy seeds *use* Radioactive Element
Broad ligament *use* Uterine Supporting Structure
Bronchial artery *use* Upper Artery
Bronchography
   see Plain Radiography, Respiratory System BB0
   see Fluoroscopy, Respiratory System BB1
Bronchoplasty
   see Repair, Respiratory System 0BQ
   see Supplement, Respiratory System 0BU
Bronchorrhaphy *see* Repair, Respiratory System 0BQ
Bronchoscopy 0BJ08ZZ
Bronchotomy *see* Drainage, Respiratory System 0B9
Bronchus Intermedius *use* Main Bronchus, Right
BRYAN® Cervical Disc System *use* Synthetic Substitute
Buccal gland *use* Buccal Mucosa
Buccinator lymph node *use* Lymphatic, Head
Buccinator muscle *use* Facial Muscle
Buckling, scleral with implant *see* Supplement, Eye 08U
Bulbospongiosus muscle *use* Perineum Muscle
Bulbourethral (Cowper's) gland *use* Urethra
Bundle of His *use* Conduction Mechanism
Bundle of Kent *use* Conduction Mechanism
Bunionectomy *see* Excision, Lower Bones 0QB
Bursectomy
   see Excision, Bursae and Ligaments 0MB
   see Resection, Bursae and Ligaments 0MT
Bursocentesis *see* Drainage, Bursae and Ligaments 0M9

▶ New   ⟹ Revised   ~~deleted~~ Deleted

B

Bursography
  see Plain Radiography, Non-Axial Upper
    Bones BP0
  see Plain Radiography, Non-Axial Lower
    Bones BQ0
Bursotomy
  see Division, Bursae and Ligaments 0M8
  see Drainage, Bursae and Ligaments
    0M9
BVS 5000 Ventricular Assist Device use
  Short-term External Heart Assist System
    in Heart and Great Vessels
Bypass
  Anterior Chamber
    Left 08133
    Right 08123
  Aorta
    Abdominal 0410
    Thoracic
      Ascending/Arch 021X
      Descending 021W
  Artery
  ▶Anterior Tibial
    ▶Left 041Q
    ▶Right 041P
    Axillary
      Left 03160
      Right 03150
    Brachial
      Left 03180
      Right 03170
    Common Carotid
      Left 031J0
      Right 031H0
    Common Iliac
      Left 041D
      Right 041C
    Coronary
      Four or More Arteries 0213
      One Artery 0210
      Three Arteries 0212
      Two Arteries 0211
    External Carotid
      Left 031N0
      Right 031M0
    External Iliac
      Left 041J
      Right 041H
    Femoral
      Left 041L
      Right 041K
    Foot
      Left 041W
      Right 041V
    Hepatic 0413
    Innominate 03120
    Internal Carotid
      Left 031L0
      Right 031K0
    Internal Iliac
      Left 041F
      Right 041E
    Intracranial 031G0
    Peroneal
      Left 041U
      Right 041T
    Popliteal
      Left 041N
      Right 041M
  ▶Posterior Tibial
    ▶Left 041S
    ▶Right 041R
    Pulmonary
      Left 021R
      Right 021Q

Bypass (*Continued*)
  Artery (*Continued*)
    Pulmonary Trunk 021P
    Radial
      Left 031C0
      Right 031B0
    Splenic 0414
    Subclavian
      Left 03140
      Right 03130
    Temporal
      Left 031T0
      Right 031S0
    Ulnar
      Left 031A0
      Right 03190
  Atrium
    Left 0217
    Right 0216
  Bladder 0T1B
  Cavity, Cranial 0W110J
  Cecum 0D1H
  Cerebral Ventricle 0016
  Colon
    Ascending 0D1K
    Descending 0D1M
    Sigmoid 0D1N
    Transverse 0D1L
  Duct
    Common Bile 0F19
    Cystic 0F18
    Hepatic
      Common 0F17
      Left 0F16
      Right 0F15
    Lacrimal
      Left 081Y
      Right 081X
    Pancreatic 0F1D
      Accessory 0F1F
  Duodenum 0D19
  Ear
    Left 091E0
    Right 091D0
  Esophagus 0D15
    Lower 0D13
    Middle 0D12
    Upper 0D11
  Fallopian Tube
    Left 0U16
    Right 0U15
  Gallbladder 0F14
  Ileum 0D1B
  Jejunum 0D1A
  Kidney Pelvis
    Left 0T14
    Right 0T13
  Pancreas 0F1G
  Pelvic Cavity 0W1J
  Peritoneal Cavity 0W1G
  Pleural Cavity
    Left 0W1B
    Right 0W19
  Spinal Canal 001U
  Stomach 0D16
  Trachea 0B11
  Ureter
    Left 0T17
    Right 0T16
  Ureters, Bilateral 0T18
  Vas Deferens
    Bilateral 0V1Q
    Left 0V1P
    Right 0V1N

Bypass (*Continued*)
  Vein
    Axillary
      Left 0518
      Right 0517
    Azygos 0510
    Basilic
      Left 051C
      Right 051B
    Brachial
      Left 051A
      Right 0519
    Cephalic
      Left 051F
      Right 051D
    Colic 0617
    Common Iliac
      Left 061D
      Right 061C
    Esophageal 0613
    External Iliac
      Left 061G
      Right 061F
    External Jugular
      Left 051Q
      Right 051P
    Face
      Left 051V
      Right 051T
    Femoral
      Left 061N
      Right 061M
    Foot
      Left 061V
      Right 061T
    Gastric 0612
    Hand
      Left 051H
      Right 051G
    Hemiazygos 0511
    Hepatic 0614
    Hypogastric
      Left 061J
      Right 061H
    Inferior Mesenteric 0616
    Innominate
      Left 0514
      Right 0513
    Internal Jugular
      Left 051N
      Right 051M
    Intracranial 051L
    Portal 0618
    Renal
      Left 061B
      Right 0619
    Saphenous
      Left 061Q
      Right 061P
    Splenic 0611
    Subclavian
      Left 0516
      Right 0515
    Superior Mesenteric 0615
    Vertebral
      Left 051S
      Right 051R
  Vena Cava
    Inferior 0610
    Superior 021V
  Ventricle
    Left 021L
    Right 021K
Bypass, cardiopulmonary 5A1221Z

▶ New   ⇒ Revised   ~~deleted~~ Deleted

C

Caesarean section *see* Extraction, Products of Conception 10D0
Calcaneocuboid joint
  use Tarsal Joint, Right
  use Tarsal Joint, Left
Calcaneocuboid ligament
  use Foot Bursa and Ligament, Right
  use Foot Bursa and Ligament, Left
Calcaneofibular ligament
  use Ankle Bursa and Ligament, Right
  use Ankle Bursa and Ligament, Left
Calcaneus
  use Tarsal, Right
  use Tarsal, Left
Cannulation
  see Bypass
  see Dilation
  see Drainage
  see Irrigation
Canthorrhaphy *see* Repair, Eye 08Q
Canthotomy *see* Release, Eye 08N
Capitate bone
  use Carpal, Right
  use Carpal, Left
Capsulectomy, lens *see* Excision, Eye 08B
Capsulorrhaphy, joint
  see Repair, Upper Joints 0RQ
  see Repair, Lower Joints 0SQ
Cardia *use* Esophagogastric Junction
Cardiac contractility modulation lead *use* Cardiac Lead in Heart and Great Vessels
Cardiac event recorder *use* Monitoring Device
Cardiac Lead
  Defibrillator
    Atrium
      Left 02H7
      Right 02H6
    Pericardium 02HN
    Vein, Coronary 02H4
    Ventricle
      Left 02HL
      Right 02HK
  Insertion of device in
    Atrium
      Left 02H7
      Right 02H6
    Pericardium 02HN
    Vein, Coronary 02H4
    Ventricle
      Left 02HL
      Right 02HK
  Pacemaker
    Atrium
      Left 02H7
      Right 02H6
    Pericardium 02HN
    Vein, Coronary 02H4
    Ventricle
      Left 02HL
      Right 02HK
  Removal of device from, Heart 02PA
  Revision of device in, Heart 02WA
Cardiac plexus *use* Nerve, Thoracic Sympathetic
Cardiac Resynchronization Defibrillator Pulse Generator
  Abdomen 0JH8
  Chest 0JH6
Cardiac Resynchronization Pacemaker Pulse Generator
  Abdomen 0JH8
  Chest 0JH6
Cardiac resynchronization therapy (CRT) lead
  use Cardiac Lead, Pacemaker in 02H
  use Cardiac Lead, Defibrillator in 02H
Cardiac Rhythm Related Device
  Insertion of device in
    Abdomen 0JH8
    Chest 0JH6

Cardiac Rhythm Related Device *(Continued)*
  Removal of device from, Subcutaneous Tissue and Fascia, Trunk 0JPT
  Revision of device in, Subcutaneous Tissue and Fascia, Trunk 0JWT
Cardiocentesis *see* Drainage, Pericardial Cavity 0W9D
Cardioesophageal junction *use* Esophagogastric Junction
Cardiolysis *see* Release, Heart and Great Vessels 02N
CardioMEMS® pressure sensor *use* Monitoring Device, Pressure Sensor in 02H
Cardiomyotomy *see* Division, Esophagogastric Junction 0D84
Cardioplegia *see* Introduction of substance in or on, Heart 3E08
Cardiorrhaphy *see* Repair, Heart and Great Vessels 02Q
Cardioversion 5A2204Z
Caregiver Training F0FZ
Caroticotympanic artery
  use Internal Carotid Artery, Right
  use Internal Carotid Artery, Left
Carotid (artery) sinus (baroreceptor) lead *use* Stimulator Lead in Upper Arteries
Carotid glomus
  use Carotid Body, Left
  use Carotid Body, Right
  use Carotid Bodies, Bilateral
Carotid sinus
  use Internal Carotid Artery, Right
  use Internal Carotid Artery, Left
Carotid sinus nerve *use* Glossopharyngeal Nerve
Carotid WALLSTENT® Monorail® Endoprosthesis *use* Intraluminal Device
Carpectomy
  see Excision, Upper Bones 0PB
  see Resection, Upper Bones 0PT
Carpometacarpal ligament
  use Hand Bursa and Ligament, Right
  use Hand Bursa and Ligament, Left
Casting *see* Immobilization
CAT scan *see* Computerized Tomography (CT Scan)
Catheterization
  see Dilation
  see Drainage
  see Insertion of device in
  see Irrigation
  Heart *see* Measurement, Cardiac 4A02
  Umbilical vein, for infusion 06H033T
Cauda equina *use* Lumbar Spinal Cord
Cauterization
  see Destruction
  see Repair
Cavernous plexus *use* Head and Neck Sympathetic Nerve
CBMA (Concentrated Bone Marrow Aspirate) *use* Concentrated Bone Marrow Aspirate
CBMA (Concentrated Bone Marrow Aspirate) injection, intramuscular XK02303
Cecectomy
  see Excision, Cecum 0DBH
  see Resection, Cecum 0DTH
Cecocolostomy
  see Bypass, Gastrointestinal System 0D1
  see Drainage, Gastrointestinal System 0D9
Cecopexy
  see Repair, Cecum 0DQH
  see Reposition, Cecum 0DSH
Cecoplication *see* Restriction, Cecum 0DVH
Cecorrhaphy *see* Repair, Cecum 0DQH
Cecostomy
  see Bypass, Cecum 0D1H
  see Drainage, Cecum 0D9H
Cecotomy *see* Drainage, Cecum 0D9H
Ceftazidime-Avibactam Anti-infective XW0
Celiac (solar) plexus *use* Abdominal Sympathetic Nerve

Celiac ganglion *use* Abdominal Sympathetic Nerve
Celiac lymph node *use* Lymphatic, Aortic
Celiac trunk *use* Celiac Artery
Central axillary lymph node
  use Lymphatic, Right Axillary
  use Lymphatic, Left Axillary
Central venous pressure *see* Measurement, Venous 4A04
Centrimag® Blood Pump *use* Short-term External Heart Assist System in Heart and Great Vessels
Cephalogram BN00ZZZ
Ceramic on ceramic bearing surface *use* Synthetic Substitute, Ceramic in 0SR
Cerclage *see* Restriction
Cerebral aqueduct (Sylvius) *use* Cerebral Ventricle
Cerebral Embolic Filtration, Dual Filter X2A5312
Cerebrum *use* Brain
Cervical esophagus *use* Esophagus, Upper
Cervical facet joint
  use Cervical Vertebral Joint
  use Cervical Vertebral Joint, 2 or more
Cervical ganglion *use* Head and Neck Sympathetic Nerve
Cervical interspinous ligament *use* Head and Neck Bursa and Ligament
Cervical intertransverse ligament *use* Head and Neck Bursa and Ligament
Cervical ligamentum flavum *use* Head and Neck Bursa and Ligament
Cervical lymph node
  use Lymphatic, Right Neck
  use Lymphatic, Left Neck
Cervicectomy
  see Excision, Cervix 0UBC
  see Resection, Cervix 0UTC
Cervicothoracic facet joint *use* Cervicothoracic Vertebral Joint
Cesarean section *see* Extraction, Products of Conception 10D0
Cesium-131 Collagen Implant *use* Radioactive Element, Cesium-131 Collagen Implant in 00H
Change device in
  Abdominal Wall 0W2FX
  Back
    Lower 0W2LX
    Upper 0W2KX
  Bladder 0T2BX
  Bone
    Facial 0N2WX
    Lower 0Q2YX
    Nasal 0N2BX
    Upper 0P2YX
  Bone Marrow 072TX
  Brain 0020X
  Breast
    Left 0H2UX
    Right 0H2TX
  Bursa and Ligament
    Lower 0M2YX
    Upper 0M2XX
  Cavity, Cranial 0W21X
  Chest Wall 0W28X
  Cisterna Chyli 072LX
  Diaphragm 0B2TX
  Duct
    Hepatobiliary 0F2BX
    Pancreatic 0F2DX
  Ear
    Left 092JX
    Right 092HX
  Epididymis and Spermatic Cord 0V2MX
  Extremity
    Lower
      Left 0Y2BX
      Right 0Y29X
    Upper
      Left 0X27X
      Right 0X26X

▶ New   ⇒ Revised   ~~deleted~~ Deleted

Change device in (Continued)
Eye
Left 0821X
Right 0820X
Face 0W22X
Fallopian Tube 0U28X
Gallbladder 0F24X
Gland
Adrenal 0G25X
Endocrine 0G2SX
Pituitary 0G20X
Salivary 0C2AX
Head 0W20X
Intestinal Tract
Lower 0D2DXUZ
Upper 0D20XUZ
Jaw
Lower 0W25X
Upper 0W24X
Joint
Lower 0S2YX
Upper 0R2YX
Kidney 0T25X
Larynx 0C2SX
Liver 0F20X
Lung
Left 0B2LX
Right 0B2KX
Lymphatic 072NX
Thoracic Duct 072KX
Mediastinum 0W2CX
Mesentery 0D2VX
Mouth and Throat 0C2YX
Muscle
Lower 0K2YX
Upper 0K2XX
Nasal Mucosa and Soft Tissue
092KX
Neck 0W26X
Nerve
Cranial 002EX
Peripheral 012YX
Omentum 0D2UX
Ovary 0U23X
Pancreas 0F2GX
Parathyroid Gland 0G2RX
Pelvic Cavity 0W2JX
Penis 0V2SX
Pericardial Cavity 0W2DX
Perineum
Female 0W2NX
Male 0W2MX
Peritoneal Cavity 0W2GX
Peritoneum 0D2WX
Pineal Body 0G21X
Pleura 0B2QX
Pleural Cavity
Left 0W2BX
Right 0W29X
Products of Conception 10207
Prostate and Seminal Vesicles 0V24X
Retroperitoneum 0W2HX
Scrotum and Tunica Vaginalis 0V28X
Sinus 092YX
Skin 0H2PX
Skull 0N20X
Spinal Canal 002UX
Spleen 072PX
Subcutaneous Tissue and Fascia
Head and Neck 0J2SX
Lower Extremity 0J2WX
Trunk 0J2TX
Upper Extremity 0J2VX
Tendon
Lower 0L2YX
Upper 0L2XX
Testis 0V2DX
Thymus 072MX
Thyroid Gland 0G2KX
Trachea 0B21
Tracheobronchial Tree 0B20X

Change device in (Continued)
Ureter 0T29X
Urethra 0T2DX
Uterus and Cervix 0U2DXHZ
Vagina and Cul-de-sac 0U2HXGZ
Vas Deferens 0V2RX
Vulva 0U2MX
Change device in or on
Abdominal Wall 2W03X
Anorectal 2Y03X5Z
Arm
Lower
Left 2W0DX
Right 2W0CX
Upper
Left 2W0BX
Right 2W0AX
Back 2W05X
Chest Wall 2W04X
Ear 2Y02X5Z
Extremity
Lower
Left 2W0MX
Right 2W0LX
Upper
Left 2W09X
Right 2W08X
Face 2W01X
Finger
Left 2W0KX
Right 2W0JX
Foot
Left 2W0TX
Right 2W0SX
Genital Tract, Female 2Y04X5Z
Hand
Left 2W0FX
Right 2W0EX
Head 2W00X
Inguinal Region
Left 2W07X
Right 2W06X
Leg
Lower
Left 2W0RX
Right 2W0QX
Upper
Left 2W0PX
Right 2W0NX
Mouth and Pharynx 2Y00X5Z
Nasal 2Y01X5Z
Neck 2W02X
Thumb
Left 2W0HX
Right 2W0GX
Toe
Left 2W0VX
Right 2W0UX
Urethra 2Y05X5Z
Chemoembolization see Introduction of
substance in or on
Chemosurgery, Skin 3E00XTZ
Chemothalamectomy see Destruction,
Thalamus 0059
Chemotherapy, Infusion for cancer see
Introduction of substance in or on
Chest x-ray see Plain Radiography, Chest
BW03
Chiropractic Manipulation
Abdomen 9WB9X
Cervical 9WB1X
Extremities
Lower 9WB6X
Upper 9WB7X
Head 9WB0X
Lumbar 9WB3X
Pelvis 9WB5X
Rib Cage 9WB8X
Sacrum 9WB4X
Thoracic 9WB2X
Choana use Nasopharynx

Cholangiogram
see Plain Radiography, Hepatobiliary System
and Pancreas BF0
see Fluoroscopy, Hepatobiliary System and
Pancreas BF1
Cholecystectomy
see Excision, Gallbladder 0FB4
see Resection, Gallbladder 0FT4
Cholecystojejunostomy
see Bypass, Hepatobiliary System and
Pancreas 0F1
see Drainage, Hepatobiliary System and
Pancreas 0F9
Cholecystopexy
see Repair, Gallbladder 0FQ4
see Reposition, Gallbladder 0FS4
Cholecystoscopy 0FJ44ZZ
Cholecystostomy
see Bypass, Gallbladder 0F14
see Drainage, Gallbladder 0F94
Cholecystotomy see Drainage, Gallbladder 0F94
Choledochectomy
see Excision, Hepatobiliary System and
Pancreas 0FB
see Resection, Hepatobiliary System and
Pancreas 0FT
Choledocholithotomy see Extirpation, Duct,
Common Bile 0FC9
Choledochoplasty
see Repair, Hepatobiliary System and
Pancreas 0FQ
see Replacement, Hepatobiliary System and
Pancreas 0FR
see Supplement, Hepatobiliary System and
Pancreas 0FU
Choledochoscopy 0FJB8ZZ
Choledochotomy see Drainage, Hepatobiliary
System and Pancreas 0F9
Cholelithotomy see Extirpation, Hepatobiliary
System and Pancreas 0FC
Chondrectomy
see Excision, Upper Joints 0RB
see Excision, Lower Joints 0SB
Knee see Excision, Lower Joints 0SB
Semilunar cartilage see Excision, Lower Joints
0SB
Chondroglossus muscle use Tongue, Palate,
Pharynx Muscle
Chorda tympani use Facial Nerve
Chordotomy see Division, Central Nervous
System and Cranial Nerves 008
Choroid plexus use Cerebral Ventricle
Choroidectomy
see Excision, Eye 08B
see Resection, Eye 08T
Ciliary body
use Eye, Right
use Eye, Left
Ciliary ganglion use Head and Neck
Sympathetic Nerve
Circle of Willis use Intracranial Artery
Circumcision 0VTTXZZ
Circumflex iliac artery
use Femoral Artery, Right
use Femoral Artery, Left
Clamp and rod internal fixation system (CRIF)
use Internal Fixation Device in Upper Bones
use Internal Fixation Device in Lower Bones
Clamping see Occlusion
Claustrum use Basal Ganglia
Claviculectomy
see Excision, Upper Bones 0PB
see Resection, Upper Bones 0PT
Claviculotomy
see Division, Upper Bones 0P8
see Drainage, Upper Bones 0P9
Clipping, aneurysm
see Occlusion using Extraluminal Device
see Restriction using Extraluminal Device
Clitorectomy, clitoridectomy
see Excision, Clitoris 0UBJ
see Resection, Clitoris 0UTJ

Clolar *use* Clofarabine
Closure
   see Occlusion
   see Repair
Clysis *see* Introduction of substance in or on
Coagulation *see* Destruction
COALESCE® radiolucent interbody fusion
   device *use* Interbody Fusion Device,
   Radiolucent Porous in New Technology
CoAxia NeuroFlo catheter *use* Intraluminal
   Device
Cobalt/chromium head and polyethylene
   socket *use* Synthetic Substitute, Metal on
   Polyethylene in 0SR
Cobalt/chromium head and socket *use*
   Synthetic Substitute, Metal in 0SR
Coccygeal body *use* Coccygeal Glomus
Coccygeus muscle
   use Trunk Muscle, Right
   use Trunk Muscle, Left
Cochlea
   use Inner Ear, Right
   use Inner Ear, Left
Cochlear implant (CI), multiple channel
   (electrode) *use* Hearing Device, Multiple
   Channel Cochlear Prosthesis in 09H
Cochlear implant (CI), single channel
   (electrode) *use* Hearing Device, Single
   Channel Cochlear Prosthesis in 09H
Cochlear Implant Treatment F0BZ0
Cochlear nerve *use* Acoustic Nerve
COGNIS® CRT-D *use* Cardiac
   Resynchronization Defibrillator Pulse
   Generator in 0JH
COHERE® radiolucent interbody fusion
   device *use* Interbody Fusion Device,
   Radiolucent Porous in New Technology
Colectomy
   see Excision, Gastrointestinal System 0DB
   see Resection, Gastrointestinal System 0DT
Collapse *see* Occlusion
Collection from
   Breast, Breast Milk 8E0HX62
   Indwelling Device
     Circulatory System
       Blood 8C02X6K
       Other Fluid 8C02X6L
     Nervous System
       Cerebrospinal Fluid 8C01X6J
       Other Fluid 8C01X6L
   Integumentary System, Breast Milk 8E0HX62
   Reproductive System, Male, Sperm 8E0VX63
Colocentesis *see* Drainage, Gastrointestinal
   System 0D9
Colofixation
   see Repair, Gastrointestinal System 0DQ
   see Reposition, Gastrointestinal System 0DS
Cololysis *see* Release, Gastrointestinal System
   0DN
Colonic Z-Stent® *use* Intraluminal Device
Colonoscopy 0DJD8ZZ
Colopexy
   see Repair, Gastrointestinal System 0DQ
   see Reposition, Gastrointestinal System 0DS
Coloplication *see* Restriction, Gastrointestinal
   System 0DV
Coloproctectomy
   see Excision, Gastrointestinal System 0DB
   see Resection, Gastrointestinal System 0DT
Coloproctostomy
   see Bypass, Gastrointestinal System 0D1
   see Drainage, Gastrointestinal System 0D9
Colopuncture *see* Drainage, Gastrointestinal
   System 0D9
Colorrhaphy *see* Repair, Gastrointestinal System
   0DQ
Colostomy
   see Bypass, Gastrointestinal System 0D1
   see Drainage, Gastrointestinal System 0D9
Colpectomy
   see Excision, Vagina 0UBG
   see Resection, Vagina 0UTG

Colpocentesis *see* Drainage, Vagina 0U9G
Colpopexy
   see Repair, Vagina 0UQG
   see Reposition, Vagina 0USG
Colpoplasty
   see Repair, Vagina 0UQG
   see Supplement, Vagina 0UUG
Colporrhaphy *see* Repair, Vagina 0UQG
Colposcopy 0UJH8ZZ
Columella *use* Nasal Mucosa and Soft Tissue
Common digital vein
   use Foot Vein, Right
   use Foot Vein, Left
Common facial vein
   use Face Vein, Right
   use Face Vein, Left
Common fibular nerve *use* Peroneal Nerve
Common hepatic artery *use* Hepatic Artery
Common iliac (subaortic) lymph node *use*
   Lymphatic, Pelvis
Common interosseous artery
   use Ulnar Artery, Right
   use Ulnar Artery, Left
Common peroneal nerve *use* Peroneal
   Nerve
Complete (SE) stent *use* Intraluminal Device
Compression *see* Restriction
   Abdominal Wall 2W13X
   Arm
     Lower
       Left 2W1DX
       Right 2W1CX
     Upper
       Left 2W1BX
       Right 2W1AX
   Back 2W15X
   Chest Wall 2W14X
   Extremity
     Lower
       Left 2W1MX
       Right 2W1LX
     Upper
       Left 2W19X
       Right 2W18X
   Face 2W11X
   Finger
     Left 2W1KX
     Right 2W1JX
   Foot
     Left 2W1TX
     Right 2W1SX
   Hand
     Left 2W1FX
     Right 2W1EX
   Head 2W10X
   Inguinal Region
     Left 2W17X
     Right 2W16X
   Leg
     Lower
       Left 2W1RX
       Right 2W1QX
     Upper
       Left 2W1PX
       Right 2W1NX
   Neck 2W12X
   Thumb
     Left 2W1HX
     Right 2W1GX
   Toe
     Left 2W1VX
     Right 2W1UX
Computer Assisted Procedure
   Extremity
     Lower
       No Qualifier 8E0YXBZ
       With Computerized Tomography
         8E0YXBG
       With Fluoroscopy 8E0YXBF
       With Magnetic Resonance Imaging
         8E0YXBH

Computer Assisted Procedure *(Continued)*
   Extremity *(Continued)*
     Upper
       No Qualifier 8E0XXBZ
       With Computerized Tomography
         8E0XXBG
       With Fluoroscopy 8E0XXBF
       With Magnetic Resonance Imaging
         8E0XXBH
   Head and Neck Region
     No Qualifier 8E09XBZ
     With Computerized Tomography 8E09XBG
     With Fluoroscopy 8E09XBF
     With Magnetic Resonance Imaging 8E09XBH
   Trunk Region
     No Qualifier 8E0WXBZ
     With Computerized Tomography 8E0WXBG
     With Fluoroscopy 8E0WXBF
     With Magnetic Resonance Imaging
       8E0WXBH
Computerized Tomography (CT Scan)
   Abdomen BW20
     Chest and Pelvis BW25
   Abdomen and Chest BW24
   Abdomen and Pelvis BW21
   Airway, Trachea BB2F
   Ankle
     Left BQ2H
     Right BQ2G
   Aorta
     Abdominal B420
       Intravascular Optical Coherence
         B420Z2Z
     Thoracic B320
       Intravascular Optical Coherence
         B320Z2Z
   Arm
     Left BP2F
     Right BP2E
   Artery
     Celiac B421
       Intravascular Optical Coherence
         B421Z2Z
     Common Carotid
       Bilateral B325
       Intravascular Optical Coherence
         B325Z2Z
     Coronary
       Bypass Graft
         Multiple B223
         Intravascular Optical Coherence
           B223Z2Z
       Multiple B221
         Intravascular Optical Coherence
           B221Z2Z
     Internal Carotid
       Bilateral B328
       Intravascular Optical Coherence
         B328Z2Z
     Intracranial B32R
       Intravascular Optical Coherence
         B32RZ2Z
     Lower Extremity
       Bilateral B42H
       Intravascular Optical Coherence
         B42HZ2Z
       Left B42G
       Intravascular Optical Coherence
         B42GZ2Z
       Right B42F
       Intravascular Optical Coherence
         B42FZ2Z
     Pelvic B42C
       Intravascular Optical Coherence
         B42CZ2Z
     Pulmonary
       Left B32T
       Intravascular Optical Coherence
         B32TZ2Z
       Right B32S
       Intravascular Optical Coherence
         B32SZ2Z

Computerized Tomography (*Continued*)
  Artery (*Continued*)
    Renal
      Bilateral B428
        Intravascular Optical Coherence B428Z2Z
      Transplant B42M
        Intravascular Optical Coherence B42MZ2Z
    Superior Mesenteric B424
      Intravascular Optical Coherence B424Z2Z
    Vertebral
      Bilateral B32G
        Intravascular Optical Coherence B32GZ2Z
  Bladder BT20
  Bone
    Facial BN25
    Temporal BN2F
  Brain B020
  Calcaneus
    Left BQ2K
    Right BQ2J
  Cerebral Ventricle B028
  Chest, Abdomen and Pelvis BW25
  Chest and Abdomen BW24
  Cisterna B027
  Clavicle
    Left BP25
    Right BP24
  Coccyx BR2F
  Colon BD24
  Ear B920
  Elbow
    Left BP2H
    Right BP2G
  Extremity
    Lower
      Left BQ2S
      Right BQ2R
    Upper
      Bilateral BP2V
      Left BP2U
      Right BP2T
  Eye
    Bilateral B827
    Left B826
    Right B825
  Femur
    Left BQ24
    Right BQ23
  Fibula
    Left BQ2C
    Right BQ2B
  Finger
    Left BP2S
    Right BP2R
  Foot
    Left BQ2M
    Right BQ2L
  Forearm
    Left BP2K
    Right BP2J
  Gland
    Adrenal, Bilateral BG22
    Parathyroid BG23
    Parotid, Bilateral B926
    Salivary, Bilateral B92D
    Submandibular, Bilateral B929
    Thyroid BG24
  Hand
    Left BP2P
    Right BP2N
  Hands and Wrists, Bilateral BP2Q
  Head BW28
  Head and Neck BW29
  Heart
    Right and Left B226
    Intravascular Optical Coherence B226Z2Z
  Hepatobiliary System, All BF2C

Computerized Tomography (*Continued*)
  Hip
    Left BQ21
    Right BQ20
  Humerus
    Left BP2B
    Right BP2A
  Intracranial Sinus B522
    Intravascular Optical Coherence B522Z2Z
  Joint
    Acromioclavicular, Bilateral BP23
    Finger
      Left BP2DZZZ
      Right BP2CZZZ
    Foot
      Left BQ2Y
      Right BQ2X
    Hand
      Left BP2DZZZ
      Right BP2CZZZ
    Sacroiliac BR2D
    Sternoclavicular
      Bilateral BP22
      Left BP21
      Right BP20
    Temporomandibular, Bilateral BN29
    Toe
      Left BQ2Y
      Right BQ2X
  Kidney
    Bilateral BT23
    Left BT22
    Right BT21
    Transplant BT29
  Knee
    Left BQ28
    Right BQ27
  Larynx B92J
  Leg
    Left BQ2F
    Right BQ2D
  Liver BF25
  Liver and Spleen BF26
  Lung, Bilateral BB24
  Mandible BN26
  Nasopharynx B92F
  Neck BW2F
  Neck and Head BW29
  Orbit, Bilateral BN23
  Oropharynx B92F
  Pancreas BF27
  Patella
    Left BQ2W
    Right BQ2V
  Pelvic Region BW2G
  Pelvis BR2C
    Chest and Abdomen BW25
  Pelvis and Abdomen BW21
  Pituitary Gland B029
  Prostate BV23
  Ribs
    Left BP2Y
    Right BP2X
  Sacrum BR2F
  Scapula
    Left BP27
    Right BP26
  Sella Turcica B029
  Shoulder
    Left BP29
    Right BP28
  Sinus
    Intracranial B522
      Intravascular Optical Coherence B522Z2Z
    Paranasal B922
  Skull BN20
  Spinal Cord B02B
  Spine
    Cervical BR20
    Lumbar BR29
    Thoracic BR27

Computerized Tomography (*Continued*)
  Spleen and Liver BF26
  Thorax BP2W
  Tibia
    Left BQ2C
    Right BQ2B
  Toe
    Left BQ2Q
    Right BQ2P
  Trachea BB2F
  Tracheobronchial Tree
    Bilateral BB29
    Left BB28
    Right BB27
  Vein
    Pelvic (Iliac)
      Left B52G
        Intravascular Optical Coherence B52GZ2Z
      Right B52F
        Intravascular Optical Coherence B52FZ2Z
    Pelvic (Iliac) Bilateral B52H
      Intravascular Optical Coherence B52HZ2Z
    Portal B52T
      Intravascular Optical Coherence B52TZ2Z
    Pulmonary
      Bilateral B52S
        Intravascular Optical Coherence B52SZ2Z
      Left B52R
        Intravascular Optical Coherence B52RZ2Z
      Right B52Q
        Intravascular Optical Coherence B52QZ2Z
    Renal
      Bilateral B52L
        Intravascular Optical Coherence B52LZ2Z
      Left B52K
        Intravascular Optical Coherence B52KZ2Z
      Right B52J
        Intravascular Optical Coherence B52JZ2Z
    Spanchnic B52T
      Intravascular Optical Coherence B52TZ2Z
  Vena Cava
    Inferior B529
      Intravascular Optical Coherence B529Z2Z
    Superior B528
      Intravascular Optical Coherence B528Z2Z
  Ventricle, Cerebral B028
  Wrist
    Left BP2M
    Right BP2L
Concentrated Bone Marrow Aspirate (CBMA) injection, intramuscular XK02303
Concerto II CRT-D *use* Cardiac Resynchronization Defibrillator Pulse Generator in 0JH
Condylectomy
  see Excision, Head and Facial Bones 0NB
  see Excision, Upper Bones 0PB
  see Excision, Lower Bones 0QB
Condyloid process
  use Mandible, Left
  use Mandible, Right
Condylotomy
  see Division, Head and Facial Bones 0N8
  see Drainage, Head and Facial Bones 0N9
  see Division, Upper Bones 0P8
  see Drainage, Upper Bones 0P9
  see Division, Lower Bones 0Q8
  see Drainage, Lower Bones 0Q9

▶ New   ⇒ Revised   ~~deleted~~ Deleted

Condylysis
   see Release, Head and Facial Bones ØNN
   see Release, Upper Bones ØPN
   see Release, Lower Bones ØQN
Conization, cervix *see* Excision, Cervix ØUBC
Conjunctivoplasty
   see Repair, Eye Ø8Q
   see Replacement, Eye Ø8R
CONSERVE® PLUS Total Resurfacing Hip
   System *use* Resurfacing Device in Lower
   Joints
Construction
   Auricle, ear *see* Replacement, Ear, Nose, Sinus
   Ø9R
   Ileal conduit *see* Bypass, Urinary System ØT1
Consulta CRT-D *use* Cardiac
   Resynchronization Defibrillator Pulse
   Generator in ØJH
Consulta CRT-P *use* Cardiac Resynchronization
   Pacemaker Pulse Generator in ØJH
Contact Radiation
   Abdomen DWY37ZZ
   Adrenal Gland DGY27ZZ
   Bile Ducts DFY27ZZ
   Bladder DTY27ZZ
   Bone, Other DPYC7ZZ
   Brain DØY07ZZ
   Brain Stem DØY17ZZ
   Breast
      Left DMY07ZZ
      Right DMY17ZZ
   Bronchus DBY17ZZ
   Cervix DUY17ZZ
   Chest DWY27ZZ
   Chest Wall DBY77ZZ
   Colon DDY57ZZ
   Diaphragm DBY87ZZ
   Duodenum DDY27ZZ
   Ear D9Y07ZZ
   Esophagus DDY07ZZ
   Eye D8Y07ZZ
   Femur DPY97ZZ
   Fibula DPYB7ZZ
   Gallbladder DFY17ZZ
   Gland
      Adrenal DGY27ZZ
      Parathyroid DGY47ZZ
      Pituitary DGY07ZZ
      Thyroid DGY57ZZ
   Glands, Salivary D9Y67ZZ
   Head and Neck DWY17ZZ
   Hemibody DWY47ZZ
   Humerus DPY67ZZ
   Hypopharynx D9Y37ZZ
   Ileum DDY47ZZ
   Jejunum DDY37ZZ
   Kidney DTY07ZZ
   Larynx D9YB7ZZ
   Liver DFY07ZZ
   Lung DBY27ZZ
   Mandible DPY37ZZ
   Maxilla DPY27ZZ
   Mediastinum DBY67ZZ
   Mouth D9Y47ZZ
   Nasopharynx D9YD7ZZ
   Neck and Head DWY17ZZ
   Nerve, Peripheral DØY77ZZ
   Nose D9Y17ZZ
   Oropharynx D9YF7ZZ
   Ovary DUY07ZZ
   Palate
      Hard D9Y87ZZ
      Soft D9Y97ZZ
   Pancreas DFY37ZZ
   Parathyroid Gland DGY47ZZ
   Pelvic Bones DPY87ZZ
   Pelvic Region DWY67ZZ
   Pineal Body DGY17ZZ
   Pituitary Gland DGY07ZZ
   Pleura DBY57ZZ

Contact Radiation *(Continued)*
   Prostate DVY07ZZ
   Radius DPY77ZZ
   Rectum DDY77ZZ
   Rib DPY57ZZ
   Sinuses D9Y77ZZ
   Skin
      Abdomen DHY87ZZ
      Arm DHY47ZZ
      Back DHY77ZZ
      Buttock DHY97ZZ
      Chest DHY67ZZ
      Face DHY27ZZ
      Leg DHYB7ZZ
      Neck DHY37ZZ
   Skull DPY07ZZ
   Spinal Cord DØY67ZZ
   Sternum DPY47ZZ
   Stomach DDY17ZZ
   Testis DVY17ZZ
   Thyroid Gland DGY57ZZ
   Tibia DPYB7ZZ
   Tongue D9Y57ZZ
   Trachea DBY07ZZ
   Ulna DPY77ZZ
   Ureter DTY17ZZ
   Urethra DTY37ZZ
   Uterus DUY27ZZ
   Whole Body DWY57ZZ
CONTAK RENEWAL® 3 RF (HE) CRT-D *use*
   Cardiac Resynchronization Defibrillator
   Pulse Generator in ØJH
Contegra Pulmonary Valved Conduit *use*
   Zooplastic Tissue in Heart and Great
   Vessels
Continuous Glucose Monitoring (CGM)
   device *use* Monitoring Device
Continuous Negative Airway Pressure
   24-96 Consecutive Hours, Ventilation
      5A09459
   Greater than 96 Consecutive Hours,
      Ventilation 5A09559
   Less than 24 Consecutive Hours, Ventilation
      5A09359
Continuous Positive Airway Pressure
   24-96 Consecutive Hours, Ventilation
      5A09457
   Greater than 96 Consecutive Hours,
      Ventilation 5A09557
   Less than 24 Consecutive Hours, Ventilation
      5A09357
Continuous renal replacement therapy (CRRT)
   5A1D90Z
Contraceptive Device
   Change device in, Uterus and Cervix
      ØU2DXHZ
   Insertion of device in
      Cervix ØUHC
      Subcutaneous Tissue and Fascia
         Abdomen ØJH8
         Chest ØJH6
         Lower Arm
            Left ØJHH
            Right ØJHG
         Lower Leg
            Left ØJHP
            Right ØJHN
         Upper Arm
            Left ØJHF
            Right ØJHD
         Upper Leg
            Left ØJHM
            Right ØJHL
      Uterus ØUH9
   Removal of device from
      Subcutaneous Tissue and Fascia
         Lower Extremity ØJPW
         Trunk ØJPT
         Upper Extremity ØJPV
      Uterus and Cervix ØUPD

Contraceptive Device *(Continued)*
   Revision of device in
      Subcutaneous Tissue and Fascia
         Lower Extremity ØJWW
         Trunk ØJWT
         Upper Extremity ØJWV
      Uterus and Cervix ØUWD
Contractility Modulation Device
   Abdomen ØJH8
   Chest ØJH6
► Control, Epistaxis *see* Control bleeding in,
   Nasal Mucosa and Soft Tissue 093K
Control bleeding in
   Abdominal Wall ØW3F
   Ankle Region
      Left ØY3L
      Right ØY3K
   Arm
      Lower
         Left ØX3F
         Right ØX3D
      Upper
         Left ØX39
         Right ØX38
   Axilla
      Left ØX35
      Right ØX34
   Back
      Lower ØW3L
      Upper ØW3K
   Buttock
      Left ØY31
      Right ØY30
   Cavity, Cranial ØW31
   Chest Wall ØW38
   Elbow Region
      Left ØX3C
      Right ØX3B
   Extremity
      Lower
         Left ØY3B
         Right ØY39
      Upper
         Left ØX37
         Right ØX36
   Face ØW32
   Femoral Region
      Left ØY38
      Right ØY37
   Foot
      Left ØY3N
      Right ØY3M
   Gastrointestinal Tract ØW3P
   Genitourinary Tract ØW3R
   Hand
      Left ØX3K
      Right ØX3J
   Head ØW30
   Inguinal Region
      Left ØY36
      Right ØY35
   Jaw
      Lower ØW35
      Upper ØW34
   Knee Region
      Left ØY3G
      Right ØY3F
   Leg
      Lower
         Left ØY3J
         Right ØY3H
      Upper
         Left ØY3D
         Right ØY3C
   Mediastinum ØW3C
► Nasal Mucosa and Soft Tissue 093K
   Neck ØW36
   Oral Cavity and Throat ØW33
   Pelvic Cavity ØW3J
   Pericardial Cavity ØW3D

► New   ⇒ Revised   ~~deleted~~ Deleted

Control bleeding in *(Continued)*
  Perineum
    Female ØW3N
    Male ØW3M
  Peritoneal Cavity ØW3G
  Pleural Cavity
    Left ØW3B
    Right ØW39
  Respiratory Tract ØW3Q
  Retroperitoneum ØW3H
  Shoulder Region
    Left ØX33
    Right ØX32
  Wrist Region
    Left ØX3H
    Right ØX3G
Conus arteriosus *use* Ventricle, Right
Conus medullaris *use* Spinal Cord,
  Lumbar
Conversion
  Cardiac rhythm 5A2204Z
  Gastrostomy to jejunostomy feeding device
    see Insertion of device in, Jejunum ØDHA
Cook Biodesign® Fistula Plug(s) *use*
  Nonautologous Tissue Substitute
Cook Biodesign® Hernia Graft(s) *use*
  Nonautologous Tissue Substitute
Cook Biodesign® Layered Graft(s) *use*
  Nonautologous Tissue Substitute
Cook Zenapro™ Layered Graft(s) *use*
  Nonautologous Tissue Substitute
Cook Zenith AAA Endovascular Graft
  use Intraluminal Device, Branched or
    Fenestrated, One or Two Arteries in Ø4V
  use Intraluminal Device, Branched or
    Fenestrated, Three or More Arteries in
    Ø4V
  use Intraluminal Device
Coracoacromial ligament
  use Shoulder Bursa and Ligament, Right
  use Shoulder Bursa and Ligament, Left
Coracobrachialis muscle
  use Upper Arm Muscle, Right
  use Upper Arm Muscle, Left
Coracoclavicular ligament
  use Shoulder Bursa and Ligament, Right
  use Shoulder Bursa and Ligament, Left
Coracohumeral ligament
  use Shoulder Bursa and Ligament, Right
  use Shoulder Bursa and Ligament, Left
Coracoid process
  use Scapula, Right
  use Scapula, Left
Cordotomy *see* Division, Central Nervous
  System and Cranial Nerves ØØ8
Core needle biopsy *see* Excision with qualifier
  Diagnostic
CoreValve transcatheter aortic valve *use*
  Zooplastic Tissue in Heart and Great
  Vessels
Cormet Hip Resurfacing System *use*
  Resurfacing Device in Lower Joints
Corniculate cartilage *use* Larynx
CoRoent® XL *use* Interbody Fusion Device in
  Lower Joints
Coronary arteriography
  see Plain Radiography, Heart B2Ø
  see Fluoroscopy, Heart B21
Corox (OTW) Bipolar Lead
  use Cardiac Lead, Pacemaker in Ø2H
  use Cardiac Lead, Defibrillator in Ø2H
Corpus callosum *use* Brain
Corpus cavernosum *use* Penis
Corpus spongiosum *use* Penis
Corpus striatum *use* Basal Ganglia
Corrugator supercilii muscle *use* Facial
  Muscle
Cortical strip neurostimulator lead *use*
  Neurostimulator Lead in Central Nervous
  System and Cranial Nerves

Costatectomy
  see Excision, Upper Bones ØPB
  see Resection, Upper Bones ØPT
Costectomy
  see Excision, Upper Bones ØPB
  see Resection, Upper Bones ØPT
Costocervical trunk
  use Subclavian Artery, Right
  use Subclavian Artery, Left
Costochondrectomy
  see Excision, Upper Bones ØPB
  see Resection, Upper Bones ØPT
Costoclavicular ligament
  use Shoulder Bursa and Ligament,
    Right
  use Shoulder Bursa and Ligament,
    Left
Costosternoplasty
  see Repair, Upper Bones ØPQ
  see Replacement, Upper Bones ØPR
  see Supplement, Upper Bones ØPU
Costotomy
  see Division, Upper Bones ØP8
  see Drainage, Upper Bones ØP9
Costotransverse joint *use* Thoracic Vertebral
  Joint
➡Costotransverse ligament *use* Rib(s) Bursa and
  Ligament
Costovertebral joint *use* Thoracic Vertebral
  Joint
➡Costoxiphoid ligament *use* Sternum Bursa and
  Ligament
Counseling
  Family, for substance abuse, Other Family
    Counseling HZ63ZZZ
  Group
    12-Step HZ43ZZZ
    Behavioral HZ41ZZZ
    Cognitive HZ40ZZZ
    Cognitive-Behavioral HZ42ZZZ
    Confrontational HZ48ZZZ
    Continuing Care HZ49ZZZ
    Infectious Disease
      Post-Test HZ4CZZZ
      Pre-Test HZ4CZZZ
    Interpersonal HZ44ZZZ
    Motivational Enhancement HZ47ZZZ
    Psychoeducation HZ46ZZZ
    Spiritual HZ4BZZZ
    Vocational HZ45ZZZ
  Individual
    12-Step HZ33ZZZ
    Behavioral HZ31ZZZ
    Cognitive HZ30ZZZ
    Cognitive-Behavioral HZ32ZZZ
    Confrontational HZ38ZZZ
    Continuing Care HZ39ZZZ
    Infectious Disease
      Post-Test HZ3CZZZ
      Pre-Test HZ3CZZZ
    Interpersonal HZ34ZZZ
    Motivational Enhancement HZ37ZZZ
    Psychoeducation HZ36ZZZ
    Spiritual HZ3BZZZ
    Vocational HZ35ZZZ
  Mental Health Services
    Educational GZ60ZZZ
    Other Counseling GZ63ZZZ
    Vocational GZ61ZZZ
Countershock, cardiac 5A2204Z
Cowper's (bulbourethral) gland
  use Urethra
CPAP (continuous positive airway
  pressure) *see* Assistance, Respiratory
  5AØ9
Craniectomy
  see Excision, Head and Facial Bones
    ØNB
  see Resection, Head and Facial Bones
    ØNT

Cranioplasty
  see Repair, Head and Facial Bones ØNQ
  see Replacement, Head and Facial Bones
    ØNR
  see Supplement, Head and Facial Bones
    ØNU
Craniotomy
  see Drainage, Central Nervous System and
    Cranial Nerves ØØ9
  see Division, Head and Facial Bones ØN8
  see Drainage, Head and Facial Bones ØN9
Creation
  Perineum
    Female ØW4NØ
    Male ØW4MØ
  Valve
    Aortic Ø24FØ
    Mitral Ø24GØ
    Tricuspid Ø24JØ
Cremaster muscle *use* Perineum Muscle
Cribriform plate
  use Ethmoid Bone, Right
  use Ethmoid Bone, Left
Cricoid cartilage *use* Trachea
Cricoidectomy *see* Excision, Larynx ØCBS
Cricothyroid artery
  use Thyroid Artery, Right
  use Thyroid Artery, Left
Cricothyroid muscle
  use Neck Muscle, Right
  use Neck Muscle, Left
Crisis Intervention GZ2ZZZZ
CRRT (Continuous renal replacement therapy)
  5A1D9ØZ
Crural fascia
  use Subcutaneous Tissue and Fascia, Right
    Upper Leg
  use Subcutaneous Tissue and Fascia, Left
    Upper Leg
Crushing, nerve
  Cranial *see* Destruction, Central Nervous
    System and Cranial Nerves ØØ5
  Peripheral *see* Destruction, Peripheral
    Nervous System Ø15
Cryoablation *see* Destruction
Cryotherapy *see* Destruction
Cryptorchidectomy
  see Excision, Male Reproductive System ØVB
  see Resection, Male Reproductive System ØVT
Cryptorchiectomy
  see Excision, Male Reproductive System ØVB
  see Resection, Male Reproductive System ØVT
Cryptotomy
  see Division, Gastrointestinal System ØD8
  see Drainage, Gastrointestinal System ØD9
CT scan *see* Computerized Tomography (CT
  Scan)
CT sialogram *see* Computerized Tomography
  (CT Scan), Ear, Nose, Mouth and Throat
  B92
Cubital lymph node
  use Lymphatic, Right Upper Extremity
  use Lymphatic, Left Upper Extremity
Cubital nerve *use* Ulnar Nerve
Cuboid bone
  use Tarsal, Right
  use Tarsal, Left
Cuboideonavicular joint
  use Tarsal Joint, Right
  use Tarsal Joint, Left
Culdocentesis *see* Drainage, Cul-de-sac
  ØU9F
Culdoplasty
  see Repair, Cul-de-sac ØUQF
  see Supplement, Cul-de-sac ØUUF
Culdoscopy ØUJH8ZZ
Culdotomy *see* Drainage, Cul-de-sac ØU9F
Culmen *use* Cerebellum
Cultured epidermal cell autograft *use*
  Autologous Tissue Substitute

Cuneiform cartilage *use* Larynx
Cuneonavicular joint
   use Tarsal Joint, Right
   use Tarsal Joint, Left
Cuneonavicular ligament
   use Foot Bursa and Ligament, Right
   use Foot Bursa and Ligament, Left
Curettage
   see Excision
   see Extraction
Cutaneous (transverse) cervical nerve *use*
   Nerve, Cervical Plexus
CVP (central venous pressure) *see*
   Measurement, Venous 4A04
Cyclodiathermy *see* Destruction, Eye Ø85
Cyclophotocoagulation *see* Destruction,
   Eye Ø85

CYPHER® Stent *use* Intraluminal Device,
   Drug-eluting in Heart and Great
   Vessels
Cystectomy
   see Excision, Bladder ØTBB
   see Resection, Bladder ØTTB
Cystocele repair *see* Repair, Subcutaneous
   Tissue and Fascia, Pelvic Region ØJQC
Cystography
   see Plain Radiography, Urinary System
     BTØ
   see Fluoroscopy, Urinary System BT1
Cystolithotomy *see* Extirpation, Bladder
   ØTCB
Cystopexy
   see Repair, Bladder ØTQB
   see Reposition, Bladder ØTSB

Cystoplasty
   see Repair, Bladder ØTQB
   see Replacement, Bladder ØTRB
   see Supplement, Bladder ØTUB
Cystorrhaphy *see* Repair, Bladder ØTQB
Cystoscopy ØTJB8ZZ
Cystostomy *see* Bypass, Bladder ØT1B
Cystostomy tube *use* Drainage Device
Cystotomy *see* Drainage, Bladder ØT9B
Cystourethrography
   see Plain Radiography, Urinary System BTØ
   see Fluoroscopy, Urinary System BT1
Cystourethroplasty
   see Repair, Urinary System ØTQ
   see Replacement, Urinary System ØTR
   see Supplement, Urinary System ØTU
Cytarabine and Daunorubicin Liposome
   Antineoplastic XWØ

▶ New   ⇒ Revised   ~~deleted~~ Deleted

D

DBS lead *use* Neurostimulator Lead in Central Nervous System and Cranial Nerves
DeBakey Left Ventricular Assist Device *use* Implantable Heart Assist System in Heart and Great Vessels
Debridement
  Excisional *see* Excision
  Non-excisional *see* Extraction
Decompression, Circulatory 6A15
Decortication, lung
  see Extirpation, Respiratory System 0BC
  see Release, Respiratory System 0BN
Deep brain neurostimulator lead *use* Neurostimulator Lead in Central Nervous System and Cranial Nerves
Deep cervical fascia
  use Subcutaneous Tissue and Fascia, Right Neck
  use Subcutaneous Tissue and Fascia, Left Neck
Deep cervical vein
  use Vertebral Vein, Right
  use Vertebral Vein, Left
Deep circumflex iliac artery
  use External Iliac Artery, Right
  use External Iliac Artery, Left
Deep facial vein
  use Face Vein, Right
  use Face Vein, Left
Deep femoral (profunda femoris) vein
  use Femoral Vein, Right
  use Femoral Vein, Left
Deep femoral artery
  use Femoral Artery, Right
  use Femoral Artery, Left
Deep Inferior Epigastric Artery Perforator Flap
  Replacement
    Bilateral 0HRV077
    Left 0HRU077
    Right 0HRT077
  Transfer
    Left 0KXG
    Right 0KXF
Deep palmar arch
  use Hand Artery, Right
  use Hand Artery, Left
Deep transverse perineal muscle *use* Perineum Muscle
Deferential artery
  use Internal Iliac Artery, Right
  use Internal Iliac Artery, Left
Defibrillator Generator
  Abdomen 0JH8
  Chest 0JH6
Defibrotide Sodium Anticoagulant XW0
Defitelio *use* Defibrotide Sodium Anticoagulant
Delivery
  Cesarean *see* Extraction, Products of Conception 10D0
  Forceps *see* Extraction, Products of Conception 10D0
  Manually assisted 10E0XZZ
  Products of Conception 10E0XZZ
  Vacuum assisted *see* Extraction, Products of Conception 10D0
Delta frame external fixator
  use External Fixation Device, Hybrid in 0PH
  use External Fixation Device, Hybrid in 0PS
  use External Fixation Device, Hybrid in 0QH
  use External Fixation Device, Hybrid in 0QS
Delta III Reverse shoulder prosthesis *use* Synthetic Substitute, Reverse Ball and Socket in 0RR

Deltoid fascia
  use Subcutaneous Tissue and Fascia, Right Upper Arm
  use Subcutaneous Tissue and Fascia, Left Upper Arm
Deltoid ligament
  use Ankle Bursa and Ligament, Right
  use Ankle Bursa and Ligament, Left
Deltoid muscle
  use Shoulder Muscle, Right
  use Shoulder Muscle, Left
Deltopectoral (infraclavicular) lymph node
  use Lymphatic, Right Upper Extremity
  use Lymphatic, Left Upper Extremity
Denervation
  Cranial nerve *see* Destruction, Central Nervous System and Cranial Nerves 005
  Peripheral nerve *see* Destruction, Peripheral Nervous System 015
Dens *use* Cervical Vertebra
Densitometry
  Plain Radiography
    Femur
      Left BQ04ZZ1
      Right BQ03ZZ1
    Hip
      Left BQ01ZZ1
      Right BQ00ZZ1
    Spine
      Cervical BR00ZZ1
      Lumbar BR09ZZ1
      Thoracic BR07ZZ1
      Whole BR0GZZ1
  Ultrasonography
    Elbow
      Left BP4HZZ1
      Right BP4GZZ1
    Hand
      Left BP4PZZ1
      Right BP4NZZ1
    Shoulder
      Left BP49ZZ1
      Right BP48ZZ1
    Wrist
      Left BP4MZZ1
      Right BP4LZZ1
Denticulate (dentate) ligament *use* Spinal Meninges
Depressor anguli oris muscle *use* Facial Muscle
Depressor labii inferioris muscle *use* Facial Muscle
Depressor septi nasi muscle *use* Facial Muscle
Depressor supercilii muscle *use* Facial Muscle
Dermabrasion *see* Extraction, Skin and Breast 0HD
Dermis *see* Skin
Descending genicular artery
  use Femoral Artery, Right
  use Femoral Artery, Left
Destruction
  Acetabulum
    Left 0Q55
    Right 0Q54
  Adenoids 0C5Q
  Ampulla of Vater 0F5C
  Anal Sphincter 0D5R
  Anterior Chamber
    Left 08533ZZ
    Right 08523ZZ
  Anus 0D5Q
  Aorta
    Abdominal 0450
    Thoracic
      Ascending/Arch 025X
      Descending 025W
  Aortic Body 0G5D
  Appendix 0D5J
  Artery
    Anterior Tibial
      Left 045Q
      Right 045P

Destruction *(Continued)*
  Artery *(Continued)*
    Axillary
      Left 0356
      Right 0355
    Brachial
      Left 0358
      Right 0357
    Celiac 0451
    Colic
      Left 0457
      Middle 0458
      Right 0456
    Common Carotid
      Left 035J
      Right 035H
    Common Iliac
      Left 045D
      Right 045C
    External Carotid
      Left 035N
      Right 035M
    External Iliac
      Left 045J
      Right 045H
    Face 035R
    Femoral
      Left 045L
      Right 045K
    Foot
      Left 045W
      Right 045V
    Gastric 0452
    Hand
      Left 035F
      Right 035D
    Hepatic 0453
    Inferior Mesenteric 045B
    Innominate 0352
    Internal Carotid
      Left 035L
      Right 035K
    Internal Iliac
      Left 045F
      Right 045E
    Internal Mammary
      Left 0351
      Right 0350
    Intracranial 035G
    Lower 045Y
    Peroneal
      Left 045U
      Right 045T
    Popliteal
      Left 045N
      Right 045M
    Posterior Tibial
      Left 045S
      Right 045R
    Pulmonary
      Left 025R
      Right 025Q
    Pulmonary Trunk 025P
    Radial
      Left 035C
      Right 035B
    Renal
      Left 045A
      Right 0459
    Splenic 0454
    Subclavian
      Left 0354
      Right 0353
    Superior Mesenteric 0455
    Temporal
      Left 035T
      Right 035S
    Thyroid
      Left 035V
      Right 035U

▶ New   ⇒ Revised   ~~deleted~~ Deleted

▶ New   ⇒ Revised   ~~deleted~~ Deleted

▶ New   ⇒ Revised   ~~deleted~~ Deleted

▶ New   ⟹ Revised   ~~deleted~~ Deleted

Direct Lateral Interbody Fusion (DLIF) device
  use Interbody Fusion Device in Lower Joints
Disarticulation *see* Detachment
Discectomy, diskectomy
  see Excision, Upper Joints ØRB
  see Resection, Upper Joints ØRT
  see Excision, Lower Joints ØSB
  see Resection, Lower Joints ØST
Discography
  see Plain Radiography, Axial Skeleton, Except Skull and Facial Bones BRØ
  see Fluoroscopy, Axial Skeleton, Except Skull and Facial Bones BR1
Distal humerus
  use Humeral Shaft, Right
  use Humeral Shaft, Left
Distal humerus, involving joint
  use Elbow Joint, Right
  use Elbow Joint, Left
Distal radioulnar joint
  use Wrist Joint, Right
  use Wrist Joint, Left
Diversion *see* Bypass
Diverticulectomy *see* Excision, Gastrointestinal System ØDB
Division
  Acetabulum
    Left ØQ85
    Right ØQ84
  Anal Sphincter ØD8R
  Basal Ganglia ØØ88
  Bladder Neck ØT8C
  Bone
    Ethmoid
      Left ØN8G
      Right ØN8F
    Frontal ØN81
    Hyoid ØN8X
    Lacrimal
      Left ØN8J
      Right ØN8H
    Nasal ØN8B
    Occipital ØN87
    Palatine
      Left ØN8L
      Right ØN8K
    Parietal
      Left ØN84
      Right ØN83
    Pelvic
      Left ØQ83
      Right ØQ82
    Sphenoid ØN8C
    Temporal
      Left ØN86
      Right ØN85
    Zygomatic
      Left ØN8N
      Right ØN8M
  Brain ØØ80
  Bursa and Ligament
    Abdomen
      Left ØM8J
      Right ØM8H
    Ankle
      Left ØM8R
      Right ØM8Q
    Elbow
      Left ØM84
      Right ØM83
    Foot
      Left ØM8T
      Right ØM8S
    Hand
      Left ØM88
      Right ØM87
    Head and Neck ØM80
    Hip
      Left ØM8M
      Right ØM8L

Division *(Continued)*
  Bursa and Ligament *(Continued)*
    Knee
      Left ØM8P
      Right ØM8N
    Lower Extremity
      Left ØM8W
      Right ØM8V
    Perineum ØM8K
    Rib(s) ØM8G
    Shoulder
      Left ØM82
      Right ØM81
    Spine
      Lower ØM8D
      Upper ØM8C
    Sternum ØM8F
    Upper Extremity
      Left ØM8B
      Right ØM89
    Wrist
      Left ØM86
      Right ØM85
  Carpal
    Left ØP8N
    Right ØP8M
  Cerebral Hemisphere ØØ87
  Chordae Tendineae Ø289
  Clavicle
    Left ØP8B
    Right ØP89
  Coccyx ØQ8S
  Conduction Mechanism Ø288
  Esophagogastric Junction ØD84
  Femoral Shaft
    Left ØQ89
    Right ØQ88
  Femur
    Lower
      Left ØQ8C
      Right ØQ8B
    Upper
      Left ØQ87
      Right ØQ86
  Fibula
    Left ØQ8K
    Right ØQ8J
  Gland, Pituitary ØG80
  Glenoid Cavity
    Left ØP88
    Right ØP87
  Humeral Head
    Left ØP8D
    Right ØP8C
  Humeral Shaft
    Left ØP8G
    Right ØP8F
  Hymen ØU8K
  Kidneys, Bilateral ØT82
  Mandible
    Left ØN8V
    Right ØN8T
  Maxilla ØN8R
  Metacarpal
    Left ØP8Q
    Right ØP8P
  Metatarsal
    Left ØQ8P
    Right ØQ8N
  Muscle
    Abdomen
      Left ØK8L
      Right ØK8K
    Facial ØK81
    Foot
      Left ØK8W
      Right ØK8V
    Hand
      Left ØK8D
      Right ØK8C

Division *(Continued)*
  Muscle *(Continued)*
    Head ØK80
    Hip
      Left ØK8P
      Right ØK8N
    Lower Arm and Wrist
      Left ØK8B
      Right ØK89
    Lower Leg
      Left ØK8T
      Right ØK8S
    Neck
      Left ØK83
      Right ØK82
    Papillary Ø28D
    Perineum ØK8M
    Shoulder
      Left ØK86
      Right ØK85
    Thorax
      Left ØK8J
      Right ØK8H
    Tongue, Palate, Pharynx ØK84
    Trunk
      Left ØK8G
      Right ØK8F
    Upper Arm
      Left ØK88
      Right ØK87
    Upper Leg
      Left ØK8R
      Right ØK8Q
  Nerve
    Abdominal Sympathetic Ø18M
    Abducens ØØ8L
    Accessory ØØ8R
    Acoustic ØØ8N
    Brachial Plexus Ø183
    Cervical Ø181
    Cervical Plexus Ø180
    Facial ØØ8M
    Femoral Ø18D
    Glossopharyngeal ØØ8P
    Head and Neck Sympathetic Ø18K
    Hypoglossal ØØ8S
    Lumbar Ø18B
    Lumbar Plexus Ø189
    Lumbar Sympathetic Ø18N
    Lumbosacral Plexus Ø18A
    Median Ø185
    Oculomotor ØØ8H
    Olfactory ØØ8F
    Optic ØØ8G
    Peroneal Ø18H
    Phrenic Ø182
    Pudendal Ø18C
    Radial Ø186
    Sacral Ø18R
    Sacral Plexus Ø18Q
    Sacral Sympathetic Ø18P
    Sciatic Ø18F
    Thoracic Ø188
    Thoracic Sympathetic Ø18L
    Tibial Ø18G
    Trigeminal ØØ8K
    Trochlear ØØ8J
    Ulnar Ø184
    Vagus ØØ8Q
  Orbit
    Left ØN8Q
    Right ØN8P
  Ovary
    Bilateral ØU82
    Left ØU81
    Right ØU80
  Pancreas ØF8G
  Patella
    Left ØQ8F
    Right ØQ8D
  Perineum, Female ØW8NXZZ

▶ New   ⇒ Revised   ~~deleted~~ Deleted

Drainage *(Continued)*
Eustachian Tube
Left 099G
Right 099F
Extremity
Lower
Left 0Y9B
Right 0Y99
Upper
Left 0X97
Right 0X96
Eye
Left 0891
Right 0890
Eyelid
Lower
Left 089R
Right 089Q
Upper
Left 089P
Right 089N
Face 0W92
Fallopian Tube
Left 0U96
Right 0U95
Fallopian Tubes, Bilateral 0U97
Femoral Region
Left 0Y98
Right 0Y97
Femoral Shaft
Left 0Q99
Right 0Q98
Femur
Lower
Left 0Q9C
Right 0Q9B
Upper
Left 0Q97
Right 0Q96
Fibula
Left 0Q9K
Right 0Q9J
Finger Nail 0H9Q
Foot
Left 0Y9N
Right 0Y9M
Gallbladder 0F94
Gingiva
Lower 0C96
Upper 0C95
Gland
Adrenal
Bilateral 0G94
Left 0G92
Right 0G93
Lacrimal
Left 089W
Right 089V
Minor Salivary 0C9J
Parotid
Left 0C99
Right 0C98
Pituitary 0G90
Sublingual
Left 0C9F
Right 0C9D
Submaxillary
Left 0C9H
Right 0C9G
Vestibular 0U9L
Glenoid Cavity
Left 0P98
Right 0P97
Glomus Jugulare 0G9C
Hand
Left 0X9K
Right 0X9J
Head 0W90
Humeral Head
Left 0P9D
Right 0P9C

Drainage *(Continued)*
Humeral Shaft
Left 0P9G
Right 0P9F
Hymen 0U9K
Hypothalamus 009A
Ileocecal Valve 0D9C
Ileum 0D9B
Inguinal Region
Left 0Y96
Right 0Y95
Intestine
Large 0D9E
Left 0D9G
Right 0D9F
Small 0D98
Iris
Left 089D
Right 089C
Jaw
Lower 0W95
Upper 0W94
Jejunum 0D9A
Joint
Acromioclavicular
Left 0R9H
Right 0R9G
Ankle
Left 0S9G
Right 0S9F
Carpal
Left 0R9R
Right 0R9Q
Carpometacarpal
Left 0R9T
Right 0R9S
Cervical Vertebral 0R91
Cervicothoracic Vertebral 0R94
Coccygeal 0S96
Elbow
Left 0R9M
Right 0R9L
Finger Phalangeal
Left 0R9X
Right 0R9W
Hip
Left 0S9B
Right 0S99
Knee
Left 0S9D
Right 0S9C
Lumbar Vertebral 0S90
Lumbosacral 0S93
Metacarpophalangeal
Left 0R9V
Right 0R9U
Metatarsal-Phalangeal
Left 0S9N
Right 0S9M
Occipital-cervical 0R90
Sacrococcygeal 0S95
Sacroiliac
Left 0S98
Right 0S97
Shoulder
Left 0R9K
Right 0R9J
Sternoclavicular
Left 0R9F
Right 0R9E
Tarsal
Left 0S9J
Right 0S9H
Tarsometatarsal
Left 0S9L
Right 0S9K
Temporomandibular
Left 0R9D
Right 0R9C
Thoracic Vertebral 0R96
Thoracolumbar Vertebral 0R9A

Drainage *(Continued)*
Joint *(Continued)*
Toe Phalangeal
Left 0S9Q
Right 0S9P
Wrist
Left 0R9P
Right 0R9N
Kidney
Left 0T91
Right 0T90
Kidney Pelvis
Left 0T94
Right 0T93
Knee Region
Left 0Y9G
Right 0Y9F
Larynx 0C9S
Leg
Lower
Left 0Y9J
Right 0Y9H
Upper
Left 0Y9D
Right 0Y9C
Lens
Left 089K
Right 089J
Lip
Lower 0C91
Upper 0C90
Liver 0F90
Left Lobe 0F92
Right Lobe 0F91
Lung
Bilateral 0B9M
Left 0B9L
Lower Lobe
Left 0B9J
Right 0B9F
Middle Lobe, Right 0B9D
Right 0B9K
Upper Lobe
Left 0B9G
Right 0B9C
Lung Lingula 0B9H
Lymphatic
Aortic 079D
Axillary
Left 0796
Right 0795
Head 0790
Inguinal
Left 079J
Right 079H
Internal Mammary
Left 0799
Right 0798
Lower Extremity
Left 079G
Right 079F
Mesenteric 079B
Neck
Left 0792
Right 0791
Pelvis 079C
Thoracic Duct 079K
Thorax 0797
Upper Extremity
Left 0794
Right 0793
Mandible
Left 0N9V
Right 0N9T
Maxilla 0N9R
Mediastinum 0W9C
Medulla Oblongata 009D
Mesentery 0D9V
Metacarpal
Left 0P9Q
Right 0P9P

▶ New   ⇒ Revised   ~~deleted~~ Deleted

Drainage *(Continued)*
Metatarsal
  Left ØQ9P
  Right ØQ9N
Muscle
  Abdomen
    Left ØK9L
    Right ØK9K
  Extraocular
    Left Ø89M
    Right Ø89L
  Facial ØK91
  Foot
    Left ØK9W
    Right ØK9V
  Hand
    Left ØK9D
    Right ØK9C
  Head ØK90
  Hip
    Left ØK9P
    Right ØK9N
  Lower Arm and Wrist
    Left ØK9B
    Right ØK99
  Lower Leg
    Left ØK9T
    Right ØK9S
  Neck
    Left ØK93
    Right ØK92
  Perineum ØK9M
  Shoulder
    Left ØK96
    Right ØK95
  Thorax
    Left ØK9J
    Right ØK9H
  Tongue, Palate, Pharynx ØK94
  Trunk
    Left ØK9G
    Right ØK9F
  Upper Arm
    Left ØK98
    Right ØK97
  Upper Leg
    Left ØK9R
    Right ØK9Q
Nasal Mucosa and Soft Tissue Ø99K
Nasopharynx Ø99N
Neck ØW96
Nerve
  Abdominal Sympathetic Ø19M
  Abducens ØØ9L
  Accessory ØØ9R
  Acoustic ØØ9N
  Brachial Plexus Ø193
  Cervical Ø191
  Cervical Plexus Ø190
  Facial ØØ9M
  Femoral Ø19D
  Glossopharyngeal ØØ9P
  Head and Neck Sympathetic Ø19K
  Hypoglossal ØØ9S
  Lumbar Ø19B
  Lumbar Plexus Ø199
  Lumbar Sympathetic Ø19N
  Lumbosacral Plexus Ø19A
  Median Ø195
  Oculomotor ØØ9H
  Olfactory ØØ9F
  Optic ØØ9G
  Peroneal Ø19H
  Phrenic Ø192
  Pudendal Ø19C
  Radial Ø196
  Sacral Ø19R
  Sacral Sympathetic Ø19P
  Sciatic Ø19F
  Thoracic Ø198
  Thoracic Sympathetic Ø19L

Drainage *(Continued)*
  Nerve *(Continued)*
    Tibial Ø19G
    Trigeminal ØØ9K
    Trochlear ØØ9J
    Ulnar Ø194
    Vagus ØØ9Q
  Nipple
    Left ØH9X
    Right ØH9W
  Omentum ØD9U
  Oral Cavity and Throat ØW93
  Orbit
    Left ØN9Q
    Right ØN9P
  Ovary
    Bilateral ØU92
    Left ØU91
    Right ØU90
  Palate
    Hard ØC92
    Soft ØC93
  Pancreas ØF9G
  Para-aortic Body ØG99
  Paraganglion Extremity ØG9F
  Parathyroid Gland ØG9R
    Inferior
      Left ØG9P
      Right ØG9N
    Multiple ØG9Q
    Superior
      Left ØG9P
      Right ØG9L
  Patella
    Left ØQ9F
    Right ØQ9D
  Pelvic Cavity ØW9J
  Penis ØV9S
  Pericardial Cavity ØW9D
  Perineum
    Female ØW9N
    Male ØW9M
  Peritoneal Cavity ØW9G
  Peritoneum ØD9W
  Phalanx
    Finger
      Left ØP9V
      Right ØP9T
    Thumb
      Left ØP9S
      Right ØP9R
    Toe
      Left ØQ9R
      Right ØQ9Q
  Pharynx ØC9M
  Pineal Body ØG91
  Pleura
    Left ØB9P
    Right ØB9N
  Pleural Cavity
    Left ØW9B
    Right ØW99
  Pons ØØ9B
  Prepuce ØV9T
  Products of Conception
    Amniotic Fluid
      Diagnostic 1Ø9Ø
      Therapeutic 1Ø9Ø
    Fetal Blood 1Ø9Ø
    Fetal Cerebrospinal Fluid 1Ø9Ø
    Fetal Fluid, Other 1Ø9Ø
    Fluid, Other 1Ø9Ø
  Prostate ØV90
  Radius
    Left ØP9J
    Right ØP9H
  Rectum ØD9P
  Retina
    Left Ø89F
    Right Ø89E

Drainage *(Continued)*
  Retinal Vessel
    Left Ø89H
    Right Ø89G
  Retroperitoneum ØW9H
  Ribs
    1 to 2 ØP91
    3 or More ØP92
  Sacrum ØQ91
  Scapula
    Left ØP96
    Right ØP95
  Sclera
    Left Ø897
    Right Ø896
  Scrotum ØV95
  Septum, Nasal Ø99M
  Shoulder Region
    Left ØX93
    Right ØX92
  Sinus
    Accessory Ø99P
    Ethmoid
      Left Ø99V
      Right Ø99U
    Frontal
      Left Ø99T
      Right Ø99S
    Mastoid
      Left Ø99C
      Right Ø99B
    Maxillary
      Left Ø99R
      Right Ø99Q
    Sphenoid
      Left Ø99X
      Right Ø99W
  Skin
    Abdomen ØH97
    Back ØH96
    Buttock ØH98
    Chest ØH95
    Ear
      Left ØH93
      Right ØH92
    Face ØH91
    Foot
      Left ØH9N
      Right ØH9M
    Hand
      Left ØH9G
      Right ØH9F
    Inguinal ØH9A
    Lower Arm
      Left ØH9E
      Right ØH9D
    Lower Leg
      Left ØH9L
      Right ØH9K
    Neck ØH94
    Perineum ØH99
    Scalp ØH90
    Upper Arm
      Left ØH9C
      Right ØH9B
    Upper Leg
      Left ØH9J
      Right ØH9H
  Skull ØN90
  Spinal Canal ØØ9U
  Spinal Cord
    Cervical ØØ9W
    Lumbar ØØ9Y
    Thoracic ØØ9X
  Spinal Meninges ØØ9T
  Spleen Ø79P
  Sternum ØP90
  Stomach ØD96
    Pylorus ØD97
  Subarachnoid Space, Intracranial ØØ95

▶ New ⇒ Revised ~~deleted~~ Deleted

743

▶ New   ⇒ Revised   ~~deleted~~ Deleted

Dressing *(Continued)*
  Leg *(Continued)*
    Upper
      Left 2W2PX4Z
      Right 2W2NX4Z
    Neck 2W22X4Z
    Thumb
      Left 2W2HX4Z
      Right 2W2GX4Z
    Toe
      Left 2W2VX4Z
      Right 2W2UX4Z
Driver stent (RX) (OTW) *use* Intraluminal
  Device
▶ Drotrecogin alfa, Infusion *see* Introduction of
  Recombinant Human-activated Protein C
Duct of Santorini *use* Duct, Pancreatic,
  Accessory
Duct of Wirsung *use* Duct, Pancreatic
Ductogram, mammary *see* Plain Radiography,
  Skin, Subcutaneous Tissue and Breast
  BH0

Ductography, mammary *see* Plain Radiography,
  Skin, Subcutaneous Tissue and Breast
  BH0
Ductus deferens
  use Vas Deferens, Right
  use Vas Deferens, Left
  use Vas Deferens, Bilateral
  use Vas Deferens
Duodenal ampulla *use* Ampulla of Vater
Duodenectomy
  see Excision, Duodenum 0DB9
  see Resection, Duodenum 0DT9
Duodenocholedochotomy *see* Drainage,
  Gallbladder 0F94
Duodenocystostomy
  see Bypass, Gallbladder 0F14
  see Drainage, Gallbladder 0F94
Duodenoenterostomy
  see Bypass, Gastrointestinal System 0D1
  see Drainage, Gastrointestinal System
  0D9
Duodenojejunal flexure *use* Jejunum

Duodenolysis *see* Release, Duodenum 0DN9
Duodenorrhaphy *see* Repair, Duodenum
  0DQ9
Duodenostomy
  see Bypass, Duodenum 0D19
  see Drainage, Duodenum 0D99
Duodenotomy *see* Drainage, Duodenum 0D99
DuraGraft® Endothelial Damage Inhibitor *use*
  Endothelial Damage Inhibitor
DuraHeart Left Ventricular Assist System *use*
  Implantable Heart Assist System in Heart
  and Great Vessels
Dural venous sinus *use* Vein, Intracranial
Dura mater, intracranial *use* Dura Mater
Dura mater, spinal *use* Spinal Meninges
Durata® Defibrillation Lead *use* Cardiac Lead,
  Defibrillator in 02H
Dynesys® Dynamic Stabilization System
  use Spinal Stabilization Device, Pedicle-Based
  in 0RH
  use Spinal Stabilization Device, Pedicle-Based
  in 0SH

E

E-Luminexx™ (Biliary) (Vascular) Stent *use* Intraluminal Device
Earlobe
  use External Ear, Right
  use External Ear, Left
  use External Ear, Bilateral
ECCO2R (Extracorporeal Carbon Dioxide Removal) 5A0920Z
Echocardiogram *see* Ultrasonography, Heart B24
Echography *see* Ultrasonography
ECMO *see* Performance, Circulatory 5A15
EDWARDS INTUITY Elite valve system *use* Zooplastic Tissue, Rapid Deployment Technique in New Technology
EEG (electroencephalogram) *see* Measurement, Central Nervous 4A00
EGD (esophagogastroduodenoscopy) 0DJ08ZZ
Eighth cranial nerve *use* Acoustic Nerve
Ejaculatory duct
  use Vas Deferens, Right
  use Vas Deferens, Left
  use Vas Deferens, Bilateral
  use Vas Deferens
EKG (electrocardiogram) *see* Measurement, Cardiac 4A02
Electrical bone growth stimulator (EBGS)
  use Bone Growth Stimulator in Head and Facial Bones
  use Bone Growth Stimulator in Upper Bones
  use Bone Growth Stimulator in Lower Bones
Electrical muscle stimulation (EMS) lead *use* Stimulator Lead in Muscles
Electrocautery
  Destruction *see* Destruction
  Repair *see* Repair
Electroconvulsive Therapy
  Bilateral-Multiple Seizure GZB3ZZZ
  Bilateral-Single Seizure GZB2ZZZ
  Electroconvulsive Therapy, Other GZB4ZZZ
  Unilateral-Multiple Seizure GZB1ZZZ
  Unilateral-Single Seizure GZB0ZZZ
Electroencephalogram (EEG) *see* Measurement, Central Nervous 4A00
Electromagnetic Therapy
  Central Nervous 6A22
  Urinary 6A21
Electronic muscle stimulator lead *use* Stimulator Lead in Muscles
Electrophysiologic stimulation (EPS) *see* Measurement, Cardiac 4A02
Electroshock therapy *see* Electroconvulsive Therapy
Elevation, bone fragments, skull *see* Reposition, Head and Facial Bones 0NS
Eleventh cranial nerve *use* Accessory Nerve
Embolectomy *see* Extirpation
Embolization
  see Occlusion
  see Restriction
Embolization coil(s) *use* Intraluminal Device
EMG (electromyogram) *see* Measurement, Musculoskeletal 4A0F
Encephalon *use* Brain
Endarterectomy
  see Extirpation, Upper Arteries 03C
  see Extirpation, Lower Arteries 04C
Endeavor® (III) (IV) (Sprint) Zotarolimus-eluting Coronary Stent System *use* Intraluminal Device, Drug-eluting in Heart and Great Vessels
Endologix AFX® Endovascular AAA System use Intraluminal Device
EndoSure® sensor *use* Monitoring Device, Pressure Sensor in 02H
ENDOTAK RELIANCE® (G) Defibrillation Lead *use* Cardiac Lead, Defibrillator in 02H

Endothelial damage inhibitor, applied to vein graft XY0VX83
Endotracheal tube (cuffed) (double-lumen) *use* Intraluminal Device, Endotracheal Airway in Respiratory System
Endurant® Endovascular Stent Graft *use* Intraluminal Device
Endurant® II AAA stent graft system *use* Intraluminal Device
Engineered Autologous Chimeric Antigen Receptor T-cell Immunotherapy XW0
Enlargement
  see Dilation
  see Repair
EnRhythm *use* Pacemaker, Dual Chamber in 0JH
Enterorrhaphy *see* Repair, Gastrointestinal System 0DQ
Enterra gastric neurostimulator *use* Stimulator Generator, Multiple Array in 0JH
Enucleation
  Eyeball *see* Resection, Eye 08T
  Eyeball with prosthetic implant *see* Replacement, Eye 08R
Ependyma *use* Cerebral Ventricle
Epic™ Stented Tissue Valve (aortic) *use* Zooplastic Tissue in Heart and Great Vessels
Epicel® cultured epidermal autograft *use* Autologous Tissue Substitute
Epidermis *use* Skin
Epididymectomy
  see Excision, Male Reproductive System 0VB
  see Resection, Male Reproductive System 0VT
Epididymoplasty
  see Repair, Male Reproductive System 0VQ
  see Supplement, Male Reproductive System 0VU
Epididymorrhaphy *see* Repair, Male Reproductive System 0VQ
Epididymotomy *see* Drainage, Male Reproductive System 0V9
Epidural space, spinal *use* Spinal Canal
Epiphysiodesis
  see Insertion of device in, Upper Bones 0PH
  see Repair, Upper Bones 0PQ
  see Insertion of device in, Lower Bones 0QH
  see Repair, Lower Bones 0QQ
Epiploic foramen *use* Peritoneum
Epiretinal Visual Prosthesis
  Left 08H105Z
  Right 08H005Z
Episiorrhaphy *see* Repair, Perineum, Female 0WQN
Episiotomy *see* Division, Perineum, Female 0W8N
Epithalamus *use* Thalamus
Epitroclear lymph node
  use Lymphatic, Right Upper Extremity
  use Lymphatic, Left Upper Extremity
EPS (electrophysiologic stimulation) *see* Measurement, Cardiac 4A02
Eptifibatide, infusion *see* Introduction of Platelet Inhibitor
ERCP (endoscopic retrograde cholangiopancreatography) *see* Fluoroscopy, Hepatobiliary System and Pancreas BF1
Erector spinae muscle
  use Trunk Muscle, Right
  use Trunk Muscle, Left
Esophageal artery *use* Upper Artery
Esophageal obturator airway (EOA) *use* Intraluminal Device, Airway in Gastrointestinal System
Esophageal plexus *use* Thoracic Sympathetic Nerve
Esophagectomy
  see Excision, Gastrointestinal System 0DB
  see Resection, Gastrointestinal System 0DT

Esophagocoloplasty
  see Repair, Gastrointestinal System 0DQ
  see Supplement, Gastrointestinal System 0DU
Esophagoenterostomy
  see Bypass, Gastrointestinal System 0D1
  see Drainage, Gastrointestinal System 0D9
Esophagoesophagostomy
  see Bypass, Gastrointestinal System 0D1
  see Drainage, Gastrointestinal System 0D9
Esophagogastrectomy
  see Excision, Gastrointestinal System 0DB
  see Resection, Gastrointestinal System 0DT
Esophagogastroduodenoscopy (EGD) 0DJ08ZZ
Esophagogastroplasty
  see Repair, Gastrointestinal System 0DQ
  see Supplement, Gastrointestinal System 0DU
Esophagogastroscopy 0DJ68ZZ
Esophagogastrostomy
  see Bypass, Gastrointestinal System 0D1
  see Drainage, Gastrointestinal System 0D9
Esophagojejunoplasty *see* Supplement, Gastrointestinal System 0DU
Esophagojejunostomy
  see Bypass, Gastrointestinal System 0D1
  see Drainage, Gastrointestinal System 0D9
Esophagomyotomy *see* Division, Esophagogastric Junction 0D84
Esophagoplasty
  see Repair, Gastrointestinal System 0DQ
  see Replacement, Esophagus 0DR5
  see Supplement, Gastrointestinal System 0DU
Esophagoplication *see* Restriction, Gastrointestinal System 0DV
Esophagorrhaphy *see* Repair, Gastrointestinal System 0DQ
Esophagoscopy 0DJ08ZZ
Esophagotomy *see* Drainage, Gastrointestinal System 0D9
Esteem® implantable hearing system *use* Hearing Device in Ear, Nose, Sinus
ESWL (extracorporeal shock wave lithotripsy) *see* Fragmentation
Ethmoidal air cell
  use Ethmoid Sinus, Right
  use Ethmoid Sinus, Left
Ethmoidectomy
  see Excision, Ear, Nose, Sinus 09B
  see Resection, Ear, Nose, Sinus 09T
  see Excision, Head and Facial Bones 0NB
  see Resection, Head and Facial Bones 0NT
Ethmoidotomy *see* Drainage, Ear, Nose, Sinus 099
Evacuation
  Hematoma *see* Extirpation
  Other Fluid *see* Drainage
Evera (XT)(S)(DR/VR) *use* Defibrillator Generator in 0JH
Everolimus-eluting coronary stent *use* Intraluminal Device, Drug-eluting in Heart and Great Vessels
Evisceration
  Eyeball *see* Resection, Eye 08T
  Eyeball with prosthetic implant *see* Replacement, Eye 08R
Ex-PRESS™ mini glaucoma shunt *use* Synthetic Substitute
Examination *see* Inspection
Exchange *see* Change device in
Excision
  Abdominal Wall 0WBF
  Acetabulum
    Left 0QB5
    Right 0QB4
  Adenoids 0CBQ
  Ampulla of Vater 0FBC
  Anal Sphincter 0DBR
  Ankle Region
    Left 0YBL
    Right 0YBK

▶ New   ⇒ Revised   ~~deleted~~ Deleted

Excision (Continued)
  Conduction Mechanism 02B8
  Conjunctiva
    Left 08BTXZ
    Right 08BSXZ
  Cord
    Bilateral 0VBH
    Left 0VBG
    Right 0VBF
  Cornea
    Left 08B9XZ
    Right 08B8XZ
  Cul-de-sac 0UBF
  Diaphragm 0BBT
  Disc
    Cervical Vertebral 0RB3
    Cervicothoracic Vertebral 0RB5
    Lumbar Vertebral 0SB2
    Lumbosacral 0SB4
    Thoracic Vertebral 0RB9
    Thoracolumbar Vertebral 0RBB
  Duct
    Common Bile 0FB9
    Cystic 0FB8
    Hepatic
      Common 0FB7
      Left 0FB6
      Right 0FB5
    Lacrimal
      Left 08BY
      Right 08BX
    Pancreatic 0FBD
      Accessory 0FBF
    Parotid
      Left 0CBC
      Right 0CBB
  Duodenum 0DB9
  Dura Mater 00B2
  Ear
    External
      Left 09B1
      Right 09B0
    External Auditory Canal
      Left 09B4
      Right 09B3
    Inner
      Left 09BE
      Right 09BD
    Middle
      Left 09B6
      Right 09B5
  Elbow Region
    Left 0XBC
    Right 0XBB
  Epididymis
    Bilateral 0VBL
    Left 0VBK
    Right 0VBJ
  Epiglottis 0CBR
  Esophagogastric Junction 0DB4
  Esophagus 0DB5
    Lower 0DB3
    Middle 0DB2
    Upper 0DB1
  Eustachian Tube
    Left 09BG
    Right 09BF
  Extremity
    Lower
      Left 0YBB
      Right 0YB9
    Upper
      Left 0XB7
      Right 0XB6
  Eye
    Left 08B1
    Right 08B0
  Eyelid
    Lower
      Left 08BR
      Right 08BQ

Excision (Continued)
  Eyelid (Continued)
    Upper
      Left 08BP
      Right 08BN
  Face 0WB2
  Fallopian Tube
    Left 0UB6
    Right 0UB5
  Fallopian Tubes, Bilateral 0UB7
  Femoral Region
    Left 0YB8
    Right 0YB7
  Femoral Shaft
    Left 0QB9
    Right 0QB8
  Femur
    Lower
      Left 0QBC
      Right 0QBB
    Upper
      Left 0QB7
      Right 0QB6
  Fibula
    Left 0QBK
    Right 0QBJ
  Finger Nail 0HBQXZ
  Floor of mouth see Excision, Oral Cavity and
      Throat 0WB3
  Foot
    Left 0YBN
    Right 0YBM
  Gallbladder 0FB4
  Gingiva
    Lower 0CB6
    Upper 0CB5
  Gland
    Adrenal
      Bilateral 0GB4
      Left 0GB2
      Right 0GB3
    Lacrimal
      Left 08BW
      Right 08BV
    Minor Salivary 0CBJ
    Parotid
      Left 0CB9
      Right 0CB8
    Pituitary 0GB0
    Sublingual
      Left 0CBF
      Right 0CBD
    Submaxillary
      Left 0CBH
      Right 0CBG
    Vestibular 0UBL
  Glenoid Cavity
    Left 0PB8
    Right 0PB7
  Glomus Jugulare 0GBC
  Hand
    Left 0XBK
    Right 0XBJ
  Head 0WB0
  Humeral Head
    Left 0PBD
    Right 0PBC
  Humeral Shaft
    Left 0PBG
    Right 0PBF
  Hymen 0UBK
  Hypothalamus 00BA
  Ileocecal Valve 0DBC
  Ileum 0DBB
  Inguinal Region
    Left 0YB6
    Right 0YB5
  Intestine
    Large 0DBE
      Left 0DBG
      Right 0DBF
    Small 0DB8

Excision (Continued)
  Iris
    Left 08BD3Z
    Right 08BC3Z
  Jaw
    Lower 0WB5
    Upper 0WB4
  Jejunum 0DBA
  Joint
    Acromioclavicular
      Left 0RBH
      Right 0RBG
    Ankle
      Left 0SBG
      Right 0SBF
    Carpal
      Left 0RBR
      Right 0RBQ
    Carpometacarpal
      Left 0RBT
      Right 0RBS
    Cervical Vertebral 0RB1
    Cervicothoracic Vertebral 0RB4
    Coccygeal 0SB6
    Elbow
      Left 0RBM
      Right 0RBL
    Finger Phalangeal
      Left 0RBX
      Right 0RBW
    Hip
      Left 0SBB
      Right 0SB9
    Knee
      Left 0SBD
      Right 0SBC
    Lumbar Vertebral 0SB0
    Lumbosacral 0SB3
    Metacarpophalangeal
      Left 0RBV
      Right 0RBU
    Metatarsal-Phalangeal
      Left 0SBN
      Right 0SBM
    Occipital-cervical 0RB0
    Sacrococcygeal 0SB5
    Sacroiliac
      Left 0SB8
      Right 0SB7
    Shoulder
      Left 0RBK
      Right 0RBJ
    Sternoclavicular
      Left 0RBF
      Right 0RBE
    Tarsal
      Left 0SBJ
      Right 0SBH
    Tarsometatarsal
      Left 0SBL
      Right 0SBK
    Temporomandibular
      Left 0RBD
      Right 0RBC
    Thoracic Vertebral 0RB6
    Thoracolumbar Vertebral 0RBA
    Toe Phalangeal
      Left 0SBQ
      Right 0SBP
    Wrist
      Left 0RBP
      Right 0RBN
  Kidney
    Left 0TB1
    Right 0TB0
  Kidney Pelvis
    Left 0TB4
    Right 0TB3
  Knee Region
    Left 0YBG
    Right 0YBF

▶ New   ⇒ Revised   ~~deleted~~ Deleted

Excision *(Continued)*
  Larynx 0CBS
  Leg
    Lower
      Left 0YBJ
      Right 0YBH
    Upper
      Left 0YBD
      Right 0YBC
  Lens
    Left 08BK3Z
    Right 08BJ3Z
  Lip
    Lower 0CB1
    Upper 0CB0
  Liver 0FB0
    Left Lobe 0FB2
    Right Lobe 0FB1
  Lung
    Bilateral 0BBM
    Left 0BBL
    Lower Lobe
      Left 0BBJ
      Right 0BBF
    Middle Lobe, Right 0BBD
    Right 0BBK
    Upper Lobe
      Left 0BBG
      Right 0BBC
  Lung Lingula 0BBH
  Lymphatic
    Aortic 07BD
    Axillary
      Left 07B6
      Right 07B5
    Head 07B0
    Inguinal
      Left 07BJ
      Right 07BH
    Internal Mammary
      Left 07B9
      Right 07B8
    Lower Extremity
      Left 07BG
      Right 07BF
    Mesenteric 07BB
    Neck
      Left 07B2
      Right 07B1
    Pelvis 07BC
    Thoracic Duct 07BK
    Thorax 07B7
    Upper Extremity
      Left 07B4
      Right 07B3
  Mandible
    Left 0NBV
    Right 0NBT
  Maxilla 0NBR
  Mediastinum 0WBC
  Medulla Oblongata 00BD
  Mesentery 0DBV
  Metacarpal
    Left 0PBQ
    Right 0PBP
  Metatarsal
    Left 0QBP
    Right 0QBN
  Muscle
    Abdomen
      Left 0KBL
      Right 0KBK
    Extraocular
      Left 08BM
      Right 08BL
    Facial 0KB1
    Foot
      Left 0KBW
      Right 0KBV
    Hand
      Left 0KBD
      Right 0KBC

Excision *(Continued)*
  Head 0KB0
  Hip
    Left 0KBP
    Right 0KBN
  Lower Arm and Wrist
    Left 0KBB
    Right 0KB9
  Lower Leg
    Left 0KBT
    Right 0KBS
  Neck
    Left 0KB3
    Right 0KB2
  Papillary 02BD
  Perineum 0KBM
  Shoulder
    Left 0KB6
    Right 0KB5
  Thorax
    Left 0KBJ
    Right 0KBH
  Tongue, Palate, Pharynx 0KB4
  Trunk
    Left 0KBG
    Right 0KBF
  Upper Arm
    Left 0KB8
    Right 0KB7
  Upper Leg
    Left 0KBR
    Right 0KBQ
  Nasal Mucosa and Soft Tissue 09BK
  Nasopharynx 09BN
  Neck 0WB6
  Nerve
    Abdominal Sympathetic 01BM
    Abducens 00BL
    Accessory 00BR
    Acoustic 00BN
    Brachial Plexus 01B3
    Cervical 01B1
    Cervical Plexus 01B0
    Facial 00BM
    Femoral 01BD
    Glossopharyngeal 00BP
    Head and Neck Sympathetic 01BK
    Hypoglossal 00BS
    Lumbar 01BB
    Lumbar Plexus 01B9
    Lumbar Sympathetic 01BN
    Lumbosacral Plexus 01BA
    Median 01B5
    Oculomotor 00BH
    Olfactory 00BF
    Optic 00BG
    Peroneal 01BH
    Phrenic 01B2
    Pudendal 01BC
    Radial 01B6
    Sacral 01BR
    Sacral Plexus 01BQ
    Sacral Sympathetic 01BP
    Sciatic 01BF
    Thoracic 01B8
    Thoracic Sympathetic 01BL
    Tibial 01BG
    Trigeminal 00BK
    Trochlear 00BJ
    Ulnar 01B4
    Vagus 00BQ
  Nipple
    Left 0HBX
    Right 0HBW
  Omentum 0DBU
  Oral Cavity and Throat 0WB3
  Orbit
    Left 0NBQ
    Right 0NBP

Excision *(Continued)*
  Ovary
    Bilateral 0UB2
    Left 0UB1
    Right 0UB0
  Palate
    Hard 0CB2
    Soft 0CB3
  Pancreas 0FBG
  Para-aortic Body 0GB9
  Paraganglion Extremity 0GBF
  Parathyroid Gland 0GBR
    Inferior
      Left 0GBP
      Right 0GBN
    Multiple 0GBQ
    Superior
      Left 0GBM
      Right 0GBL
  Patella
    Left 0QBF
    Right 0QBD
  Penis 0VBS
  Pericardium 02BN
  Perineum
    Female 0WBN
    Male 0WBM
  Peritoneum 0DBW
  Phalanx
    Finger
      Left 0PBV
      Right 0PBT
    Thumb
      Left 0PBS
      Right 0PBR
    Toe
      Left 0QBR
      Right 0QBQ
  Pharynx 0CBM
  Pineal Body 0GB1
  Pleura
    Left 0BBP
    Right 0BBN
  Pons 00BB
  Prepuce 0VBT
  Prostate 0VB0
  Radius
    Left 0PBJ
    Right 0PBH
  Rectum 0DBP
  Retina
    Left 08BF3Z
    Right 08BE3Z
  Retroperitoneum 0WBH
  Ribs
    1 to 2 0PB1
    3 or More 0PB2
  Sacrum 0QB1
  Scapula
    Left 0PB6
    Right 0PB5
  Sclera
    Left 08B7XZ
    Right 08B6XZ
  Scrotum 0VB5
  Septum
    Atrial 02B5
    Nasal 09BM
    Ventricular 02BM
  Shoulder Region
    Left 0XB3
    Right 0XB2
  Sinus
    Accessory 09BP
    Ethmoid
      Left 09BV
      Right 09BU
    Frontal
      Left 09BT
      Right 09BS

▶ New ⮕ Revised ~~deleted~~ Deleted

Excision *(Continued)*
Vein *(Continued)*
Upper Ø5BY
Vertebral
Left Ø5BS
Right Ø5BR
Vena Cava
Inferior Ø6BØ
Superior Ø2BV
Ventricle
Left Ø2BL
Right Ø2BK
Vertebra
Cervical ØPB3
Lumbar ØQBØ
Thoracic ØPB4
Vesicle
Bilateral ØVB3
Left ØVB2
Right ØVB1
Vitreous
Left Ø8B53Z
Right Ø8B43Z
Vocal Cord
Left ØCBV
Right ØCBT
Vulva ØUBM
Wrist Region
Left ØXBH
Right ØXBG
EXCLUDER® AAA Endoprosthesis
use Intraluminal Device, Branched or Fenestrated, One or Two Arteries in Ø4V
use Intraluminal Device, Branched or Fenestrated, Three or More Arteries in Ø4V
use Intraluminal Device
EXCLUDER® IBE Endoprosthesis use Intraluminal Device, Branched or Fenestrated, One or Two Arteries in Ø4V
Exclusion, Left atrial appendage (LAA) *see* Occlusion, Atrium, Left Ø2L7
Exercise, rehabilitation *see* Motor Treatment, Rehabilitation FØ7
Exploration *see* Inspection
Express® (LD) Premounted Stent System *use* Intraluminal Device
Express® Biliary SD Monorail® Premounted Stent System *use* Intraluminal Device
Express® SD Renal Monorail® Premounted Stent System *use* Intraluminal Device
Extensor carpi radialis muscle
use Lower Arm and Wrist Muscle, Right
use Lower Arm and Wrist Muscle, Left
Extensor carpi ulnaris muscle
use Lower Arm and Wrist Muscle, Right
use Lower Arm and Wrist Muscle, Left
Extensor digitorum brevis muscle
use Foot Muscle, Right
use Foot Muscle, Left
Extensor digitorum longus muscle
use Lower Leg Muscle, Right
use Lower Leg Muscle, Left
Extensor hallucis brevis muscle
use Foot Muscle, Right
use Foot Muscle, Left
Extensor hallucis longus muscle
use Lower Leg Muscle, Right
use Lower Leg Muscle, Left
External anal sphincter *use* Anal Sphincter
External auditory meatus
use External Auditory Canal, Right
use External Auditory Canal, Left
External fixator
use External Fixation Device in Head and Facial Bones
use External Fixation Device in Upper Bones
use External Fixation Device in Lower Bones
use External Fixation Device in Upper Joints
use External Fixation Device in Lower Joints
External maxillary artery *use* Face Artery
External naris *use* Nasal Mucosa and Soft Tissue
External oblique aponeurosis *use* Subcutaneous Tissue and Fascia, Trunk
External oblique muscle
use Abdomen Muscle, Right
use Abdomen Muscle, Left
External popliteal nerve *use* Peroneal Nerve
External pudendal artery
use Femoral Artery, Right
use Femoral Artery, Left
External pudendal vein
use Saphenous Vein, Right
use Saphenous Vein, Left
External urethral sphincter *use* Urethra
Extirpation
Acetabulum
Left ØQC5
Right ØQC4
Adenoids ØCCQ
Ampulla of Vater ØFCC
Anal Sphincter ØDCR
Anterior Chamber
Left Ø8C3
Right Ø8C2
Anus ØDCQ
Aorta
Abdominal Ø4CØ
Thoracic
Ascending/Arch Ø2CX
Descending Ø2CW
Aortic Body ØGCD
Appendix ØDCJ
Artery
Anterior Tibial
Left Ø4CQ
Right Ø4CP
Axillary
Left Ø3C6
Right Ø3C5
Brachial
Left Ø3C8
Right Ø3C7
Celiac Ø4C1
Colic
Left Ø4C7
Middle Ø4C8
Right Ø4C6
Common Carotid
Left Ø3CJ
Right Ø3CH
Common Iliac
Left Ø4CD
Right Ø4CC
Coronary
Four or More Arteries Ø2C3
One Artery Ø2CØ
Three Arteries Ø2C2
Two Arteries Ø2C1
External Carotid
Left Ø3CN
Right Ø3CM
External Iliac
Left Ø4CJ
Right Ø4CH
Face Ø3CR
Femoral
Left Ø4CL
Right Ø4CK
Foot
Left Ø4CW
Right Ø4CV
Gastric Ø4C2
Hand
Left Ø3CF
Right Ø3CD
Hepatic Ø4C3
Inferior Mesenteric Ø4CB
Innominate Ø3C2
Extirpation *(Continued)*
Artery *(Continued)*
Internal Carotid
Left Ø3CL
Right Ø3CK
Internal Iliac
Left Ø4CF
Right Ø4CE
Internal Mammary
Left Ø3C1
Right Ø3CØ
Intracranial Ø3CG
Lower Ø4CY
Peroneal
Left Ø4CU
Right Ø4CT
Popliteal
Left Ø4CN
Right Ø4CM
Posterior Tibial
Left Ø4CS
Right Ø4CR
Pulmonary
Left Ø2CR
Right Ø2CQ
Pulmonary Trunk Ø2CP
Radial
Left Ø3CC
Right Ø3CB
Renal
Left Ø4CA
Right Ø4C9
Splenic Ø4C4
Subclavian
Left Ø3C4
Right Ø3C3
Superior Mesenteric Ø4C5
Temporal
Left Ø3CT
Right Ø3CS
Thyroid
Left Ø3CV
Right Ø3CU
Ulnar
Left Ø3CA
Right Ø3C9
Upper Ø3CY
Vertebral
Left Ø3CQ
Right Ø3CP
Atrium
Left Ø2C7
Right Ø2C6
Auditory Ossicle
Left Ø9CA
Right Ø9C9
Basal Ganglia ØØC8
Bladder ØTCB
Bladder Neck ØTCC
Bone
Ethmoid
Left ØNCG
Right ØNCF
Frontal ØNC1
Hyoid ØNCX
Lacrimal
Left ØNCJ
Right ØNCH
Nasal ØNCB
Occipital ØNC7
Palatine
Left ØNCL
Right ØNCK
Parietal
Left ØNC4
Right ØNC3
Pelvic
Left ØQC3
Right ØQC2
Sphenoid ØNCC

E

▶ New   ⟹ Revised   ~~deleted~~ Deleted

Extirpation *(Continued)*
Joint
  Acromioclavicular
    Left ØRCH
    Right ØRCG
  Ankle
    Left ØSCG
    Right ØSCF
  Carpal
    Left ØRCR
    Right ØRCQ
  Carpometacarpal
    Left ØRCT
    Right ØRCS
  Cervical Vertebral ØRC1
  Cervicothoracic Vertebral ØRC4
  Coccygeal ØSC6
  Elbow
    Left ØRCM
    Right ØRCL
  Finger Phalangeal
    Left ØRCX
    Right ØRCW
  Hip
    Left ØSCB
    Right ØSC9
  Knee
    Left ØSCD
    Right ØSCC
  Lumbar Vertebral ØSCØ
  Lumbosacral ØSC3
  Metacarpophalangeal
    Left ØRCV
    Right ØRCU
  Metatarsal-Phalangeal
    Left ØSCN
    Right ØSCM
  Occipital-cervical ØRCØ
  Sacrococcygeal ØSC5
  Sacroiliac
    Left ØSC8
    Right ØSC7
  Shoulder
    Left ØRCK
    Right ØRCJ
  Sternoclavicular
    Left ØRCF
    Right ØRCE
  Tarsal
    Left ØSCJ
    Right ØSCH
  Tarsometatarsal
    Left ØSCL
    Right ØSCK
  Temporomandibular
    Left ØRCD
    Right ØRCC
  Thoracic Vertebral ØRC6
  Thoracolumbar Vertebral ØRCA
  Toe Phalangeal
    Left ØSCQ
    Right ØSCP
  Wrist
    Left ØRCP
    Right ØRCN
Kidney
  Left ØTC1
  Right ØTCØ
Kidney Pelvis
  Left ØTC4
  Right ØTC3
Larynx ØCCS
Lens
  Left Ø8CK
  Right Ø8CJ
Lip
  Lower ØCC1
  Upper ØCCØ
Liver ØFCØ
  Left Lobe ØFC2
  Right Lobe ØFC1

Extirpation *(Continued)*
Lung
  Bilateral ØBCM
  Left ØBCL
  Lower Lobe
    Left ØBCJ
    Right ØBCF
  Middle Lobe, Right ØBCD
  Right ØBCK
  Upper Lobe
    Left ØBCG
    Right ØBCC
Lung Lingula ØBCH
Lymphatic
  Aortic Ø7CD
  Axillary
    Left Ø7C6
    Right Ø7C5
  Head Ø7CØ
  Inguinal
    Left Ø7CJ
    Right Ø7CH
  Internal Mammary
    Left Ø7C9
    Right Ø7C8
  Lower Extremity
    Left Ø7CG
    Right Ø7CF
  Mesenteric Ø7CB
  Neck
    Left Ø7C2
    Right Ø7C1
  Pelvis Ø7CC
  Thoracic Duct Ø7CK
  Thorax Ø7C7
  Upper Extremity
    Left Ø7C4
    Right Ø7C3
Mandible
  Left ØNCV
  Right ØNCT
Maxilla ØNCR
Mediastinum ØWCC
Medulla Oblongata ØØCD
Mesentery ØDCV
Metacarpal
  Left ØPCQ
  Right ØPCP
Metatarsal
  Left ØQCP
  Right ØQCN
Muscle
  Abdomen
    Left ØKCL
    Right ØKCK
  Extraocular
    Left Ø8CM
    Right Ø8CL
  Facial ØKC1
  Foot
    Left ØKCW
    Right ØKCV
  Hand
    Left ØKCD
    Right ØKCC
  Head ØKCØ
  Hip
    Left ØKCP
    Right ØKCN
  Lower Arm and Wrist
    Left ØKCB
    Right ØKC9
  Lower Leg
    Left ØKCT
    Right ØKCS
  Neck
    Left ØKC3
    Right ØKC2
  Papillary Ø2CD
  Perineum ØKCM

Extirpation *(Continued)*
Lymphatic *(Continued)*
  Shoulder
    Left ØKC6
    Right ØKC5
  Thorax
    Left ØKCJ
    Right ØKCH
  Tongue, Palate, Pharynx ØKC4
  Trunk
    Left ØKCG
    Right ØKCF
  Upper Arm
    Left ØKC8
    Right ØKC7
  Upper Leg
    Left ØKCR
    Right ØKCQ
Nasal Mucosa and Soft Tissue Ø9CK
Nasopharynx Ø9CN
Nerve
  Abdominal Sympathetic Ø1CM
  Abducens ØØCL
  Accessory ØØCR
  Acoustic ØØCN
  Brachial Plexus Ø1C3
  Cervical Ø1C1
  Cervical Plexus Ø1CØ
  Facial ØØCM
  Femoral Ø1CD
  Glossopharyngeal ØØCP
  Head and Neck Sympathetic Ø1CK
  Hypoglossal ØØCS
  Lumbar Ø1CB
  Lumbar Plexus Ø1C9
  Lumbar Sympathetic Ø1CN
  Lumbosacral Plexus Ø1CA
  Median Ø1C5
  Oculomotor ØØCH
  Olfactory ØØCF
  Optic ØØCG
  Peroneal Ø1CH
  Phrenic Ø1C2
  Pudendal Ø1CC
  Radial Ø1C6
  Sacral Ø1CR
  Sacral Plexus Ø1CQ
  Sacral Sympathetic Ø1CP
  Sciatic Ø1CF
  Thoracic Ø1C8
  Thoracic Sympathetic Ø1CL
  Tibial Ø1CG
  Trigeminal ØØCK
  Trochlear ØØCJ
  Ulnar Ø1C4
  Vagus ØØCQ
Nipple
  Left ØHCX
  Right ØHCW
Omentum ØDCU
Oral Cavity and Throat ØWC3
Orbit
  Left ØNCQ
  Right ØNCP
Orbital Atherectomy Technology X2C
Ovary
  Bilateral ØUC2
  Left ØUC1
  Right ØUCØ
Palate
  Hard ØCC2
  Soft ØCC3
Pancreas ØFCG
Para-aortic Body ØGC9
Paraganglion Extremity ØGCF
Parathyroid Gland ØGCR
  Inferior
    Left ØGCP
    Right ØGCN
  Multiple ØGCQ

▶ New　⇨ Revised　~~deleted~~ Deleted

▶ New   ⇒ Revised   ~~deleted~~ Deleted

F

Face lift see Alteration, Face 0W02
Facet replacement spinal stabilization device
  use Spinal Stabilization Device, Facet
    Replacement in 0RH
  use Spinal Stabilization Device, Facet
    Replacement in 0SH
Facial artery use Face Artery
Factor Xa Inhibitor Reversal Agent, Andexanet
  Alfa use Andexanet Alfa, Factor Xa
    Inhibitor Reversal Agent
False vocal cord use Larynx
Falx cerebri use Dura Mater
Fascia lata
  use Subcutaneous Tissue and Fascia, Right
    Upper Leg
  use Subcutaneous Tissue and Fascia, Left
    Upper Leg
Fasciaplasty, fascioplasty
  see Repair, Subcutaneous Tissue and Fascia 0JQ
  see Replacement, Subcutaneous Tissue and
    Fascia 0JR
Fasciectomy
  see Excision, Subcutaneous Tissue and Fascia
    0JB
Fasciorrhaphy see Repair, Subcutaneous Tissue
    and Fascia 0JQ
Fasciotomy
  see Division, Subcutaneous Tissue and Fascia
    0J8
  see Drainage, Subcutaneous Tissue and Fascia
    0J9
  see Release
Feeding Device
  Change device in
    Lower 0D2DXUZ
    Upper 0D20XUZ
  Insertion of device in
    Duodenum 0DH9
    Esophagus 0DH5
    Ileum 0DHB
    Intestine, Small 0DH8
    Jejunum 0DHA
    Stomach 0DH6
  Removal of device from
    Esophagus 0DP5
    Intestinal Tract
      Lower 0DPD
      Upper 0DP0
    Stomach 0DP6
  Revision of device in
    Intestinal Tract
      Lower 0DWD
      Upper 0DW0
    Stomach 0DW6
Femoral head
  use Upper Femur, Right
  use Upper Femur, Left
Femoral lymph node
  use Lymphatic, Right Lower Extremity
  use Lymphatic, Left Lower Extremity
Femoropatellar joint
  use Knee Joint, Right
  use Knee Joint, Left
  use Knee Joint, Femoral Surface, Right
  use Knee Joint, Femoral Surface, Left
Femorotibial joint
  use Knee Joint, Right
  use Knee Joint, Left
  use Knee Joint, Tibial Surface, Right
  use Knee Joint, Tibial Surface, Left
Fibular artery
  use Peroneal Artery, Right
  use Peroneal Artery, Left
Fibularis brevis muscle
  use Lower Leg Muscle, Right
  use Lower Leg Muscle, Left
Fibularis longus muscle
  use Lower Leg Muscle, Right
  use Lower Leg Muscle, Left

Fifth cranial nerve use Trigeminal Nerve
Filum terminale use Spinal Meninges
Fimbriectomy
  see Excision, Female Reproductive System 0UB
  see Resection, Female Reproductive System
    0UT
Fine needle aspiration
  ➠ Fluid or gas see Drainage
  ▶ Tissue biopsy
    ▶ see Extraction
    ▶ see Excision
First cranial nerve use Olfactory Nerve
First intercostal nerve use Brachial
    Plexus
Fistulization
  see Bypass
  see Drainage
  see Repair
Fitting
  Arch bars, for fracture reduction see
    Reposition, Mouth and Throat 0CS
  Arch bars, for immobilization see
    Immobilization, Face 2W31
  Artificial limb see Device Fitting,
    Rehabilitation F0D
  Hearing aid see Device Fitting, Rehabilitation
    F0D
  Ocular prosthesis F0DZ8UZ
  Prosthesis, limb see Device Fitting,
    Rehabilitation F0D
  Prosthesis, ocular F0DZ8UZ
Fixation, bone
  External, with fracture reduction see
    Reposition
  External, without fracture reduction see
    Insertion
  Internal, with fracture reduction see
    Reposition
  Internal, without fracture reduction see
    Insertion
FLAIR® Endovascular Stent Graft use
    Intraluminal Device
Flexible Composite Mesh use Synthetic
    Substitute
Flexor carpi radialis muscle
  use Lower Arm and Wrist Muscle, Right
  use Lower Arm and Wrist Muscle, Left
Flexor carpi ulnaris muscle
  use Lower Arm and Wrist Muscle, Right
  use Lower Arm and Wrist Muscle, Left
Flexor digitorum brevis muscle
  use Foot Muscle, Right
  use Foot Muscle, Left
Flexor digitorum longus muscle
  use Lower Leg Muscle, Right
  use Lower Leg Muscle, Left
Flexor hallucis brevis muscle
  use Foot Muscle, Right
  use Foot Muscle, Left
Flexor hallucis longus muscle
  use Lower Leg Muscle, Right
  use Lower Leg Muscle, Left
Flexor pollicis longus muscle
  use Lower Arm and Wrist Muscle, Right
  use Lower Arm and Wrist Muscle, Left
Fluoroscopy
  Abdomen and Pelvis BW11
  Airway, Upper BB1DZZZ
  Ankle
    Left BQ1H
    Right BQ1G
  Aorta
    Abdominal B410
      Laser, Intraoperative B410
    Thoracic B310
      Laser, Intraoperative B310
    Thoraco-Abdominal B31P
      Laser, Intraoperative B31P
  Aorta and Bilateral Lower Extremity Arteries
    B41D
    Laser, Intraoperative B41D

Fluoroscopy (Continued)
  Arm
    Left BP1FZZZ
    Right BP1EZZZ
  Artery
    Brachiocephalic-Subclavian
      Right B311
        Laser, Intraoperative B311
    Bronchial B31L
      Laser, Intraoperative B31L
    Bypass Graft, Other B21F
    Cervico-Cerebral Arch B31Q
      Laser, Intraoperative B31Q
    Common Carotid
      Bilateral B315
        Laser, Intraoperative B315
      Left B314
        Laser, Intraoperative B314
      Right B313
        Laser, Intraoperative B313
    Coronary
      Bypass Graft
        Multiple B213
          Laser, Intraoperative B213
        Single B212
          Laser, Intraoperative B212
      Multiple B211
        Laser, Intraoperative B211
      Single B210
        Laser, Intraoperative B210
    External Carotid
      Bilateral B31C
        Laser, Intraoperative B31C
      Left B31B
        Laser, Intraoperative B31B
      Right B319
        Laser, Intraoperative B319
    Hepatic B412
      Laser, Intraoperative B412
    Inferior Mesenteric B415
      Laser, Intraoperative B415
    Intercostal B31L
      Laser, Intraoperative B31L
    Internal Carotid
      Bilateral B318
        Laser, Intraoperative B318
      Left B317
        Laser, Intraoperative B317
      Right B316
        Laser, Intraoperative B316
    Internal Mammary Bypass Graft
      Left B218
      Right B217
    Intra-Abdominal
      Other B41B
        Laser, Intraoperative B41B
    Intracranial B31R
      Laser, Intraoperative B31R
    Lower
      Other B41J
        Laser, Intraoperative B41J
    Lower Extremity
      Bilateral and Aorta B41D
        Laser, Intraoperative B41D
      Left B41G
        Laser, Intraoperative B41G
      Right B41F
        Laser, Intraoperative B41F
    Lumbar B419
      Laser, Intraoperative B419
    Pelvic B41C
      Laser, Intraoperative B41C
    Pulmonary
      Left B31T
        Laser, Intraoperative B31T
      Right B31S
        Laser, Intraoperative B31S
    Pulmonary Trunk B31U
      Laser, Intraoperative B31U
    Renal
      Bilateral B418
        Laser, Intraoperative B418

▶ New   ➠ Revised   ~~deleted~~ Deleted

▶ New   ⇒ Revised   ~~deleted~~ Deleted

Fluoroscopy *(Continued)*
  Vena Cava
    Inferior B519
    Superior B518
  Wrist
    Left BP1M
    Right BP1L
Fluoroscopy, laser intraoperative
  see Fluoroscopy, Heart B21
  see Fluoroscopy, Upper Arteries B31
  see Fluoroscopy, Lower Arteries B41
Flushing *see* Irrigation
Foley catheter *use* Drainage Device
Fontan completion procedure Stage II *see*
    Bypass, Vena Cava, Inferior 0610
Foramen magnum *use* Occipital Bone
Foramen of Monro (intraventricular) *use*
    Cerebral Ventricle
Foreskin *use* Prepuce
Formula™ Balloon-Expandable Renal
    Stent System *use* Intraluminal
    Device
Fossa of Rosenmuller *use* Nasopharynx
Fourth cranial nerve *use* Nerve, Trochlear
Fourth ventricle *use* Cerebral Ventricle
Fovea
  use Retina, Right
  use Retina, Left
Fragmentation
  Ampulla of Vater 0FFC
  Anus 0DFQ
  Appendix 0DFJ
  Bladder 0TFB
  Bladder Neck 0TFC
  Bronchus
    Lingula 0BF9
    Lower Lobe
      Left 0BFB
      Right 0BF6
    Main
      Left 0BF7
      Right 0BF3
    Middle Lobe, Right 0BF5
    Upper Lobe
      Left 0BF8
      Right 0BF4
  Carina 0BF2
  Cavity, Cranial 0WF1
  Cecum 0DFH
  Cerebral Ventricle 00F6
  Colon
    Ascending 0DFK
    Descending 0DFM
    Sigmoid 0DFN
    Transverse 0DFL
  Duct
    Common Bile 0FF9
    Cystic 0FF8
    Hepatic
      Common 0FF7
      Left 0FF6
      Right 0FF5
    Pancreatic 0FFD
      Accessory 0FFF
    Parotid
      Left 0CFC
      Right 0CFB
  Duodenum 0DF9
  Epidural Space, Intracranial 00F3
  Esophagus 0DF5
  Fallopian Tube
    Left 0UF6
    Right 0UF5
  Fallopian Tubes, Bilateral 0UF7
  Gallbladder 0FF4
  Gastrointestinal Tract 0WFP
  Genitourinary Tract 0WFR
  Ileum 0DFB

Fragmentation *(Continued)*
  Intestine
    Large 0DFE
      Left 0DFG
      Right 0DFF
    Small 0DF8
  Jejunum 0DFA
  Kidney Pelvis
    Left 0TF4
    Right 0TF3
  Mediastinum 0WFC
  Oral Cavity and Throat 0WF3
  Pelvic Cavity 0WFJ
  Pericardial Cavity 0WFD
  Pericardium 02FN
  Peritoneal Cavity 0WFG
  Pleural Cavity
    Left 0WFB
    Right 0WF9
  Rectum 0DFP
  Respiratory Tract 0WFQ
  Spinal Canal 00FU
  Stomach 0DF6
  Subarachnoid Space, Intracranial 00F5
  Subdural Space, Intracranial 00F4
  Trachea 0BF1
  Ureter
    Left 0TF7
    Right 0TF6
  Urethra 0TFD
  Uterus 0UF9
  Vitreous
    Left 08F5
    Right 08F4
Freestyle (Stentless) Aortic Root Bioprosthesis
    use Zooplastic Tissue in Heart and Great
    Vessels
Frenectomy
  see Excision, Mouth and Throat 0CB
  see Resection, Mouth and Throat 0CT
Frenoplasty, frenuloplasty
  see Repair, Mouth and Throat 0CQ
  see Replacement, Mouth and Throat 0CR
  see Supplement, Mouth and Throat 0CU
Frenotomy
  see Drainage, Mouth and Throat 0C9
  see Release, Mouth and Throat 0CN
Frenulotomy
  see Drainage, Mouth and Throat 0C9
  see Release, Mouth and Throat 0CN
Frenulum labii inferioris *use* Lower Lip
Frenulum labii superioris *use* Upper Lip
Frenulum linguae *use* Tongue
Frenulumectomy
  see Excision, Mouth and Throat 0CB
  see Resection, Mouth and Throat 0CT
Frontal lobe *use* Cerebral Hemisphere
Frontal vein
  use Face Vein, Right
  use Face Vein, Left
Fulguration *see* Destruction
Fundoplication, gastroesophageal *see*
    Restriction, Esophagogastric Junction
    0DV4
Fundus uteri *use* Uterus
Fusion
  Acromioclavicular
    Left 0RGH
    Right 0RGG
  Ankle
    Left 0SGG
    Right 0SGF
  Carpal
    Left 0RGR
    Right 0RGQ
  Carpometacarpal
    Left 0RGT
    Right 0RGS

Fusion *(Continued)*
  Cervical Vertebral 0RG1
    2 or more 0RG2
      Interbody Fusion Device
        Nanotextured Surface XRG2092
        Radiolucent Porous XRG20F3
      Interbody Fusion Device
        Nanotextured Surface XRG1092
        Radiolucent Porous XRG10F3
  Cervicothoracic Vertebral 0RG4
      Interbody Fusion Device
        Nanotextured Surface XRG4092
        Radiolucent Porous XRG40F3
  Coccygeal 0SG6
  Elbow
    Left 0RGM
    Right 0RGL
  Finger Phalangeal
    Left 0RGX
    Right 0RGW
  Hip
    Left 0SGB
    Right 0SG9
  Knee
    Left 0SGD
    Right 0SGC
  Lumbar Vertebral 0SG0
    2 or more 0SG1
      Interbody Fusion Device
        Nanotextured Surface XRGC092
        Radiolucent Porous XRGC0F3
      Interbody Fusion Device
        Nanotextured Surface XRGB092
        Radiolucent Porous XRGB0F3
  Lumbosacral 0SG3
      Interbody Fusion Device
        Nanotextured Surface XRGD092
        Radiolucent Porous XRGD0F3
  Metacarpophalangeal
    Left 0RGV
    Right 0RGU
  Metatarsal-Phalangeal
    Left 0SGN
    Right 0SGM
  Occipital-cervical 0RG0
      Interbody Fusion Device
        Nanotextured Surface XRG0092
        Radiolucent Porous XRG00F3
  Sacrococcygeal 0SG5
  Sacroiliac
    Left 0SG8
    Right 0SG7
  Shoulder
    Left 0RGK
    Right 0RGJ
  Sternoclavicular
    Left 0RGF
    Right 0RGE
  Tarsal
    Left 0SGJ
    Right 0SGH
  Tarsometatarsal
    Left 0SGL
    Right 0SGK
  Temporomandibular
    Left 0RGD
    Right 0RGC
  Thoracic Vertebral 0RG6
    2 to 7 0RG7
      Interbody Fusion Device
        Nanotextured Surface XRG7092
        Radiolucent Porous XRG70F3
    8 or more 0RG8
      Interbody Fusion Device
        Nanotextured Surface XRG8092
        Radiolucent Porous XRG80F3
      Interbody Fusion Device
        Nanotextured Surface XRG6092
        Radiolucent Porous XRG60F3

▶ New   ⇒ Revised   ~~deleted~~ Deleted

G

Gait training *see* Motor Treatment, Rehabilitation F07
Galea aponeurotica *use* Subcutaneous Tissue and Fascia, Scalp
GammaTile™ *use* Radioactive Element, Cesium-131 Collagen Implant in 00H
Ganglion impar (ganglion of Walther) *use* Sacral Sympathetic Nerve
Ganglionectomy
    Destruction of lesion *see* Destruction
    Excision of lesion *see* Excision
Gasserian ganglion *use* Trigeminal Nerve
Gastrectomy
    Partial *see* Excision, Stomach 0DB6
    Total *see* Resection, Stomach 0DT6
    Vertical (sleeve) *see* Excision, Stomach 0DB6
Gastric electrical stimulation (GES) lead *use* Stimulator Lead in Gastrointestinal System
Gastric lymph node *use* Lymphatic, Aortic
Gastric pacemaker lead *use* Stimulator Lead in Gastrointestinal System
Gastric plexus *see* Abdominal Sympathetic Nerve
Gastrocnemius muscle
    use Lower Leg Muscle, Right
    use Lower Leg Muscle, Left
Gastrocolic ligament *use* Omentum
Gastrocolic omentum *use* Omentum
Gastrocolostomy
    see Bypass, Gastrointestinal System 0D1
    see Drainage, Gastrointestinal System 0D9
Gastroduodenal artery *use* Hepatic Artery
Gastroduodenectomy
    see Excision, Gastrointestinal System 0DB
    see Resection, Gastrointestinal System 0DT
Gastroduodenoscopy 0DJ08ZZ
Gastroenteroplasty
    see Repair, Gastrointestinal System 0DQ
    see Supplement, Gastrointestinal System 0DU
Gastroenterostomy
    see Bypass, Gastrointestinal System 0D1
    see Drainage, Gastrointestinal System 0D9
Gastroesophageal (GE) junction *use* Esophagogastric Junction
Gastrogastrostomy
    see Bypass, Stomach 0D16
    see Drainage, Stomach 0D96
Gastrohepatic omentum *use* Omentum
Gastrojejunostomy
    see Bypass, Stomach 0D16
    see Drainage, Stomach 0D96
Gastrolysis *see* Release, Stomach 0DN6
Gastropexy
    see Repair, Stomach 0DQ6
    see Reposition, Stomach 0DS6
Gastrophrenic ligament *use* Omentum
Gastroplasty
    see Repair, Stomach 0DQ6
    see Supplement, Stomach 0DU6
Gastroplication *see* Restriction, Stomach 0DV6
Gastropylorectomy *see* Excision, Gastrointestinal System 0DB

Gastrorrhaphy *see* Repair, Stomach 0DQ6
Gastroscopy 0DJ68ZZ
Gastrosplenic ligament *use* Omentum
Gastrostomy
    see Bypass, Stomach 0D16
    see Drainage, Stomach 0D96
Gastrotomy *see* Drainage, Stomach 0D96
Gemellus muscle
    use Hip Muscle, Right
    use Hip Muscle, Left
Geniculate ganglion *use* Facial Nerve
Geniculate nucleus *use* Thalamus
Genioglossus muscle *use* Tongue, Palate, Pharynx Muscle
Genioplasty *see* Alteration, Jaw, Lower 0W05
Genitofemoral nerve *use* Lumbar Plexus
▶GIAPREZA(tm) *use* Synthetic Human Angiotensin II
Gingivectomy *see* Excision, Mouth and Throat 0CB
Gingivoplasty
    see Repair, Mouth and Throat 0CQ
    see Replacement, Mouth and Throat 0CR
    see Supplement, Mouth and Throat 0CU
Glans penis *use* Prepuce
Glenohumeral joint
    use Shoulder Joint, Right
    use Shoulder Joint, Left
Glenohumeral ligament
    use Shoulder Bursa and Ligament, Right
    use Shoulder Bursa and Ligament, Left
Glenoid fossa (of scapula)
    use Glenoid Cavity, Right
    use Glenoid Cavity, Left
Glenoid ligament (labrum)
    use Shoulder Joint, Right
    use Shoulder Joint, Left
Globus pallidus *use* Basal Ganglia
Glomectomy
    see Excision, Endocrine System 0GB
    see Resection, Endocrine System 0GT
Glossectomy
    see Excision, Tongue 0CB7
    see Resection, Tongue 0CT7
Glossoepiglottic fold *use* Epiglottis
Glossopexy
    see Repair, Tongue 0CQ7
    see Reposition, Tongue 0CS7
Glossoplasty
    see Repair, Tongue 0CQ7
    see Replacement, Tongue 0CR7
    see Supplement, Tongue 0CU7
Glossorrhaphy *see* Repair, Tongue 0CQ7
Glossotomy *see* Drainage, Tongue 0C97
Glottis *use* Larynx
Gluteal Artery Perforator Flap
    Replacement
        Bilateral 0HRV079
        Left 0HRU079
        Right 0HRT079
    Transfer
        Left 0KXG
        Right 0KXF

Gluteal lymph node *use* Lymphatic, Pelvis
Gluteal vein
    use Hypogastric Vein, Right
    use Hypogastric Vein, Left
Gluteus maximus muscle
    use Hip Muscle, Right
    use Hip Muscle, Left
Gluteus medius muscle
    use Hip Muscle, Right
    use Hip Muscle, Left
Gluteus minimus muscle
    use Hip Muscle, Right
    use Hip Muscle, Left
GORE EXCLUDER® AAA Endoprosthesis
    use Intraluminal Device, Branched or Fenestrated, One or Two Arteries in 04V
    use Intraluminal Device, Branched or Fenestrated, Three or More Arteries in 04V
    use Intraluminal Device
GORE EXCLUDER® IBE Endoprosthesis
    use Intraluminal Device, Branched or Fenestrated, One or Two Arteries in 04V
GORE TAG® Thoracic Endoprosthesis *use* Intraluminal Device
GORE® DUALMESH® *use* Synthetic Substitute
Gracilis muscle
    use Upper Leg Muscle, Right
    use Upper Leg Muscle, Left
Graft
    see Replacement
    see Supplement
Great auricular nerve *use* Lumbar Plexus
Great cerebral vein *use* Intracranial Vein
Great(er) saphenous vein
    use Saphenous Vein, Right
    use Saphenous Vein, Left
Greater alar cartilage *use* Nasal Mucosa and Soft Tissue
Greater occipital nerve *use* Cervical Nerve
Greater Omentum *use* Omentum
Greater splanchnic nerve *use* Thoracic Sympathetic Nerve
Greater superficial petrosal nerve *use* Facial Nerve
Greater trochanter
    use Upper Femur, Right
    use Upper Femur, Left
Greater tuberosity
    use Humeral Head, Right
    use Humeral Head, Left
Greater vestibular (Bartholin's) gland *use* Vestibular Gland
Greater wing *use* Sphenoid Bone
Guedel airway *use* Intraluminal Device, Airway in Mouth and Throat
Guidance, catheter placement
    EKG *see* Measurement, Physiological Systems 4A0
    Fluoroscopy *see* Fluoroscopy, Veins B51
    Ultrasound *see* Ultrasonography, Veins B54

▶ New   ⇒ Revised   ~~deleted~~ Deleted

H

Hallux
  use Toe, 1st, Right
  use Toe, 1st, Left
Hamate bone
  use Carpal, Right
  use Carpal, Left
Hancock Bioprosthesis (aortic) (mitral) valve
  use Zooplastic Tissue in Heart and Great
    Vessels
Hancock Bioprosthetic Valved Conduit use
  Zooplastic Tissue in Heart and Great Vessels
Harvesting, stem cells see Pheresis, Circulatory
  6A55
Head of fibula
  use Fibula, Right
  use Fibula, Left
Hearing Aid Assessment F14Z
Hearing Assessment F13Z
Hearing Device
  Bone Conduction
    Left 09HE
    Right 09HD
  Insertion of device in
    Left 0NH6[034]SZ
    Right 0NH5[034]SZ
  Multiple Channel Cochlear Prosthesis
    Left 09HE
    Right 09HD
  Removal of device from, Skull 0NP0
  Revision of device in, Skull 0NW0
  Single Channel Cochlear Prosthesis
    Left 09HE
    Right 09HD
Hearing Treatment F09Z
Heart Assist System
  Implantable
    Insertion of device in, Heart 02HA
    Removal of device from, Heart 02PA
    Revision of device in, Heart 02WA
  Short-term External
    Insertion of device in, Heart 02HA
    Removal of device from, Heart 02PA
    Revision of device in, Heart 02WA
HeartMate 3™ LVAS use Implantable Heart
  Assist System in Heart and Great Vessels
HeartMate II® Left Ventricular Assist Device
  (LVAD) use Implantable Heart Assist
  System in Heart and Great Vessels
HeartMate XVE® Left Ventricular Assist
  Device (LVAD) use Implantable Heart
  Assist System in Heart and Great Vessels
HeartMate® implantable heart assist system
  see Insertion of device in, Heart 02HA
Helix
  use External Ear, Right
  use External Ear, Left
  use External Ear, Bilateral
Hematopoietic cell transplant (HCT) see
  Transfusion, Circulatory 302
Hemicolectomy see Resection, Gastrointestinal
  System 0DT
Hemicystectomy see Excision, Urinary System
  0TB
Hemigastrectomy see Excision, Gastrointestinal
  System 0DB
Hemiglossectomy see Excision, Mouth and
  Throat 0CB
Hemilaminectomy
  see Excision, Upper Bones 0PB
  see Excision, Lower Bones 0QB
Hemilaminotomy
  see Release, Central Nervous System 00N
  see Release, Peripheral Nervous System 01N
  see Drainage, Upper Bones 0P9
  see Excision, Upper Bones 0PB
  see Release, Upper Bones 0PN
  see Drainage, Lower Bones 0Q9
  see Excision, Lower Bones 0QB
  see Release, Lower Bones 0QN

Hemilaryngectomy see Excision, Larynx
  0CBS
Hemimandibulectomy see Excision, Head
  and Facial Bones 0NB
Hemimaxillectomy see Excision, Head and
  Facial Bones 0NB
Hemipylorectomy see Excision, Gastrointestinal
  System 0DB
Hemispherectomy
  see Excision, Central Nervous System and
    Cranial Nerves 00B
  see Resection, Central Nervous System and
    Cranial Nerves 00T
Hemithyroidectomy
  see Excision, Endocrine System 0GB
  see Resection, Endocrine System 0GT
Hemodialysis see Performance, Urinary
  5A1D
Hemolung© Respiratory Assist System (RAS)
  5A0920Z
Hepatectomy
  see Excision, Hepatobiliary System and
    Pancreas 0FB
  see Resection, Hepatobiliary System and
    Pancreas 0FT
Hepatic artery proper use Hepatic Artery
Hepatic flexure use Transverse Colon
Hepatic lymph node use Aortic Lymphatic
Hepatic plexus use Abdominal Sympathetic
  Nerve
Hepatic portal vein use Portal Vein
Hepaticoduodenostomy
  see Bypass, Hepatobiliary System and
    Pancreas 0F1
  see Drainage, Hepatobiliary System and
    Pancreas 0F9
Hepaticotomy see Drainage, Hepatobiliary
  System and Pancreas 0F9
Hepatocholedochostomy see Drainage, Duct,
  Common Bile 0F99
Hepatogastric ligament use Omentum
Hepatopancreatic ampulla use Ampulla of
  Vater
Hepatopexy
  see Repair, Hepatobiliary System and
    Pancreas 0FQ
  see Reposition, Hepatobiliary System and
    Pancreas 0FS
Hepatorrhaphy see Repair, Hepatobiliary
  System and Pancreas 0FQ
Hepatotomy see Drainage, Hepatobiliary
  System and Pancreas 0F9
Herculink (RX) Elite Renal Stent System use
  Intraluminal Device
Herniorrhaphy
  see Repair, Anatomical Regions, General
    0WQ
  see Repair, Anatomical Regions, Lower
    Extremities 0YQ
  ➡ With synthetic substitute
    see Supplement, Anatomical Regions,
      General 0WU
    see Supplement, Anatomical Regions,
      Lower Extremities 0YU
Hip (joint) liner use Liner in Lower Joints
Holter monitoring 4A12X45
Holter valve ventricular shunt use Synthetic
  Substitute
▶ Human angiotensin II, synthetic use Synthetic
  Human Angiotensin II
Humeroradial joint
  use Elbow Joint, Right
  use Elbow Joint, Left
Humeroulnar joint
  use Elbow Joint, Right
  use Elbow Joint, Left
Humerus, distal
  use Humeral Shaft, Right
  use Humeral Shaft, Left
Hydrocelectomy see Excision, Male
  Reproductive System 0VB

Hydrotherapy
  Assisted exercise in pool see Motor Treatment,
    Rehabilitation F07
  Whirlpool see Activities of Daily Living
    Treatment, Rehabilitation F08
Hymenectomy
  see Excision, Hymen 0UBK
  see Resection, Hymen 0UTK
Hymenoplasty
  see Repair, Hymen 0UQK
  see Supplement, Hymen 0UUK
Hymenorrhaphy see Repair, Hymen 0UQK
Hymenotomy
  see Division, Hymen 0U8K
  see Drainage, Hymen 0U9K
Hyoglossus muscle use Tongue, Palate, Pharynx
  Muscle
Hyoid artery
  use Thyroid Artery, Right
  use Thyroid Artery, Left
Hyperalimentation see Introduction of
  substance in or on
Hyperbaric oxygenation
  Decompression sickness treatment see
    Decompression, Circulatory
    6A15
  Wound treatment see Assistance,
    Circulatory 5A05
Hyperthermia
  Radiation Therapy
    Abdomen DWY38ZZ
    Adrenal Gland DGY28ZZ
    Bile Ducts DFY28ZZ
    Bladder DTY28ZZ
    Bone, Other DPYC8ZZ
    Bone Marrow D7Y08ZZ
    Brain D0Y08ZZ
    Brain Stem D0Y18ZZ
    Breast
      Left DMY08ZZ
      Right DMY18ZZ
    Bronchus DBY18ZZ
    Cervix DUY18ZZ
    Chest DWY28ZZ
    Chest Wall DBY78ZZ
    Colon DDY58ZZ
    Diaphragm DBY88ZZ
    Duodenum DDY28ZZ
    Ear D9Y08ZZ
    Esophagus DDY08ZZ
    Eye D8Y08ZZ
    Femur DPY98ZZ
    Fibula DPYB8ZZ
    Gallbladder DFY18ZZ
    Gland
      Adrenal DGY28ZZ
      Parathyroid DGY48ZZ
      Pituitary DGY08ZZ
      Thyroid DGY58ZZ
    Glands, Salivary D9Y68ZZ
    Head and Neck DWY18ZZ
    Hemibody DWY48ZZ
    Humerus DPY68ZZ
    Hypopharynx D9Y38ZZ
    Ileum DDY48ZZ
    Jejunum DDY38ZZ
    Kidney DTY08ZZ
    Larynx D9YB8ZZ
    Liver DFY08ZZ
    Lung DBY28ZZ
    Lymphatics
      Abdomen D7Y68ZZ
      Axillary D7Y48ZZ
      Inguinal D7Y88ZZ
      Neck D7Y38ZZ
      Pelvis D7Y78ZZ
      Thorax D7Y58ZZ
    Mandible DPY38ZZ
    Maxilla DPY28ZZ
    Mediastinum DBY68ZZ
    Mouth D9Y48ZZ

Hyperthermia *(Continued)*
    Radiation Therapy *(Continued)*
        Nasopharynx D9YD8ZZ
        Neck and Head DWY18ZZ
        Nerve, Peripheral D0Y78ZZ
        Nose D9Y18ZZ
        Oropharynx D9YF8ZZ
        Ovary DUY08ZZ
        Palate
            Hard D9Y88ZZ
            Soft D9Y98ZZ
        Pancreas DFY38ZZ
        Parathyroid Gland DGY48ZZ
        Pelvic Bones DPY88ZZ
        Pelvic Region DWY68ZZ
        Pineal Body DGY18ZZ
        Pituitary Gland DGY08ZZ
        Pleura DBY58ZZ
        Prostate DVY08ZZ
        Radius DPY78ZZ
        Rectum DDY78ZZ
        Rib DPY58ZZ
        Sinuses D9Y78ZZ
        Skin
            Abdomen DHY88ZZ
            Arm DHY48ZZ
            Back DHY78ZZ
            Buttock DHY98ZZ
            Chest DHY68ZZ
            Face DHY28ZZ

Hyperthermia *(Continued)*
    Radiation Therapy *(Continued)*
        Skin *(Continued)*
            Leg DHYB8ZZ
            Neck DHY38ZZ
        Skull DPY08ZZ
        Spinal Cord D0Y68ZZ
        Spleen D7Y28ZZ
        Sternum DPY48ZZ
        Stomach DDY18ZZ
        Testis DVY18ZZ
        Thymus D7Y18ZZ
        Thyroid Gland DGY58ZZ
        Tibia DPYB8ZZ
        Tongue D9Y58ZZ
        Trachea DBY08ZZ
        Ulna DPY78ZZ
        Ureter DTY18ZZ
        Urethra DTY38ZZ
        Uterus DUY28ZZ
        Whole Body DWY58ZZ
    Whole Body 6A3Z
Hypnosis GZFZZZZ
Hypogastric artery
    use Internal Iliac Artery, Right
    use Internal Iliac Artery, Left
Hypopharynx *use* Pharynx
Hypophysectomy
    see Excision, Gland, Pituitary 0GB0
    see Resection, Gland, Pituitary 0GT0

Hypophysis *use* Gland, Pituitary
Hypothalamotomy *see* Destruction, Thalamus 0059
Hypothenar muscle
    use Hand Muscle, Right
    use Hand Muscle, Left
Hypothermia, Whole Body 6A4Z
Hysterectomy
    ⮕Supracervical *see* Resection, Uterus 0UT9
    ⮕Total *see* Resection, Uterus 0UT9
Hysterolysis *see* Release, Uterus 0UN9
Hysteropexy
    see Repair, Uterus 0UQ9
    see Reposition, Uterus 0US9
Hysteroplasty
    see Repair, Uterus 0UQ9
Hysterorrhaphy *see* Repair, Uterus 0UQ9
Hysteroscopy 0UJD8ZZ
Hysterotomy
    see Drainage, Uterus 0U99
Hysterotrachelectomy
    see Resection, Uterus 0UT9
    see Resection, Cervix 0UTC
Hysterotracheloplasty
    see Repair, Uterus 0UQ9
Hysterotrachelorrhaphy *see* Repair, Uterus 0UQ9

▶ New   ⮕ Revised   ~~deleted~~ Deleted

I

IABP (Intra-aortic balloon pump) *see* Assistance, Cardiac 5A02
IAEMT (Intraoperative anesthetic effect monitoring and titration) *see* Monitoring, Central Nervous 4A10
Idarucizumab, Dabigatran Reversal Agent XW0
IHD (Intermittent hemodialysis) 5A1D70Z
Ileal artery *use* Superior Mesenteric Artery
Ileectomy
  see Excision, Ileum 0DBB
  see Resection, Ileum 0DTB
Ileocolic artery *use* Superior Mesenteric Artery
Ileocolic vein *use* Colic Vein
Ileopexy
  see Repair, Ileum 0DQB
  see Reposition, Ileum 0DSB
Ileorrhaphy *see* Repair, Ileum 0DQB
Ileoscopy 0DJD8ZZ
Ileostomy
  see Bypass, Ileum 0D1B
  see Drainage, Ileum 0D9B
Ileotomy *see* Drainage, Ileum 0D9B
Ileoureterostomy *see* Bypass, Bladder 0T1B
Iliac crest
  use Pelvic Bone, Right
  use Pelvic Bone, Left
Iliac fascia
  use Subcutaneous Tissue and Fascia, Right Upper Leg
  use Subcutaneous Tissue and Fascia, Left Upper Leg
Iliac lymph node *use* Lymphatic, Pelvis
Iliacus muscle
  use Hip Muscle, Right
  use Hip Muscle, Left
Iliofemoral ligament
  use Hip Bursa and Ligament, Right
  use Hip Bursa and Ligament, Left
Iliohypogastric nerve *use* Lumbar Plexus
Ilioinguinal nerve *use* Lumbar Plexus
Iliolumbar artery
  use Internal Iliac Artery, Right
  use Internal Iliac Artery, Left
Iliolumbar ligament *use* Lower Spine Bursa and Ligament
Iliotibial tract (band)
  use Subcutaneous Tissue and Fascia, Right Upper Leg
  use Subcutaneous Tissue and Fascia, Left Upper Leg
Ilium
  use Pelvic Bone, Right
  use Pelvic Bone, Left
Ilizarov external fixator
  use External Fixation Device, Ring in 0PH
  use External Fixation Device, Ring in 0PS
  use External Fixation Device, Ring in 0QH
  use External Fixation Device, Ring in 0QS
Ilizarov-Vecklich device
  use External Fixation Device, Limb Lengthening in 0PH
  use External Fixation Device, Limb Lengthening in 0QH
Imaging, diagnostic
  see Plain Radiography
  see Fluoroscopy
  see Computerized Tomography (CT Scan)
  see Magnetic Resonance Imaging (MRI)
  see Ultrasonography
Immobilization
  Abdominal Wall 2W33X
  Arm
    Lower
      Left 2W3DX
      Right 2W3CX
    Upper
      Left 2W3BX
      Right 2W3AX

Immobilization *(Continued)*
  Back 2W35X
  Chest Wall 2W34X
  Extremity
    Lower
      Left 2W3MX
      Right 2W3LX
    Upper
      Left 2W39X
      Right 2W38X
  Face 2W31X
  Finger
    Left 2W3KX
    Right 2W3JX
  Foot
    Left 2W3TX
    Right 2W3SX
  Hand
    Left 2W3FX
    Right 2W3EX
  Head 2W30X
  Inguinal Region
    Left 2W37X
    Right 2W36X
  Leg
    Lower
      Left 2W3RX
      Right 2W3QX
    Upper
      Left 2W3PX
      Right 2W3NX
  Neck 2W32X
  Thumb
    Left 2W3HX
    Right 2W3GX
  Toe
    Left 2W3VX
    Right 2W3UX
Immunization *see* Introduction of Serum, Toxoid, and Vaccine
Immunotherapy *see* Introduction of Immunotherapeutic Substance
Immunotherapy, antineoplastic
  Interferon *see* Introduction of Low-dose Interleukin-2
  Interleukin-2 of high-dose *see* Introduction, High-dose Interleukin-2
  Interleukin-2, low-dose *see* Introduction of Low-dose Interleukin-2
  Monoclonal antibody *see* Introduction of Monoclonal Antibody
  Proleukin, high-dose *see* Introduction of High-dose Interleukin-2
  Proleukin, low-dose *see* Introduction of Low-dose Interleukin-2
Impella® heart pump *use* Short-term External Heart Assist System in Heart and Great Vessels
Impeller Pump
  Continuous, Output 5A0221D
  Intermittent, Output 5A0211D
Implantable cardioverter-defibrillator (ICD) *use* Defibrillator Generator in 0JH
Implantable drug infusion pump (anti-spasmodic) (chemotherapy) (pain) *use* Infusion Device, Pump in Subcutaneous Tissue and Fascia
Implantable glucose monitoring device *use* Monitoring Device
Implantable hemodynamic monitor (IHM) *use* Monitoring Device, Hemodynamic in 0JH
Implantable hemodynamic monitoring system (IHMS) *use* Monitoring Device, Hemodynamic in 0JH
Implantable Miniature Telescope™ (IMT) use Synthetic Substitute, Intraocular Telescope in 08R
Implantation
  see Replacement
  see Insertion

Implanted (venous) (access) port *use* Vascular Access Device, Totally Implantable in Subcutaneous Tissue and Fascia
IMV (intermittent mandatory ventilation) *see* Assistance, Respiratory 5A09
In Vitro Fertilization 8E0ZXY1
Incision, abscess *see* Drainage
Incudectomy
  see Excision, Ear, Nose, Sinus 09B
  see Resection, Ear, Nose, Sinus 09T
Incudopexy
  see Repair, Ear, Nose, Sinus 09Q
  see Reposition, Ear, Nose, Sinus 09S
Incus
  use Ossicle, Auditory, Right
  use Ossicle, Auditory, Left
Induction of labor
  Artificial rupture of membranes *see* Drainage, Pregnancy 109
  Oxytocin *see* Introduction of Hormone
InDura, intrathecal catheter (1P) (spinal) *use* Infusion Device
Inferior cardiac nerve *use* Thoracic Sympathetic Nerve
Inferior cerebellar vein *use* Intracranial Vein
Inferior cerebral vein *use* Intracranial Vein
Inferior epigastric artery
  use External Iliac Artery, Right
  use External Iliac Artery, Left
Inferior epigastric lymph node *use* Lymphatic, Pelvis
Inferior genicular artery
  use Popliteal Artery, Right
  use Popliteal Artery, Left
Inferior gluteal artery
  use Internal Iliac Artery, Right
  use Internal Iliac Artery, Left
Inferior gluteal nerve *use* Sacral Plexus Nerve
Inferior hypogastric plexus *use* Abdominal Sympathetic Nerve
Inferior labial artery *use* Face Artery
Inferior longitudinal muscle *use* Tongue, Palate, Pharynx Muscle
Inferior mesenteric ganglion *use* Abdominal Sympathetic Nerve
Inferior mesenteric lymph node *use* Mesenteric Lymphatic
Inferior mesenteric plexus *use* Abdominal Sympathetic Nerve
Inferior oblique muscle
  use Extraocular Muscle, Right
  use Extraocular Muscle, Left
Inferior pancreaticoduodenal artery *use* Superior Mesenteric Artery
Inferior phrenic artery *use* Abdominal Aorta
Inferior rectus muscle
  use Extraocular Muscle, Right
  use Extraocular Muscle, Left
Inferior suprarenal artery
  use Renal Artery, Right
  use Renal Artery, Left
Inferior tarsal plate
  use Lower Eyelid, Right
  use Lower Eyelid, Left
Inferior thyroid vein
  use Innominate Vein, Right
  use Innominate Vein, Left
Inferior tibiofibular joint
  use Ankle Joint, Right
  use Ankle Joint, Left
Inferior turbinate *use* Nasal Turbinate
Inferior ulnar collateral artery
  use Brachial Artery, Right
  use Brachial Artery, Left
Inferior vesical artery
  use Internal Iliac Artery, Right
  use Internal Iliac Artery, Left
Infraauricular lymph node *use* Lymphatic, Head
Infraclavicular (deltopectoral) lymph node
  use Lymphatic, Right Upper Extremity
  use Lymphatic, Left Upper Extremity

▶ New   ⇒ Revised   ~~deleted~~ Deleted

Infrahyoid muscle
　use Neck Muscle, Right
　use Neck Muscle, Left
Infraparotid lymph node *use* Lymphatic, Head
Infraspinatus fascia
　use Subcutaneous Tissue and Fascia, Right
　　Upper Arm
　use Subcutaneous Tissue and Fascia, Left
　　Upper Arm
Infraspinatus muscle
　use Shoulder Muscle, Right
　use Shoulder Muscle, Left
Infundibulopelvic ligament *use* Uterine
　　Supporting Structure
Infusion *see* Introduction of substance in or on
Infusion Device, Pump
　Insertion of device in
　　Abdomen 0JH8
　　Back 0JH7
　　Chest 0JH6
　　Lower Arm
　　　Left 0JHH
　　　Right 0JHG
　　Lower Leg
　　　Left 0JHP
　　　Right 0JHN
　　Trunk 0JHT
　　Upper Arm
　　　Left 0JHF
　　　Right 0JHD
　　Upper Leg
　　　Left 0JHM
　　　Right 0JHL
　Removal of device from
　　Lower Extremity 0JPW
　　Trunk 0JPT
　　Upper Extremity 0JPV
　Revision of device in
　　Lower Extremity 0JWW
　　Trunk 0JWT
　　Upper Extremity 0JWV
Infusion, glucarpidase
　Central vein 3E043GQ
　Peripheral vein 3E033GQ
Inguinal canal
　use Inguinal Region, Right
　use Inguinal Region, Left
　use Inguinal Region, Bilateral
Inguinal triangle
　see Inguinal Region, Right
　see Inguinal Region, Left
　see Inguinal Region, Bilateral
Injection *see* Introduction of substance in or on
Injection reservoir, port *use* Vascular Access
　　Device, Reservoir in Subcutaneous Tissue
　　and Fascia
Injection reservoir, pump *use* Infusion Device,
　　Pump in Subcutaneous Tissue and Fascia
Injection, Concentrated Bone Marrow Aspirate
　　(CBMA), intramuscular XK02303
Insemination, artificial 3E0P7LZ
Insertion
　Antimicrobial envelope *see* Introduction of
　　Anti-infective
　Aqueous drainage shunt
　　see Bypass, Eye 081
　　see Drainage, Eye 089
　Products of Conception 10H0
　Spinal Stabilization Device
　　see Insertion of device in, Upper Joints 0RH
　　see Insertion of device in, Lower Joints 0SH
Insertion of device in
　Abdominal Wall 0WHF
　Acetabulum
　　Left 0QH5
　　Right 0QH4
　Anal Sphincter 0DHR
　Ankle Region
　　Left 0YHL
　　Right 0YHK
　Anus 0DHQ

Insertion of device in (*Continued*)
　Aorta
　　Abdominal 04H0
　　Thoracic
　　　Ascending/Arch 02HX
　　　Descending 02HW
　Arm
　　Lower
　　　Left 0XHF
　　　Right 0XHD
　　Upper
　　　Left 0XH9
　　　Right 0XH8
　Artery
　　Anterior Tibial
　　　Left 04HQ
　　　Right 04HP
　　Axillary
　　　Left 03H6
　　　Right 03H5
　　Brachial
　　　Left 03H8
　　　Right 03H7
　　Celiac 04H1
　　Colic
　　　Left 04H7
　　　Middle 04H8
　　　Right 04H6
　　Common Carotid
　　　Left 03HJ
　　　Right 03HH
　　Common Iliac
　　　Left 04HD
　　　Right 04HC
　　External Carotid
　　　Left 03HN
　　　Right 03HM
　　External Iliac
　　　Left 04HJ
　　　Right 04HH
　　Face 03HR
　　Femoral
　　　Left 04HL
　　　Right 04HK
　　Foot
　　　Left 04HW
　　　Right 04HV
　　Gastric 04H2
　　Hand
　　　Left 03HF
　　　Right 03HD
　　Hepatic 04H3
　　Inferior Mesenteric 04HB
　　Innominate 03H2
　　Internal Carotid
　　　Left 03HL
　　　Right 03HK
　　Internal Iliac
　　　Left 04HF
　　　Right 04HE
　　Internal Mammary
　　　Left 03H1
　　　Right 03H0
　　Intracranial 03HG
　　Lower 04HY
　　Peroneal
　　　Left 04HU
　　　Right 04HT
　　Popliteal
　　　Left 04HN
　　　Right 04HM
　　Posterior Tibial
　　　Left 04HS
　　　Right 04HR
　　Pulmonary
　　　Left 02HR
　　　Right 02HQ
　　Pulmonary Trunk 02HP
　　Radial
　　　Left 03HC
　　　Right 03HB

Insertion of device in (*Continued*)
　Artery (*Continued*)
　　Renal
　　　Left 04HA
　　　Right 04H9
　　Splenic 04H4
　　Subclavian
　　　Left 03H4
　　　Right 03H3
　　Superior Mesenteric 04H5
　　Temporal
　　　Left 03HT
　　　Right 03HS
　　Thyroid
　　　Left 03HV
　　　Right 03HU
　　Ulnar
　　　Left 03HA
　　　Right 03H9
　　Upper 03HY
　　Vertebral
　　　Left 03HQ
　　　Right 03HP
　Atrium
　　Left 02H7
　　Right 02H6
　Axilla
　　Left 0XH5
　　Right 0XH4
　Back
　　Lower 0WHL
　　Upper 0WHK
　Bladder 0THB
　Bladder Neck 0THC
　Bone
　　Ethmoid
　　　Left 0NHG
　　　Right 0NHF
　　Facial 0NHW
　　Frontal 0NH1
　　Hyoid 0NHX
　　Lacrimal
　　　Left 0NHJ
　　　Right 0NHH
　　Lower 0QHY
　　Nasal 0NHB
　　Occipital 0NH7
　　Palatine
　　　Left 0NHL
　　　Right 0NHK
　　Parietal
　　　Left 0NH4
　　　Right 0NH3
　　Pelvic
　　　Left 0QH3
　　　Right 0QH2
　　Sphenoid 0NHC
　　Temporal
　　　Left 0NH6
　　　Right 0NH5
　　Upper 0PHY
　　Zygomatic
　　　Left 0NHN
　　　Right 0NHM
　Brain 00H0
　Breast
　　Bilateral 0HHV
　　Left 0HHU
　　Right 0HHT
　Bronchus
　　Lingula 0BH9
　　Lower Lobe
　　　Left 0BHB
　　　Right 0BH6
　　Main
　　　Left 0BH7
　　　Right 0BH3
　　Middle Lobe, Right 0BH5
　　Upper Lobe
　　　Left 0BH8
　　　Right 0BH4

▶ New　⇒ Revised　~~deleted~~ Deleted

▶ New   ⇒ Revised   ~~deleted~~ Deleted

Inspection *(Continued)*
Epididymis and Spermatic Cord 0VJM
Extremity
Lower
Left 0YJB
Right 0YJ9
Upper
Left 0XJ7
Right 0XJ6
Eye
Left 08J1XZZ
Right 08J0XZZ
Face 0WJ2
Fallopian Tube 0UJ8
Femoral Region
Bilateral 0YJE
Left 0YJ8
Right 0YJ7
Finger Nail 0HJQXZZ
Foot
Left 0YJN
Right 0YJM
Gallbladder 0FJ4
Gastrointestinal Tract 0WJP
Genitourinary Tract 0WJR
Gland
Adrenal 0GJ5
Endocrine 0GJS
Pituitary 0GJ0
Salivary 0CJA
Great Vessel 02JY
Hand
Left 0XJK
Right 0XJJ
Head 0WJ0
Heart 02JA
Inguinal Region
Bilateral 0YJA
Left 0YJ6
Right 0YJ5
Intestinal Tract
Lower 0DJD
Upper 0DJ0
Jaw
Lower 0WJ5
Upper 0WJ4
Joint
Acromioclavicular
Left 0RJH
Right 0RJG
Ankle
Left 0SJG
Right 0SJF
Carpal
Left 0RJR
Right 0RJQ
Carpometacarpal
Left 0RJT
Right 0RJS
Cervical Vertebral 0RJ1
Cervicothoracic Vertebral 0RJ4
Coccygeal 0SJ6
Elbow
Left 0RJM
Right 0RJL
Finger Phalangeal
Left 0RJX
Right 0RJW
Hip
Left 0SJB
Right 0SJ9
Knee
Left 0SJD
Right 0SJC
Lumbar Vertebral 0SJ0
Lumbosacral 0SJ3
Metacarpophalangeal
Left 0RJV
Right 0RJU
Metatarsal-Phalangeal
Left 0SJN
Right 0SJM

Inspection *(Continued)*
Joint *(Continued)*
Occipital-cervical 0RJ0
Sacrococcygeal 0SJ5
Sacroiliac
Left 0SJ8
Right 0SJ7
Shoulder
Left 0RJK
Right 0RJJ
Sternoclavicular
Left 0RJF
Right 0RJE
Tarsal
Left 0SJJ
Right 0SJH
Tarsometatarsal
Left 0SJL
Right 0SJK
Temporomandibular
Left 0RJD
Right 0RJC
Thoracic Vertebral 0RJ6
Thoracolumbar Vertebral 0RJA
Toe Phalangeal
Left 0SJQ
Right 0SJP
Wrist
Left 0RJP
Right 0RJN
Kidney 0TJ5
Knee Region
Left 0YJG
Right 0YJF
Larynx 0CJS
Leg
Lower
Left 0YJJ
Right 0YJH
Upper
Left 0YJD
Right 0YJC
Lens
Left 08JKXZZ
Right 08JJXZZ
Liver 0FJ0
Lung
Left 0BJL
Right 0BJK
Lymphatic 07JN
Thoracic Duct 07JK
Mediastinum 0WJC
Mesentery 0DJV
Mouth and Throat 0CJY
Muscle
Extraocular
Left 08JM
Right 08JL
Lower 0KJY
Upper 0KJX
Nasal Mucosa and Soft Tissue
09JK
Neck 0WJ6
Nerve
Cranial 00JE
Peripheral 01JY
Omentum 0DJU
Oral Cavity and Throat 0WJ3
Ovary 0UJ3
Pancreas 0FJG
Parathyroid Gland 0GJR
Pelvic Cavity 0WJD
Penis 0VJS
Pericardial Cavity 0WJD
Perineum
Female 0WJN
Male 0WJM
Peritoneal Cavity 0WJG
Peritoneum 0DJW
Pineal Body 0GJ1
Pleura 0BJQ

Inspection *(Continued)*
Pleural Cavity
Left 0WJB
Right 0WJ9
Products of Conception 10J0
Ectopic 10J2
Retained 10J1
Prostate and Seminal Vesicles 0VJ4
Respiratory Tract 0WJQ
Retroperitoneum 0WJH
Scrotum and Tunica Vaginalis 0VJ8
Shoulder Region
Left 0XJ3
Right 0XJ2
Sinus 09JY
Skin 0HJPXZZ
Skull 0NJ0
Spinal Canal 00JU
Spinal Cord 00JV
Spleen 07JP
Stomach 0DJ6
Subcutaneous Tissue and Fascia
Head and Neck 0JJS
Lower Extremity 0JJW
Trunk 0JJT
Upper Extremity 0JJV
Tendon
Lower 0LJY
Upper 0LJX
Testis 0VJD
Thymus 07JM
Thyroid Gland 0GJK
Toe Nail 0HJRXZZ
Trachea 0BJ1
Tracheobronchial Tree 0BJ0
Tympanic Membrane
Left 09J8
Right 09J7
Ureter 0TJ9
Urethra 0TJD
Uterus and Cervix 0UJD
Vagina and Cul-de-sac 0UJH
Vas Deferens 0VJR
Vein
Lower 06JY
Upper 05JY
Vulva 0UJM
Wall
Abdominal 0WJF
Chest 0WJ8
Wrist Region
Left 0XJH
Right 0XJG
Instillation *see* Introduction of substance in or on
Insufflation *see* Introduction of substance in or on
Interatrial septum *use* Atrial Septum
Interbody fusion (spine) cage
use Interbody Fusion Device in Upper Joints
use Interbody Fusion Device in Lower Joints
Interbody Fusion Device
Nanotextured Surface
Cervical Vertebral XRG1092
2 or more XRG2092
Cervicothoracic Vertebral XRG4092
Lumbar Vertebral XRGB092
2 or more XRGC092
Lumbosacral XRGD092
Occipital-cervical XRG0092
Thoracic Vertebral XRG6092
2 to 7 XRG7092
8 or more XRG8092
Thoracolumbar Vertebral XRGA092
Radiolucent Porous
Cervical Vertebral XRG10F3
2 or more XRG20F3
Cervicothoracic Vertebral XRG40F3
Lumbar Vertebral XRGB0F3
2 or more XRGC0F3
Lumbosacral XRGD0F3

▶ New　⇒ Revised　~~deleted~~ Deleted

▶ New ⇒ Revised ~~deleted~~ Deleted

▶ New   ⇒ Revised   ~~deleted~~ Deleted

▶ New ⇒ Revised ~~deleted~~ Deleted

Introduction of substance in or on (Continued)
  Spinal Canal 3E0R3GC
    Analgesics 3E0R3NZ
    Anesthetic Agent 3E0R3BZ
    Anti-infective 3E0R32
    Anti-inflammatory 3E0R33Z
    Antineoplastic 3E0R30
    Destructive Agent 3E0R3TZ
    Diagnostic Substance, Other 3E0R3KZ
    Electrolytic Substance 3E0R37Z
    Gas 3E0R
    Hypnotics 3E0R3NZ
    Nutritional Substance 3E0R36Z
    Radioactive Substance 3E0R3HZ
    Sedatives 3E0R3NZ
    Stem Cells
      Embryonic 3E0R
      Somatic 3E0R
    Water Balance Substance 3E0R37Z
  Subcutaneous Tissue 3E013GC
    Analgesics 3E013NZ
    Anesthetic Agent 3E013BZ
    Anti-infective 3E01
    Anti-inflammatory 3E0133Z
    Antineoplastic 3E0130
    Destructive Agent 3E013TZ
    Diagnostic Substance, Other 3E013KZ
    Electrolytic Substance 3E0137Z
    Hormone 3E013V
    Hypnotics 3E013NZ
    Nutritional Substance 3E0136Z
    Radioactive Substance 3E013HZ
    Sedatives 3E013NZ
    Serum 3E0134Z
    Toxoid 3E0134Z
    Vaccine 3E0134Z
    Water Balance Substance 3E0137Z
  Vein
    Central 3E04
      Analgesics 3E04
      Anesthetic, Intracirculatory 3E04
      Anti-infective 3E04
      Anti-inflammatory 3E04
      Antiarrhythmic 3E04
      Antineoplastic 3E04
      Destructive Agent 3E04
      Diagnostic Substance, Other 3E04
      Electrolytic Substance 3E04
      Hormone 3E04
      Hypnotics 3E04
      Immunotherapeutic 3E04
      Nutritional Substance 3E04

Introduction of substance in or on (Continued)
  Vein (Continued)
    Central (Continued)
      Platelet Inhibitor 3E04
      Radioactive Substance 3E04
      Sedatives 3E04
      Serum 3E04
      Thrombolytic 3E04
      Toxoid 3E04
      Vaccine 3E04
      Vasopressor 3E04
      Water Balance Substance 3E04
    Peripheral 3E03
      Analgesics 3E03
      Anesthetic, Intracirculatory 3E03
      Anti-infective 3E03
      Anti-inflammatory 3E03
      Antiarrhythmic 3E03
      Antineoplastic 3E03
      Destructive Agent 3E03
      Diagnostic Substance, Other 3E03
      Electrolytic Substance 3E03
      Hormone 3E03
      Hypnotics 3E03
      Immunotherapeutic 3E03
      Islet Cells, Pancreatic 3E03
      Nutritional Substance 3E03
      Platelet Inhibitor 3E03
      Radioactive Substance 3E03
      Sedatives 3E03
      Serum 3E03
      Thrombolytic 3E03
      Toxoid 3E03
      Vaccine 3E03
      Vasopressor 3E03
      Water Balance Substance 3E03
Intubation
  Airway
    see Insertion of device in, Trachea 0BH1
    see Insertion of device in, Mouth and
      Throat 0CHY
    see Insertion of device in, Esophagus
      0DH5
  Drainage device see Drainage
  Feeding Device see Insertion of device in,
    Gastrointestinal System 0DH
INTUITY Elite valve system, EDWARDS
  use Zooplastic Tissue, Rapid Deployment
    Technique in New Technology
IPPB (intermittent positive pressure
  breathing) see Assistance, Respiratory
  5A09

Iridectomy
  see Excision, Eye 08B
  see Resection, Eye 08T
Iridoplasty
  see Repair, Eye 08Q
  see Replacement, Eye 08R
  see Supplement, Eye 08U
Iridotomy see Drainage, Eye 089
Irrigation
  Biliary Tract, Irrigating Substance 3E1J
  Brain, Irrigating Substance 3E1Q38Z
  Cranial Cavity, Irrigating Substance 3E1Q38Z
  Ear, Irrigating Substance 3E1B
  Epidural Space, Irrigating Substance 3E1S38Z
  Eye, Irrigating Substance 3E1C
  Gastrointestinal Tract
    Lower, Irrigating Substance 3E1H
    Upper, Irrigating Substance 3E1G
  Genitourinary Tract, Irrigating Substance
    3E1K
  Irrigating Substance 3C1ZX8Z
  Joint, Irrigating Substance 3E1U38Z
  Mucous Membrane, Irrigating Substance
    3E10
  Nose, Irrigating Substance 3E19
  Pancreatic Tract, Irrigating Substance 3E1J
  Pericardial Cavity, Irrigating Substance
    3E1Y38Z
  Peritoneal Cavity
    Dialysate 3E1M39Z
    Irrigating Substance 3E1M38Z
  Pleural Cavity, Irrigating Substance 3E1L38Z
  Reproductive
    Female, Irrigating Substance 3E1P
    Male, Irrigating Substance 3E1N
  Respiratory Tract, Irrigating Substance 3E1F
  Skin, Irrigating Substance 3E10
  Spinal Canal, Irrigating Substance 3E1R38Z
Isavuconazole Anti-infective XW0
Ischiatic nerve use Sciatic Nerve
Ischiocavernosus muscle use Perineum Muscle
Ischiofemoral ligament
  use Hip Bursa and Ligament, Right
  use Hip Bursa and Ligament, Left
Ischium
  use Pelvic Bone, Right
  use Pelvic Bone, Left
Isolation 8E0ZXY6
Isotope Administration, Whole Body
  DWY5G
Itrel (3) (4) neurostimulator use Stimulator
  Generator, Single Array in 0JH

J

Jejunal artery *use* Superior Mesenteric Artery
Jejunectomy
  see Excision, Jejunum ØDBA
  see Resection, Jejunum ØDTA
Jejunocolostomy
  see Bypass, Gastrointestinal System ØD1
  see Drainage, Gastrointestinal System ØD9
Jejunopexy
  see Repair, Jejunum ØDQA
  see Reposition, Jejunum ØDSA
Jejunostomy
  see Bypass, Jejunum ØD1A
  see Drainage, Jejunum ØD9A
Jejunotomy *see* Drainage, Jejunum ØD9A
Joint fixation plate
  use Internal Fixation Device in Upper Joints
  use Internal Fixation Device in Lower Joints
Joint liner (insert) *use* Liner in Lower Joints
Joint spacer (antibiotic)
  use Spacer in Upper Joints
  use Spacer in Lower Joints
Jugular body *use* Glomus Jugulare
Jugular lymph node
  use Lymphatic, Right Neck
  use Lymphatic, Left Neck

K

Kappa *use* Pacemaker, Dual Chamber in ØJH
Kcentra *use* 4-Factor Prothrombin Complex
  Concentrate
Keratectomy, kerectomy
  see Excision, Eye Ø8B
  see Resection, Eye Ø8T
Keratocentesis *see* Drainage, Eye Ø89
Keratoplasty
  see Repair, Eye Ø8Q
  see Replacement, Eye Ø8R
  see Supplement, Eye Ø8U
Keratotomy
  see Drainage, Eye Ø89
  see Repair, Eye Ø8Q
Kirschner wire (K-wire)
  use Internal Fixation Device in Head and
    Facial Bones
  use Internal Fixation Device in Upper Bones
  use Internal Fixation Device in Lower Bones
  use Internal Fixation Device in Upper Joints
  use Internal Fixation Device in Lower Joints
Knee (implant) insert *use* Liner in Lower Joints
KUB x-ray *see* Plain Radiography, Kidney,
  Ureter and Bladder BTØ4
Kuntscher nail
  use Internal Fixation Device, Intramedullary
    in Upper Bones
  use Internal Fixation Device, Intramedullary
    in Lower Bones
▶KYMRIAH *use* Engineered Autologous
  Chimeric Antigen Receptor T-cell
  Immunotherapy

L

Labia majora *use* Vulva
Labia minora *use* Vulva
Labial gland
  use Upper Lip
  use Lower Lip
Labiectomy
  see Excision, Female Reproductive System
    ØUB
  see Resection, Female Reproductive System
    ØUT
Lacrimal canaliculus
  use Lacrimal Duct, Right
  use Lacrimal Duct, Left
Lacrimal punctum
  use Lacrimal Duct, Right
  use Lacrimal Duct, Left

Lacrimal sac
  use Lacrimal Duct, Right
  use Lacrimal Duct, Left
LAGB (laparoscopic adjustable gastric
  banding)
  Initial procedure ØDV64CZ
▶Surgical correction *use* Revision of device in,
  Stomach ØDW6
Laminectomy
  see Release, Central Nervous System and
    Cranial Nerves ØØN
  see Release, Peripheral Nervous System Ø1N
  see Excision, Upper Bones ØPB
  see Excision, Lower Bones ØQB
Laminotomy
  see Release, Central Nervous System ØØN
  see Release, Peripheral Nervous System
    Ø1N
  see Drainage, Upper Bones ØP9
  see Excision, Upper Bones ØPB
  see Release, Upper Bones ØPN
  see Drainage, Lower Bones ØQ9
  see Excision, Lower Bones ØQB
  see Release, Lower Bones ØQN
LAP-BAND® adjustable gastric banding
  system *use* Extraluminal Device
Laparoscopic-assisted transanal pull-through
  see Excision, Gastrointestinal System ØDB
  see Resection, Gastrointestinal System ØDT
Laparoscopy *see* Inspection
Laparotomy
  Drainage *see* Drainage, Peritoneal Cavity
    ØW9G
  Exploratory *see* Inspection, Peritoneal *use*
    Nerve, Lumbar Plexus ØWJG
Laryngectomy
  see Excision, Larynx ØCBS
  see Resection, Larynx ØCTS
Laryngocentesis *see* Drainage, Larynx ØC9S
Laryngogram *see* Fluoroscopy, Larynx B91J
Laryngopexy
  see Repair, Larynx ØCQS
Laryngopharynx *use* Pharynx
Laryngoplasty
  see Repair, Larynx ØCQS
  see Replacement, Larynx ØCRS
  see Supplement, Larynx ØCUS
Laryngorrhaphy *see* Repair, Larynx ØCQS
Laryngoscopy ØCJS8ZZ
Laryngotomy *see* Drainage, Larynx ØC9S
Laser Interstitial Thermal Therapy
  Adrenal Gland DGY2KZZ
  Anus DDY8KZZ
  Bile Ducts DFY2KZZ
  Brain DØY0KZZ
  Brain Stem DØY1KZZ
  Breast
    Left DMY0KZZ
    Right DMY1KZZ
  Bronchus DBY1KZZ
  Chest Wall DBY7KZZ
  Colon DDY5KZZ
  Diaphragm DBY8KZZ
  Duodenum DDY2KZZ
  Esophagus DDY0KZZ
  Gallbladder DFY1KZZ
  Gland
    Adrenal DGY2KZZ
    Parathyroid DGY4KZZ
    Pituitary DGY0KZZ
    Thyroid DGY5KZZ
  Ileum DDY4KZZ
  Jejunum DDY3KZZ
  Liver DFY0KZZ
  Lung DBY2KZZ
  Mediastinum DBY6KZZ
  Nerve, Peripheral DØY7KZZ
  Pancreas DFY3KZZ
  Parathyroid Gland DGY4KZZ
  Pineal Body DGY1KZZ
  Pituitary Gland DGY0KZZ

Laser Interstitial Thermal Therapy
  (Continued)
  Pleura DBY5KZZ
  Prostate DVY0KZZ
  Rectum DDY7KZZ
  Spinal Cord DØY6KZZ
  Stomach DDY1KZZ
  Thyroid Gland DGY5KZZ
  Trachea DBY0KZZ
Lateral (brachial) lymph node
  use Lymphatic, Right Axillary
  use Lymphatic, Left Axillary
Lateral canthus
  use Upper Eyelid, Right
  use Upper Eyelid, Left
Lateral collateral ligament (LCL)
  use Knee Bursa and Ligament, Right
  use Knee Bursa and Ligament, Left
Lateral condyle of femur
  use Lower Femur, Right
  use Lower Femur, Left
Lateral condyle of tibia
  use Tibia, Right
  use Tibia, Left
Lateral cuneiform bone
  use Tarsal, Right
  use Tarsal, Left
Lateral epicondyle of femur
  use Lower Femur, Right
  use Lower Femur, Left
Lateral epicondyle of humerus
  use Humeral Shaft, Right
  use Humeral Shaft, Left
Lateral femoral cutaneous nerve *use* Lumbar
  Plexus
Lateral malleolus
  use Fibula, Right
  use Fibula, Left
Lateral meniscus
  use Knee Joint, Right
  use Knee Joint, Left
Lateral nasal cartilage *use* Nasal Mucosa and
  Soft Tissue
Lateral plantar artery
  use Foot Artery, Right
  use Foot Artery, Left
Lateral plantar nerve *use* Tibial Nerve
Lateral rectus muscle
  use Extraocular Muscle, Right
  use Extraocular Muscle, Left
Lateral sacral artery
  use Internal Iliac Artery, Right
  use Internal Iliac Artery, Left
Lateral sacral vein
  use Hypogastric Vein, Right
  use Hypogastric Vein, Left
Lateral sural cutaneous nerve *use* Peroneal
  Nerve
Lateral tarsal artery
  use Foot Artery, Right
  use Foot Artery, Left
Lateral temporomandibular ligament *use* Head
  and Neck Bursa and Ligament
Lateral thoracic artery
  use Axillary Artery, Right
  use Axillary Artery, Left
Latissimus dorsi muscle
  use Trunk Muscle, Right
  use Trunk Muscle, Left
Latissimus Dorsi Myocutaneous Flap
  Replacement
    Bilateral ØHRV075
    Left ØHRU075
    Right ØHRT075
  Transfer
    Left ØKXG
    Right ØKXF
Lavage
  see Irrigation
▶Bronchial alveolar, diagnostic *see* Drainage,
  Respiratory System ØB9

▶ New   ▥ Revised   ~~deleted~~ Deleted

Least splanchnic nerve *use* Thoracic
  Sympathetic Nerve
Left ascending lumbar vein *use* Hemiazygos
  Vein
Left atrioventricular valve *use* Mitral Valve
Left auricular appendix *use* Atrium, Left
Left colic vein *use* Colic Vein
Left coronary sulcus *use* Heart, Left
Left gastric artery *use* Gastric Artery
Left gastroepiploic artery *use* Splenic Artery
Left gastroepiploic vein *use* Splenic Vein
Left inferior phrenic vein *use* Renal Vein, Left
Left inferior pulmonary vein *use* Pulmonary
  Vein, Left
Left jugular trunk *use* Thoracic Duct
Left lateral ventricle *use* Cerebral Ventricle
Left ovarian vein *use* Renal Vein, Left
Left second lumbar vein *use* Renal Vein, Left
Left subclavian trunk *use* Thoracic Duct
Left subcostal vein *use* Hemiazygos Vein
Left superior pulmonary vein *use* Pulmonary
  Vein, Left
Left suprarenal vein *use* Renal Vein, Left
Left testicular vein *use* Renal Vein, Left
Lengthening
  Bone, with device *see* Insertion of Limb
    Lengthening Device
  Muscle, by incision *see* Division, Muscles 0K8
  Tendon, by incision *see* Division, Tendons 0L8
Leptomeninges, intracranial *use* Cerebral
  Meninges
Leptomeninges, spinal *use* Spinal Meninges
Lesser alar cartilage *use* Nasal Mucosa and Soft
  Tissue
Lesser occipital nerve *use* Cervical Plexus
Lesser Omentum *use* Omentum
Lesser saphenous vein
  use Saphenous Vein, Right
  use Saphenous Vein, Left
Lesser splanchnic nerve *use* Thoracic
  Sympathetic Nerve
Lesser trochanter
  use Upper Femur, Right
  use Upper Femur, Left
Lesser tuberosity
  use Humeral Head, Right
  use Humeral Head, Left
Lesser wing *use* Sphenoid Bone
Leukopheresis, therapeutic *see* Pheresis,
  Circulatory 6A55
Levator anguli oris muscle *use* Facial Muscle
Levator ani muscle *use* Perineum Muscle
Levator labii superioris alaeque nasi muscle
  use Facial Muscle
Levator labii superioris muscle *use* Facial
  Muscle
Levator palpebrae superioris muscle
  use Upper Eyelid, Right
  use Upper Eyelid, Left
Levator scapulae muscle
  use Neck Muscle, Right
  use Neck Muscle, Left
Levator veli palatini muscle *use* Tongue, Palate,
  Pharynx Muscle
Levatores costarum muscle
  use Thorax Muscle, Right
  use Thorax Muscle, Left

LifeStent® (Flexstar) (XL) Vascular Stent
  System *use* Intraluminal Device
Ligament of head of fibula
  use Knee Bursa and Ligament, Right
  use Knee Bursa and Ligament, Left
Ligament of the lateral malleolus
  use Ankle Bursa and Ligament, Right
  use Ankle Bursa and Ligament, Left
▶Ligamentum flavum, cervical *use* Head and
  Neck Bursa and Ligament
▶Ligamentum flavum, lumbar *use* Lower Spine
  Bursa and Ligament
▶Ligamentum flavum, thoracic *use* Upper Spine
  Bursa and Ligament
~~Ligamentum flavum~~
Ligation *see* Occlusion
Ligation, hemorrhoid *see* Occlusion, Lower
  Veins, Hemorrhoidal Plexus
Light Therapy GZJZZZZ
Liner
  Removal of device from
    Hip
      Left 0SPB09Z
      Right 0SP909Z
    Knee
      Left 0SPD09Z
      Right 0SPC09Z
  Revision of device in
    Hip
      Left 0SWB09Z
      Right 0SW909Z
    Knee
      Left 0SWD09Z
      Right 0SWC09Z
  Supplement
    Hip
      Left 0SUB09Z
        Acetabular Surface 0SUE09Z
        Femoral Surface 0SUS09Z
      Right 0SU909Z
        Acetabular Surface 0SUA09Z
        Femoral Surface 0SUR09Z
    Knee
      Left 0SUD09
        Femoral Surface 0SUU09Z
        Tibial Surface 0SUW09Z
      Right 0SUC09
        Femoral Surface 0SUT09Z
        Tibial Surface 0SUV09Z
Lingual artery
  use Artery, External Carotid, Right
  use Artery, External Carotid, Left
Lingual tonsil *use* Pharynx
Lingulectomy, lung
  see Excision, Lung Lingula 0BBH
  see Resection, Lung Lingula 0BTH
Lithotripsy
  see Fragmentation
➠With removal of fragments *see*
  Extirpation
LITT (laser interstitial thermal therapy)
  see Laser Interstitial Thermal
  Therapy
LIVIAN™ CRT-D *use* Cardiac
  Resynchronization Defibrillator Pulse
  Generator in 0JH

Lobectomy
  see Excision, Central Nervous System and
    Cranial Nerves 00B
  see Excision, Respiratory System 0BB
  see Resection, Respiratory System 0BT
  see Excision, Hepatobiliary System and
    Pancreas 0FB
  see Resection, Hepatobiliary System and
    Pancreas 0FT
  see Excision, Endocrine System 0GB
  see Resection, Endocrine System 0GT
Lobotomy *see* Division, Brain 0080
Localization
  see Map
  see Imaging
Locus ceruleus *use* Pons
Long thoracic nerve *use* Brachial Plexus
Loop ileostomy *see* Bypass, Ileum 0D1B
Loop recorder, implantable *use* Monitoring
  Device
Lower GI series *see* Fluoroscopy, Colon
  BD14
Lumbar artery *use* Abdominal Aorta
Lumbar facet joint *use* Lumbar Vertebral
  Joint
Lumbar ganglion *use* Lumbar Sympathetic
  Nerve
Lumbar lymph node *use* Lymphatic, Aortic
Lumbar lymphatic trunk *use* Cisterna Chyli
Lumbar splanchnic nerve *use* Lumbar
  Sympathetic Nerve
Lumbosacral facet joint *use* Lumbosacral
  Joint
Lumbosacral trunk *use* Lumbar Nerve
Lumpectomy
  see Excision
Lunate bone
  use Carpal, Right
  use Carpal, Left
Lunotriquetral ligament
  use Hand Bursa and Ligament, Right
  use Hand Bursa and Ligament, Left
Lymphadenectomy
  see Excision, Lymphatic and Hemic Systems
    07B
  see Resection, Lymphatic and Hemic Systems
    07T
Lymphadenotomy *see* Drainage, Lymphatic and
  Hemic Systems 079
Lymphangiectomy
  see Excision, Lymphatic and Hemic Systems
    07B
  see Resection, Lymphatic and Hemic Systems
    07T
Lymphangiogram *see* Plain Radiography,
  Lymphatic System B70
Lymphangioplasty
  see Repair, Lymphatic and Hemic Systems
    07Q
  see Supplement, Lymphatic and Hemic
    Systems 07U
Lymphangiorrhaphy *see* Repair, Lymphatic and
  Hemic Systems 07Q
Lymphangiotomy *see* Drainage, Lymphatic and
  Hemic Systems 079
Lysis *see* Release

M

Macula
use Retina, Right
use Retina, Left
MAGEC® Spinal Bracing and Distraction
    System *use* Magnetically Controlled
    Growth Rod(s) in New Technology
Magnet extraction, ocular foreign body *see*
    Extirpation, Eye 08C
Magnetic Resonance Imaging (MRI)
Abdomen BW30
Ankle
    Left BQ3H
    Right BQ3G
Aorta
    Abdominal B430
    Thoracic B330
Arm
    Left BP3F
    Right BP3E
Artery
    Celiac B431
    Cervico-Cerebral Arch B33Q
    Common Carotid, Bilateral B335
    Coronary
        Bypass Graft, Multiple B233
        Multiple B231
    Internal Carotid, Bilateral B338
    Intracranial B33R
    Lower Extremity
        Bilateral B43H
        Left B43G
        Right B43F
    Pelvic B43C
    Renal, Bilateral B438
    Spinal B33M
    Superior Mesenteric B434
    Upper Extremity
        Bilateral B33K
        Left B33J
        Right B33H
    Vertebral, Bilateral B33G
Bladder BT30
Brachial Plexus BW3P
Brain B030
Breast
    Bilateral BH32
    Left BH31
    Right BH30
Calcaneus
    Left BQ3K
    Right BQ3J
Chest BW33Y
Coccyx BR3F
Connective Tissue
    Lower Extremity BL31
    Upper Extremity BL30
Corpora Cavernosa BV30
Disc
    Cervical BR31
    Lumbar BR33
    Thoracic BR32
Ear B930
Elbow
    Left BP3H
    Right BP3G
Eye
    Bilateral B837
    Left B836
    Right B835
Femur
    Left BQ34
    Right BQ33
Fetal Abdomen BY33
Fetal Extremity BY35
Fetal Head BY30
Fetal Heart BY31
Fetal Spine BY34
Fetal Thorax BY32
Fetus, Whole BY36

Magnetic Resonance Imaging (MRI)
    (Continued)
Foot
    Left BQ3M
    Right BQ3L
Forearm
    Left BP3K
    Right BP3J
Gland
    Adrenal, Bilateral BG32
    Parathyroid BG33
    Parotid, Bilateral B936
    Salivary, Bilateral B93D
    Submandibular, Bilateral B939
    Thyroid BG34
Head BW38
Heart, Right and Left B236
Hip
    Left BQ31
    Right BQ30
Intracranial Sinus B532
Joint
    Finger
        Left BP3D
        Right BP3C
    Hand
        Left BP3D
        Right BP3C
    Temporomandibular, Bilateral BN39
Kidney
    Bilateral BT33
    Left BT32
    Right BT31
    Transplant BT39
Knee
    Left BQ38
    Right BQ37
Larynx B93J
Leg
    Left BQ3F
    Right BQ3D
Liver BF35
Liver and Spleen BF36
Lung Apices BB3G
Nasopharynx B93F
Neck BW3F
Nerve
    Acoustic B03C
    Brachial Plexus BW3P
Oropharynx B93F
Ovary
    Bilateral BU35
    Left BU34
    Right BU33
Ovary and Uterus BU3C
Pancreas BF37
Patella
    Left BQ3W
    Right BQ3V
Pelvic Region BW3G
Pelvis BR3C
Pituitary Gland B039
Plexus, Brachial BW3P
Prostate BV33
Retroperitoneum BW3H
Sacrum BR3F
Scrotum BV34
Sella Turcica B039
Shoulder
    Left BP39
    Right BP38
Sinus
    Intracranial B532
    Paranasal B932
Spinal Cord B03B
Spine
    Cervical BR30
    Lumbar BR39
    Thoracic BR37
Spleen and Liver BF36

Magnetic Resonance Imaging (MRI)
    (Continued)
Subcutaneous Tissue
    Abdomen BH3H
    Extremity
        Lower BH3J
        Upper BH3F
    Head BH3D
    Neck BH3D
    Pelvis BH3H
    Thorax BH3G
Tendon
    Lower Extremity BL33
    Upper Extremity BL32
Testicle
    Bilateral BV37
    Left BV36
    Right BV35
Toe
    Left BQ3Q
    Right BQ3P
Uterus BU36
    Pregnant BU3B
Uterus and Ovary BU3C
Vagina BU39
Vein
    Cerebellar B531
    Cerebral B531
    Jugular, Bilateral B535
    Lower Extremity
        Bilateral B53D
        Left B53C
        Right B53B
    Other B53V
    Pelvic (Iliac) Bilateral B53H
    Portal B53T
    Pulmonary, Bilateral B53S
    Renal, Bilateral B53L
    Spanchnic B53T
    Upper Extremity
        Bilateral B53P
        Left B53N
        Right B53M
Vena Cava
    Inferior B539
    Superior B538
Wrist
    Left BP3M
    Right BP3L
Magnetically Controlled Growth Rod(s)
    Cervical XNS3
    Lumbar XNS0
    Thoracic XNS4
Malleotomy *see* Drainage, Ear, Nose, Sinus 099
Malleus
    use Auditory Ossicle, Right
    use Auditory Ossicle, Left
Mammaplasty, mammoplasty
    see Alteration, Skin and Breast 0H0
    see Repair, Skin and Breast 0HQ
    see Replacement, Skin and Breast 0HR
    see Supplement, Skin and Breast 0HU
Mammary duct
    use Breast, Right
    use Breast, Left
    use Breast, Bilateral
Mammary gland
    use Breast, Right
    use Breast, Left
    use Breast, Bilateral
Mammectomy
    see Excision, Skin and Breast 0HB
    see Resection, Skin and Breast 0HT
Mammillary body *use* Hypothalamus
Mammography *see* Plain Radiography, Skin,
    Subcutaneous Tissue and Breast BH0
Mammotomy *see* Drainage, Skin and Breast 0H9
Mandibular nerve *use* Trigeminal Nerve
Mandibular notch
    use Mandible, Right
    use Mandible, Left

▶ New   ⇒ Revised   ~~deleted~~ Deleted

▶ New   ⇒ Revised   ~~deleted~~ Deleted

Meditation 8E0ZXY5
Medtronic Endurant® II AAA stent graft
   system *use* Intraluminal Device
Meissner's (submucous) plexus *use* Abdominal
   Sympathetic Nerve
Melody® transcatheter pulmonary valve
   use Zooplastic Tissue in Heart and Great
   Vessels
Membranous urethra *use* Urethra
Meningeorrhaphy
   see Repair, Cerebral Meninges 00Q1
   see Repair, Spinal Meninges 00QT
Meniscectomy, knee
   see Excision, Joint, Knee, Right 0SBC
   see Excision, Joint, Knee, Left 0SBD
Mental foramen
   use Mandible, Right
   use Mandible, Left
Mentalis muscle *use* Facial Muscle
Mentoplasty *see* Alteration, Jaw, Lower 0W05
Mesenterectomy *see* Excision, Mesentery
   0DBV
Mesenteriorrhaphy, mesenterorrhaphy *see*
   Repair, Mesentery 0DQV
Mesenteriplication *see* Repair, Mesentery
   0DQV
Mesoappendix *use* Mesentery
Mesocolon *use* Mesentery
Metacarpal ligament
   use Hand Bursa and Ligament, Right
   use Hand Bursa and Ligament, Left
Metacarpophalangeal ligament
   use Hand Bursa and Ligament, Right
   use Hand Bursa and Ligament, Left
Metal on metal bearing surface *use* Synthetic
   Substitute, Metal in 0SR
Metatarsal ligament
   use Foot Bursa and Ligament, Right
   use Foot Bursa and Ligament, Left
Metatarsectomy
   see Excision, Lower Bones 0QB
   see Resection, Lower Bones 0QT
Metatarsophalangeal (MTP) joint
   use Metatarsal-Phalangeal Joint, Right
   use Metatarsal-Phalangeal Joint, Left
Metatarsophalangeal ligament
   use Foot Bursa and Ligament, Right
   use Foot Bursa and Ligament, Left
Metathalamus *use* Thalamus
Micro-Driver stent (RX) (OTW) *use*
   Intraluminal Device
MicroMed HeartAssist *use* Implantable
   Heart Assist System in Heart and Great
   Vessels
Micrus CERECYTE microcoil *use* Intraluminal
   Device, Bioactive in Upper Arteries
Midcarpal joint
   use Carpal Joint, Right
   use Carpal Joint, Left
Middle cardiac nerve *use* Thoracic Sympathetic
   Nerve
Middle cerebral artery *use* Intracranial Artery
Middle cerebral vein *use* Intracranial Vein
Middle colic vein *use* Colic Vein
Middle genicular artery
   use Popliteal Artery, Right
   use Popliteal Artery, Left
Middle hemorrhoidal vein
   use Hypogastric Vein, Right
   use Hypogastric Vein, Left
Middle rectal artery
   use Internal Iliac Artery, Right
   use Internal Iliac Artery, Left
Middle suprarenal artery *use* Abdominal
   Aorta
Middle temporal artery
   use Temporal Artery, Right
   use Temporal Artery, Left
Middle turbinate *use* Nasal Turbinate

MIRODERM™ Biologic Wound Matrix *use*
   Skin Substitute, Porcine Liver Derived in
   New Technology
MitraClip valve repair system *use* Synthetic
   Substitute
Mitral annulus *use* Mitral Valve
Mitroflow® Aortic Pericardial Heart Valve *use*
   Zooplastic Tissue in Heart and Great Vessels
Mobilization, adhesions *see* Release
Molar gland *use* Buccal Mucosa
Monitoring
   Arterial
      Flow
         Coronary 4A13
         Peripheral 4A13
         Pulmonary 4A13
      Pressure
         Coronary 4A13
         Peripheral 4A13
         Pulmonary 4A13
      Pulse
         Coronary 4A13
         Peripheral 4A13
         Pulmonary 4A13
      Saturation, Peripheral 4A13
      Sound, Peripheral 4A13
   Cardiac
      Electrical Activity 4A12
         Ambulatory 4A12X45
         No Qualifier 4A12X4Z
      Output 4A12
      Rate 4A12
      Rhythm 4A12
      Sound 4A12
      Total Activity, Stress 4A12XM4
      Vascular Perfusion, Indocyanine Green
         Dye 4A12XSH
   Central Nervous
      Conductivity 4A10
      Electrical Activity
         Intraoperative 4A10
         No Qualifier 4A10
      Pressure 4A100BZ
         Intracranial 4A10
      Saturation, Intracranial 4A10
      Temperature, Intracranial 4A10
   Gastrointestinal
      Motility 4A1B
      Pressure 4A1B
      Secretion 4A1B
      Vascular Perfusion, Indocyanine Green
         Dye 4A1BXSH
   Intraoperative Knee Replacement Sensor
      XR2
   Lymphatic
      Flow 4A16
      Pressure 4A16
   Peripheral Nervous
      Conductivity
         Motor 4A11
         Sensory 4A11
      Electrical Activity Intraoperative 4A11
      No Qualifier 4A11
   Products of Conception
      Cardiac
         Electrical Activity 4A1H
         Rate 4A1H
         Rhythm 4A1H
         Sound 4A1H
      Nervous
         Conductivity 4A1J
         Electrical Activity 4A1J
         Pressure 4A1J
   Respiratory
      Capacity 4A19
      Flow 4A19
      Rate 4A19
      Resistance 4A19
      Volume 4A19

Monitoring *(Continued)*
   Skin and Breast, Vascular Perfusion,
      Indocyanine Green Dye 4A1GXSH
   Sleep 4A1ZXQZ
   Temperature 4A1Z
   Urinary
      Contractility 4A1D
      Flow 4A1D
      Pressure 4A1D
      Resistance 4A1D
      Volume 4A1D
   Venous
      Flow
         Central 4A14
         Peripheral 4A14
         Portal 4A14
         Pulmonary 4A14
      Pressure
         Central 4A14
         Peripheral 4A14
         Portal 4A14
         Pulmonary 4A14
      Pulse
         Central 4A14
         Peripheral 4A14
         Portal 4A14
         Pulmonary 4A14
      Saturation
         Central 4A14
         Portal 4A14
         Pulmonary 4A14
Monitoring Device, Hemodynamic
   Abdomen 0JH8
   Chest 0JH6
Mosaic Bioprosthesis (aortic) (mitral) valve
   use Zooplastic Tissue in Heart and Great
   Vessels
Motor Function Assessment F01
Motor Treatment F07
MR Angiography
   see Magnetic Resonance Imaging (MRI),
      Heart B23
   see Magnetic Resonance Imaging (MRI),
      Upper Arteries B33
   see Magnetic Resonance Imaging (MRI),
      Lower Arteries B43
MULTI-LINK (VISION)(MINI-VISION)
   (ULTRA) Coronary Stent System *use*
   Intraluminal Device
Multiple sleep latency test 4A0ZXQZ
Musculocutaneous nerve *use* Brachial Plexus
   Nerve
Musculopexy
   see Repair, Muscles 0KQ
   see Reposition, Muscles 0KS
Musculophrenic artery
   use Internal Mammary Artery, Right
   use Internal Mammary Artery, Left
Musculoplasty
   see Repair, Muscles 0KQ
   see Supplement, Muscles 0KU
Musculorrhaphy *see* Repair, Muscles
   0KQ
Musculospiral nerve *use* Radial Nerve
Myectomy
   see Excision, Muscles 0KB
   see Resection, Muscles 0KT
Myelencephalon *use* Medulla Oblongata
Myelogram
   CT *see* Computerized Tomography (CT Scan),
      Central Nervous System B02
   MRI *see* Magnetic Resonance Imaging (MRI),
      Central Nervous System B03
Myenteric (Auerbach's) plexus *use* Abdominal
   Sympathetic Nerve
Myocardial Bridge Release *see* Release, Artery,
   Coronary
Myomectomy *see* Excision, Female
   Reproductive System 0UB

Myometrium *use* Uterus
Myopexy
  see Repair, Muscles ØKQ
  see Reposition, Muscles ØKS
Myoplasty
  see Repair, Muscles ØKQ
  see Supplement, Muscles ØKU
Myorrhaphy *see* Repair, Muscles ØKQ

Myoscopy *see* Inspection, Muscles ØKJ
Myotomy
  see Division, Muscles ØK8
  see Drainage, Muscles ØK9
Myringectomy
  see Excision, Ear, Nose, Sinus Ø9B
  see Resection, Ear, Nose, Sinus Ø9T

Myringoplasty
  see Repair, Ear, Nose, Sinus Ø9Q
  see Replacement, Ear, Nose, Sinus Ø9R
  see Supplement, Ear, Nose, Sinus Ø9U
Myringostomy *see* Drainage, Ear, Nose, Sinus Ø99
Myringotomy *see* Drainage, Ear, Nose, Sinus Ø99

N

New Technology *(Continued)*
▶Synthetic Human Angiotensin II XWØ
  Uridine Triacetate XWØDX82
Ninth cranial nerve *use* Glossopharyngeal
  Nerve
Nitinol framed polymer mesh *use* Synthetic
  Substitute
Non-tunneled central venous catheter *use*
  Infusion Device
Nonimaging Nuclear Medicine Assay
  Bladder, Kidneys and Ureters CT63
  Blood C763
  Kidneys, Ureters and Bladder CT63
  Lymphatics and Hematologic System
    C76YYZZ
  Ureters, Kidneys and Bladder CT63
  Urinary System CT6YYZZ
Nonimaging Nuclear Medicine Probe
  Abdomen CW5Ø
  Abdomen and Chest CW54
  Abdomen and Pelvis CW51
  Brain CØ5Ø
  Central Nervous System CØ5YYZZ
  Chest CW53
  Chest and Abdomen CW54
  Chest and Neck CW56

Nonimaging Nuclear Medicine Probe
    (Continued)
  Extremity
    Lower CP5PZZZ
    Upper CP5NZZZ
  Head and Neck CW5B
  Heart C25YYZZ
    Right and Left C256
  Lymphatics
    Head C75J
    Head and Neck C755
    Lower Extremity C75P
    Neck C75K
    Pelvic C75D
    Trunk C75M
    Upper Chest C75L
    Upper Extremity C75N
  Lymphatics and Hematologic System
    C75YYZZ
  Musculoskeletal System, Other
    CP5YYZZ
  Neck and Chest CW56
  Neck and Head CW5B
  Pelvic Region CW5J
  Pelvis and Abdomen CW51
  Spine CP55ZZZ

Nonimaging Nuclear Medicine Uptake
  Endocrine System CG4YYZZ
  Gland, Thyroid CG42
Nostril *use* Nasal Mucosa and Soft Tissue
Novacor Left Ventricular Assist Device *use*
    Implantable Heart Assist System in Heart
    and Great Vessels
Novation® Ceramic AHS® (Articulation Hip
    System) *use* Synthetic Substitute, Ceramic
    in ØSR
Nuclear medicine
  see Planar Nuclear Medicine Imaging
  see Tomographic (Tomo) Nuclear Medicine
    Imaging
  see Positron Emission Tomographic (PET)
    Imaging
  see Nonimaging Nuclear Medicine Uptake
  see Nonimaging Nuclear Medicine Probe
  see Nonimaging Nuclear Medicine Assay
  see Systemic Nuclear Medicine Therapy
Nuclear scintigraphy *see* Nuclear Medicine
Nutrition, concentrated substances
  Enteral infusion 3EØG36Z
  Parenteral (peripheral) infusion *see*
    Introduction of Nutritional Substance

N

O

Obliteration *see* Destruction
Obturator artery
   use Internal Iliac Artery, Right
   use Internal Iliac Artery, Left
Obturator lymph node *use* Lymphatic, Pelvis
Obturator muscle
   use Hip Muscle, Right
   use Hip Muscle, Left
Obturator nerve *use* Lumbar Plexus
Obturator vein
   use Hypogastric Vein, Right
   use Hypogastric Vein, Left
Obtuse margin *use* Heart, Left
Occipital artery
   use External Carotid Artery, Right
   use External Carotid Artery, Left
Occipital lobe *use* Cerebral Hemisphere
Occipital lymph node
   use Lymphatic, Right Neck
   use Lymphatic, Left Neck
Occipitofrontalis muscle *use* Facial Muscle
Occlusion
  Ampulla of Vater ØFLC
  Anus ØDLQ
  Aorta
    Abdominal 04LØ
    Thoracic, Descending 02LW3DJ
  Artery
    Anterior Tibial
      Left 04LQ
      Right 04LP
    Axillary
      Left 03L6
      Right 03L5
    Brachial
      Left 03L8
      Right 03L7
    Celiac 04L1
    Colic
      Left 04L7
      Middle 04L8
      Right 04L6
    Common Carotid
      Left 03LJ
      Right 03LH
    Common Iliac
      Left 04LD
      Right 04LC
    External Carotid
      Left 03LN
      Right 03LM
    External Iliac
      Left 04LJ
      Right 04LH
    Face 03LR
    Femoral
      Left 04LL
      Right 04LK
    Foot
      Left 04LW
      Right 04LV
    Gastric 04L2
    Hand
      Left 03LF
      Right 03LD
    Hepatic 04L3
    Inferior Mesenteric 04LB
    Innominate 03L2
    Internal Carotid
      Left 03LL
      Right 03LK
    Internal Iliac
      Left 04LF
      Right 04LE
    Internal Mammary
      Left 03L1
      Right 03LØ
    Intracranial 03LG

Occlusion *(Continued)*
  Artery *(Continued)*
    Lower 04LY
    Peroneal
      Left 04LU
      Right 04LT
    Popliteal
      Left 04LN
      Right 04LM
    Posterior Tibial
      Left 04LS
      Right 04LR
    Pulmonary
      Left 02LR
      Right 02LQ
    Pulmonary Trunk 02LP
    Radial
      Left 03LC
      Right 03LB
    Renal
      Left 04LA
      Right 04L9
    Splenic 04L4
    Subclavian
      Left 03L4
      Right 03L3
    Superior Mesenteric 04L5
    Temporal
      Left 03LT
      Right 03LS
    Thyroid
      Left 03LV
      Right 03LU
    Ulnar
      Left 03LA
      Right 03L9
    Upper 03LY
    Vertebral
      Left 03LQ
      Right 03LP
  Atrium, Left 02L7
  Bladder ØTLB
  Bladder Neck ØTLC
  Bronchus
    Lingula ØBL9
    Lower Lobe
      Left ØBLB
      Right ØBL6
    Main
      Left ØBL7
      Right ØBL3
    Middle Lobe, Right ØBL5
    Upper Lobe
      Left ØBL8
      Right ØBL4
  Carina ØBL2
  Cecum ØDLH
  Cisterna Chyli 07LL
  Colon
    Ascending ØDLK
    Descending ØDLM
    Sigmoid ØDLN
    Transverse ØDLL
  Cord
    Bilateral ØVLH
    Left ØVLG
    Right ØVLF
  Cul-de-sac ØULF
  Duct
    Common Bile ØFL9
    Cystic ØFL8
    Hepatic
      Common ØFL7
      Left ØFL6
      Right ØFL5
    Lacrimal
      Left 08LY
      Right 08LX
    Pancreatic ØFLD
      Accessory ØFLF

Occlusion *(Continued)*
  Duct *(Continued)*
    Parotid
      Left ØCLC
      Right ØCLB
  Duodenum ØDL9
  Esophagogastric Junction ØDL4
  Esophagus ØDL5
    Lower ØDL3
    Middle ØDL2
    Upper ØDL1
  Fallopian Tube
    Left ØUL6
    Right ØUL5
  Fallopian Tubes, Bilateral ØUL7
  Ileocecal Valve ØDLC
  Ileum ØDLB
  Intestine
    Large ØDLE
      Left ØDLG
      Right ØDLF
    Small ØDL8
  Jejunum ØDLA
  Kidney Pelvis
    Left ØTL4
    Right ØTL3
  Left atrial appendage (LAA) *see* Occlusion,
    Atrium, Left 02L7
  Lymphatic
    Aortic 07LD
    Axillary
      Left 07L6
      Right 07L5
    Head 07LØ
    Inguinal
      Left 07LJ
      Right 07LH
    Internal Mammary
      Left 07L9
      Right 07L8
    Lower Extremity
      Left 07LG
      Right 07LF
    Mesenteric 07LB
    Neck
      Left 07L2
      Right 07L1
    Pelvis 07LC
    Thoracic Duct 07LK
    Thorax 07L7
    Upper Extremity
      Left 07L4
      Right 07L3
  Rectum ØDLP
  Stomach ØDL6
    Pylorus ØDL7
  Trachea ØBL1
  Ureter
    Left ØTL7
    Right ØTL6
  Urethra ØTLD
  Vagina ØULG
  Valve, Pulmonary 02LH
  Vas Deferens
    Bilateral ØVLQ
    Left ØVLP
    Right ØVLN
  Vein
    Axillary
      Left 05L8
      Right 05L7
    Azygos 05LØ
    Basilic
      Left 05LC
      Right 05LB
    Brachial
      Left 05LA
      Right 05L9
    Cephalic
      Left 05LF
      Right 05LD

▶ New   ⇛ Revised   ~~deleted~~ Deleted

Occlusion (Continued)
Vein (Continued)
Colic 06L7
Common Iliac
Left 06LD
Right 06LC
Esophageal 06L3
External Iliac
Left 06LG
Right 06LF
External Jugular
Left 05LQ
Right 05LP
Face
Left 05LV
Right 05LT
Femoral
Left 06LN
Right 06LM
Foot
Left 06LV
Right 06LT
Gastric 06L2
Hand
Left 05LH
Right 05LG
Hemiazygos 05L1
Hepatic 06L4
Hypogastric
Left 06LJ
Right 06LH
Inferior Mesenteric 06L6
Innominate
Left 05L4
Right 05L3
Internal Jugular
Left 05LN
Right 05LM
Intracranial 05LL
Lower 06LY
Portal 06L8
Pulmonary
Left 02LT
Right 02LS
Renal
Left 06LB
Right 06L9
Saphenous
Left 06LQ
Right 06LP
Splenic 06L1
Subclavian
Left 05L6
Right 05L5
Superior Mesenteric 06L5
Upper 05LY
Vertebral
Left 05LS
Right 05LR
Vena Cava
Inferior 06L0
Superior 02LV
Occlusion, REBOA (resuscitative
endovascular balloon occlusion
of the aorta)
02LW3DJ
04L03DJ
Occupational therapy see Activities of Daily
Living Treatment, Rehabilitation F08
Odentectomy
see Excision, Mouth and Throat 0CB
see Resection, Mouth and Throat 0CT
Odontoid process use Cervical Vertebra
Olecranon bursa
use Elbow Bursa and Ligament, Right
use Elbow Bursa and Ligament, Left
Olecranon process
use Ulna, Right
use Ulna, Left
Olfactory bulb use Olfactory Nerve

Omentectomy, omentumectomy
see Excision, Gastrointestinal System 0DB
see Resection, Gastrointestinal System 0DT
Omentofixation see Repair, Gastrointestinal
System 0DQ
Omentoplasty
see Repair, Gastrointestinal System 0DQ
see Replacement, Gastrointestinal System
0DR
see Supplement, Gastrointestinal System
0DU
Omentorrhaphy see Repair, Gastrointestinal
System 0DQ
Omentotomy see Drainage, Gastrointestinal
System 0D9
Omnilink Elite Vascular Balloon Expandable
Stent System use Intraluminal Device
Onychectomy
see Excision, Skin and Breast 0HB
see Resection, Skin and Breast 0HT
Onychoplasty
see Repair, Skin and Breast 0HQ
see Replacement, Skin and Breast 0HR
Onychotomy see Drainage, Skin and Breast
0H9
Oophorectomy
see Excision, Female Reproductive System
0UB
see Resection, Female Reproductive System
0UT
Oophoropexy
see Repair, Female Reproductive System 0UQ
see Reposition, Female Reproductive System
0US
Oophoroplasty
see Repair, Female Reproductive System 0UQ
see Supplement, Female Reproductive System
0UU
Oophororrhaphy see Repair, Female
Reproductive System 0UQ
Oophorostomy see Drainage, Female
Reproductive System 0U9
Oophorotomy
see Division, Female Reproductive System
0U8
see Drainage, Female Reproductive System
0U9
Oophorrhaphy see Repair, Female Reproductive
System 0UQ
Open Pivot (mechanical) valve use Synthetic
Substitute
Open Pivot Aortic Valve Graft (AVG) use
Synthetic Substitute
Ophthalmic artery use Intracranial Artery
Ophthalmic nerve use Trigeminal Nerve
Ophthalmic vein use Intracranial Vein
Opponensplasty
Tendon replacement see Replacement,
Tendons 0LR
Tendon transfer see Transfer, Tendons 0LX
Optic chiasma use Optic Nerve
Optic disc
use Retina, Right
use Retina, Left
Optic foramen use Sphenoid Bone
Optical coherence tomography, intravascular
see Computerized Tomography (CT Scan)
Optimizer™ III implantable pulse generator
use Contractility Modulation Device in
0JH
Orbicularis oculi muscle
use Upper Eyelid, Right
use Upper Eyelid, Left
Orbicularis oris muscle use Facial Muscle
Orbital Atherectomy Technology X2C
Orbital fascia use Subcutaneous Tissue and
Fascia, Face
Orbital portion of ethmoid bone
use Orbit, Right
use Orbit, Left

Orbital portion of frontal bone
use Orbit, Right
use Orbit, Left
Orbital portion of lacrimal bone
use Orbit, Right
use Orbit, Left
Orbital portion of maxilla
use Orbit, Right
use Orbit, Left
Orbital portion of palatine bone
use Orbit, Right
use Orbit, Left
Orbital portion of sphenoid bone
use Orbit, Right
use Orbit, Left
Orbital portion of zygomatic bone
use Orbit, Right
use Orbit, Left
Orchectomy, orchidectomy, orchiectomy
see Excision, Male Reproductive System
0VB
see Resection, Male Reproductive System
0VT
Orchidoplasty, orchioplasty
see Repair, Male Reproductive System 0VQ
see Replacement, Male Reproductive System
0VR
see Supplement, Male Reproductive System
0VU
Orchidorrhaphy, orchiorrhaphy see Repair,
Male Reproductive System 0VQ
Orchidotomy, orchiotomy, orchotomy see
Drainage, Male Reproductive System
0V9
Orchiopexy
see Repair, Male Reproductive System 0VQ
see Reposition, Male Reproductive System
0VS
Oropharyngeal airway (OPA) use Intraluminal
Device, Airway in Mouth and Throat
Oropharynx use Pharynx
Ossiculectomy
see Excision, Ear, Nose, Sinus 09B
see Resection, Ear, Nose, Sinus 09T
Ossiculotomy see Drainage, Ear, Nose, Sinus
099
Ostectomy
see Excision, Head and Facial Bones 0NB
see Resection, Head and Facial Bones 0NT
see Excision, Upper Bones 0PB
see Resection, Upper Bones 0PT
see Excision, Lower Bones 0QB
see Resection, Lower Bones 0QT
Osteoclasis
see Division, Head and Facial Bones 0N8
see Division, Upper Bones 0P8
see Division, Lower Bones 0Q8
Osteolysis
see Release, Head and Facial Bones 0NN
see Release, Upper Bones 0PN
see Release, Lower Bones 0QN
Osteopathic Treatment
Abdomen 7W09X
Cervical 7W01X
Extremity
Lower 7W06X
Upper 7W07X
Head 7W00X
Lumbar 7W03X
Pelvis 7W05X
Rib Cage 7W08X
Sacrum 7W04X
Thoracic 7W02X
Osteopexy
see Repair, Head and Facial Bones 0NQ
see Reposition, Head and Facial Bones 0NS
see Repair, Upper Bones 0PQ
see Reposition, Upper Bones 0PS
see Repair, Lower Bones 0QQ
see Reposition, Lower Bones 0QS

Osteoplasty
   see Repair, Head and Facial Bones ØNQ
   see Replacement, Head and Facial Bones ØNR
   see Supplement, Head and Facial Bones ØNU
   see Repair, Upper Bones ØPQ
   see Replacement, Upper Bones ØPR
   see Supplement, Upper Bones ØPU
   see Repair, Lower Bones ØQQ
   see Replacement, Lower Bones ØQR
   see Supplement, Lower Bones ØQU
Osteorrhaphy
   see Repair, Head and Facial Bones ØNQ
   see Repair, Upper Bones ØPQ
   see Repair, Lower Bones ØQQ
Osteotomy, ostotomy
   see Division, Head and Facial Bones ØN8
   see Drainage, Head and Facial Bones ØN9
   see Division, Upper Bones ØP8
   see Drainage, Upper Bones ØP9
   see Division, Lower Bones ØQ8
   see Drainage, Lower Bones ØQ9
Otic ganglion *use* Head and Neck Sympathetic
   Nerve

Otoplasty
   see Repair, Ear, Nose, Sinus Ø9Q
   see Replacement, Ear, Nose, Sinus Ø9R
   see Supplement, Ear, Nose, Sinus Ø9U
Otoscopy *see* Inspection, Ear, Nose, Sinus Ø9J
Oval window
   use Middle Ear, Right
   use Middle Ear, Left
Ovarian artery *use* Abdominal Aorta
Ovarian ligament *use* Uterine Supporting
   Structure
Ovariectomy
   see Excision, Female Reproductive System
     ØUB
   see Resection, Female Reproductive System
     ØUT
Ovariocentesis *see* Drainage, Female
   Reproductive System ØU9
Ovariopexy
   see Repair, Female Reproductive System
     ØUQ
   see Reposition, Female Reproductive System
     ØUS

Ovariotomy
   see Division, Female Reproductive System
     ØU8
   see Drainage, Female Reproductive System
     ØU9
Ovatio™ CRT-D *use* Cardiac Resynchronization
   Defibrillator Pulse Generator in ØJH
Oversewing
   Gastrointestinal ulcer *see* Repair,
     Gastrointestinal System ØDQ
   Pleural bleb *see* Repair, Respiratory System
     ØBQ
Oviduct
   use Fallopian Tube, Right
   use Fallopian Tube, Left
Oximetry, Fetal pulse 10H073Z
OXINIUM *use* Synthetic Substitute, Oxidized
   Zirconium on Polyethylene in ØSR
Oxygenation
   Extracorporeal membrane (ECMO) *see*
     Performance, Circulatory 5A15
   Hyperbaric *see* Assistance, Circulatory 5A05
   Supersaturated *see* Assistance, Circulatory
     5A05

▶ New   ⇒ Revised   ~~deleted~~ Deleted

P

Pacemaker
  Dual Chamber
    Abdomen ØJH8
    Chest ØJH6
  Intracardiac
    Insertion of device in
      Atrium
        Left 02H7
        Right 02H6
      Vein, Coronary 02H4
      Ventricle
        Left 02HL
        Right 02HK
    Removal of device from, Heart 02PA
    Revision of device in, Heart 02WA
  Single Chamber
    Abdomen ØJH8
    Chest ØJH6
  Single Chamber Rate Responsive
    Abdomen ØJH8
    Chest ØJH6
Packing
  Abdominal Wall 2W43X5Z
  Anorectal 2Y43X5Z
  Arm
    Lower
      Left 2W4DX5Z
      Right 2W4CX5Z
    Upper
      Left 2W4BX5Z
      Right 2W4AX5Z
  Back 2W45X5Z
  Chest Wall 2W44X5Z
  Ear 2Y42X5Z
  Extremity
    Lower
      Left 2W4MX5Z
      Right 2W4LX5Z
    Upper
      Left 2W49X5Z
      Right 2W48X5Z
  Face 2W41X5Z
  Finger
    Left 2W4KX5Z
    Right 2W4JX5Z
  Foot
    Left 2W4TX5Z
    Right 2W4SX5Z
  Genital Tract, Female 2Y44X5Z
  Hand
    Left 2W4FX5Z
    Right 2W4EX5Z
  Head 2W40X5Z
  Inguinal Region
    Left 2W47X5Z
    Right 2W46X5Z
  Leg
    Lower
      Left 2W4RX5Z
      Right 2W4QX5Z
    Upper
      Left 2W4PX5Z
      Right 2W4NX5Z
  Mouth and Pharynx 2Y40X5Z
  Nasal 2Y41X5Z
  Neck 2W42X5Z
  Thumb
    Left 2W4HX5Z
    Right 2W4GX5Z
  Toe
    Left 2W4VX5Z
    Right 2W4UX5Z
  Urethra 2Y45X5Z
Paclitaxel-eluting coronary stent
  use Intraluminal Device, Drug-eluting in Heart and Great Vessels

Paclitaxel-eluting peripheral stent
  use Intraluminal Device, Drug-eluting in Upper Arteries
  use Intraluminal Device, Drug-eluting in Lower Arteries
Palatine gland *use* Buccal Mucosa
Palatine tonsil *use* Tonsils
Palatine uvula *use* Uvula
Palatoglossal muscle *use* Tongue, Palate, Pharynx Muscle
Palatopharyngeal muscle *use* Tongue, Palate, Pharynx Muscle
Palatoplasty
  see Repair, Mouth and Throat ØCQ
  see Replacement, Mouth and Throat ØCR
  see Supplement, Mouth and Throat ØCU
Palatorrhaphy *see* Repair, Mouth and Throat ØCQ
Palmar (volar) digital vein
  use Hand Vein, Right
  use Hand Vein, Left
Palmar (volar) metacarpal vein
  use Hand Vein, Right
  use Hand Vein, Left
Palmar cutaneous nerve
  use Radial Nerve
  use Median Nerve
Palmar fascia (aponeurosis)
  use Subcutaneous Tissue and Fascia, Right Hand
  use Subcutaneous Tissue and Fascia, Left Hand
Palmar interosseous muscle
  use Hand Muscle, Right
  use Hand Muscle, Left
Palmar ulnocarpal ligament
  use Wrist Bursa and Ligament, Right
  use Wrist Bursa and Ligament, Left
Palmaris longus muscle
  use Lower Arm and Wrist Muscle, Right
  use Lower Arm and Wrist Muscle, Left
Pancreatectomy
  see Excision, Pancreas ØFB
  see Resection, Pancreas ØFTG
Pancreatic artery *use* Splenic Artery
Pancreatic plexus *use* Abdominal Sympathetic Nerve
Pancreatic vein *use* Splenic Vein
Pancreaticoduodenostomy *see* Bypass, Hepatobiliary System and Pancreas ØF1
Pancreaticosplenic lymph node *use* Lymphatic, Aortic
Pancreatogram, endoscopic retrograde *see* Fluoroscopy, Pancreatic Duct BF18
Pancreatolithotomy *see* Extirpation, Pancreas ØFCG
Pancreatotomy
  see Division, Pancreas ØF8G
  see Drainage, Pancreas ØF9G
Panniculectomy
  see Excision, Skin, Abdomen ØHB7
  see Excision, Abdominal Wall ØWBF
Paraaortic lymph node *use* Lymphatic, Aortic
Paracentesis
  Eye *see* Drainage, Eye 089
  Peritoneal Cavity *see* Drainage, Peritoneal Cavity ØW9G
  Tympanum *see* Drainage, Ear, Nose, Sinus 099
Pararectal lymph node *use* Lymphatic, Mesenteric
Parasternal lymph node *use* Lymphatic, Thorax
Parathyroidectomy
  see Excision, Endocrine System ØGB
  see Resection, Endocrine System ØGT
Paratracheal lymph node *use* Lymphatic, Thorax
Paraurethral (Skene's) gland *use* Vestibular Gland
Parenteral nutrition, total *see* Introduction of Nutritional Substance
Parietal lobe *use* Cerebral Hemisphere
Parotid lymph node *use* Lymphatic, Head
Parotid plexus *use* Facial Nerve

Parotidectomy
  see Excision, Mouth and Throat ØCB
  see Resection, Mouth and Throat ØCT
Pars flaccida
  use Tympanic Membrane, Right
  use Tympanic Membrane, Left
Partial joint replacement
  Hip *see* Replacement, Lower Joints ØSR
  Knee *see* Replacement, Lower Joints ØSR
  Shoulder *see* Replacement, Upper Joints ØRR
Partially absorbable mesh *use* Synthetic Substitute
➡ **Patch, blood, spinal** 3E0R3GC
Patellapexy
  see Repair, Lower Bones ØQQ
  see Reposition, Lower Bones ØQS
Patellaplasty
  see Repair, Lower Bones ØQQ
  see Replacement, Lower Bones ØQR
  see Supplement, Lower Bones ØQU
Patellar ligament
  use Knee Bursa and Ligament, Right
  use Knee Bursa and Ligament, Left
Patellar tendon
  use Knee Tendon, Right
  use Knee Tendon, Left
Patellectomy
  see Excision, Lower Bones ØQB
  see Resection, Lower Bones ØQT
Patellofemoral joint
  use Knee Joint, Right
  use Knee Joint, Left
  use Knee Joint, Femoral Surface, Right
  use Knee Joint, Femoral Surface, Left
Pectineus muscle
  use Upper Leg Muscle, Right
  use Upper Leg Muscle, Left
Pectoral (anterior) lymph node
  use Lymphatic, Right Axillary
  use Lymphatic, Left Axillary
Pectoral fascia *use* Subcutaneous Tissue and Fascia, Chest
Pectoralis major muscle
  use Thorax Muscle, Right
  use Thorax Muscle, Left
Pectoralis minor muscle
  use Thorax Muscle, Right
  use Thorax Muscle, Left
Pedicle-based dynamic stabilization device
  use Spinal Stabilization Device, Pedicle-Based in ØRH
  use Spinal Stabilization Device, Pedicle-Based in ØSH
PEEP (positive end expiratory pressure) *see* Assistance, Respiratory 5A09
PEG (percutaneous endoscopic gastrostomy) ØDH63UZ
PEJ (percutaneous endoscopic jejunostomy) ØDHA3UZ
Pelvic splanchnic nerve
  use Abdominal Sympathetic Nerve
  use Sacral Sympathetic Nerve
Penectomy
  see Excision, Male Reproductive System ØVB
  see Resection, Male Reproductive System ØVT
Penile urethra *use* Urethra
Perceval sutureless valve *use* Zooplastic Tissue, Rapid Deployment Technique in New Technology
Percutaneous endoscopic gastrojejunostomy (PEG/J) tube *use* Feeding Device in Gastrointestinal System
Percutaneous endoscopic gastrostomy (PEG) tube *use* Feeding Device in Gastrointestinal System
Percutaneous nephrostomy catheter *use* Drainage Device
Percutaneous transluminal coronary angioplasty (PTCA) *see* Dilation, Heart and Great Vessels 027

▶ New   ⇒ Revised   ~~deleted~~ Deleted

Performance
  Biliary
    Multiple, Filtration 5A1C60Z
    Single, Filtration 5A1C00Z
  Cardiac
    Continuous
      Output 5A1221Z
      Pacing 5A1223Z
    Intermittent, Pacing 5A1213Z
    Single, Output, Manual 5A12012
  ▶Circulatory
    ▶Central Membrane 5A1522F
    ▶Peripheral Veno-arterial Membrane
      5A1522G
    ▶Peripheral Veno-venous Membrane
      5A1522H
    ~~Circulatory, Continuous, Oxygenation,~~
      ~~Membrane 5A15223~~
  Respiratory
    24-96 Consecutive Hours, Ventilation
      5A1945Z
    Greater than 96 Consecutive Hours,
      Ventilation 5A1955Z
    Less than 24 Consecutive Hours,
      Ventilation 5A1935Z
    Single, Ventilation, Nonmechanical
      5A19054
  Urinary
    Continuous, Greater than 18 hours per day,
      Filtration 5A1D90Z
    Intermittent, Less than 6 Hours Per Day,
      Filtration 5A1D70Z
    Prolonged Intermittent, 6-18 hours per day,
      Filtration 5A1D80Z
Perfusion see Introduction of substance in or on
Perfusion, donor organ
  Heart 6AB50BZ
  Kidney(s) 6ABT0BZ
  Liver 6ABF0BZ
  Lung(s) 6ABB0BZ
Pericardiectomy
  see Excision, Pericardium 02BN
  see Resection, Pericardium 02TN
Pericardiocentesis
  see Drainage, Cavity, Pericardial 0W9D
Pericardiolysis see Release, Pericardium
  02NN
Pericardiophrenic artery
  use Internal Mammary Artery, Right
  use Internal Mammary Artery, Left
Pericardioplasty
  see Repair, Pericardium 02QN
  see Replacement, Pericardium 02RN
  see Supplement, Pericardium 02UN
Pericardiorrhaphy see Repair, Pericardium
  02QN
Pericardiostomy see Drainage, Cavity,
  Pericardial 0W9D
Pericardiotomy see Drainage, Cavity, Pericardial
  0W9D
Perimetrium use Uterus
Peripheral parenteral nutrition see Introduction
  of Nutritional Substance
Peripherally inserted central catheter (PICC)
  use Infusion Device
Peritoneal dialysis 3E1M39Z
Peritoneocentesis
  see Drainage, Peritoneum 0D9W
  see Drainage, Cavity, Peritoneal 0W9G
Peritoneoplasty
  see Repair, Peritoneum 0DQW
  see Replacement, Peritoneum 0DRW
  see Supplement, Peritoneum 0DUW
Peritoneoscopy 0DJW4ZZ
Peritoneotomy see Drainage, Peritoneum 0D9W
Peritoneumectomy
  see Excision, Peritoneum 0DBW
Peroneus brevis muscle
  use Lower Leg Muscle, Right
  use Lower Leg Muscle, Left

Peroneus longus muscle
  use Lower Leg Muscle, Right
  use Lower Leg Muscle, Left
Pessary ring use Intraluminal Device, Pessary in
  Female Reproductive System
PET scan see Positron Emission Tomographic
  (PET) Imaging
Petrous part of temporal bone
  use Temporal Bone, Right
  use Temporal Bone, Left
Phacoemulsification, lens
  With IOL implant see Replacement, Eye 08R
  Without IOL implant see Extraction, Eye 08D
Phalangectomy
  see Excision, Upper Bones 0PB
  see Resection, Upper Bones 0PT
  see Excision, Lower Bones 0QB
  see Resection, Lower Bones 0QT
Phallectomy
  see Excision, Penis 0VBS
  see Resection, Penis 0VTS
Phalloplasty
  see Repair, Penis 0VQS
  see Supplement, Penis 0VUS
Phallotomy see Drainage, Penis 0V9S
Pharmacotherapy, for substance abuse
  Antabuse HZ93ZZZ
  Bupropion HZ97ZZZ
  Clonidine HZ96ZZZ
  Levo-alpha-acetyl-methadol (LAAM)
    HZ92ZZZ
  Methadone Maintenance HZ91ZZZ
  Naloxone HZ95ZZZ
  Naltrexone HZ94ZZZ
  Nicotine Replacement HZ90ZZZ
  Psychiatric Medication HZ98ZZZ
  Replacement Medication, Other HZ99ZZZ
Pharyngeal constrictor muscle use Tongue,
  Palate, Pharynx Muscle
Pharyngeal plexus use Vagus Nerve
Pharyngeal recess use Nasopharynx
Pharyngeal tonsil use Adenoids
Pharyngogram see Fluoroscopy, Pharynx
  B91G
Pharyngoplasty
  see Repair, Mouth and Throat 0CQ
  see Replacement, Mouth and Throat 0CR
  see Supplement, Mouth and Throat 0CU
Pharyngorrhaphy see Repair, Mouth and Throat
  0CQ
Pharyngotomy see Drainage, Mouth and Throat
  0C9
Pharyngotympanic tube
  use Eustachian Tube, Right
  use Eustachian Tube, Left
Pheresis
  Erythrocytes 6A55
  Leukocytes 6A55
  Plasma 6A55
  Platelets 6A55
  Stem Cells
    Cord Blood 6A55
    Hematopoietic 6A55
Phlebectomy
  see Excision, Upper Veins 05B
  see Extraction, Upper Veins 05D
  see Excision, Lower Veins 06B
  see Extraction, Lower Veins 06D
Phlebography
  see Plain Radiography, Veins B50
  Impedance 4A04X51
Phleborrhaphy
  see Repair, Upper Veins 05Q
  see Repair, Lower Veins 06Q
Phlebotomy
  see Drainage, Upper Veins 059
  see Drainage, Lower Veins 069
Photocoagulation
➥For Destruction see Destruction
➥For Repair see Repair

Photopheresis, therapeutic see Phototherapy,
  Circulatory 6A65
Phototherapy
  Circulatory 6A65
  Skin 6A60
  Ultraviolet light see Ultraviolet Light
    Therapy, Physiological Systems 6A8
Phrenectomy, phrenoneurectomy see Excision,
  Nerve, Phrenic 01B2
Phrenemphraxis see Destruction, Nerve,
  Phrenic 0152
Phrenic nerve stimulator generator use
  Stimulator Generator in Subcutaneous
  Tissue and Fascia
Phrenic nerve stimulator lead use
  Diaphragmatic Pacemaker Lead in
  Respiratory System
Phreniclasis see Destruction, Nerve, Phrenic
  0152
Phrenicoexeresis see Extraction, Nerve, Phrenic
  01D2
Phrenicotomy see Division, Nerve, Phrenic
  0182
Phrenicotripsy see Destruction, Nerve, Phrenic
  0152
Phrenoplasty
  see Repair, Respiratory System 0BQ
  see Supplement, Respiratory System 0BU
Phrenotomy see Drainage, Respiratory System
  0B9
Physiatry see Motor Treatment, Rehabilitation
  F07
Physical medicine see Motor Treatment,
  Rehabilitation F07
Physical therapy see Motor Treatment,
  Rehabilitation F07
PHYSIOMESH™ Flexible Composite Mesh use
  Synthetic Substitute
Pia mater, intracranial use Cerebral Meninges
Pia mater, spinal use Spinal Meninges
Pinealectomy
  see Excision, Pineal Body 0GB1
  see Resection, Pineal Body 0GT1
Pinealoscopy 0GJ14ZZ
Pinealotomy see Drainage, Pineal Body 0G91
Pinna
  use External Ear, Right
  use External Ear, Left
  use External Ear, Bilateral
Pipeline™ Embolization device (PED) use
  Intraluminal Device
Piriform recess (sinus) use Pharynx
Piriformis muscle
  use Hip Muscle, Right
  use Hip Muscle, Left
PIRRT (Prolonged intermittent renal
  replacement therapy) 5A1D80Z
Pisiform bone
  use Carpal, Right
  use Carpal, Left
Pisohamate ligament
  use Hand Bursa and Ligament, Right
  use Hand Bursa and Ligament, Left
Pisometacarpal ligament
  use Hand Bursa and Ligament, Right
  use Hand Bursa and Ligament, Left
Pituitectomy
  see Excision, Gland, Pituitary 0GB0
  see Resection, Gland, Pituitary 0GT0
Plain film radiology see Plain Radiography
Plain Radiography
  Abdomen BW00ZZZ
  Abdomen and Pelvis BW01ZZZ
  Abdominal Lymphatic
    Bilateral B701
    Unilateral B700
  Airway, Upper BB0DZZZ
  Ankle
    Left BQ0H
    Right BQ0G

▶ New   ➥ Revised   ~~deleted~~ Deleted

▶ New   ⮕ Revised   ~~deleted~~ Deleted

▶ New   ⇛ Revised   ~~deleted~~ Deleted

Plaque Radiation (*Continued*)
Chest DWY2FZZ
Chest Wall DBY7FZZ
Colon DDY5FZZ
Diaphragm DBY8FZZ
Duodenum DDY2FZZ
Ear D9Y0FZZ
Esophagus DDY0FZZ
Eye D8Y0FZZ
Femur DPY9FZZ
Fibula DPYBFZZ
Gallbladder DFY1FZZ
Gland
    Adrenal DGY2FZZ
    Parathyroid DGY4FZZ
    Pituitary DGY0FZZ
    Thyroid DGY5FZZ
Glands, Salivary D9Y6FZZ
Head and Neck DWY1FZZ
Hemibody DWY4FZZ
Humerus DPY6FZZ
Ileum DDY4FZZ
Jejunum DDY3FZZ
Kidney DTY0FZZ
Larynx D9YBFZZ
Liver DFY0FZZ
Lung DBY2FZZ
Lymphatics
    Abdomen D7Y6FZZ
    Axillary D7Y4FZZ
    Inguinal D7Y8FZZ
    Neck D7Y3FZZ
    Pelvis D7Y7FZZ
    Thorax D7Y5FZZ
Mandible DPY3FZZ
Maxilla DPY2FZZ
Mediastinum DBY6FZZ
Mouth D9Y4FZZ
Nasopharynx D9YDFZZ
Neck and Head DWY1FZZ
Nerve, Peripheral D0Y7FZZ
Nose D9Y1FZZ
Ovary DUY0FZZ
Palate
    Hard D9Y8FZZ
    Soft D9Y9FZZ
Pancreas DFY3FZZ
Parathyroid Gland DGY4FZZ
Pelvic Bones DPY8FZZ
Pelvic Region DWY6FZZ
Pharynx D9YCFZZ
Pineal Body DGY1FZZ
Pituitary Gland DGY0FZZ
Pleura DBY5FZZ
Prostate DVY0FZZ
Radius DPY7FZZ
Rectum DDY7FZZ
Rib DPY5FZZ
Sinuses D9Y7FZZ
Skin
    Abdomen DHY8FZZ
    Arm DHY4FZZ
    Back DHY7FZZ
    Buttock DHY9FZZ
    Chest DHY6FZZ
    Face DHY2FZZ
    Foot DHYCFZZ
    Hand DHY5FZZ
    Leg DHYBFZZ
    Neck DHY3FZZ
Skull DPY0FZZ
Spinal Cord D0Y6FZZ
Spleen D7Y2FZZ
Sternum DPY4FZZ
Stomach DDY1FZZ
Testis DVY1FZZ
Thymus D7Y1FZZ
Thyroid Gland DGY5FZZ
Tibia DPYBFZZ

Plaque Radiation (*Continued*)
Tongue D9Y5FZZ
Trachea DBY0FZZ
Ulna DPY7FZZ
Ureter DTY1FZZ
Urethra DTY3FZZ
Uterus DUY2FZZ
Whole Body DWY5FZZ
Plasmapheresis, therapeutic *see* Pheresis,
    Physiological Systems 6A5
Plateletpheresis, therapeutic *see* Pheresis,
    Physiological Systems 6A5
Platysma muscle
    use Neck Muscle, Right
    use Neck Muscle, Left
▶Plazomicin Anti-infective XW0
Pleurectomy
    see Excision, Respiratory System 0BB
    see Resection, Respiratory System 0BT
Pleurocentesis *see* Drainage, Anatomical
    Regions, General 0W9
Pleurodesis, pleurosclerosis
⇒Chemical Injection *see* Introduction of
        substance in or on, Pleural Cavity 3E0L
    Surgical *see* Destruction, Respiratory System
        0B5
Pleurolysis *see* Release, Respiratory System 0BN
Pleuroscopy 0BJQ4ZZ
Pleurotomy *see* Drainage, Respiratory System
    0B9
Plica semilunaris
    use Conjunctiva, Right
    use Conjunctiva, Left
Plication *see* Restriction
Pneumectomy
    see Excision, Respiratory System 0BB
    see Resection, Respiratory System 0BT
Pneumocentesis *see* Drainage, Respiratory
    System 0B9
Pneumogastric nerve *use* Vagus Nerve
Pneumolysis *see* Release, Respiratory System
    0BN
Pneumonectomy *see* Resection, Respiratory
    System 0BT
Pneumonolysis *see* Release, Respiratory System
    0BN
Pneumonopexy
    see Repair, Respiratory System 0BQ
    see Reposition, Respiratory System 0BS
Pneumonorrhaphy *see* Repair, Respiratory
    System 0BQ
Pneumonotomy *see* Drainage, Respiratory
    System 0B9
Pneumotaxic center *use* Pons
Pneumotomy *see* Drainage, Respiratory System
    0B9
Pollicization *see* Transfer, Anatomical Regions,
    Upper Extremities 0XX
Polyethylene socket *use* Synthetic Substitute,
    Polyethylene in 0SR
Polymethylmethacrylate (PMMA) *use*
    Synthetic Substitute
Polypectomy, gastrointestinal *see* Excision,
    Gastrointestinal System 0DB
Polypropylene mesh *use* Synthetic Substitute
Polysomnogram 4A1ZXQZ
Pontine tegmentum *use* Pons
Popliteal ligament
    use Knee Bursa and Ligament, Right
    use Knee Bursa and Ligament, Left
Popliteal lymph node
    use Lymphatic, Right Lower Extremity
    use Lymphatic, Left Lower Extremity
Popliteal vein
    use Femoral Vein, Right
    use Femoral Vein, Left
Popliteus muscle
    use Lower Leg Muscle, Right
    use Lower Leg Muscle, Left

Porcine (bioprosthetic) valve *use* Zooplastic
    Tissue in Heart and Great Vessels
Positive end expiratory pressure *see*
    Performance, Respiratory 5A19
Positron Emission Tomographic (PET)
        Imaging
    Brain C030
    Bronchi and Lungs CB32
    Central Nervous System C03YYZZ
    Heart C23YYZZ
    Lungs and Bronchi CB32
    Myocardium C23G
    Respiratory System CB3YYZZ
    Whole Body CW3NYZZ
Positron emission tomography *see* Positron
    Emission Tomographic (PET) Imaging
Postauricular (mastoid) lymph node
    use Lymphatic, Right Neck
    use Lymphatic, Left Neck
Postcava *use* Inferior Vena Cava
Posterior (subscapular) lymph node
    use Lymphatic, Right Axillary
    use Lymphatic, Left Axillary
Posterior auricular artery
    use External Carotid Artery, Right
    use External Carotid Artery, Left
Posterior auricular nerve *use* Facial Nerve
Posterior auricular vein
    use External Jugular Vein, Right
    use External Jugular Vein, Left
Posterior cerebral artery *use* Intracranial
    Artery
Posterior chamber
    use Eye, Right
    use Eye, Left
Posterior circumflex humeral artery
    use Axillary Artery, Right
    use Axillary Artery, Left
Posterior communicating artery *use* Intracranial
    Artery
Posterior cruciate ligament (PCL)
    use Knee Bursa and Ligament, Right
    use Knee Bursa and Ligament, Left
Posterior facial (retromandibular) vein
    use Face Vein, Right
    use Face Vein, Left
Posterior femoral cutaneous nerve *use* Sacral
    Plexus Nerve
Posterior inferior cerebellar artery (PICA) *use*
    Intracranial Artery
Posterior interosseous nerve *use* Radial
    Nerve
Posterior labial nerve *use* Pudendal Nerve
Posterior scrotal nerve *use* Pudendal
    Nerve
Posterior spinal artery
    use Vertebral Artery, Right
    use Vertebral Artery, Left
Posterior tibial recurrent artery
    use Anterior Tibial Artery, Right
    use Anterior Tibial Artery, Left
Posterior ulnar recurrent artery
    use Ulnar Artery, Right
    use Ulnar Artery, Left
Posterior vagal trunk *use* Vagus Nerve
PPN (peripheral parenteral nutrition) *see*
    Introduction of Nutritional Substance
Preauricular lymph node *use* Lymphatic,
    Head
Precava *use* Superior Vena Cava
Prepatellar bursa
    use Knee Bursa and Ligament, Right
    use Knee Bursa and Ligament, Left
Preputiotomy *see* Drainage, Male Reproductive
    System 0V9
Pressure support ventilation *see* Performance,
    Respiratory 5A19
PRESTIGE® Cervical Disc *use* Synthetic
    Substitute

Pretracheal fascia
  use Subcutaneous Tissue and Fascia, Right Neck
  use Subcutaneous Tissue and Fascia, Left Neck
Prevertebral fascia
  use Subcutaneous Tissue and Fascia, Right Neck
  use Subcutaneous Tissue and Fascia, Left Neck
PrimeAdvanced neurostimulator (SureScan) (MRI Safe) *use* Stimulator Generator, Multiple Array in ØJH
Princeps pollicis artery
  use Hand Artery, Right
  use Hand Artery, Left
Probing, duct
  Diagnostic *see* Inspection
  Dilation *see* Dilation
PROCEED™ Ventral Patch *use* Synthetic Substitute
Procerus muscle *use* Facial Muscle
Proctectomy
  see Excision, Rectum ØDBP
  see Resection, Rectum ØDTP
Proctoclysis *see* Introduction of substance in or on, Gastrointestinal Tract, Lower 3EØH
Proctocolectomy
  see Excision, Gastrointestinal System ØDB
  see Resection, Gastrointestinal System ØDT
Proctocolpoplasty
  see Repair, Gastrointestinal System ØDQ
  see Supplement, Gastrointestinal System ØDU
Proctoperineoplasty
  see Repair, Gastrointestinal System ØDQ
  see Supplement, Gastrointestinal System ØDU
Proctoperineorrhaphy *see* Repair, Gastrointestinal System ØDQ
Proctopexy
  see Repair, Rectum ØDQP
  see Reposition, Rectum ØDSP
Proctoplasty
  see Repair, Rectum ØDQP
  see Supplement, Rectum ØDUP
Proctorrhaphy *see* Repair, Rectum ØDQP
Proctoscopy ØDJD8ZZ
Proctosigmoidectomy
  see Excision, Gastrointestinal System ØDB
  see Resection, Gastrointestinal System ØDT
Proctosigmoidoscopy ØDJD8ZZ
Proctostomy *see* Drainage, Rectum ØD9P
Proctotomy *see* Drainage, Rectum ØD9P
Prodisc-C *use* Synthetic Substitute
Prodisc-L *use* Synthetic Substitute
Production, atrial septal defect *see* Excision, Septum, Atrial Ø2B5
Profunda brachii
  use Brachial Artery, Right
  use Brachial Artery, Left
Profunda femoris (deep femoral) vein
  use Femoral Vein, Right
  use Femoral Vein, Left
PROLENE Polypropylene Hernia System (PHS) *use* Synthetic Substitute
Pronator quadratus muscle
  use Lower Arm and Wrist Muscle, Right
  use Lower Arm and Wrist Muscle, Left
Pronator teres muscle
  use Lower Arm and Wrist Muscle, Right
  use Lower Arm and Wrist Muscle, Left
Prostatectomy
  see Excision, Prostate ØVBØ
  see Resection, Prostate ØVTØ
Prostatic urethra *use* Urethra
Prostatomy, prostatotomy *see* Drainage, Prostate ØV9Ø

Protecta XT CRT-D *use* Cardiac Resynchronization Defibrillator Pulse Generator in ØJH
Protecta XT DR (XT VR) *use* Defibrillator Generator in ØJH
Protégé® RX Carotid Stent System *use* Intraluminal Device
Proximal radioulnar joint
  use Elbow Joint, Right
  use Elbow Joint, Left
Psoas muscle
  use Hip Muscle, Right
  use Hip Muscle, Left
PSV (pressure support ventilation) *see* Performance, Respiratory 5A19
Psychoanalysis GZ54ZZZ
Psychological Tests
  Cognitive Status GZ14ZZZ
  Developmental GZ10ZZZ
  Intellectual and Psychoeducational GZ12ZZZ
  Neurobehavioral Status GZ14ZZZ
  Neuropsychological GZ13ZZZ
  Personality and Behavioral GZ11ZZZ
Psychotherapy
  Family, Mental Health Services GZ72ZZZ
  Group
    GZHZZZZ
    Mental Health Services GZHZZZZ
  Individual
    see Psychotherapy, Individual, Mental Health Services
    for substance abuse
      12-Step HZ53ZZZ
      Behavioral HZ51ZZZ
      Cognitive HZ50ZZZ
      Cognitive-Behavioral HZ52ZZZ
      Confrontational HZ58ZZZ
      Interactive HZ55ZZZ
      Interpersonal HZ54ZZZ
      Motivational Enhancement HZ57ZZZ
      Psychoanalysis HZ5BZZZ
      Psychodynamic HZ5CZZZ
      Psychoeducation HZ56ZZZ
      Psychophysiological HZ5DZZZ
      Supportive HZ59ZZZ
    Mental Health Services
      Behavioral GZ51ZZZ
      Cognitive GZ52ZZZ
      Cognitive-Behavioral GZ58ZZZ
      Interactive GZ50ZZZ
      Interpersonal GZ53ZZZ
      Psychoanalysis GZ54ZZZ
      Psychodynamic GZ55ZZZ
      Psychophysiological GZ59ZZZ
      Supportive GZ56ZZZ
PTCA (percutaneous transluminal coronary angioplasty) *see* Dilation, Heart and Great Vessels Ø27
Pterygoid muscle *use* Head Muscle
Pterygoid process *use* Sphenoid Bone
Pterygopalatine (sphenopalatine) ganglion *use* Head and Neck Sympathetic Nerve
Pubis
  use Pelvic Bone, Right
  use Pelvic Bone, Left
Pubofemoral ligament
  use Hip Bursa and Ligament, Right
  use Hip Bursa and Ligament, Left
Pudendal nerve *use* Sacral Plexus
Pull-through, laparoscopic-assisted transanal
  see Excision, Gastrointestinal System ØDB
  see Resection, Gastrointestinal System ØDT
Pull-through, rectal *see* Resection, Rectum ØDTP
Pulmoaortic canal *use* Pulmonary Artery, Left

Pulmonary annulus *use* Pulmonary Valve
Pulmonary artery wedge monitoring *see* Monitoring, Arterial 4A13
Pulmonary plexus
  use Vagus Nerve
  use Thoracic Sympathetic Nerve
Pulmonic valve *use* Pulmonary Valve
Pulpectomy *see* Excision, Mouth and Throat ØCB
Pulverization *see* Fragmentation
Pulvinar *use* Thalamus
Pump reservoir *use* Infusion Device, Pump in Subcutaneous Tissue and Fascia
Punch biopsy *see* Excision with qualifier Diagnostic
Puncture *see* Drainage
Puncture, lumbar *see* Drainage, Spinal Canal ØØ9U
Pyelography
  see Plain Radiography, Urinary System BTØ
  see Fluoroscopy, Urinary System BT1
Pyeloileostomy, urinary diversion *see* Bypass, Urinary System ØT1
Pyeloplasty
  see Repair, Urinary System ØTQ
  see Replacement, Urinary System ØTR
  see Supplement, Urinary System ØTU
Pyelorrhaphy *see* Repair, Urinary System ØTQ
Pyeloscopy ØTJ58ZZ
Pyelostomy
  see Bypass, Urinary System ØT1
  see Drainage, Urinary System ØT9
Pyelotomy *see* Drainage, Urinary System ØT9
Pylorectomy
  see Excision, Stomach, Pylorus ØDB7
  see Resection, Stomach, Pylorus ØDT7
Pyloric antrum *use* Stomach, Pylorus
Pyloric canal *use* Stomach, Pylorus
Pyloric sphincter *use* Stomach, Pylorus
Pylorodiosis *see* Dilation, Stomach, Pylorus ØD77
Pylorogastrectomy
  see Excision, Gastrointestinal System ØDB
  see Resection, Gastrointestinal System ØDT
Pyloroplasty
  see Repair, Stomach, Pylorus ØDQ7
  see Supplement, Stomach, Pylorus ØDU7
Pyloroscopy ØDJ68ZZ
Pylorotomy *see* Drainage, Stomach, Pylorus ØD97
Pyramidalis muscle
  use Abdomen Muscle, Right
  use Abdomen Muscle, Left

Q

Quadrangular cartilage *use* Nasal Septum
Quadrant resection of breast *see* Excision, Skin and Breast ØHB
Quadrate lobe *use* Liver
Quadratus femoris muscle
  use Hip Muscle, Right
  use Hip Muscle, Left
Quadratus lumborum muscle
  use Trunk Muscle, Right
  use Trunk Muscle, Left
Quadratus plantae muscle
  use Foot Muscle, Right
  use Foot Muscle, Left
Quadriceps (femoris)
  use Upper Leg Muscle, Right
  use Upper Leg Muscle, Left
Quarantine 8EØZXY6

▶ New   ⇒ Revised   ~~deleted~~ Deleted

R

Radial collateral carpal ligament
  use Wrist Bursa and Ligament, Right
  use Wrist Bursa and Ligament, Left
Radial collateral ligament
  use Elbow Bursa and Ligament, Right
  use Elbow Bursa and Ligament, Left
Radial notch
  use Ulna, Right
  use Ulna, Left
Radial recurrent artery
  use Radial Artery, Right
  use Radial Artery, Left
Radial vein
  use Brachial Vein, Right
  use Brachial Vein, Left
Radialis indicis
  use Hand Artery, Right
  use Hand Artery, Left
Radiation Therapy
  see Beam Radiation
  see Brachytherapy
  see Stereotactic Radiosurgery
Radiation treatment *see* Radiation
    Therapy
Radiocarpal joint
  use Wrist Joint, Right
  use Wrist Joint, Left
Radiocarpal ligament
  use Wrist Bursa and Ligament, Right
  use Wrist Bursa and Ligament, Left
Radiography *see* Plain Radiography
Radiology, analog *see* Plain Radiography
Radiology, diagnostic *see* Imaging,
    Diagnostic
Radioulnar ligament
  use Wrist Bursa and Ligament, Right
  use Wrist Bursa and Ligament, Left
Range of motion testing *see* Motor
    Function Assessment, Rehabilitation
    F01
REALIZE® Adjustable Gastric Band *use*
    Extraluminal Device
Reattachment
  Abdominal Wall 0WMF0ZZ
  Ampulla of Vater 0FMC
  Ankle Region
    Left 0YML0ZZ
    Right 0YMK0ZZ
  Arm
    Lower
      Left 0XMF0ZZ
      Right 0XMD0ZZ
    Upper
      Left 0XM90ZZ
      Right 0XM80ZZ
  Axilla
    Left 0XM50ZZ
    Right 0XM40ZZ
  Back
    Lower 0WML0ZZ
    Upper 0WMK0ZZ
  Bladder 0TMB
  Bladder Neck 0TMC
  Breast
    Bilateral 0HMVXZZ
    Left 0HMUXZZ
    Right 0HMTXZZ
  Bronchus
    Lingula 0BM90ZZ
    Lower Lobe
      Left 0BMB0ZZ
      Right 0BM60ZZ
    Main
      Left 0BM70ZZ
      Right 0BM30ZZ
    Middle Lobe, Right 0BM50ZZ
    Upper Lobe
      Left 0BM80ZZ
      Right 0BM40ZZ

Reattachment *(Continued)*
  Bursa and Ligament
    Abdomen
      Left 0MMJ
      Right 0MMH
    Ankle
      Left 0MMR
      Right 0MMQ
    Elbow
      Left 0MM4
      Right 0MM3
    Foot
      Left 0MMT
      Right 0MMS
    Hand
      Left 0MM8
      Right 0MM7
    Head and Neck 0MM0
    Hip
      Left 0MMM
      Right 0MML
    Knee
      Left 0MMP
      Right 0MMN
    Lower Extremity
      Left 0MMW
      Right 0MMV
    Perineum 0MMK
    Rib(s) 0MMG
    Shoulder
      Left 0MM2
      Right 0MM1
    Spine
      Lower 0MMD
      Upper 0MMC
    Sternum 0MMF
    Upper Extremity
      Left 0MMB
      Right 0MM9
    Wrist
      Left 0MM6
      Right 0MM5
  Buttock
    Left 0YM10ZZ
    Right 0YM00ZZ
  Carina 0BM20ZZ
  Cecum 0DMH
  Cervix 0UMC
  Chest Wall 0WM80ZZ
  Clitoris 0UMJXZZ
  Colon
    Ascending 0DMK
    Descending 0DMM
    Sigmoid 0DMN
    Transverse 0DML
  Cord
    Bilateral 0VMH
    Left 0VMG
    Right 0VMF
  Cul-de-sac 0UMF
  Diaphragm 0BMT0ZZ
  Duct
    Common Bile 0FM9
    Cystic 0FM8
    Hepatic
      Common 0FM7
      Left 0FM6
      Right 0FM5
    Pancreatic 0FMD
      Accessory 0FMF
  Duodenum 0DM9
  Ear
    Left 09M1XZZ
    Right 09M0XZZ
  Elbow Region
    Left 0XMC0ZZ
    Right 0XMB0ZZ
  Esophagus 0DM5
  Extremity
    Lower
      Left 0YMB0ZZ
      Right 0YM90ZZ

Reattachment *(Continued)*
  Extremity *(Continued)*
    Upper
      Left 0XM70ZZ
      Right 0XM60ZZ
  Eyelid
    Lower
      Left 08MRXZZ
      Right 08MQXZZ
    Upper
      Left 08MPXZZ
      Right 08MNXZZ
  Face 0WM20ZZ
  Fallopian Tube
    Left 0UM6
    Right 0UM5
  Fallopian Tubes, Bilateral 0UM7
  Femoral Region
    Left 0YM80ZZ
    Right 0YM70ZZ
  Finger
    Index
      Left 0XMP0ZZ
      Right 0XMN0ZZ
    Little
      Left 0XMW0ZZ
      Right 0XMV0ZZ
    Middle
      Left 0XMR0ZZ
      Right 0XMQ0ZZ
    Ring
      Left 0XMT0ZZ
      Right 0XMS0ZZ
  Foot
    Left 0YMN0ZZ
    Right 0YMM0ZZ
  Forequarter
    Left 0XM10ZZ
    Right 0XM00ZZ
  Gallbladder 0FM4
  Gland
    Adrenal
      Left 0GM2
      Right 0GM3
  Hand
    Left 0XMK0ZZ
    Right 0XMJ0ZZ
  Hindquarter
    Bilateral 0YM40ZZ
    Left 0YM30ZZ
    Right 0YM20ZZ
  Hymen 0UMK
  Ileum 0DMB
  Inguinal Region
    Left 0YM60ZZ
    Right 0YM50ZZ
  Intestine
    Large 0DME
      Left 0DMG
      Right 0DMF
    Small 0DM8
  Jaw
    Lower 0WM50ZZ
    Upper 0WM40ZZ
  Jejunum 0DMA
  Kidney
    Left 0TM1
    Right 0TM0
  Kidney Pelvis
    Left 0TM4
    Right 0TM3
  Kidneys, Bilateral 0TM2
  Knee Region
    Left 0YMG0ZZ
    Right 0YMF0ZZ
  Leg
    Lower
      Left 0YMJ0ZZ
      Right 0YMH0ZZ
    Upper
      Left 0YMD0ZZ
      Right 0YMC0ZZ

Reattachment *(Continued)*
Lip
Lower 0CM10ZZ
Upper 0CM00ZZ
Liver 0FM0
Left Lobe 0FM2
Right Lobe 0FM1
Lung
Left 0BML0ZZ
Lower Lobe
Left 0BMJ0ZZ
Right 0BMF0ZZ
Middle Lobe, Right 0BMD0ZZ
Right 0BMK0ZZ
Upper Lobe
Left 0BMG0ZZ
Right 0BMC0ZZ
Lung Lingula 0BMH0ZZ
Muscle
Abdomen
Left 0KML
Right 0KMK
Facial 0KM1
Foot
Left 0KMW
Right 0KMV
Hand
Left 0KMD
Right 0KMC
Head 0KM0
Hip
Left 0KMP
Right 0KMN
Lower Arm and Wrist
Left 0KMB
Right 0KM9
Lower Leg
Left 0KMT
Right 0KMS
Neck
Left 0KM3
Right 0KM2
Perineum 0KMM
Shoulder
Left 0KM6
Right 0KM5
Thorax
Left 0KMJ
Right 0KMH
Tongue, Palate, Pharynx 0KM4
Trunk
Left 0KMG
Right 0KMF
Upper Arm
Left 0KM8
Right 0KM7
Upper Leg
Left 0KMR
Right 0KMQ
Nasal Mucosa and Soft Tissue 09MKXZZ
Neck 0WM60ZZ
Nipple
Left 0HMXXZZ
Right 0HMWXZZ
Ovary
Bilateral 0UM2
Left 0UM1
Right 0UM0
Palate, Soft 0CM30ZZ
Pancreas 0FMG
Parathyroid Gland 0GMR
Inferior
Left 0GMP
Right 0GMN
Multiple 0GMQ
Superior
Left 0GMM
Right 0GML
Penis 0VMSXZZ
Perineum
Female 0WMN0ZZ
Male 0WMM0ZZ

Reattachment *(Continued)*
Rectum 0DMP
Scrotum 0VM5XZZ
Shoulder Region
Left 0XM30ZZ
Right 0XM20ZZ
Skin
Abdomen 0HM7XZZ
Back 0HM6XZZ
Buttock 0HM8XZZ
Chest 0HM5XZZ
Ear
Left 0HM3XZZ
Right 0HM2XZZ
Face 0HM1XZZ
Foot
Left 0HMNXZZ
Right 0HMMXZZ
Hand
Left 0HMGXZZ
Right 0HMFXZZ
Inguinal 0HMAXZZ
Lower Arm
Left 0HMEXZZ
Right 0HMDXZZ
Lower Leg
Left 0HMLXZZ
Right 0HMKXZZ
Neck 0HM4XZZ
Perineum 0HM9XZZ
Scalp 0HM0XZZ
Upper Arm
Left 0HMCXZZ
Right 0HMBXZZ
Upper Leg
Left 0HMJXZZ
Right 0HMHXZZ
Stomach 0DM6
Tendon
Abdomen
Left 0LMG
Right 0LMF
Ankle
Left 0LMT
Right 0LMS
Foot
Left 0LMW
Right 0LMV
Hand
Left 0LM8
Right 0LM7
Head and Neck 0LM0
Hip
Left 0LMK
Right 0LMJ
Knee
Left 0LMR
Right 0LMQ
Lower Arm and Wrist
Left 0LM6
Right 0LM5
Lower Leg
Left 0LMP
Right 0LMN
Perineum 0LMH
Shoulder
Left 0LM2
Right 0LM1
Thorax
Left 0LMD
Right 0LMC
Trunk
Left 0LMB
Right 0LM9
Upper Arm
Left 0LM4
Right 0LM3
Upper Leg
Left 0LMM
Right 0LML

Reattachment *(Continued)*
Testis
Bilateral 0VMC
Left 0VMB
Right 0VM9
Thumb
Left 0XMM0ZZ
Right 0XML0ZZ
Thyroid Gland
Left Lobe 0GMG
Right Lobe 0GMH
Toe
1st
Left 0YMQ0ZZ
Right 0YMP0ZZ
2nd
Left 0YMS0ZZ
Right 0YMR0ZZ
3rd
Left 0YMU0ZZ
Right 0YMT0ZZ
4th
Left 0YMW0ZZ
Right 0YMV0ZZ
5th
Left 0YMY0ZZ
Right 0YMX0ZZ
Tongue 0CM70ZZ
Tooth
Lower 0CMX
Upper 0CMW
Trachea 0BM10ZZ
Tunica Vaginalis
Left 0VM7
Right 0VM6
Ureter
Left 0TM7
Right 0TM6
Ureters, Bilateral 0TM8
Urethra 0TMD
Uterine Supporting Structure 0UM4
Uterus 0UM9
Uvula 0CMN0ZZ
Vagina 0UMG
Vulva 0UMMXZZ
Wrist Region
Left 0XMH0ZZ
Right 0XMG0ZZ
REBOA (resuscitative endovascular balloon occlusion of the aorta)
02LW3DJ
04L03DJ
Rebound HRD® (Hernia Repair Device) *use* Synthetic Substitute
Recession
see Repair
see Reposition
Reclosure, disrupted abdominal wall
0WQFXZZ
Reconstruction
see Repair
see Replacement
see Supplement
Rectectomy
see Excision, Rectum 0DBP
see Resection, Rectum 0DTP
Rectocele repair
see Repair, Subcutaneous Tissue and Fascia, Pelvic Region 0JQC
Rectopexy
see Repair, Gastrointestinal System 0DQ
see Reposition, Gastrointestinal System 0DS
Rectoplasty
see Repair, Gastrointestinal System 0DQ
see Supplement, Gastrointestinal System 0DU
Rectorrhaphy *see* Repair, Gastrointestinal System 0DQ
Rectoscopy 0DJD8ZZ
Rectosigmoid junction *use* Colon, Sigmoid

▶ New   ⇒ Revised   ~~deleted~~ Deleted

Rectosigmoidectomy
  see Excision, Gastrointestinal System ØDB
  see Resection, Gastrointestinal System ØDT
Rectostomy *see* Drainage, Rectum ØD9P
Rectotomy *see* Drainage, Rectum ØD9P
Rectus abdominis muscle
  use Abdomen Muscle, Right
  use Abdomen Muscle, Left
Rectus femoris muscle
  use Upper Leg Muscle, Right
  use Upper Leg Muscle, Left
Recurrent laryngeal nerve *use* Vagus Nerve
Reduction
  Dislocation *see* Reposition
  Fracture *see* Reposition
  Intussusception, intestinal *see* Reposition,
    Gastrointestinal System ØDS
  Mammoplasty *see* Excision, Skin and Breast
    ØHB
  Prolapse *see* Reposition
  Torsion *see* Reposition
  Volvulus, gastrointestinal *see* Reposition,
    Gastrointestinal System ØDS
Refusion *see* Fusion
Rehabilitation
  see Speech Assessment, Rehabilitation FØØ
  see Motor Function Assessment,
    Rehabilitation FØ1
  see Activities of Daily Living Assessment,
    Rehabilitation FØ2
  see Speech Treatment, Rehabilitation FØ6
  see Motor Treatment, Rehabilitation FØ7
  see Activities of Daily Living Treatment,
    Rehabilitation FØ8
  see Hearing Treatment, Rehabilitation FØ9
  see Cochlear Implant Treatment,
    Rehabilitation FØB
  see Vestibular Treatment, Rehabilitation FØC
  see Device Fitting, Rehabilitation FØD
  see Caregiver Training, Rehabilitation FØF
Reimplantation
  see Reattachment
  see Reposition
  see Transfer
Reinforcement
  see Repair
  see Supplement
Relaxation, scar tissue *see* Release
Release
  Acetabulum
    Left ØQN5
    Right ØQN4
  Adenoids ØCNQ
  Ampulla of Vater ØFNC
  Anal Sphincter ØDNR
  Anterior Chamber
    Left Ø8N33ZZ
    Right Ø8N23ZZ
  Anus ØDNQ
  Aorta
    Abdominal Ø4NØ
    Thoracic
      Ascending/Arch Ø2NX
      Descending Ø2NW
  Aortic Body ØGND
  Appendix ØDNJ
  Artery
    Anterior Tibial
      Left Ø4NQ
      Right Ø4NP
    Axillary
      Left Ø3N6
      Right Ø3N5
    Brachial
      Left Ø3N8
      Right Ø3N7
    Celiac Ø4N1
    Colic
      Left Ø4N7
      Middle Ø4N8
      Right Ø4N6

Release *(Continued)*
  Artery *(Continued)*
    Common Carotid
      Left Ø3NJ
      Right Ø3NH
    Common Iliac
      Left Ø4ND
      Right Ø4NC
    Coronary
      Four or More Arteries Ø2N3
      One Artery Ø2NØ
      Three Arteries Ø2N2
      Two Arteries Ø2N1
    External Carotid
      Left Ø3NN
      Right Ø3NM
    External Iliac
      Left Ø4NJ
      Right Ø4NH
    Face Ø3NR
    Femoral
      Left Ø4NL
      Right Ø4NK
    Foot
      Left Ø4NW
      Right Ø4NV
    Gastric Ø4N2
    Hand
      Left Ø3NF
      Right Ø3ND
    Hepatic Ø4N3
    Inferior Mesenteric Ø4NB
    Innominate Ø3N2
    Internal Carotid
      Left Ø3NL
      Right Ø3NK
    Internal Iliac
      Left Ø4NF
      Right Ø4NE
    Internal Mammary
      Left Ø3N1
      Right Ø3NØ
    Intracranial Ø3NG
    Lower Ø4NY
    Peroneal
      Left Ø4NU
      Right Ø4NT
    Popliteal
      Left Ø4NN
      Right Ø4NM
    Posterior Tibial
      Left Ø4NS
      Right Ø4NR
    Pulmonary
      Left Ø2NR
      Right Ø2NQ
    Pulmonary Trunk Ø2NP
    Radial
      Left Ø3NC
      Right Ø3NB
    Renal
      Left Ø4NA
      Right Ø4N9
    Splenic Ø4N4
    Subclavian
      Left Ø3N4
      Right Ø3N3
    Superior Mesenteric Ø4N5
    Temporal
      Left Ø3NT
      Right Ø3NS
    Thyroid
      Left Ø3NV
      Right Ø3NU
    Ulnar
      Left Ø3NA
      Right Ø3N9
    Upper Ø3NY
    Vertebral
      Left Ø3NQ
      Right Ø3NP

Release *(Continued)*
  Atrium
    Left Ø2N7
    Right Ø2N6
  Auditory Ossicle
    Left Ø9NA
    Right Ø9N9
  Basal Ganglia ØØN8
  Bladder ØTNB
  Bladder Neck ØTNC
  Bone
    Ethmoid
      Left ØNNG
      Right ØNNF
    Frontal ØNN1
    Hyoid ØNNX
    Lacrimal
      Left ØNNJ
      Right ØNNH
    Nasal ØNNB
    Occipital ØNN7
    Palatine
      Left ØNNL
      Right ØNNK
    Parietal
      Left ØNN4
      Right ØNN3
    Pelvic
      Left ØQN3
      Right ØQN2
    Sphenoid ØNNC
    Temporal
      Left ØNN6
      Right ØNN5
    Zygomatic
      Left ØNNN
      Right ØNNM
  Brain ØØNØ
  Breast
    Bilateral ØHNV
    Left ØHNU
    Right ØHNT
  Bronchus
    Lingula ØBN9
    Lower Lobe
      Left ØBNB
      Right ØBN6
    Main
      Left ØBN7
      Right ØBN3
    Middle Lobe, Right ØBN5
    Upper Lobe
      Left ØBN8
      Right ØBN4
  Buccal Mucosa ØCN4
  Bursa and Ligament
    Abdomen
      Left ØMNJ
      Right ØMNH
    Ankle
      Left ØMNR
      Right ØMNQ
    Elbow
      Left ØMN4
      Right ØMN3
    Foot
      Left ØMNT
      Right ØMNS
    Hand
      Left ØMN8
      Right ØMN7
    Head and Neck ØMNØ
    Hip
      Left ØMNM
      Right ØMNL
    Knee
      Left ØMNP
      Right ØMNN
    Lower Extremity
      Left ØMNW
      Right ØMNV

Release *(Continued)*
  Bursa and Ligament *(Continued)*
    Perineum ØMNK
    Rib(s) ØMNG
    Shoulder
      Left ØMN2
      Right ØMN1
    Spine
      Lower ØMND
      Upper ØMNC
    Sternum ØMNF
    Upper Extremity
      Left ØMNB
      Right ØMN9
    Wrist
      Left ØMN6
      Right ØMN5
  Carina ØBN2
  Carotid Bodies, Bilateral ØGN8
  Carotid Body
    Left ØGN6
    Right ØGN7
  Carpal
    Left ØPNN
    Right ØPNM
  Cecum ØDNH
  Cerebellum ØØNC
  Cerebral Hemisphere ØØN7
  Cerebral Meninges ØØN1
  Cerebral Ventricle ØØN6
  Cervix ØUNC
  Chordae Tendineae Ø2N9
  Choroid
    Left Ø8NB
    Right Ø8NA
  Cisterna Chyli Ø7NL
  Clavicle
    Left ØPNB
    Right ØPN9
  Clitoris ØUNJ
  Coccygeal Glomus ØGNB
  Coccyx ØQNS
  Colon
    Ascending ØDNK
    Descending ØDNM
    Sigmoid ØDNN
    Transverse ØDNL
  Conduction Mechanism Ø2N8
  Conjunctiva
    Left Ø8NTXZZ
    Right Ø8NSXZZ
  Cord
    Bilateral ØVNH
    Left ØVNG
    Right ØVNF
  Cornea
    Left Ø8N9XZZ
    Right Ø8N8XZZ
  Cul-de-sac ØUNF
  Diaphragm ØBNT
  Disc
    Cervical Vertebral ØRN3
    Cervicothoracic Vertebral ØRN5
    Lumbar Vertebral ØSN2
    Lumbosacral ØSN4
    Thoracic Vertebral ØRN9
    Thoracolumbar Vertebral ØRNB
  Duct
    Common Bile ØFN9
    Cystic ØFN8
    Hepatic
      Common ØFN7
      Left ØFN6
      Right ØFN5
    Lacrimal
      Left Ø8NY
      Right Ø8NX
    Pancreatic ØFND
      Accessory ØFNF

Release *(Continued)*
  Duct *(Continued)*
    Parotid
      Left ØCNC
      Right ØCNB
  Duodenum ØDN9
  Dura Mater ØØN2
  Ear
    External
      Left Ø9N1
      Right Ø9NØ
    External Auditory Canal
      Left Ø9N4
      Right Ø9N3
    Inner
      Left Ø9NE
      Right Ø9ND
    Middle
      Left Ø9N6
      Right Ø9N5
  Epididymis
    Bilateral ØVNL
    Left ØVNK
    Right ØVNJ
  Epiglottis ØCNR
  Esophagogastric Junction ØDN4
  Esophagus ØDN5
    Lower ØDN3
    Middle ØDN2
    Upper ØDN1
  Eustachian Tube
    Left Ø9NG
    Right Ø9NF
  Eye
    Left Ø8N1XZZ
    Right Ø8NØXZZ
  Eyelid
    Lower
      Left Ø8NR
      Right Ø8NQ
    Upper
      Left Ø8NP
      Right Ø8NN
  Fallopian Tube
    Left ØUN6
    Right ØUN5
  Fallopian Tubes, Bilateral ØUN7
  Femoral Shaft
    Left ØQN9
    Right ØQN8
  Femur
    Lower
      Left ØQNC
      Right ØQNB
    Upper
      Left ØQN7
      Right ØQN6
  Fibula
    Left ØQNK
    Right ØQNJ
  Finger Nail ØHNQXZZ
  Gallbladder ØFN4
  Gingiva
    Lower ØCN6
    Upper ØCN5
  Gland
    Adrenal
      Bilateral ØGN4
      Left ØGN2
      Right ØGN3
    Lacrimal
      Left Ø8NW
      Right Ø8NV
    Minor Salivary ØCNJ
    Parotid
      Left ØCN9
      Right ØCN8
    Pituitary ØGNØ

Release *(Continued)*
  Gland *(Continued)*
    Sublingual
      Left ØCNF
      Right ØCND
    Submaxillary
      Left ØCNH
      Right ØCNG
    Vestibular ØUNL
  Glenoid Cavity
    Left ØPN8
    Right ØPN7
  Glomus Jugulare ØGNC
  Humeral Head
    Left ØPND
    Right ØPNC
  Humeral Shaft
    Left ØPNG
    Right ØPNF
  Hymen ØUNK
  Hypothalamus ØØNA
  Ileocecal Valve ØDNC
  Ileum ØDNB
  Intestine
    Large ØDNE
      Left ØDNG
      Right ØDNF
    Small ØDN8
  Iris
    Left Ø8ND3ZZ
    Right Ø8NC3ZZ
  Jejunum ØDNA
  Joint
    Acromioclavicular
      Left ØRNH
      Right ØRNG
    Ankle
      Left ØSNG
      Right ØSNF
    Carpal
      Left ØRNR
      Right ØRNQ
    Carpometacarpal
      Left ØRNT
      Right ØRNS
    Cervical Vertebral ØRN1
    Cervicothoracic Vertebral ØRN4
    Coccygeal ØSN6
    Elbow
      Left ØRNM
      Right ØRNL
    Finger Phalangeal
      Left ØRNX
      Right ØRNW
    Hip
      Left ØSNB
      Right ØSN9
    Knee
      Left ØSND
      Right ØSNC
    Lumbar Vertebral ØSNØ
    Lumbosacral ØSN3
    Metacarpophalangeal
      Left ØRNV
      Right ØRNU
    Metatarsal-Phalangeal
      Left ØSNN
      Right ØSNM
    Occipital-cervical ØRNØ
    Sacrococcygeal ØSN5
    Sacroiliac
      Left ØSN8
      Right ØSN7
    Shoulder
      Left ØRNK
      Right ØRNJ
    Sternoclavicular
      Left ØRNF
      Right ØRNE

Release *(Continued)*
Scapula
  Left 0PN6
  Right 0PN5
Sclera
  Left 08N7XZZ
  Right 08N6XZZ
Scrotum 0VN5
Septum
  Atrial 02N5
  Nasal 09NM
  Ventricular 02NM
Sinus
  Accessory 09NP
  Ethmoid
    Left 09NV
    Right 09NU
  Frontal
    Left 09NT
    Right 09NS
  Mastoid
    Left 09NC
    Right 09NB
  Maxillary
    Left 09NR
    Right 09NQ
  Sphenoid
    Left 09NX
    Right 09NW
Skin
  Abdomen 0HN7XZZ
  Back 0HN6XZZ
  Buttock 0HN8XZZ
  Chest 0HN5XZZ
  Ear
    Left 0HN3XZZ
    Right 0HN2XZZ
  Face 0HN1XZZ
  Foot
    Left 0HNNXZZ
    Right 0HNMXZZ
  Hand
    Left 0HNGXZZ
    Right 0HNFXZZ
  Inguinal 0HNAXZZ
  Lower Arm
    Left 0HNEXZZ
    Right 0HNDXZZ
  Lower Leg
    Left 0HNLXZZ
    Right 0HNKXZZ
  Neck 0HN4XZZ
  Perineum 0HN9XZZ
  Scalp 0HN0XZZ
  Upper Arm
    Left 0HNCXZZ
    Right 0HNBXZZ
  Upper Leg
    Left 0HNJXZZ
    Right 0HNHXZZ
Spinal Cord
  Cervical 00NW
  Lumbar 00NY
  Thoracic 00NX
Spinal Meninges 00NT
Spleen 07NP
Sternum 0PN0
Stomach 0DN6
  Pylorus 0DN7
Subcutaneous Tissue and Fascia
  Abdomen 0JN8
  Back 0JN7
  Buttock 0JN9
  Chest 0JN6
  Face 0JN1
  Foot
    Left 0JNR
    Right 0JNQ
  Hand
    Left 0JNK
    Right 0JNJ

Release *(Continued)*
Subcutaneous Tissue and Fascia
  (Continued)
  Lower Arm
    Left 0JNH
    Right 0JNG
  Lower Leg
    Left 0JNP
    Right 0JNN
  Neck
    Left 0JN5
    Right 0JN4
  Pelvic Region 0JNC
  Perineum 0JNB
  Scalp 0JN0
  Upper Arm
    Left 0JNF
    Right 0JND
  Upper Leg
    Left 0JNM
    Right 0JNL
Tarsal
  Left 0QNM
  Right 0QNL
Tendon
  Abdomen
    Left 0LNG
    Right 0LNF
  Ankle
    Left 0LNT
    Right 0LNS
  Foot
    Left 0LNW
    Right 0LNV
  Hand
    Left 0LN8
    Right 0LN7
  Head and Neck 0LN0
  Hip
    Left 0LNK
    Right 0LNJ
  Knee
    Left 0LNR
    Right 0LNQ
  Lower Arm and Wrist
    Left 0LN6
    Right 0LN5
  Lower Leg
    Left 0LNP
    Right 0LNN
  Perineum 0LNH
  Shoulder
    Left 0LN2
    Right 0LN1
  Thorax
    Left 0LND
    Right 0LNC
  Trunk
    Left 0LNB
    Right 0LN9
  Upper Arm
    Left 0LN4
    Right 0LN3
  Upper Leg
    Left 0LNM
    Right 0LNL
Testis
  Bilateral 0VNC
  Left 0VNB
  Right 0VN9
Thalamus 00N9
Thymus 07NM
Thyroid Gland 0GNK
  Left Lobe 0GNG
  Right Lobe 0GNH
Tibia
  Left 0QNH
  Right 0QNG
Toe Nail 0HNRXZZ
Tongue 0CN7
Tonsils 0CNP

Release *(Continued)*
Tooth
  Lower 0CNX
  Upper 0CNW
Trachea 0BN1
Tunica Vaginalis
  Left 0VN7
  Right 0VN6
Turbinate, Nasal 09NL
Tympanic Membrane
  Left 09N8
  Right 09N7
Ulna
  Left 0PNL
  Right 0PNK
Ureter
  Left 0TN7
  Right 0TN6
Urethra 0TND
Uterine Supporting Structure
  0UN4
Uterus 0UN9
Uvula 0CNN
Vagina 0UNG
Valve
  Aortic 02NF
  Mitral 02NG
  Pulmonary 02NH
  Tricuspid 02NJ
Vas Deferens
  Bilateral 0VNQ
  Left 0VNP
  Right 0VNN
Vein
  Axillary
    Left 05N8
    Right 05N7
  Azygos 05N0
  Basilic
    Left 05NC
    Right 05NB
  Brachial
    Left 05NA
    Right 05N9
  Cephalic
    Left 05NF
    Right 05ND
  Colic 06N7
  Common Iliac
    Left 06ND
    Right 06NC
  Coronary 02N4
  Esophageal 06N3
  External Iliac
    Left 06NG
    Right 06NF
  External Jugular
    Left 05NQ
    Right 05NP
  Face
    Left 05NV
    Right 05NT
  Femoral
    Left 06NN
    Right 06NM
  Foot
    Left 06NV
    Right 06NT
  Gastric 06N2
  Hand
    Left 05NH
    Right 05NG
  Hemiazygos 05N1
  Hepatic 06N4
  Hypogastric
    Left 06NJ
    Right 06NH
  Inferior Mesenteric 06N6
  Innominate
    Left 05N4
    Right 05N3

▶ New   ⇒ Revised   ~~deleted~~ Deleted

Removal of device from *(Continued)*
  Joint *(Continued)*
    Hip *(Continued)*
      Right 0SP9
        Acetabular Surface 0SPA
        Femoral Surface 0SPR
     Knee
      Left 0SPD
        Femoral Surface 0SPU
        Tibial Surface 0SPW
      Right 0SPC
        Femoral Surface 0SPT
        Tibial Surface 0SPV
    Lumbar Vertebral 0SP0
    Lumbosacral 0SP3
    Metacarpophalangeal
     Left 0RPV
     Right 0RPU
    Metatarsal-Phalangeal
     Left 0SPN
     Right 0SPM
    Occipital-cervical 0RP0
    Sacrococcygeal 0SP5
    Sacroiliac
     Left 0SP8
     Right 0SP7
    Shoulder
     Left 0RPK
     Right 0RPJ
    Sternoclavicular
     Left 0RPF
     Right 0RPE
    Tarsal
     Left 0SPJ
     Right 0SPH
    Tarsometatarsal
     Left 0SPL
     Right 0SPK
    Temporomandibular
     Left 0RPD
     Right 0RPC
    Thoracic Vertebral 0RP6
    Thoracolumbar Vertebral 0RPA
    Toe Phalangeal
     Left 0SPQ
     Right 0SPP
    Wrist
     Left 0RPP
     Right 0RPN
  Kidney 0TP5
  Larynx 0CPS
  Lens
   Left 08PK3
   Right 08PJ3
  Liver 0FP0
  Lung
   Left 0BPL
   Right 0BPK
  Lymphatic 07PN
   Thoracic Duct 07PK
  Mediastinum 0WPC
  Mesentery 0DPV
  Metacarpal
   Left 0PPQ
   Right 0PPP
  Metatarsal
   Left 0QPP
   Right 0QPN
  Mouth and Throat 0CPY
  Muscle
   Extraocular
    Left 08PM
    Right 08PL
   Lower 0KPY
   Upper 0KPX
  Nasal Mucosa and Soft Tissue 09PK
  Neck 0WP6
  Nerve
   Cranial 00PE
   Peripheral 01PY
  Omentum 0DPU

Removal of device from *(Continued)*
  Ovary 0UP3
  Pancreas 0FPG
  Parathyroid Gland 0GPR
  Patella
   Left 0QPF
   Right 0QPD
  Pelvic Cavity 0WPJ
  Penis 0VPS
  Pericardial Cavity 0WPD
  Perineum
   Female 0WPN
   Male 0WPM
  Peritoneal Cavity 0WPG
  Peritoneum 0DPW
  Phalanx
   Finger
    Left 0PPV
    Right 0PPT
   Thumb
    Left 0PPS
    Right 0PPR
   Toe
    Left 0QPR
    Right 0QPQ
  Pineal Body 0GP1
  Pleura 0BPQ
  Pleural Cavity
   Left 0WPB
   Right 0WP9
  Products of Conception 10P0
  Prostate and Seminal Vesicles 0VP4
  Radius
   Left 0PPJ
   Right 0PPH
  Rectum 0DPP
  Respiratory Tract 0WPQ
  Retroperitoneum 0WPH
  Ribs
   1 to 2 0PP1
   3 or More 0PP2
  Sacrum 0QP1
  Scapula
   Left 0PP6
   Right 0PP5
  Scrotum and Tunica Vaginalis 0VP8
  Sinus 09PY
  Skin 0HPPX
  Skull 0NP0
  Spinal Canal 00PU
  Spinal Cord 00PV
  Spleen 07PP
  Sternum 0PP0
  Stomach 0DP6
  Subcutaneous Tissue and Fascia
   Head and Neck 0JPS
   Lower Extremity 0JPW
   Trunk 0JPT
   Upper Extremity 0JPV
  Tarsal
   Left 0QPM
   Right 0QPL
  Tendon
   Lower 0LPY
   Upper 0LPX
  Testis 0VPD
  Thymus 07PM
  Thyroid Gland 0GPK
  Tibia
   Left 0QPH
   Right 0QPG
  Toe Nail 0HPRX
  Trachea 0BP1
  Tracheobronchial Tree 0BP0
  Tympanic Membrane
   Left 09P8
   Right 09P7
  Ulna
   Left 0PPL
   Right 0PPK
  Ureter 0TP9

Removal of device from *(Continued)*
  Urethra 0TPD
  Uterus and Cervix 0UPD
  Vagina and Cul-de-sac 0UPH
  Vas Deferens 0VPR
  Vein
   Azygos 05P0
   Innominate
    Left 05P4
    Right 05P3
   Lower 06PY
   Upper 05PY
  Vertebra
   Cervical 0PP3
   Lumbar 0QP0
   Thoracic 0PP4
  Vulva 0UPM
Renal calyx
  use Kidney, Right
  use Kidney, Left
  use Kidneys, Bilateral
  use Kidney
Renal capsule
  use Kidney, Right
  use Kidney, Left
  use Kidneys, Bilateral
  use Kidney
Renal cortex
  use Kidney, Right
  use Kidney, Left
  use Kidneys, Bilateral
  use Kidney
Renal dialysis *see* Performance, Urinary 5A1D
Renal plexus *use* Abdominal Sympathetic Nerve
Renal segment
  use Kidney, Right
  use Kidney, Left
  use Kidneys, Bilateral
  use Kidney
Renal segmental artery
  use Renal Artery, Right
  use Renal Artery, Left
Reopening, operative site
  Control of bleeding *see* Control bleeding in
  Inspection only *see* Inspection
Repair
  Abdominal Wall 0WQF
  Acetabulum
   Left 0QQ5
   Right 0QQ4
  Adenoids 0CQQ
  Ampulla of Vater 0FQC
  Anal Sphincter 0DQR
  Ankle Region
   Left 0YQL
   Right 0YQK
  Anterior Chamber
   Left 08Q33ZZ
   Right 08Q23ZZ
  Anus 0DQQ
  Aorta
   Abdominal 04Q0
   Thoracic
    Ascending/Arch 02QX
    Descending 02QW
  Aortic Body 0GQD
  Appendix 0DQJ
  Arm
   Lower
    Left 0XQF
    Right 0XQD
   Upper
    Left 0XQ9
    Right 0XQ8
  Artery
   Anterior Tibial
    Left 04QQ
    Right 04QP
   Axillary
    Left 03Q6
    Right 03Q5

▶ New   ⇒ Revised   ~~deleted~~ Deleted

Repair *(Continued)*
Disc
  Cervical Vertebral 0RQ3
  Cervicothoracic Vertebral 0RQ5
  Lumbar Vertebral 0SQ2
  Lumbosacral 0SQ4
  Thoracic Vertebral 0RQ9
  Thoracolumbar Vertebral 0RQB
Duct
  Common Bile 0FQ9
  Cystic 0FQ8
  Hepatic
    Common 0FQ7
    Left 0FQ6
    Right 0FQ5
  Lacrimal
    Left 08QY
    Right 08QX
  Pancreatic 0FQD
    Accessory 0FQF
  Parotid
    Left 0CQC
    Right 0CQB
Duodenum 0DQ9
Dura Mater 00Q2
Ear
  External
    Bilateral 09Q2
    Left 09Q1
    Right 09Q0
  External Auditory Canal
    Left 09Q4
    Right 09Q3
  Inner
    Left 09QE
    Right 09QD
  Middle
    Left 09Q6
    Right 09Q5
Elbow Region
  Left 0XQC
  Right 0XQB
Epididymis
  Bilateral 0VQL
  Left 0VQK
  Right 0VQJ
Epiglottis 0CQR
Esophagogastric Junction 0DQ4
Esophagus 0DQ5
  Lower 0DQ3
  Middle 0DQ2
  Upper 0DQ1
Eustachian Tube
  Left 09QG
  Right 09QF
Extremity
  Lower
    Left 0YQB
    Right 0YQ9
  Upper
    Left 0XQ7
    Right 0XQ6
Eye
  Left 08Q1XZZ
  Right 08Q0XZZ
Eyelid
  Lower
    Left 08QR
    Right 08QQ
  Upper
    Left 08QP
    Right 08QN
Face 0WQ2
Fallopian Tube
  Left 0UQ6
  Right 0UQ5
Fallopian Tubes, Bilateral 0UQ7
Femoral Region
  Bilateral 0YQE
  Left 0YQ8
  Right 0YQ7

Repair *(Continued)*
Femoral Shaft
  Left 0QQ9
  Right 0QQ8
Femur
  Lower
    Left 0QQC
    Right 0QQB
  Upper
    Left 0QQ7
    Right 0QQ6
Fibula
  Left 0QQK
  Right 0QQJ
Finger
  Index
    Left 0XQP
    Right 0XQN
  Little
    Left 0XQW
    Right 0XQV
  Middle
    Left 0XQR
    Right 0XQQ
  Ring
    Left 0XQT
    Right 0XQS
Finger Nail 0HQQXZZ
Floor of mouth *see* Repair, Oral Cavity and
    Throat 0WQ3
Foot
  Left 0YQN
  Right 0YQM
Gallbladder 0FQ4
Gingiva
  Lower 0CQ6
  Upper 0CQ5
Gland
  Adrenal
    Bilateral 0GQ4
    Left 0GQ2
    Right 0GQ3
  Lacrimal
    Left 08QW
    Right 08QV
  Minor Salivary 0CQJ
  Parotid
    Left 0CQ9
    Right 0CQ8
  Pituitary 0GQ0
  Sublingual
    Left 0CQF
    Right 0CQD
  Submaxillary
    Left 0CQH
    Right 0CQG
  Vestibular 0UQL
Glenoid Cavity
  Left 0PQ8
  Right 0PQ7
Glomus Jugulare 0GQC
Hand
  Left 0XQK
  Right 0XQJ
Head 0WQ0
Heart 02QA
  Left 02QC
  Right 02QB
Humeral Head
  Left 0PQD
  Right 0PQC
Humeral Shaft
  Left 0PQG
  Right 0PQF
Hymen 0UQK
Hypothalamus 00QA
Ileocecal Valve 0DQC
Ileum 0DQB
Inguinal Region
  Bilateral 0YQA
  Left 0YQ6
  Right 0YQ5

Repair *(Continued)*
Intestine
  Large 0DQE
    Left 0DQG
    Right 0DQF
  Small 0DQ8
Iris
  Left 08QD3ZZ
  Right 08QC3ZZ
Jaw
  Lower 0WQ5
  Upper 0WQ4
Jejunum 0DQA
Joint
  Acromioclavicular
    Left 0RQH
    Right 0RQG
  Ankle
    Left 0SQG
    Right 0SQF
  Carpal
    Left 0RQR
    Right 0RQQ
  Carpometacarpal
    Left 0RQT
    Right 0RQS
  Cervical Vertebral 0RQ1
  Cervicothoracic Vertebral 0RQ4
  Coccygeal 0SQ6
  Elbow
    Left 0RQM
    Right 0RQL
  Finger Phalangeal
    Left 0RQX
    Right 0RQW
  Hip
    Left 0SQB
    Right 0SQ9
  Knee
    Left 0SQD
    Right 0SQC
  Lumbar Vertebral 0SQ0
  Lumbosacral 0SQ3
  Metacarpophalangeal
    Left 0RQV
    Right 0RQU
  Metatarsal-Phalangeal
    Left 0SQN
    Right 0SQM
  Occipital-cervical 0RQ0
  Sacrococcygeal 0SQ5
  Sacroiliac
    Left 0SQ8
    Right 0SQ7
  Shoulder
    Left 0RQK
    Right 0RQJ
  Sternoclavicular
    Left 0RQF
    Right 0RQE
  Tarsal
    Left 0SQJ
    Right 0SQH
  Tarsometatarsal
    Left 0SQL
    Right 0SQK
  Temporomandibular
    Left 0RQD
    Right 0RQC
  Thoracic Vertebral 0RQ6
  Thoracolumbar Vertebral
    0RQA
  Toe Phalangeal
    Left 0SQQ
    Right 0SQP
  Wrist
    Left 0RQP
    Right 0RQN
Kidney
  Left 0TQ1
  Right 0TQ0

▶ New   ➡ Revised   ~~deleted~~ Deleted

▶ New   ⇒ Revised   ~~deleted~~ Deleted

Repair (Continued)

Sinus
  Accessory Ø9QP
  Ethmoid
    Left Ø9QV
    Right Ø9QU
  Frontal
    Left Ø9QT
    Right Ø9QS
  Mastoid
    Left Ø9QC
    Right Ø9QB
  Maxillary
    Left Ø9QR
    Right Ø9QQ
  Sphenoid
    Left Ø9QX
    Right Ø9QW
Skin
  Abdomen ØHQ7XZZ
  Back ØHQ6XZZ
  Buttock ØHQ8XZZ
  Chest ØHQ5XZZ
  Ear
    Left ØHQ3XZZ
    Right ØHQ2XZZ
  Face ØHQ1XZZ
  Foot
    Left ØHQNXZZ
    Right ØHQMXZZ
  Hand
    Left ØHQGXZZ
    Right ØHQFXZZ
  Inguinal ØHQAXZZ
  Lower Arm
    Left ØHQEXZZ
    Right ØHQDXZZ
  Lower Leg
    Left ØHQLXZZ
    Right ØHQKXZZ
  Neck ØHQ4XZZ
  Perineum ØHQ9XZZ
  Scalp ØHQ0XZZ
  Upper Arm
    Left ØHQCXZZ
    Right ØHQBXZZ
  Upper Leg
    Left ØHQJXZZ
    Right ØHQHXZZ
Skull ØNQØ
Spinal Cord
  Cervical ØØQW
  Lumbar ØØQY
  Thoracic ØØQX
Spinal Meninges ØØQT
Spleen Ø7QP
Sternum ØPQØ
Stomach ØDQ6
  Pylorus ØDQ7
Subcutaneous Tissue and Fascia
  Abdomen ØJQ8
  Back ØJQ7
  Buttock ØJQ9
  Chest ØJQ6
  Face ØJQ1
  Foot
    Left ØJQR
    Right ØJQQ
  Hand
    Left ØJQK
    Right ØJQJ
  Lower Arm
    Left ØJQH
    Right ØJQG
  Lower Leg
    Left ØJQP
    Right ØJQN
  Neck
    Left ØJQ5
    Right ØJQ4

Repair (Continued)

Subcutaneous Tissue and Fascia (Continued)
  Pelvic Region ØJQC
  Perineum ØJQB
  Scalp ØJQØ
  Upper Arm
    Left ØJQF
    Right ØJQD
  Upper Leg
    Left ØJQM
    Right ØJQL
Tarsal
  Left ØQQM
  Right ØQQL
Tendon
  Abdomen
    Left ØLQG
    Right ØLQF
  Ankle
    Left ØLQT
    Right ØLQS
  Foot
    Left ØLQW
    Right ØLQV
  Hand
    Left ØLQ8
    Right ØLQ7
  Head and Neck ØLQØ
  Hip
    Left ØLQK
    Right ØLQJ
  Knee
    Left ØLQR
    Right ØLQQ
  Lower Arm and Wrist
    Left ØLQ6
    Right ØLQ5
  Lower Leg
    Left ØLQP
    Right ØLQN
  Perineum ØLQH
  Shoulder
    Left ØLQ2
    Right ØLQ1
  Thorax
    Left ØLQD
    Right ØLQC
  Trunk
    Left ØLQB
    Right ØLQ9
  Upper Arm
    Left ØLQ4
    Right ØLQ3
  Upper Leg
    Left ØLQM
    Right ØLQL
Testis
  Bilateral ØVQC
  Left ØVQB
  Right ØVQ9
Thalamus ØØQ9
Thumb
  Left ØXQM
  Right ØXQL
Thymus Ø7QM
Thyroid Gland ØGQK
  Left Lobe ØGQG
  Right Lobe ØGQH
Thyroid Gland Isthmus ØGQJ
Tibia
  Left ØQQH
  Right ØQQG
Toe
  1st
    Left ØYQQ
    Right ØYQP
  2nd
    Left ØYQS
    Right ØYQR
  3rd
    Left ØYQU
    Right ØYQT

Repair (Continued)

Toe (Continued)
  4th
    Left ØYQW
    Right ØYQV
  5th
    Left ØYQY
    Right ØYQX
Toe Nail ØHQRXZZ
Tongue ØCQ7
Tonsils ØCQP
Tooth
  Lower ØCQX
  Upper ØCQW
Trachea ØBQ1
Tunica Vaginalis
  Left ØVQ7
  Right ØVQ6
Turbinate, Nasal Ø9QL
Tympanic Membrane
  Left Ø9Q8
  Right Ø9Q7
Ulna
  Left ØPQL
  Right ØPQK
Ureter
  Left ØTQ7
  Right ØTQ6
Urethra ØTQD
Uterine Supporting Structure ØUQ4
Uterus ØUQ9
Uvula ØCQN
Vagina ØUQG
Valve
  Aortic Ø2QF
  Mitral Ø2QG
  Pulmonary Ø2QH
  Tricuspid Ø2QJ
Vas Deferens
  Bilateral ØVQQ
  Left ØVQP
  Right ØVQN
Vein
  Axillary
    Left Ø5Q8
    Right Ø5Q7
  Azygos Ø5QØ
  Basilic
    Left Ø5QC
    Right Ø5QB
  Brachial
    Left Ø5QA
    Right Ø5Q9
  Cephalic
    Left Ø5QF
    Right Ø5QD
  Colic Ø6Q7
  Common Iliac
    Left Ø6QD
    Right Ø6QC
  Coronary Ø2Q4
  Esophageal Ø6Q3
  External Iliac
    Left Ø6QG
    Right Ø6QF
  External Jugular
    Left Ø5QQ
    Right Ø5QP
  Face
    Left Ø5QV
    Right Ø5QT
  Femoral
    Left Ø6QN
    Right Ø6QM
  Foot
    Left Ø6QV
    Right Ø6QT
  Gastric Ø6Q2
  Hand
    Left Ø5QH
    Right Ø5QG

Repair *(Continued)*
Vein *(Continued)*
Hemiazygos 05Q1
Hepatic 06Q4
Hypogastric
Left 06QJ
Right 06QH
Inferior Mesenteric 06Q6
Innominate
Left 05Q4
Right 05Q3
Internal Jugular
Left 05QN
Right 05QM
Intracranial 05QL
Lower 06QY
Portal 06Q8
Pulmonary
Left 02QT
Right 02QS
Renal
Left 06QB
Right 06Q9
Saphenous
Left 06QQ
Right 06QP
Splenic 06Q1
Subclavian
Left 05Q6
Right 05Q5
Superior Mesenteric 06Q5
Upper 05QY
Vertebral
Left 05QS
Right 05QR
Vena Cava
Inferior 06Q0
Superior 02QV
Ventricle
Left 02QL
Right 02QK
Vertebra
Cervical 0PQ3
Lumbar 0QQ0
Thoracic 0PQ4
Vesicle
Bilateral 0VQ3
Left 0VQ2
Right 0VQ1
Vitreous
Left 08Q53ZZ
Right 08Q43ZZ
Vocal Cord
Left 0CQV
Right 0CQT
Vulva 0UQM
Wrist Region
Left 0XQH
Right 0XQG
Repair, obstetric laceration, periurethral
0UQMXZZ
Replacement
Acetabulum
Left 0QR5
Right 0QR4
Ampulla of Vater 0FRC
Anal Sphincter 0DRR
Aorta
Abdominal 04R0
Thoracic
Ascending/Arch 02RX
Descending 02RW
Artery
Anterior Tibial
Left 04RQ
Right 04RP
Axillary
Left 03R6
Right 03R5
Brachial
Left 03R8
Right 03R7

Replacement *(Continued)*
Artery *(Continued)*
Celiac 04R1
Colic
Left 04R7
Middle 04R8
Right 04R6
Common Carotid
Left 03RJ
Right 03RH
Common Iliac
Left 04RD
Right 04RC
External Carotid
Left 03RN
Right 03RM
External Iliac
Left 04RJ
Right 04RH
Face 03RR
Femoral
Left 04RL
Right 04RK
Foot
Left 04RW
Right 04RV
Gastric 04R2
Hand
Left 03RF
Right 03RD
Hepatic 04R3
Inferior Mesenteric 04RB
Innominate 03R2
Internal Carotid
Left 03RL
Right 03RK
Internal Iliac
Left 04RF
Right 04RE
Internal Mammary
Left 03R1
Right 03R0
Intracranial 03RG
Lower 04RY
Peroneal
Left 04RU
Right 04RT
Popliteal
Left 04RN
Right 04RM
Posterior Tibial
Left 04RS
Right 04RR
Pulmonary
Left 02RR
Right 02RQ
Pulmonary Trunk 02RP
Radial
Left 03RC
Right 03RB
Renal
Left 04RA
Right 04R9
Splenic 04R4
Subclavian
Left 03R4
Right 03R3
Superior Mesenteric 04R5
Temporal
Left 03RT
Right 03RS
Thyroid
Left 03RV
Right 03RU
Ulnar
Left 03RA
Right 03R9
Upper 03RY
Vertebral
Left 03RQ
Right 03RP

Replacement *(Continued)*
Atrium
Left 02R7
Right 02R6
Auditory Ossicle
Left 09RA0
Right 09R90
Bladder 0TRB
Bladder Neck 0TRC
Bone
Ethmoid
Left 0NRG
Right 0NRF
Frontal 0NR1
Hyoid 0NRX
Lacrimal
Left 0NRJ
Right 0NRH
Nasal 0NRB
Occipital 0NR7
Palatine
Left 0NRL
Right 0NRK
Parietal
Left 0NR4
Right 0NR3
Pelvic
Left 0QR3
Right 0QR2
Sphenoid 0NRC
Temporal
Left 0NR6
Right 0NR5
Zygomatic
Left 0NRN
Right 0NRM
Breast
Bilateral 0HRV
Left 0HRU
Right 0HRT
Bronchus
Lingula 0BR9
Lower Lobe
Left 0BRB
Right 0BR6
Main
Left 0BR7
Right 0BR3
Middle Lobe, Right 0BR5
Upper Lobe
Left 0BR8
Right 0BR4
Buccal Mucosa 0CR4
Bursa and Ligament
Abdomen
Left 0MRJ
Right 0MRH
Ankle
Left 0MRR
Right 0MRQ
Elbow
Left 0MR4
Right 0MR3
Foot
Left 0MRT
Right 0MRS
Hand
Left 0MR8
Right 0MR7
Head and Neck 0MR0
Hip
Left 0MRM
Right 0MRL
Knee
Left 0MRP
Right 0MRN
Lower Extremity
Left 0MRW
Right 0MRV
Perineum 0MRK
Rib(s) 0MRG

▶ New   ⇒ Revised   ~~deleted~~ Deleted

Replacement *(Continued)*
  Muscle *(Continued)*
    Upper Arm
      Left 0KR8
      Right 0KR7
    Upper Leg
      Left 0KRR
      Right 0KRQ
  Nasal Mucosa and Soft Tissue 09RK
  Nasopharynx 09RN
  Nerve
    Abducens 00RL
    Accessory 00RR
    Acoustic 00RN
    Cervical 01R1
    Facial 00RM
    Femoral 01RD
    Glossopharyngeal 00RP
    Hypoglossal 00RS
    Lumbar 01RB
    Median 01R5
    Oculomotor 00RH
    Olfactory 00RF
    Optic 00RG
    Peroneal 01RH
    Phrenic 01R2
    Pudendal 01RC
    Radial 01R6
    Sacral 01RR
    Sciatic 01RF
    Thoracic 01R8
    Tibial 01RG
    Trigeminal 00RK
    Trochlear 00RJ
    Ulnar 01R4
    Vagus 00RQ
  Nipple
    Left 0HRX
    Right 0HRW
  Omentum 0DRU
  Orbit
    Left 0NRQ
    Right 0NRP
  Palate
    Hard 0CR2
    Soft 0CR3
  Patella
    Left 0QRF
    Right 0QRD
  Pericardium 02RN
  Peritoneum 0DRW
  Phalanx
    Finger
      Left 0PRV
      Right 0PRT
    Thumb
      Left 0PRS
      Right 0PRR
    Toe
      Left 0QRR
      Right 0QRQ
  Pharynx 0CRM
  Radius
    Left 0PRJ
    Right 0PRH
  Retinal Vessel
    Left 08RH3
    Right 08RG3
  Ribs
    1 to 2 0PR1
    3 or More 0PR2
  Sacrum 0QR1
  Scapula
    Left 0PR6
    Right 0PR5
  Sclera
    Left 08R7X
    Right 08R6X
  Septum
    Atrial 02R5
    Nasal 09RM
    Ventricular 02RM

Replacement *(Continued)*
  Skin
    Abdomen 0HR7
    Back 0HR6
    Buttock 0HR8
    Chest 0HR5
    Ear
      Left 0HR3
      Right 0HR2
    Face 0HR1
    Foot
      Left 0HRN
      Right 0HRM
    Hand
      Left 0HRG
      Right 0HRF
    Inguinal 0HRA
    Lower Arm
      Left 0HRE
      Right 0HRD
    Lower Leg
      Left 0HRL
      Right 0HRK
    Neck 0HR4
    Perineum 0HR9
    Scalp 0HR0
    Upper Arm
      Left 0HRC
      Right 0HRB
    Upper Leg
      Left 0HRJ
      Right 0HRH
  Skin Substitute, Porcine Liver
    Derived XHRPXL2
  Skull 0NR0
  Spinal Meninges 00RT
  Sternum 0PR0
  Subcutaneous Tissue and
    Fascia
    Abdomen 0JR8
    Back 0JR7
    Buttock 0JR9
    Chest 0JR6
    Face 0JR1
    Foot
      Left 0JRR
      Right 0JRQ
    Hand
      Left 0JRK
      Right 0JRJ
    Lower Arm
      Left 0JRH
      Right 0JRG
    Lower Leg
      Left 0JRP
      Right 0JRN
    Neck
      Left 0JR5
      Right 0JR4
    Pelvic Region 0JRC
    Perineum 0JRB
    Scalp 0JR0
    Upper Arm
      Left 0JRF
      Right 0JRD
    Upper Leg
      Left 0JRM
      Right 0JRL
  Tarsal
    Left 0QRM
    Right 0QRL
  Tendon
    Abdomen
      Left 0LRG
      Right 0LRF
    Ankle
      Left 0LRT
      Right 0LRS
    Foot
      Left 0LRW
      Right 0LRV

Replacement *(Continued)*
  Subcutaneous Tissue and Fascia *(Continued)*
    Hand
      Left 0LR8
      Right 0LR7
    Head and Neck 0LR0
    Hip
      Left 0LRK
      Right 0LRJ
    Knee
      Left 0LRR
      Right 0LRQ
    Lower Arm and Wrist
      Left 0LR6
      Right 0LR5
    Lower Leg
      Left 0LRP
      Right 0LRN
    Perineum 0LRH
    Shoulder
      Left 0LR2
      Right 0LR1
    Thorax
      Left 0LRD
      Right 0LRC
    Trunk
      Left 0LRB
      Right 0LR9
    Upper Arm
      Left 0LR4
      Right 0LR3
    Upper Leg
      Left 0LRM
      Right 0LRL
  Testis
    Bilateral 0VRC0JZ
    Left 0VRB0JZ
    Right 0VR90JZ
  Thumb
    Left 0XRM
    Right 0XRL
  Tibia
    Left 0QRH
    Right 0QRG
  Toe Nail 0HRRX
  Tongue 0CR7
  Tooth
    Lower 0CRX
    Upper 0CRW
  Trachea 0BR1
  Turbinate, Nasal 09RL
  Tympanic Membrane
    Left 09R8
    Right 09R7
  Ulna
    Left 0PRL
    Right 0PRK
  Ureter
    Left 0TR7
    Right 0TR6
  Urethra 0TRD
  Uvula 0CRN
  Valve
    Aortic 02RF
    Mitral 02RG
    Pulmonary 02RH
    Tricuspid 02RJ
  Vein
    Axillary
      Left 05R8
      Right 05R7
    Azygos 05R0
    Basilic
      Left 05RC
      Right 05RB
    Brachial
      Left 05RA
      Right 05R9
    Cephalic
      Left 05RF
      Right 05RD

▶ New   ⇒ Revised   ~~deleted~~ Deleted

Replacement *(Continued)*
  Vein *(Continued)*
    Colic 06R7
    Common Iliac
      Left 06RD
      Right 06RC
    Esophageal 06R3
    External Iliac
      Left 06RG
      Right 06RF
    External Jugular
      Left 05RQ
      Right 05RP
    Face
      Left 05RV
      Right 05RT
    Femoral
      Left 06RN
      Right 06RM
    Foot
      Left 06RV
      Right 06RT
    Gastric 06R2
    Hand
      Left 05RH
      Right 05RG
    Hemiazygos 05R1
    Hepatic 06R4
    Hypogastric
      Left 06RJ
      Right 06RH
    Inferior Mesenteric 06R6
    Innominate
      Left 05R4
      Right 05R3
    Internal Jugular
      Left 05RN
      Right 05RM
    Intracranial 05RL
    Lower 06RY
    Portal 06R8
    Pulmonary
      Left 02RT
      Right 02RS
    Renal
      Left 06RB
      Right 06R9
    Saphenous
      Left 06RQ
      Right 06RP
    Splenic 06R1
    Subclavian
      Left 05R6
      Right 05R5
    Superior Mesenteric 06R5
    Upper 05RY
    Vertebral
      Left 05RS
      Right 05RR
  Vena Cava
    Inferior 06R0
    Superior 02RV
  Ventricle
    Left 02RL
    Right 02RK
  Vertebra
    Cervical 0PR3
    Lumbar 0QR0
    Thoracic 0PR4
  Vitreous
    Left 08R53
    Right 08R43
  Vocal Cord
    Left 0CRV
    Right 0CRT
  Zooplastic Tissue, Rapid Deployment
    Technique X2RF
Replacement, hip
  Partial or total *see* Replacement, Lower Joints
    0SR
  Resurfacing only *see* Supplement, Lower
    Joints 0SU

Replantation *see* Reposition
Replantation, scalp *see* Reattachment, Skin,
  Scalp 0HM0
Reposition
  Acetabulum
    Left 0QS5
    Right 0QS4
  Ampulla of Vater 0FSC
  Anus 0DSQ
  Aorta
    Abdominal 04S0
    Thoracic
      Ascending/Arch 02SX0ZZ
      Descending 02SW0ZZ
  Artery
    Anterior Tibial
      Left 04SQ
      Right 04SP
    Axillary
      Left 03S6
      Right 03S5
    Brachial
      Left 03S8
      Right 03S7
    Celiac 04S1
    Colic
      Left 04S7
      Middle 04S8
      Right 04S6
    Common Carotid
      Left 03SJ
      Right 03SH
    Common Iliac
      Left 04SD
      Right 04SC
    Coronary
      One Artery 02S00ZZ
      Two Arteries 02S10ZZ
    External Carotid
      Left 03SN
      Right 03SM
    External Iliac
      Left 04SJ
      Right 04SH
    Face 03SR
    Femoral
      Left 04SL
      Right 04SK
    Foot
      Left 04SW
      Right 04SV
    Gastric 04S2
    Hand
      Left 03SF
      Right 03SD
    Hepatic 04S3
    Inferior Mesenteric 04SB
    Innominate 03S2
    Internal Carotid
      Left 03SL
      Right 03SK
    Internal Iliac
      Left 04SF
      Right 04SE
    Internal Mammary
      Left 03S1
      Right 03S0
    Intracranial 03SG
    Lower 04SY
    Peroneal
      Left 04SU
      Right 04ST
    Popliteal
      Left 04SN
      Right 04SM
    Posterior Tibial
      Left 04SS
      Right 04SR
    Pulmonary
      Left 02SR0ZZ
      Right 02SQ0ZZ

Reposition *(Continued)*
  Artery *(Continued)*
    Pulmonary Trunk 02SP0ZZ
    Radial
      Left 03SC
      Right 03SB
    Renal
      Left 04SA
      Right 04S9
    Splenic 04S4
    Subclavian
      Left 03S4
      Right 03S3
    Superior Mesenteric 04S5
    Temporal
      Left 03ST
      Right 03SS
    Thyroid
      Left 03SV
      Right 03SU
    Ulnar
      Left 03SA
      Right 03S9
    Upper 03SY
    Vertebral
      Left 03SQ
      Right 03SP
  Auditory Ossicle
    Left 09SA
    Right 09S9
  Bladder 0TSB
  Bladder Neck 0TSC
  Bone
    Ethmoid
      Left 0NSG
      Right 0NSF
    Frontal 0NS1
    Hyoid 0NSX
    Lacrimal
      Left 0NSJ
      Right 0NSH
    Nasal 0NSB
    Occipital 0NS7
    Palatine
      Left 0NSL
      Right 0NSK
    Parietal
      Left 0NS4
      Right 0NS3
    Pelvic
      Left 0QS3
      Right 0QS2
    Sphenoid 0NSC
    Temporal
      Left 0NS6
      Right 0NS5
    Zygomatic
      Left 0NSN
      Right 0NSM
  Breast
    Bilateral 0HSV0ZZ
    Left 0HSU0ZZ
    Right 0HST0ZZ
  Bronchus
    Lingula 0BS90ZZ
    Lower Lobe
      Left 0BSB0ZZ
      Right 0BS60ZZ
    Main
      Left 0BS70ZZ
      Right 0BS30ZZ
    Middle Lobe, Right 0BS50ZZ
    Upper Lobe
      Left 0BS80ZZ
      Right 0BS40ZZ
  Bursa and Ligament
    Abdomen
      Left 0MSJ
      Right 0MSH
    Ankle
      Left 0MSR
      Right 0MSQ

▶ New   ⬙ Revised   ~~deleted~~ Deleted

Reposition *(Continued)*
  Muscle *(Continued)*
    Hand
      Left ØKSD
      Right ØKSC
    Head ØKS0
    Hip
      Left ØKSP
      Right ØKSN
    Lower Arm and Wrist
      Left ØKSB
      Right ØKS9
    Lower Leg
      Left ØKST
      Right ØKSS
    Neck
      Left ØKS3
      Right ØKS2
    Perineum ØKSM
    Shoulder
      Left ØKS6
      Right ØKS5
    Thorax
      Left ØKSJ
      Right ØKSH
    Tongue, Palate, Pharynx ØKS4
    Trunk
      Left ØKSG
      Right ØKSF
    Upper Arm
      Left ØKS8
      Right ØKS7
    Upper Leg
      Left ØKSR
      Right ØKSQ
  Nasal Mucosa and Soft Tissue 09SK
  Nerve
    Abducens 00SL
    Accessory 00SR
    Acoustic 00SN
    Brachial Plexus 01S3
    Cervical 01S1
    Cervical Plexus 01S0
    Facial 00SM
    Femoral 01SD
    Glossopharyngeal 00SP
    Hypoglossal 00SS
    Lumbar 01SB
    Lumbar Plexus 01S9
    Lumbosacral Plexus 01SA
    Median 01S5
    Oculomotor 00SH
    Olfactory 00SF
    Optic 00SG
    Peroneal 01SH
    Phrenic 01S2
    Pudendal 01SC
    Radial 01S6
    Sacral 01SR
    Sacral Plexus 01SQ
    Sciatic 01SF
    Thoracic 01S8
    Tibial 01SG
    Trigeminal 00SK
    Trochlear 00SJ
    Ulnar 01S4
    Vagus 00SQ
  Nipple
    Left ØHSXXZZ
    Right ØHSWXZZ
  Orbit
    Left ØNSQ
    Right ØNSP
  Ovary
    Bilateral ØUS2
    Left ØUS1
    Right ØUS0
  Palate
    Hard ØCS2
    Soft ØCS3
  Pancreas ØFSG

Reposition *(Continued)*
  Parathyroid Gland ØGSR
    Inferior
      Left ØGSP
      Right ØGSN
    Multiple ØGSQ
    Superior
      Left ØGSM
      Right ØGSL
  Patella
    Left ØQSF
    Right ØQSD
  Phalanx
    Finger
      Left ØPSV
      Right ØPST
    Thumb
      Left ØPSS
      Right ØPSR
    Toe
      Left ØQSR
      Right ØQSQ
  Products of Conception 10S0
    Ectopic 10S2
  Radius
    Left ØPSJ
    Right ØPSH
  Rectum ØDSP
  Retinal Vessel
    Left 08SH3ZZ
    Right 08SG3ZZ
  Ribs
    1 to 2 ØPS1
    3 or More ØPS2
  Sacrum ØQS1
  Scapula
    Left ØPS6
    Right ØPS5
  Septum, Nasal 09SM
  Sesamoid Bone(s) 1st Toe
      see Reposition, Metatarsal, Right
        ØQSN
      see Reposition, Metatarsal, Left ØQSP
  Skull ØNS0
  Spinal Cord
    Cervical 00SW
    Lumbar 00SY
    Thoracic 00SX
  Spleen 07SP0ZZ
  Sternum ØPS0
  Stomach ØDS6
  Tarsal
    Left ØQSM
    Right ØQSL
  Tendon
    Abdomen
      Left ØLSG
      Right ØLSF
    Ankle
      Left ØLST
      Right ØLSS
    Foot
      Left ØLSW
      Right ØLSV
    Hand
      Left ØLS8
      Right ØLS7
    Head and Neck ØLS0
    Hip
      Left ØLSK
      Right ØLSJ
    Knee
      Left ØLSR
      Right ØLSQ
    Lower Arm and Wrist
      Left ØLS6
      Right ØLS5
    Lower Leg
      Left ØLSP
      Right ØLSN
    Perineum ØLSH

Reposition *(Continued)*
  Tendon *(Continued)*
    Shoulder
      Left ØLS2
      Right ØLS1
    Thorax
      Left ØLSD
      Right ØLSC
    Trunk
      Left ØLSB
      Right ØLS9
    Upper Arm
      Left ØLS4
      Right ØLS3
    Upper Leg
      Left ØLSM
      Right ØLSL
  Testis
    Bilateral ØVSC
    Left ØVSB
    Right ØVS9
  Thymus 07SM0ZZ
  Thyroid Gland
    Left Lobe ØGSG
    Right Lobe ØGSH
  Tibia
    Left ØQSH
    Right ØQSG
  Tongue ØCS7
  Tooth
    Lower ØCSX
    Upper ØCSW
  Trachea ØBS10ZZ
  Turbinate, Nasal 09SL
  Tympanic Membrane
    Left 09S8
    Right 09S7
  Ulna
    Left ØPSL
    Right ØPSK
  Ureter
    Left ØTS7
    Right ØTS6
  Ureters, Bilateral ØTS8
  Urethra ØTSD
  Uterine Supporting Structure
    ØUS4
  Uterus ØUS9
  Uvula ØCSN
  Vagina ØUSG
  Vein
    Axillary
      Left 05S8
      Right 05S7
    Azygos 05S0
    Basilic
      Left 05SC
      Right 05SB
    Brachial
      Left 05SA
      Right 05S9
    Cephalic
      Left 05SF
      Right 05SD
    Colic 06S7
    Common Iliac
      Left 06SD
      Right 06SC
    Esophageal 06S3
    External Iliac
      Left 06SG
      Right 06SF
    External Jugular
      Left 05SQ
      Right 05SP
    Face
      Left 05SV
      Right 05ST
    Femoral
      Left 06SN
      Right 06SM

▶ New   ⇒ Revised   ~~deleted~~ Deleted

▶ New   ⇒ Revised   ~~deleted~~ Deleted

Resection *(Continued)*
  Eye
    Left 08T1XZZ
    Right 08T0XZZ
  Eyelid
    Lower
      Left 08TR
      Right 08TQ
    Upper
      Left 08TP
      Right 08TN
  Fallopian Tube
    Left 0UT6
    Right 0UT5
  Fallopian Tubes, Bilateral 0UT7
  Femoral Shaft
    Left 0QT90ZZ
    Right 0QT80ZZ
  Femur
    Lower
      Left 0QTC0ZZ
      Right 0QTB0ZZ
    Upper
      Left 0QT70ZZ
      Right 0QT60ZZ
  Fibula
    Left 0QTK0ZZ
    Right 0QTJ0ZZ
  Finger Nail 0HTQXZZ
  Gallbladder 0FT4
  Gland
    Adrenal
      Bilateral 0GT4
      Left 0GT2
      Right 0GT3
    Lacrimal
      Left 08TW
      Right 08TV
    Minor Salivary 0CTJ0ZZ
    Parotid
      Left 0CT90ZZ
      Right 0CT80ZZ
    Pituitary 0GT0
    Sublingual
      Left 0CTF0ZZ
      Right 0CTD0ZZ
    Submaxillary
      Left 0CTH0ZZ
      Right 0CTG0ZZ
    Vestibular 0UTL
  Glenoid Cavity
    Left 0PT80ZZ
    Right 0PT70ZZ
  Glomus Jugulare 0GTC
  Humeral Head
    Left 0PTD0ZZ
    Right 0PTC0ZZ
  Humeral Shaft
    Left 0PTG0ZZ
    Right 0PTF0ZZ
  Hymen 0UTK
  Ileocecal Valve 0DTC
  Ileum 0DTB
  Intestine
    Large 0DTE
      Left 0DTG
      Right 0DTF
    Small 0DT8
  Iris
    Left 08TD3ZZ
    Right 08TC3ZZ
  Jejunum 0DTA
  Joint
    Acromioclavicular
      Left 0RTH0ZZ
      Right 0RTG0ZZ
    Ankle
      Left 0STG0ZZ
      Right 0STF0ZZ

Resection *(Continued)*
  Joint *(Continued)*
    Carpal
      Left 0RTR0ZZ
      Right 0RTQ0ZZ
    Carpometacarpal
      Left 0RTT0ZZ
      Right 0RTS0ZZ
    Cervicothoracic Vertebral
      0RT40ZZ
    Coccygeal 0ST60ZZ
    Elbow
      Left 0RTM0ZZ
      Right 0RTL0ZZ
    Finger Phalangeal
      Left 0RTX0ZZ
      Right 0RTW0ZZ
    Hip
      Left 0STB0ZZ
      Right 0ST90ZZ
    Knee
      Left 0STD0ZZ
      Right 0STC0ZZ
    Metacarpophalangeal
      Left 0RTV0ZZ
      Right 0RTU0ZZ
    Metatarsal-Phalangeal
      Left 0STN0ZZ
      Right 0STM0ZZ
    Sacrococcygeal 0ST50ZZ
    Sacroiliac
      Left 0ST80ZZ
      Right 0ST70ZZ
    Shoulder
      Left 0RTK0ZZ
      Right 0RTJ0ZZ
    Sternoclavicular
      Left 0RTF0ZZ
      Right 0RTE0ZZ
    Tarsal
      Left 0STJ0ZZ
      Right 0STH0ZZ
    Tarsometatarsal
      Left 0STL0ZZ
      Right 0STK0ZZ
    Temporomandibular
      Left 0RTD0ZZ
      Right 0RTC0ZZ
    Toe Phalangeal
      Left 0STQ0ZZ
      Right 0STP0ZZ
    Wrist
      Left 0RTP0ZZ
      Right 0RTN0ZZ
  Kidney
    Left 0TT1
    Right 0TT0
  Kidney Pelvis
    Left 0TT4
    Right 0TT3
  Kidneys, Bilateral 0TT2
  Larynx 0CTS
  Lens
    Left 08TK3ZZ
    Right 08TJ3ZZ
  Lip
    Lower 0CT1
    Upper 0CT0
  Liver 0FT0
    Left Lobe 0FT2
    Right Lobe 0FT1
  Lung
    Bilateral 0BTM
    Left 0BTL
    Lower Lobe
      Left 0BTJ
      Right 0BTF
    Middle Lobe, Right 0BTD
    Right 0BTK

Resection *(Continued)*
  Lung *(Continued)*
    Upper Lobe
      Left 0BTG
      Right 0BTC
  Lung Lingula 0BTH
  Lymphatic
    Aortic 07TD
    Axillary
      Left 07T6
      Right 07T5
    Head 07T0
    Inguinal
      Left 07TJ
      Right 07TH
    Internal Mammary
      Left 07T9
      Right 07T8
    Lower Extremity
      Left 07TG
      Right 07TF
    Mesenteric 07TB
    Neck
      Left 07T2
      Right 07T1
    Pelvis 07TC
    Thoracic Duct 07TK
    Thorax 07T7
    Upper Extremity
      Left 07T4
      Right 07T3
  Mandible
    Left 0NTV0ZZ
    Right 0NTT0ZZ
  Maxilla 0NTR0ZZ
  Metacarpal
    Left 0PTQ0ZZ
    Right 0PTP0ZZ
  Metatarsal
    Left 0QTP0ZZ
    Right 0QTN0ZZ
  Muscle
    Abdomen
      Left 0KTL
      Right 0KTK
    Extraocular
      Left 08TM
      Right 08TL
    Facial 0KT1
    Foot
      Left 0KTW
      Right 0KTV
    Hand
      Left 0KTD
      Right 0KTC
    Head 0KT0
    Hip
      Left 0KTP
      Right 0KTN
    Lower Arm and Wrist
      Left 0KTB
      Right 0KT9
    Lower Leg
      Left 0KTT
      Right 0KTS
    Neck
      Left 0KT3
      Right 0KT2
    Papillary 02TD
    Perineum 0KTM
    Shoulder
      Left 0KT6
      Right 0KT5
    Thorax
      Left 0KTJ
      Right 0KTH
    Tongue, Palate, Pharynx 0KT4
    Trunk
      Left 0KTG
      Right 0KTF

▶ New   ⇒ Revised   ~~deleted~~ Deleted

Resection *(Continued)*
 Muscle *(Continued)*
  Upper Arm
   Left 0KT8
   Right 0KT7
  Upper Leg
   Left 0KTR
   Right 0KTQ
 Nasal Mucosa and Soft Tissue
  09TK
 Nasopharynx 09TN
 Nipple
  Left 0HTXXZZ
  Right 0HTWXZZ
 Omentum 0DTU
 Orbit
  Left 0NTQ0ZZ
  Right 0NTP0ZZ
 Ovary
  Bilateral 0UT2
  Left 0UT1
  Right 0UT0
 Palate
  Hard 0CT2
  Soft 0CT3
 Pancreas 0FTG
 Para-aortic Body 0GT9
 Paraganglion Extremity 0GTF
 Parathyroid Gland 0GTR
  Inferior
   Left 0GTP
   Right 0GTN
  Multiple 0GTQ
  Superior
   Left 0GTM
   Right 0GTL
 Patella
  Left 0QTF0ZZ
  Right 0QTD0ZZ
 Penis 0VTS
 Pericardium 02TN
 Phalanx
  Finger
   Left 0PTV0ZZ
   Right 0PTT0ZZ
  Thumb
   Left 0PTS0ZZ
   Right 0PTR0ZZ
  Toe
   Left 0QTR0ZZ
   Right 0QTQ0ZZ
 Pharynx 0CTM
 Pineal Body 0GT1
 Prepuce 0VTT
 Products of Conception, Ectopic 10T2
 Prostate 0VT0
 Radius
  Left 0PTJ0ZZ
  Right 0PTH0ZZ
 Rectum 0DTP
 Ribs
  1 to 2 0PT10ZZ
  3 or More 0PT20ZZ
 Scapula
  Left 0PT60ZZ
  Right 0PT50ZZ
 Scrotum 0VT5
 Septum
  Atrial 02T5
  Nasal 09TM
  Ventricular 02TM
 Sinus
  Accessory 09TP
  Ethmoid
   Left 09TV
   Right 09TU
  Frontal
   Left 09TT
   Right 09TS

Resection *(Continued)*
  Mastoid
   Left 09TC
   Right 09TB
  Maxillary
   Left 09TR
   Right 09TQ
  Sphenoid
   Left 09TX
   Right 09TW
 Spleen 07TP
 Sternum 0PT00ZZ
 Stomach 0DT6
  Pylorus 0DT7
 Tarsal
  Left 0QTM0ZZ
  Right 0QTL0ZZ
 Tendon
  Abdomen
   Left 0LTG
   Right 0LTF
  Ankle
   Left 0LTT
   Right 0LTS
  Foot
   Left 0LTW
   Right 0LTV
  Hand
   Left 0LT8
   Right 0LT7
  Head and Neck 0LT0
  Hip
   Left 0LTK
   Right 0LTJ
  Knee
   Left 0LTR
   Right 0LTQ
  Lower Arm and Wrist
   Left 0LT6
   Right 0LT5
  Lower Leg
   Left 0LTP
   Right 0LTN
  Perineum 0LTH
  Shoulder
   Left 0LT2
   Right 0LT1
  Thorax
   Left 0LTD
   Right 0LTC
  Trunk
   Left 0LTB
   Right 0LT9
  Upper Arm
   Left 0LT4
   Right 0LT3
  Upper Leg
   Left 0LTM
   Right 0LTL
 Testis
  Bilateral 0VTC
  Left 0VTB
  Right 0VT9
 Thymus 07TM
 Thyroid Gland 0GTK
  Left Lobe 0GTG
  Right Lobe 0GTH
 Thyroid Gland Isthmus 0GTJ
 Tibia
  Left 0QTH0ZZ
  Right 0QTG0ZZ
 Toe Nail 0HTRXZZ
 Tongue 0CT7
 Tonsils 0CTP
 Tooth
  Lower 0CTX0Z
  Upper 0CTW0Z
 Trachea 0BT1

Resection *(Continued)*
 Tunica Vaginalis
  Left 0VT7
  Right 0VT6
 Turbinate, Nasal 09TL
 Tympanic Membrane
  Left 09T8
  Right 09T7
 Ulna
  Left 0PTL0ZZ
  Right 0PTK0ZZ
 Ureter
  Left 0TT7
  Right 0TT6
 Urethra 0TTD
 Uterine Supporting Structure 0UT4
 Uterus 0UT9
 Uvula 0CTN
 Vagina 0UTG
 Valve, Pulmonary 02TH
 Vas Deferens
  Bilateral 0VTQ
  Left 0VTP
  Right 0VTN
 Vesicle
  Bilateral 0VT3
  Left 0VT2
  Right 0VT1
 Vitreous
  Left 08T53ZZ
  Right 08T43ZZ
 Vocal Cord
  Left 0CTV
  Right 0CTT
 Vulva 0UTM
Resection, Left ventricular outflow tract
  obstruction (LVOT) *see* Dilation, Ventricle,
  Left 027L
Resection, Subaortic membrane (Left
  ventricular outflow tract obstruction) *see*
  Dilation, Ventricle, Left 027L
Restoration, Cardiac, Single, Rhythm 5A2204Z
RestoreAdvanced neurostimulator (SureScan)
  (MRI Safe) *use* Stimulator Generator,
  Multiple Array Rechargeable in 0JH
RestoreSensor neurostimulator (SureScan)
  (MRI Safe) *use* Stimulator Generator,
  Multiple Array Rechargeable in 0JH
RestoreUltra neurostimulator (SureScan)
  (MRI Safe) *use* Stimulator Generator,
  Multiple Array Rechargeable in 0JH
Restriction
 Ampulla of Vater 0FVC
 Anus 0DVQ
 Aorta
  Abdominal 04V0
   Ascending/Arch, Intraluminal Device,
    Branched or Fenestrated
    02VX
   Descending, Intraluminal Device,
    Branched or Fenestrated 02VW
  Thoracic
   Intraluminal Device, Branched or
    Fenestrated 04V0
 Artery
  Anterior Tibial
   Left 04VQ
   Right 04VP
  Axillary
   Left 03V6
   Right 03V5
  Brachial
   Left 03V8
   Right 03V7
  Celiac 04V1
  Colic
   Left 04V7
   Middle 04V8
   Right 04V6

▶ New   ⇒ Revised   ~~deleted~~ Deleted

Restriction *(Continued)*
  Vein *(Continued)*
    Subclavian
      Left Ø5V6
      Right Ø5V5
    Superior Mesenteric
      Ø6V5
    Upper Ø5VY
    Vertebral
      Left Ø5VS
      Right Ø5VR
  Vena Cava
    Inferior Ø6VØ
    Superior Ø2VV
Resurfacing Device
  Removal of device from
    Left ØSPBØBZ
    Right ØSP9ØBZ
  Revision of device in
    Left ØSWBØBZ
    Right ØSW9ØBZ
  Supplement
    Left ØSUBØBZ
      Acetabular Surface ØSUEØBZ
      Femoral Surface ØSUSØBZ
    Right ØSU9ØBZ
      Acetabular Surface ØSUAØBZ
      Femoral Surface ØSURØBZ
Resuscitation
  Cardiopulmonary *see* Assistance, Cardiac
    5AØ2
  Cardioversion 5A22Ø4Z
  Defibrillation 5A22Ø4Z
  Endotracheal intubation *see* Insertion of
    device in, Trachea ØBH1
  External chest compression 5A12Ø12
  Pulmonary 5A19Ø54
Resuscitative endovascular balloon occlusion
  of the aorta (REBOA)
    Ø2LW3DJ
    Ø4LØ3DJ
Resuture, Heart valve prosthesis *see* Revision
  of device in, Heart and Great Vessels
  Ø2W
Retained placenta, manual removal *see*
  Extraction, Products of Conception,
  Retained 1ØD1
Retraining
  Cardiac *see* Motor Treatment, Rehabilitation
    FØ7
  Vocational *see* Activities of Daily Living
    Treatment, Rehabilitation FØ8
Retrogasserian rhizotomy *see* Division, Nerve,
  Trigeminal ØØ8K
▶ Retroperitoneal cavity *use* Retroperitoneum
Retroperitoneal lymph node *use* Lymphatic,
  Aortic
Retroperitoneal space *use* Retroperitoneum
Retropharyngeal lymph node
  use Lymphatic, Right Neck
  use Lymphatic, Left Neck
Retropubic space *use* Pelvic Cavity
Reveal (DX) (XT) *use* Monitoring Device
Reverse total shoulder replacement *see*
  Replacement, Upper Joints ØRR
Reverse® Shoulder Prosthesis *use* Synthetic
  Substitute, Reverse Ball and Socket in
  ØRR
Revision
  Correcting a portion of existing device *see*
    Revision of device in
  Removal of device without replacement *see*
    Removal of device from
  Replacement of existing device
    see Removal of device from
    see Root operation to place new device,
      e.g., Insertion, Replacement,
      Supplement

Revision of device in
  Abdominal Wall ØWWF
  Acetabulum
    Left ØQW5
    Right ØQW4
  Anal Sphincter ØDWR
  Anus ØDWQ
  Artery
    Lower Ø4WY
    Upper Ø3WY
  Auditory Ossicle
    Left Ø9WA
    Right Ø9W9
  Back
    Lower ØWWL
    Upper ØWWK
  Bladder ØTWB
  Bone
    Facial ØNWW
    Lower ØQWY
    Nasal ØNWB
    Pelvic
      Left ØQW3
      Right ØQW2
    Upper ØPWY
  Bone Marrow Ø7WT
  Brain ØØWØ
  Breast
    Left ØHWU
    Right ØHWT
  Bursa and Ligament
    Lower ØMWY
    Upper ØMWX
  Carpal
    Left ØPWN
    Right ØPWM
  Cavity, Cranial ØWW1
  Cerebral Ventricle ØØW6
  Chest Wall ØWW8
  Cisterna Chyli Ø7WL
  Clavicle
    Left ØPWB
    Right ØPW9
  Coccyx ØQWS
  Diaphragm ØBWT
  Disc
    Cervical Vertebral ØRW3
    Cervicothoracic Vertebral ØRW5
    Lumbar Vertebral ØSW2
    Lumbosacral ØSW4
    Thoracic Vertebral ØRW9
    Thoracolumbar Vertebral ØRWB
  Duct
    Hepatobiliary ØFWB
    Pancreatic ØFWD
    Thoracic Ø7WK
  Ear
    Inner
      Left Ø9WE
      Right Ø9WD
    Left Ø9WJ
    Right Ø9WH
  Epididymis and Spermatic Cord ØVWM
  Esophagus ØDW5
  Extremity
    Lower
      Left ØYWB
      Right ØYW9
    Upper
      Left ØXW7
      Right ØXW6
  Eye
    Left Ø8W1
    Right Ø8WØ
  Face ØWW2
  Fallopian Tube ØUW8
  Femoral Shaft
    Left ØQW9
    Right ØQW8

Revision of device in *(Continued)*
  Femur
    Lower
      Left ØQWC
      Right ØQWB
    Upper
      Left ØQW7
      Right ØQW6
  Fibula
    Left ØQWK
    Right ØQWJ
  Finger Nail ØHWQX
  Gallbladder ØFW4
  Gastrointestinal Tract ØWWP
  Genitourinary Tract ØWWR
  Gland
    Adrenal ØGW5
    Endocrine ØGWS
    Pituitary ØGWØ
    Salivary ØCWA
  Glenoid Cavity
    Left ØPW8
    Right ØPW7
  Great Vessel Ø2WY
  Hair ØHWSX
  Head ØWWØ
  Heart Ø2WA
  Humeral Head
    Left ØPWD
    Right ØPWC
  Humeral Shaft
    Left ØPWG
    Right ØPWF
  Intestinal Tract
    Lower ØDWD
    Upper ØDWØ
  Intestine
    Large ØDWE
    Small ØDW8
  Jaw
    Lower ØWW5
    Upper ØWW4
  Joint
    Acromioclavicular
      Left ØRWH
      Right ØRWG
    Ankle
      Left ØSWG
      Right ØSWF
    Carpal
      Left ØRWR
      Right ØRWQ
    Carpometacarpal
      Left ØRWT
      Right ØRWS
    Cervical Vertebral ØRW1
    Cervicothoracic Vertebral ØRW4
    Coccygeal ØSW6
    Elbow
      Left ØRWM
      Right ØRWL
    Finger Phalangeal
      Left ØRWX
      Right ØRWW
    Hip
      Left ØSWB
        Acetabular Surface ØSWE
        Femoral Surface ØSWS
      Right ØSW9
        Acetabular Surface ØSWA
        Femoral Surface ØSWR
    Knee
      Left ØSWD
        Femoral Surface ØSWU
        Tibial Surface ØSWW
      Right ØSWC
        Femoral Surface ØSWT
        Tibial Surface ØSWV

R

▶ New   ➡ Revised   ~~deleted~~ Deleted

Risorius muscle *use* Facial Muscle
RNS System lead *use* Neurostimulator Lead
    in Central Nervous System and Cranial
    Nerves
RNS system neurostimulator generator *use*
    Neurostimulator Generator in Head and
    Facial Bones
Robotic Assisted Procedure
   Extremity
      Lower 8E0Y
      Upper 8E0X

Robotic Assisted Procedure *(Continued)*
   Head and Neck Region 8E09
   Trunk Region 8E0W
▶Robotic Waterjet Ablation, Destruction,
   Prostate XV508A4
Rotation of fetal head
   Forceps 10S07ZZ
   Manual 10S0XZZ
Round ligament of uterus *use* Uterine
   Supporting Structure

Round window
   use Inner Ear, Right
   use Inner Ear, Left
Roux-en-Y operation
   see Bypass, Gastrointestinal System 0D1
   see Bypass, Hepatobiliary System and
      Pancreas 0F1
Rupture
   Adhesions *see* Release
   Fluid collection *see* Drainage

S

Sacral ganglion *use* Sacral Sympathetic Nerve
Sacral lymph node *use* Lymphatic, Pelvis
Sacral nerve modulation (SNM) lead *use* Stimulator Lead in Urinary System
Sacral neuromodulation lead *use* Stimulator Lead in Urinary System
Sacral splanchnic nerve *use* Sacral Sympathetic Nerve
Sacrectomy *see* Excision, Lower Bones 0QB
Sacrococcygeal ligament *use* Lower Spine Bursa and Ligament
Sacrococcygeal symphysis *use* Sacrococcygeal Joint
Sacroiliac ligament *use* Lower Spine Bursa and Ligament
Sacrospinous ligament *use* Lower Spine Bursa and Ligament
Sacrotuberous ligament *use* Lower Spine Bursa and Ligament
Salpingectomy
    see Excision, Female Reproductive System 0UB
    see Resection, Female Reproductive System 0UT
Salpingolysis *see* Release, Female Reproductive System 0UN
Salpingopexy
    see Repair, Female Reproductive System 0UQ
    see Reposition, Female Reproductive System 0US
Salpingopharyngeus muscle *use* Tongue, Palate, Pharynx Muscle
Salpingoplasty
    see Repair, Female Reproductive System 0UQ
    see Supplement, Female Reproductive System 0UU
Salpingorrhaphy *see* Repair, Female Reproductive System 0UQ
Salpingoscopy 0UJ88ZZ
Salpingostomy *see* Drainage, Female Reproductive System 0U9
Salpingotomy *see* Drainage, Female Reproductive System 0U9
Salpinx
    use Fallopian Tube, Right
    use Fallopian Tube, Left
Saphenous nerve *use* Femoral Nerve
SAPIEN transcatheter aortic valve *use* Zooplastic Tissue in Heart and Great Vessels
Sartorius muscle
    use Upper Leg Muscle, Right
    use Upper Leg Muscle, Left
Scalene muscle
    use Neck Muscle, Right
    use Neck Muscle, Left
Scan
    Computerized Tomography (CT) *see* Computerized Tomography (CT Scan)
    Radioisotope *see* Planar Nuclear Medicine Imaging
Scaphoid bone
    use Carpal, Right
    use Carpal, Left
Scapholunate ligament
    use Hand Bursa and Ligament, Right
    use Hand Bursa and Ligament, Left
Scaphotrapezium ligament
    use Hand Bursa and Ligament, Right
    use Hand Bursa and Ligament, Left
Scapulectomy
    see Excision, Upper Bones 0PB
    see Resection, Upper Bones 0PT
Scapulopexy
    see Repair, Upper Bones 0PQ
    see Reposition, Upper Bones 0PS
Scarpa's (vestibular) ganglion *use* Acoustic Nerve
Sclerectomy *see* Excision, Eye 08B

Sclerotherapy, mechanical *see* Destruction
▶Sclerotherapy, via injection of sclerosing agent *see* Introduction, Destructive Agent
Sclerotomy *see* Drainage, Eye 089
Scrotectomy
    see Excision, Male Reproductive System 0VB
    see Resection, Male Reproductive System 0VT
Scrotoplasty
    see Repair, Male Reproductive System 0VQ
    see Supplement, Male Reproductive System 0VU
Scrotorrhaphy *see* Repair, Male Reproductive System 0VQ
Scrotomy *see* Drainage, Male Reproductive System 0V9
Sebaceous gland *use* Skin
Second cranial nerve *use* Optic Nerve
Section, cesarean *see* Extraction, Pregnancy 10D
Secura (DR) (VR) *use* Defibrillator Generator in 0JH
Sella turcica *use* Sphenoid Bone
Semicircular canal
    use Inner Ear, Right
    use Inner Ear, Left
Semimembranosus muscle
    use Upper Leg Muscle, Right
    use Upper Leg Muscle, Left
Semitendinosus muscle
    use Upper Leg Muscle, Right
    use Upper Leg Muscle, Left
Seprafilm *use* Adhesion Barrier
Septal cartilage *use* Nasal Septum
Septectomy
    see Excision, Heart and Great Vessels 02B
    see Resection, Heart and Great Vessels 02T
    see Excision, Ear, Nose, Sinus 09B
    see Resection, Ear, Nose, Sinus 09T
Septoplasty
    see Repair, Heart and Great Vessels 02Q
    see Replacement, Heart and Great Vessels 02R
    see Supplement, Heart and Great Vessels 02U
    see Repair, Ear, Nose, Sinus 09Q
    see Replacement, Ear, Nose, Sinus 09R
    see Reposition, Ear, Nose, Sinus 09S
    see Supplement, Ear, Nose, Sinus 09U
Septostomy, balloon atrial 02163Z7
Septotomy *see* Drainage, Ear, Nose, Sinus 099
Sequestrectomy, bone *see* Extirpation
Serratus anterior muscle
    use Thorax Muscle, Right
    use Thorax Muscle, Left
Serratus posterior muscle
    use Trunk Muscle, Right
    use Trunk Muscle, Left
Seventh cranial nerve *use* Facial Nerve
Sheffield hybrid external fixator
    use External Fixation Device, Hybrid in 0PH
    use External Fixation Device, Hybrid in 0PS
    use External Fixation Device, Hybrid in 0QH
    use External Fixation Device, Hybrid in 0QS
Sheffield ring external fixator
    use External Fixation Device, Ring in 0PH
    use External Fixation Device, Ring in 0PS
    use External Fixation Device, Ring in 0QH
    use External Fixation Device, Ring in 0QS
Shirodkar cervical cerclage 0UVC7ZZ
Shock Wave Therapy, Musculoskeletal 6A93
Short gastric artery *use* Splenic Artery
Shortening
    see Excision
    see Repair
    see Reposition
Shunt creation *see* Bypass
Sialoadenectomy
    Complete *see* Resection, Mouth and Throat 0CT
    Partial *see* Excision, Mouth and Throat 0CB
Sialodochoplasty
    see Repair, Mouth and Throat 0CQ
    see Replacement, Mouth and Throat 0CR
    see Supplement, Mouth and Throat 0CU

Sialoectomy
    see Excision, Mouth and Throat 0CB
    see Resection, Mouth and Throat 0CT
Sialography *see* Plain Radiography, Ear, Nose, Mouth and Throat B90
Sialolithotomy *see* Extirpation, Mouth and Throat 0CC
Sigmoid artery *use* Inferior Mesenteric Artery
Sigmoid flexure *use* Sigmoid Colon
Sigmoid vein *use* Inferior Mesenteric Vein
Sigmoidectomy
    see Excision, Gastrointestinal System 0DB
    see Resection, Gastrointestinal System 0DT
Sigmoidorrhaphy *see* Repair, Gastrointestinal System 0DQ
Sigmoidoscopy 0DJD8ZZ
Sigmoidotomy *see* Drainage, Gastrointestinal System 0D9
Single lead pacemaker (atrium) (ventricle) *use* Pacemaker, Single Chamber in 0JH
Single lead rate responsive pacemaker (atrium) (ventricle) *use* Pacemaker, Single Chamber Rate Responsive in 0JH
Sinoatrial node *use* Conduction Mechanism
Sinogram
    Abdominal Wall *see* Fluoroscopy, Abdomen and Pelvis BW11
    Chest Wall *see* Plain Radiography, Chest BW03
    Retroperitoneum *see* Fluoroscopy, Abdomen and Pelvis BW11
Sinus venosus *use* Atrium, Right
Sinusectomy
    see Excision, Ear, Nose, Sinus 09B
    see Resection, Ear, Nose, Sinus 09T
Sinusoscopy 09JY4ZZ
Sinusotomy *see* Drainage, Ear, Nose, Sinus 099
Sirolimus-eluting coronary stent *use* Intraluminal Device, Drug-eluting in Heart and Great Vessels
Sixth cranial nerve *use* Abducens Nerve
Size reduction, breast *see* Excision, Skin and Breast 0HB
SJM Biocor® Stented Valve System *use* Zooplastic Tissue in Heart and Great Vessels
Skene's (paraurethral) gland *use* Vestibular Gland
Skin Substitute, Porcine Liver Derived, Replacement XHRPXL2
Sling
    Fascial, orbicularis muscle (mouth) *see* Supplement, Muscle, Facial 0KU1
    Levator muscle, for urethral suspension *see* Reposition, Bladder Neck 0TSC
    Pubococcygeal, for urethral suspension *see* Reposition, Bladder Neck 0TSC
    Rectum *see* Reposition, Rectum 0DSP
Small bowel series *see* Fluoroscopy, Bowel, Small BD13
Small saphenous vein
    use Saphenous Vein, Right
    use Saphenous Vein, Left
Snaring, polyp, colon *see* Excision, Gastrointestinal System 0DB
Solar (celiac) plexus *use* Abdominal Sympathetic Nerve
Soleus muscle
    use Lower Leg Muscle, Right
    use Lower Leg Muscle, Left
Spacer
    Insertion of device in
        Disc
            Lumbar Vertebral 0SH2
            Lumbosacral 0SH4
        Joint
            Acromioclavicular
                Left 0RHH
                Right 0RHG
            Ankle
                Left 0SHG
                Right 0SHF

▶ New   ⫸ Revised   ~~deleted~~ Deleted

Spinal Stabilization Device (*Continued*)
  Interspinous Process (*Continued*)
    Thoracic Vertebral ØRH6
    Thoracolumbar Vertebral ØRHA
  Pedicle-Based
    Cervical Vertebral ØRH1
    Cervicothoracic Vertebral ØRH4
    Lumbar Vertebral ØSHØ
    Lumbosacral ØSH3
    Occipital-cervical ØRHØ
    Thoracic Vertebral ØRH6
    Thoracolumbar Vertebral ØRHA
Spinous process
  use Cervical Vertebra
  use Thoracic Vertebra
  use Lumbar Vertebra
Spiral ganglion *use* Acoustic Nerve
Spiration IBV™ Valve System *use* Intraluminal Device, Endobronchial Valve in Respiratory System
Splenectomy
  see Excision, Lymphatic and Hemic Systems Ø7B
  see Resection, Lymphatic and Hemic Systems Ø7T
Splenic flexure *use* Transverse Colon
Splenic plexus *use* Abdominal Sympathetic Nerve
Splenius capitis muscle *use* Head Muscle
Splenius cervicis muscle
  use Neck Muscle, Right
  use Neck Muscle, Left
Splenolysis *see* Release, Lymphatic and Hemic Systems Ø7N
Splenopexy
  see Repair, Lymphatic and Hemic Systems Ø7Q
  see Reposition, Lymphatic and Hemic Systems Ø7S
Splenoplasty *see* Repair, Lymphatic and Hemic Systems Ø7Q
Splenorrhaphy *see* Repair, Lymphatic and Hemic Systems Ø7Q
Splenotomy *see* Drainage, Lymphatic and Hemic Systems Ø79
Splinting, musculoskeletal *see* Immobilization, Anatomical Regions 2W3
SPY system intravascular fluorescence angiography *see* Monitoring, Physiological Systems 4A1
Stapedectomy
  see Excision, Ear, Nose, Sinus Ø9B
  see Resection, Ear, Nose, Sinus Ø9T
Stapediolysis *see* Release, Ear, Nose, Sinus Ø9N
Stapedioplasty
  see Repair, Ear, Nose, Sinus Ø9Q
  see Replacement, Ear, Nose, Sinus Ø9R
  see Supplement, Ear, Nose, Sinus Ø9U
Stapedotomy *see* Drainage, Ear, Nose, Sinus Ø99
Stapes
  use Auditory Ossicle, Right
  use Auditory Ossicle, Left
▶**Static Spacer (Antibiotic)** *use* Spacer in Lower Joints
STELARA® *use* Other New Technology Therapeutic Substance
Stellate ganglion *use* Head and Neck Sympathetic Nerve
Stem cell transplant *see* Transfusion, Circulatory 3Ø2
Stensen's duct
  use Parotid Duct, Right
  use Parotid Duct, Left
Stent, intraluminal (cardiovascular) (gastrointestinal)(hepatobiliary)(urinary) *use* Intraluminal Device
▶**Stent retriever thrombectomy** *see* Extirpation, Upper Arteries Ø3C

Stented tissue valve *use* Zooplastic Tissue in Heart and Great Vessels
Stereotactic Radiosurgery
  Abdomen DW23
  Adrenal Gland DG22
  Bile Ducts DF22
  Bladder DT22
  Bone Marrow D72Ø
  Brain DØ2Ø
  Brain Stem DØ21
  Breast
    Left DM2Ø
    Right DM21
  Bronchus DB21
  Cervix DU21
  Chest DW22
  Chest Wall DB27
  Colon DD25
  Diaphragm DB28
  Duodenum DD22
  Ear D92Ø
  Esophagus DD2Ø
  Eye D82Ø
  Gallbladder DF21
  Gamma Beam
    Abdomen DW23JZZ
    Adrenal Gland DG22JZZ
    Bile Ducts DF22JZZ
    Bladder DT22JZZ
    Bone Marrow D72ØJZZ
    Brain DØ2ØJZZ
    Brain Stem DØ21JZZ
    Breast
      Left DM2ØJZZ
      Right DM21JZZ
    Bronchus DB21JZZ
    Cervix DU21JZZ
    Chest DW22JZZ
    Chest Wall DB27JZZ
    Colon DD25JZZ
    Diaphragm DB28JZZ
    Duodenum DD22JZZ
    Ear D92ØJZZ
    Esophagus DD2ØJZZ
    Eye D82ØJZZ
    Gallbladder DF21JZZ
    Gland
      Adrenal DG22JZZ
      Parathyroid DG24JZZ
      Pituitary DG2ØJZZ
      Thyroid DG25JZZ
    Glands, Salivary D926JZZ
    Head and Neck DW21JZZ
    Ileum DD24JZZ
    Jejunum DD23JZZ
    Kidney DT2ØJZZ
    Larynx D92BJZZ
    Liver DF2ØJZZ
    Lung DB22JZZ
    Lymphatics
      Abdomen D726JZZ
      Axillary D724JZZ
      Inguinal D728JZZ
      Neck D723JZZ
      Pelvis D727JZZ
      Thorax D725JZZ
    Mediastinum DB26JZZ
    Mouth D924JZZ
    Nasopharynx D92DJZZ
    Neck and Head DW21JZZ
    Nerve, Peripheral DØ27JZZ
    Nose D921JZZ
    Ovary DU2ØJZZ
    Palate
      Hard D928JZZ
      Soft D929JZZ
    Pancreas DF23JZZ
    Parathyroid Gland DG24JZZ
    Pelvic Region DW26JZZ
    Pharynx D92CJZZ

Stereotactic Radiosurgery (*Continued*)
  Gamma Beam (*Continued*)
    Pineal Body DG21JZZ
    Pituitary Gland DG2ØJZZ
    Pleura DB25JZZ
    Prostate DV2ØJZZ
    Rectum DD27JZZ
    Sinuses D927JZZ
    Spinal Cord DØ26JZZ
    Spleen D722JZZ
    Stomach DD21JZZ
    Testis DV21JZZ
    Thymus D721JZZ
    Thyroid Gland DG25JZZ
    Tongue D925JZZ
    Trachea DB2ØJZZ
    Ureter DT21JZZ
    Urethra DT23JZZ
    Uterus DU22JZZ
  Gland
    Adrenal DG22
    Parathyroid DG24
    Pituitary DG2Ø
    Thyroid DG25
  Glands, Salivary D926
  Head and Neck DW21
  Ileum DD24
  Jejunum DD23
  Kidney DT2Ø
  Larynx D92B
  Liver DF2Ø
  Lung DB22
  Lymphatics
    Abdomen D726
    Axillary D724
    Inguinal D728
    Neck D723
    Pelvis D727
    Thorax D725
  Mediastinum DB26
  Mouth D924
  Nasopharynx D92D
  Neck and Head DW21
  Nerve, Peripheral DØ27
  Nose D921
  Other Photon
    Abdomen DW23DZZ
    Adrenal Gland DG22DZZ
    Bile Ducts DF22DZZ
    Bladder DT22DZZ
    Bone Marrow D72ØDZZ
    Brain DØ2ØDZZ
    Brain Stem DØ21DZZ
    Breast
      Left DM2ØDZZ
      Right DM21DZZ
    Bronchus DB21DZZ
    Cervix DU21DZZ
    Chest DW22DZZ
    Chest Wall DB27DZZ
    Colon DD25DZZ
    Diaphragm DB28DZZ
    Duodenum DD22DZZ
    Ear D92ØDZZ
    Esophagus DD2ØDZZ
    Eye D82ØDZZ
    Gallbladder DF21DZZ
    Gland
      Adrenal DG22DZZ
      Parathyroid DG24DZZ
      Pituitary DG2ØDZZ
      Thyroid DG25DZZ
    Glands, Salivary D926DZZ
    Head and Neck DW21DZZ
    Ileum DD24DZZ
    Jejunum DD23DZZ
    Kidney DT2ØDZZ
    Larynx D92BDZZ
    Liver DF2ØDZZ
    Lung DB22DZZ

▶ New   ⟹ Revised   ~~deleted~~ Deleted

S

▶ New   ⇒ Revised   ~~deleted~~ Deleted

Styloglossus muscle *use* Tongue, Palate, Pharynx Muscle
Stylomandibular ligament *use* Head and Neck Bursa and Ligament
Stylopharyngeus muscle *use* Tongue, Palate, Pharynx Muscle
Subacromial bursa
  use Shoulder Bursa and Ligament, Right
  use Shoulder Bursa and Ligament, Left
Subaortic (common iliac) lymph node *use* Lymphatic, Pelvis
Subarachnoid space, spinal *use* Spinal Canal
Subclavicular (apical) lymph node
  use Lymphatic, Right Axillary
  use Lymphatic, Left Axillary
Subclavius muscle
  use Thorax Muscle, Right
  use Thorax Muscle, Left
Subclavius nerve *use* Brachial Plexus Nerve
Subcostal artery *use* Upper Artery
Subcostal muscle
  use Thorax Muscle, Right
  use Thorax Muscle, Left
Subcostal nerve *use* Thoracic Nerve
Subcutaneous injection reservoir, port
  use Vascular Access Device, Totally Implantable in Subcutaneous Tissue and Fascia
Subcutaneous injection reservoir, pump *use* Infusion Device, Pump in Subcutaneous Tissue and Fascia
Subdermal progesterone implant *use* Contraceptive Device in Subcutaneous Tissue and Fascia
Subdural space, spinal *use* Spinal Canal
Submandibular ganglion
  use Head and Neck Sympathetic Nerve
  use Facial Nerve
Submandibular gland
  use Submaxillary Gland, Right
  use Submaxillary Gland, Left
Submandibular lymph node *use* Lymphatic, Head
Submaxillary ganglion *use* Head and Neck Sympathetic Nerve
Submaxillary lymph node *use* Lymphatic, Head
Submental artery *use* Face Artery
Submental lymph node *use* Lymphatic, Head
Submucous (Meissner's) plexus *use* Abdominal Sympathetic Nerve
Suboccipital nerve *use* Cervical Nerve
Suboccipital venous plexus
  use Vertebral Vein, Right
  use Vertebral Vein, Left
Subparotid lymph node *use* Lymphatic, Head
Subscapular (posterior) lymph node
  use Lymphatic, Right Axillary
  use Lymphatic, Left Axillary
Subscapular aponeurosis
  use Subcutaneous Tissue and Fascia, Right Upper Arm
  use Subcutaneous Tissue and Fascia, Left Upper Arm
Subscapular artery
  use Axillary Artery, Right
  use Axillary Artery, Left
Subscapularis muscle
  use Shoulder Muscle, Right
  use Shoulder Muscle, Left
Substance Abuse Treatment
  Counseling
    Family, for substance abuse, Other Family Counseling HZ63ZZZ
    Group
      12-Step HZ43ZZZ
      Behavioral HZ41ZZZ
      Cognitive HZ40ZZZ
      Cognitive-Behavioral HZ42ZZZ
      Confrontational HZ48ZZZ
      Continuing Care HZ49ZZZ

Substance Abuse Treatment *(Continued)*
  Counseling *(Continued)*
    Group *(Continued)*
      Infectious Disease
        Post-Test HZ4CZZZ
        Pre-Test HZ4CZZZ
      Interpersonal HZ44ZZZ
      Motivational Enhancement HZ47ZZZ
      Psychoeducation HZ46ZZZ
      Spiritual HZ4BZZZ
      Vocational HZ45ZZZ
    Individual
      12-Step HZ33ZZZ
      Behavioral HZ31ZZZ
      Cognitive HZ30ZZZ
      Cognitive-Behavioral HZ32ZZZ
      Confrontational HZ38ZZZ
      Continuing Care HZ39ZZZ
      Infectious Disease
        Post-Test HZ3CZZZ
        Pre-Test HZ3CZZZ
      Interpersonal HZ34ZZZ
      Motivational Enhancement HZ37ZZZ
      Psychoeducation HZ36ZZZ
      Spiritual HZ3BZZZ
      Vocational HZ35ZZZ
  Detoxification Services, for substance abuse HZ2ZZZZ
  Medication Management
    Antabuse HZ83ZZZ
    Bupropion HZ87ZZZ
    Clonidine HZ86ZZZ
    Levo-alpha-acetyl-methadol (LAAM) HZ82ZZZ
    Methadone Maintenance HZ81ZZZ
    Naloxone HZ85ZZZ
    Naltrexone HZ84ZZZ
    Nicotine Replacement HZ80ZZZ
    Other Replacement Medication HZ89ZZZ
    Psychiatric Medication HZ88ZZZ
  Pharmacotherapy
    Antabuse HZ93ZZZ
    Bupropion HZ97ZZZ
    Clonidine HZ96ZZZ
    Levo-alpha-acetyl-methadol (LAAM) HZ92ZZZ
    Methadone Maintenance HZ91ZZZ
    Naloxone HZ95ZZZ
    Naltrexone HZ94ZZZ
    Nicotine Replacement HZ90ZZZ
    Psychiatric Medication HZ98ZZZ
    Replacement Medication, Other HZ99ZZZ
  Psychotherapy
    12-Step HZ53ZZZ
    Behavioral HZ51ZZZ
    Cognitive HZ50ZZZ
    Cognitive-Behavioral HZ52ZZZ
    Confrontational HZ58ZZZ
    Interactive HZ55ZZZ
    Interpersonal HZ54ZZZ
    Motivational Enhancement HZ57ZZZ
    Psychoanalysis HZ5BZZZ
    Psychodynamic HZ5CZZZ
    Psychoeducation HZ56ZZZ
    Psychophysiological HZ5DZZZ
    Supportive HZ59ZZZ
Substantia nigra *use* Basal Ganglia
Subtalar (talocalcaneal) joint
  use Tarsal Joint, Right
  use Tarsal Joint, Left
Subtalar ligament
  use Foot Bursa and Ligament, Right
  use Foot Bursa and Ligament, Left
Subthalamic nucleus *use* Basal Ganglia
Suction curettage (D&C), nonobstetric *see* Extraction, Endometrium 0UDB
Suction curettage, obstetric post-delivery *see* Extraction, Products of Conception, Retained 10D1

Superficial circumflex iliac vein
  use Saphenous Vein, Right
  use Saphenous Vein, Left
Superficial epigastric artery
  use Femoral Artery, Right
  use Femoral Artery, Left
Superficial epigastric vein
  use Saphenous Vein, Right
  use Saphenous Vein, Left
Superficial Inferior Epigastric Artery Flap
  Replacement
    Bilateral 0HRV078
    Left 0HRU078
    Right 0HRT078
  Transfer
    Left 0KXG
    Right 0KXF
Superficial palmar arch
  use Hand Artery, Right
  use Hand Artery, Left
Superficial palmar venous arch
  use Hand Vein, Right
  use Hand Vein, Left
Superficial temporal artery
  use Temporal Artery, Right
  use Temporal Artery, Left
Superficial transverse perineal muscle *use* Perineum Muscle
Superior cardiac nerve *use* Thoracic Sympathetic Nerve
Superior cerebellar vein *use* Intracranial Vein
Superior cerebral vein *use* Intracranial Vein
Superior clunic (cluneal) nerve *use* Lumbar Nerve
Superior epigastric artery
  use Internal Mammary Artery, Right
  use Internal Mammary Artery, Left
Superior genicular artery
  use Popliteal Artery, Right
  use Popliteal Artery, Left
Superior gluteal artery
  use Internal Iliac Artery, Right
  use Internal Iliac Artery, Left
Superior gluteal nerve *use* Lumbar Plexus Nerve
Superior hypogastric plexus *use* Abdominal Sympathetic Nerve
Superior labial artery *use* Face Artery
Superior laryngeal artery
  use Thyroid Artery, Right
  use Thyroid Artery, Left
Superior laryngeal nerve *use* Vagus Nerve
Superior longitudinal muscle *use* Tongue, Palate, Pharynx Muscle
Superior mesenteric ganglion *use* Abdominal Sympathetic Nerve
Superior mesenteric lymph node *use* Lymphatic, Mesenteric
Superior mesenteric plexus *use* Abdominal Sympathetic Nerve
Superior oblique muscle
  use Extraocular Muscle, Right
  use Extraocular Muscle, Left
Superior olivary nucleus *use* Pons
Superior rectal artery *use* Inferior Mesenteric Artery
Superior rectal vein *use* Inferior Mesenteric Vein
Superior rectus muscle
  use Extraocular Muscle, Right
  use Extraocular Muscle, Left
Superior tarsal plate
  use Upper Eyelid, Right
  use Upper Eyelid, Left
Superior thoracic artery
  use Axillary Artery, Right
  use Axillary Artery, Left
Superior thyroid artery
  use External Carotid Artery, Right
  use External Carotid Artery, Left
  use Thyroid Artery, Right
  use Thyroid Artery, Left

▶ New   ⇒ Revised   ~~deleted~~ Deleted

Superior turbinate *use* Nasal Turbinate
Superior ulnar collateral artery
   use Brachial Artery, Right
   use Brachial Artery, Left
▶Supersaturated Oxygen therapy
  ▶5A0512C
  ▶5A0522C
Supplement
  Abdominal Wall 0WUF
  Acetabulum
    Left 0QU5
    Right 0QU4
  Ampulla of Vater 0FUC
  Anal Sphincter 0DUR
  Anus 0DUQ
  Ankle Region
    Left 0YUL
    Right 0YUK
  Anus 0DUQ
  Aorta
    Abdominal 04U0
    Thoracic
      Ascending/Arch 02UX
      Descending 02UW
  Arm
    Lower
      Left 0XUF
      Right 0XUD
    Upper
      Left 0XU9
      Right 0XU8
  Artery
    Anterior Tibial
      Left 04UQ
      Right 04UP
    Axillary
      Left 03U6
      Right 03U5
    Brachial
      Left 03U8
      Right 03U7
    Celiac 04U1
    Colic
      Left 04U7
      Middle 04U8
      Right 04U6
    Common Carotid
      Left 03UJ
      Right 03UH
    Common Iliac
      Left 04UD
      Right 04UC
    External Carotid
      Left 03UN
      Right 03UM
    External Iliac
      Left 04UJ
      Right 04UH
    Face 03UR
    Femoral
      Left 04UL
      Right 04UK
    Foot
      Left 04UW
      Right 04UV
    Gastric 04U2
    Hand
      Left 03UF
      Right 03UD
    Hepatic 04U3
    Inferior Mesenteric 04UB
    Innominate 03U2
    Internal Carotid
      Left 03UL
      Right 03UK
    Internal Iliac
      Left 04UF
      Right 04UE
    Internal Mammary
      Left 03U1
      Right 03U0
    Intracranial 03UG

Supplement *(Continued)*
  Artery *(Continued)*
    Lower 04UY
    Peroneal
      Left 04UU
      Right 04UT
    Popliteal
      Left 04UN
      Right 04UM
    Posterior Tibial
      Left 04US
      Right 04UR
    Pulmonary
      Left 02UR
      Right 02UQ
    Pulmonary Trunk 02UP
    Radial
      Left 03UC
      Right 03UB
    Renal
      Left 04UA
      Right 04U9
    Splenic 04U4
    Subclavian
      Left 03U4
      Right 03U3
    Superior Mesenteric 04U5
    Temporal
      Left 03UT
      Right 03US
    Thyroid
      Left 03UV
      Right 03UU
    Ulnar
      Left 03UA
      Right 03U9
    Upper 03UY
    Vertebral
      Left 03UQ
      Right 03UP
  Atrium
    Left 02U7
    Right 02U6
  Auditory Ossicle
    Left 09UA
    Right 09U9
  Axilla
    Left 0XU5
    Right 0XU4
  Back
    Lower 0WUL
    Upper 0WUK
  Bladder 0TUB
  Bladder Neck 0TUC
  Bone
    Ethmoid
      Left 0NUG
      Right 0NUF
    Frontal 0NU1
    Hyoid 0NUX
    Lacrimal
      Left 0NUJ
      Right 0NUH
    Nasal 0NUB
    Occipital 0NU7
    Palatine
      Left 0NUL
      Right 0NUK
    Parietal
      Left 0NU4
      Right 0NU3
    Pelvic
      Left 0QU3
      Right 0QU2
    Sphenoid 0NUC
    Temporal
      Left 0NU6
      Right 0NU5
    Zygomatic
      Left 0NUN
      Right 0NUM

Supplement *(Continued)*
  Breast
    Bilateral 0HUV
    Left 0HUU
    Right 0HUT
  Bronchus
    Lingula 0BU9
    Lower Lobe
      Left 0BUB
      Right 0BU6
    Main
      Left 0BU7
      Right 0BU3
    Middle Lobe, Right 0BU5
    Upper Lobe
      Left 0BU8
      Right 0BU4
  Buccal Mucosa 0CU4
  Bursa and Ligament
    Abdomen
      Left 0MUJ
      Right 0MUH
    Ankle
      Left 0MUR
      Right 0MUQ
    Elbow
      Left 0MU4
      Right 0MU3
    Foot
      Left 0MUT
      Right 0MUS
    Hand
      Left 0MU8
      Right 0MU7
    Head and Neck 0MU0
    Hip
      Left 0MUM
      Right 0MUL
    Knee
      Left 0MUP
      Right 0MUN
    Lower Extremity
      Left 0MUW
      Right 0MUV
    Perineum 0MUK
    Rib(s) 0MUG
    Shoulder
      Left 0MU2
      Right 0MU1
    Spine
      Lower 0MUD
      Upper 0MUC
    Sternum 0MUF
    Upper Extremity
      Left 0MUB
      Right 0MU9
    Wrist
      Left 0MU6
      Right 0MU5
  Buttock
    Left 0YU1
    Right 0YU0
  Carina 0BU2
  Carpal
    Left 0PUN
    Right 0PUM
  Cecum 0DUH
  Cerebral Meninges 00U1
  Cerebral Ventricle 00U6
  Chest Wall 0WU8
  Chordae Tendineae 02U9
  Cisterna Chyli 07UL
  Clavicle
    Left 0PUB
    Right 0PU9
  Clitoris 0UUJ
  Coccyx 0QUS
  Colon
    Ascending 0DUK
    Descending 0DUM
    Sigmoid 0DUN
    Transverse 0DUL

▶ New   ⇒ Revised   ~~deleted~~ Deleted

S

▶ New   ⇒ Revised   ~~deleted~~ Deleted

T

Takedown
 Arteriovenous shunt *see* Removal of device from, Upper Arteries 03P
 Arteriovenous shunt, with creation of new shunt *see* Bypass, Upper Arteries 031
 Stoma
  see Excision
  see Reposition
Talent® Converter *use* Intraluminal Device
Talent® Occluder *use* Intraluminal Device
Talent® Stent Graft (abdominal) (thoracic) *use* Intraluminal Device
Talocalcaneal (subtalar) joint
 use Tarsal Joint, Right
 use Tarsal Joint, Left
Talocalcaneal ligament
 use Foot Bursa and Ligament, Right
 use Foot Bursa and Ligament, Left
Talocalcaneonavicular joint
 use Tarsal Joint, Right
 use Tarsal Joint, Left
Talocalcaneonavicular ligament
 use Foot Bursa and Ligament, Right
 use Foot Bursa and Ligament, Left
Talocrural joint
 use Ankle Joint, Right
 use Ankle Joint, Left
Talofibular ligament
 use Ankle Bursa and Ligament, Right
 use Ankle Bursa and Ligament, Left
Talus bone
 use Tarsal, Right
 use Tarsal, Left
TandemHeart® System *use* Short-term External Heart Assist System in Heart and Great Vessels
Tarsectomy
 see Excision, Lower Bones 0QB
 see Resection, Lower Bones 0QT
Tarsometatarsal ligament
 use Foot Bursa and Ligament, Right
 use Foot Bursa and Ligament, Left
Tarsorrhaphy *see* Repair, Eye 08Q
Tattooing
 Cornea 3E0CXMZ
 Skin *see* Introduction of substance in or on Skin 3E00
TAXUS® Liberté® Paclitaxel-eluting Coronary Stent System *use* Intraluminal Device, Drug-eluting in Heart and Great Vessels
➠**TBNA (transbronchial needle aspiration)**
 ▶Fluid or gas *see* Drainage, Respiratory System 0B9
 ▶Tissue biopsy *see* Extraction, Respiratory System 0BD
Telemetry
 4A12X4Z
 Ambulatory 4A12X45
Temperature gradient study 4A0ZXKZ
Temporal lobe *use* Cerebral Hemisphere
Temporalis muscle *use* Head Muscle
Temporoparietalis muscle *use* Head Muscle
Tendolysis *see* Release, Tendons 0LN
Tendonectomy
 see Excision, Tendons 0LB
 see Resection, Tendons 0LT
Tendonoplasty, tenoplasty
 see Repair, Tendons 0LQ
 see Replacement, Tendons 0LR
 see Supplement, Tendons 0LU
Tendorrhaphy *see* Repair, Tendons 0LQ
Tendototomy
 see Division, Tendons 0L8
 see Drainage, Tendons 0L9
Tenectomy, tenonectomy
 see Excision, Tendons 0LB
 see Resection, Tendons 0LT
Tenolysis *see* Release, Tendons 0LN

Tenontorrhaphy *see* Repair, Tendons 0LQ
Tenontotomy
 see Division, Tendons 0L8
 see Drainage, Tendons 0L9
Tenorrhaphy *see* Repair, Tendons 0LQ
Tenosynovectomy
 see Excision, Tendons 0LB
 see Resection, Tendons 0LT
Tenotomy
 see Division, Tendons 0L8
 see Drainage, Tendons 0L9
Tensor fasciae latae muscle
 use Hip Muscle, Right
 use Hip Muscle, Left
Tensor veli palatini muscle *use* Tongue, Palate, Pharynx Muscle
Tenth cranial nerve *use* Vagus Nerve
Tentorium cerebelli *use* Dura Mater
Teres major muscle
 use Shoulder Muscle, Right
 use Shoulder Muscle, Left
Teres minor muscle
 use Shoulder Muscle, Right
 use Shoulder Muscle, Left
Termination of pregnancy
 Aspiration curettage 10A07ZZ
 Dilation and curettage 10A07ZZ
 Hysterotomy 10A00ZZ
 Intra-amniotic injection 10A03ZZ
 Laminaria 10A07ZW
 Vacuum 10A07Z6
Testectomy
 see Excision, Male Reproductive System 0VB
 see Resection, Male Reproductive System 0VT
Testicular artery *use* Abdominal Aorta
Testing
 Glaucoma 4A07XBZ
 Hearing *see* Hearing Assessment, Diagnostic Audiology F13
 Mental health *see* Psychological Tests
 Muscle function, electromyography (EMG) *see* Measurement, Musculoskeletal 4A0F
 Muscle function, manual *see* Motor Function Assessment, Rehabilitation F01
 Neurophysiologic monitoring, intra-operative *see* Monitoring, Physiological Systems 4A1
 Range of motion *see* Motor Function Assessment, Rehabilitation F01
 Vestibular function *see* Vestibular Assessment, Diagnostic Audiology F15
Thalamectomy *see* Excision, Thalamus 00B9
Thalamotomy
 see Drainage, Thalamus 0099
Thenar muscle
 use Hand Muscle, Right
 use Hand Muscle, Left
Therapeutic Massage
 Musculoskeletal System 8E0KX1Z
 Reproductive System
  Prostate 8E0VX1C
  Rectum 8E0VX1D
Therapeutic occlusion coil(s) *use* Intraluminal Device
Thermography 4A0ZXKZ
Thermotherapy, prostate *see* Destruction, Prostate 0V50
Third cranial nerve *use* Oculomotor Nerve
Third occipital nerve *use* Cervical Nerve
Third ventricle *use* Cerebral Ventricle
Thoracectomy *see* Excision, Anatomical Regions, General 0WB
Thoracentesis *see* Drainage, Anatomical Regions, General 0W9
Thoracic aortic plexus *use* Thoracic Sympathetic Nerve
Thoracic esophagus *use* Esophagus, Middle
Thoracic facet joint *use* Thoracic Vertebral Joint
Thoracic ganglion *use* Thoracic Sympathetic Nerve

Thoracoacromial artery
 use Axillary Artery, Right
 use Axillary Artery, Left
Thoracocentesis *see* Drainage, Anatomical Regions, General 0W9
Thoracolumbar facet joint *use* Thoracolumbar Vertebral Joint
Thoracoplasty
 see Repair, Anatomical Regions, General 0WQ
 see Supplement, Anatomical Regions, General 0WU
Thoracostomy tube *use* Drainage Device
Thoracostomy, for lung collapse *see* Drainage, Respiratory System 0B9
Thoracotomy *see* Drainage, Anatomical Regions, General 0W9
Thoratec IVAD (Implantable Ventricular Assist Device) *use* Implantable Heart Assist System in Heart and Great Vessels
Thoratec Paracorporeal Ventricular Assist Device *use* Short-term External Heart Assist System in Heart and Great Vessels
Thrombectomy *see* Extirpation
Thymectomy
 see Excision, Lymphatic and Hemic Systems 07B
 see Resection, Lymphatic and Hemic Systems 07T
Thymopexy
 see Repair, Lymphatic and Hemic Systems 07Q
 see Reposition, Lymphatic and Hemic Systems 07S
Thymus gland *use* Thymus
Thyroarytenoid muscle
 use Neck Muscle, Right
 use Neck Muscle, Left
Thyrocervical trunk
 use Thyroid Artery, Right
 use Thyroid Artery, Left
Thyroid cartilage *use* Larynx
Thyroidectomy
 see Excision, Endocrine System 0GB
 see Resection, Endocrine System 0GT
Thyroidorrhaphy *see* Repair, Endocrine System 0GQ
Thyroidoscopy 0GJK4ZZ
Thyroidotomy *see* Drainage, Endocrine System 0G9
Tibial insert *use* Liner in Lower Joints
Tibialis anterior muscle
 use Lower Leg Muscle, Right
 use Lower Leg Muscle, Left
Tibialis posterior muscle
 use Lower Leg Muscle, Right
 use Lower Leg Muscle, Left
Tibiofemoral joint
 use Knee Joint, Right
 use Knee Joint, Left
 use Knee Joint, Tibial Surface, Right
 use Knee Joint, Tibial Surface, Left
▶**Tisagenlecleucel** *use* Engineered Autologous Chimeric Antigen Receptor T-cell Immunotherapy
Tissue bank graft *use* Nonautologous Tissue Substitute
Tissue Expander
 Insertion of device in
  Breast
   Bilateral 0HHV
   Left 0HHU
   Right 0HHT
  Nipple
   Left 0HHX
   Right 0HHW
  Subcutaneous Tissue and Fascia
   Abdomen 0JH8
   Back 0JH7
   Buttock 0JH9
   Chest 0JH6
   Face 0JH1

Transfusion *(Continued)*
  Artery *(Continued)*
    Central *(Continued)*
      Globulin 3026
      Plasma
        Fresh 3026
        Frozen 3026
      Plasma Cryoprecipitate 3026
      Serum Albumin 3026
      Stem Cells
        Cord Blood 3026
        Hematopoietic 3026
    Peripheral
      Antihemophilic Factors 3025
      Blood
        Platelets 3025
        Red Cells 3025
          Frozen 3025
        White Cells 3025
        Whole 3025
      Bone Marrow 3025
      Factor IX 3025
      Fibrinogen 3025
      Globulin 3025
      Plasma
        Fresh 3025
        Frozen 3025
      Plasma Cryoprecipitate 3025
      Serum Albumin 3025
      Stem Cells
        Cord Blood 3025
        Hematopoietic 3025
  Products of Conception
    Antihemophilic Factors 3027
    Blood
      Platelets 3027
      Red Cells 3027
        Frozen 3027
      White Cells 3027
      Whole 3027
    Factor IX 3027
    Fibrinogen 3027
    Globulin 3027
    Plasma
      Fresh 3027
      Frozen 3027
    Plasma Cryoprecipitate 3027
    Serum Albumin 3027
  Vein
    4-Factor Prothrombin Complex
      Concentrate 3028[03]B1
    Central
      Antihemophilic Factors 3024
      Blood
        Platelets 3024
        Red Cells 3024
          Frozen 3024
        White Cells 3024
        Whole 3024
      Bone Marrow 3024
      Factor IX 3024
      Fibrinogen 3024
      Globulin 3024
      Plasma
        Fresh 3024
        Frozen 3024
      Plasma Cryoprecipitate 3024
      Serum Albumin 3024
      Stem Cells
        Cord Blood 3024
        Embryonic 3024
        Hematopoietic 3024
    Peripheral
      Antihemophilic Factors 3023
      Blood
        Platelets 3023
        Red Cells 3023
          Frozen 3023
        White Cells 3023
        Whole 3023
      Bone Marrow 3023
      Factor IX 3023

Transfusion *(Continued)*
  Vein *(Continued)*
    Peripheral *(Continued)*
      Globulin 3023
      Plasma
        Fresh 3023
        Frozen 3023
      Plasma Cryoprecipitate 3023
      Serum Albumin 3023
      Stem Cells
        Cord Blood 3023
        Embryonic 3023
        Hematopoietic 3023
Transplant *see* Transplantation
Transplantation
  Bone marrow *see* Transfusion, Circulatory 302
  Esophagus 0DY50Z
  Face 0WY20Z
  Hand
    Left 0XYK0Z
    Right 0XYJ0Z
  Heart 02YA0Z
  Hematopoietic cell *see* Transfusion,
    Circulatory 302
  Intestine
    Large 0DYE0Z
    Small 0DY80Z
  Kidney
    Left 0TY10Z
    Right 0TY00Z
  Liver 0FY00Z
  Lung
    Bilateral 0BYM0Z
    Left 0BYL0Z
    Lower Lobe
      Left 0BYJ0Z
      Right 0BYF0Z
    Middle Lobe, Right 0BYD0Z
    Right 0BYK0Z
    Upper Lobe
      Left 0BYG0Z
      Right 0BYC0Z
  Lung Lingula 0BYH0Z
  Ovary
    Left 0UY10Z
    Right 0UY00Z
  Pancreas 0FYG0Z
  Products of Conception 10Y0
  Spleen 07YP0Z
  Stem cell *see* Transfusion, Circulatory 302
  Stomach 0DY60Z
  Thymus 07YM0Z
  ▶ Uterus 0UY90Z
Transposition
  see Bypass
  see Reposition
  see Transfer
Transversalis fascia *use* Subcutaneous Tissue
  and Fascia, Trunk
Transverse (cutaneous) cervical nerve *use*
  Cervical Plexus
Transverse acetabular ligament
  use Hip Bursa and Ligament, Right
  use Hip Bursa and Ligament, Left
Transverse facial artery
  use Temporal Artery, Right
  use Temporal Artery, Left
Transverse foramen *use* Cervical Vertebra
Transverse humeral ligament
  use Shoulder Bursa and Ligament, Right
  use Shoulder Bursa and Ligament, Left
Transverse ligament of atlas *use* Head and
  Neck Bursa and Ligament
Transverse process
  use Cervical Vertebra
  use Thoracic Vertebra
  use Lumbar Vertebra
Transverse Rectus Abdominis Myocutaneous
  Flap
  Replacement
    Bilateral 0HRV076
    Left 0HRU076
    Right 0HRT076

Transverse Rectus Abdominis Myocutaneous
  Flap *(Continued)*
  Transfer
    Left 0KXL
    Right 0KXK
Transverse scapular ligament
  use Shoulder Bursa and Ligament, Right
  use Shoulder Bursa and Ligament, Left
Transverse thoracis muscle
  use Thorax Muscle, Right
  use Thorax Muscle, Left
Transversospinalis muscle
  use Trunk Muscle, Right
  use Trunk Muscle, Left
Transversus abdominis muscle
  use Abdomen Muscle, Right
  use Abdomen Muscle, Left
Trapezium bone
  use Carpal, Right
  use Carpal, Left
Trapezius muscle
  use Trunk Muscle, Right
  use Trunk Muscle, Left
Trapezoid bone
  use Carpal, Right
  use Carpal, Left
Triceps brachii muscle
  use Upper Arm Muscle, Right
  use Upper Arm Muscle, Left
Tricuspid annulus *use* Tricuspid Valve
Trifacial nerve *use* Trigeminal Nerve
Trifecta™ Valve (aortic) *use* Zooplastic Tissue
  in Heart and Great Vessels
Trigone of bladder *use* Bladder
Trimming, excisional *see* Excision
Triquetral bone
  use Carpal, Right
  use Carpal, Left
Trochanteric bursa
  use Hip Bursa and Ligament, Right
  use Hip Bursa and Ligament, Left
TUMT (Transurethral microwave
  thermotherapy of prostate) 0V507ZZ
TUNA (transurethral needle ablation of
  prostate) 0V507ZZ
Tunneled central venous catheter *use* Vascular
  Access Device, Tunneled in Subcutaneous
  Tissue and Fascia
Tunneled spinal (intrathecal) catheter *use*
  Infusion Device
Turbinectomy
  see Excision, Ear, Nose, Sinus 09B
  see Resection, Ear, Nose, Sinus 09T
Turbinoplasty
  see Repair, Ear, Nose, Sinus 09Q
  see Replacement, Ear, Nose, Sinus 09R
  see Supplement, Ear, Nose, Sinus 09U
Turbinotomy
  see Division, Ear, Nose, Sinus 098
  see Drainage, Ear, Nose, Sinus 099
TURP (transurethral resection of prostate)
  see Excision, Prostate 0VB0
  see Resection, Prostate 0VT0
Twelfth cranial nerve *use* Hypoglossal Nerve
Two lead pacemaker *use* Pacemaker, Dual
  Chamber in 0JH
Tympanic cavity
  use Middle Ear, Right
  use Middle Ear, Left
Tympanic nerve *use* Glossopharyngeal Nerve
Tympanic part of temoporal bone
  use Temporal Bone, Right
  use Temporal Bone, Left
Tympanogram *see* Hearing Assessment,
  Diagnostic Audiology F13
Tympanoplasty
  see Repair, Ear, Nose, Sinus 09Q
  see Replacement, Ear, Nose, Sinus 09R
  see Supplement, Ear, Nose, Sinus 09U
Tympanosympathectomy *see* Excision, Nerve,
  Head and Neck Sympathetic 01BK
Tympanotomy *see* Drainage, Ear, Nose, Sinus 099

▶ New   ⟹ Revised   ~~deleted~~ Deleted

▶ New   ⇒ Revised   ~~deleted~~ Deleted

Ultrasonography (Continued)
  Vena Cava
    Inferior, Intravascular B549ZZ3
    Superior, Intravascular B548ZZ3
  Wrist
    Left, Densitometry BP4MZZ1
    Right, Densitometry BP4LZZ1
Ultrasound bone healing system
  use Bone Growth Stimulator in Head and
      Facial Bones
  use Bone Growth Stimulator in Upper Bones
  use Bone Growth Stimulator in Lower Bones
Ultrasound Therapy
  Heart 6A75
  No Qualifier 6A75
  Vessels
    Head and Neck 6A75
    Other 6A75
    Peripheral 6A75
Ultraviolet Light Therapy, Skin 6A80
Umbilical artery
  use Internal Iliac Artery, Right
  use Internal Iliac Artery, Left
  use Lower Artery
Uniplanar external fixator
  use External Fixation Device, Monoplanar in
      0PH
  use External Fixation Device, Monoplanar
      in 0PS
  use External Fixation Device, Monoplanar in
      0QH
  use External Fixation Device, Monoplanar
      in 0QS
Upper GI series *see* Fluoroscopy,
    Gastrointestinal, Upper BD15
Ureteral orifice
  use Ureter, Left
  use Ureter
  use Ureter, Right
  use Ureters, Bilateral
Ureterectomy
  see Excision, Urinary System 0TB
  see Resection, Urinary System 0TT

Ureterocolostomy *see* Bypass, Urinary System
    0T1
Ureterocystostomy *see* Bypass, Urinary System
    0T1
Ureteroenterostomy *see* Bypass, Urinary System
    0T1
Ureteroileostomy *see* Bypass, Urinary System
    0T1
Ureterolithotomy *see* Extirpation, Urinary
    System 0TC
Ureterolysis *see* Release, Urinary System 0TN
Ureteroneocystostomy
  see Bypass, Urinary System 0T1
  see Reposition, Urinary System 0TS
Ureteropelvic junction (UPJ)
  use Kidney Pelvis, Right
  use Kidney Pelvis, Left
Ureteropexy
  see Repair, Urinary System 0TQ
  see Reposition, Urinary System 0TS
Ureteroplasty
  see Repair, Urinary System 0TQ
  see Replacement, Urinary System 0TR
  see Supplement, Urinary System 0TU
Ureteroplication *see* Restriction, Urinary
    System 0TV
Ureteropyelography *see* Fluoroscopy, Urinary
    System BT1
Ureterorrhaphy *see* Repair, Urinary System
    0TQ
Ureteroscopy 0TJ98ZZ
Ureterostomy
  see Bypass, Urinary System 0T1
  see Drainage, Urinary System 0T9
Ureterotomy *see* Drainage, Urinary System
    0T9
Ureteroureterostomy *see* Bypass, Urinary
    System 0T1
Ureterovesical orifice
  use Ureter, Right
  use Ureter, Left
  use Ureters, Bilateral
  use Ureter

Urethral catheterization, indwelling
    0T9B70Z
Urethrectomy
  see Excision, Urethra 0TBD
  see Resection, Urethra 0TTD
Urethrolithotomy *see* Extirpation, Urethra
    0TCD
Urethrolysis *see* Release, Urethra 0TND
Urethropexy
  see Repair, Urethra 0TQD
  see Reposition, Urethra 0TSD
Urethroplasty
  see Repair, Urethra 0TQD
  see Replacement, Urethra 0TRD
  see Supplement, Urethra 0TUD
Urethrorrhaphy *see* Repair, Urethra 0TQD
Urethroscopy 0TJD8ZZ
Urethrotomy *see* Drainage, Urethra 0T9D
Uridine Triacetate XW0DX82
Urinary incontinence stimulator lead *use*
    Stimulator Lead in Urinary System
Urography *see* Fluoroscopy, Urinary System
    BT1
Ustekinumab *use* Other New Technology
    Therapeutic Substance
Uterine Artery
  use Internal Iliac Artery, Right
  use Internal Iliac Artery, Left
Uterine artery embolization (UAE) *see*
    Occlusion, Lower Arteries 04L
Uterine cornu *use* Uterus
Uterine tube
  use Fallopian Tube, Right
  use Fallopian Tube, Left
Uterine vein
  use Hypogastric Vein, Right
  use Hypogastric Vein, Left
Uvulectomy
  see Excision, Uvula 0CBN
  see Resection, Uvula 0CTN
Uvulorrhaphy *see* Repair, Uvula 0CQN
Uvulotomy *see* Drainage, Uvula 0C9N

▶ New   ⇒ Revised   ~~deleted~~ Deleted

V

Vaccination *see* Introduction of Serum, Toxoid, and Vaccine
Vacuum extraction, obstetric 10D07Z6
Vaginal artery
  use Internal Iliac Artery, Right
  use Internal Iliac Artery, Left
Vaginal pessary *use* Intraluminal Device, Pessary in Female Reproductive System
Vaginal vein
  use Hypogastric Vein, Right
  use Hypogastric Vein, Left
Vaginectomy
  see Excision, Vagina 0UBG
  see Resection, Vagina 0UTG
Vaginofixation
  see Repair, Vagina 0UQG
  see Reposition, Vagina 0USG
Vaginoplasty
  see Repair, Vagina 0UQG
  see Supplement, Vagina 0UUG
Vaginorrhaphy *see* Repair, Vagina 0UQG
Vaginoscopy 0UJH8ZZ
Vaginotomy *see* Drainage, Female Reproductive System 0U9
Vagotomy *see* Division, Nerve, Vagus 008Q
Valiant Thoracic Stent Graft *use* Intraluminal Device
Valvotomy, valvulotomy
  see Division, Heart and Great Vessels 028
  see Release, Heart and Great Vessels 02N
Valvuloplasty
  see Repair, Heart and Great Vessels 02Q
  see Replacement, Heart and Great Vessels 02R
  see Supplement, Heart and Great Vessels 02U
Valvuloplasty, Alfieri Stitch *see* Restriction, Valve, Mitral 02VG
Vascular Access Device
  Totally Implantable
    Insertion of device in
      Abdomen 0JH8
      Chest 0JH6
      Lower Arm
        Left 0JHH
        Right 0JHG
      Lower Leg
        Left 0JHP
        Right 0JHN
      Upper Arm
        Left 0JHF
        Right 0JHD
      Upper Leg
        Left 0JHM
        Right 0JHL
    Removal of device from
      Lower Extremity 0JPW
      Trunk 0JPT
      Upper Extremity 0JPV
    Revision of device in
      Lower Extremity 0JWW
      Trunk 0JWT
      Upper Extremity 0JWV
  Tunneled
    Insertion of device in
      Abdomen 0JH8
      Chest 0JH6
      Lower Arm
        Left 0JHH
        Right 0JHG
      Lower Leg
        Left 0JHP
        Right 0JHN
      Upper Arm
        Left 0JHF
        Right 0JHD
      Upper Leg
        Left 0JHM
        Right 0JHL
    Removal of device from
      Lower Extremity 0JPW
      Trunk 0JPT
      Upper Extremity 0JPV

Vascular Access Device *(Continued)*
  Tunneled *(Continued)*
    Revision of device in
      Lower Extremity 0JWW
      Trunk 0JWT
      Upper Extremity 0JWV
Vasectomy *see* Excision, Male Reproductive System 0VB
Vasography
  see Plain Radiography, Male Reproductive System BV0
  see Fluoroscopy, Male Reproductive System BV1
Vasoligation *see* Occlusion, Male Reproductive System 0VL
Vasorrhaphy *see* Repair, Male Reproductive System 0VQ
Vasostomy *see* Bypass, Male Reproductive System 0V1
Vasotomy
  Drainage *see* Drainage, Male Reproductive System 0V9
  With ligation *see* Occlusion, Male Reproductive System 0VL
Vasovasostomy *see* Repair, Male Reproductive System 0VQ
Vastus intermedius muscle
  use Upper Leg Muscle, Right
  use Upper Leg Muscle, Left
Vastus lateralis muscle
  use Upper Leg Muscle, Right
  use Upper Leg Muscle, Left
Vastus medialis muscle
  use Upper Leg Muscle, Right
  use Upper Leg Muscle, Left
VCG (vectorcardiogram) *see* Measurement, Cardiac 4A02
Vectra® Vascular Access Graft *use* Vascular Access Device, Tunneled in Subcutaneous Tissue and Fascia
Venectomy
  see Excision, Upper Veins 05B
  see Excision, Lower Veins 06B
Venography
  see Plain Radiography, Veins B50
  see Fluoroscopy, Veins B51
Venorrhaphy
  see Repair, Upper Veins 05Q
  see Repair, Lower Veins 06Q
Venotripsy
  see Occlusion, Upper Veins 05L
  see Occlusion, Lower Veins 06L
Ventricular fold *use* Larynx
Ventriculoatriostomy *see* Bypass, Central Nervous System and Cranial Nerves 001
Ventriculocisternostomy *see* Bypass, Central Nervous System and Cranial Nerves 001
Ventriculogram, cardiac
  Combined left and right heart *see* Fluoroscopy, Heart, Right and Left B216
  Left ventricle *see* Fluoroscopy, Heart, Left B215
  Right ventricle *see* Fluoroscopy, Heart, Right B214
Ventriculopuncture, through previously implanted catheter 8C01X6J
Ventriculoscopy 00J04ZZ
Ventriculostomy
  External drainage *see* Drainage, Cerebral Ventricle 0096
  Internal shunt *see* Bypass, Cerebral Ventricle 0016
Ventriculovenostomy *see* Bypass, Cerebral Ventricle 0016
Ventrio™ Hernia Patch *use* Synthetic Substitute
VEP (visual evoked potential) 4A07X0Z
Vermiform appendix *use* Appendix
Vermilion border
  use Upper Lip
  use Lower Lip
Versa *use* Pacemaker, Dual Chamber in 0JH

Version, obstetric
  External 10S0XZZ
  Internal 10S07ZZ
Vertebral arch
  use Cervical Vertebra
  use Thoracic Vertebra
  use Lumbar Vertebra
Vertebral body
  use Cervical Vertebra
  use Thoracic Vertebra
  use Lumbar Vertebra
Vertebral canal *use* Spinal Canal
Vertebral foramen
  use Cervical Vertebra
  use Thoracic Vertebra
  use Lumbar Vertebra
Vertebral lamina
  use Cervical Vertebra
  use Thoracic Vertebra
  use Lumbar Vertebra
Vertebral pedicle
  use Cervical Vertebra
  use Thoracic Vertebra
  use Lumbar Vertebra
Vesical vein
  use Hypogastric Vein, Right
  use Hypogastric Vein, Left
Vesicotomy *see* Drainage, Urinary System 0T9
Vesiculectomy
  see Excision, Male Reproductive System 0VB
  see Resection, Male Reproductive System 0VT
Vesiculogram, seminal *see* Plain Radiography, Male Reproductive System BV0
Vesiculotomy *see* Drainage, Male Reproductive System 0V9
Vestibular (Scarpa's) ganglion *use* Acoustic Nerve
Vestibular Assessment F15Z
Vestibular nerve *use* Acoustic Nerve
Vestibular Treatment F0C
Vestibulocochlear nerve *use* Acoustic Nerve
VH-IVUS (virtual histology intravascular ultrasound) *see* Ultrasonography, Heart B24
Virchow's (supraclavicular) lymph node
  use Lymphatic, Right Neck
  use Lymphatic, Left Neck
Virtuoso (II) (DR) (VR) *use* Defibrillator Generator in 0JH
Vistogard® *use* Uridine Triacetate
Vitrectomy
  see Excision, Eye 08B
  see Resection, Eye 08T
Vitreous body
  use Vitreous, Right
  use Vitreous, Left
Viva (XT)(S) *use* Cardiac Resynchronization Defibrillator Pulse Generator in 0JH
Vocal fold
  use Vocal Cord, Right
  use Vocal Cord, Left
Vocational
  Assessment *see* Activities of Daily Living Assessment, Rehabilitation F02
  Retraining *see* Activities of Daily Living Treatment, Rehabilitation F08
Volar (palmar) digital vein
  use Hand Vein, Right
  use Hand Vein, Left
Volar (palmar) metacarpal vein
  use Hand Vein, Right
  use Hand Vein, Left
Vomer bone *use* Nasal Septum
Vomer of nasal septum *use* Nasal Bone
Voraxaze *use* Glucarpidase
Vulvectomy
  see Excision, Female Reproductive System 0UB
  see Resection, Female Reproductive System 0UT
VYXEOS™ *use* Cytarabine and Daunorubicin Liposome Antineoplastic

W

WALLSTENT® Endoprosthesis *use*
Intraluminal Device
Washing *see* Irrigation
Wedge resection, pulmonary *see* Excision,
Respiratory System 0BB
Window *see* Drainage
Wiring, dental 2W31X9Z

X

Xact Carotid Stent System *use* Intraluminal
Device
X-ray *see* Plain Radiography
X-STOP® Spacer
use Spinal Stabilization Device, Interspinous
Process in 0RH
use Spinal Stabilization Device, Interspinous
Process in 0SH
Xenograft *use* Zooplastic Tissue in Heart and
Great Vessels
XIENCE Everolimus Eluting Coronary Stent
System *use* Intraluminal Device, Drug-
eluting in Heart and Great Vessels
Xiphoid process *use* Sternum
XLIF® System *use* Interbody Fusion Device in
Lower Joints

Y

Yoga Therapy 8E0ZXY4

Z

Z-plasty, skin for scar contracture *see* Release,
Skin and Breast 0HN
Zenith AAA Endovascular Graft
use Intraluminal Device, Branched or
Fenestrated, One or Two Arteries in 04V
use Intraluminal Device, Branched or
Fenestrated, Three or More Arteries in
04V
use Intraluminal Device
Zenith Flex® AAA Endovascular Graft *use*
Intraluminal Device
Zenith TX2® TAA Endovascular Graft *use*
Intraluminal Device
Zenith® Renu™ AAA Ancillary Graft *use*
Intraluminal Device
Zilver® PTX® (paclitaxel) Drug-Eluting
Peripheral Stent
use Intraluminal Device, Drug-eluting in
Upper Arteries
use Intraluminal Device, Drug-eluting in
Lower Arteries

Zimmer® NexGen® LPS Mobile Bearing Knee
use Synthetic Substitute
Zimmer® NexGen® LPS-Flex Mobile Knee *use*
Synthetic Substitute
ZINPLAVA™ *use* Bezlotoxumab Monoclonal
Antibody
Zonule of Zinn
use Lens, Right
use Lens, Left
Zooplastic Tissue, Rapid Deployment
Technique, Replacement X2RF
Zotarolimus-eluting coronary stent *use*
Intraluminal Device, Drug-eluting in Heart
and Great Vessels
Zygomatic process of frontal bone *use* Frontal
Bone
Zygomatic process of temporal bone
use Temporal Bone, Right
use Temporal Bone, Left
Zygomaticus muscle *use* Facial Muscle
Zyvox *use* Oxazolidinones

▶ New ⟫ Revised ~~deleted~~ Deleted

Appendices

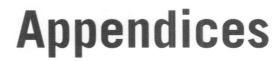

DEFINITIONS

SECTION-CHARACTER

DEFINITIONS

SECTION Ø - MEDICAL AND SURGICAL
CHARACTER 3 - OPERATION

Alteration	**Definition:** Modifying the anatomic structure of a body part without affecting the function of the body part **Explanation:** Principal purpose is to improve appearance **Includes/Examples:** Face lift, breast augmentation
Bypass	**Definition:** Altering the route of passage of the contents of a tubular body part **Explanation:** Rerouting contents of a body part to a downstream area of the normal route, to a similar route and body part, or to an abnormal route and dissimilar body part. Includes one or more anastomoses, with or without the use of a device **Includes/Examples:** Coronary artery bypass, colostomy formation
Change	**Definition:** Taking out or off a device from a body part and putting back an identical or similar device in or on the same body part without cutting or puncturing the skin or a mucous membrane **Explanation:** All CHANGE procedures are coded using the approach EXTERNAL **Includes/Examples:** Urinary catheter change, gastrostomy tube change
Control	**Definition:** Stopping, or attempting to stop, postprocedural or other acute bleeding **Explanation:** The site of the bleeding is coded as an anatomical region and not to a specific body part **Includes/Examples:** Control of post-prostatectomy hemorrhage, control of intracranial subdural hemorrhage, control of bleeding duodenal ulcer, control of retroperitoneal hemorrhage
Creation	**Definition:** Putting in or on biological or synthetic material to form a new body part that to the extent possible replicates the anatomic structure or function of an absent body part **Explanation:** Used for gender reassignment surgery and corrective procedures in individuals with congenital anomalies **Includes/Examples:** Creation of vagina in a male, creation of right and left atrioventricular valve from common atrioventricular valve
Destruction	**Definition:** Physical eradication of all or a portion of a body part by the direct use of energy, force, or a destructive agent **Explanation:** None of the body part is physically taken out **Includes/Examples:** Fulguration of rectal polyp, cautery of skin lesion
Detachment	**Definition:** Cutting off all or a portion of the upper or lower extremities **Explanation:** The body part value is the site of the detachment, with a qualifier if applicable to further specify the level where the extremity was detached **Includes/Examples:** Below knee amputation, disarticulation of shoulder
Dilation	**Definition:** Expanding an orifice or the lumen of a tubular body part **Explanation:** The orifice can be a natural orifice or an artificially created orifice. Accomplished by stretching a tubular body part using intraluminal pressure or by cutting part of the orifice or wall of the tubular body part **Includes/Examples:** Percutaneous transluminal angioplasty, internal urethrotomy
Division	**Definition:** Cutting into a body part, without draining fluids and/or gases from the body part, in order to separate or transect a body part **Explanation:** All or a portion of the body part is separated into two or more portions **Includes/Examples:** Spinal cordotomy, osteotomy
Drainage	**Definition:** Taking or letting out fluids and/or gases from a body part **Explanation:** The qualifier DIAGNOSTIC is used to identify drainage procedures that are biopsies **Includes/Examples:** Thoracentesis, incision and drainage
Excision	**Definition:** Cutting out or off, without replacement, a portion of a body part **Explanation:** The qualifier DIAGNOSTIC is used to identify excision procedures that are biopsies **Includes/Examples:** Partial nephrectomy, liver biopsy
Extirpation	**Definition:** Taking or cutting out solid matter from a body part **Explanation:** The solid matter may be an abnormal byproduct of a biological function or a foreign body; it may be imbedded in a body part or in the lumen of a tubular body part. The solid matter may or may not have been previously broken into pieces **Includes/Examples:** Thrombectomy, choledocholithotomy
Extraction	**Definition:** Pulling or stripping out or off all or a portion of a body part by the use of force **Explanation:** The qualifier DIAGNOSTIC is used to identify extraction procedures that are biopsies **Includes/Examples:** Dilation and curettage, vein stripping

SECTION Ø - MEDICAL AND SURGICAL
CHARACTER 3 - OPERATION

Fragmentation	**Definition:** Breaking solid matter in a body part into pieces **Explanation:** Physical force (e.g., manual, ultrasonic) applied directly or indirectly is used to break the solid matter into pieces. The solid matter may be an abnormal byproduct of a biological function or a foreign body. The pieces of solid matter are not taken out **Includes/Examples:** Extracorporeal shockwave lithotripsy, transurethral lithotripsy
Fusion	**Definition:** Joining together portions of an articular body part rendering the articular body part immobile **Explanation:** The body part is joined together by fixation device, bone graft, or other means **Includes/Examples:** Spinal fusion, ankle arthrodesis
Insertion	**Definition:** Putting in a nonbiological appliance that monitors, assists, performs, or prevents a physiological function but does not physically take the place of a body part **Includes/Examples:** Insertion of radioactive implant, insertion of central venous catheter
Inspection	**Definition:** Visually and/or manually exploring a body part **Explanation:** Visual exploration may be performed with or without optical instrumentation. Manual exploration may be performed directly or through intervening body layers **Includes/Examples:** Diagnostic arthroscopy, exploratory laparotomy
Map	**Definition:** Locating the route of passage of electrical impulses and/or locating functional areas in a body part **Explanation:** Applicable only to the cardiac conduction mechanism and the central nervous system **Includes/Examples:** Cardiac mapping, cortical mapping
Occlusion	**Definition:** Completely closing an orifice or the lumen of a tubular body part **Explanation:** The orifice can be a natural orifice or an artificially created orifice **Includes/Examples:** Fallopian tube ligation, ligation of inferior vena cava
Reattachment	**Definition:** Putting back in or on all or a portion of a separated body part to its normal location or other suitable location **Explanation:** Vascular circulation and nervous pathways may or may not be reestablished **Includes/Examples:** Reattachment of hand, reattachment of avulsed kidney

Release	**Definition:** Freeing a body part from an abnormal physical constraint by cutting or by the use of force **Explanation:** Some of the restraining tissue may be taken out but none of the body part is taken out **Includes/Examples:** Adhesiolysis, carpal tunnel release
Removal	**Definition:** Taking out or off a device from a body part **Explanation:** If a device is taken out and a similar device put in without cutting or puncturing the skin or mucous membrane, the procedure is coded to the root operation CHANGE. Otherwise, the procedure for taking out a device is coded to the root operation REMOVAL **Includes/Examples:** Drainage tube removal, cardiac pacemaker removal
Repair	**Definition:** Restoring, to the extent possible, a body part to its normal anatomic structure and function **Explanation:** Used only when the method to accomplish the repair is not one of the other root operations **Includes/Examples:** Colostomy takedown, suture of laceration
Replacement	**Definition:** Putting in or on biological or synthetic material that physically takes the place and/or function of all or a portion of a body part **Explanation:** The body part may have been taken out or replaced, or may be taken out, physically eradicated, or rendered nonfunctional during the Replacement procedure. A Removal procedure is coded for taking out the device used in a previous replacement procedure **Includes/Examples:** Total hip replacement, bone graft, free skin graft
Reposition	**Definition:** Moving to its normal location, or other suitable location, all or a portion of a body part **Explanation:** The body part is moved to a new location from an abnormal location, or from a normal location where it is not functioning correctly. The body part may or may not be cut out or off to be moved to the new location **Includes/Examples:** Reposition of undescended testicle, fracture reduction
Resection	**Definition:** Cutting out or off, without replacement, all of a body part **Includes/Examples:** Total nephrectomy, total lobectomy of lung

SECTION Ø - MEDICAL AND SURGICAL
CHARACTER 3 - OPERATION

Restriction	**Definition:** Partially closing an orifice or the lumen of a tubular body part **Explanation:** The orifice can be a natural orifice or an artificially created orifice **Includes/Examples:** Esophagogastric fundoplication, cervical cerclage
Revision	**Definition:** Correcting, to the extent possible, a portion of a malfunctioning device or the position of a displaced device **Explanation:** Revision can include correcting a malfunctioning or displaced device by taking out or putting in components of the device such as a screw or pin **Includes/Examples:** Adjustment of position of pacemaker lead, recementing of hip prosthesis
Supplement	**Definition:** Putting in or on biological or synthetic material that physically reinforces and/or augments the function of a portion of a body part **Explanation:** The biological material is non-living, or is living and from the same individual. The body part may have been previously replaced, and the Supplement procedure is performed to physically reinforce and/or augment the function of the replaced body part **Includes/Examples:** Herniorrhaphy using mesh, free nerve graft, mitral valve ring annuloplasty, put a new acetabular liner in a previous hip replacement

Transfer	**Definition:** Moving, without taking out, all or a portion of a body part to another location to take over the function of all or a portion of a body part **Explanation:** The body part transferred remains connected to its vascular and nervous supply **Includes/Examples:** Tendon transfer, skin pedicle flap transfer
Transplantation	**Definition:** Putting in or on all or a portion of a living body part taken from another individual or animal to physically take the place and/or function of all or a portion of a similar body part **Explanation:** The native body part may or may not be taken out, and the transplanted body part may take over all or a portion of its function **Includes/Examples:** Kidney transplant, heart transplant

SECTION Ø - MEDICAL AND SURGICAL
CHARACTER 4 - BODY PART

1st Toe, Left 1st Toe, Right	**Includes:** Hallux
Abdomen Muscle, Left Abdomen Muscle, Right	**Includes:** External oblique muscle Internal oblique muscle Pyramidalis muscle Rectus abdominis muscle Transversus abdominis muscle
Abdominal Aorta	**Includes:** Inferior phrenic artery Lumbar artery Median sacral artery Middle suprarenal artery Ovarian artery Testicular artery

Abdominal Sympathetic Nerve	**Includes:** Abdominal aortic plexus Auerbach's (myenteric) plexus Celiac (solar) plexus Celiac ganglion Gastric plexus Hepatic plexus Inferior hypogastric plexus Inferior mesenteric ganglion Inferior mesenteric plexus Meissner's (submucous) plexus Myenteric (Auerbach's) plexus Pancreatic plexus Pelvic splanchnic nerve Renal plexus Solar (celiac) plexus Splenic plexus Submucous (Meissner's) plexus Superior hypogastric plexus Superior mesenteric ganglion Superior mesenteric plexus Suprarenal plexus

SECTION 0 - MEDICAL AND SURGICAL
CHARACTER 4 - BODY PART

Abducens Nerve	**Includes:** Sixth cranial nerve
Accessory Nerve	**Includes:** Eleventh cranial nerve
Acoustic Nerve	**Includes:** Cochlear nerve Eighth cranial nerve Scarpa's (vestibular) ganglion Spiral ganglion Vestibular (Scarpa's) ganglion Vestibular nerve Vestibulocochlear nerve
Adenoids	**Includes:** Pharyngeal tonsil
Adrenal Gland Adrenal Gland, Left Adrenal Gland, Right Adrenal Glands, Bilateral	**Includes:** Suprarenal gland
Ampulla of Vater	**Includes:** Duodenal ampulla Hepatopancreatic ampulla
Anal Sphincter	**Includes:** External anal sphincter Internal anal sphincter
Ankle Bursa and Ligament, Left Ankle Bursa and Ligament, Right	**Includes:** Calcaneofibular ligament Deltoid ligament Ligament of the lateral malleolus Talofibular ligament
Ankle Joint, Left Ankle Joint, Right	**Includes:** Inferior tibiofibular joint Talocrural joint
Anterior Chamber, Left Anterior Chamber, Right	**Includes:** Aqueous humour
Anterior Tibial Artery, Left Anterior Tibial Artery, Right	**Includes:** Anterior lateral malleolar artery Anterior medial malleolar artery Anterior tibial recurrent artery Dorsalis pedis artery Posterior tibial recurrent artery
Anus	**Includes:** Anal orifice

Aortic Valve	**Includes:** Aortic annulus
Appendix	**Includes:** Vermiform appendix
Atrial Septum	**Includes:** Interatrial septum
Atrium, Left	**Includes:** Atrium pulmonale Left auricular appendix
Atrium, Right	**Includes:** Atrium dextrum cordis Right auricular appendix Sinus venosus
Auditory Ossicle, Left Auditory Ossicle, Right	**Includes:** Incus Malleus Stapes
Axillary Artery, Left Axillary Artery, Right	**Includes:** Anterior circumflex humeral artery Lateral thoracic artery Posterior circumflex humeral artery Subscapular artery Superior thoracic artery Thoracoacromial artery
Azygos Vein	**Includes:** Right ascending lumbar vein Right subcostal vein
Basal Ganglia	**Includes:** Basal nuclei Claustrum Corpus striatum Globus pallidus Substantia nigra Subthalamic nucleus
Basilic Vein, Left Basilic Vein, Right	**Includes:** Median antebrachial vein Median cubital vein
Bladder	**Includes:** Trigone of bladder
Brachial Artery, Left Brachial Artery, Right	**Includes:** Inferior ulnar collateral artery Profunda brachii Superior ulnar collateral artery

SECTION Ø - MEDICAL AND SURGICAL
CHARACTER 4 - BODY PART

Brachial Plexus	**Includes:** Axillary nerve Dorsal scapular nerve First intercostal nerve Long thoracic nerve Musculocutaneous nerve Subclavius nerve Suprascapular nerve
Brachial Vein, Left Brachial Vein, Right	**Includes:** Radial vein Ulnar vein
Brain	**Includes:** Cerebrum Corpus callosum Encephalon
Breast, Bilateral Breast, Left Breast, Right	**Includes:** Mammary duct Mammary gland
Buccal Mucosa	**Includes:** Buccal gland Molar gland Palatine gland
Carotid Bodies, Bilateral Carotid Body, Left Carotid Body, Right	**Includes:** Carotid glomus
Carpal Joint, Left Carpal Joint, Right	**Includes:** Intercarpal joint Midcarpal joint
Carpal, Left Carpal, Right	**Includes:** Capitate bone Hamate bone Lunate bone Pisiform bone Scaphoid bone Trapezium bone Trapezoid bone Triquetral bone
Celiac Artery	**Includes:** Celiac trunk
Cephalic Vein, Left Cephalic Vein, Right	**Includes:** Accessory cephalic vein
Cerebellum	**Includes:** Culmen
Cerebral Hemisphere	**Includes:** Frontal lobe Occipital lobe Parietal lobe Temporal lobe

Cerebral Meninges	**Includes:** Arachnoid mater, intracranial Leptomeninges, intracranial Pia mater, intracranial
Cerebral Ventricle	**Includes:** Aqueduct of Sylvius Cerebral aqueduct (Sylvius) Choroid plexus Ependyma Foramen of Monro (intraventricular) Fourth ventricle Interventricular foramen (Monro) Left lateral ventricle Right lateral ventricle Third ventricle
Cervical Nerve	**Includes:** Greater occipital nerve Spinal nerve, cervical Suboccipital nerve Third occipital nerve
Cervical Plexus	**Includes:** Ansa cervicalis Cutaneous (transverse) cervical nerve Great auricular nerve Lesser occipital nerve Supraclavicular nerve Transverse (cutaneous) cervical nerve
Cervical Vertebra	**Includes:** Dens Odontoid process Spinous process Transverse foramen Transverse process Vertebral body Vertebral arch Vertebral foramen Vertebral lamina Vertebral pedicle
Cervical Vertebral Joint	**Includes:** Atlantoaxial joint Cervical facet joint

Cervical Vertebral
    Joints, 2 or
    more
	Includes:
	Cervical facet joint

Cervicothoracic Vertebral Joint	**Includes:** Cervicothoracic facet joint
Cisterna Chyli	**Includes:** Intestinal lymphatic trunk Lumbar lymphatic trunk
Coccygeal Glomus	**Includes:** Coccygeal body

SECTION Ø - MEDICAL AND SURGICAL
CHARACTER 4 - BODY PART

Colic Vein	**Includes:** Ileocolic vein Left colic vein Middle colic vein Right colic vein
Conduction Mechanism	**Includes:** Atrioventricular node Bundle of His Bundle of Kent Sinoatrial node
Conjunctiva, Left Conjunctiva, Right	**Includes:** Plica semilunaris
Dura Mater	**Includes:** Diaphragma sellae Dura mater, intracranial Falx cerebri Tentorium cerebelli
Elbow Bursa and Ligament, Left Elbow Bursa and Ligament, Right	**Includes:** Annular ligament Olecranon bursa Radial collateral ligament Ulnar collateral ligament
Elbow Joint, Left Elbow Joint, Right	**Includes:** Distal humerus, involving joint Humeroradial joint Humeroulnar joint Proximal radioulnar joint
Epidural Space, Intracranial	**Includes:** Extradural space, intracranial
Epiglottis	**Includes:** Glossoepiglottic fold
Esophagogastric Junction	**Includes:** Cardia Cardioesophageal junction Gastroesophageal (GE) junction
Esophagus, Lower	**Includes:** Abdominal esophagus
Esophagus, Middle	**Includes:** Thoracic esophagus
Esophagus, Upper	**Includes:** Cervical esophagus
Ethmoid Bone, Left Ethmoid Bone, Right	**Includes:** Cribriform plate
Ethmoid Sinus, Left Ethmoid Sinus, Right	**Includes:** Ethmoidal air cell
Eustachian Tube, Left Eustachian Tube, Right	**Includes:** Auditory tube Pharyngotympanic tube
External Auditory Canal, Left External Auditory Canal, Right	**Includes:** External auditory meatus
External Carotid Artery, Left External Carotid Artery, Right	**Includes:** Ascending pharyngeal artery Internal maxillary artery Lingual artery Maxillary artery Occipital artery Posterior auricular artery Superior thyroid artery
External Ear, Bilateral External Ear, Left External Ear, Right	**Includes:** Antihelix Antitragus Auricle Earlobe Helix Pinna Tragus
External Iliac Artery, Left External Iliac Artery, Right	**Includes:** Deep circumflex iliac artery Inferior epigastric artery
External Jugular Vein, Left External Jugular Vein, Right	**Includes:** Posterior auricular vein
Extraocular Muscle, Left Extraocular Muscle, Right	**Includes:** Inferior oblique muscle Inferior rectus muscle Lateral rectus muscle Medial rectus muscle Superior oblique muscle Superior rectus muscle
Eye, Left Eye, Right	**Includes:** Ciliary body Posterior chamber
Face Artery	**Includes:** Angular artery Ascending palatine artery External maxillary artery Facial artery Inferior labial artery Submental artery Superior labial artery

SECTION Ø - MEDICAL AND SURGICAL
CHARACTER 4 - BODY PART

Face Vein, Left Face Vein, Right	**Includes:** Angular vein Anterior facial vein Common facial vein Deep facial vein Frontal vein Posterior facial (retromandibular) vein Supraorbital vein
Facial Muscle	**Includes:** Buccinator muscle Corrugator supercilii muscle Depressor anguli oris muscle Depressor labii inferioris muscle Depressor septi nasi muscle Depressor supercilii muscle Levator anguli oris muscle Levator labii superioris alaeque nasi muscle Levator labii superioris muscle Mentalis muscle Nasalis muscle Occipitofrontalis muscle Orbicularis oris muscle Procerus muscle Risorius muscle Zygomaticus muscle
Facial Nerve	**Includes:** Chorda tympani Geniculate ganglion Greater superficial petrosal nerve Nerve to the stapedius Parotid plexus Posterior auricular nerve Seventh cranial nerve Submandibular ganglion
Fallopian Tube, Left Fallopian Tube, Right	**Includes:** Oviduct Salpinx Uterine tube
Femoral Artery, Left Femoral Artery, Right	**Includes:** Circumflex iliac artery Deep femoral artery Descending genicular artery External pudendal artery Superficial epigastric artery
Femoral Nerve	**Includes:** Anterior crural nerve Saphenous nerve
Femoral Shaft, Left Femoral Shaft, Right	**Includes:** Body of femur

Femoral Vein, Left Femoral Vein, Right	**Includes:** Deep femoral (profunda femoris) vein Popliteal vein Profunda femoris (deep femoral) vein
Fibula, Left Fibula, Right	**Includes:** Body of fibula Head of fibula Lateral malleolus
Finger Nail	**Includes:** Nail bed Nail plate
Finger Phalangeal Joint, Left Finger Phalangeal Joint, Right	**Includes:** Interphalangeal (IP) joint
Foot Artery, Left Foot Artery, Right	**Includes:** Arcuate artery Dorsal metatarsal artery Lateral plantar artery Lateral tarsal artery Medial plantar artery
Foot Bursa and Ligament, Left Foot Bursa and Ligament, Right	**Includes:** Calcaneocuboid ligament Cuneonavicular ligament Intercuneiform ligament Interphalangeal ligament Metatarsal ligament Metatarsophalangeal ligament Subtalar ligament Talocalcaneal ligament Talocalcaneonavicular ligament Tarsometatarsal ligament
Foot Muscle, Left Foot Muscle, Right	**Includes:** Abductor hallucis muscle Adductor hallucis muscle Extensor digitorum brevis muscle Extensor hallucis brevis muscle Flexor digitorum brevis muscle Flexor hallucis brevis muscle Quadratus plantae muscle
Foot Vein, Left Foot Vein, Right	**Includes:** Common digital vein Dorsal metatarsal vein Dorsal venous arch Plantar digital vein Plantar metatarsal vein Plantar venous arch
Frontal Bone	**Includes:** Zygomatic process of frontal bone

SECTION Ø - MEDICAL AND SURGICAL
CHARACTER 4 - BODY PART

Gastric Artery	**Includes:** Left gastric artery Right gastric artery
Glenoid Cavity, Left Glenoid Cavity, Right	**Includes:** Glenoid fossa (of scapula)
Glomus Jugulare	**Includes:** Jugular body
Glossopharyngeal Nerve	**Includes:** Carotid sinus nerve Ninth cranial nerve Tympanic nerve
Hand Artery, Left Hand Artery, Right	**Includes:** Deep palmar arch Princeps pollicis artery Radialis indicis Superficial palmar arch
Hand Bursa and Ligament, Left Hand Bursa and Ligament, Right	**Includes:** Carpometacarpal ligament Intercarpal ligament Interphalangeal ligament Lunotriquetral ligament Metacarpal ligament Metacarpophalangeal ligament Pisohamate ligament Pisometacarpal ligament Scapholunate ligament Scaphotrapezium ligament
Hand Muscle, Left Hand Muscle, Right	**Includes:** Hypothenar muscle Palmar interosseous muscle Thenar muscle
Hand Vein, Left Hand Vein, Right	**Includes:** Dorsal metacarpal vein Palmar (volar) digital vein Palmar (volar) metacarpal vein Superficial palmar venous arch Volar (palmar) digital vein Volar (palmar) metacarpal vein
Head and Neck Bursa and Ligament	**Includes:** Alar ligament of axis Cervical interspinous ligament Cervical intertransverse ligament Cervical ligamentum flavum Interspinous ligament, cervical Intertransverse ligament, cervical Lateral temporomandibular ligament Ligamentum flavum, cervical Sphenomandibular ligament Stylomandibular ligament Transverse ligament of atlas

Head and Neck Sympathetic Nerve	**Includes:** Cavernous plexus Cervical ganglion Ciliary ganglion Internal carotid plexus Otic ganglion Pterygopalatine (sphenopalatine) ganglion Sphenopalatine (pterygopalatine) ganglion Stellate ganglion Submandibular ganglion Submaxillary ganglion
Head Muscle	**Includes:** Auricularis muscle Masseter muscle Pterygoid muscle Splenius capitis muscle Temporalis muscle Temporoparietalis muscle
Heart, Left	**Includes:** Left coronary sulcus Obtuse margin
Heart, Right	**Includes:** Right coronary sulcus
Hemiazygos Vein	**Includes** Left ascending lumbar vein Left subcostal vein
Hepatic Artery	**Includes:** Common hepatic artery Gastroduodenal artery Hepatic artery proper
Hip Bursa and Ligament, Left Hip Bursa and Ligament, Right	**Includes:** Iliofemoral ligament Ischiofemoral ligament Pubofemoral ligament Transverse acetabular ligament Trochanteric bursa
Hip Joint, Left Hip Joint, Right	**Includes:** Acetabulofemoral joint
Hip Muscle, Left Hip Muscle, Right	**Includes:** Gemellus muscle Gluteus maximus muscle Gluteus medius muscle Gluteus minimus muscle Iliacus muscle Obturator muscle Piriformis muscle Psoas muscle Quadratus femoris muscle Tensor fasciae latae muscle

SECTION Ø - MEDICAL AND SURGICAL
CHARACTER 4 - BODY PART

Humeral Head, Left Humeral Head, Right	**Includes:** Greater tuberosity Lesser tuberosity Neck of humerus (anatomical) (surgical)
Humeral Shaft, Left Humeral Shaft, Right	**Includes:** Distal humerus Humerus, distal Lateral epicondyle of humerus Medial epicondyle of humerus
Hypogastric Vein, Left Hypogastric Vein, Right	**Includes:** Gluteal vein Internal iliac vein Internal pudendal vein Lateral sacral vein Middle hemorrhoidal vein Obturator vein Uterine vein Vaginal vein Vesical vein
Hypoglossal Nerve	**Includes:** Twelfth cranial nerve
Hypothalamus	**Includes:** Mammillary body
Inferior Mesenteric Artery	**Includes:** Sigmoid artery Superior rectal artery
Inferior Mesenteric Vein	**Includes:** Sigmoid vein Superior rectal vein
Inferior Vena Cava	**Includes:** Postcava Right inferior phrenic vein Right ovarian vein Right second lumbar vein Right suprarenal vein Right testicular vein
Inguinal Region, Bilateral Inguinal Region, Left Inguinal Region, Right	**Includes:** Inguinal canal Inguinal triangle
Inner Ear, Left Inner Ear, Right	**Includes:** Bony labyrinth Bony vestibule Cochlea Round window Semicircular canal

Innominate Artery	**Includes:** Brachiocephalic artery Brachiocephalic trunk
Innominate Vein, Left Innominate Vein, Right	**Includes:** Brachiocephalic vein Inferior thyroid vein
Internal Carotid Artery, Left Internal Carotid Artery, Right	**Includes:** Caroticotympanic artery Carotid sinus
Internal Iliac Artery, Left Internal Iliac Artery, Right	**Includes:** Deferential artery Hypogastric artery Iliolumbar artery Inferior gluteal artery Inferior vesical artery Internal pudendal artery Lateral sacral artery Middle rectal artery Obturator artery Superior gluteal artery Umbilical artery Uterine Artery Vaginal artery
Internal Mammary Artery, Left Internal Mammary Artery, Right	**Includes:** Anterior intercostal artery Internal thoracic artery Musculophrenic artery Pericardiophrenic artery Superior epigastric artery
Intracranial Artery	**Includes:** Anterior cerebral artery Anterior choroidal artery Anterior communicating artery Basilar artery Circle of Willis Internal carotid artery, intracranial portion Middle cerebral artery Ophthalmic artery Posterior cerebral artery Posterior communicating artery Posterior inferior cerebellar artery (PICA)

SECTION Ø - MEDICAL AND SURGICAL
CHARACTER 4 - BODY PART

Intracranial Vein	**Includes:** Anterior cerebral vein Basal (internal) cerebral vein Dural venous sinus Great cerebral vein Inferior cerebellar vein Inferior cerebral vein Internal (basal) cerebral vein Middle cerebral vein Ophthalmic vein Superior cerebellar vein Superior cerebral vein
Jejunum	**Includes:** Duodenojejunal flexure
Kidney	**Includes:** Renal calyx Renal capsule Renal cortex Renal segment
Kidney Pelvis, Left Kidney Pelvis, Right	**Includes:** Ureteropelvic junction (UPJ)
Kidney, Left Kidney, Right Kidneys, Bilateral	**Includes:** Renal calyx Renal capsule Renal cortex Renal segment
Knee Bursa and Ligament, Left Knee Bursa and Ligament, Right	**Includes:** Anterior cruciate ligament (ACL) Lateral collateral ligament (LCL) Ligament of head of fibula Medial collateral ligament (MCL) Patellar ligament Popliteal ligament Posterior cruciate ligament (PCL) Prepatellar bursa
Knee Joint, Femoral Surface, Left Knee Joint, Femoral Surface, Right	**Includes:** Femoropatellar joint Patellofemoral joint
Knee Joint, Left Knee Joint, Right	**Includes:** Femoropatellar joint Femorotibial joint Lateral meniscus Medial meniscus Patellofemoral joint Tibiofemoral joint

Knee Joint, Tibial Surface, Left Knee Joint, Tibial Surface, Right	**Includes:** Femorotibial joint Tibiofemoral joint
Knee Tendon, Left Knee Tendon, Right	**Includes:** Patellar tendon
Lacrimal Duct, Left Lacrimal Duct, Right	**Includes:** Lacrimal canaliculus Lacrimal punctum Lacrimal sac Nasolacrimal duct
Larynx	**Includes:** Aryepiglottic fold Arytenoid cartilage Corniculate cartilage Cuneiform cartilage False vocal cord Glottis Rima glottidis Thyroid cartilage Ventricular fold
Lens, Left Lens, Right	**Includes:** Zonule of Zinn
Liver	**Includes:** Quadrate lobe
Lower Arm and Wrist Muscle, Left Lower Arm and Wrist Muscle, Right	**Includes:** Anatomical snuffbox Brachioradialis muscle Extensor carpi radialis muscle Extensor carpi ulnaris muscle Flexor carpi radialis muscle Flexor carpi ulnaris muscle Flexor pollicis longus muscle Palmaris longus muscle Pronator quadratus muscle Pronator teres muscle
Lower Artery	**Includes:** Umbilical artery
Lower Eyelid, Left Lower Eyelid, Right	**Includes:** Inferior tarsal plate Medial canthus
Lower Femur, Left Lower Femur, Right	**Includes:** Lateral condyle of femur Lateral epicondyle of femur Medial condyle of femur Medial epicondyle of femur

SECTION Ø - MEDICAL AND SURGICAL
CHARACTER 4 - BODY PART

Body Part	Includes
Lower Leg Muscle, Left Lower Leg Muscle, Right	**Includes:** Extensor digitorum longus muscle Extensor hallucis longus muscle Fibularis brevis muscle Fibularis longus muscle Flexor digitorum longus muscle Flexor hallucis longus muscle Gastrocnemius muscle Peroneus brevis muscle Peroneus longus muscle Popliteus muscle Soleus muscle Tibialis anterior muscle Tibialis posterior muscle
Lower Leg Tendon, Left Lower Leg Tendon, Right	**Includes:** Achilles tendon
Lower Lip	**Includes:** Frenulum labii inferioris Labial gland Vermilion border
Lower Spine Bursa and Ligament	**Includes:** Iliolumbar ligament Interspinous ligament, lumbar Intertransverse ligament, lumbar Ligamentum flavum, lumbar Sacrococcygeal ligament Sacroiliac ligament Sacrospinous ligament Sacrotuberous ligament Supraspinous ligament
Lumbar Nerve	**Includes:** Lumbosacral trunk Spinal nerve, lumbar Superior clunic (cluneal) nerve
Lumbar Plexus	**Includes:** Accessory obturator nerve Genitofemoral nerve Iliohypogastric nerve Ilioinguinal nerve Lateral femoral cutaneous nerve Obturator nerve Superior gluteal nerve
Lumbar Spinal Cord	**Includes:** Cauda equina Conus medullaris
Lumbar Sympathetic Nerve	**Includes:** Lumbar ganglion Lumbar splanchnic nerve

Body Part	Includes
Lumbar Vertebra	**Includes:** Spinous process Transverse process Vertebral arch Vertebral body Vertebral foramen Vertebral lamina Vertebral pedicle
Lumbar Vertebral Joint	**Includes:** Lumbar facet joint
Lumbosacral Joint	**Includes:** Lumbosacral facet joint
Lymphatic, Aortic	**Includes:** Celiac lymph node Gastric lymph node Hepatic lymph node Lumbar lymph node Pancreaticosplenic lymph node Paraaortic lymph node Retroperitoneal lymph node
Lymphatic, Head	**Includes:** Buccinator lymph node Infraauricular lymph node Infraparotid lymph node Parotid lymph node Preauricular lymph node Submandibular lymph node Submaxillary lymph node Submental lymph node Subparotid lymph node Suprahyoid lymph node
Lymphatic, Left Axillary	**Includes:** Anterior (pectoral) lymph node Apical (subclavicular) lymph node Brachial (lateral) lymph node Central axillary lymph node Lateral (brachial) lymph node Pectoral (anterior) lymph node Posterior (subscapular) lymph node Subclavicular (apical) lymph node Subscapular (posterior) lymph node
Lymphatic, Left Lower Extremity	**Includes:** Femoral lymph node Popliteal lymph node
Lymphatic, Left Neck	**Includes:** Cervical lymph node Jugular lymph node Mastoid (postauricular) lymph node Occipital lymph node Postauricular (mastoid) lymph node Retropharyngeal lymph node Supraclavicular (Virchow's) lymph node Virchow's (supraclavicular) lymph node

SECTION Ø - MEDICAL AND SURGICAL
CHARACTER 4 - BODY PART

Lymphatic, Left Upper Extremity	**Includes:** Cubital lymph node Deltopectoral (infraclavicular) lymph node Epitrochlear lymph node Infraclavicular (deltopectoral) lymph node Supratrochlear lymph node
Lymphatic, Mesenteric	**Includes:** Inferior mesenteric lymph node Pararectal lymph node Superior mesenteric lymph node
Lymphatic, Pelvis	**Includes:** Common iliac (subaortic) lymph node Gluteal lymph node Iliac lymph node Inferior epigastric lymph node Obturator lymph node Sacral lymph node Subaortic (common iliac) lymph node Suprainguinal lymph node
Lymphatic, Right Axillary	**Includes:** Anterior (pectoral) lymph node Apical (subclavicular) lymph node Brachial (lateral) lymph node Central axillary lymph node Lateral (brachial) lymph node Pectoral (anterior) lymph node Posterior (subscapular) lymph node Subclavicular (apical) lymph node Subscapular (posterior) lymph node
Lymphatic, Right Lower Extremity	**Includes:** Femoral lymph node Popliteal lymph node
Lymphatic, Right Neck	**Includes:** Cervical lymph node Jugular lymph node Mastoid (postauricular) lymph node Occipital lymph node Postauricular (mastoid) lymph node Retropharyngeal lymph node Right jugular trunk Right lymphatic duct Right subclavian trunk Supraclavicular (Virchow's) lymph node Virchow's (supraclavicular) lymph node
Lymphatic, Right Upper Extremity	**Includes:** Cubital lymph node Deltopectoral (infraclavicular) lymph node Epitrochlear lymph node Infraclavicular (deltopectoral) lymph node Supratrochlear lymph node

Lymphatic, Thorax	**Includes:** Intercostal lymph node Mediastinal lymph node Parasternal lymph node Paratracheal lymph node Tracheobronchial lymph node
Main Bronchus, Right	**Includes:** Bronchus Intermedius Intermediate bronchus
Mandible, Left Mandible, Right	**Includes:** Alveolar process of mandible Condyloid process Mandibular notch Mental foramen
Mastoid Sinus, Left Mastoid Sinus, Right	**Includes:** Mastoid air cells
Maxilla	**Includes:** Alveolar process of maxilla
Maxillary Sinus, Left Maxillary Sinus, Right	**Includes:** Antrum of Highmore
Median Nerve	**Includes:** Anterior interosseous nerve Palmar cutaneous nerve
Mediastinum	**Includes:** Mediastinal cavity Mediastinal space
Medulla Oblongata	**Includes:** Myelencephalon
Mesentery	**Includes:** Mesoappendix Mesocolon
Metatarsal-Phalangeal Joint, Left Metatarsal-Phalangeal Joint, Right	**Includes:** Metatarsophalangeal (MTP) joint
Middle Ear, Left Middle Ear, Right	**Includes:** Oval window Tympanic cavity
Minor Salivary Gland	**Includes:** Anterior lingual gland
Mitral Valve	**Includes:** Bicuspid valve Left atrioventricular valve Mitral annulus
Nasal Bone	**Includes:** Vomer of nasal septum

SECTION Ø - MEDICAL AND SURGICAL
CHARACTER 4 - BODY PART

Nasal Mucosa and Soft Tissue	**Includes:** Columella External naris Greater alar cartilage Internal naris Lateral nasal cartilage Lesser alar cartilage Nasal cavity Nostril
Nasal Septum	**Includes:** Quadrangular cartilage Septal cartilage Vomer bone
Nasal Turbinate	**Includes:** Inferior turbinate Middle turbinate Nasal concha Superior turbinate
Nasopharynx	**Includes:** Choana Fossa of Rosenmuller Pharyngeal recess Rhinopharynx
Neck Muscle, Left Neck Muscle, Right	**Includes:** Anterior vertebral muscle Arytenoid muscle Cricothyroid muscle Infrahyoid muscle Levator scapulae muscle Platysma muscle Scalene muscle Splenius cervicis muscle Sternocleidomastoid muscle Suprahyoid muscle Thyroarytenoid muscle
Nipple, Left Nipple, Right	**Includes:** Areola
Occipital Bone	**Includes:** Foramen magnum
Oculomotor Nerve	**Includes:** Third cranial nerve
Olfactory Nerve	**Includes:** First cranial nerve Olfactory bulb
Omentum	**Includes:** Gastrocolic ligament Gastrocolic omentum Gastrohepatic omentum Gastrophrenic ligament Gastrosplenic ligament Greater Omentum Hepatogastric ligament Lesser Omentum

Optic Nerve	**Includes:** Optic chiasma Second cranial nerve
Orbit, Left Orbit, Right	**Includes:** Bony orbit Orbital portion of ethmoid bone Orbital portion of frontal bone Orbital portion of lacrimal bone Orbital portion of maxilla Orbital portion of palatine bone Orbital portion of sphenoid bone Orbital portion of zygomatic bone
Pancreatic Duct	**Includes:** Duct of Wirsung
Pancreatic Duct, Accessory	**Includes:** Duct of Santorini
Parotid Duct, Left Parotid Duct, Right	**Includes:** Stensen's duct
Pelvic Bone, Left Pelvic Bone, Right	**Includes:** Iliac crest Ilium Ischium Pubis
Pelvic Cavity	**Includes:** Retropubic space
Penis	**Includes:** Corpus cavernosum Corpus spongiosum
Perineum Muscle	**Includes:** Bulbospongiosus muscle Cremaster muscle Deep transverse perineal muscle Ischiocavernosus muscle Levator ani muscle Superficial transverse perineal muscle
Peritoneum	**Includes:** Epiploic foramen
Peroneal Artery, Left Peroneal Artery, Right	**Includes:** Fibular artery
Peroneal Nerve	**Includes:** Common fibular nerve Common peroneal nerve External popliteal nerve Lateral sural cutaneous nerve

SECTION Ø - MEDICAL AND SURGICAL
CHARACTER 4 - BODY PART

Pharynx	**Includes:** Base of Tongue Hypopharynx Laryngopharynx Lingual tonsil Oropharynx Piriform recess (sinus) Tongue, base of
Phrenic Nerve	**Includes:** Accessory phrenic nerve
Pituitary Gland	**Includes:** Adenohypophysis Hypophysis Neurohypophysis
Pons	**Includes:** Apneustic center Basis pontis Locus ceruleus Pneumotaxic center Pontine tegmentum Superior olivary nucleus
Popliteal Artery, Left Popliteal Artery, Right	**Includes:** Inferior genicular artery Middle genicular artery Superior genicular artery Sural artery
Portal Vein	**Includes:** Hepatic portal vein
Prepuce	**Includes:** Foreskin Glans penis
Pudendal Nerve	**Includes:** Posterior labial nerve Posterior scrotal nerve
Pulmonary Artery, Left	**Includes:** Arterial canal (duct) Botallo's duct Pulmoaortic canal
Pulmonary Valve	**Includes:** Pulmonary annulus Pulmonic valve
Pulmonary Vein, Left	**Includes:** Left inferior pulmonary vein Left superior pulmonary vein
Pulmonary Vein, Right	**Includes:** Right inferior pulmonary vein Right superior pulmonary vein
Radial Artery, Left Radial Artery, Right	**Includes:** Radial recurrent artery

Radial Nerve	**Includes:** Dorsal digital nerve Musculospiral nerve Palmar cutaneous nerve Posterior interosseous nerve
Radius, Left Radius, Right	**Includes:** Ulnar notch
Rectum	**Includes:** Anorectal junction
Renal Artery, Left Renal Artery, Right	**Includes:** Inferior suprarenal artery Renal segmental artery
Renal Vein, Left	**Includes:** Left inferior phrenic vein Left ovarian vein Left second lumbar vein Left suprarenal vein Left testicular vein
Retina, Left Retina, Right	**Includes:** Fovea Macula Optic disc
Retroperitoneum	**Includes:** Retroperitoneal cavity Retroperitoneal space
Rib(s) Bursa and Ligament	**Includes:** Costoxiphoid ligament
Sacral Nerve	**Includes:** Spinal nerve, sacral
Sacral Plexus	**Includes:** Inferior gluteal nerve Posterior femoral cutaneous nerve Pudendal nerve
Sacral Sympathetic Nerve	**Includes:** Ganglion impar (ganglion of Walther) Pelvic splanchnic nerve Sacral ganglion Sacral splanchnic nerve
Sacrococcygeal Joint	**Includes:** Sacrococcygeal symphysis
Saphenous Vein, Left Saphenous Vein, Right	**Includes:** External pudendal vein Great(er) saphenous vein Lesser saphenous vein Small saphenous vein Superficial circumflex iliac vein Superficial epigastric vein

SECTION Ø - MEDICAL AND SURGICAL
CHARACTER 4 - BODY PART

Scapula, Left Scapula, Right	**Includes:** Acromion (process) Coracoid process
Sciatic Nerve	**Includes:** Ischiatic nerve
Shoulder Bursa and Ligament, Left Shoulder Bursa and Ligament, Right	**Includes:** Acromioclavicular ligament Coracoacromial ligament Coracoclavicular ligament Coracohumeral ligament Costoclavicular ligament Glenohumeral ligament Interclavicular ligament Sternoclavicular ligament Subacromial bursa Transverse humeral ligament Transverse scapular ligament
Shoulder Joint, Left Shoulder Joint, Right	**Includes:** Glenohumeral joint Glenoid ligament (labrum)
Shoulder Muscle, Left Shoulder Muscle, Right	**Includes:** Deltoid muscle Infraspinatus muscle Subscapularis muscle Supraspinatus muscle Teres major muscle Teres minor muscle
Sigmoid Colon	**Includes:** Rectosigmoid junction Sigmoid flexure
Skin	**Includes:** Dermis Epidermis Sebaceous gland Sweat gland
Sphenoid Bone	**Includes:** Greater wing Lesser wing Optic foramen Pterygoid process Sella turcica
Spinal Canal	**Includes:** Epidural space, spinal Extradural space, spinal Subarachnoid space, spinal Subdural space, spinal Vertebral canal

Spinal Meninges	**Includes:** Arachnoid mater, spinal Denticulate (dentate) ligament Dura mater, spinal Filum terminale Leptomeninges, spinal Pia mater, spinal
Spleen	**Includes:** Accessory spleen
Splenic Artery	**Includes:** Left gastroepiploic artery Pancreatic artery Short gastric artery
Splenic Vein	**Includes:** Left gastroepiploic vein Pancreatic vein
Sternum	**Includes:** Manubrium Suprasternal notch Xiphoid process
Sternum Bursa and Ligament	**Includes:** Costoxiphoid ligament Sternocostal ligament
Stomach, Pylorus	**Includes:** Pyloric antrum Pyloric canal Pyloric sphincter
Subclavian Artery, Left Subclavian Artery, Right	**Includes:** Costocervical trunk Dorsal scapular artery Internal thoracic artery
Subcutaneous Tissue and Fascia, Chest	**Includes:** Pectoral fascia
Subcutaneous Tissue and Fascia, Face	**Includes:** Masseteric fascia Orbital fascia
Subcutaneous Tissue and Fascia, Left Foot	**Includes:** Plantar fascia (aponeurosis)
Subcutaneous Tissue and Fascia, Left Hand	**Includes:** Palmar fascia (aponeurosis)
Subcutaneous Tissue and Fascia, Left Lower Arm	**Includes:** Antebrachial fascia Bicipital aponeurosis

APPENDIX A

SECTION Ø - MEDICAL AND SURGICAL
CHARACTER 4 - BODY PART

Subcutaneous Tissue and Fascia, Left Neck	**Includes:** Deep cervical fascia Pretracheal fascia Prevertebral fascia
Subcutaneous Tissue and Fascia, Left Upper Arm	**Includes:** Axillary fascia Deltoid fascia Infraspinatus fascia Subscapular aponeurosis Supraspinatus fascia
Subcutaneous Tissue and Fascia, Left Upper Leg	**Includes:** Crural fascia Fascia lata Iliac fascia Iliotibial tract (band)
Subcutaneous Tissue and Fascia, Right Foot	**Includes:** Plantar fascia (aponeurosis)
Subcutaneous Tissue and Fascia, Right Hand	**Includes:** Palmar fascia (aponeurosis)
Subcutaneous Tissue and Fascia, Right Lower Arm	**Includes:** Antebrachial fascia Bicipital aponeurosis
Subcutaneous Tissue and Fascia, Right Neck	**Includes:** Deep cervical fascia Pretracheal fascia Prevertebral fascia
Subcutaneous Tissue and Fascia, Right Upper Arm	**Includes:** Axillary fascia Deltoid fascia Infraspinatus fascia Subscapular aponeurosis Supraspinatus fascia
Subcutaneous Tissue and Fascia, Right Upper Leg	**Includes:** Crural fascia Fascia lata Iliac fascia Iliotibial tract (band)
Subcutaneous Tissue and Fascia, Scalp	**Includes:** Galea aponeurotica
Subcutaneous Tissue and Fascia, Trunk	**Includes:** External oblique aponeurosis Transversalis fascia
Submaxillary Gland, Left Submaxillary Gland, Right	**Includes:** Submandibular gland

Superior Mesenteric Artery	**Includes:** Ileal artery Ileocolic artery Inferior pancreaticoduodenal artery Jejunal artery
Superior Mesenteric Vein	**Includes:** Right gastroepiploic vein
Superior Vena Cava	**Includes:** Precava
Tarsal Joint, Left Tarsal Joint, Right	**Includes:** Calcaneocuboid joint Cuboideonavicular joint Cuneonavicular joint Intercuneiform joint Subtalar (talocalcaneal) joint Talocalcaneal (subtalar) joint Talocalcaneonavicular joint
Tarsal, Left Tarsal, Right	**Includes:** Calcaneus Cuboid bone Intermediate cuneiform bone Lateral cuneiform bone Medial cuneiform bone Navicular bone Talus bone
Temporal Artery, Left Temporal Artery, Right	**Includes:** Middle temporal artery Superficial temporal artery Transverse facial artery
Temporal Bone, Left Temporal Bone, Right	**Includes:** Mastoid process Petrous part of temporal bone Tympanic part of temporal bone Zygomatic process of temporal bone
Thalamus	**Includes:** Epithalamus Geniculate nucleus Metathalamus Pulvinar
Thoracic Aorta, Ascending/Arch	**Includes:** Aortic arch Ascending aorta
Thoracic Duct	**Includes:** Left jugular trunk Left subclavian trunk
Thoracic Nerve	**Includes:** Intercostal nerve Intercostobrachial nerve Spinal nerve, thoracic Subcostal nerve

SECTION Ø - MEDICAL AND SURGICAL
CHARACTER 4 - BODY PART

Thoracic Sympathetic Nerve	**Includes:** Cardiac plexus Esophageal plexus Greater splanchnic nerve Inferior cardiac nerve Least splanchnic nerve Lesser splanchnic nerve Middle cardiac nerve Pulmonary plexus Superior cardiac nerve Thoracic aortic plexus Thoracic ganglion	**Tibial Nerve**	**Includes:** Lateral plantar nerve Medial plantar nerve Medial popliteal nerve Medial sural cutaneous nerve
		Toe Nail	**Includes:** Nail bed Nail plate
Thoracic Vertebra	**Includes:** Spinous process Transverse process Vertebral arch Vertebral body Vertebral foramen Vertebral lamina Vertebral pedicle	**Toe Phalangeal Joint, Left** **Toe Phalangeal Joint, Right**	**Includes:** Interphalangeal (IP) joint
		Tongue	**Includes:** Frenulum linguae
Thoracic Vertebral Joint	**Includes:** Costotransverse joint Costovertebral joint Thoracic facet joint	**Tongue, Palate, Pharynx Muscle**	**Includes:** Chrondroglossus muscle Genioglossus muscle Hyoglossus muscle Inferior longitudinal muscle Levator veli palatini muscle Palatoglossal muscle Palatopharyngeal muscle Pharyngeal constrictor muscle Salpingopharyngeus muscle Styloglossus muscle Stylopharyngeus muscle Superior longitudinal muscle Tensor veli palatini muscle
Thoracolumbar Vertebral Joint	**Includes:** Thoracolumbar facet joint		
Thorax Muscle, Left **Thorax Muscle, Right**	**Includes:** Intercostal muscle Levatores costarum muscle Pectoralis major muscle Pectoralis minor muscle Serratus anterior muscle Subclavius muscle Subcostal muscle Transverse thoracis muscle		
		Tonsils	**Includes:** Palatine tonsil
		Trachea	**Includes:** Cricoid cartilage
		Transverse Colon	**Includes:** Hepatic flexure Splenic flexure
Thymus	**Includes:** Thymus gland	**Tricuspid Valve**	**Includes:** Right atrioventricular valve Tricuspid annulus
Thyroid Artery, Left **Thyroid Artery, Right**	**Includes:** Cricothyroid artery Hyoid artery Sternocleidomastoid artery Superior laryngeal artery Superior thyroid artery Thyrocervical trunk	**Trigeminal Nerve**	**Includes:** Fifth cranial nerve Gasserian ganglion Mandibular nerve Maxillary nerve Ophthalmic nerve Trifacial nerve
Tibia, Left **Tibia, Right**	**Includes:** Lateral condyle of tibia Medial condyle of tibia Medial malleolus	**Trochlear Nerve**	**Includes:** Fourth cranial nerve

SECTION 0 - MEDICAL AND SURGICAL
CHARACTER 4 - BODY PART

Trunk Muscle, Left Trunk Muscle, Right	**Includes:** Coccygeus muscle Erector spinae muscle Interspinalis muscle Intertransversarius muscle Latissimus dorsi muscle Quadratus lumborum muscle Rhomboid major muscle Rhomboid minor muscle Serratus posterior muscle Transversospinalis muscle Trapezius muscle
Tympanic Membrane, Left Tympanic Membrane, Right	**Includes:** Pars flaccida
Ulna, Left Ulna, Right	**Includes:** Olecranon process Radial notch
Ulnar Artery, Left Ulnar Artery, Right	**Includes:** Anterior ulnar recurrent artery Common interosseous artery Posterior ulnar recurrent artery
Ulnar Nerve	**Includes:** Cubital nerve
Upper Arm Muscle, Left Upper Arm Muscle, Right	**Includes:** Biceps brachii muscle Brachialis muscle Coracobrachialis muscle Triceps brachii muscle
Upper Artery	**Includes:** Aortic intercostal artery Bronchial artery Esophageal artery Subcostal artery
Upper Eyelid, Left Upper Eyelid, Right	**Includes:** Lateral canthus Levator palpebrae superioris muscle Orbicularis oculi muscle Superior tarsal plate
Upper Femur, Left Upper Femur, Right	**Includes:** Femoral head Greater trochanter Lesser trochanter Neck of femur

Upper Leg Muscle, Left Upper Leg Muscle, Right	**Includes:** Adductor brevis muscle Adductor longus muscle Adductor magnus muscle Biceps femoris muscle Gracilis muscle Pectineus muscle Quadriceps (femoris) Rectus femoris muscle Sartorius muscle Semimembranosus muscle Semitendinosus muscle Vastus intermedius muscle Vastus lateralis muscle Vastus medialis muscle
Upper Lip	**Includes:** Frenulum labii superioris Labial gland Vermilion border
Upper Spine Bursa and Ligament	**Includes:** Interspinous ligament, thoracic Intertransverse ligament, thoracic Ligamentum flavum, thoracic Supraspinous ligament
Ureter Ureter, Left Ureter, Right Ureters, Bilateral	**Includes:** Ureteral orifice Ureterovesical orifice
Urethra	**Includes:** Bulbourethral (Cowper's) gland Cowper's (bulbourethral) gland External urethral sphincter Internal urethral sphincter Membranous urethra Penile urethra Prostatic urethra
Uterine Supporting Structure	**Includes:** Broad ligament Infundibulopelvic ligament Ovarian ligament Round ligament of uterus
Uterus	**Includes:** Fundus uteri Myometrium Perimetrium Uterine cornu
Uvula	**Includes:** Palatine uvula

SECTION Ø - MEDICAL AND SURGICAL
CHARACTER 4 - BODY PART

Vagus Nerve	**Includes:** Anterior vagal trunk Pharyngeal plexus Pneumogastric nerve Posterior vagal trunk Pulmonary plexus Recurrent laryngeal nerve Superior laryngeal nerve Tenth cranial nerve
Vas Deferens Vas Deferens, Bilateral Vas Deferens, Left Vas Deferens, Right	**Includes:** Ductus deferens Ejaculatory duct
Ventricle, Right	**Includes:** Conus arteriosus
Ventricular Septum	**Includes:** Interventricular septum

Vertebral Artery,
  Left
Vertebral Artery,
  Right
	Includes:
	Anterior spinal artery
	Posterior spinal artery

Vertebral Vein, Left Vertebral Vein, Right	**Includes:** Deep cervical vein Suboccipital venous plexus

Vestibular Gland	**Includes:** Bartholin's (greater vestibular) gland Greater vestibular (Bartholin's) gland Paraurethral (Skene's) gland Skene's (paraurethral) gland
Vitreous, Left Vitreous, Right	**Includes:** Vitreous body
Vocal Cord, Left Vocal Cord, Right	**Includes:** Vocal fold
Vulva	**Includes:** Labia majora Labia minora

Wrist Bursa and
  Ligament, Left
Wrist Bursa and
  Ligament, Right
	Includes:
	Palmar ulnocarpal ligament
	Radial collateral carpal ligament
	Radiocarpal ligament
	Radioulnar ligament
	Ulnar collateral carpal ligament

Wrist Joint, Left Wrist Joint, Right	**Includes:** Distal radioulnar joint Radiocarpal joint

SECTION Ø - MEDICAL AND SURGICAL
CHARACTER 5 - APPROACH

External	**Definition:** Procedures performed directly on the skin or mucous membrane and procedures performed indirectly by the application of external force through the skin or mucous membrane
Open	**Definition:** Cutting through the skin or mucous membrane and any other body layers necessary to expose the site of the procedure
Percutaneous	**Definition:** Entry, by puncture or minor incision, of instrumentation through the skin or mucous membrane and any other body layers necessary to reach the site of the procedure
Percutaneous Endoscopic	**Definition:** Entry, by puncture or minor incision, of instrumentation through the skin or mucous membrane and any other body layers necessary to reach and visualize the site of the procedure

Via Natural or Artificial Opening	**Definition:** Entry of instrumentation through a natural or artificial external opening to reach the site of the procedure
Via Natural or Artificial Opening Endoscopic	**Definition:** Entry of instrumentation through a natural or artificial external opening to reach and visualize the site of the procedure
Via Natural or Artificial Opening With Percutaneous Endoscopic Assistance	**Definition:** Entry of instrumentation through a natural or artificial external opening and entry, by puncture or minor incision, of instrumentation through the skin or mucous membrane and any other body layers necessary to aid in the performance of the procedure

SECTION 0 - MEDICAL AND SURGICAL
CHARACTER 6 - DEVICE

Articulating Spacer in Lower Joints	**Includes:** Articulating Spacer (Antibiotic) Spacer, Articulating (Antibiotic)
Artificial Sphincter in Gastrointestinal System	**Includes:** Artificial anal sphincter (AAS) Artificial bowel sphincter (neosphincter)
Artificial Sphincter in Urinary System	**Includes:** AMS 800® Urinary Control System Artificial urinary sphincter (AUS)
Autologous Arterial Tissue in Heart and Great Vessels	**Includes:** Autologous artery graft
Autologous Arterial Tissue in Lower Arteries	**Includes:** Autologous artery graft
Autologous Arterial Tissue in Lower Veins	**Includes:** Autologous artery graft
Autologous Arterial Tissue in Upper Arteries	**Includes:** Autologous artery graft
Autologous Arterial Tissue in Upper Veins	**Includes:** Autologous artery graft
Autologous Tissue Substitute	**Includes:** Autograft Cultured epidermal cell autograft Epicel® cultured epidermal autograft
Autologous Venous Tissue in Heart and Great Vessels	**Includes:** Autologous vein graft
Autologous Venous Tissue in Lower Arteries	**Includes:** Autologous vein graft
Autologous Venous Tissue in Lower Veins	**Includes:** Autologous vein graft
Autologous Venous Tissue in Upper Arteries	**Includes:** Autologous vein graft
Autologous Venous Tissue in Upper Veins	**Includes:** Autologous vein graft
Bone Growth Stimulator in Head and Facial Bones	**Includes:** Electrical bone growth stimulator (EBGS) Ultrasonic osteogenic stimulator Ultrasound bone healing system
Bone Growth Stimulator in Lower Bones	**Includes:** Electrical bone growth stimulator (EBGS) Ultrasonic osteogenic stimulator Ultrasound bone healing system
Bone Growth Stimulator in Upper Bones	**Includes:** Electrical bone growth stimulator (EBGS) Ultrasonic osteogenic stimulator Ultrasound bone healing system
Cardiac Lead in Heart and Great Vessels	**Includes:** Cardiac contractility modulation lead
Cardiac Lead, Defibrillator for Insertion in Heart and Great Vessels	**Includes:** ACUITY™ Steerable Lead Attain Ability® lead Attain StarFix® (OTW) lead Cardiac resynchronization therapy (CRT) lead Corox (OTW) Bipolar Lead Durata® Defibrillation Lead ENDOTAK RELIANCE® (G) Defibrillation Lead
Cardiac Lead, Pacemaker for Insertion in Heart and Great Vessels	**Includes:** ACUITY™ Steerable Lead Attain Ability® Lead Attain StarFix® (OTW) lead Cardiac resynchronization therapy (CRT) lead Corox (OTW) Bipolar Lead
Cardiac Resynchronization Defibrillator Pulse Generator for Insertion in Subcutaneous Tissue and Fascia	**Includes:** COGNIS® CRT-D Concerto II CRT-D Consulta CRT-D CONTAK RENEWAL® 3 RF (HE) CRT-D LIVIAN™ CRT-D Maximo II DR CRT-D Ovatio™ CRT-D Protecta XT CRT-D Viva (XT)(S)
Cardiac Resynchronization Pacemaker Pulse Generator for Insertion in Subcutaneous Tissue and Fascia	**Includes:** Consulta CRT-P Stratos LV Synchra CRT-P
Contraceptive Device in Female Reproductive System	**Includes:** Intrauterine device (IUD)
Contraceptive Device in Subcutaneous Tissue and Fascia	**Includes:** Subdermal progesterone implant
Contractility Modulation Device for Insertion in Subcutaneous Tissue and Fascia	**Includes:** Optimizer™ III implantable pulse generator

SECTION Ø - MEDICAL AND SURGICAL
CHARACTER 6 - DEVICE

Defibrillator Generator for Insertion in Subcutaneous Tissue and Fascia	**Includes:** Implantable cardioverter-defibrillator (ICD) Maximo II DR (VR) Protecta XT DR (XT VR) Secura (DR) (VR) Evera (XT)(S)(DR/VR) Virtuoso (II) (DR) (VR)
Diaphragmatic Pacemaker Lead in Respiratory System	**Includes:** Phrenic nerve stimulator lead
Drainage Device	**Includes:** Cystostomy tube Foley catheter Percutaneous nephrostomy catheter Thoracostomy tube
External Fixation Device in Head and Facial Bones	**Includes:** External fixator
External Fixation Device in Lower Bones	**Includes:** External fixator
External Fixation Device in Lower Joints	**Includes:** External fixator
External Fixation Device in Upper Bones	**Includes:** External fixator
External Fixation Device in Upper Joints	**Includes:** External fixator
External Fixation Device, Hybrid for Insertion in Upper Bones	**Includes:** Delta frame external fixator Sheffield hybrid external fixator
External Fixation Device, Hybrid for Insertion in Lower Bones	**Includes:** Delta frame external fixator Sheffield hybrid external fixator
External Fixation Device, Hybrid for Reposition in Upper Bones	**Includes:** Delta frame external fixator Sheffield hybrid external fixator
External Fixation Device, Hybrid for Reposition in Lower Bones	**Includes:** Delta frame external fixator Sheffield hybrid external fixator
External Fixation Device, Limb Lengthening for Insertion in Upper Bones	**Includes:** Ilizarov-Vecklich device
External Fixation Device, Limb Lengthening for Insertion in Lower Bones	**Includes:** Ilizarov-Vecklich device
External Fixation Device, Monoplanar for Insertion in Upper Bones	**Includes:** Uniplanar external fixator
External Fixation Device, Monoplanar for Insertion in Lower Bones	**Includes:** Uniplanar external fixator
External Fixation Device, Monoplanar for Reposition in Upper Bones	**Includes:** Uniplanar external fixator
External Fixation Device, Monoplanar for Reposition in Lower Bones	**Includes:** Uniplanar external fixator
External Fixation Device, Ring for Insertion in Upper Bones	**Includes:** Ilizarov external fixator Sheffield ring external fixator
External Fixation Device, Ring for Insertion in Lower Bones	**Includes:** Ilizarov external fixator Sheffield ring external fixator
External Fixation Device, Ring for Reposition in Upper Bones	**Includes:** Ilizarov external fixator Sheffield ring external fixator
External Fixation Device, Ring for Reposition in Lower Bones	**Includes:** Ilizarov external fixator Sheffield ring external fixator
Extraluminal Device	**Includes:** AtriClip LAA Exclusion System LAP-BAND® adjustable gastric banding system REALIZE® Adjustable Gastric Band
Feeding Device in Gastrointestinal System	**Includes:** Percutaneous endoscopic gastrojejunostomy (PEG/J) tube Percutaneous endoscopic gastrostomy (PEG) tube

SECTION Ø - MEDICAL AND SURGICAL
CHARACTER 6 - DEVICE

Hearing Device in Ear, Nose, Sinus	**Includes:** Esteem® implantable hearing system		Interbody Fusion Device in Upper Joints	**Includes:** BAK/C® Interbody Cervical Fusion System Interbody fusion (spine) cage
Hearing Device in Head and Facial Bones	**Includes:** Bone anchored hearing device		Internal Fixation Device in Head and Facial Bones	**Includes:** Bone screw (interlocking) (lag) (pedicle) (recessed) Kirschner wire (K-wire) Neutralization plate
Hearing Device, Bone Conduction for Insertion in Ear, Nose, Sinus	**Includes:** Bone anchored hearing device		Internal Fixation Device in Lower Bones	**Includes:** Bone screw (interlocking) (lag) (pedicle) (recessed) Clamp and rod internal fixation system (CRIF) Kirschner wire (K-wire) Neutralization plate
Hearing Device, Multiple Channel Cochlear Prosthesis for Insertion in Ear, Nose, Sinus	**Includes:** Cochlear implant (CI), multiple channel (electrode)		Internal Fixation Device in Lower Joints	**Includes:** Fusion screw (compression) (lag) (locking) Joint fixation plate Kirschner wire (K-wire)
Hearing Device, Single Channel Cochlear Prosthesis for Insertion in Ear, Nose, Sinus	**Includes:** Cochlear implant (CI), single channel (electrode)		Internal Fixation Device in Upper Bones	**Includes:** Bone screw (interlocking) (lag) (pedicle) (recessed) Clamp and rod internal fixation system (CRIF) Kirschner wire (K-wire) Neutralization plate
Implantable Heart Assist System in Heart and Great Vessels	**Includes:** Berlin Heart Ventricular Assist Device DeBakey Left Ventricular Assist Device DuraHeart Left Ventricular Assist System HeartMate 3™ LVAS HeartMate II® Left Ventricular Assist Device (LVAD) HeartMate XVE® Left Ventricular Assist Device (LVAD) MicroMed HeartAssist Novacor Left Ventricular Assist Device Thoratec IVAD (Implantable Ventricular Assist Device)		Internal Fixation Device in Upper Joints	**Includes:** Fusion screw (compression) (lag) (locking) Joint fixation plate Kirschner wire (K-wire)
			Internal Fixation Device, Intramedullary in Lower Bones	**Includes:** Intramedullary (IM) rod (nail) Intramedullary skeletal kinetic distractor (ISKD) Kuntscher nail
Infusion Device	**Includes:** Ascenda Intrathecal Catheter InDura, intrathecal catheter (1P) (spinal) Non-tunneled central venous catheter Peripherally inserted central catheter (PICC) Tunneled spinal (intrathecal) catheter		Internal Fixation Device, Intramedullary in Upper Bones	**Includes:** Intramedullary (IM) rod (nail) Intramedullary skeletal kinetic distractor (ISKD) Kuntscher nail
Infusion Device, Pump in Subcutaneous Tissue and Fascia	**Includes:** Implantable drug infusion pump (anti-spasmodic) (chemotherapy) (pain) Injection reservoir, pump Pump reservoir Subcutaneous injection reservoir, pump SynchroMed pump		Internal Fixation Device, Rigid Plate for Insertion in Upper Bones	**Includes:** Titanium Sternal Fixation System (TSFS)
Interbody Fusion Device in Lower Joints	**Includes:** Axial Lumbar Interbody Fusion System AxiaLIF® System CoRoent® XL Direct Lateral Interbody Fusion (DLIF) device EXtreme Lateral Interbody Fusion (XLIF) device Interbody fusion (spine) cage XLIF® System		Internal Fixation Device, Rigid Plate for Reposition in Upper Bones	**Includes:** Titanium Sternal Fixation System (TSFS)

SECTION Ø - MEDICAL AND SURGICAL
CHARACTER 6 - DEVICE

Intraluminal Device	**Includes:**
	Absolute Pro Vascular (OTW) Self-Expanding
	   Stent System
	Acculink (RX) Carotid Stent System
	AFX® Endovascular AAA System
	AneuRx® AAA Advantage®
	Assurant (Cobalt) stent
	Carotid WALLSTENT® Monorail® Endoprosthesis
	CoAxia NeuroFlo catheter
	Colonic Z-Stent®
	Complete (SE) stent
	Cook Zenith AAA Endovascular Graft
	Driver stent (RX) (OTW)
	E-Luminexx™ (Biliary) (Vascular) Stent
	Embolization coil(s)
	Endologix AFX® Endovascular AAA System
	Endurant® Endovascular Stent Graft
	Endurant® II AAA stent graft system
	EXCLUDER® AAA Endoprosthesis
	Express® (LD) Premounted Stent System
	Express® Biliary SD Monorail® Premounted
	   Stent System
	Express® SD Renal Monorail® Premounted
	   Stent System
	FLAIR® Endovascular Stent Graft
	Formula™ Balloon-Expandable Renal Stent
	   System
	GORE EXCLUDER® AAA Endoprosthesis
	GORE TAG® Thoracic Endoprosthesis
	Herculink (RX) Elite Renal Stent System
	LifeStent® (Flexstar) (XL) Vascular Stent System
	Medtronic Endurant® II AAA stent graft system
	Micro-Driver stent (RX) (OTW)
	MULTI-LINK (VISION)(MINI-VISION)(ULTRA)
	   Coronary Stent System
	Omnilink Elite Vascular Balloon Expandable
	   Stent System
	Pipeline™ Embolization device (PED)
	Protégé® RX Carotid Stent System
	Stent, intraluminal (cardiovascular)
	   (gastrointestinal)(hepatobiliary)(urinary)
	Talent® Converter
	Talent® Occluder
	Talent® Stent Graft (abdominal) (thoracic)
	Therapeutic occlusion coil(s)
	Ultraflex™ Precision Colonic Stent System
	Valiant Thoracic Stent Graft
	WALLSTENT® Endoprosthesis
	Xact Carotid Stent System
	Zenith AAA Endovascular Graft
	Zenith Flex® AAA Endovascular Graft
	Zenith® Renu™ AAA Ancillary Graft
	Zenith TX2® TAA Endovascular Graft

Intraluminal Device, Airway in Ear, Nose, Sinus	**Includes:** Nasopharyngeal airway (NPA)

Intraluminal Device, Airway in Gastrointestinal System	**Includes:** Esophageal obturator airway (EOA)
Intraluminal Device, Airway in Mouth and Throat	**Includes:** Guedel airway Oropharyngeal airway (OPA)
Intraluminal Device, Bioactive in Upper Arteries	**Includes:** Bioactive embolization coil(s) Micrus CERECYTE microcoil
Intraluminal Device, Branched or Fenestrated, One or Two Arteries for Restriction in Lower Arteries	**Includes:** Cook Zenith AAA Endovascular Graft EXCLUDER® AAA Endoprosthesis EXCLUDER® IBE Endoprosthesis GORE EXCLUDER® AAA Endoprosthesis GORE EXCLUDER® IBE Endoprosthesis Zenith AAA Endovascular Graft
Intraluminal Device, Branched or Fenestrated, Three or More Arteries for Restriction in Lower Arteries	**Includes:** Cook Zenith AAA Endovascular Graft EXCLUDER® AAA Endoprosthesis GORE EXCLUDER® AAA Endoprosthesis Zenith AAA Endovascular Graft

Intraluminal Device,
Drug-eluting in
Heart and Great
Vessels
	Includes:
	CYPHER® Stent
	Endeavor® (III) (IV) (Sprint) Zotarolimus-
	   eluting Coronary Stent System
	Everolimus-eluting coronary stent
	Paclitaxel-eluting coronary stent
	Sirolimus-eluting coronary stent
	TAXUS® Liberté® Paclitaxel-eluting Coronary
	   Stent System
	XIENCE Everolimus Eluting Coronary Stent
	   System
	Zotarolimus-eluting coronary stent

Intraluminal Device, Drug-eluting in Lower Arteries	**Includes:** Paclitaxel-eluting peripheral stent Zilver® PTX® (paclitaxel) Drug-Eluting Peripheral Stent
Intraluminal Device, Drug-eluting in Upper Arteries	**Includes:** Paclitaxel-eluting peripheral stent Zilver® PTX® (paclitaxel) Drug-Eluting Peripheral Stent
Intraluminal Device, Endobronchial Valve in Respiratory System	**Includes:** Spiration IBV™ Valve System
Intraluminal Device, Endotracheal Airway in Respiratory System	**Includes:** Endotracheal tube (cuffed) (double-lumen)

SECTION Ø - MEDICAL AND SURGICAL
CHARACTER 6 - DEVICE

Intraluminal Device, Pessary in Female Reproductive System	**Includes:** Pessary ring Vaginal pessary	**Pacemaker, Dual Chamber for Insertion in Subcutaneous Tissue and Fascia**	**Includes:** Advisa (MRI) EnRhythm Kappa Revo MRI™ SureScan® pacemaker Two lead pacemaker Versa
Liner in Lower Joints	**Includes:** Acetabular cup Hip (joint) liner Joint liner (insert) Knee (implant) insert Tibial insert	**Pacemaker, Single Chamber for Insertion in Subcutaneous Tissue and Fascia**	**Includes:** Single lead pacemaker (atrium) (ventricle)
Monitoring Device	**Includes:** Blood glucose monitoring system Cardiac event recorder Continuous Glucose Monitoring (CGM) device Implantable glucose monitoring device Loop recorder, implantable Reveal (DX) (XT)	**Pacemaker, Single Chamber Rate Responsive for Insertion in Subcutaneous Tissue and Fascia**	**Includes:** Single lead rate responsive pacemaker (atrium) (ventricle)
Monitoring Device, Hemodynamic for Insertion in Subcutaneous Tissue and Fascia	**Includes:** Implantable hemodynamic monitor (IHM) Implantable hemodynamic monitoring system (IHMS)	**Radioactive Element**	**Includes:** Brachytherapy seeds
Monitoring Device, Pressure Sensor for Insertion in Heart and Great Vessels	**Includes:** CardioMEMS® pressure sensor EndoSure® sensor	**Radioactive Element, Cesium-131 Collagen Implant for Insertion in Central Nervous System and Cranial Nerves**	Cesium-131 Collagen Implant GammaTile™
Neurostimulator Lead in Central Nervous System and Cranial Nerves	**Includes:** Cortical strip neurostimulator lead DBS lead Deep brain neurostimulator lead RNS System lead Spinal cord neurostimulator lead	**Resurfacing Device in Lower Joints**	**Includes:** CONSERVE® PLUS Total Resurfacing Hip System Cormet Hip Resurfacing System
Neurostimulator Lead in Peripheral Nervous System	**Includes:** InterStim® Therapy lead	**Short-term External Heart Assist System in Heart and Great Vessels**	Biventricular external heart assist system BVS 5ØØØ Ventricular Assist Device Centrimag® Blood Pump Impella® heart pump TandemHeart® System Thoratec Paracorporeal Ventricular Assist Device
Neurostimulator Generator in Head and Facial Bones	**Includes:** RNS system neurostimulator generator	**Spacer in Lower Joints**	**Includes:** Joint spacer (antibiotic)
Nonautologous Tissue Substitute	**Includes:** Acellular Hydrated Dermis Bone bank bone graft Cook Biodesign® Fistula Plug(s) Cook Biodesign® Hernia Graft(s) Cook Biodesign® Layered Graft(s) Cook Zenapro™ Layered Graft(s) Tissue bank graft	**Spacer in Upper Joints**	**Includes:** Joint spacer (antibiotic) Spacer, static (antibiotic) Static spacer (antibiotic)
		Spinal Stabilization Device, Facet Replacement for Insertion in Upper Joints	**Includes:** Facet replacement spinal stabilization device
		Spinal Stabilization Device, Facet Replacement for Insertion in Lower Joints	**Includes:** Facet replacement spinal stabilization device

SECTION Ø - MEDICAL AND SURGICAL
CHARACTER 6 - DEVICE

Spinal Stabilization Device, Interspinous Process for Insertion in Upper Joints	**Includes:** Interspinous process spinal stabilization device X-STOP® Spacer
Spinal Stabilization Device, Interspinous Process for Insertion in Lower Joints	**Includes:** Interspinous process spinal stabilization device X-STOP® Spacer
Spinal Stabilization Device, Pedicle-Based for Insertion in Upper Joints	**Includes:** Dynesys® Dynamic Stabilization System Pedicle-based dynamic stabilization device
Spinal Stabilization Device, Pedicle-Based for Insertion in Lower Joints	**Includes:** Dynesys® Dynamic Stabilization System Pedicle-based dynamic stabilization device
Stimulator Generator in Subcutaneous Tissue and Fascia	**Includes:** Baroreflex Activation Therapy® (BAT®) Diaphragmatic pacemaker generator Mark IV Breathing Pacemaker System Phrenic nerve stimulator generator Rheos® System device
Stimulator Generator, Multiple Array for Insertion in Subcutaneous Tissue and Fascia	**Includes:** Activa PC neurostimulator Enterra gastric neurostimulator Neurostimulator generator, multiple channel PrimeAdvanced neurostimulator (SureScan) (MRI Safe)
Stimulator Generator, Multiple Array Rechargeable for Insertion in Subcutaneous Tissue and Fascia	**Includes:** Activa RC neurostimulator Neurostimulator generator, multiple channel rechargeable RestoreAdvanced neurostimulator (SureScan) (MRI Safe) RestoreSensor neurostimulator (SureScan) (MRI Safe) RestoreUltra neurostimulator (SureScan) (MRI Safe)
Stimulator Generator, Single Array for Insertion in Subcutaneous Tissue and Fascia	**Includes:** Activa SC neurostimulator InterStim® Therapy neurostimulator Itrel (3) (4) neurostimulator Neurostimulator generator, single channel
Stimulator Generator, Single Array Rechargeable for Insertion in Subcutaneous Tissue and Fascia	**Includes:** Neurostimulator generator, single channel rechargeable
Stimulator Lead in Gastrointestinal System	**Includes:** Gastric electrical stimulation (GES) lead Gastric pacemaker lead
Stimulator Lead in Muscles	**Includes:** Electrical muscle stimulation (EMS) lead Electronic muscle stimulator lead Neuromuscular electrical stimulation (NEMS) lead
Stimulator Lead in Upper Arteries	**Includes:** Baroreflex Activation Therapy® (BAT®) Carotid (artery) sinus (baroreceptor) lead Rheos® System lead
Stimulator Lead in Urinary System	**Includes:** Sacral nerve modulation (SNM) lead Sacral neuromodulation lead Urinary incontinence stimulator lead
Synthetic Substitute	**Includes:** AbioCor® Total Replacement Heart AMPLATZER® Muscular VSD Occluder Annuloplasty ring Bard® Composix® (E/X) (LP) mesh Bard® Composix® Kugel® patch Bard® Dulex™ mesh Bard® Ventralex™ hernia patch BRYAN® Cervical Disc System Ex-PRESS™ mini glaucoma shunt Flexible Composite Mesh GORE® DUALMESH® Holter valve ventricular shunt MitraClip valve repair system Nitinol framed polymer mesh Open Pivot (mechanical) valve Open Pivot Aortic Valve Graft (AVG) Partially absorbable mesh PHYSIOMESH™ Flexible Composite Mesh Polymethylmethacrylate (PMMA) Polypropylene mesh PRESTIGE® Cervical Disc PROCEED™ Ventral Patch Prodisc-C Prodisc-L PROLENE Polypropylene Hernia System (PHS) Rebound HRD® (Hernia Repair Device) SynCardia Total Artificial Heart Total artificial (replacement) heart ULTRAPRO Hernia System (UHS) ULTRAPRO Partially Absorbable Lightweight Mesh ULTRAPRO Plug Ventrio™ Hernia Patch Zimmer® NexGen® LPS Mobile Bearing Knee Zimmer® NexGen® LPS-Flex Mobile Knee

SECTION Ø - MEDICAL AND SURGICAL
CHARACTER 6 - DEVICE

Synthetic Substitute, Ceramic for Replacement in Lower Joints	**Includes:** Ceramic on ceramic bearing surface Novation® Ceramic AHS® (Articulation Hip System)
Synthetic Substitute, Intraocular Telescope for Replacement in Eye	**Includes:** Implantable Miniature Telescope™ (IMT)
Synthetic Substitute, Metal for Replacement in Lower Joints	**Includes:** Cobalt/chromium head and socket Metal on metal bearing surface
Synthetic Substitute, Metal on Polyethylene for Replacement in Lower Joints	**Includes:** Cobalt/chromium head and polyethylene socket
Synthetic Substitute, Oxidized Zirconium on Polyethylene for Replacement in Lower Joints	OXINIUM
Synthetic Substitute, Polyethylene for Replacement in Lower Joints	**Includes:** Polyethylene socket
Synthetic Substitute, Reverse Ball and Socket for Replacement in Upper Joints	**Includes:** Delta III Reverse shoulder prosthesis Reverse® Shoulder Prosthesis
Tissue Expander in Skin and Breast	**Includes:** Tissue expander (inflatable) (injectable)

Tissue Expander in Subcutaneous Tissue and Fascia	**Includes:** Tissue expander (inflatable) (injectable)
Tracheostomy Device in Respiratory System	**Includes:** Tracheostomy tube
Vascular Access Device, Totally Implantable in Subcutaneous Tissue and Fascia	**Includes:** Implanted (venous) (access) port Injection reservoir, port Subcutaneous injection reservoir, port
Vascular Access Device, Tunneled in Subcutaneous Tissue and Fascia	**Includes:** Tunneled central venous catheter Vectra® Vascular Access Graft
Zooplastic Tissue in Heart and Great Vessels	**Includes:** 3f (Aortic) Bioprosthesis valve Bovine pericardial valve Bovine pericardium graft Contegra Pulmonary Valved Conduit CoreValve transcatheter aortic valve Epic™ Stented Tissue Valve (aortic) Freestyle (Stentless) Aortic Root Bioprosthesis Hancock Bioprosthesis (aortic) (mitral) valve Hancock Bioprosthetic Valved Conduit Melody® transcatheter pulmonary valve Mitroflow® Aortic Pericardial Heart Valve Mosaic Bioprosthesis (aortic) (mitral) valve Porcine (bioprosthetic) valve SAPIEN transcatheter aortic valve SJM Biocor® Stented Valve System Stented tissue valve Trifecta™ Valve (aortic) Xenograft

SECTION 1 - OBSTETRICS
CHARACTER 3 - OPERATION

Abortion	**Definition:** Artificially terminating a pregnancy
Change	**Definition:** Taking out or off a device from a body part and putting back an identical or similar device in or on the same body part without cutting or puncturing the skin or a mucous membrane
Delivery	**Definition:** Assisting the passage of the products of conception from the genital canal
Drainage	**Definition:** Taking or letting out fluids and/or gases from a body part by the use of force

Extraction	**Definition:** Pulling or stripping out or off all or a portion of a body part
Insertion	**Definition:** Putting in a nonbiological appliance that monitors, assists, performs, or prevents a physiological function but does not physically take the place of a body part
Inspection	**Definition:** Visually and/or manually exploring a body part **Explanation:** Visual exploration may be performed with or without optical instrumentation. Manual exploration may be performed directly or through intervening body layers

SECTION 1 - OBSTETRICS
CHARACTER 3 - OPERATION

Removal	**Definition:** Taking out or off a device from a body part, region or orifice **Explanation:** If a device is taken out and a similar device put in without cutting or puncturing the skin or mucous membrane, the procedure is coded to the root operation CHANGE. Otherwise, the procedure for taking out a device is coded to the root operation REMOVAL
Repair	**Definition:** Restoring, to the extent possible, a body part to its normal anatomic structure and function **Explanation:** Used only when the method to accomplish the repair is not one of the other root operations

Reposition	**Definition:** Moving to its normal location or other suitable location all or a portion of a body part **Explanation:** The body part is moved to a new location from an abnormal location, or from a normal location where it is not functioning correctly. The body part may or may not be cut out or off to be moved to the new location
Resection	**Definition:** Cutting out or off, without replacement, all of a body part
Transplantation	**Definition:** Putting in or on all or a portion of a living body part taken from another individual or animal to physically take the place and/or function of all or a portion of a similar body part **Explanation:** The native body part may or may not be taken out, and the transplanted body part may take over all or a portion of its function

SECTION 1 - OBSTETRICS
CHARACTER 5 - APPROACH

External	**Definition:** Procedures performed directly on the skin or mucous membrane and procedures performed indirectly by the application of external force through the skin or mucous membrane
Open	**Definition:** Cutting through the skin or mucous membrane and any other body layers necessary to expose the site of the procedure
Percutaneous	**Definition:** Entry, by puncture or minor incision, of instrumentation through the skin or mucous membrane and any other body layers necessary to reach the site of the procedure

Percutaneous Endoscopic	**Definition:** Entry, by puncture or minor incision, of instrumentation through the skin or mucous membrane and any other body layers necessary to reach and visualize the site of the procedure
Via Natural or Artificial Opening	**Definition:** Entry of instrumentation through a natural or artificial external opening to reach the site of the procedure
Via Natural or Artificial Opening Endoscopic	**Definition:** Entry of instrumentation through a natural or artificial external opening to reach and visualize the site of the procedure

SECTION 2 - PLACEMENT
CHARACTER 3 - OPERATION

Change	**Definition:** Taking out or off a device from a body part and putting back an identical or similar device in or on the same body part without cutting or puncturing the skin or a mucous membrane
Compression	**Definition:** Putting pressure on a body region
Dressing	**Definition:** Putting material on a body region for protection

Immobilization	**Definition:** Limiting or preventing motion of a body region
Packing	**Definition:** Putting material in a body region or orifice
Removal	**Definition:** Taking out or off a device from a body part
Traction	**Definition:** Exerting a pulling force on a body region in a distal direction

SECTION 2; 3, CHARACTER 5; 3; 5; 6

SECTION 2 - PLACEMENT
CHARACTER 5 - APPROACH

External	**Definition:** Procedures performed directly on the skin or mucous membrane and procedures performed indirectly by the application of external force through the skin or mucous membrane

SECTION 3 - ADMINISTRATION
CHARACTER 3 - OPERATION

Introduction	**Definition:** Putting in or on a therapeutic, diagnostic, nutritional, physiological, or prophylactic substance except blood or blood products

Irrigation	**Definition:** Putting in or on a cleansing substance
Transfusion	**Definition:** Putting in blood or blood products

SECTION 3 - ADMINISTRATION
CHARACTER 5 - APPROACH

External	**Definition:** Procedures performed directly on the skin or mucous membrane and procedures performed indirectly by the application of external force through the skin or mucous membrane
Open	**Definition:** Cutting through the skin or mucous membrane and any other body layers necessary to expose the site of the procedure
Percutaneous	**Definition:** Entry, by puncture or minor incision, of instrumentation through the skin or mucous membrane and any other body layers necessary to reach the site of the procedure

Percutaneous Endoscopic	**Definition:** Entry, by puncture or minor incision, of instrumentation through the skin or mucous membrane and any other body layers necessary to reach and visualize the site of the procedure
Via Natural or Artificial Opening	**Definition:** Entry of instrumentation through a natural or artificial external opening to reach the site of the procedure
Via Natural or Artificial Opening Endoscopic	**Definition:** Entry of instrumentation through a natural or artificial external opening to reach and visualize the site of the procedure

SECTION 3 - ADMINISTRATION
CHARACTER 6 - SUBSTANCE

4-Factor Prothrombin Complex Concentrate	**Includes:** Kcentra
Adhesion Barrier	**Includes:** Seprafilm
Anti-Infective Envelope	**Includes:** AIGISRx Antibacterial Envelope Antimicrobial envelope
Clofarabine	**Includes:** Clolar
Glucarpidase	**Includes:** Voraxaze

Human B-type Natriuretic Peptide	**Includes:** Nesiritide
Other Thrombolytic	**Includes:** Tissue Plasminogen Activator (tPA)(r-tPA)
Oxazolidinones	**Includes:** Zyvox
Recombinant Bone Morphogenetic Protein	**Includes:** Bone morphogenetic protein 2 (BMP 2) rhBMP-2

SECTION 4 - MEASUREMENT AND MONITORING
CHARACTER 3 - OPERATION

Measurement	**Definition:** Determining the level of a physiological or physical function at a point in time

Monitoring	**Definition:** Determining the level of a physiological or physical function repetitively over a period of time

SECTION 4 - MEASUREMENT AND MONITORING
CHARACTER 5 - APPROACH

External	**Definition:** Procedures performed directly on the skin or mucous membrane and procedures performed indirectly by the application of external force through the skin or mucous membrane
Open	**Definition:** Cutting through the skin or mucous membrane and any other body layers necessary to expose the site of the procedure
Percutaneous	**Definition:** Entry, by puncture or minor incision, of instrumentation through the skin or mucous membrane and any other body layers necessary to reach the site of the procedure

Percutaneous Endoscopic	**Definition:** Entry, by puncture or minor incision, of instrumentation through the skin or mucous membrane and any other body layers necessary to reach and visualize the site of the procedure
Via Natural or Artificial Opening	**Definition:** Entry of instrumentation through a natural or artificial external opening to reach the site of the procedure
Via Natural or Artificial Opening Endoscopic	**Definition:** Entry of instrumentation through a natural or artificial external opening to reach and visualize the site of the procedure

SECTION 5 - EXTRACORPOREAL OR SYSTEMIC ASSISTANCE AND PERFORMANCE
CHARACTER 3 - OPERATION

Assistance	**Definition:** Taking over a portion of a physiological function by extracorporeal means
Performance	**Definition:** Completely taking over a physiological function by extracorporeal means

Restoration	**Definition:** Returning, or attempting to return, a physiological function to its original state by extracorporeal means.

SECTION 6 - EXTRACORPOREAL OR SYSTEMIC THERAPIES
CHARACTER 3 - OPERATION

Atmospheric Control	**Definition:** Extracorporeal control of atmospheric pressure and composition
Decompression	**Definition:** Extracorporeal elimination of undissolved gas from body fluids
Electromagnetic Therapy	**Definition:** Extracorporeal treatment by electromagnetic rays
Hyperthermia	**Definition:** Extracorporeal raising of body temperature
Hypothermia	**Definition:** Extracorporeal lowering of body temperature
Perfusion	**Definition:** Extracorporeal treatment by diffusion of therapeutic fluid

Pheresis	**Definition:** Extracorporeal separation of blood products
Phototherapy	**Definition:** Extracorporeal treatment by light rays
Shock Wave Therapy	**Definition:** Extracorporeal treatment by shock waves
Ultrasound Therapy	**Definition:** Extracorporeal treatment by ultrasound
Ultraviolet Light Therapy	**Definition:** Extracorporeal treatment by ultraviolet light

SECTION 7 - OSTEOPATHIC
CHARACTER 3 - OPERATION

Treatment	**Definition:** Manual treatment to eliminate or alleviate somatic dysfunction and related disorders

SECTION 7 - OSTEOPATHIC
CHARACTER 5 - APPROACH

External	**Definition:** Procedures performed directly on the skin or mucous membrane and procedures performed indirectly by the application of external force through the skin or mucous membrane

SECTION 8 - OTHER PROCEDURES
CHARACTER 3 - OPERATION

Other Procedures	**Definition:** Methodologies which attempt to remediate or cure a disorder or disease

SECTION 8 - OTHER PROCEDURES
CHARACTER 5 - APPROACH

External	**Definition:** Procedures performed directly on the skin or mucous membrane and procedures performed indirectly by the application of external force through the skin or mucous membrane
Percutaneous	**Definition:** Entry, by puncture or minor incision, of instrumentation through the skin or mucous membrane and any other body layers necessary to reach the site of the procedure
Percutaneous Endoscopic	**Definition:** Entry, by puncture or minor incision, of instrumentation through the skin or mucous membrane and any other body layers necessary to reach and visualize the site of the procedure

Via Natural or Artificial Opening	**Definition:** Entry of instrumentation through a natural or artificial external opening to reach the site of the procedure
Via Natural or Artificial Opening Endoscopic	**Definition:** Entry of instrumentation through a natural or artificial external opening to reach and visualize the site of the procedure

SECTION 9 - CHIROPRACTIC
CHARACTER 3 - OPERATION

Manipulation	**Definition:** Manual procedure that involves a directed thrust to move a joint past the physiological range of motion, without exceeding the anatomical limit

SECTION 9 - CHIROPRACTIC
CHARACTER 5 - APPROACH

External	**Definition:** Procedures performed directly on the skin or mucous membrane and procedures performed indirectly by the application of external force through the skin or mucous membrane

SECTION B - IMAGING
CHARACTER 3 - TYPE

Computerized Tomography (CT Scan)	**Definition:** Computer reformatted digital display of multiplanar images developed from the capture of multiple exposures of external ionizing radiation	Plain Radiography	**Definition:** Planar display of an image developed from the capture of external ionizing radiation on photographic or photoconductive plate
Fluoroscopy	**Definition:** Single plane or bi-plane real time display of an image developed from the capture of external ionizing radiation on a fluorescent screen. The image may also be stored by either digital or analog means	Ultrasonography	**Definition:** Real time display of images of anatomy or flow information developed from the capture of reflected and attenuated high frequency sound waves
Magnetic Resonance Imaging (MRI)	**Definition:** Computer reformatted digital display of multiplanar images developed from the capture of radiofrequency signals emitted by nuclei in a body site excited within a magnetic field		

SECTION C - NUCLEAR MEDICINE
CHARACTER 3 - TYPE

Nonimaging Nuclear Medicine Assay	**Definition:** Introduction of radioactive materials into the body for the study of body fluids and blood elements, by the detection of radioactive emissions	Planar Nuclear Medicine Imaging	**Definition:** Introduction of radioactive materials into the body for single plane display of images developed from the capture of radioactive emissions
Nonimaging Nuclear Medicine Probe	**Definition:** Introduction of radioactive materials into the body for the study of distribution and fate of certain substances by the detection of radioactive emissions; or, alternatively, measurement of absorption of radioactive emissions from an external source	Positron Emission Tomographic (PET) Imaging	**Definition:** Introduction of radioactive materials into the body for three dimensional display of images developed from the simultaneous capture, 18Ø degrees apart, of radioactive emissions
Nonimaging Nuclear Medicine Uptake	**Definition:** Introduction of radioactive materials into the body for measurements of organ function, from the detection of radioactive emissions	Systemic Nuclear Medicine Therapy	**Definition:** Introduction of unsealed radioactive materials into the body for treatment
		Tomographic (Tomo) Nuclear Medicine Imaging	**Definition:** Introduction of radioactive materials into the body for three dimensional display of images developed from the capture of radioactive emissions

SECTION F - PHYSICAL REHABILITATION AND DIAGNOSTIC AUDIOLOGY
CHARACTER 3 - TYPE

Activities of Daily Living Assessment	**Definition:** Measurement of functional level for activities of daily living	Hearing Treatment	**Definition:** Application of techniques to improve, augment, or compensate for hearing and related functional impairment
Activities of Daily Living Treatment	**Definition:** Exercise or activities to facilitate functional competence for activities of daily living	Motor and/or Nerve Function Assessment	**Definition:** Measurement of motor, nerve, and related functions
Caregiver Training	**Definition:** Training in activities to support patient's optimal level of function	Motor Treatment	**Definition:** Exercise or activities to increase or facilitate motor function
Cochlear Implant Treatment	**Definition:** Application of techniques to improve the communication abilities of individuals with cochlear implant	Speech Assessment	**Definition:** Measurement of speech and related functions
Device Fitting	**Definition:** Fitting of a device designed to facilitate or support achievement of a higher level of function	Speech Treatment	**Definition:** Application of techniques to improve, augment, or compensate for speech and related functional impairment
Hearing Aid Assessment	**Definition:** Measurement of the appropriateness and/or effectiveness of a hearing device	Vestibular Assessment	**Definition:** Measurement of the vestibular system and related functions
Hearing Assessment	**Definition:** Measurement of hearing and related functions	Vestibular Treatment	**Definition:** Application of techniques to improve, augment, or compensate for vestibular and related functional impairment

SECTION F - PHYSICAL REHABILITATION AND DIAGNOSTIC AUDIOLOGY
CHARACTER 5 - TYPE QUALIFIER

Acoustic Reflex Decay	**Definition:** Measures reduction in size/strength of acoustic reflex over time **Includes/Examples:** Includes site of lesion test	Alternate Binaural or Monaural Loudness Balance	**Definition:** Determines auditory stimulus parameter that yields the same objective sensation **Includes/Examples:** Sound intensities that yield same loudness perception
Acoustic Reflex Patterns	**Definition:** Defines site of lesion based upon presence/absence of acoustic reflexes with ipsilateral vs. contralateral stimulation	Anthropometric Characteristics	**Definition:** Measures edema, body fat composition, height, weight, length and girth
Acoustic Reflex Threshold	**Definition:** Determines minimal intensity that acoustic reflex occurs with ipsilateral and/or contralateral stimulation	Aphasia (Assessment)	**Definition:** Measures expressive and receptive speech and language function including reading and writing
Aerobic Capacity and Endurance	**Definition:** Measures autonomic responses to positional changes; perceived exertion, dyspnea or angina during activity; performance during exercise protocols; standard vital signs; and blood gas analysis or oxygen consumption	Aphasia (Treatment)	**Definition:** Applying techniques to improve, augment, or compensate for receptive/expressive language impairments
		Articulation/Phonology (Assessment)	**Definition:** Measures speech production

SECTION F - PHYSICAL REHABILITATION AND DIAGNOSTIC AUDIOLOGY
CHARACTER 5 - TYPE QUALIFIER

Articulation/Phonology (Treatment)	**Definition:** Applying techniques to correct, improve, or compensate for speech productive impairment
Assistive Listening Device	**Definition:** Assists in use of effective and appropriate assistive listening device/system
Assistive Listening System/Device Selection	**Definition:** Measures the effectiveness and appropriateness of assistive listening systems/devices
Assistive, Adaptive,Supportive or Protective Devices	**Explanation:** Devices to facilitate or support achievement of a higher level of function in wheelchair mobility; bed mobility; transfer or ambulation ability; bath and showering ability; dressing; grooming; personal hygiene; play or leisure
Auditory Evoked Potentials	**Definition:** Measures electric responses produced by the VIIIth cranial nerve and brainstem following auditory stimulation
Auditory Processing (Assessment)	**Definition:** Evaluates ability to receive and process auditory information and comprehension of spoken language
Auditory Processing (Treatment)	**Definition:** Applying techniques to improve the receiving and processing of auditory information and comprehension of spoken language
Augmentative/ Alternative Communication System (Assessment)	**Definition:** Determines the appropriateness of aids, techniques, symbols, and/or strategies to augment or replace speech and enhance communication **Includes/Examples:** Includes the use of telephones, writing equipment, emergency equipment, and TDD
Augmentative/ Alternative Communication System (Treatment)	**Includes/Examples:** Includes augmentative communication devices and aids
Aural Rehabilitation	**Definition:** Applying techniques to improve the communication abilities associated with hearing loss
Aural Rehabilitation Status	**Definition:** Measures impact of a hearing loss including evaluation of receptive and expressive communication skills

Bathing/Showering	**Includes/Examples:** Includes obtaining and using supplies; soaping, rinsing, and drying body parts; maintaining bathing position; and transferring to and from bathing positions
Bathing/Showering Techniques	**Definition:** Activities to facilitate obtaining and using supplies, soaping, rinsing and drying body parts, maintaining bathing position, and transferring to and from bathing positions
Bed Mobility (Assessment)	**Definition:** Transitional movement within bed
Bed Mobility (Treatment)	**Definition:** Exercise or activities to facilitate transitional movements within bed
Bedside Swallowing and Oral Function	**Includes/Examples:** Bedside swallowing includes assessment of sucking, masticating, coughing, and swallowing. Oral function includes assessment of musculature for controlled movements, structures and functions to determine coordination and phonation
Bekesy Audiometry	**Definition:** Uses an instrument that provides a choice of discrete or continuously varying pure tones; choice of pulsed or continuous signal
Binaural Electroacoustic Hearing Aid Check	**Definition:** Determines mechanical and electroacoustic function of bilateral hearing aids using hearing aid test box
Binaural Hearing Aid (Assessment)	**Definition:** Measures the candidacy, effectiveness, and appropriateness of hearing aids **Explanation:** Measures bilateral fit
Binaural Hearing Aid (Treatment)	**Explanation:** Assists in achieving maximum understanding and performance
Bithermal, Binaural Caloric Irrigation	**Definition:** Measures the rhythmic eye movements stimulated by changing the temperature of the vestibular system
Bithermal, Monaural Caloric Irrigation	**Definition:** Measures the rhythmic eye movements stimulated by changing the temperature of the vestibular system in one ear

SECTION F - PHYSICAL REHABILITATION AND DIAGNOSTIC AUDIOLOGY
CHARACTER 5 - TYPE QUALIFIER

Brief Tone Stimuli	**Definition:** Measures specific central auditory process
Cerumen Management	**Definition:** Includes examination of external auditory canal and tympanic membrane and removal of cerumen from external ear canal
Cochlear Implant	**Definition:** Measures candidacy for cochlear implant
Cochlear Implant Rehabilitation	**Definition:** Applying techniques to improve the communication abilities of individuals with cochlear implant; includes programming the device, providing patients/families with information
Communicative/ Cognitive Integration Skills (Assessment)	**Definition:** Measures ability to use higher cortical functions **Includes/Examples:** Includes orientation, recognition, attention span, initiation and termination of activity, memory, sequencing, categorizing, concept formation, spatial operations, judgment, problem solving, generalization and pragmatic communication
Communicative/ Cognitive Integration Skills (Treatment)	**Definition:** Activities to facilitate the use of higher cortical functions **Includes/Examples:** Includes level of arousal, orientation, recognition, attention span, initiation and termination of activity, memory sequencing, judgment and problem solving, learning and generalization, and pragmatic communication
Computerized Dynamic Posturography	**Definition:** Measures the status of the peripheral and central vestibular system and the sensory/motor component of balance; evaluates the efficacy of vestibular rehabilitation
Conditioned Play Audiometry	**Definition:** Behavioral measures using nonspeech and speech stimuli to obtain frequency-specific and ear-specific information on auditory status from the patient **Explanation:** Obtains speech reception threshold by having patient point to pictures of spondaic words
Coordination/Dexterity (Assessment)	**Definition:** Measures large and small muscle groups for controlled goal-directed movements **Explanation:** Dexterity includes object manipulation
Coordination/Dexterity (Treatment)	**Definition:** Exercise or activities to facilitate gross coordination and fine coordination
Cranial Nerve Integrity	**Definition:** Measures cranial nerve sensory and motor functions, including tastes, smell and facial expression
Dichotic Stimuli	**Definition:** Measures specific central auditory process
Distorted Speech	**Definition:** Measures specific central auditory process
Dix-Hallpike Dynamic	**Definition:** Measures nystagmus following Dix-Hallpike maneuver
Dressing	**Includes/Examples:** Includes selecting clothing and accessories, obtaining clothing from storage, dressing and, fastening and adjusting clothing and shoes, and applying and removing personal devices, prosthesis or orthosis
Dressing Techniques	**Definition:** Activities to facilitate selecting clothing and accessories, dressing and undressing, adjusting clothing and shoes, applying and removing devices, prostheses or orthoses
Dynamic Orthosis	**Includes/Examples:** Includes customized and prefabricated splints, inhibitory casts, spinal and other braces, and protective devices; allows motion through transfer of movement from other body parts or by use of outside forces
Ear Canal Probe Microphone	**Definition:** Real ear measures
Ear Protector Attentuation	**Definition:** Measures ear protector fit and effectiveness
Electrocochleography	**Definition:** Measures the VIIIth cranial nerve action potential
Environmental, Home and Work Barriers	**Definition:** Measures current and potential barriers to optimal function, including safety hazards, access problems and home or office design

SECTION F - PHYSICAL REHABILITATION AND DIAGNOSTIC AUDIOLOGY
CHARACTER 5 - TYPE QUALIFIER

Ergonomics and Body Mechanics	**Definition:** Ergonomic measurement of job tasks, work hardening or work conditioning needs; functional capacity; and body mechanics
Eustachian Tube Function	**Definition:** Measures eustachian tube function and patency of eustachian tube
Evoked Otoacoustic Emissions, Diagnostic	**Definition:** Measures auditory evoked potentials in a diagnostic format
Evoked Otoacoustic Emissions, Screening	**Definition:** Measures auditory evoked potentials in a screening format
Facial Nerve Function	**Definition:** Measures electrical activity of the VIIth cranial nerve (facial nerve)
Feeding/Eating (Assessment)	**Includes/Examples:** Includes setting up food, selecting and using utensils and tableware, bringing food or drink to mouth, cleaning face, hands, and clothing, and management of alternative methods of nourishment
Feeding/Eating (Treatment)	**Definition:** Exercise or activities to facilitate setting up food, selecting and using utensils and tableware, bringing food or drink to mouth, cleaning face, hands, and clothing, and management of alternative methods of nourishment
Filtered Speech	**Definition:** Uses high or low pass filtered speech stimuli to assess central auditory processing disorders, site of lesion testing
Fluency (Assessment)	**Definition:** Measures speech fluency or stuttering
Fluency (Treatment)	**Definition:** Applying techniques to improve and augment fluent speech
Gait and/or Balance	**Definition:** Measures biomechanical, arthrokinematic and other spatial and temporal characteristics of gait and balance
Gait Training/ Functional Ambulation	**Definition:** Exercise or activities to facilitate ambulation on a variety of surfaces and in a variety of environments
Grooming/Personal Hygiene (Assessment)	**Includes/Examples:** Includes ability to obtain and use supplies in a sequential fashion, general grooming, oral hygiene, toilet hygiene, personal care devices, including care for artificial airways

Grooming/Personal Hygiene (Treatment)	**Definition:** Activities to facilitate obtaining and using supplies in a sequential fashion: general grooming, oral hygiene, toilet hygiene, cleaning body, and personal care devices, including artificial airways
Hearing and Related Disorders Counseling	**Definition:** Provides patients/families/ caregivers with information, support, referrals to facilitate recovery from a communication disorder **Includes/Examples:** Includes strategies for psychosocial adjustment to hearing loss for clients and families/caregivers
Hearing and Related Disorders Prevention	**Definition:** Provides patients/families/ caregivers with information and support to prevent communication disorders
Hearing Screening	**Definition:** Pass/refer measures designed to identify need for further audiologic assessment
Home Management (Assessment)	**Definition:** Obtaining and maintaining personal and household possessions and environment **Includes/Examples:** Includes clothing care, cleaning, meal preparation and cleanup, shopping, money management, household maintenance, safety procedures, and childcare/parenting
Home Management (Treatment)	**Definition:** Activities to facilitate obtaining and maintaining personal household possessions and environment **Includes/Examples:** Includes clothing care, cleaning, meal preparation and clean-up, shopping, money management, household maintenance, safety procedures, childcare/ parenting
Instrumental Swallowing and Oral Function	**Definition:** Measures swallowing function using instrumental diagnostic procedures **Explanation:** Methods include videofluoroscopy, ultrasound, manometry, endoscopy
Integumentary Integrity	**Includes/Examples:** Includes burns, skin conditions, ecchymosis, bleeding, blisters, scar tissue, wounds and other traumas, tissue mobility, turgor and texture

SECTION F - PHYSICAL REHABILITATION AND DIAGNOSTIC AUDIOLOGY

CHARACTER 5 - TYPE QUALIFIER

Manual Therapy Techniques	**Definition:** Techniques in which the therapist uses his/her hands to administer skilled movements **Includes/Examples:** Includes connective tissue massage, joint mobilization and manipulation, manual lymph drainage, manual traction, soft tissue mobilization and manipulation
Masking Patterns	**Definition:** Measures central auditory processing status
Monaural Electroacoustic Hearing Aid Check	**Definition:** Determines mechanical and electroacoustic function of one hearing aid using hearing aid test box
Monaural Hearing Aid (Assessment)	**Definition:** Measures the candidacy, effectiveness, and appropriateness of a hearing aid **Explanation:** Measures unilateral fit
Monaural Hearing Aid (Treatment)	**Explanation:** Assists in achieving maximum understanding and performance
Motor Function (Assessment)	**Definition:** Measures the body's functional and versatile movement patterns **Includes/Examples:** Includes motor assessment scales, analysis of head, trunk and limb movement, and assessment of motor learning
Motor Function (Treatment)	**Definition:** Exercise or activities to facilitate crossing midline, laterality, bilateral integration, praxis, neuromuscular relaxation, inhibition, facilitation, motor function and motor learning
Motor Speech (Assessment)	**Definition:** Measures neurological motor aspects of speech production
Motor Speech (Treatment)	**Definition:** Applying techniques to improve and augment the impaired neurological motor aspects of speech production
Muscle Performance (Assessment)	**Definition:** Measures muscle strength, power and endurance using manual testing, dynamometry or computer-assisted electromechanical muscle test; functional muscle strength, power and endurance; muscle pain, tone, or soreness; or pelvic-floor musculature **Explanation:** Muscle endurance refers to the ability to contract a muscle repeatedly over time
Muscle Performance (Treatment)	**Definition:** Exercise or activities to increase the capacity of a muscle to do work in terms of strength, power, and/or endurance **Explanation:** Muscle strength is the force exerted to overcome resistance in one maximal effort. Muscle power is work produced per unit of time, or the product of strength and speed. Muscle endurance is the ability to contract a muscle repeatedly over time
Neuromotor Development	**Definition:** Measures motor development, righting and equilibrium reactions, and reflex and equilibrium reactions
Non-invasive Instrumental Status	**Definition:** Instrumental measures of oral, nasal, vocal, and velopharyngeal functions as they pertain to speech production
Nonspoken Language (Assessment)	**Definition:** Measures nonspoken language (print, sign, symbols) for communication
Nonspoken Language (Treatment)	**Definition:** Applying techniques that improve, augment, or compensate spoken communication
Oral Peripheral Mechanism	**Definition:** Structural measures of face, jaw, lips, tongue, teeth, hard and soft palate, pharynx as related to speech production
Orofacial Myofunctional (Assessment)	**Definition:** Measures orofacial myofunctional patterns for speech and related functions
Orofacial Myofunctional (Treatment)	**Definition:** Applying techniques to improve, alter, or augment impaired orofacial myofunctional patterns and related speech production errors
Oscillating Tracking	**Definition:** Measures ability to visually track
Pain	**Definition:** Measures muscle soreness, pain and soreness with joint movement, and pain perception **Includes/Examples:** Includes questionnaires, graphs, symptom magnification scales or visual analog scales
Perceptual Processing (Assessment)	**Definition:** Measures stereognosis, kinesthesia, body schema, right-left discrimination, form constancy, position in space, visual closure, figure-ground, depth perception, spatial relations and topographical orientation

SECTION F - PHYSICAL REHABILITATION AND DIAGNOSTIC AUDIOLOGY

CHARACTER 5 - TYPE QUALIFIER

Perceptual Processing (Treatment)	**Definition:** Exercise and activities to facilitate perceptual processing **Explanation:** Includes stereognosis, kinesthesia, body schema, right-left discrimination, form constancy, position in space, visual closure, figure-ground, depth perception, spatial relations, and topographical orientation **Includes/Examples:** Includes stereognosis, kinesthesia, body schema, right-left discrimination, form constancy, position in space, visual closure, figure-ground, depth perception, spatial relations, and topographical orientation
Performance Intensity Phonetically Balanced Speech Discrimination	**Definition:** Measures word recognition over varying intensity levels
Postural Control	**Definition:** Exercise or activities to increase postural alignment and control
Prosthesis	**Definition:** Artificial substitutes for missing body parts that augment performance or function **Includes/Examples:** Limb prosthesis, ocular prosthesis
Psychosocial Skills (Assessment)	**Definition:** The ability to interact in society and to process emotions **Includes/Examples:** Includes psychological (values, interests, self-concept); social (role performance, social conduct, interpersonal skills, self expression); self-management (coping skills, time management, self-control)
Psychosocial Skills (Treatment)	**Definition:** The ability to interact in society and to process emotions **Includes/Examples:** Includes psychological (values, interests, self-concept); social (role performance, social conduct, interpersonal skills, self expression); self-management (coping skills, time management, self-control)
Pure Tone Audiometry, Air	**Definition:** Air-conduction pure tone threshold measures with appropriate masking
Pure Tone Audiometry, Air and Bone	**Definition:** Air-conduction and bone-conduction pure tone threshold measures with appropriate masking

Pure Tone Stenger	**Definition:** Measures unilateral nonorganic hearing loss based on simultaneous presentation of pure tones of differing volume
Range of Motion and Joint Integrity	**Definition:** Measures quantity, quality, grade, and classification of joint movement and/or mobility **Explanation:** Range of Motion is the space, distance or angle through which movement occurs at a joint or series of joints. Joint integrity is the conformance of joints to expected anatomic, biomechanical and kinematic norms
Range of Motion and Joint Mobility	**Definition:** Exercise or activities to increase muscle length and joint mobility
Receptive/Expressive Language (Assessment)	**Definition:** Measures receptive and expressive language
Receptive/Expressive Language (Treatment)	**Definition:** Applying techniques tot improve and augment receptive/expressive language
Reflex Integrity	**Definition:** Measures the presence, absence, or exaggeration of developmentally appropriate, pathologic or normal reflexes
Select Picture Audiometry	**Definition:** Establishes hearing threshold levels for speech using pictures
Sensorineural Acuity Level	**Definition:** Measures sensorineural acuity masking presented via bone conduction
Sensory Aids	**Definition:** Determines the appropriateness of a sensory prosthetic device, other than a hearing aid or assistive listening system/device
Sensory Awareness/ Processing/Integrity	**Includes/Examples:** Includes light touch, pressure, temperature, pain, sharp/dull, proprioception, vestibular, visual, auditory, gustatory, and olfactory
Short Increment Sensitivity Index	**Definition:** Measures the ear's ability to detect small intensity changes; site of lesion test requiring a behavioral response
Sinusoidal Vertical Axis Rotational	**Definition:** Measures nystagmus following rotation
Somatosensory Evoked Potentials	**Definition:** Measures neural activity from sites throughout the body

APPENDIX A

SECTION F - PHYSICAL REHABILITATION AND DIAGNOSTIC AUDIOLOGY
CHARACTER 5 - TYPE QUALIFIER

Speech and/or Language Screening	**Definition:** Identifies need for further speech and/or language evaluation
Speech Threshold	**Definition:** Measures minimal intensity needed to repeat spondaic words
Speech-Language Pathology and Related Disorders Counseling	**Definition:** Provides patients/families with information, support, referrals to facilitate recovery from a communication disorder
Speech-Language Pathology and Related Disorders Prevention	**Definition:** Applying techniques to avoid or minimize onset and/or development of a communication disorder
Speech/Word Recognition	**Definition:** Measures ability to repeat/identify single syllable words; scores given as a percentage; includes word recognition/speech discrimination
Staggered Spondaic Word	**Definition:** Measures central auditory processing site of lesion based upon dichotic presentation of spondaic words
Static Orthosis	**Includes/Examples:** Includes customized and prefabricated splints, inhibitory casts, spinal and other braces, and protective devices; has no moving parts, maintains joint(s) in desired position
Stenger	**Definition:** Measures unilateral nonorganic hearing loss based on simultaneous presentation of signals of differing volume
Swallowing Dysfunction	**Definition:** Activities to improve swallowing function in coordination with respiratory function **Includes/Examples:** Includes function and coordination of sucking, mastication, coughing, swallowing
Synthetic Sentence Identification	**Definition:** Measures central auditory dysfunction using identification of third order approximations of sentences and competing messages
Temporal Ordering of Stimuli	**Definition:** Measures specific central auditory process

Therapeutic Exercise	**Definition:** Exercise or activities to facilitate sensory awareness, sensory processing, sensory integration, balance training, conditioning, reconditioning **Includes/Examples:** Includes developmental activities, breathing exercises, aerobic endurance activities, aquatic exercises, stretching and ventilatory muscle training
Tinnitus Masker (Assessment)	**Definition:** Determines candidacy for tinnitus masker
Tinnitus Masker (Treatment)	**Explanation:** Used to verify physical fit, acoustic appropriateness, and benefit; assists in achieving maximum benefit
Tone Decay	**Definition:** Measures decrease in hearing sensitivity to a tone; site of lesion test requiring a behavioral response
Transfer	**Definition:** Transitional movement from one surface to another
Transfer Training	**Definition:** Exercise or activities to facilitate movement from one surface to another
Tympanometry	**Definition:** Measures the integrity of the middle ear; measures ease at which sound flows through the tympanic membrane while air pressure against the membrane is varied
Unithermal Binaural Screen	**Definition:** Measures the rhythmic eye movements stimulated by changing the temperature of the vestibular system in both ears using warm water, screening format
Ventilation, Respiration and Circulation	**Definition:** Measures ventilatory muscle strength, power and endurance, pulmonary function and ventilatory mechanics **Includes/Examples:** Includes ability to clear airway, activities that aggravate or relieve edema, pain, dyspnea or other symptoms, chest wall mobility, cardiopulmonary response to performance of ADL and IAD, cough and sputum, standard vital signs

SECTION F - PHYSICAL REHABILITATION AND DIAGNOSTIC AUDIOLOGY
CHARACTER 5 - TYPE QUALIFIER

Vestibular	**Definition:** Applying techniques to compensate for balance disorders; includes habituation, exercise therapy, and balance retraining
Visual Motor Integration (Assessment)	**Definition:** Coordinating the interaction of information from the eyes with body movement during activity
Visual Motor Integration (Treatment)	**Definition:** Exercise or activities to facilitate coordinating the interaction of information from eyes with body movement during activity
Visual Reinforcement Audiometry	**Definition:** Behavioral measures using nonspeech and speech stimuli to obtain frequency/ear-specific information on auditory status **Includes/Examples:** Includes a conditioned response of looking toward a visual reinforcer (e.g., lights, animated toy) every time auditory stimuli are heard
Vocational Activities and Functional Community or Work Reintegration Skills (Assessment)	**Definition:** Measures environmental, home, work (job/school/play) barriers that keep patients from functioning optimally in their environment **Includes/Examples:** Includes assessment of vocational skill and interests, environment of work (job/school/play), injury potential and injury prevention or reduction, ergonomic stressors, transportation skills, and ability to access and use community resources
Vocational Activities and Functional Community or Work Reintegration Skills (Treatment)	**Definition:** Activities to facilitate vocational exploration, body mechanics training, job acquisition, and environmental or work (job/school/play) task adaptation **Includes/Examples:** Includes injury prevention and reduction, ergonomic stressor reduction, job coaching and simulation, work hardening and conditioning, driving training, transportation skills, and use of community resources
Voice (Assessment)	**Definition:** Measures vocal structure, function and production
Voice (Treatment)	**Definition:** Applying techniques to improve voice and vocal function
Voice Prosthetic (Assessment)	**Definition:** Determines the appropriateness of voice prosthetic/adaptive device to enhance or facilitate communication
Voice Prosthetic (Treatment)	**Includes/Examples:** Includes electrolarynx, and other assistive, adaptive, supportive devices
Wheelchair Mobility (Assessment)	**Definition:** Measures fit and functional abilities within wheelchair in a variety of environments
Wheelchair Mobility (Treatment)	**Definition:** Management, maintenance and controlled operation of a wheelchair, scooter or other device, in and on a variety of surfaces and environments
Wound Management	**Includes/Examples:** Includes non-selective and selective debridement (enzymes, autolysis, sharp debridement), dressings (wound coverings, hydrogel, vacuum-assisted closure), topical agents, etc.

APPENDIX A

SECTION G - MENTAL HEALTH
CHARACTER 3 - TYPE

Biofeedback	**Definition:** Provision of information from the monitoring and regulating of physiological processes in conjunction with cognitive-behavioral techniques to improve patient functioning or well-being **Includes/Examples:** Includes EEG, blood pressure, skin temperature or peripheral blood flow, ECG, electrooculogram, EMG, respirometry or capnometry, GSR/EDR, perineometry to monitor/regulate bowel/bladder activity, electrogastrogram to monitor/regulate gastric motility
Counseling	**Definition:** The application of psychological methods to treat an individual with normal developmental issues and psychological problems in order to increase function, improve well-being, alleviate distress, maladjustment or resolve crises
Crisis Intervention	**Definition:** Treatment of a traumatized, acutely disturbed or distressed individual for the purpose of short-term stabilization **Includes/Examples:** Includes defusing, debriefing, counseling, psychotherapy and/or coordination of care with other providers or agencies
Electroconvulsive Therapy	**Definition:** The application of controlled electrical voltages to treat a mental health disorder **Includes/Examples:** Includes appropriate sedation and other preparation of the individual
Family Psychotherapy	**Definition:** Treatment that includes one or more family members of an individual with a mental health disorder by behavioral, cognitive, psychoanalytic, psychodynamic or psychophysiological means to improve functioning or well-being **Explanation:** Remediation of emotional or behavioral problems presented by one or more family members in cases where psychotherapy with more than one family member is indicated

Group Psychotherapy	**Definition:** Treatment of two or more individuals with a mental health disorder by behavioral, cognitive, psychoanalytic, psychodynamic or psychophysiological means to improve functioning or well-being
Hypnosis	**Definition:** Induction of a state of heightened suggestibility by auditory, visual and tactile techniques to elicit an emotional or behavioral response
Individual Psychotherapy	**Definition:** Treatment of an individual with a mental health disorder by behavioral, cognitive, psychoanalytic, psychodynamic or psychophysiological means to improve functioning or well-being
Light Therapy	**Definition:** Application of specialized light treatments to improve functioning or well-being
Medication Management	**Definition:** Monitoring and adjusting the use of medications for the treatment of a mental health disorder
Narcosynthesis	**Definition:** Administration of intravenous barbiturates in order to release suppressed or repressed thoughts
Psychological Tests	**Definition:** The administration and interpretation of standardized psychological tests and measurement instruments for the assessment of psychological function

SECTION G - MENTAL HEALTH
CHARACTER 4 - QUALIFIER

Behavioral	**Definition:** Primarily to modify behavior **Includes/Examples:** Includes modeling and role playing, positive reinforcement of target behaviors, response cost, and training of self-management skills
Cognitive	**Definition:** Primarily to correct cognitive distortions and errors
Cognitive-Behavioral	**Definition:** Combining cognitive and behavioral treatment strategies to improve functioning **Explanation:** Maladaptive responses are examined to determine how cognitions relate to behavior patterns in response to an event. Uses learning principles and information-processing models
Developmental	**Definition:** Age-normed developmental status of cognitive, social and adaptive behavior skills
Intellectual and Psychoeducational	**Definition:** Intellectual abilities, academic achievement and learning capabilities (including behaviors and emotional factors affecting learning)
Interactive	**Definition:** Uses primarily physical aids and other forms of non-oral interaction with a patient who is physically, psychologically or developmentally unable to use ordinary language for communication **Includes/Examples:** Includes the use of toys in symbolic play
Interpersonal	**Definition:** Helps an individual make changes in interpersonal behaviors to reduce psychological dysfunction **Includes/Examples:** Includes exploratory techniques, encouragement of affective expression, clarification of patient statements, analysis of communication patterns, use of therapy relationship and behavior change techniques
Neurobehavioral and Cognitive Status	**Definition:** Includes neurobehavioral status exam, interview(s), and observation for the clinical assessment of thinking, reasoning and judgment, acquired knowledge, attention, memory, visual spatial abilities, language functions, and planning

Neuropsychological	**Definition:** Thinking, reasoning and judgment, acquired knowledge, attention, memory, visual spatial abilities, language functions, planning
Personality and Behavioral	**Definition:** Mood, emotion, behavior, social functioning, psychopathological conditions, personality traits and characteristics
Psychoanalysis	**Definition:** Methods of obtaining a detailed account of past and present mental and emotional experiences to determine the source and eliminate or diminish the undesirable effects of unconscious conflicts **Explanation:** Accomplished by making the individual aware of their existence, origin, and inappropriate expression in emotions and behavior
Psychodynamic	**Definition:** Exploration of past and present emotional experiences to understand motives and drives using insight-oriented techniques to reduce the undesirable effects of internal conflicts on emotions and behavior **Explanation:** Techniques include empathetic listening, clarifying self-defeating behavior patterns, and exploring adaptive alternatives
Psychophysiological	**Definition:** Monitoring and alteration of physiological processes to help the individual associate physiological reactions combined with cognitive and behavioral strategies to gain improved control of these processes to help the individual cope more effectively
Supportive	**Definition:** Formation of therapeutic relationship primarily for providing emotional support to prevent further deterioration in functioning during periods of particular stress **Explanation:** Often used in conjunction with other therapeutic approaches
Vocational	**Definition:** Exploration of vocational interests, aptitudes and required adaptive behavior skills to develop and carry out a plan for achieving a successful vocational placement **Includes/Examples:** Includes enhancing work related adjustment and/or pursuing viable options in training education or preparation

SECTION H - SUBSTANCE ABUSE TREATMENT
CHARACTER 3 - TYPE

Detoxification Services	**Definition:** Detoxification from alcohol and/or drugs **Explanation:** Not a treatment modality, but helps the patient stabilize physically and psychologically until the body becomes free of drugs and the effects of alcohol
Family Counseling	**Definition:** The application of psychological methods that includes one or more family members to treat an individual with addictive behavior **Explanation:** Provides support and education for family members of addicted individuals. Family member participation is seen as a critical area of substance abuse treatment
Group Counseling	**Definition:** The application of psychological methods to treat two or more individuals with addictive behavior **Explanation:** Provides structured group counseling sessions and healing power through the connection with others

Individual Counseling	**Definition:** The application of psychological methods to treat an individual with addictive behavior **Explanation:** Comprised of several different techniques, which apply various strategies to address drug addiction
Individual Psychotherapy	**Definition:** Treatment of an individual with addictive behavior by behavioral, cognitive, psychoanalytic, psychodynamic or psychophysiological means
Medication Management	**Definition:** Monitoring and adjusting the use of replacement medications for the treatment of addiction
Pharmacotherapy	**Definition:** The use of replacement medications for the treatment of addiction

SECTION X - NEW TECHNOLOGY
CHARACTER 3 - OPERATION

Assistance	**Definition:** Taking over a portion of a physiological function by extracorporeal means
Destruction	**Definition:** Physical eradication of all or a portion of a body part by the direct use of energy, force, or a destructive agent **Explanation:** None of the body part is physically taken out **Includes/Examples:** Fulguration of rectal polyp, cautery of skin lesion
Extirpation	**Definition:** Taking or cutting out solid matter from a body part **Explanation:** The solid matter may be an abnormal byproduct of a biological function or foreign body; it may be imbedded in a body part or in the lumen of a tubular body part. The solid matter may or may not have been previously broken into pieces. **Includes/Examples:** Thrombectomy, choledocholithotomy
Fusion	**Definition:** Joining together portions of an articular body part rendering the articular body part immobile **Explanation:** The body part is joined together by fixation device, bone graft, or other means **Includes/Examples:** Spinal fusion, ankle arthrodesis

Introduction	**Definition:** Putting in or on a therapeutic, diagnostic, nutritional, physiological, or prophylactic substance except blood or blood products
Monitoring	**Definition:** Determining the level of a physiological or physical function repetitively over a period of time
Replacement	**Definition:** Putting in or on biological or synthetic material that physically takes the place and/or function of all or a portion of a body part **Explanation:** The body part may have been taken out or replaced, or may be taken out, physically eradicated, or rendered nonfunctional during the Replacement procedure. A Removal procedure is coded for taking out the device used in a previous replacement procedure **Includes/Examples:** Total hip replacement, bone graft, free skin graft
Reposition	**Definition:** Moving to its normal location, or other suitable location, all or a portion of a body part **Explanation:** The body part is moved to a new location from an abnormal location, or from a normal location where it is not functioning correctly. The body part may or may not be cut out or off to be moved to the new location **Includes/Examples:** Reposition of undescended testicle, fracture reduction

SECTION X - NEW TECHNOLOGY
CHARACTER 5 - APPROACH

External	**Definition:** Procedures performed directly on the skin or mucous membrane and procedures performed indirectly by the application of external force through the skin or mucous membrane
Open	**Definition:** Cutting through the skin or mucous membrane and any other body layers necessary to expose the site of the procedure
Percutaneous	**Definition:** Entry, by puncture or minor incision, of instrumentation through the skin or mucous membrane and any other body layers necessary to reach the site of the procedure

Percutaneous Endoscopic	**Definition:** Entry, by puncture or minor incision, of instrumentation through the skin or mucous membrane and any other body layers necessary to reach and visualize the site of the procedure
Via Natural or Artificial Opening Endoscopic	**Definition:** Entry of instrumentation through a natural or artificial external opening to reach and visualize the site of the procedure

SECTION X - NEW TECHNOLOGY
CHARACTER 6 - DEVICE / SUBSTANCE / TECHNOLOGY

Andexanet Alfa, Factor Xa Inhibitor Reversal Agent	Factor Xa Inhibitor Reversal Agent, Andexanet Alfa
Bezlotoxumab Monoclonal Antibody	ZINPLAVA™
Concentrated Bone Marrow Aspirate	CBMA (Concentrated Bone Marrow Aspirate)
Cytarabine and Daunorubicin Liposome Antineoplastic	VYXEOS™
Defibrotide Sodium Anticoagulant	Defitelio
Endothelial Damage Inhibitor	DuraGraft® Endothelial Damage Inhibitor
Engineered Autologous Chimeric Antigen Receptor T-cell Immunotherapy	Axicabtagene Ciloeucel KYMRIAH Tisagenlecleucel
Interbody Fusion Device, Nanotextured Surface in New Technology	nanoLOCK™ interbody fusion device

Interbody Fusion Device, Radiolucent Porous in New Technology	COALESCE® radiolucent interbody fusion device COHERE® radiolucent interbody fusion device
Magnetically Controlled Growth Rod(s) in New Technology	MAGEC® Spinal Bracing and Distraction System Spinal growth rods, magnetically controlled
Other New Technology Therapeutic Substance	STELARA® Ustekinumab
Synthetic Human Angiotensin II	Angiotensin II GIAPREZA™ Human angiotensin II, synthetic
Skin Substitute, Porcine Liver Derived in New Technology	MIRODERM™ Biologic Wound Matrix
Uridine Triacetate	Vistogard®
Zooplastic Tissue, Rapid Deployment Technique in New Technology	EDWARDS INTUITY Elite valve system INTUITY Elite valve system, EDWARDS Perceval sutureless valve Sutureless valve, Perceval

BODY PART KEY

Abdominal aortic plexus	**Use:** Abdominal Sympathetic Nerve
Abdominal esophagus	**Use:** Esophagus, Lower
Abductor hallucis muscle	**Use:** Foot Muscle, Right Foot Muscle, Left
Accessory cephalic vein	**Use:** Cephalic Vein, Right Cephalic Vein, Left
Accessory obturator nerve	**Use:** Lumbar Plexus
Accessory phrenic nerve	**Use:** Phrenic Nerve
Accessory spleen	**Use:** Spleen
Acetabulofemoral joint	**Use:** Hip Joint, Right Hip Joint, Left
Achilles tendon	**Use:** Lower Leg Tendon, Right Lower Leg Tendon, Left
Acromioclavicular ligament	**Use:** Shoulder Bursa and Ligament, Right Shoulder Bursa and Ligament, Left
Acromion (process)	**Use:** Scapula, Right Scapula, Left
Adductor brevis muscle	**Use:** Upper Leg Muscle, Right Upper Leg Muscle, Left
Adductor hallucis muscle	**Use:** Foot Muscle, Right Foot Muscle, Left
Adductor longus muscle Adductor magnus muscle	**Use:** Upper Leg Muscle, Right Upper Leg Muscle, Left
Adenohypophysis	**Use:** Pituitary Gland
Alar ligament of axis	**Use:** Head and Neck Bursa and Ligament
Alveolar process of mandible	**Use:** Mandible, Right Mandible, Left

Alveolar process of maxilla	**Use:** Maxilla
Anal orifice	**Use:** Anus
Anatomical snuffbox	**Use:** Lower Arm and Wrist Muscle, Right Lower Arm and Wrist Muscle, Left
Angular artery	**Use:** Face Artery
Angular vein	**Use:** Face Vein, Right Face Vein, Left
Annular ligament	**Use:** Elbow Bursa and Ligament, Right Elbow Bursa and Ligament, Left
Anorectal junction	**Use:** Rectum
Ansa cervicalis	**Use:** Cervical Plexus
Antebrachial fascia	**Use:** Subcutaneous Tissue and Fascia, Right Lower Arm Subcutaneous Tissue and Fascia, Left Lower Arm
Anterior (pectoral) lymph node	**Use:** Lymphatic, Right Axillary Lymphatic, Left Axillary
Anterior cerebral artery	**Use:** Intracranial Artery
Anterior cerebral vein	**Use:** Intracranial Vein
Anterior choroidal artery	**Use:** Intracranial Artery
Anterior circumflex humeral artery	**Use:** Axillary Artery, Right Axillary Artery, Left
Anterior communicating artery	**Use:** Intracranial Artery
Anterior cruciate ligament (ACL)	**Use:** Knee Bursa and Ligament, Right Knee Bursa and Ligament, Left
Anterior crural nerve	**Use:** Femoral Nerve

BODY PART KEY

Anterior facial vein	**Use:** Face Vein, Right Face Vein, Left
Anterior intercostal artery	**Use:** Internal Mammary Artery, Right Internal Mammary Artery, Left
Anterior interosseous nerve	**Use:** Median Nerve
Anterior lateral malleolar artery	**Use:** Anterior Tibial Artery, Right Anterior Tibial Artery, Left
Anterior lingual gland	**Use:** Minor Salivary Gland
Anterior medial malleolar artery	**Use:** Anterior Tibial Artery, Right Anterior Tibial Artery, Left
Anterior spinal artery	**Use:** Vertebral Artery, Right Vertebral Artery, Left
Anterior tibial recurrent artery	**Use:** Anterior Tibial Artery, Right Anterior Tibial Artery, Left
Anterior ulnar recurrent artery	**Use:** Ulnar Artery, Right Ulnar Artery, Left
Anterior vagal trunk	**Use:** Vagus Nerve
Anterior vertebral muscle	**Use:** Neck Muscle, Right Neck Muscle, Left
Antihelix Antitragus	**Use:** External Ear, Right External Ear, Left External Ear, Bilateral
Antrum of Highmore	**Use:** Maxillary Sinus, Right Maxillary Sinus, Left
Aortic annulus	**Use:** Aortic Valve
Aortic arch	**Use:** Thoracic Aorta, Ascending/Arch
Aortic intercostal artery	**Use:** Upper Artery
Apical (subclavicular) lymph node	**Use:** Lymphatic, Right Axillary Lymphatic, Left Axillary
Apneustic center	**Use:** Pons
Aqueduct of Sylvius	**Use:** Cerebral Ventricle
Aqueous humour	**Use:** Anterior Chamber, Right Anterior Chamber, Left
Arachnoid mater	**Use:** Cerebral Meninges Spinal Meninges
Arcuate artery	**Use:** Foot Artery, Right Foot Artery, Left
Areola	**Use:** Nipple, Right Nipple, Left
Arterial canal (duct)	**Use:** Pulmonary Artery, Left
Aryepiglottic fold Arytenoid cartilage	**Use:** Larynx
Arytenoid muscle	**Use:** Neck Muscle, Right Neck Muscle, Left
Ascending aorta	**Use:** Thoracic Aorta, Ascending/Arch
Ascending palatine artery	**Use:** Face Artery
Ascending pharyngeal artery	**Use:** External Carotid Artery, Right External Carotid Artery, Left
Atlantoaxial joint	**Use:** Cervical Vertebral Joint
Atrioventricular node	**Use:** Conduction Mechanism
Atrium dextrum cordis	**Use:** Atrium, Right
Atrium pulmonale	**Use:** Atrium, Left
Auditory tube	**Use:** Eustachian Tube, Right Eustachian Tube, Left
Auerbach's (myenteric) plexus	**Use:** Abdominal Sympathetic Nerve

BODY PART KEY

Auricle	**Use:** External Ear, Right External Ear, Left External Ear, Bilateral
Auricularis muscle	**Use:** Head Muscle
Axillary fascia	**Use:** Subcutaneous Tissue and Fascia, Right Upper Arm Subcutaneous Tissue and Fascia, Left Upper Arm
Axillary nerve	**Use:** Brachial Plexus
Bartholin's (greater vestibular) gland	**Use:** Vestibular Gland
Basal (internal) cerebral vein	**Use:** Intracranial Vein
Basal nuclei	**Use:** Basal Ganglia
Base of Tongue	**Use:** Pharynx
Basilar artery	**Use:** Intracranial Artery
Basis pontis	**Use:** Pons
Biceps brachii muscle	**Use:** Upper Arm Muscle, Right Upper Arm Muscle, Left
Biceps femoris muscle	**Use:** Upper Leg Muscle, Right Upper Leg Muscle, Left
Bicipital aponeurosis	**Use:** Subcutaneous Tissue and Fascia, Right Lower Arm Subcutaneous Tissue and Fascia, Left Lower Arm
Bicuspid valve	**Use:** Mitral Valve
Body of femur	**Use:** Femoral Shaft, Right Femoral Shaft, Left
Body of fibula	**Use:** Fibula, Right Fibula, Left
Bony labyrinth	**Use:** Inner Ear, Right Inner Ear, Left
Bony orbit	**Use:** Orbit, Right Orbit, Left
Bony vestibule	**Use:** Inner Ear, Right Inner Ear, Left
Botallo's duct	**Use:** Pulmonary Artery, Left
Brachial (lateral) lymph node	**Use:** Lymphatic, Right Axillary Lymphatic, Left Axillary
Brachialis muscle	**Use:** Upper Arm Muscle, Right Upper Arm Muscle, Left
Brachiocephalic artery Brachiocephalic trunk	**Use:** Innominate Artery
Brachiocephalic vein	**Use:** Innominate Vein, Right Innominate Vein, Left
Brachioradialis muscle	**Use:** Lower Arm and Wrist Muscle, Right Lower Arm and Wrist Muscle, Left
Broad ligament	**Use:** Uterine Supporting Structure
Bronchial artery	**Use:** Upper Artery
Bronchus Intermedius	**Use:** Main Bronchus, Right
Buccal gland	**Use:** Buccal Mucosa
Buccinator lymph node	**Use:** Lymphatic, Head
Buccinator muscle	**Use:** Facial Muscle
Bulbospongiosus muscle	**Use:** Perineum Muscle
Bulbourethral (Cowper's) gland	**Use:** Urethra
Bundle of His Bundle of Kent	**Use:** Conduction Mechanism
Calcaneocuboid joint	**Use:** Tarsal Joint, Right Tarsal Joint, Left
Calcaneocuboid ligament	**Use:** Foot Bursa and Ligament, Right Foot Bursa and Ligament, Left

BODY PART KEY

Calcaneofibular ligament	**Use:** Ankle Bursa and Ligament, Right Ankle Bursa and Ligament, Left
Calcaneus	**Use:** Tarsal, Right Tarsal, Left
Capitate bone	**Use:** Carpal, Right Carpal, Left
Cardia	**Use:** Esophagogastric Junction
Cardiac plexus	**Use:** Thoracic Sympathetic Nerve
Cardioesophageal junction	**Use:** Esophagogastric Junction
Caroticotympanic artery	**Use:** Internal Carotid Artery, Right Internal Carotid Artery, Left
Carotid glomus	**Use:** Carotid Body, Left Carotid Body, Right Carotid Bodies, Bilateral
Carotid sinus	**Use:** Internal Carotid Artery, Right Internal Carotid Artery, Left
Carotid sinus nerve	**Use:** Glossopharyngeal Nerve
Carpometacarpal ligament	**Use:** Hand Bursa and Ligament, Right Hand Bursa and Ligament, Left
Cauda equina	**Use:** Lumbar Spinal Cord
Cavernous plexus	**Use:** Head and Neck Sympathetic Nerve
Celiac (solar) plexus Celiac ganglion	**Use:** Abdominal Sympathetic Nerve
Celiac lymph node	**Use:** Lymphatic, Aortic
Celiac trunk	**Use:** Celiac Artery
Central axillary lymph node	**Use:** Lymphatic, Right Axillary Lymphatic, Left Axillary
Cerebral aqueduct (Sylvius)	**Use:** Cerebral Ventricle
Cerebrum	**Use:** Brain
Cervical esophagus	**Use:** Esophagus, Upper
Cervical facet joint	**Use:** Cervical Vertebral Joint Cervical Vertebral Joints, 2 or more
Cervical ganglion	**Use:** Head and Neck Sympathetic Nerve
Cervical interspinous ligament Cervical intertransverse ligament Cervical ligamentum flavum	**Use:** Head and Neck Bursa and Ligament
Cervical lymph node	**Use:** Lymphatic, Right Neck Lymphatic, Left Neck
Cervicothoracic facet joint	**Use:** Cervicothoracic Vertebral Joint
Choana	**Use:** Nasopharynx
Chondroglossus muscle	**Use:** Tongue, Palate, Pharynx Muscle
Chorda tympani	**Use:** Facial Nerve
Choroid plexus	**Use:** Cerebral Ventricle
Ciliary body	**Use:** Eye, Right Eye, Left
Ciliary ganglion	**Use:** Head and Neck Sympathetic Nerve
Circle of Willis	**Use:** Intracranial Artery
Circumflex iliac artery	**Use:** Femoral Artery, Right Femoral Artery, Left
Claustrum	**Use:** Basal Ganglia
Coccygeal body	**Use:** Coccygeal Glomus
Coccygeus muscle	**Use:** Trunk Muscle, Right Trunk Muscle, Left
Cochlea	**Use:** Inner Ear, Right Inner Ear, Left

BODY PART KEY

Cochlear nerve	**Use:** Acoustic Nerve
Columella	**Use:** Nasal Mucosa and Soft Tissue
Common digital vein	**Use:** Foot Vein, Right / Foot Vein, Left
Common facial vein	**Use:** Face Vein, Right / Face Vein, Left
Common fibular nerve	**Use:** Peroneal Nerve
Common hepatic artery	**Use:** Hepatic Artery
Common iliac (subaortic) lymph node	**Use:** Lymphatic, Pelvis
Common interosseous artery	**Use:** Ulnar Artery, Right / Ulnar Artery, Left
Common peroneal nerve	**Use:** Peroneal Nerve
Condyloid process	**Use:** Mandible, Right / Mandible, Left
Conus arteriosus	**Use:** Ventricle, Right
Conus medullaris	**Use:** Lumbar Spinal Cord
Coracoacromial ligament	**Use:** Shoulder Bursa and Ligament, Right / Shoulder Bursa and Ligament, Left
Coracobrachialis muscle	**Use:** Upper Arm Muscle, Right / Upper Arm Muscle, Left
Coracoclavicular ligament / Coracohumeral ligament	**Use:** Shoulder Bursa and Ligament, Right / Shoulder Bursa and Ligament, Left
Coracoid process	**Use:** Scapula, Right / Scapula, Left
Corniculate cartilage	**Use:** Larynx
Corpus callosum	**Use:** Brain
Corpus cavernosum / Corpus spongiosum	**Use:** Penis
Corpus striatum	**Use:** Basal Ganglia
Corrugator supercilii muscle	**Use:** Facial Muscle
Costocervical trunk	**Use:** Subclavian Artery, Right / Subclavian Artery, Left
Costoclavicular ligament	**Use:** Shoulder Bursa and Ligament, Right / Shoulder Bursa and Ligament, Left
Costotransverse joint	**Use:** Thoracic Vertebral Joint / Thoracic Vertebral Joints, 2 to 7 / Thoracic Vertebral Joints, 8 or more
Costotransverse ligament	**Use:** Sternum Bursa and Ligament / Rib(s) Bursa and Ligament
Costovertebral joint	**Use:** Thoracic Vertebral Joint / Thoracic Vertebral Joints, 2 to 7 / Thoracic Vertebral Joints, 8 or more
Costoxiphoid ligament	**Use:** Sternum Bursa and Ligament / Rib(s) Bursa and Ligament
Cowper's (bulbourethral) gland	**Use:** Urethra
Cremaster muscle	**Use:** Perineum Muscle
Cribriform plate	**Use:** Ethmoid Bone, Right / Ethmoid Bone, Left
Cricoid cartilage	**Use:** Trachea
Cricothyroid artery	**Use:** Thyroid Artery, Right / Thyroid Artery, Left
Cricothyroid muscle	**Use:** Neck Muscle, Right / Neck Muscle, Left

BODY PART KEY

Crural fascia	**Use:** Subcutaneous Tissue and Fascia, Right Upper Leg Subcutaneous Tissue and Fascia, Left Upper Leg
Cubital lymph node	**Use:** Lymphatic, Right Upper Extremity Lymphatic, Left Upper Extremity
Cubital nerve	**Use:** Ulnar Nerve
Cuboid bone	**Use:** Tarsal, Right Tarsal, Left
Cuboideonavicular joint	**Use:** Tarsal Joint, Right Tarsal Joint, Left
Culmen	**Use:** Cerebellum
Cuneiform cartilage	**Use:** Larynx
Cuneonavicular joint	**Use:** Tarsal Joint, Right Tarsal Joint, Left
Cuneonavicular ligament	**Use:** Foot Bursa and Ligament, Right Foot Bursa and Ligament, Left
Cutaneous (transverse) cervical nerve	**Use:** Cervical Plexus
Deep cervical fascia	**Use:** Subcutaneous Tissue and Fascia, Right Neck Subcutaneous Tissue and Fascia, Left Neck
Deep cervical vein	**Use:** Vertebral Vein, Right Vertebral Vein, Left
Deep circumflex iliac artery	**Use:** External Iliac Artery, Right External Iliac Artery, Left
Deep facial vein	**Use:** Face Vein, Right Face Vein, Left
Deep femoral (profunda femoris) vein	**Use:** Femoral Vein, Right Femoral Vein, Left
Deep femoral artery	**Use:** Femoral Artery, Right Femoral Artery, Left

Deep palmar arch	**Use:** Hand Artery, Right Hand Artery, Left
Deep transverse perineal muscle	**Use:** Perineum Muscle
Deferential artery	**Use:** Internal Iliac Artery, Right Internal Iliac Artery, Left
Deltoid fascia	**Use:** Subcutaneous Tissue and Fascia, Right Upper Arm Subcutaneous Tissue and Fascia, Left Upper Arm
Deltoid ligament	**Use:** Ankle Bursa and Ligament, Right Ankle Bursa and Ligament, Left
Deltoid muscle	**Use:** Shoulder Muscle, Right Shoulder Muscle, Left
Deltopectoral (infraclavicular) lymph node	**Use:** Lymphatic, Right Upper Extremity Lymphatic, Left Upper Extremity
Dens	**Use:** Cervical Vertebra
Denticulate (dentate) ligament	**Use:** Spinal Cord
Depressor anguli oris muscle Depressor labii inferioris muscle Depressor septi nasi muscle Depressor supercilii muscle	**Use:** Facial Muscle
Dermis	**Use:** Skin
Descending genicular artery	**Use:** Femoral Artery, Right Femoral Artery, Left
Diaphragma sellae	**Use:** Dura Mater
Distal humerus	**Use:** Humeral Shaft, Right Humeral Shaft, Left
Distal humerus, involving joint	**Use:** Elbow Joint, Right Elbow Joint, Left
Distal radioulnar joint	**Use:** Wrist Joint, Right Wrist Joint, Left
Dorsal digital nerve	**Use:** Radial Nerve

BODY PART KEY

Dorsal metacarpal vein	**Use:** Hand Vein, Right Hand Vein, Left
Dorsal metatarsal artery	**Use:** Foot Artery, Right Foot Artery, Left
Dorsal metatarsal vein	**Use:** Foot Vein, Right Foot Vein, Left
Dorsal scapular artery	**Use:** Subclavian Artery, Right Subclavian Artery, Left
Dorsal scapular nerve	**Use:** Brachial Plexus
Dorsal venous arch	**Use:** Foot Vein, Right Foot Vein, Left
Dorsalis pedis artery	**Use:** Anterior Tibial Artery, Right Anterior Tibial Artery, Left
Duct of Santorini	**Use:** Pancreatic Duct, Accessory
Duct of Wirsung	**Use:** Pancreatic Duct
Ductus deferens	**Use:** Vas Deferens, Right Vas Deferens, Left Vas Deferens, Bilateral Vas Deferens
Duodenal ampulla	**Use:** Ampulla of Vater
Duodenojejunal flexure	**Use:** Jejunum
Dura mater, intracranial	**Use:** Dura Mater
Dura mater, spinal	**Use:** Spinal Meninges
Dural venous sinus	**Use:** Intracranial Vein
Earlobe	**Use:** External Ear, Right External Ear, Left External Ear, Bilateral
Eighth cranial nerve	**Use:** Acoustic Nerve

Ejaculatory duct	**Use:** Vas Deferens, Right Vas Deferens, Left Vas Deferens, Bilateral Vas Deferens
Eleventh cranial nerve	**Use:** Accessory Nerve
Encephalon	**Use:** Brain
Ependyma	**Use:** Cerebral Ventricle
Epidermis	**Use:** Skin
Epidural space, spinal	**Use:** Spinal Canal
Epiploic foramen	**Use:** Peritoneum
Epithalamus	**Use:** Thalamus
Epitrochlear lymph node	**Use:** Lymphatic, Right Upper Extremity Lymphatic, Left Upper Extremity
Erector spinae muscle	**Use:** Trunk Muscle, Right Trunk Muscle, Left
Esophageal artery	**Use:** Upper Artery
Esophageal plexus	**Use:** Thoracic Sympathetic Nerve
Ethmoidal air cell	**Use:** Ethmoid Sinus, Right Ethmoid Sinus, Left
Extensor carpi radialis muscle Extensor carpi ulnaris muscle	**Use:** Lower Arm and Wrist Muscle, Right Lower Arm and Wrist Muscle, Left
Extensor digitorum brevis muscle	**Use:** Foot Muscle, Right Foot Muscle, Left
Extensor digitorum longus muscle	**Use:** Lower Leg Muscle, Right Lower Leg Muscle, Left
Extensor hallucis brevis muscle	**Use:** Foot Muscle, Right Foot Muscle, Left

BODY PART KEY

Extensor hallucis longus muscle	**Use:** Lower Leg Muscle, Right Lower Leg Muscle, Left
External anal sphincter	**Use:** Anal Sphincter
External auditory meatus	**Use:** External Auditory Canal, Right External Auditory Canal, Left
External maxillary artery	**Use:** Face Artery
External naris	**Use:** Nasal Mucosa and Soft Tissue
External oblique aponeurosis	**Use:** Subcutaneous Tissue and Fascia, Trunk
External oblique muscle	**Use:** Abdomen Muscle, Right Abdomen Muscle, Left
External popliteal nerve	**Use:** Peroneal Nerve
External pudendal artery	**Use:** Femoral Artery, Right Femoral Artery, Left
External pudendal vein	**Use:** Saphenous Vein, Right Saphenous Vein, Left
External urethral sphincter	**Use:** Urethra
Extradural space, intracranial	**Use:** Epidural Space, Intracranial
Extradural space, spinal	**Use:** Spinal Canal
Facial artery	**Use:** Face Artery
False vocal cord	**Use:** Larynx
Falx cerebri	**Use:** Dura Mater
Fascia lata	**Use:** Subcutaneous Tissue and Fascia, Right Upper Leg Subcutaneous Tissue and Fascia, Left Upper Leg
Femoral head	**Use:** Upper Femur, Right Upper Femur, Left

Femoral lymph node	**Use:** Lymphatic, Right Lower Extremity Lymphatic, Left Lower Extremity
Femoropatellar joint Femorotibial joint	**Use:** Knee Joint, Right Knee Joint, Left
Fibular artery	**Use:** Peroneal Artery, Right Peroneal Artery, Left
Fibularis brevis muscle Fibularis longus muscle	**Use:** Lower Leg Muscle, Right Lower Leg Muscle, Left
Fifth cranial nerve	**Use:** Trigeminal Nerve
Filum terminale	**Use:** Spinal Meninges
First cranial nerve	**Use:** Olfactory Nerve
First intercostal nerve	**Use:** Brachial Plexus
Flexor carpi radialis muscle Flexor carpi ulnaris muscle	**Use:** Lower Arm and Wrist Muscle, Right Lower Arm and Wrist Muscle, Left
Flexor digitorum brevis muscle	**Use:** Foot Muscle, Right Foot Muscle, Left
Flexor digitorum longus muscle	**Use:** Lower Leg Muscle, Right Lower Leg Muscle, Left
Flexor hallucis brevis muscle	**Use:** Foot Muscle, Right Foot Muscle, Left
Flexor hallucis longus muscle	**Use:** Lower Leg Muscle, Right Lower Leg Muscle, Left
Flexor pollicis longus muscle	**Use:** Lower Arm and Wrist Muscle, Right Lower Arm and Wrist Muscle, Left
Foramen magnum	**Use:** Occipital Bone
Foramen of Monro (intraventricular)	**Use:** Cerebral Ventricle
Foreskin	**Use:** Prepuce
Fossa of Rosenmuller	**Use:** Nasopharynx

BODY PART KEY

Fourth cranial nerve	**Use:** Trochlear Nerve	Gemellus muscle	**Use:** Hip Muscle, Right Hip Muscle, Left
Fourth ventricle	**Use:** Cerebral Ventricle	Geniculate ganglion	**Use:** Facial Nerve
Fovea	**Use:** Retina, Right Retina, Left	Geniculate nucleus	**Use:** Thalamus
Frenulum labii inferioris	**Use:** Lower Lip	Genioglossus muscle	**Use:** Tongue, Palate, Pharynx Muscle
Frenulum labii superioris	**Use:** Upper Lip	Genitofemoral nerve	**Use:** Lumbar Plexus
Frenulum linguae	**Use:** Tongue	Glans penis	**Use:** Prepuce
Frontal lobe	**Use:** Cerebral Hemisphere	Glenohumeral joint	**Use:** Shoulder Joint, Right Shoulder Joint, Left
Frontal vein	**Use:** Face Vein, Right Face Vein, Left	Glenohumeral ligament	**Use:** Shoulder Bursa and Ligament, Right Shoulder Bursa and Ligament, Left
Fundus uteri	**Use:** Uterus	Glenoid fossa (of scapula)	**Use:** Glenoid Cavity, Right Glenoid Cavity, Left
Galea aponeurotica	**Use:** Subcutaneous Tissue and Fascia, Scalp	Glenoid ligament (labrum)	**Use:** Shoulder Bursa and Ligament, Right Shoulder Bursa and Ligament, Left
Ganglion impar (ganglion of Walther)	**Use:** Sacral Sympathetic Nerve	Globus pallidus	**Use:** Basal Ganglia
Gasserian ganglion	**Use:** Trigeminal Nerve	Glossoepiglottic fold	**Use:** Epiglottis
Gastric lymph node	**Use:** Lymphatic, Aortic	Glottis	**Use:** Larynx
Gastric plexus	**Use:** Abdominal Sympathetic Nerve	Gluteal lymph node	**Use:** Lymphatic, Pelvis
Gastrocnemius muscle	**Use:** Lower Leg Muscle, Right Lower Leg Muscle, Left	Gluteal vein	**Use:** Hypogastric Vein, Right Hypogastric Vein, Left
Gastrocolic ligament Gastrocolic omentum	**Use:** Omentum	Gluteus maximus muscle Gluteus medius muscle Gluteus minimus muscle	**Use:** Hip Muscle, Right Hip Muscle, Left
Gastroduodenal artery	**Use:** Hepatic Artery	Gracilis muscle	**Use:** Upper Leg Muscle, Right Upper Leg Muscle, Left
Gastroesophageal (GE) junction	**Use:** Esophagogastric Junction		
Gastrohepatic omentum Gastrophrenic ligament Gastrosplenic ligament	**Use:** Omentum		

BODY PART KEY

Great auricular nerve	**Use:** Cervical Plexus
Great cerebral vein	**Use:** Intracranial Vein
Greater saphenous vein	**Use:** Saphenous Vein, Right Saphenous Vein, Left
Greater alar cartilage	**Use:** Nasal Mucosa and Soft Tissue
Greater occipital nerve	**Use:** Cervical Nerve
Greater Omentum	**Use:** Omentum
Greater splanchnic nerve	**Use:** Thoracic Sympathetic Nerve
Greater superficial petrosal nerve	**Use:** Facial Nerve
Greater trochanter	**Use:** Upper Femur, Right Upper Femur, Left
Greater tuberosity	**Use:** Humeral Head, Right Humeral Head, Left
Greater vestibular (Bartholin's) gland	**Use:** Vestibular Gland
Greater wing	**Use:** Sphenoid Bone
Hallux	**Use:** 1st Toe, Right 1st Toe, Left
Hamate bone	**Use:** Carpal, Right Carpal, Left
Head of fibula	**Use:** Fibula, Right Fibula, Left
Helix	**Use:** External Ear, Right External Ear, Left External Ear, Bilateral
Hepatic artery proper	**Use:** Hepatic Artery
Hepatic flexure	**Use:** Transverse Colon
Hepatic lymph node	**Use:** Lymphatic, Aortic
Hepatic plexus	**Use:** Abdominal Sympathetic Nerve
Hepatic portal vein	**Use:** Portal Vein
Hepatogastric ligament	**Use:** Omentum
Hepatopancreatic ampulla	**Use:** Ampulla of Vater
Humeroradial joint Humeroulnar joint	**Use:** Elbow Joint, Right Elbow Joint, Left
Humerus, distal	**Use:** Humeral Shaft, Right Humeral Shaft, Left
Hyoglossus muscle	**Use:** Tongue, Palate, Pharynx Muscle
Hyoid artery	**Use:** Thyroid Artery, Right Thyroid Artery, Left
Hypogastric artery	**Use:** Internal Iliac Artery, Right Internal Iliac Artery, Left
Hypopharynx	**Use:** Pharynx
Hypophysis	**Use:** Pituitary Gland
Hypothenar muscle	**Use:** Hand Muscle, Right Hand Muscle, Left
Ileal artery Ileocolic artery	**Use:** Superior Mesenteric Artery
Ileocolic vein	**Use:** Colic Vein
Iliac crest	**Use:** Pelvic Bone, Right Pelvic Bone, Left

Iliac fascia	**Use:**
	Subcutaneous Tissue and Fascia,
	   Right Upper Leg
	Subcutaneous Tissue and Fascia,
	   Left Upper Leg

BODY PART KEY

Iliac lymph node	**Use:** Lymphatic, Pelvis
Iliacus muscle	**Use:** Hip Muscle, Right Hip Muscle, Left
Iliofemoral ligament	**Use:** Hip Bursa and Ligament, Right Hip Bursa and Ligament, Left
Iliohypogastric nerve Ilioinguinal nerve	**Use:** Lumbar Plexus
Iliolumbar artery	**Use:** Internal Iliac Artery, Right Internal Iliac Artery, Left
Iliolumbar ligament	**Use:** Lower Spine Bursa and Ligament

Iliotibial tract (band)	**Use:**
	Subcutaneous Tissue and Fascia,
	    Right Upper Leg
	Subcutaneous Tissue and Fascia,
	    Left Upper Leg

Ilium	**Use:** Pelvic Bone, Right Pelvic Bone, Left
Incus	**Use:** Auditory Ossicle, Right Auditory Ossicle, Left
Inferior cardiac nerve	**Use:** Thoracic Sympathetic Nerve
Inferior cerebellar vein Inferior cerebral vein	**Use:** Intracranial Vein
Inferior epigastric artery	**Use:** External Iliac Artery, Right External Iliac Artery, Left
Inferior epigastric lymph node	**Use:** Lymphatic, Pelvis
Inferior genicular artery	**Use:** Popliteal Artery, Right Popliteal Artery, Left
Inferior gluteal artery	**Use:** Internal Iliac Artery, Right Internal Iliac Artery, Left
Inferior gluteal nerve	**Use:** Sacral Plexus

Inferior hypogastric plexus	**Use:** Abdominal Sympathetic Nerve
Inferior labial artery	**Use:** Face Artery
Inferior longitudinal muscle	**Use:** Tongue, Palate, Pharynx Muscle
Inferior mesenteric ganglion	**Use:** Abdominal Sympathetic Nerve
Inferior mesenteric lymph node	**Use:** Lymphatic, Mesenteric
Inferior mesenteric plexus	**Use:** Abdominal Sympathetic Nerve
Inferior oblique muscle	**Use:** Extraocular Muscle, Right Extraocular Muscle, Left
Inferior pancreaticoduodenal artery	**Use:** Superior Mesenteric Artery
Inferior phrenic artery	**Use:** Abdominal Aorta
Inferior rectus muscle	**Use:** Extraocular Muscle, Right Extraocular Muscle, Left
Inferior suprarenal artery	**Use:** Renal Artery, Right Renal Artery, Left
Inferior tarsal plate	**Use:** Lower Eyelid, Right Lower Eyelid, Left
Inferior thyroid vein	**Use:** Innominate Vein, Right Innominate Vein, Left
Inferior tibiofibular joint	**Use:** Ankle Joint, Right Ankle Joint, Left
Inferior turbinate	**Use:** Nasal Turbinate
Inferior ulnar collateral artery	**Use:** Brachial Artery, Right Brachial Artery, Left
Inferior vesical artery	**Use:** Internal Iliac Artery, Right Internal Iliac Artery, Left

BODY PART KEY

Infraauricular lymph node	**Use:** Lymphatic, Head
Infraclavicular (deltopectoral) lymph node	**Use:** Lymphatic, Right Upper Extremity Lymphatic, Left Upper Extremity
Infrahyoid muscle	**Use:** Neck Muscle, Right Neck Muscle, Left
Infraparotid lymph node	**Use:** Lymphatic, Head
Infraspinatus fascia	**Use:** Subcutaneous Tissue and Fascia, Right Upper Arm Subcutaneous Tissue and Fascia, Left Upper Arm
Infraspinatus muscle	**Use:** Shoulder Muscle, Right Shoulder Muscle, Left
Infundibulopelvic ligament	**Use:** Uterine Supporting Structure
Inguinal canal Inguinal triangle	**Use:** Inguinal Region, Right Inguinal Region, Left Inguinal Region, Bilateral
Interatrial septum	**Use:** Atrial Septum
Intercarpal joint	**Use:** Carpal Joint, Right Carpal Joint, Left
Intercarpal ligament	**Use:** Hand Bursa and Ligament, Right Hand Bursa and Ligament, Left
Interclavicular ligament	**Use:** Shoulder Bursa and Ligament, Right Shoulder Bursa and Ligament, Left
Intercostal lymph node	**Use:** Lymphatic, Thorax
Intercostal muscle	**Use:** Thorax Muscle, Right Thorax Muscle, Left
Intercostal nerve Intercostobrachial nerve	**Use:** Thoracic Nerve
Intercuneiform joint	**Use:** Tarsal Joint, Right Tarsal Joint, Left

Intercuneiform ligament	**Use:** Foot Bursa and Ligament, Right Foot Bursa and Ligament, Left
Intermediate bronchus	**Use:** Main Bronchus, Right
Intermediate cuneiform bone	**Use:** Tarsal, Right Tarsal, Left
Internal (basal) cerebral vein	**Use:** Intracranial Vein
Internal anal sphincter	**Use:** Anal Sphincter
Internal carotid artery, intracranial portion	**Use:** Intracranial Artery
Internal carotid plexus	**Use:** Head and Neck Sympathetic Nerve
Internal iliac vein	**Use:** Hypogastric Vein, Right Hypogastric Vein, Left
Internal maxillary artery	**Use:** External Carotid Artery, Right External Carotid Artery, Left
Internal naris	**Use:** Nasal Mucosa and Soft Tissue
Internal oblique muscle	**Use:** Abdomen Muscle, Right Abdomen Muscle, Left
Internal pudendal artery	**Use:** Internal Iliac Artery, Right Internal Iliac Artery, Left
Internal pudendal vein	**Use:** Hypogastric Vein, Right Hypogastric Vein, Left
Internal thoracic artery	**Use:** Internal Mammary Artery, Right Internal Mammary Artery, Left Subclavian Artery, Right Subclavian Artery, Left
Internal urethral sphincter	**Use:** Urethra
Interphalangeal (IP) joint	**Use:** Finger Phalangeal Joint, Right Finger Phalangeal Joint, Left Toe Phalangeal Joint, Right Toe Phalangeal Joint, Left

BODY PART KEY

Interphalangeal ligament	**Use:** Hand Bursa and Ligament, Right Hand Bursa and Ligament, Left Foot Bursa and Ligament, Right Foot Bursa and Ligament, Left
Interspinalis muscle	**Use:** Trunk Muscle, Right Trunk Muscle, Left
Interspinous ligament	**Use:** Head and Neck Bursa and Ligament Upper Spine Bursa and Ligament Lower Spine Bursa and Ligament
Intertransversarius muscle	**Use:** Trunk Muscle, Right Trunk Muscle, Left
Intertransverse ligament	**Use:** Upper Spine Bursa and Ligament Lower Spine Bursa and Ligament
Interventricular foramen (Monro)	**Use:** Cerebral Ventricle
Interventricular septum	**Use:** Ventricular Septum
Intestinal lymphatic trunk	**Use:** Cisterna Chyli
Ischiatic nerve	**Use:** Sciatic Nerve
Ischiocavernosus muscle	**Use:** Perineum Muscle
Ischiofemoral ligament	**Use:** Hip Bursa and Ligament, Right Hip Bursa and Ligament, Left
Ischium	**Use:** Pelvic Bone, Right Pelvic Bone, Left
Jejunal artery	**Use:** Superior Mesenteric Artery
Jugular body	**Use:** Glomus Jugulare
Jugular lymph node	**Use:** Lymphatic, Right Neck Lymphatic, Left Neck
Labia majora Labia minora	**Use:** Vulva
Labial gland	**Use:** Upper Lip Lower Lip

Lacrimal canaliculus Lacrimal punctum Lacrimal sac	**Use:** Lacrimal Duct, Right Lacrimal Duct, Left
Laryngopharynx	**Use:** Pharynx
Lateral (brachial) lymph node	**Use:** Lymphatic, Right Axillary Lymphatic, Left Axillary
Lateral canthus	**Use:** Upper Eyelid, Right Upper Eyelid, Left
Lateral collateral ligament (LCL)	**Use:** Knee Bursa and Ligament, Right Knee Bursa and Ligament, Left
Lateral condyle of femur	**Use:** Lower Femur, Right Lower Femur, Left
Lateral condyle of tibia	**Use:** Tibia, Right Tibia, Left
Lateral cuneiform bone	**Use:** Tarsal, Right Tarsal, Left
Lateral epicondyle of femur	**Use:** Lower Femur, Right Lower Femur, Left
Lateral epicondyle of humerus	**Use:** Humeral Shaft, Right Humeral Shaft, Left
Lateral femoral cutaneous nerve	**Use:** Lumbar Plexus
Lateral malleolus	**Use:** Fibula, Right Fibula, Left
Lateral meniscus	**Use:** Knee Joint, Right Knee Joint, Left
Lateral nasal cartilage	**Use:** Nasal Mucosa and Soft Tissue
Lateral plantar artery	**Use:** Foot Artery, Right Foot Artery, Left
Lateral plantar nerve	**Use:** Tibial Nerve
Lateral rectus muscle	**Use:** Extraocular Muscle, Right Extraocular Muscle, Left

BODY PART KEY

Lateral sacral artery	**Use:** Internal Iliac Artery, Right Internal Iliac Artery, Left
Lateral sacral vein	**Use:** Hypogastric Vein, Right Hypogastric Vein, Left
Lateral sural cutaneous nerve	**Use:** Peroneal Nerve
Lateral tarsal artery	**Use:** Foot Artery, Right Foot Artery, Left
Lateral temporomandibular ligament	**Use:** Head and Neck Bursa and Ligament
Lateral thoracic artery	**Use:** Axillary Artery, Right Axillary Artery, Left
Latissimus dorsi muscle	**Use:** Trunk Muscle, Right Trunk Muscle, Left
Least splanchnic nerve	**Use:** Thoracic Sympathetic Nerve
Left ascending lumbar vein	**Use:** Hemiazygos Vein
Left atrioventricular valve	**Use:** Mitral Valve
Left auricular appendix	**Use:** Atrium, Left
Left colic vein	**Use:** Colic Vein
Left coronary sulcus	**Use:** Heart, Left
Left gastric artery	**Use:** Gastric Artery
Left gastroepiploic artery	**Use:** Splenic Artery
Left gastroepiploic vein	**Use:** Splenic Vein
Left inferior phrenic vein	**Use:** Renal Vein, Left
Left inferior pulmonary vein	**Use:** Pulmonary Vein, Left
Left jugular trunk	**Use:** Thoracic Duct

Left lateral ventricle	**Use:** Cerebral Ventricle
Left ovarian vein Left second lumbar vein	**Use:** Renal Vein, Left
Left subclavian trunk	**Use:** Thoracic Duct
Left subcostal vein	**Use:** Hemiazygos Vein
Left superior pulmonary vein	**Use:** Pulmonary Vein, Left
Left suprarenal vein Left testicular vein	**Use:** Renal Vein, Left
Leptomeninges, intracranial	**Use:** Cerebral Meninges
Leptomeninges, spinal	**Use:** Spinal Meninges
Lesser alar cartilage	**Use:** Nasal Mucosa and Soft Tissue
Lesser occipital nerve	**Use:** Cervical Plexus
Lesser Omentum	**Use:** Omentum
Lesser saphenous vein	**Use:** Saphenous Vein, Right Saphenous Vein, Left
Lesser splanchnic nerve	**Use:** Thoracic Sympathetic Nerve
Lesser trochanter	**Use:** Upper Femur, Right Upper Femur, Left
Lesser tuberosity	**Use:** Humeral Head, Right Humeral Head, Left
Lesser wing	**Use:** Sphenoid Bone
Levator anguli oris muscle	**Use:** Facial Muscle
Levator ani muscle	**Use:** Perineum Muscle
Levator labii superioris alaeque nasi muscle Levator labii superioris muscle	**Use:** Facial Muscle

BODY PART KEY

Levator palpebrae superioris muscle	**Use:** Upper Eyelid, Right Upper Eyelid, Left
Levator scapulae muscle	**Use:** Neck Muscle, Right Neck Muscle, Left
Levator veli palatini muscle	**Use:** Tongue, Palate, Pharynx Muscle
Levatores costarum muscle	**Use:** Thorax Muscle, Right Thorax Muscle, Left
Ligament of head of fibula	**Use:** Knee Bursa and Ligament, Right Knee Bursa and Ligament, Left
Ligament of the lateral malleolus	**Use:** Ankle Bursa and Ligament, Right Ankle Bursa and Ligament, Left
Ligamentum flavum	**Use:** Upper Spine Bursa and Ligament Lower Spine Bursa and Ligament
Lingual artery	**Use:** External Carotid Artery, Right External Carotid Artery, Left
Lingual tonsil	**Use:** Pharynx
Locus ceruleus	**Use:** Pons
Long thoracic nerve	**Use:** Brachial Plexus
Lumbar artery	**Use:** Abdominal Aorta
Lumbar facet joint	**Use:** Lumbar Vertebral Joint Lumbar Vertebral Joints, 2 or more
Lumbar ganglion	**Use:** Lumbar Sympathetic Nerve
Lumbar lymph node	**Use:** Lymphatic, Aortic
Lumbar lymphatic trunk	**Use:** Cisterna Chyli
Lumbar splanchnic nerve	**Use:** Lumbar Sympathetic Nerve
Lumbosacral facet joint	**Use:** Lumbosacral Joint

Lumbosacral trunk	**Use:** Lumbar Nerve
Lunate bone	**Use:** Carpal, Right Carpal, Left
Lunotriquetral ligament	**Use:** Hand Bursa and Ligament, Right Hand Bursa and Ligament, Left
Macula	**Use:** Retina, Right Retina, Left
Malleus	**Use:** Auditory Ossicle, Right Auditory Ossicle, Left
Mammary duct Mammary gland	**Use:** Breast, Right Breast, Left Breast, Bilateral
Mammillary body	**Use:** Hypothalamus
Mandibular nerve	**Use:** Trigeminal Nerve
Mandibular notch	**Use:** Mandible, Right Mandible, Left
Manubrium	**Use:** Sternum
Masseter muscle	**Use:** Head Muscle
Masseteric fascia	**Use:** Subcutaneous Tissue and Fascia, Face
Mastoid (postauricular) lymph node	**Use:** Lymphatic, Right Neck Lymphatic, Left Neck
Mastoid air cells	**Use:** Mastoid Sinus, Right Mastoid Sinus, Left
Mastoid process	**Use:** Temporal Bone, Right Temporal Bone, Left
Maxillary artery	**Use:** External Carotid Artery, Right External Carotid Artery, Left
Maxillary nerve	**Use:** Trigeminal Nerve

BODY PART KEY

Medial canthus	**Use:** Lower Eyelid, Right Lower Eyelid, Left
Medial collateral ligament (MCL)	**Use:** Knee Bursa and Ligament, Right Knee Bursa and Ligament, Left
Medial condyle of femur	**Use:** Lower Femur, Right Lower Femur, Left
Medial condyle of tibia	**Use:** Tibia, Right Tibia, Left
Medial cuneiform bone	**Use:** Tarsal, Right Tarsal, Left
Medial epicondyle of femur	**Use:** Lower Femur, Right Lower Femur, Left
Medial epicondyle of humerus	**Use:** Humeral Shaft, Right Humeral Shaft, Left
Medial malleolus	**Use:** Tibia, Right Tibia, Left
Medial meniscus	**Use:** Knee Joint, Right Knee Joint, Left
Medial plantar artery	**Use:** Foot Artery, Right Foot Artery, Left
Medial plantar nerve Medial popliteal nerve	**Use:** Tibial Nerve
Medial rectus muscle	**Use:** Extraocular Muscle, Right Extraocular Muscle, Left
Medial sural cutaneous nerve	**Use:** Tibial Nerve
Median antebrachial vein Median cubital vein	**Use:** Basilic Vein, Right Basilic Vein, Left
Median sacral artery	**Use:** Abdominal Aorta
Mediastinal lymph node	**Use:** Lymphatic, Thorax
Meissner's (submucous) plexus	**Use:** Abdominal Sympathetic Nerve

Membranous urethra	**Use:** Urethra
Mental foramen	**Use:** Mandible, Right Mandible, Left
Mentalis muscle	**Use:** Facial Muscle
Mesoappendix Mesocolon	**Use:** Mesentery
Metacarpal ligament Metacarpophalangeal ligament	**Use:** Hand Bursa and Ligament, Right Hand Bursa and Ligament, Left
Metatarsal ligament	**Use:** Foot Bursa and Ligament, Right Foot Bursa and Ligament, Left
Metatarsophalangeal (MTP) joint	**Use:** Metatarsal-Phalangeal Joint, Right Metatarsal-Phalangeal Joint, Left
Metatarsophalangeal ligament	**Use:** Foot Bursa and Ligament, Right Foot Bursa and Ligament, Left
Metathalamus	**Use:** Thalamus
Midcarpal joint	**Use:** Carpal Joint, Right Carpal Joint, Left
Middle cardiac nerve	**Use:** Thoracic Sympathetic Nerve
Middle cerebral artery	**Use:** Intracranial Artery
Middle cerebral vein	**Use:** Intracranial Vein
Middle colic vein	**Use:** Colic Vein
Middle genicular artery	**Use:** Popliteal Artery, Right Popliteal Artery, Left
Middle hemorrhoidal vein	**Use:** Hypogastric Vein, Right Hypogastric Vein, Left
Middle rectal artery	**Use:** Internal Iliac Artery, Right Internal Iliac Artery, Left
Middle suprarenal artery	**Use:** Abdominal Aorta

BODY PART KEY

Middle temporal artery	**Use:** Temporal Artery, Right Temporal Artery, Left
Middle turbinate	**Use:** Nasal Turbinate
Mitral annulus	**Use:** Mitral Valve
Molar gland	**Use:** Buccal Mucosa
Musculocutaneous nerve	**Use:** Brachial Plexus
Musculophrenic artery	**Use:** Internal Mammary Artery, Right Internal Mammary Artery, Left
Musculospiral nerve	**Use:** Radial Nerve
Myelencephalon	**Use:** Medulla Oblongata
Myenteric (Auerbach's) plexus	**Use:** Abdominal Sympathetic Nerve
Myometrium	**Use:** Uterus
Nail bed Nail plate	**Use:** Finger Nail Toe Nail
Nasal cavity	**Use:** Nasal Mucosa and Soft Tissue
Nasal concha	**Use:** Nasal Turbinate
Nasalis muscle	**Use:** Facial Muscle
Nasolacrimal duct	**Use:** Lacrimal Duct, Right Lacrimal Duct, Left
Navicular bone	**Use:** Tarsal, Right Tarsal, Left
Neck of femur	**Use:** Upper Femur, Right Upper Femur, Left
Neck of humerus (anatomical) (surgical)	**Use:** Humeral Head, Right Humeral Head, Left
Nerve to the stapedius	**Use:** Facial Nerve

Neurohypophysis	**Use:** Pituitary Gland
Ninth cranial nerve	**Use:** Glossopharyngeal Nerve
Nostril	**Use:** Nasal Mucosa and Soft Tissue
Obturator artery	**Use:** Internal Iliac Artery, Right Internal Iliac Artery, Left
Obturator lymph node	**Use:** Lymphatic, Pelvis
Obturator muscle	**Use:** Hip Muscle, Right Hip Muscle, Left
Obturator nerve	**Use:** Lumbar Plexus
Obturator vein	**Use:** Hypogastric Vein, Right Hypogastric Vein, Left
Obtuse margin	**Use:** Heart, Left
Occipital artery	**Use:** External Carotid Artery, Right External Carotid Artery, Left
Occipital lobe	**Use:** Cerebral Hemisphere
Occipital lymph node	**Use:** Lymphatic, Right Neck Lymphatic, Left Neck
Occipitofrontalis muscle	**Use:** Facial Muscle
Odontoid process	**Use:** Cervical Vertebra
Olecranon bursa	**Use:** Elbow Bursa and Ligament, Right Elbow Bursa and Ligament, Left
Olecranon process	**Use:** Ulna, Right Ulna, Left
Olfactory bulb	**Use:** Olfactory Nerve
Ophthalmic artery	**Use:** Intracranial Artery
Ophthalmic nerve	**Use:** Trigeminal Nerve

BODY PART KEY

Ophthalmic vein	**Use:** Intracranial Vein
Optic chiasma	**Use:** Optic Nerve
Optic disc	**Use:** Retina, Right Retina, Left
Optic foramen	**Use:** Sphenoid Bone
Orbicularis oculi muscle	**Use:** Upper Eyelid, Right Upper Eyelid, Left
Orbicularis oris muscle	**Use:** Facial Muscle
Orbital fascia	**Use:** Subcutaneous Tissue and Fascia, Face
Orbital portion of ethmoid bone Orbital portion of frontal bone Orbital portion of lacrimal bone Orbital portion of maxilla Orbital portion of palatine bone Orbital portion of sphenoid bone Orbital portion of zygomatic bone	**Use:** Orbit, Right Orbit, Left
Oropharynx	**Use:** Pharynx
Otic ganglion	**Use:** Head and Neck Sympathetic Nerve
Oval window	**Use:** Middle Ear, Right Middle Ear, Left
Ovarian artery	**Use:** Abdominal Aorta
Ovarian ligament	**Use:** Uterine Supporting Structure
Oviduct	**Use:** Fallopian Tube, Right Fallopian Tube, Left
Palatine gland	**Use:** Buccal Mucosa
Palatine tonsil	**Use:** Tonsils
Palatine uvula	**Use:** Uvula
Palatoglossal muscle Palatopharyngeal muscle	**Use:** Tongue, Palate, Pharynx Muscle

Palmar (volar) digital vein Palmar (volar) metacarpal vein	**Use:** Hand Vein, Right Hand Vein, Left
Palmar cutaneous nerve	**Use:** Median Nerve Radial Nerve
Palmar fascia (aponeurosis)	**Use:** Subcutaneous Tissue and Fascia, Right Hand Subcutaneous Tissue and Fascia, Left Hand
Palmar interosseous muscle	**Use:** Hand Muscle, Right Hand Muscle, Left
Palmar ulnocarpal ligament	**Use:** Wrist Bursa and Ligament, Right Wrist Bursa and Ligament, Left
Palmaris longus muscle	**Use:** Lower Arm and Wrist Muscle, Right Lower Arm and Wrist Muscle, Left
Pancreatic artery	**Use:** Splenic Artery
Pancreatic plexus	**Use:** Abdominal Sympathetic Nerve
Pancreatic vein	**Use:** Splenic Vein
Pancreaticosplenic lymph node Paraaortic lymph node	**Use:** Lymphatic, Aortic
Pararectal lymph node	**Use:** Lymphatic, Mesenteric
Parasternal lymph node Paratracheal lymph node	**Use:** Lymphatic, Thorax
Paraurethral (Skene's) gland	**Use:** Vestibular Gland
Parietal lobe	**Use:** Cerebral Hemisphere
Parotid lymph node	**Use:** Lymphatic, Head
Parotid plexus	**Use:** Facial Nerve
Pars flaccida	**Use:** Tympanic Membrane, Right Tympanic Membrane, Left
Patellar ligament	**Use:** Knee Bursa and Ligament, Right Knee Bursa and Ligament, Left

BODY PART KEY

Patellar tendon	**Use:** Knee Tendon, Right Knee Tendon, Left
Pectineus muscle	**Use:** Upper Leg Muscle, Right Upper Leg Muscle, Left
Pectoral (anterior) lymph node	**Use:** Lymphatic, Right Axillary Lymphatic, Left Axillary
Pectoral fascia	**Use:** Subcutaneous Tissue and Fascia, Chest
Pectoralis major muscle Pectoralis minor muscle	**Use:** Thorax Muscle, Right Thorax Muscle, Left
Pelvic splanchnic nerve	**Use:** Abdominal Sympathetic Nerve Sacral Sympathetic Nerve
Penile urethra	**Use:** Urethra
Pericardiophrenic artery	**Use:** Internal Mammary Artery, Right Internal Mammary Artery, Left
Perimetrium	**Use:** Uterus
Peroneus brevis muscle Peroneus longus muscle	**Use:** Lower Leg Muscle, Right Lower Leg Muscle, Left
Petrous part of temporal bone	**Use:** Temporal Bone, Right Temporal Bone, Left
Pharyngeal constrictor muscle	**Use:** Tongue, Palate, Pharynx Muscle
Pharyngeal plexus	**Use:** Vagus Nerve
Pharyngeal recess	**Use:** Nasopharynx
Pharyngeal tonsil	**Use:** Adenoids
Pharyngotympanic tube	**Use:** Eustachian Tube, Right Eustachian Tube, Left
Pia mater, intracranial	**Use:** Cerebral Meninges
Pia mater, spinal	**Use:** Spinal Meninges

Pinna	**Use:** External Ear, Right External Ear, Left External Ear, Bilateral
Piriform recess (sinus)	**Use:** Pharynx
Piriformis muscle	**Use:** Hip Muscle, Right Hip Muscle, Left
Pisiform bone	**Use:** Carpal, Right Carpal, Left
Pisohamate ligament Pisometacarpal ligament	**Use:** Hand Bursa and Ligament, Right Hand Bursa and Ligament, Left
Plantar digital vein	**Use:** Foot Vein, Right Foot Vein, Left

Plantar fascia (aponeurosis)	**Use:**
	Subcutaneous Tissue and Fascia,
	  Right Foot
	Subcutaneous Tissue and Fascia,
	  Left Foot

Plantar metatarsal vein Plantar venous arch	**Use:** Foot Vein, Right Foot Vein, Left
Platysma muscle	**Use:** Neck Muscle, Right Neck Muscle, Left
Plica semilunaris	**Use:** Conjunctiva, Right Conjunctiva, Left
Pneumogastric nerve	**Use:** Vagus Nerve
Pneumotaxic center Pontine tegmentum	**Use:** Pons
Popliteal ligament	**Use:** Knee Bursa and Ligament, Right Knee Bursa and Ligament, Left
Popliteal lymph node	**Use:** Lymphatic, Right Lower Extremity Lymphatic, Left Lower Extremity
Popliteal vein	**Use:** Femoral Vein, Right Femoral Vein, Left
Popliteus muscle	**Use:** Lower Leg Muscle, Right Lower Leg Muscle, Left

BODY PART KEY

Postauricular (mastoid) lymph node	**Use:** Lymphatic, Right Neck Lymphatic, Left Neck
Postcava	**Use:** Inferior Vena Cava
Posterior (subscapular) lymph node	**Use:** Lymphatic, Right Axillary Lymphatic, Left Axillary
Posterior auricular artery	**Use:** External Carotid Artery, Right External Carotid Artery, Left
Posterior auricular nerve	**Use:** Facial Nerve
Posterior auricular vein	**Use:** External Jugular Vein, Right External Jugular Vein, Left
Posterior cerebral artery	**Use:** Intracranial Artery
Posterior chamber	**Use:** Eye, Right Eye, Left
Posterior circumflex humeral artery	**Use:** Axillary Artery, Right Axillary Artery, Left
Posterior communicating artery	**Use:** Intracranial Artery
Posterior cruciate ligament (PCL)	**Use:** Knee Bursa and Ligament, Right Knee Bursa and Ligament, Left
Posterior facial (retromandibular) vein	**Use:** Face Vein, Right Face Vein, Left
Posterior femoral cutaneous nerve	**Use:** Sacral Plexus
Posterior inferior cerebellar artery (PICA)	**Use:** Intracranial Artery
Posterior interosseous nerve	**Use:** Radial Nerve
Posterior labial nerve Posterior scrotal nerve	**Use:** Pudendal Nerve
Posterior spinal artery	**Use:** Vertebral Artery, Right Vertebral Artery, Left
Posterior tibial recurrent artery	**Use:** Anterior Tibial Artery, Right Anterior Tibial Artery, Left

Posterior ulnar recurrent artery	**Use:** Ulnar Artery, Right Ulnar Artery, Left
Posterior vagal trunk	**Use:** Vagus Nerve
Preauricular lymph node	**Use:** Lymphatic, Head
Precava	**Use:** Superior Vena Cava
Prepatellar bursa	**Use:** Knee Bursa and Ligament, Right Knee Bursa and Ligament, Left

Pretracheal fascia
Prevertebral fascia
	Use:
	Subcutaneous Tissue and Fascia,
	  Right Neck
	Subcutaneous Tissue and Fascia,
	  Left Neck

Princeps pollicis artery	**Use:** Hand Artery, Right Hand Artery, Left
Procerus muscle	**Use:** Facial Muscle
Profunda brachii	**Use:** Brachial Artery, Right Brachial Artery, Left
Profunda femoris (deep femoral) vein	**Use:** Femoral Vein, Right Femoral Vein, Left
Pronator quadratus muscle Pronator teres muscle	**Use:** Lower Arm and Wrist Muscle, Right Lower Arm and Wrist Muscle, Left
Prostatic urethra	**Use:** Urethra
Proximal radioulnar joint	**Use:** Elbow Joint, Right Elbow Joint, Left
Psoas muscle	**Use:** Hip Muscle, Right Hip Muscle, Left
Pterygoid muscle	**Use:** Head Muscle
Pterygoid process	**Use:** Sphenoid Bone
Pterygopalatine (sphenopalatine) ganglion	**Use:** Head and Neck Sympathetic Nerve

BODY PART KEY

Pubis	**Use:** Pelvic Bone, Right Pelvic Bone, Left
Pubofemoral ligament	**Use:** Hip Bursa and Ligament, Right Hip Bursa and Ligament, Left
Pudendal nerve	**Use:** Sacral Plexus
Pulmoaortic canal	**Use:** Pulmonary Artery, Left
Pulmonary annulus	**Use:** Pulmonary Valve
Pulmonary plexus	**Use:** Vagus Nerve Thoracic Sympathetic Nerve
Pulmonic valve	**Use:** Pulmonary Valve
Pulvinar	**Use:** Thalamus
Pyloric antrum Pyloric canal Pyloric sphincter	**Use:** Stomach, Pylorus
Pyramidalis muscle	**Use:** Abdomen Muscle, Right Abdomen Muscle, Left
Quadrangular cartilage	**Use:** Nasal Septum
Quadrate lobe	**Use:** Liver
Quadratus femoris muscle	**Use:** Hip Muscle, Right Hip Muscle, Left
Quadratus lumborum muscle	**Use:** Trunk Muscle, Right Trunk Muscle, Left
Quadratus plantae muscle	**Use:** Foot Muscle, Right Foot Muscle, Left
Quadriceps (femoris)	**Use:** Upper Leg Muscle, Right Upper Leg Muscle, Left
Radial collateral carpal ligament	**Use:** Wrist Bursa and Ligament, Right Wrist Bursa and Ligament, Left
Radial collateral ligament	**Use:** Elbow Bursa and Ligament, Right Elbow Bursa and Ligament, Left

Radial notch	**Use:** Ulna, Right Ulna, Left
Radial recurrent artery	**Use:** Radial Artery, Right Radial Artery, Left
Radial vein	**Use:** Brachial Vein, Right Brachial Vein, Left
Radialis indicis	**Use:** Hand Artery, Right Hand Artery, Left
Radiocarpal joint	**Use:** Wrist Joint, Right Wrist Joint, Left
Radiocarpal ligament Radioulnar ligament	**Use:** Wrist Bursa and Ligament, Right Wrist Bursa and Ligament, Left
Rectosigmoid junction	**Use:** Sigmoid Colon
Rectus abdominis muscle	**Use:** Abdomen Muscle, Right Abdomen Muscle, Left
Rectus femoris muscle	**Use:** Upper Leg Muscle, Right Upper Leg Muscle, Left
Recurrent laryngeal nerve	**Use:** Vagus Nerve
Renal calyx Renal capsule Renal cortex	**Use:** Kidney, Right Kidney, Left Kidneys, Bilateral Kidney
Renal plexus	**Use:** Abdominal Sympathetic Nerve
Renal segment	**Use:** Kidney, Right Kidney, Left Kidneys, Bilateral Kidney
Renal segmental artery	**Use:** Renal Artery, Right Renal Artery, Left
Retroperitoneal lymph node	**Use:** Lymphatic, Aortic
Retroperitoneal space	**Use:** Retroperitoneum

BODY PART KEY

Retropharyngeal lymph node	**Use:** Lymphatic, Right Neck Lymphatic, Left Neck
Retropubic space	**Use:** Pelvic Cavity
Rhinopharynx	**Use:** Nasopharynx
Rhomboid major muscle Rhomboid minor muscle	**Use:** Trunk Muscle, Right Trunk Muscle, Left
Right ascending lumbar vein	**Use:** Azygos Vein
Right atrioventricular valve	**Use:** Tricuspid Valve
Right auricular appendix	**Use:** Atrium, Right
Right colic vein	**Use:** Colic Vein
Right coronary sulcus	**Use:** Heart, Right
Right gastric artery	**Use:** Gastric Artery
Right gastroepiploic vein	**Use:** Superior Mesenteric Vein
Right inferior phrenic vein	**Use:** Inferior Vena Cava
Right inferior pulmonary vein	**Use:** Pulmonary Vein, Right
Right jugular trunk	**Use:** Lymphatic, Right Neck
Right lateral ventricle	**Use:** Cerebral Ventricle
Right lymphatic duct	**Use:** Lymphatic, Right Neck
Right ovarian vein Right second lumbar vein	**Use:** Inferior Vena Cava
Right subclavian trunk	**Use:** Lymphatic, Right Neck
Right subcostal vein	**Use:** Azygos Vein
Right superior pulmonary vein	**Use:** Pulmonary Vein, Right
Right suprarenal vein Right testicular vein	**Use:** Inferior Vena Cava

Rima glottidis	**Use:** Larynx
Risorius muscle	**Use:** Facial Muscle
Round ligament of uterus	**Use:** Uterine Supporting Structure
Round window	**Use:** Inner Ear, Right Inner Ear, Left
Sacral ganglion	**Use:** Sacral Sympathetic Nerve
Sacral lymph node	**Use:** Lymphatic, Pelvis
Sacral splanchnic nerve	**Use:** Sacral Sympathetic Nerve
Sacrococcygeal ligament	**Use:** Lower Spine Bursa and Ligament
Sacrococcygeal symphysis	**Use:** Sacrococcygeal Joint
Sacroiliac ligament Sacrospinous ligament Sacrotuberous ligament	**Use:** Lower Spine Bursa and Ligament
Salpingopharyngeus muscle	**Use:** Tongue, Palate, Pharynx Muscle
Salpinx	**Use:** Fallopian Tube, Right Fallopian Tube, Left
Saphenous nerve	**Use:** Femoral Nerve
Sartorius muscle	**Use:** Upper Leg Muscle, Right Upper Leg Muscle, Left
Scalene muscle	**Use:** Neck Muscle, Right Neck Muscle, Left
Scaphoid bone	**Use:** Carpal, Right Carpal, Left
Scapholunate ligament Scaphotrapezium ligament	**Use:** Hand Bursa and Ligament, Right Hand Bursa and Ligament, Left
Scarpa's (vestibular) ganglion	**Use:** Acoustic Nerve
Sebaceous gland	**Use:** Skin

BODY PART KEY

Second cranial nerve	**Use:** Optic Nerve
Sella turcica	**Use:** Sphenoid Bone
Semicircular canal	**Use:** Inner Ear, Right Inner Ear, Left
Semimembranosus muscle Semitendinosus muscle	**Use:** Upper Leg Muscle, Right Upper Leg Muscle, Left
Septal cartilage	**Use:** Nasal Septum
Serratus anterior muscle	**Use:** Thorax Muscle, Right Thorax Muscle, Left
Serratus posterior muscle	**Use:** Trunk Muscle, Right Trunk Muscle, Left
Seventh cranial nerve	**Use:** Facial Nerve
Short gastric artery	**Use:** Splenic Artery
Sigmoid artery	**Use:** Inferior Mesenteric Artery
Sigmoid flexure	**Use:** Sigmoid Colon
Sigmoid vein	**Use:** Inferior Mesenteric Vein
Sinoatrial node	**Use:** Conduction Mechanism
Sinus venosus	**Use:** Atrium, Right
Sixth cranial nerve	**Use:** Abducens Nerve
Skene's (paraurethral) gland	**Use:** Vestibular Gland
Small saphenous vein	**Use:** Saphenous Vein, Right Saphenous Vein, Left
Solar (celiac) plexus	**Use:** Abdominal Sympathetic Nerve
Soleus muscle	**Use:** Lower Leg Muscle, Right Lower Leg Muscle, Left

Sphenomandibular ligament	**Use:** Head and Neck Bursa and Ligament
Sphenopalatine (pterygopalatine) ganglion	**Use:** Head and Neck Sympathetic Nerve
Spinal nerve, cervical	**Use:** Cervical Nerve
Spinal nerve, lumbar	**Use:** Lumbar Nerve
Spinal nerve, sacral	**Use:** Sacral Nerve
Spinal nerve, thoracic	**Use:** Thoracic Nerve
Spinous process	**Use:** Cervical Vertebra Thoracic Vertebra Lumbar Vertebra
Spiral ganglion	**Use:** Acoustic Nerve
Splenic flexure	**Use:** Transverse Colon
Splenic plexus	**Use:** Abdominal Sympathetic Nerve
Splenius capitis muscle	**Use:** Head Muscle
Splenius cervicis muscle	**Use:** Neck Muscle, Right Neck Muscle, Left
Stapes	**Use:** Auditory Ossicle, Right Auditory Ossicle, Left
Stellate ganglion	**Use:** Head and Neck Sympathetic Nerve
Stensen's duct	**Use:** Parotid Duct, Right Parotid Duct, Left
Sternoclavicular ligament	**Use:** Shoulder Bursa and Ligament, Right Shoulder Bursa and Ligament, Left
Sternocleidomastoid artery	**Use:** Thyroid Artery, Right Thyroid Artery, Left

BODY PART KEY

Sternocleidomastoid muscle	**Use:** Neck Muscle, Right Neck Muscle, Left
Sternocostal ligament	**Use:** Sternum Bursa and Ligament Rib(s) Bursa and Ligament
Styloglossus muscle	**Use:** Tongue, Palate, Pharynx Muscle
Stylomandibular ligament	**Use:** Head and Neck Bursa and Ligament
Stylopharyngeus muscle	**Use:** Tongue, Palate, Pharynx Muscle
Subacromial bursa	**Use:** Shoulder Bursa and Ligament, Right Shoulder Bursa and Ligament, Left
Subaortic (common iliac) lymph node	**Use:** Lymphatic, Pelvis
Subarachnoid space, spinal	**Use:** Spinal Canal
Subclavicular (apical) lymph node	**Use:** Lymphatic, Right Axillary Lymphatic, Left Axillary
Subclavius muscle	**Use:** Thorax Muscle, Right Thorax Muscle, Left
Subclavius nerve	**Use:** Brachial Plexus
Subcostal artery	**Use:** Upper Artery
Subcostal muscle	**Use:** Thorax Muscle, Right Thorax Muscle, Left
Subcostal nerve	**Use:** Thoracic Nerve
Subdural space, spinal	**Use:** Spinal Canal
Submandibular ganglion	**Use:** Facial Nerve Head and Neck Sympathetic Nerve
Submandibular gland	**Use:** Submaxillary Gland, Right Submaxillary Gland, Left

Submandibular lymph node	**Use:** Lymphatic, Head
Submaxillary ganglion	**Use:** Head and Neck Sympathetic Nerve
Submaxillary lymph node	**Use:** Lymphatic, Head
Submental artery	**Use:** Face Artery
Submental lymph node	**Use:** Lymphatic, Head
Submucous (Meissner's) plexus	**Use:** Abdominal Sympathetic Nerve
Suboccipital nerve	**Use:** Cervical Nerve
Suboccipital venous plexus	**Use:** Vertebral Vein, Right Vertebral Vein, Left
Subparotid lymph node	**Use:** Lymphatic, Head
Subscapular (posterior) lymph node	**Use:** Lymphatic, Right Axillary Lymphatic, Left Axillary
Subscapular aponeurosis	**Use:** Subcutaneous Tissue and Fascia, Right Upper Arm Subcutaneous Tissue and Fascia, Left Upper Arm
Subscapular artery	**Use:** Axillary Artery, Right Axillary Artery, Left
Subscapularis muscle	**Use:** Shoulder Muscle, Right Shoulder Muscle, Left
Substantia nigra	**Use:** Basal Ganglia
Subtalar (talocalcaneal) joint	**Use:** Tarsal Joint, Right Tarsal Joint, Left
Subtalar ligament	**Use:** Foot Bursa and Ligament, Right Foot Bursa and Ligament, Left
Subthalamic nucleus	**Use:** Basal Ganglia
Superficial circumflex iliac vein	**Use:** Saphenous Vein, Right Saphenous Vein, Left

BODY PART KEY

Superficial epigastric artery	**Use:** Femoral Artery, Right Femoral Artery, Left
Superficial epigastric vein	**Use:** Saphenous Vein, Right Saphenous Vein, Left
Superficial palmar arch	**Use:** Hand Artery, Right Hand Artery, Left
Superficial palmar venous arch	**Use:** Hand Vein, Right Hand Vein, Left
Superficial temporal artery	**Use:** Temporal Artery, Right Temporal Artery, Left
Superficial transverse perineal muscle	**Use:** Perineum Muscle
Superior cardiac nerve	**Use:** Thoracic Sympathetic Nerve
Superior cerebellar vein Superior cerebral vein	**Use:** Intracranial Vein
Superior clunic (cluneal) nerve	**Use:** Lumbar Nerve
Superior epigastric artery	**Use:** Internal Mammary Artery, Right Internal Mammary Artery, Left
Superior genicular artery	**Use:** Popliteal Artery, Right Popliteal Artery, Left
Superior gluteal artery	**Use:** Internal Iliac Artery, Right Internal Iliac Artery, Left
Superior gluteal nerve	**Use:** Lumbar Plexus
Superior hypogastric plexus	**Use:** Abdominal Sympathetic Nerve
Superior labial artery	**Use:** Face Artery
Superior laryngeal artery	**Use:** Thyroid Artery, Right Thyroid Artery, Left
Superior laryngeal nerve	**Use:** Vagus Nerve
Superior longitudinal muscle	**Use:** Tongue, Palate, Pharynx Muscle

Superior mesenteric ganglion	**Use:** Abdominal Sympathetic Nerve
Superior mesenteric lymph node	**Use:** Lymphatic, Mesenteric
Superior mesenteric plexus	**Use:** Abdominal Sympathetic Nerve
Superior oblique muscle	**Use:** Extraocular Muscle, Right Extraocular Muscle, Left
Superior olivary nucleus	**Use:** Pons
Superior rectal artery	**Use:** Inferior Mesenteric Artery
Superior rectal vein	**Use:** Inferior Mesenteric Vein
Superior rectus muscle	**Use:** Extraocular Muscle, Right Extraocular Muscle, Left
Superior tarsal plate	**Use:** Upper Eyelid, Right Upper Eyelid, Left
Superior thoracic artery	**Use:** Axillary Artery, Right Axillary Artery, Left
Superior thyroid artery	**Use:** External Carotid Artery, Right External Carotid Artery, Left Thyroid Artery, Right Thyroid Artery, Left
Superior turbinate	**Use:** Nasal Turbinate
Superior ulnar collateral artery	**Use:** Brachial Artery, Right Brachial Artery, Left
Supraclavicular (Virchow's) lymph node	**Use:** Lymphatic, Right Neck Lymphatic, Left Neck
Supraclavicular nerve	**Use:** Cervical Plexus
Suprahyoid lymph node	**Use:** Lymphatic, Head
Suprahyoid muscle	**Use:** Neck Muscle, Right Neck Muscle, Left

BODY PART KEY

Suprainguinal lymph node	**Use:** Lymphatic, Pelvis
Supraorbital vein	**Use:** Face Vein, Right Face Vein, Left
Suprarenal gland	**Use:** Adrenal Gland, Left Adrenal Gland, Right Adrenal Glands, Bilateral Adrenal Gland
Suprarenal plexus	**Use:** Abdominal Sympathetic Nerve
Suprascapular nerve	**Use:** Brachial Plexus
Supraspinatus fascia	**Use:** Subcutaneous Tissue and Fascia, Right Upper Arm Subcutaneous Tissue and Fascia, Left Upper Arm
Supraspinatus muscle	**Use:** Shoulder Muscle, Right Shoulder Muscle, Left
Supraspinous ligament	**Use:** Upper Spine Bursa and Ligament Lower Spine Bursa and Ligament
Suprasternal notch	**Use:** Sternum
Supratrochlear lymph node	**Use:** Lymphatic, Right Upper Extremity Lymphatic, Left Upper Extremity
Sural artery	**Use:** Popliteal Artery, Right Popliteal Artery, Left
Sweat gland	**Use:** Skin
Talocalcaneal (subtalar) joint	**Use:** Tarsal Joint, Right Tarsal Joint, Left
Talocalcaneal ligament	**Use:** Foot Bursa and Ligament, Right Foot Bursa and Ligament, Left
Talocalcaneonavicular joint	**Use:** Tarsal Joint, Right Tarsal Joint, Left
Talocalcaneonavicular ligament	**Use:** Foot Bursa and Ligament, Right Foot Bursa and Ligament, Left

Talocrural joint	**Use:** Ankle Joint, Right Ankle Joint, Left
Talofibular ligament	**Use:** Ankle Bursa and Ligament, Right Ankle Bursa and Ligament, Left
Talus bone	**Use:** Tarsal, Right Tarsal, Left
Tarsometatarsal ligament	**Use:** Foot Bursa and Ligament, Right Foot Bursa and Ligament, Left
Temporal lobe	**Use:** Cerebral Hemisphere
Temporalis muscle Temporoparietalis muscle	**Use:** Head Muscle
Tensor fasciae latae muscle	**Use:** Hip Muscle, Right Hip Muscle, Left
Tensor veli palatini muscle	**Use:** Tongue, Palate, Pharynx Muscle
Tenth cranial nerve	**Use:** Vagus Nerve
Tentorium cerebelli	**Use:** Dura Mater
Teres major muscle Teres minor muscle	**Use:** Shoulder Muscle, Right Shoulder Muscle, Left
Testicular artery	**Use:** Abdominal Aorta
Thenar muscle	**Use:** Hand Muscle, Right Hand Muscle, Left
Third cranial nerve	**Use:** Oculomotor Nerve
Third occipital nerve	**Use:** Cervical Nerve
Third ventricle	**Use:** Cerebral Ventricle
Thoracic aortic plexus	**Use:** Thoracic Sympathetic Nerve
Thoracic esophagus	**Use:** Esophagus, Middle

BODY PART KEY

Thoracic facet joint	**Use:** Thoracic Vertebral Joint Thoracic Vertebral Joints, 2 to 7 Thoracic Vertebral Joints, 8 or more
Thoracic ganglion	**Use:** Thoracic Sympathetic Nerve
Thoracoacromial artery	**Use:** Axillary Artery, Right Axillary Artery, Left
Thoracolumbar facet joint	**Use:** Thoracolumbar Vertebral Joint
Thymus gland	**Use:** Thymus
Thyroarytenoid muscle	**Use:** Neck Muscle, Right Neck Muscle, Left
Thyrocervical trunk	**Use:** Thyroid Artery, Right Thyroid Artery, Left
Thyroid cartilage	**Use:** Larynx
Tibialis anterior muscle Tibialis posterior muscle	**Use:** Lower Leg Muscle, Right Lower Leg Muscle, Left
Tibiofemoral joint	**Use:** Knee Joint, Right Knee Joint, Left Knee Joint, Tibial Surface, Right Knee Joint, Tibial Surface, Left
Tongue, base of	**Use:** Pharynx
Tracheobronchial lymph node	**Use:** Lymphatic, Thorax
Tragus	**Use:** External Ear, Right External Ear, Left External Ear, Bilateral
Transversalis fascia	**Use:** Subcutaneous Tissue and Fascia, Trunk
Transverse (cutaneous) cervical nerve	**Use:** Cervical Plexus
Transverse acetabular ligament	**Use:** Hip Bursa and Ligament, Right Hip Bursa and Ligament, Left

Transverse facial artery	**Use:** Temporal Artery, Right Temporal Artery, Left
Transverse foramen	**Use:** Cervical Vertebra
Transverse humeral ligament	**Use:** Shoulder Bursa and Ligament, Right Shoulder Bursa and Ligament, Left
Transverse ligament of atlas	**Use:** Head and Neck Bursa and Ligament
Transverse process	**Use:** Cervical Vertebra Thoracic Vertebra Lumbar Vertebra
Transverse scapular ligament	**Use:** Shoulder Bursa and Ligament, Right Shoulder Bursa and Ligament, Left
Transverse thoracis muscle	**Use:** Thorax Muscle, Right Thorax Muscle, Left
Transversospinalis muscle	**Use:** Trunk Muscle, Right Trunk Muscle, Left
Transversus abdominis muscle	**Use:** Abdomen Muscle, Right Abdomen Muscle, Left
Trapezium bone	**Use:** Carpal, Right Carpal, Left
Trapezius muscle	**Use:** Trunk Muscle, Right Trunk Muscle, Left
Trapezoid bone	**Use:** Carpal, Right Carpal, Left
Triceps brachii muscle	**Use:** Upper Arm Muscle, Right Upper Arm Muscle, Left
Tricuspid annulus	**Use:** Tricuspid Valve
Trifacial nerve	**Use:** Trigeminal Nerve
Trigone of bladder	**Use:** Bladder

BODY PART KEY

Triquetral bone	**Use:** Carpal, Right Carpal, Left
Trochanteric bursa	**Use:** Hip Bursa and Ligament, Right Hip Bursa and Ligament, Left
Twelfth cranial nerve	**Use:** Hypoglossal Nerve
Tympanic cavity	**Use:** Middle Ear, Right Middle Ear, Left
Tympanic nerve	**Use:** Glossopharyngeal Nerve
Tympanic part of temporal bone	**Use:** Temporal Bone, Right Temporal Bone, Left
Ulnar collateral carpal ligament	**Use:** Wrist Bursa and Ligament, Right Wrist Bursa and Ligament, Left
Ulnar collateral ligament	**Use:** Elbow Bursa and Ligament, Right Elbow Bursa and Ligament, Left
Ulnar notch	**Use:** Radius, Right Radius, Left
Ulnar vein	**Use:** Brachial Vein, Right Brachial Vein, Left
Umbilical artery	**Use:** Internal Iliac Artery, Right Internal Iliac Artery, Left Lower Artery
Ureteral orifice	**Use:** Ureter, Right Ureter, Left Ureters, Bilateral Ureter
Ureteropelvic junction (UPJ)	**Use:** Kidney Pelvis, Right Kidney Pelvis, Left
Ureterovesical orifice	**Use:** Ureter, Right Ureter, Left Ureters, Bilateral Ureter

Uterine artery	**Use:** Internal Iliac Artery, Right Internal Iliac Artery, Left
Uterine cornu	**Use:** Uterus
Uterine tube	**Use:** Fallopian Tube, Right Fallopian Tube, Left
Uterine vein	**Use:** Hypogastric Vein, Right Hypogastric Vein, Left
Vaginal artery	**Use:** Internal Iliac Artery, Right Internal Iliac Artery, Left
Vaginal vein	**Use:** Hypogastric Vein, Right Hypogastric Vein, Left
Vastus intermedius muscle Vastus lateralis muscle Vastus medialis muscle	**Use:** Upper Leg Muscle, Right Upper Leg Muscle, Left
Ventricular fold	**Use:** Larynx
Vermiform appendix	**Use:** Appendix
Vermilion border	**Use:** Upper Lip Lower Lip
Vertebral arch Vertebral body	**Use:** Cervical Vertebra Thoracic Vertebra Lumbar Vertebra
Vertebral canal	**Use:** Spinal Canal
Vertebral foramen Vertebral lamina Vertebral pedicle	**Use:** Cervical Vertebra Thoracic Vertebra Lumbar Vertebra
Vesical vein	**Use:** Hypogastric Vein, Right Hypogastric Vein, Left
Vestibular (Scarpa's) ganglion Vestibular nerve Vestibulocochlear nerve	**Use:** Acoustic Nerve
Virchow's (supraclavicular) lymph node	**Use:** Lymphatic, Right Neck Lymphatic, Left Neck

BODY PART KEY

Vitreous body	**Use:** Vitreous, Right Vitreous, Left
Vocal fold	**Use:** Vocal Cord, Right Vocal Cord, Left
Volar (palmar) digital vein Volar (palmar) metacarpal vein	**Use:** Hand Vein, Right Hand Vein, Left
Vomer bone	**Use:** Nasal Septum
Vomer of nasal septum	**Use:** Nasal Bone

Xiphoid process	**Use:** Sternum
Zonule of Zinn	**Use:** Lens, Right Lens, Left
Zygomatic process of frontal bone	**Use:** Frontal Bone
Zygomatic process of temporal bone	**Use:** Temporal Bone, Right Temporal Bone, Left
Zygomaticus muscle	**Use:** Facial Muscle

DEVICE KEY

3f (Aortic) Bioprosthesis valve	**Use:** Zooplastic Tissue in Heart and Great Vessels		Artificial bowel sphincter (neosphincter)	**Use:** Artificial Sphincter in Gastrointestinal System
AbioCor® Total Replacement Heart	**Use:** Synthetic Substitute		Artificial urinary sphincter (AUS)	**Use:** Artificial Sphincter in Urinary System
Acellular Hydrated Dermis	**Use:** Nonautologous Tissue Substitute		Assurant (Cobalt) stent	**Use:** Intraluminal Device
Acetabular cup	**Use:** Liner in Lower Joints		AtriClip LAA Exclusion System	**Use:** Extraluminal Device
Activa PC neurostimulator	**Use:** Stimulator Generator, Multiple Array for Insertion in Subcutaneous Tissue and Fascia		Attain Ability® lead	**Use:** Cardiac Lead, Pacemaker for Insertion in Heart and Great Vessels Cardiac Lead, Defibrillator for Insertion in Heart and Great Vessels
Activa RC neurostimulator	**Use:** Stimulator Generator, Multiple Array Rechargeable for Insertion in Subcutaneous Tissue and Fascia		Attain StarFix® (OTW) lead	**Use:** Cardiac Lead, Pacemaker for Insertion in Heart and Great Vessels Cardiac Lead, Defibrillator for Insertion in Heart and Great Vessels
Activa SC neurostimulator	**Use:** Stimulator Generator, Single Array for Insertion in Subcutaneous Tissue and Fascia		Autograft	**Use:** Autologous Tissue Substitute
ACUITY™ Steerable Lead	**Use:** Cardiac Lead, Pacemaker for Insertion in Heart and Great Vessels Cardiac Lead, Defibrillator for Insertion in Heart and Great Vessels		Autologous artery graft	**Use:** Autologous Arterial Tissue in Heart and Great Vessels Autologous Arterial Tissue in Upper Arteries Autologous Arterial Tissue in Lower Arteries Autologous Arterial Tissue in Upper Veins Autologous Arterial Tissue in Lower Veins
Advisa (MRI)	**Use:** Pacemaker, Dual Chamber for Insertion in Subcutaneous Tissue and Fascia			
AFX® Endovascular AAA System	**Use:** Intraluminal Device		Autologous vein graft	**Use:** Autologous Venous Tissue in Heart and Great Vessels Autologous Venous Tissue in Upper Arteries Autologous Venous Tissue in Lower Arteries Autologous Venous Tissue in Upper Veins Autologous Venous Tissue in Lower Veins
AMPLATZER® Muscular VSD Occluder	**Use:** Synthetic Substitute			
AMS 800® Urinary Control System	**Use:** Artificial Sphincter in Urinary System			
AneuRx® AAA Advantage®	**Use:** Intraluminal Device			
Annuloplasty ring	**Use:** Synthetic Substitute			
Artificial anal sphincter (AAS)	**Use:** Artificial Sphincter in Gastrointestinal System		Axial Lumbar Interbody Fusion System	**Use:** Interbody Fusion Device in Lower Joints

DEVICE KEY

AxiaLIF® System	**Use:** Interbody Fusion Device in Lower Joints
BAK/C® Interbody Cervical Fusion System	**Use:** Interbody Fusion Device in Upper Joints
Bard® Composix® (E/X) (LP) mesh	**Use:** Synthetic Substitute
Bard® Composix® Kugel® patch	**Use:** Synthetic Substitute
Bard® Dulex™ mesh	**Use:** Synthetic Substitute
Bard® Ventralex™ hernia patch	**Use:** Synthetic Substitute
Baroreflex Activation Therapy® (BAT®)	**Use:** Stimulator Lead in Upper Arteries Cardiac Rhythm Related Device in Subcutaneous Tissue and Fascia
Berlin Heart Ventricular Assist Device	**Use:** Implantable Heart Assist System in Heart and Great Vessels
Bioactive embolization coil(s)	**Use:** Intraluminal Device, Bioactive in Upper Arteries
Biventricular external heart assist system	**Use:** Short-term External Heart Assist System in Heart and Great Vessels
Blood glucose monitoring system	**Use:** Monitoring Device
Bone anchored hearing device	**Use:** Hearing Device, Bone Conduction for Insertion in Ear, Nose, Sinus Hearing Device in Head and Facial Bones
Bone bank bone graft	**Use:** Nonautologous Tissue Substitute
Bone screw (interlocking) (lag) (pedicle) (recessed)	**Use:** Internal Fixation Device in Head and Facial Bones Internal Fixation Device in Upper Bones Internal Fixation Device in Lower Bones
Bovine pericardial valve	**Use:** Zooplastic Tissue in Heart and Great Vessels
Bovine pericardium graft	**Use:** Zooplastic Tissue in Heart and Great Vessels
Brachytherapy seeds	**Use:** Radioactive Element
BRYAN® Cervical Disc System	**Use:** Synthetic Substitute
BVS 5000 Ventricular Assist Device	**Use:** Short-term External Heart Assist System in Heart and Great Vessels
Cardiac contractility modulation lead	**Use:** Cardiac Lead in Heart and Great Vessels
Cardiac event recorder	**Use:** Monitoring Device
Cardiac resynchronization therapy (CRT) lead	**Use:** Cardiac Lead, Pacemaker for Insertion in Heart and Great Vessels Cardiac Lead, Defibrillator for Insertion in Heart and Great Vessels
CardioMEMS® pressure sensor	**Use:** Monitoring Device, Pressure Sensor for Insertion in Heart and Great Vessels
Carotid (artery) sinus (baroreceptor) lead	**Use:** Stimulator Lead in Upper Arteries
Carotid WALLSTENT® Monorail® Endoprosthesis	**Use:** Intraluminal Device
Centrimag® Blood Pump	**Use:** Short-term External Heart Assist System in Heart and Great Vessels
Ceramic on ceramic bearing surface	**Use:** Synthetic Substitute, Ceramic for Replacement in Lower Joints
Cesium-131 Collagen Implant	**Use:** Radioactive Element, Cesium-131 Collagen Implant for Insertion in Central Nervous System and Cranial Nerves
Clamp and rod internal fixation system (CRIF)	**Use:** Internal Fixation Device in Upper Bones Internal Fixation Device in Lower Bones

DEVICE KEY

COALESCE® radiolucent interbody fusion device	**Use:** Interbody Fusion Device, Radiolucent Porous in New Technology
CoAxia NeuroFlo catheter	**Use:** Intraluminal Device
Cobalt/chromium head and polyethylene socket	**Use:** Synthetic Substitute, Metal on Polyethylene for Replacement in Lower Joints
Cobalt/chromium head and socket	**Use:** Synthetic Substitute, Metal for Replacement in Lower Joints
Cochlear implant (CI), multiple channel (electrode)	**Use:** Hearing Device, Multiple Channel Cochlear Prosthesis for Insertion in Ear, Nose, Sinus
Cochlear implant (CI), single channel (electrode)	**Use:** Hearing Device, Single Channel Cochlear Prosthesis for Insertion in Ear, Nose, Sinus
COGNIS® CRT-D	**Use:** Cardiac Resynchronization Defibrillator Pulse Generator for Insertion in Subcutaneous Tissue and Fascia
COHERE® radiolucent interbody fusion device	**Use:** Interbody Fusion Device, Radiolucent Porous in New Technology
Colonic Z-Stent®	**Use:** Intraluminal Device
Complete (SE) stent	**Use:** Intraluminal Device
Concerto II CRT-D	**Use:** Cardiac Resynchronization Defibrillator Pulse Generator for Insertion in Subcutaneous Tissue and Fascia
CONSERVE® PLUS Total Resurfacing Hip System	**Use:** Resurfacing Device in Lower Joints
Consulta CRT-D	**Use:** Cardiac Resynchronization Defibrillator Pulse Generator for Insertion in Subcutaneous Tissue and Fascia

Consulta CRT-P	**Use:** Cardiac Resynchronization Pacemaker Pulse Generator for Insertion in Subcutaneous Tissue and Fascia
CONTAK RENEWAL® 3 RF (HE) CRT-D	**Use:** Cardiac Resynchronization Defibrillator Pulse Generator for Insertion in Subcutaneous Tissue and Fascia
Contegra Pulmonary Valved Conduit	**Use:** Zooplastic Tissue in Heart and Great Vessels
Continuous Glucose Monitoring (CGM) device	**Use:** Monitoring Device
Cook Biodesign® Fistula Plug(s)	**Use:** Nonautologous Tissue Substitute
Cook Biodesign® Hernia Graft(s)	**Use:** Nonautologous Tissue Substitute
Cook Biodesign® Layered Graft(s)	**Use:** Nonautologous Tissue Substitute
Cook Zenapro™ Layered Graft(s)	**Use:** Nonautologous Tissue Substitute
Cook Zenith AAA Endovascular Graft	**Use:** Intraluminal Device, Branched or Fenestrated, One or Two Arteries for Restriction in Lower Arteries Intraluminal Device, Branched or Fenestrated, Three or More Arteries for Restriction in Lower Arteries Intraluminal Device
CoreValve transcatheter aortic valve	**Use:** Zooplastic Tissue in Heart and Great Vessels
Cormet Hip Resurfacing System	**Use:** Resurfacing Device in Lower Joints
CoRoent® XL	**Use:** Interbody Fusion Device in Lower Joints
Corox (OTW) Bipolar Lead	**Use:** Cardiac Lead, Pacemaker for Insertion in Heart and Great Vessels Cardiac Lead, Defibrillator for Insertion in Heart and Great Vessels

DEVICE KEY

Cortical strip neurostimulator lead	**Use:** Neurostimulator Lead in Central Nervous System and Cranial Nerves
Cultured epidermal cell autograft	**Use:** Autologous Tissue Substitute
CYPHER® Stent	**Use:** Intraluminal Device, Drug-eluting in Heart and Great Vessels
Cystostomy tube	**Use:** Drainage Device
DBS lead	**Use:** Neurostimulator Lead in Central Nervous System and Cranial Nerves
DeBakey Left Ventricular Assist Device	**Use:** Implantable Heart Assist System in Heart and Great Vessels
Deep brain neurostimulator lead	**Use:** Neurostimulator Lead in Central Nervous System and Cranial Nerves
Delta frame external fixator	**Use:** External Fixation Device, Hybrid for Insertion in Upper Bones External Fixation Device, Hybrid for Reposition in Upper Bones External Fixation Device, Hybrid for Insertion in Lower Bones External Fixation Device, Hybrid for Reposition in Lower Bones
Delta III Reverse shoulder prosthesis	**Use:** Synthetic Substitute, Reverse Ball and Socket for Replacement in Upper Joints
Diaphragmatic pacemaker generator	**Use:** Stimulator Generator in Subcutaneous Tissue and Fascia
Direct Lateral Interbody Fusion (DLIF) device	**Use:** Interbody Fusion Device in Lower Joints
Driver stent (RX) (OTW)	**Use:** Intraluminal Device
DuraHeart Left Ventricular Assist System	**Use:** Implantable Heart Assist System in Heart and Great Vessels

Durata® Defibrillation Lead	**Use:** Cardiac Lead, Defibrillator for Insertion in Heart and Great Vessels
Dynesys® Dynamic Stabilization System	**Use:** Spinal Stabilization Device, Pedicle-Based for Insertion in Upper Joints Spinal Stabilization Device, Pedicle-Based for Insertion in Lower Joints
E-Luminexx™ (Biliary) (Vascular) Stent	**Use:** Intraluminal Device
EDWARDS INTUITY Elite valve system	**Use:** Zooplastic Tissue, Rapid Deployment Technique in New Technology
Electrical bone growth stimulator (EBGS)	**Use:** Bone Growth Stimulator in Head and Facial Bones Bone Growth Stimulator in Upper Bones Bone Growth Stimulator in Lower Bones
Electrical muscle stimulation (EMS) lead	**Use:** Stimulator Lead in Muscles
Electronic muscle stimulator lead	**Use:** Stimulator Lead in Muscles
Embolization coil(s)	**Use:** Intraluminal Device
Endeavor® (III) (IV) (Sprint) Zotarolimus-eluting Coronary Stent System	**Use:** Intraluminal Device, Drug-eluting in Heart and Great Vessels
Endologix AFX® Endovascular AAA System	**Use:** Intraluminal Device
EndoSure® sensor	**Use:** Monitoring Device, Pressure Sensor for Insertion in Heart and Great Vessels
ENDOTAK RELIANCE® (G) Defibrillation Lead	**Use:** Cardiac Lead, Defibrillator for Insertion in Heart and Great Vessels
Endotracheal tube (cuffed) (double-lumen)	**Use:** Intraluminal Device, Endotracheal Airway in Respiratory System
Endurant® Endovascular Stent Graft	**Use:** Intraluminal Device

DEVICE KEY

Endurant® II AAA stent graft system	**Use:** Intraluminal Device
EnRhythm	**Use:** Pacemaker, Dual Chamber for Insertion in Subcutaneous Tissue and Fascia
Enterra gastric neurostimulator	**Use:** Stimulator Generator, Multiple Array for Insertion in Subcutaneous Tissue and Fascia
Epic™ Stented Tissue Valve (aortic)	**Use:** Zooplastic Tissue in Heart and Great Vessels
Epicel® cultured epidermal autograft	**Use:** Autologous Tissue Substitute
Esophageal obturator airway (EOA)	**Use:** Intraluminal Device, Airway in Gastrointestinal System
Esteem® implantable hearing system	**Use:** Hearing Device in Ear, Nose, Sinus
Everolimus-eluting coronary stent	**Use:** Intraluminal Device, Drug-eluting in Heart and Great Vessels
Ex-PRESS™ mini glaucoma shunt	**Use:** Synthetic Substitute
EXCLUDER® AAA Endoprosthesis	**Use:** Intraluminal Device, Branched or Fenestrated, One or Two Arteries for Restriction in Lower Arteries Intraluminal Device, Branched or Fenestrated, Three or More Arteries for Restriction in Lower Arteries
EXCLUDER® IBE Endoprosthesis	**Use:** Intraluminal Device, Branched or Fenestrated, One or Two Arteries for Restriction in Lower Arteries
Express® (LD) Premounted Stent System	**Use:** Intraluminal Device
Express® Biliary SD Monorail® Premounted Stent System	**Use:** Intraluminal Device
Express® SD Renal Monorail® Premounted Stent System	**Use:** Intraluminal Device

External fixator	**Use:** External Fixation Device in Head and Facial Bones External Fixation Device in Upper Bones External Fixation Device in Lower Bones External Fixation Device in Upper Joints External Fixation Device in Lower Joints
EXtreme Lateral Interbody Fusion (XLIF) device	**Use:** Interbody Fusion Device in Lower Joints
Facet replacement spinal stabilization device	**Use:** Spinal Stabilization Device, Facet Replacement for Insertion in Upper Joints Spinal Stabilization Device, Facet Replacement for Insertion in Lower Joints
FLAIR® Endovascular Stent Graft	**Use:** Intraluminal Device
Flexible Composite Mesh	**Use:** Synthetic Substitute
Foley catheter	**Use:** Drainage Device
Formula™ Balloon-Expandable Renal Stent System	**Use:** Intraluminal Device
Freestyle (Stentless) Aortic Root Bioprosthesis	**Use:** Zooplastic Tissue in Heart and Great Vessels
Fusion screw (compression) (lag) (locking)	**Use:** Internal Fixation Device in Upper Joints Internal Fixation Device in Lower Joints
GammaTile™	**Use:** Radioactive Element, Cesium-131 Collagen Implant for Insertion in Central Nervous System and Cranial Nerves
Gastric electrical stimulation (GES) lead	**Use:** Stimulator Lead in Gastrointestinal System
Gastric pacemaker lead	**Use:** Stimulator Lead in Gastrointestinal System

DEVICE KEY

GORE EXCLUDER® AAA Endoprosthesis	**Use:** Intraluminal Device, Branched or Fenestrated, One or Two Arteries for Restriction in Lower Arteries
GORE EXCLUDER® IBE Endoprosthesis	**Use:** Intraluminal Device, Branched or Fenestrated, One or Two Arteries for Restriction in Lower Arteries
GORE TAG® Thoracic Endoprosthesis	**Use:** Intraluminal Device
GORE® DUALMESH®	**Use:** Synthetic Substitute
Guedel airway	**Use:** Intraluminal Device, Airway in Mouth and Throat
Hancock Bioprosthesis (aortic) (mitral) valve	**Use:** Zooplastic Tissue in Heart and Great Vessels
Hancock Bioprosthetic Valved Conduit	**Use:** Zooplastic Tissue in Heart and Great Vessels
HeartMate 3™ LVAS	**Use:** Implantable Heart Assist System in Heart and Great Vessels
HeartMate II® Left Ventricular Assist Device (LVAD)	**Use:** Implantable Heart Assist System in Heart and Great Vessels
HeartMate XVE® Left Ventricular Assist Device (LVAD)	**Use:** Implantable Heart Assist System in Heart and Great Vessels
Hip (joint) liner	**Use:** Liner in Lower Joints
Holter valve ventricular shunt	**Use:** Synthetic Substitute
Ilizarov external fixator	**Use:** External Fixation Device, Ring for Insertion in Upper Bones External Fixation Device, Ring for Reposition in Upper Bones External Fixation Device, Ring for Insertion in Lower Bones External Fixation Device, Ring for Reposition in Lower Bones

Ilizarov-Vecklich device	**Use:** External Fixation Device, Limb Lengthening for Insertion in Upper Bones External Fixation Device, Limb Lengthening for Insertion in Lower Bones
Impella® heart pump	**Use:** Short-term External Heart Assist System in Heart and Great Vessels
Implantable cardioverter-defibrillator (ICD)	**Use:** Defibrillator Generator for Insertion in Subcutaneous Tissue and Fascia
Implantable drug infusion pump (anti-spasmodic) (chemotherapy) (pain)	**Use:** Infusion Device, Pump in Subcutaneous Tissue and Fascia
Implantable glucose monitoring device	**Use:** Monitoring Device
Implantable hemodynamic monitor (IHM)	**Use:** Monitoring Device, Hemodynamic for Insertion in Subcutaneous Tissue and Fascia
Implantable hemodynamic monitoring system (IHMS)	**Use:** Monitoring Device, Hemodynamic for Insertion in Subcutaneous Tissue and Fascia
Implantable Miniature Telescope™ (IMT)	**Use:** Synthetic Substitute, Intraocular Telescope for Replacement in Eye
Implanted (venous) (access) port	**Use:** Vascular Access Device, Totally Implantable in Subcutaneous Tissue and Fascia
InDura, intrathecal catheter (1P) (spinal)	**Use:** Infusion Device
Injection reservoir, port	**Use:** Vascular Access Device, Totally Implantable in Subcutaneous Tissue and Fascia
Injection reservoir, pump	**Use:** Infusion Device, Pump in Subcutaneous Tissue and Fascia

DEVICE KEY

Interbody fusion (spine) cage	**Use:** Interbody Fusion Device in Upper Joints Interbody Fusion Device in Lower Joints
Interspinous process spinal stabilization device	**Use:** Spinal Stabilization Device, Interspinous Process for Insertion in Upper Joints Spinal Stabilization Device, Interspinous Process for Insertion in Lower Joints
InterStim® Therapy lead	**Use:** Neurostimulator Lead in Peripheral Nervous System
InterStim® Therapy neurostimulator	**Use:** Stimulator Generator, Single Array for Insertion in Subcutaneous Tissue and Fascia
Intramedullary (IM) rod (nail)	**Use:** Internal Fixation Device, Intramedullary in Upper Bones Internal Fixation Device, Intramedullary in Lower Bones
Intramedullary skeletal kinetic distractor (ISKD)	**Use:** Internal Fixation Device, Intramedullary in Upper Bones Internal Fixation Device, Intramedullary in Lower Bones
Intrauterine device (IUD)	**Use:** Contraceptive Device in Female Reproductive System
INTUITY Elite valve system, EDWARDS	**Use:** Zooplastic Tissue, Rapid Deployment Technique in New Technology
Itrel (3) (4) neurostimulator	**Use:** Stimulator Generator, Single Array for Insertion in Subcutaneous Tissue and Fascia
Joint fixation plate	**Use:** Internal Fixation Device in Upper Joints Internal Fixation Device in Lower Joints
Joint liner (insert)	**Use:** Liner in Lower Joints
Joint spacer (antibiotic)	**Use:** Spacer in Upper Joints Spacer in Lower Joints

Kappa	**Use:** Pacemaker, Dual Chamber for Insertion in Subcutaneous Tissue and Fascia
Kinetra® neurostimulator	**Use:** Stimulator Generator, Multiple Array for Insertion in Subcutaneous Tissue and Fascia
Kirschner wire (K-wire)	**Use:** Internal Fixation Device in Head and Facial Bones Internal Fixation Device in Upper Bones Internal Fixation Device in Lower Bones Internal Fixation Device in Upper Joints Internal Fixation Device in Lower Joints
Knee (implant) insert	**Use:** Liner in Lower Joints
Kuntscher nail	**Use:** Internal Fixation Device, Intramedullary in Upper Bones Internal Fixation Device, Intramedullary in Lower Bones
LAP-BAND® adjustable gastric banding system	**Use:** Extraluminal Device
LifeStent® (Flexstar) (XL) Vascular Stent System	**Use:** Intraluminal Device
LIVIAN™ CRT-D	**Use:** Cardiac Resynchronization Defibrillator Pulse Generator for Insertion in Subcutaneous Tissue and Fascia
Loop recorder, implantable	**Use:** Monitoring Device
MAGEC® Spinal Bracing and Distraction System	**Use:** Magnetically Controlled Growth Rod(s) in New Technology
Mark IV Breathing Pacemaker System	Stimulator Generator in Subcutaneous Tissue and Fascia
Maximo II DR (VR)	**Use:** Defibrillator Generator for Insertion in Subcutaneous Tissue and Fascia
Maximo II DR CRT-D	**Use:** Cardiac Resynchronization Defibrillator Pulse Generator for Insertion in Subcutaneous Tissue and Fascia

DEVICE KEY

Medtronic Endurant® II AAA stent graft system	**Use:** Intraluminal Device
Melody® transcatheter pulmonary valve	**Use:** Zooplastic Tissue in Heart and Great Vessels
Metal on metal bearing surface	**Use:** Synthetic Substitute, Metal for Replacement in Lower Joints
Micro-Driver stent (RX) (OTW)	**Use:** Intraluminal Device
Micrus CERECYTE microcoil	**Use:** Intraluminal Device, Bioactive in Upper Arteries
MIRODERM™ Biologic Wound Matrix	**Use:** Skin Substitute, Porcine Liver Derived in New Technology
MitraClip valve repair system	**Use:** Synthetic Substitute
Mitroflow® Aortic Pericardial Heart Valve	**Use:** Zooplastic Tissue in Heart and Great Vessels
Mosaic Bioprosthesis (aortic) (mitral) valve	**Use:** Zooplastic Tissue in Heart and Great Vessels
MULTI-LINK (VISION)(MINIVISION) (ULTRA) Coronary Stent System	**Use:** Intraluminal Device
nanoLOCK™ interbody fusion device	**Use:** Interbody Fusion Device, Nanotextured Surface in New Technology
Nasopharyngeal airway (NPA)	**Use:** Intraluminal Device, Airway in Ear, Nose, Sinus
Neuromuscular electrical stimulation (NEMS) lead	**Use:** Stimulator Lead in Muscles
Neurostimulator generator, multiple channel	**Use:** Stimulator Generator, Multiple Array for Insertion in Subcutaneous Tissue and Fascia
Neurostimulator generator, multiple channel rechargeable	**Use:** Stimulator Generator, Multiple Array Rechargeable for Insertion in Subcutaneous Tissue and Fascia

Neurostimulator generator, single channel	**Use:** Stimulator Generator, Single Array for Insertion in Subcutaneous Tissue and Fascia
Neurostimulator generator, single channel rechargeable	**Use:** Stimulator Generator, Single Array Rechargeable for Insertion in Subcutaneous Tissue and Fascia
Neutralization plate	**Use:** Internal Fixation Device in Head and Facial Bones; Internal Fixation Device in Upper Bones; Internal Fixation Device in Lower Bones
Nitinol framed polymer mesh	**Use:** Synthetic Substitute
Non-tunneled central venous catheter	**Use:** Infusion Device
Novacor Left Ventricular Assist Device	**Use:** Implantable Heart Assist System in Heart and Great Vessels
Novation® Ceramic AHS® (Articulation Hip System)	**Use:** Synthetic Substitute, Ceramic for Replacement in Lower Joints
Optimizer™ III implantable pulse generator	**Use:** Contractility Modulation Device for Insertion in Subcutaneous Tissue and Fascia
Oropharyngeal airway (OPA)	**Use:** Intraluminal Device, Airway in Mouth and Throat
Ovatio™ CRT-D	**Use:** Cardiac Resynchronization Defibrillator Pulse Generator for Insertion in Subcutaneous Tissue and Fascia
OXINIUM	**Use:** Synthetic Substitute, Oxidized Zirconium on Polyethylene for Replacement in Lower Joints
Paclitaxel-eluting coronary stent	**Use:** Intraluminal Device, Drug-eluting in Heart and Great Vessels
Paclitaxel-eluting peripheral stent	**Use:** Intraluminal Device, Drug-eluting in Upper Arteries; Intraluminal Device, Drug-eluting in Lower Arteries

DEVICE KEY

Partially absorbable mesh	**Use:** Synthetic Substitute
Pedicle-based dynamic stabilization device	**Use:** Spinal Stabilization Device, Pedicle-Based for Insertion in Upper Joints Spinal Stabilization Device, Pedicle-Based for Insertion in Lower Joints
Perceval sutureless valve	**Use:** Zooplastic Tissue, Rapid Deployment Technique in New Technology
Percutaneous endoscopic gastrojejunostomy (PEG/J) tube	**Use:** Feeding Device in Gastrointestinal System
Percutaneous endoscopic gastrostomy (PEG) tube	**Use:** Feeding Device in Gastrointestinal System
Percutaneous nephrostomy catheter	**Use:** Drainage Device
Peripherally inserted central catheter (PICC)	**Use:** Infusion Device
Pessary ring	**Use:** Intraluminal Device, Pessary in Female Reproductive System
Phrenic nerve stimulator generator	**Use:** Stimulator Generator in Subcutaneous Tissue and Fascia
Phrenic nerve stimulator lead	**Use:** Diaphragmatic Pacemaker Lead in Respiratory System
PHYSIOMESH™ Flexible Composite Mesh	**Use:** Synthetic Substitute
Pipeline™ Embolization device (PED)	**Use:** Intraluminal Device
Polyethylene socket	**Use:** Synthetic Substitute, Polyethylene for Replacement in Lower Joints
Polymethylmethacrylate (PMMA)	**Use:** Synthetic Substitute
Polypropylene mesh	**Use:** Synthetic Substitute
Porcine (bioprosthetic) valve	**Use:** Zooplastic Tissue in Heart and Great Vessels

PRESTIGE® Cervical Disc	**Use:** Synthetic Substitute
PrimeAdvanced neurostimulator	**Use:** Stimulator Generator, Multiple Array for Insertion in Subcutaneous Tissue and Fascia
PROCEED™ Ventral Patch	**Use:** Synthetic Substitute
Prodisc-C	**Use:** Synthetic Substitute
Prodisc-L	**Use:** Synthetic Substitute
PROLENE Polypropylene Hernia System (PHS)	**Use:** Synthetic Substitute
Protecta XT CRT-D	**Use:** Cardiac Resynchronization Defibrillator Pulse Generator for Insertion in Subcutaneous Tissue and Fascia
Protecta XT DR (XT VR)	**Use:** Defibrillator Generator for Insertion in Subcutaneous Tissue and Fascia
Protégé® RX Carotid Stent System	**Use:** Intraluminal Device
Pump reservoir	**Use:** Infusion Device, Pump in Subcutaneous Tissue and Fascia
PVAD™ Ventricular Assist Device	**Use:** External Heart Assist System in Heart and Great Vessels
REALIZE® Adjustable Gastric Band	**Use:** Extraluminal Device
Rebound HRD® (Hernia Repair Device)	**Use:** Synthetic Substitute
RestoreAdvanced neurostimulator	**Use:** Stimulator Generator, Multiple Array Rechargeable for Insertion in Subcutaneous Tissue and Fascia
RestoreSensor neurostimulator	**Use:** Stimulator Generator, Multiple Array Rechargeable for Insertion in Subcutaneous Tissue and Fascia

DEVICE KEY

RestoreUltra neurostimulator	**Use:** Stimulator Generator, Multiple Array Rechargeable for Insertion in Subcutaneous Tissue and Fascia
Reveal (DX) (XT)	**Use:** Monitoring Device
Reverse® Shoulder Prosthesis	**Use:** Synthetic Substitute, Reverse Ball and Socket for Replacement in Upper Joints
Revo MRI™ SureScan® pacemaker	**Use:** Pacemaker, Dual Chamber for Insertion in Subcutaneous Tissue and Fascia
Rheos® System device	**Use:** Cardiac Rhythm Related Device in Subcutaneous Tissue and Fascia
Rheos® System lead	**Use:** Stimulator Lead in Upper Arteries
RNS System lead	**Use:** Neurostimulator Lead in Central Nervous System and Cranial Nerves
RNS system neurostimulator generator	**Use:** Neurostimulator Generator in Head and Facial Bones
Sacral nerve modulation (SNM) lead	**Use:** Stimulator Lead in Urinary System
Sacral neuromodulation lead	**Use:** Stimulator Lead in Urinary System
SAPIEN transcatheter aortic valve	**Use:** Zooplastic Tissue in Heart and Great Vessels
Secura (DR) (VR)	**Use:** Defibrillator Generator for Insertion in Subcutaneous Tissue and Fascia
Sheffield hybrid external fixator	**Use:** External Fixation Device, Hybrid for Insertion in Upper Bones External Fixation Device, Hybrid for Reposition in Upper Bones External Fixation Device, Hybrid for Insertion in Lower Bones External Fixation Device, Hybrid for Reposition in Lower Bones
Sheffield ring external fixator	**Use:** External Fixation Device, Ring for Insertion in Upper Bones External Fixation Device, Ring for Reposition in Upper Bones External Fixation Device, Ring for Insertion in Lower Bones External Fixation Device, Ring for Reposition in Lower Bones
Single lead pacemaker (atrium) (ventricle)	**Use:** Pacemaker, Single Chamber for Insertion in Subcutaneous Tissue and Fascia
Single lead rate responsive pacemaker (atrium) (ventricle)	**Use:** Pacemaker, Single Chamber Rate Responsive for Insertion in Subcutaneous Tissue and Fascia
Sirolimus-eluting coronary stent	**Use:** Intraluminal Device, Drug-eluting in Heart and Great Vessels
SJM Biocor® Stented Valve System	**Use:** Zooplastic Tissue in Heart and Great Vessels
Soletra® neurostimulator	**Use:** Stimulator Generator, Single Array for Insertion in Subcutaneous Tissue and Fascia
Spinal cord neurostimulator lead	**Use:** Neurostimulator Lead in Central Nervous System and Cranial Nerves
Spinal growth rods, magnetically controlled	**Use:** Magnetically Controlled Growth Rod(s) in New Technology
Spiration IBV™ Valve System	**Use:** Intraluminal Device, Endobronchial Valve in Respiratory System
Stent (angioplasty) (embolization)	**Use:** Intraluminal Device
Stented tissue valve	**Use:** Zooplastic Tissue in Heart and Great Vessels
Stratos LV	**Use:** Cardiac Resynchronization Pacemaker Pulse Generator for Insertion in Subcutaneous Tissue and Fascia

DEVICE KEY

Subcutaneous injection reservoir, port	**Use:** Vascular Access Device, Totally Implantable in Subcutaneous Tissue and Fascia
Subcutaneous injection reservoir, pump	**Use:** Infusion Device, Pump in Subcutaneous Tissue and Fascia
Subdermal progesterone implant	**Use:** Contraceptive Device in Subcutaneous Tissue and Fascia
Sutureless valve, Perceval	**Use:** Zooplastic Tissue, Rapid Deployment Technique in New Technology
SynCardia Total Artificial Heart	**Use:** Synthetic Substitute
Synchra CRT-P	**Use:** Cardiac Resynchronization Pacemaker Pulse Generator for Insertion in Subcutaneous Tissue and Fascia
Talent® Converter	**Use:** Intraluminal Device
Talent® Occluder	**Use:** Intraluminal Device
Talent® Stent Graft (abdominal) (thoracic)	**Use:** Intraluminal Device
TandemHeart® System	**Use:** Short-term External Heart Assist System in Heart and Great Vessels
TAXUS® Liberté® Paclitaxel-eluting Coronary Stent System	**Use:** Intraluminal Device, Drug-eluting in Heart and Great Vessels
Therapeutic occlusion coil(s)	**Use:** Intraluminal Device
Thoracostomy tube	**Use:** Drainage Device
Thoratec IVAD (Implantable Ventricular Assist Device)	**Use:** Implantable Heart Assist System in Heart and Great Vessels
Thoratec Paracorporeal Ventricular Assist Device	**Use:** Short-term External Heart Assist System in Heart and Great Vessels
Tibial insert	**Use:** Liner in Lower Joints

Tissue bank graft	**Use:** Nonautologous Tissue Substitute
Tissue expander (inflatable) (injectable)	**Use:** Tissue Expander in Skin and Breast Tissue Expander in Subcutaneous Tissue and Fascia
Titanium Sternal Fixation System (TSFS)	**Use:** Internal Fixation Device, Rigid Plate for Insertion in Upper Bones Internal Fixation Device, Rigid Plate for Reposition in Upper Bones
Total artificial (replacement) heart	**Use:** Synthetic Substitute
Tracheostomy tube	**Use:** Tracheostomy Device in Respiratory System
Trifecta™ Valve (aortic)	**Use:** Zooplastic Tissue in Heart and Great Vessels
Tunneled central venous catheter	**Use:** Vascular Access Device, Tunneled in Subcutaneous Tissue and Fascia
Tunneled spinal (intrathecal) catheter	**Use:** Infusion Device
Two lead pacemaker	**Use:** Pacemaker, Dual Chamber for Insertion in Subcutaneous Tissue and Fascia
Ultraflex™ Precision Colonic Stent System	**Use:** Intraluminal Device
ULTRAPRO Hernia System (UHS)	**Use:** Synthetic Substitute
ULTRAPRO Partially Absorbable Lightweight Mesh	**Use:** Synthetic Substitute
ULTRAPRO Plug	**Use:** Synthetic Substitute
Ultrasonic osteogenic stimulator	**Use:** Bone Growth Stimulator in Head and Facial Bones Bone Growth Stimulator in Upper Bones Bone Growth Stimulator in Lower Bones

DEVICE KEY

Ultrasound bone healing system	**Use:** Bone Growth Stimulator in Head and Facial Bones Bone Growth Stimulator in Upper Bones Bone Growth Stimulator in Lower Bones
Uniplanar external fixator	**Use:** External Fixation Device, Monoplanar for Insertion in Upper Bones External Fixation Device, Monoplanar for Reposition in Upper Bones External Fixation Device, Monoplanar for Insertion in Lower Bones External Fixation Device, Monoplanar for Reposition in Lower Bones
Urinary incontinence stimulator lead	**Use:** Stimulator Lead in Urinary System
Vaginal pessary	**Use:** Intraluminal Device, Pessary in Female Reproductive System
Valiant Thoracic Stent Graft	**Use:** Intraluminal Device
Vectra® Vascular Access Graft	**Use:** Vascular Access Device, Tunneled in Subcutaneous Tissue and Fascia
Ventrio™ Hernia Patch	**Use:** Synthetic Substitute
Versa	**Use:** Pacemaker, Dual Chamber for Insertion in Subcutaneous Tissue and Fascia
Virtuoso (II) (DR) (VR)	**Use:** Defibrillator Generator for Insertion in Subcutaneous Tissue and Fascia

WALLSTENT® Endoprosthesis	**Use:** Intraluminal Device
X-STOP® Spacer	**Use:** Spinal Stabilization Device, Interspinous Process for Insertion in Upper Joints Spinal Stabilization Device, Interspinous Process for Insertion in Lower Joints
Xenograft	**Use:** Zooplastic Tissue in Heart and Great Vessels
XIENCE V Everolimus Eluting Coronary Stent System	**Use:** Intraluminal Device, Drug-eluting in Heart and Great Vessels
XLIF® System	**Use:** Interbody Fusion Device in Lower Joints
Zenith Flex® AAA Endovascular Graft	**Use:** Intraluminal Device
Zenith TX2® TAA Endovascular Graft	**Use:** Intraluminal Device
Zenith® Renu™ AAA Ancillary Graft	**Use:** Intraluminal Device
Zilver® PTX® (paclitaxel) Drug-Eluting Peripheral Stent	**Use:** Intraluminal Device, Drug-eluting in Upper Arteries Intraluminal Device, Drug-eluting in Lower Arteries
Zimmer® NexGen® LPS Mobile Bearing Knee	**Use:** Synthetic Substitute
Zimmer® NexGen® LPS-Flex Mobile Knee	**Use:** Synthetic Substitute
Zotarolimus-eluting coronary stent	**Use:** Intraluminal Device, Drug-eluting in Heart and Great Vessels

SUBSTANCE KEY

Term	ICD-10-PCS Value
AIGISRx Antibacterial Envelope Antimicrobial envelope	**Use:** Anti-Infective Envelope
Axicabtagene Ciloeucel	**Use:** Engineered Autologous Chimeric Antigen Receptor T-cell Immunotherapy
Bone morphogenetic protein 2 (BMP 2)	**Use:** Recombinant Bone Morphogenetic Protein
CBMA (Concentrated Bone Marrow Aspirate)	**Use:** Concentrated Bone Marrow Aspirate
Clolar	**Use:** Clofarabine
Defitelio	**Use:** Defibrotide Sodium Anticoagulant
DuraGraft® Endothelial Damage Inhibitor	**Use:** Endothelial Damage Inhibitor
Factor Xa Inhibitor Reversal Agent, Andexanet Alfa	**Use:** Andexanet Alfa, Factor Xa Inhibitor Reversal Agent
Kcentra	**Use:** 4-Factor Prothrombin Complex Concentrate
Nesiritide	**Use:** Human B-type Natriuretic Peptide

Term	ICD-10-PCS Value
rhBMP-2	**Use:** Recombinant Bone Morphogenetic Protein
Seprafilm	**Use:** Adhesion Barrier
STELARA®	**Use:** Other New Technology Therapeutic Substance
Tissue Plasminogen Activator (tPA) (rtPA)	**Use:** Other Thrombolytic
Ustekinumab	**Use:** Other New Technology Therapeutic Substance
Vistogard®	**Use:** Uridine Triacetate
Voraxaze	**Use:** Glucarpidase
VYXEOS™	**Use:** Cytarabine and Daunorubicin Liposome Antineoplastic
ZINPLAVA™	**Use:** Bezlotoxumab Monoclonal Antibody
Zyvox	**Use:** Oxazolidinones

Appendix D: Substance Key

Specific Device	for Operation	in Body System	General Device
Autologous Arterial Tissue	All applicable	Heart and Great Vessels Lower Arteries Lower Veins Upper Arteries Upper Veins	**7** Autologous Tissue Substitute
Autologous Venous Tissue	All applicable	Heart and Great Vessels Lower Arteries Lower Veins Upper Arteries Upper Veins	**7** Autologous Tissue Substitute
Cardiac Lead, Defibrillator	Insertion	Heart and Great Vessels	**M** Cardiac Lead
Cardiac Lead, Pacemaker	Insertion	Heart and Great Vessels	**M** Cardiac Lead
Cardiac Resynchronization Defibrillator Pulse Generator	Insertion	Subcutaneous Tissue and Fascia	**P** Cardiac Rhythm Related Device
Cardiac Resynchronization Pacemaker Pulse Generator	Insertion	Subcutaneous Tissue and Fascia	**P** Cardiac Rhythm Related Device
Contractility Modulation Device	Insertion	Subcutaneous Tissue and Fascia	**P** Cardiac Rhythm Related Device
Defibrillator Generator	Insertion	Subcutaneous Tissue and Fascia	**P** Cardiac Rhythm Related Device
Epiretinal Visual Prosthesis	All applicable	Eye	**J** Synthetic Substitute
External Fixation Device, Hybrid	Insertion	Lower Bones Upper Bones	**5** External Fixation Device
External Fixation Device, Hybrid	Reposition	Lower Bones Upper Bones	**5** External Fixation Device
External Fixation Device, Limb Lengthening	Insertion	Lower Bones Upper Bones	**5** External Fixation Device
External Fixation Device, Monoplanar	Insertion	Lower Bones Upper Bones	**5** External Fixation Device
External Fixation Device, Monoplanar	Reposition	Lower Bones Upper Bones	**5** External Fixation Device
External Fixation Device, Ring	Insertion	Lower Bones Upper Bones	**5** External Fixation Device
External Fixation Device, Ring	Reposition	Lower Bones Upper Bones	**5** External Fixation Device
Hearing Device, Bone Conduction	Insertion	Ear, Nose, Sinus	**S** Hearing Device
Hearing Device, Multiple Channel Cochlear Prosthesis	Insertion	Ear, Nose, Sinus	**S** Hearing Device
Hearing Device, Single Channel Cochlear Prosthesis	Insertion	Ear, Nose, Sinus	**S** Hearing Device
Internal Fixation Device, Intramedullary	All applicable	Lower Bones Upper Bones	**4** Internal Fixation Device
Internal Fixation Device, Rigid Plate	Insertion	Upper Bones	**4** Internal Fixation Device
Internal Fixation Device, Rigid Plate	Reposition	Upper Bones	**4** Internal Fixation Device
Intraluminal Device, Pessary	All applicable	Female Reproductive System	**D** Intraluminal Device

DEVICE AGGREGATION TABLE

Specific Device	for Operation	in Body System	General Device
Intraluminal Device, Airway	All applicable	Ear, Nose, Sinus Gastrointestinal System Mouth and Throat	**D** Intraluminal Device
Intraluminal Device, Bioactive	All applicable	Upper Arteries	**D** Intraluminal Device
Intraluminal Device, Branched or Fenestrated, One or Two Arteries	Restriction	Heart and Great Vessels Lower Arteries	**D** Intraluminal Device
Intraluminal Device, Branched or Fenestrated, Three or More Arteries	Restriction	Heart and Great Vessels Lower Arteries	**D** Intraluminal Device
Intraluminal Device, Drug-eluting	All applicable	Heart and Great Vessels Lower Arteries Upper Arteries	**D** Intraluminal Device
Intraluminal Device, Drug-eluting, Four or More	All applicable	Heart and Great Vessels Lower Arteries Upper Arteries	**D** Intraluminal Device
Intraluminal Device, Drug-eluting, Three	All applicable	Heart and Great Vessels Lower Arteries Upper Arteries	**D** Intraluminal Device
Intraluminal Device, Drug-eluting, Two	All applicable	Heart and Great Vessels Lower Arteries Upper Arteries	**D** Intraluminal Device
Intraluminal Device, Endobronchial Valve	All applicable	Respiratory System	**D** Intraluminal Device
Intraluminal Device, Endotracheal Airway	All applicable	Respiratory System	**D** Intraluminal Device
Intraluminal Device, Four or More	All applicable	Heart and Great Vessels Lower Arteries Upper Arteries	**D** Intraluminal Device
Intraluminal Device, Radioactive	All applicable	Heart and Great Vessels	**D** Intraluminal Device
Intraluminal Device, Three	All applicable	Heart and Great Vessels Lower Arteries Upper Arteries	**D** Intraluminal Device
Intraluminal Device, Two	All applicable	Heart and Great Vessels Lower Arteries Upper Arteries	**D** Intraluminal Device
Monitoring Device, Hemodynamic	Insertion	Subcutaneous Tissue and Fascia	**2** Monitoring Device
Monitoring Device, Pressure Sensor	Insertion	Heart and Great Vessels	**2** Monitoring Device
Pacemaker, Dual Chamber	Insertion	Subcutaneous Tissue and Fascia	**P** Cardiac Rhythm Related Device
Pacemaker, Single Chamber	Insertion	Subcutaneous Tissue and Fascia	**P** Cardiac Rhythm Related Device
Pacemaker, Single Chamber Rate Responsive	Insertion	Subcutaneous Tissue and Fascia	**P** Cardiac Rhythm Related Device
Spinal Stabilization Device, Facet Replacement	Insertion	Lower Joints Upper Joints	**4** Internal Fixation Device
Spinal Stabilization Device, Interspinous Process	Insertion	Lower Joints Upper Joints	**4** Internal Fixation Device
Spinal Stabilization Device, Pedicle-Based	Insertion	Lower Joints Upper Joints	**4** Internal Fixation Device

DEVICE AGGREGATION TABLE

Specific Device	for Operation	in Body System	General Device
Stimulator Generator, Multiple Array	Insertion	Subcutaneous Tissue and Fascia	**M** Stimulator Generator
Stimulator Generator, Multiple Array Rechargeable	Insertion	Subcutaneous Tissue and Fascia	**M** Stimulator Generator
Stimulator Generator, Single Array	Insertion	Subcutaneous Tissue and Fascia	**M** Stimulator Generator
Stimulator Generator, Single Array Rechargeable	Insertion	Subcutaneous Tissue and Fascia	**M** Stimulator Generator
Synthetic Substitute, Ceramic	Replacement	Lower Joints	**J** Synthetic Substitute
Synthetic Substitute, Ceramic on Polyethylene	Replacement	Lower Joints	**J** Synthetic Substitute
Synthetic Substitute, Intraocular Telescope	Replacement	Eye	**J** Synthetic Substitute
Synthetic Substitute, Metal	Replacement	Lower Joints	**J** Synthetic Substitute
Synthetic Substitute, Metal on Polyethylene	Replacement	Lower Joints	**J** Synthetic Substitute
Synthetic Substitute, Oxidized Zirconium on Polyethylene	Replacement	Lower Joints	**J** Synthetic Substitute
Synthetic Substitute, Polyethylene	Replacement	Lower Joints	**J** Synthetic Substitute
Synthetic Substitute, Reverse Ball and Socket	Replacement	Upper Joints	**J** Synthetic Substitute

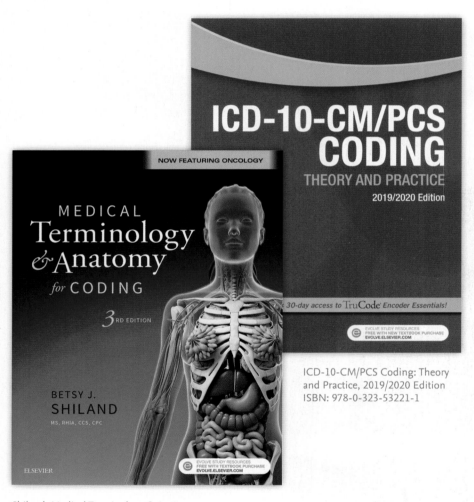

Trust Elsevier to take you through the levels *of* CODING SUCCESS

STEP4: PROFESSIONAL

STEP3: CERTIFY

STEP2: PRACTICE

STEP1: LEARN

With the resources you need for every level of coding success, we are with you every step of your coding career. From beginning to advanced, from the classroom to the workplace, from application to certification, the Step Series products are your guides to greater opportunities and successful career advancement.

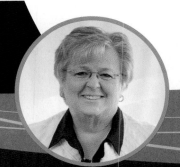

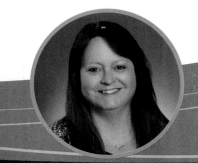

Keep climbing with the most trusted names in medical coding.

Carol J. Buck, MS, CPC, CCS-P | *Jackie Grass Koesterman, CPC*

TRUST ELSEVIER to provide you complete curriculum solution

CONTENT

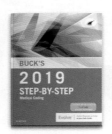 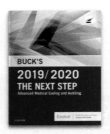 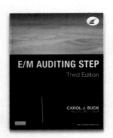

978-0-323-58219-3   978-0-323-58261-2   978-1-4557-5199-0

STUDY TOOLS

Create a customized portfolio to show employers

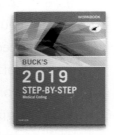 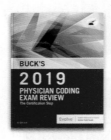 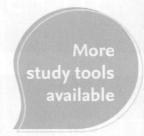

More study tools available

978-0-323-58251-3   978-0-323-58257-5

SIMULATIONS

COURSES

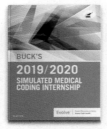 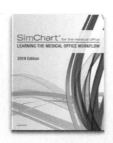 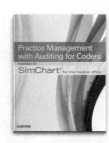 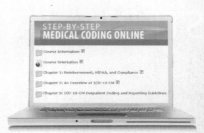

978-0-323-60873-2   978-0-323-64197-5   978-0-323-43011-1   978-0-323-60874-9